A WELLNESS WAY OF LIFE

A WELLNESS WAY OF LIFE

Ninth Edition

GWEN ROBBINS / **DEBBIE POWERS** / **SHARON BURGESS**

Ball State University

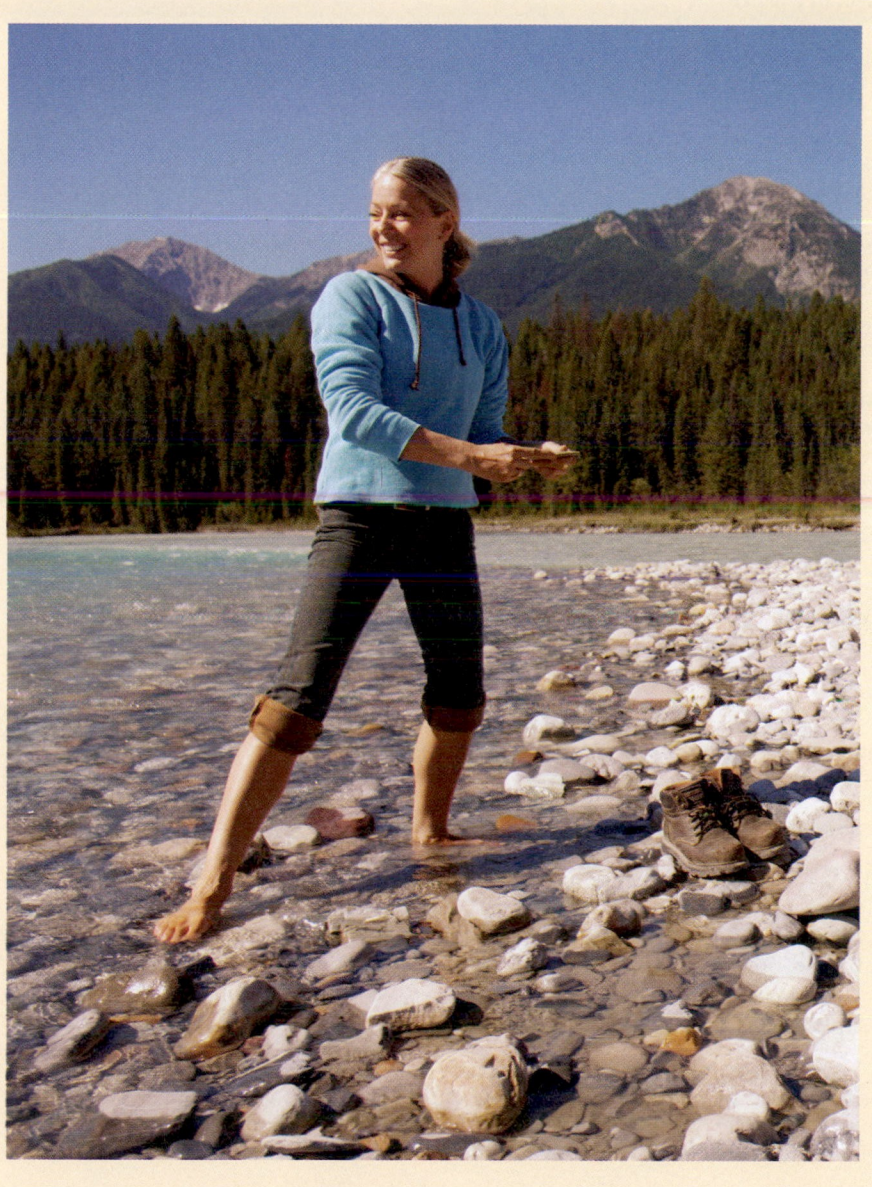

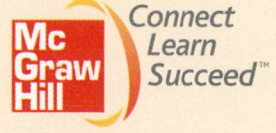

Connect
Learn
Succeed™

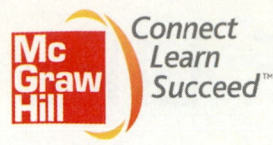

Published by McGraw-Hill, a business unit of The McGraw-Hill Companies, Inc., 1221 Avenue of the Americas, New York, NY, 10020. Copyright © 2011 by The McGraw-Hill Companies, Inc. All rights reserved. No part of this publication may be reproduced or distributed in any form or by any means, or stored in a database or retrieval system, without the prior written consent of The McGraw-Hill Companies, Inc., including, but not limited to, in any network or other electronic storage or transmission, or broadcast for distance learning. Some ancillaries, including electronic and print components, may not be available to customers outside the United States.

This book is printed on acid-free paper.

1 2 3 4 5 6 7 8 9 0 RJE/RJE 0 9 8 7 6 5 4 3 2 1 0

ISBN   978-0-07-352383-5
MHID   0-07-352383-6

Vice President, Editorial: *Mike Ryan*
Editorial Director: *Beth Mejia*
Executive Editor: *Christopher Johnson*
Marketing Manager: *Caroline McGillen*
Director of Development: *Kathleen Engelberg*
Developmental Editor: *Gary O' Brien, VanBrien & Associates*
Production Editors: *Melissa Williams/Jill Eccher*
Manuscript Editor: *Kay Mikel*
Media Project Managers: *Thomas Brierly/Andrea Helmbolt*
Cover Design: *Allister Fein/Brian Salisbury*
Interior Design: *Pam Verros*
Photo Research: *Nora Agbayani*
Buyer: *Sherry Kane*
Composition: *Aptara®, Inc.*
Printing: *Printed on #45 New Era Matte by R.R. Donnelley & Sons*

Cover Photo: © Fancy Photography/VEER.

The credits section for this book begins on page C-1 and is considered an extension of the copyright page.

Library of Congress Cataloging-in-Publication Data

Robbins, Gwen.
A wellness way of life / Gwen Robbins, Debbie Powers, Sharon Burgess.—9th ed.
    p. cm.
Includes bibliographical references and index.
ISBN-13: 978-0-07-352383-5 (alk. paper)
ISBN-10: 0-07-352383-6 (alk. paper)
  I. Health.   II. Powers, Debbie.   II. Burgess, Sharon.   III. Title.
    RA776.R63 2011
    613-dc22
                                                    2010044534

The Internet addresses listed in the text were accurate at the time of publication. The inclusion of a website does not indicate an endorsement by the authors of McGraw-Hill, and McGraw-Hill does not guarantee the accuracy of the information presented at these sites.

www.mhhe.com

BRIEF CONTENTS

CONTENTS

CHAPTER 4 Maximizing Cardiorespiratory Fitness   97

CHAPTER 16

Exploring Lifetime Wellness Issues   551

PREFACE

A WELLNESS WAY OF LIFE
invites you to become

Informed... Inspired... Connected...

A Wellness Way of Life **informs** you about wellness . . . **inspires** you to choose healthy behaviors . . . and **connects** you to the tools that make change possible.

Be Informed

Based on solid research, *A Wellness Way of Life* makes sense of the array of the confusing and sometimes contradictory health information that bombards us everyday. The authors minimize technical jargon and present health topics and issues in a clear and accessible way. *A Wellness Way of Life* gives you accurate, up-to-date information about exercise, nutrition, stress, heart disease, weight management, and much more. Knowledge is power, and *A Wellness Way of Life* empowers you with the knowledge you need to make smart health decisions.

New to this edition is a feature called "Think About It," designed to give you practice in thinking critically, applying your knowledge, and writing about factors that influence your wellness. These activities appear in the book and as online activities that you can submit directly to your instructor.

Be Inspired

Knowledge alone is not enough to change behavior. Many people know what to do but just don't do it! To make lifestyle changes, you need to take knowledge and move into action. *A Wellness Way of Life* not only gives you the "do's and don'ts" but also presents the content in a way that is motivating and inspiring. It is a "how to" book that helps you bridge the gap between knowledge and action.

Supporting the applied approach and behavior change focus in this edition are two new and enhanced features. "What Stage of Change Are You In?" behavior change flow charts help you identify your stage of change relative to each health topic. And new "Tips for Behavior Change" boxes, also

THINK ABOUT IT

Rather than relying on long-term behavioral strategies, many people look for a "quick fix." Liposuction and gastric bypass surgery are commonly utilized for weight loss, and medications are used to control high cholesterol and hypertension. However, resorting to surgeries and pharmaceutical drugs can be risky and expensive. What are the pros and cons of these "quick fix" approaches versus developing self-managed lifestyle skills to address chronic health conditions? Why do so many people fail to take charge of their own health?

connect Go online to Connect to complete this activity. http://connect.mcgraw-hill.com

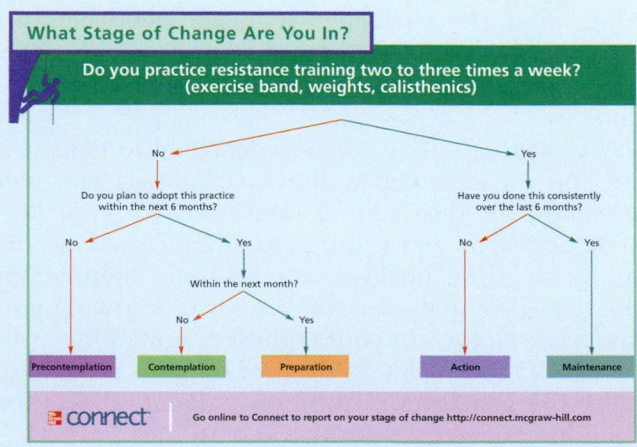

What Stage of Change Are You In?

Do you practice resistance training two to three times a week? (exercise band, weights, calisthenics)

connect Go online to Connect to report on your stage of change http://connect.mcgraw-hill.com

appearing in each chapter, offer specific strategies to help you make a behavior change or stick with one you've already made. In this edition, the chapter lab activities, which are also available online in *Connect,* are now linked to the appropriate section in the text to support your understanding and learning.

Be Connected

A Wellness Way of Life sets the stage for behavior change by providing a wealth of useful tools that help you move into action and apply new information to your life. In addition, the 9th edition is accompanied by *Connect Fitness and Wellness,* a powerful new set of online, interactive tools. This online learning system includes interactive fitness labs and health assessments, video activities, quizzes, a behavior change workbook, and a fitness and nutrition log. *Connect Fitness and Wellness* not only helps you master the content and get a better grade but also helps you develop the skills for leading a more balanced and fulfilling life.

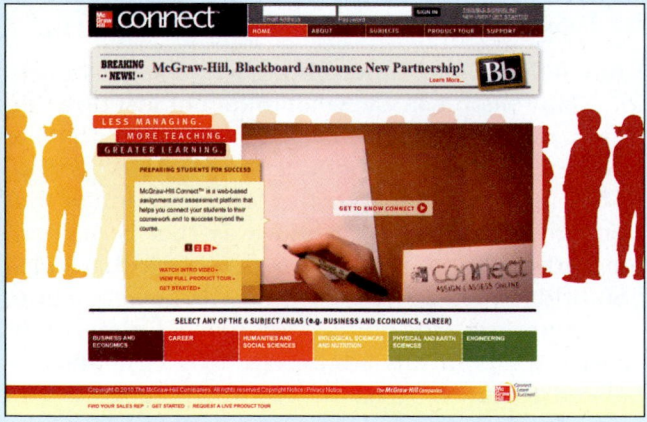

A Wellness Way of Life

There is no better feeling than knowing that you are empowered to take charge of your health—and to resist cultural norms that encourage unhealthy choices.

A Wellness Way of Life is designed to help you become an informed wellness consumer. You will be empowered to take responsibility for your lifestyle decisions and inspired to embrace the opportunity to make positive choices for a lifetime. In doing so, you will discover the joy of knowing you are working toward your highest potential for wellness. And you will also discover that this proactive, take charge attitude becomes a habitual way of thinking and acting—truly a way of life!

◆ NEW TO THIS EDITION

Based on the idea of self-responsibility and self-empowerment, *A Wellness Way of Life* gives students practical information about how to make good decisions that will positively affect their well-being throughout their lives. It is action-based and presents wellness as a dynamic, lifelong process. Here are highlights of this ninth edition:

✓ Chapter's Lab Activities, now linked to the appropriate sections in the text, better aid and support student learning.
✓ Students can more readily assess their own stage of change with enhanced Behavior Change Flow Charts....What Stage of Change Are You In?
✓ All Behavior Change Flow Charts are now presented earlier in the chapter, allowing students to assess their status before reading chapter content.
✓ Tips for Behavior Change Boxes help students evaluate how to progress to the next stage from their current stage of change.
✓ Updated Internet Resources and Bibliography direct students to additional sources for further information.
✓ Many new and updated photos in each chapter make the material relevant and understandable to students.
✓ URLs direct students to online videos and websites that enhance and supplement textbook information.
✓ Updated data and references in each chapter reflect the latest research.

Chapter 1

✓ Updated leading causes of death
✓ More emphasis on prevention of chronic diseases
✓ Expanded emphasis on health-care costs
✓ Introduced *Healthy People 2020*
✓ Updated Diversity Issues

Chapter 2

✓ Expanded information on how to stay motivated
✓ New Top Ten List: "S's for Success in Changing a Behavior"
✓ New Internet Resources
✓ New Lab Activity 2-4: "Using the S's for Success in Changing Your Behavior"

Chapter 3

✓ Added U.S. Health and Human Services Physical Activity Guidelines for Americans
✓ URLs referenced for alternate fitness tests online: BMI, home body fat test
✓ URL for 3- and 7-site skinfold test instructions to calculate body composition
✓ URL for strength test calculators used to estimate one rep max for leg press and bench press.
✓ Updated Healthy People 2020 physical activity objectives
✓ Step test norms added for 12-inch step
✓ New frequently asked questions

Chapter 4

✓ The latest Department of Health and Human Services Physical Activity Guidelines for Americans have been added
✓ New box illustrates how to apply the new DHHS physical activity guidelines (Example: "Physical Activity Workouts to Meet DHHS Guidelines)
✓ New information on how endorphins improve mental health
✓ Expanded information on how moderate exercise enhances the immune system
✓ Expanded "exercise and cancer" section
✓ Updated statistics throughout chapter

Chapter 5

✓ Information on the benefits of dynamic stretching
✓ Examples of dynamic stretching exercises
✓ URLs for videos for dynamic stretching techniques, basic Tai Chi, back exercises, seated stretches, and the Hatha Yoga Sun Salutation
✓ Directions for seated stretches
✓ A new lab using seated stretches
✓ A new lab using partner stretches
✓ Updated line illustrations

Chapter 6

✓ Strength training myths and facts
✓ URLs for videos for weight training with free weights, weight training with machines, elastic resistance exercises, abdominal and core strengthening exercises, Pilates, hip & thigh exercises, upper body exercises, stability ball exercises
✓ Updated line illustrations
✓ Directions for exercises have been added under each illustration.

Chapter 7

✓ The latest Department of Health and Human Services Physical Activity Guidelines for Older Adults have been added
✓ New information on the Guidelines for Exercise During Pregnancy
✓ Added information in the Pregnancy section includes information on weight training during pregnancy
✓ New Frequently Asked Question: Is it true that most of your body heat is lost through your head?
✓ Expanded table of caffeine content now includes the new "extra small" (2 oz.) energy drinks
✓ Updated statistics throughout chapter

Chapter 8

✓ Added information on balance training for ankle sprain rehabilitation
✓ New internet resources include URLs for videos on ankle injuries, back pain, bursitis, calf muscle strain, knee injuries, iliotibial band syndrome, increasing knee stability, patello-femoral pain and the "virtual MD" who can help with injury diagnosis
✓ Lab 8-1 on common treatments for injuries and when to see a physician has been revised

Chapter 9

✓ Added latest information on how exercise affects telomere length and increases longevity
✓ Expanded coverage of the increased risk of cardiovascular disease and post-menopausal women includes the latest research
✓ New Frequently Asked Question: How can I take control of my heart health?
✓ Revised and updated Lab Activity 9-1: "Are You at Risk for Heart Disease?"
✓ Revised and updated Lab Activity 9-4: "Are You at Risk for Diabetes?"
✓ Updated statistics throughout the chapter

Chapter 10

✓ The beginning of the chapter has been streamlined so students can move more quickly to the content on managing stress
✓ New subheading: The Relaxation Response
✓ New subheading: The Six Strategies for Stress Management
✓ Updated statistics throughout the chapter

Chapter 11

✓ Reference to the new *2010 Dietary Guidelines*
✓ New information on the impact of excessive sugar intake
✓ Updated information on organic foods
✓ New information on artificial sweeteners
✓ New Internet Resources
✓ Lab 11-2, focusing on personal diet analysis using MyPyramid, has been revised

Chapter 12

✓ Updated statistics on obesity and overweight
✓ Updated Diversity Issues
✓ New Table 12-3 on the calories and sugar in energy and coffee drinks
✓ Research on the leptin/brain connection
✓ Updated diet plan chart
✓ Information on portion control
✓ New Internet Resources

Chapter 13

✓ Updated graphs show cancer data for the most deadly cancers and racial disparities
✓ Screening guidelines added for skin and testicular cancers
✓ Revised cancer morbidity and mortality statistics throughout chapter
✓ More information on HPV related to preventing cervical cancer
✓ Information on vitamin D and cancer prevention
✓ Lab 13-3 on preventing cancer through dietary choices has been revised
✓ Added URLs for videos on breast cancer screening, mammography, skin cancer prevention, the skin self-exam, the sigmoidoscopy test, vitamin D and cancer reduction, treating cervical cancer, prostate cancer, and breast cancer

Chapter 14

✓ New section: Alcohol Poisoning
✓ New Frequently Asked Question: Are E-Cigarettes Safe?
✓ Table 14-5, Percentage of Blood Alcohol Content (BAC), now has separate BAC for men and women instead of BAC for weight only to be used by both genders
✓ Coverage of the newest method of making methamphetamine called the "shake and bake" method

✓ Coverage of the newest way of securing ammonia nitrate for making small recipes of methamphetamine, using instant cold packs or dry ice packs
✓ New photo to show instant cold packs
✓ Expanded information on medical marijuana in FAQ
✓ Lab Activity 14-1, Alcohol: High Risk vs. Low Risk, has been totally redesigned for easier student use and comprehension
✓ Updated statistics throughout the chapter

Chapter 15

✓ Updated graphs showing frequency of STD transmission by type of STD
✓ Updated graphs on AIDS/HIV incidence with latest CDC survey data
✓ New data on heterosexual transmission of HIV
✓ Information on immunizations to prevent HPV
✓ Tips on STD testing for partners
✓ New Lab Activity 15-3 with additional questions for class discussion
✓ URLs for videos on STD awareness, HPV, syphilis, chlamydia, gonorrhea, genital warts, HIV and AIDS, the hepatitis B vaccine, AIDS and pregnancy, drug resistant gonorrhea, getting tested for STDs, and how to use a condom (female and male).

Chapter 16

✓ Updated statistics on automobile safety
✓ Expanded information on rising health-care costs
✓ Updated information on wellness trends and challenges
✓ New Internet Resources

◆ ACKNOWLEDGMENTS

We are thankful to the instructors who reviewed the previous edition of *A Wellness Way of Life* and offered helpful suggestions for improvement. Their knowledge and insights are reflected throughout the pages of this book.

Gwendolyn Francavillo
Gallaudet University

Charlotte Koehler
University of South Carolina Upstate

Erin Nitschke
Sheridan College

David Sarrette
Bainbridge College

Pebbles Turbeville
Saint Andrews Presbyterian College

Lynette Gard
University of St. Francis

Toni LaSala
William Paterson University

Stefanie Latham
Oklahoma City University

Sarah Thompson
Binghamton University

We are grateful to the following individuals for their assistance in the development of this book:

Sam Minor II, Department of Art, College of Fine Arts, Ball State University for artwork.
Edgar Self, John Huffer, Ann Wasson, Gwen Robbins, and Debbie Powers for photography.
Katherine Barnet, Jill Robbins, Jeff Robbins, Jim Powers, Margaret Phillips, Boung Jin Kang, Chris Powers, Melissa Smith, Kelley Jarvis, Erika Hogan, Karlyn Rent, Jamie Troxell, and Lowell Faison for modeling for photographs.
Brian Dietz, Program Advisor, Ball State University, for consultation on higher education alcohol programming.

Carol Foust, professor at Colorado State University-Pueblo, for her consultation on spiritual health issues.
Jesse Neal, Investigator and Director, Muncie and Delaware County Drug Task Force, for consultation on illegal drugs.

A very generous thank you goes to the dedicated Ball State University Physical Fitness and Wellness faculty for their vigorous commitment to quality teaching.

Special recognition is extended to Dr. Marilyn Buck, Associate Provost; Dr. Terry S. King, Provost and Vice President for Academic Affairs; and Dr. JoAnn M. Gora, President of Ball State University, for their continuing support of the fitness/wellness program at Ball State University. We are fortunate to have administrators who have the vision to recognize that participating in a fitness/wellness program will have a positive impact on students' lives now and in the future.

We dedicate this ninth edition to the students-past, present, and future. We wish you a lifetime of wellness.

Gwen Robbins
Debbie Powers
Sharon Burgess

CHAPTER 1

Understanding Wellness

STUDY QUESTIONS

You will have successfully mastered this chapter if you can answer the following:

1. What are the top three causes of death in the United States?
2. Can you define *healthy life expectancy* and explain why it is low in the United States compared with other industrialized countries?
3. Can you name the largest contributing factor affecting longevity?
4. What are the four overarching goals of the publication *Healthy People 2020?*
5. What are five lifestyle practices that can reduce the risk of chronic diseases and enhance wellness?
6. What is the definition of *wellness?*
7. Can you identify the seven dimensions of wellness and give three examples within each dimension?
8. Can you list and describe the six factors that influence growth in wellness?
9. What are four examples of ways society supports wellness and four examples of ways society detracts from wellness?

You will find the answers as you read this chapter.

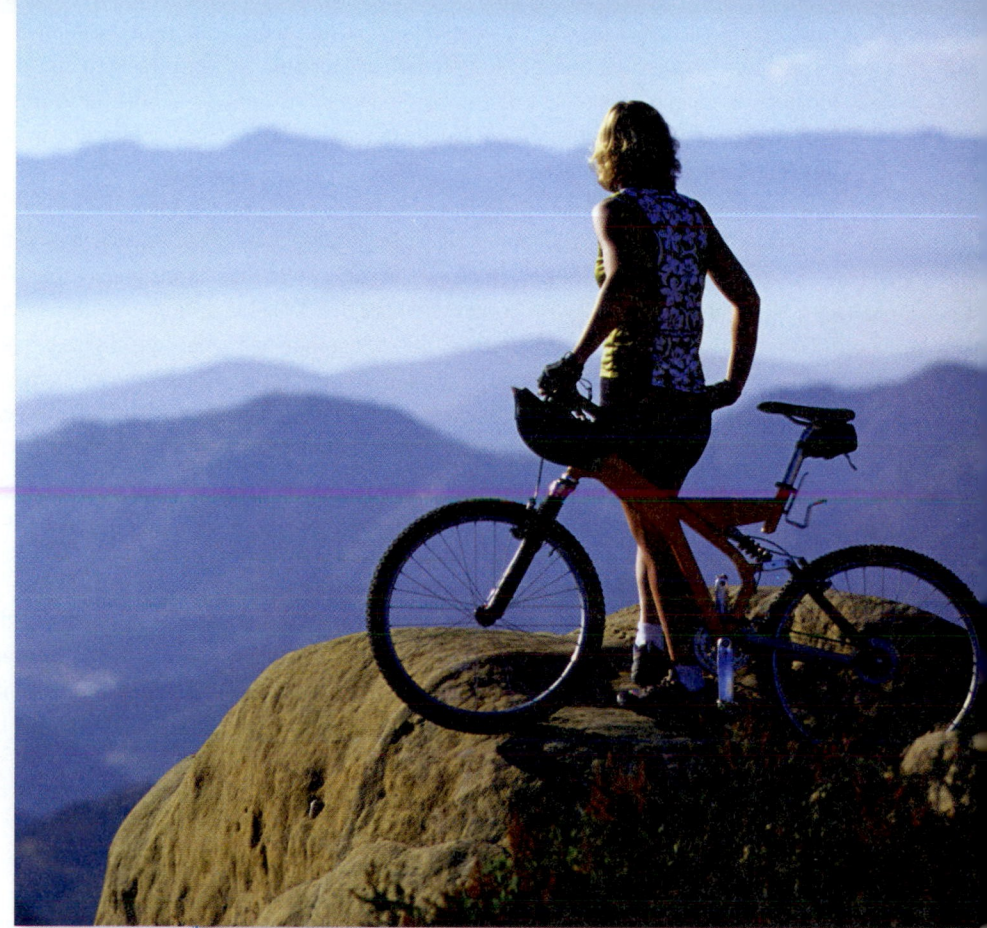

> *Life is not merely to be alive, but to be well.*
>
> —Martial

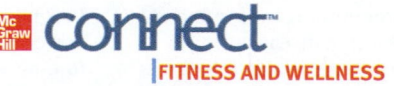

FITNESS AND WELLNESS

http://connect.mcgraw-hill.com

As Rob lay in the coronary care unit, his eyes surveyed the various tubes and wires connected to his tired body. The nightmare of the last 24 hours was over, but the pain and confusion lingered.

"How can this be? I'm only 49 years old. How could I have had a heart attack? What if I die? What about my wife? My son? My daughter? I've just become a grandpa. I was given a big promotion at work. Why now?" Rob's mind drifted.

"But I'm an athlete! Well, I *was* an athlete back in high school. Once I started college, there was no time for sports or exercise. Started smoking, too. Figured I'd stop when the deadlines subsided, but the stresses never ended. Drank too much, too; partied a lot. Still like a couple of drinks to end the day. I always thought I'd lose those extra 30 pounds—always next year, always a New Year's resolution. Diet? Too busy. Vending machines, hot dog stands, snacks in front of the TV, fast food. No time. Too much to do. Money to make. A lot of stress. Can't stop now. There'll be time later."

Rob's mind drifted back to his room. He could faintly hear his doctor's voice—"Stop smoking . . . Change in lifestyle . . . More fruits and vegetables . . . Start exercising . . . Cholesterol is 280 . . . Break old habits." Rob thought, "How I wish I could turn back the clock!"

This story is too common in the United States. More than half of all deaths in this country are attributed to coronary heart disease and stroke. Although most heart attacks occur after middle age, many people are afflicted far too young. Table 1-1 lists the leading causes of death in the United States. One hundred years ago the leading causes of death were infectious diseases such as tuberculosis, polio, diphtheria, pneumonia, and influenza and various diseases of infancy. Advances in medicine, the discovery of antibiotics, and improved sanitation diminished the incidence of these ravaging diseases and increased the average life span. Through scientific discovery, technology, industrial growth, and automation, the entire American lifestyle has changed. We use remote controls to change television channels and open garage doors. Appliances wash our clothes, dishes, and teeth. We ride vehicles to work, to school, and even while playing golf. "Surfing the Net" is much more popular than surfing the ocean. We allow ourselves to be bused and trucked, elevated and escalated, and then wonder why we get fat and are out of shape. This so-called good life has created sedentary living, changes in eating habits (fast foods, increased fats and sweets, processed foods), stress, alcohol and drug abuse, and obesity. Although social scientists predicted in the 1960s that technology would create a future of abundant leisure time, in actuality, most of us face an unrelenting pace of increased expectations and demands. Chronic hurrying has created chronic stress. Life has gotten out of balance for many. As Mahatma Gandhi once said, "There is more to life than increasing its speed."

The harsh truth is that a high percentage of disease and disability affecting the American people is preventable, a consequence of unwise behavior and lifestyle choices. The decision to smoke, for instance, is responsible for one of every five deaths in the United States each year. With the rapidly increasing obesity rate, health officials predict that obesity will soon surpass tobacco as the leading contributor to premature death in the United States. Instead of infectious diseases, we now die of **chronic diseases**—diseases that develop over many years and are heavily influenced by lifestyle. Examples of chronic diseases are heart disease, cancer, stroke, type 2 diabetes, atherosclerosis, obesity, and osteoporosis. Chronic diseases account not only for 70 percent of all deaths in the United States but also cause major limitations in daily living for 1 out of 10 Americans.

If you are like most young people, you underestimate your future risk of chronic diseases. Studies show that many young adults already possess several risk factors that can lead to these lifestyle diseases. Underestimation of your risk is of substantial concern because *action* should be an outcome of your health knowledge. After

TABLE 1-1   *Leading Causes of Death in the United States*

Rank	All Ages	Ages 15–24	Ages 25–44	Ages 45–64
1.	Heart disease	Accidents	Accidents	Cancer
2.	Cancer*	Assault (Homicide)	Cancer	Heart disease
3.	Stroke	Suicide	Heart disease	Accidents
4.	Chronic respiratory diseases	Cancer	Suicide	Chronic respiratory diseases
5.	Accidents	Heart disease	Assault (Homicide)	Diabetes mellitus
6.	Alzheimer's disease	Congenital abnormalities	HIV	Stroke
7.	Diabetes mellitus	Stroke	Chronic liver disease and cirrhosis	Chronic liver disease and cirrhosis
8.	Pneumonia and influenza	Pregnancy, childbirth	Stroke	Suicide
9.	Kidney disease	Systemic blood infections	Diabetes mellitus	Systemic blood infections
10.	Systemic blood infections	Pneumonia and influenza	Systemic blood infections	Kidney disease

*Among people under age 85, cancer is the leading cause of death.

Source: Centers for Disease Control and Prevention. National Center for Health Statistics. *National Vital Statistics Reports*, Vol. 58, August 2009.

all, the truly educated individual understands cause and effect. Nevertheless, many young adults are much more interested in the present than the future. Good health is often taken for granted until it is lost. You make choices every day that either increase or decrease your risk for developing chronic diseases.

This chapter introduces you to the concept of high-level wellness. You will see that wellness living and healthy lifestyle interventions that begin early in life can shape your health destiny and lead to a vibrant life.

◆ HEALTHY LIFE EXPECTANCY AND THE COSTS

Life expectancy in the United States is 77.9 years (75.3 years for men and 80.4 years for women). The World Health Organization (WHO) calculates **healthy life expectancy** in 191 countries. Healthy life expectancy is the number of years a person is expected to live in *good* health. This number is obtained by subtracting years spent in poor health from overall life expectancy. The United States ranks twenty-ninth in the world using this measurement, with an average of 69.3 years of healthy life expectancy. Japan ranks number one with a healthy life expectancy of 75.0 years.

The ranking of the United States is surprisingly low in light of its status as a country with one of the best medical care systems in the world. The WHO report indicates that Americans die earlier and spend more time disabled than do people in most other advanced countries. Several factors are cited in the WHO report to explain why the United States ranks relatively low among wealthy nations:

1. Some groups, such as American Indians, rural African Americans, and the inner-city poor, have extremely poor health that is more characteristic of a poor developing country than of a rich industrialized one.
2. The HIV epidemic causes a higher proportion of death and disability in the United States than in other developed countries.
3. The United States is one of the leading countries for cancers because of the high incidence of tobacco use.
4. The United States has a high incidence of coronary heart disease.
5. The United States has a fairly high level of violence, especially homicides, compared with other industrialized countries.

In contrast, the United States spends more than twice as much for health care than any other nation. Yet we are among the sickest in the world! As chronic diseases rob more Americans of their lives or their quality of life, it is also wreaking havoc on our nation's economy. National health care expenditures in the United States are $2.5 trillion and are rising every year. Seventy-five percent of this spending is for patients with chronic diseases. If current policies and conditions hold true, by the year 2018 this amount will jump to $4.3 trillion. Smoking alone costs our society billions annually in health care costs and lost productivity (and causes more than 400,000 premature deaths). Cardiovascular diseases cost more than $300 billion annually, and the financial burden of obesity rivals that of smoking. In fact, for the first time in history, experts predict a decline in life expectancy in the United States in the twenty-first century due to the rising prevalence of obesity. During the last several years, expenditures for prescription drugs have grown at a faster rate than has any other type of health cost. Unfortunately, not enough of the health care expenditures go toward prevention. America is terrific at expensive, heroic care but very poor at low-cost preventive care! Health advocate Dr. Andrew Weil concurs that a radical transformation from

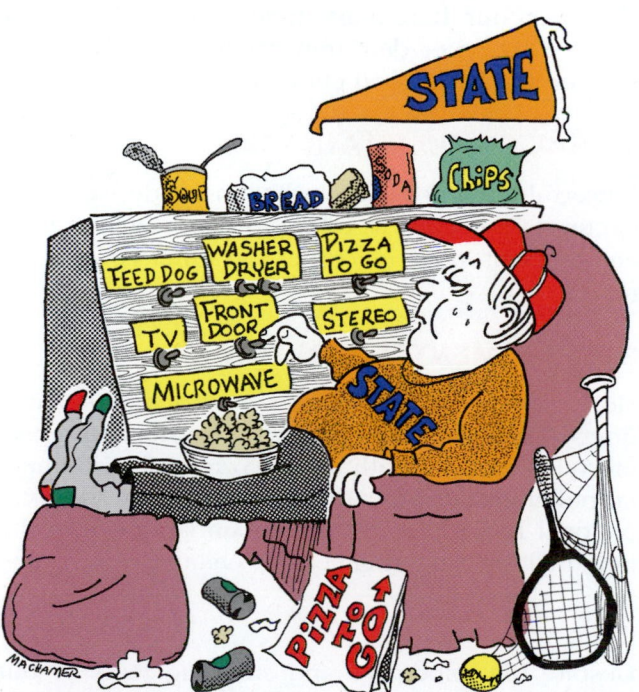

The "good life"?

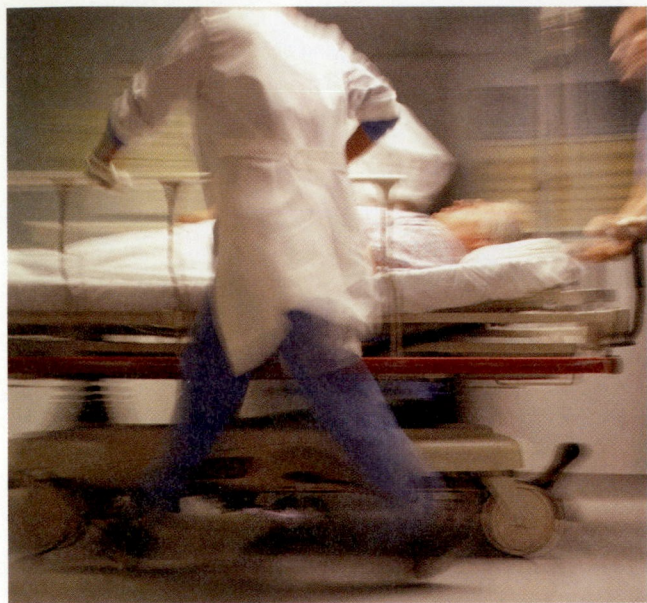

Cardiovascular diseases, the number one killer of both men and women, are considered "lifestyle" diseases.

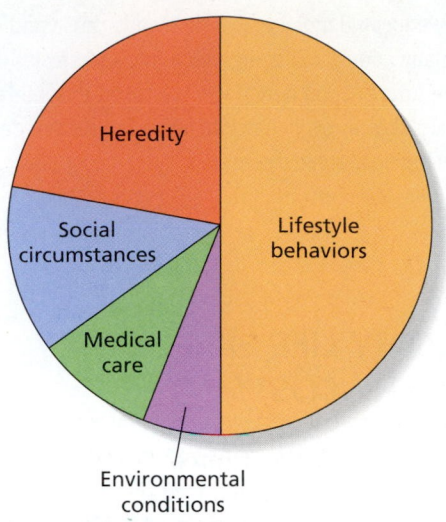

FIGURE 1-1   **Factors affecting longevity.**
Our longevity is affected by a combination of factors.
SOURCE: Adapted from McGinnis, J. M., *American Journal of Health Promotion* 18 (Nov./Dec. 2003): 146–150

disease *intervention* to disease *prevention* is the only way to make health care cost effective.

This burden will continue to grow as the population ages. By 2011, if trends continue, health care costs will double. According to government statistics, as much as two-thirds of disability and death up to age 65 would be preventable in whole or in part if we applied what we know about the effects of lifestyle on premature illness and death. You may be thinking "but we all have to die sometime!" Of course that is true. But we are born to last nearly 100 years, and not meant to suffer from chronic diseases in our 40s and 50s. Former U.S. surgeon general C. Everett Koop states, "We are in an era of self-induced premature deaths."

Determinants of Health and Longevity

As a result of the curative focus of our health care system, a majority of our health care dollars are spent on procedures for patching people up after the damage has been done. Since billions of dollars are spent to treat the results of bad eating and drinking habits, sedentary living, stress, and smoking, our system probably should be renamed "sickness care" rather than "health care." Because of the medical procedures, drugs, and technologies currently available, many people have become complacent about their health habits. They think they can be "bailed out" by medical science.

A range of factors underlie one's susceptibility and predisposition to ill health. (See Figure 1-1.) Rather than working independently, all of these

factors interact. It is important to understand how these factors work in combinations and affect each other. Nevertheless, the largest contributing factor is lifestyle behaviors.

HEREDITY

Predisposition to health or disease begins at conception. Each of us has cellular codes that dictate our size, shape, personality, and biological limits. However, our hereditary tendencies are strongly affected by other determinants like social circumstances and behavioral choices.

SOCIAL CIRCUMSTANCES

Powerful influences on our health are derived from circumstances such as education, income, housing, employment, poverty, crime, and other community forces.

ENVIRONMENTAL CONDITIONS

Home, work, and community environments sometimes present us not only with barriers to active lifestyles but also with toxic hazards. Environmental pollutants, chemical contaminants, radon, occupational hazards, and tobacco smoke all have the potential for triggering cellular changes.

MEDICAL CARE

Despite the expensive and stunning feats of our medical care system, the contribution of medical treatment to overall gains in the function and quality of life has been limited in recent years. Whereas the introduction of antibiotics and improved sanitation in the early 1900s increased our life span by more than 60 percent, modern-day medical treatments and technologies have had far less dramatic impact.

LIFESTYLE BEHAVIORS

In the United States, lifestyle behaviors represent the single most controllable influence over our health prospects. The daily choices we make with respect to diet, physical activity, stress management, tobacco and alcohol use, sexual practices, and safety issues are the most important determinants of well-being. It has been well documented that the top three lifestyle contributors to premature deaths in the United States are

1. Tobacco use
2. Poor diet
3. Lack of exercise

These are often designated as the "actual" causes of death in contrast to the "leading" causes of death listed in Table 1-1. As people learn more about the effect of behavioral factors, we hope they will accept the personal responsibility for making changes in their lifestyle and find joy in discovering how much power they truly have in determining their health destiny.

The Power of Prevention

Surveys show that two in three Americans underestimate the impact of chronic diseases on the number of premature deaths and overall health care costs. Because the vast majority of chronic diseases can be prevented or managed, it is essential to empower individual responsibility. This involves aggressive health promotion. **Health promotion** is the science and art of helping people change their lifestyle to move toward a state of optimal health. Health promotion involves systematic efforts by organizations to create healthy policies and supportive environments as well as the reorienting of health services to include more than clinical and curative care. Lifestyle change is motivated not by knowledge alone but also by supportive social environments and the availability of facilitative services. Examples of health promotion programs are weight-loss workshops, smoking cessation clinics, and stress management seminars. Laws and policies such as those prohibiting drunk driving, those curtailing pollution, and those establishing smoke-free businesses and restaurants also assist in health promotion.

Because the preventive aspects of health have become more publicized, research studies involving

diet and exercise often become instant headlines (e.g., Which is better . . . butter or margarine? Coffee or tea? Protein or carbohydrate?). Sometimes the information is reported only partially, resulting in confusion, contradiction, and even sensationalism. Bewildered and wary, many Americans reject or ignore many legitimate health pronouncements. It is a challenge to recognize legitimate health pronouncements. Being educated about wellness will empower you to make informed decisions and distinguish between legitimate health pronouncements and fads and illegitimate assertions. Regardless of the messages, a majority of Americans today continue to be sedentary and overweight. Stress levels, blood cholesterol readings, and blood sugars continue to soar. Though the relationship between lifestyle and health is clear, adopting healthy lifestyle habits can be challenging in our environment where fast food is everywhere, we ride rather than walk, and we sit rather than play. But the good news is it can be done and it does make a difference in health, longevity, and vitality.

Healthy People 2020

Every 10 years the government establishes health goals for the nation. Created in the 1970s, *Healthy People* is a national crusade for health promotion. Its objectives set an agenda for getting Americans to live longer, healthier lives. The U.S. Department of Health and Human Services reassesses these goals every 10 years and issues a report card on the progress made in the previous decade. *Healthy People 2020* is the most recent road map for improving the health of all people in the United States. *Healthy People 2020* is committed to four overarching goals:

1. Attain high-quality, longer lives free of preventable disease, disability, injury, and premature death.
2. Achieve health equity, eliminate disparities, and improve the health of all groups.
3. Create social and physical environments that promote good health for all.
4. Promote quality of life, health development, and healthy behaviors across all life stages.

To achieve these lofty goals, specific objectives have been targeted for the year 2020 in areas such as chronic diseases, environmental health, nutrition and weight status, physical activity and fitness, injury and violence prevention, and social determinants of health, among many others. The specific objectives and reports on progress toward each can be found at www.healthypeople.gov.

How are we doing at reaching these goals? By many measures, not so hot. Whereas raising childhood vaccination rates, lowering cancer death rates, increasing seat belt use, and reducing work injuries show improvement, we are failing in the main objectives. Blood pressures, consumption of healthy foods, obesity rates, and exercise habits are far from their recommended national goals.

Because of the diversity and varying needs of Americans, reaching each goal is a challenge. (See Diversity Issues.) Goals are only dreams without action plans. That is where federal agencies, state organizations, local communities, businesses, schools, families, and you enter the picture. The health of the nation is improved with coordinated efforts that begin with individual action and personal responsibility. The federal government is playing a leadership role in cultivating a culture of healthier, life-enhancing habits for all Americans, regardless of income, race, sex, or other status. We must do our part to help.

A companion document to *Healthy People 2020* is *Healthy Campus 2020,* which establishes national health objectives for the nation's colleges and universities. The health indicators in this document are similar to *Healthy People 2020* in regard to physical activity, overweight and obesity, tobacco use, and other practices. The goal of both documents is to motivate people into personal action. Surveys reveal that since 1990 young adults ages 18–24 from all racial and ethnic groups show a larger increase in several risk behaviors than all other age groups in the United States. Those risk behaviors are increases in tobacco use (especially among women), obesity, inactivity, and low vegetable and fruit intake. This is a particular public health concern because this is the age when independent lifelong habits are established. Young adults, apparently believing they are immune from risk, are not too far from entering the ages of high chronic disease burden. Most of the proposals in these two government documents are linked to everyday practices, so it is up to each of us to develop strategies for incorporating healthy habits into our daily lives. Look at the Top 10 "Lifestyle Practices That Enhance Wellness." How many of these habits do you practice?

There is nothing extreme or magical in this list. It shifts the main responsibility for health to the individual rather than relegating the individual to a position of passivity amid excessive surgeries,

> *"The United States cannot effectively address escalating health-care costs without addressing the problem of chronic diseases."*
> —Centers for Disease Control and Prevention

THINK ABOUT IT

Lifestyle behaviors represent the most controllable influence over one's health. As a result, some employers are considering increasing health insurance premiums for employees who smoke, are overweight, or have high blood pressure. Other employers are considering paying bonuses for those who exercise regularly and maintain a healthy weight. What is your reaction to these workplace trends? What are the factors to consider in implementing such programs?

connect

Go online to Connect to complete this activity.
http://connect.mcgraw-hill.com

medications, and medical tests. One physician has summarized the issue by stating, "One of my frustrations in medicine was having people come to me expecting way too much of me and not expecting anything of themselves."

To evaluate your personal lifestyle habits, look to *Healthy Lifestyle: A Self-Assessment,* Lab Activity 1-1.

TOP 10 LIST

Lifestyle Practices That Enhance Wellness

1. Exercise aerobically at least four to five times per week.
2. Eliminate all tobacco products.
3. Limit animal fats, cholesterol, trans fats, and saturated fats in the diet.
4. Eat five to nine daily servings of fruits and vegetables and include other high-fiber foods and whole grains every day in the diet.
5. Assess personal stressors and practice stress management techniques, including maintaining a strong social support system.
6. Limit the consumption of alcohol to no more than one drink (women) or two drinks (men) per day.
7. Pursue and maintain a healthy weight.
8. Fasten seat belts.
9. Practice safer sex habits.
10. Balance work, social, and personal time, including getting 7 to 9 hours of sleep every night.

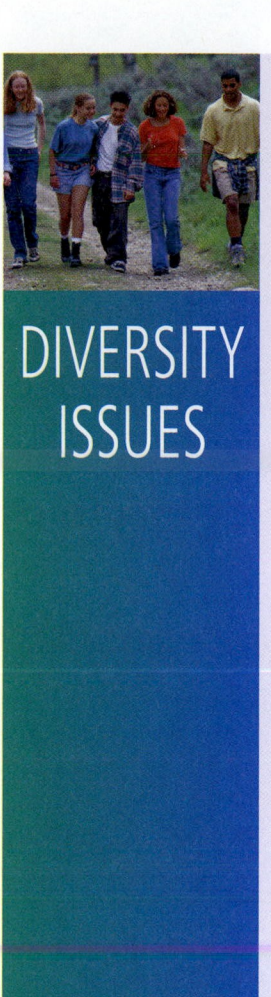

DIVERSITY ISSUES

Health Disparities Among Americans

Although the diversity of the American population may be one of our nation's greatest assets, diversity also presents a range of health improvement challenges. Causes for these disparities could be variances in education and income levels, accessibility to health care, health insurance coverage, cultural preferences and influences, and discrimination. African Americans, American Indians, Alaska Natives, Asian Americans, Hispanics, and Pacific Islanders are more likely than whites to have poor health and to die prematurely, as the following examples illustrate:

- **Breast and cervical cancers.** Although death rates from breast cancer are declining steadily, they remain higher among black women than among white women. African American women are more than twice as likely to die of cervical cancer than white women. Women of racial and ethnic minorities also are less likely than white women to get regular Pap tests.
- **Cardiovascular disease.** Age-adjusted death rates for diseases of the heart were 30 percent higher for African Americans than for whites; death rates for stroke were 41 percent higher. Furthermore, the risk of heart failure among African Americans under age 50 is 20 times that of whites.

- **Diabetes.** Compared with white adults, American Indians and Alaska Natives are 2.3 times, African Americans are 1.6 times, and Hispanics are 1.5 times more likely to have diagnosed diabetes.
- **HIV/AIDS.** Although African Americans and Hispanics represent only 24 percent of the U.S. population, they account for roughly 82 percent of pediatric AIDS cases and 69 percent of both AIDS cases and new HIV infections among adults.
- **Obesity.** The prevalence of obesity is higher among African American women at every age compared with every other gender and racial or ethnic group. Hispanic men have higher obesity rates than any other group of men.
- **Prostate cancer.** African American men die from prostate cancer at more than twice the rate of other men.
- **Life expectancy.** The life expectancy for African Americans (males and females combined) is 4.6 years less than for whites (73.7 years versus 78.3 years). White females have the highest life expectancy, followed, in order, by African American females, white males, and African American males.

Source: Centers for Disease Control and Prevention, National Center for Health Statistics

Understanding Risks

Often in this book we talk about risks. In an effort to prevent disease and promote health, it is important to identify the factors that cause disease and injury. From this process, probabilities are determined as to the chances for occurrence. Like placing a bet at a racetrack, identifying risks is a way of quoting the odds. No one can promise you that doing something or refraining from doing it will keep you safe or that doing one thing will kill you. You must draw your own conclusions from the evidence. There is no such thing as absolute safety, and so you can choose only to widen or to narrow your risk margins with your habits.

One ongoing study has resulted in much of the information we have about the risk factors associated with several chronic diseases. The people of Framingham, Massachusetts, a community 18 miles west of Boston, have been studied and charted since 1950. The Framingham Study, as it has become known, has resulted in information about how heredity, environment, medical care, and lifestyle factors affect heart disease and well-being. A comprehensive longitudinal study such as this, in contrast to a short-term, isolated study involving only a few people, results in reputable data pertaining to risks. So although the risk of most chronic diseases can't be totally eliminated, it can be significantly reduced using information from studies such as this. We hope you are thinking beyond mere "risk avoidance" to a life full of enrichment, self-fulfillment, and satisfaction. This dramatic shift in emphasis toward self-responsibility and an expanded quality of life has evolved into a concept called *wellness*.

HIGH-LEVEL WELLNESS

In 1948 the World Health Organization defined **health** as "a state of complete physical, mental and social well-being and not merely the absence of disease or infirmity." In the late 1950s Dr. Halbert Dunn

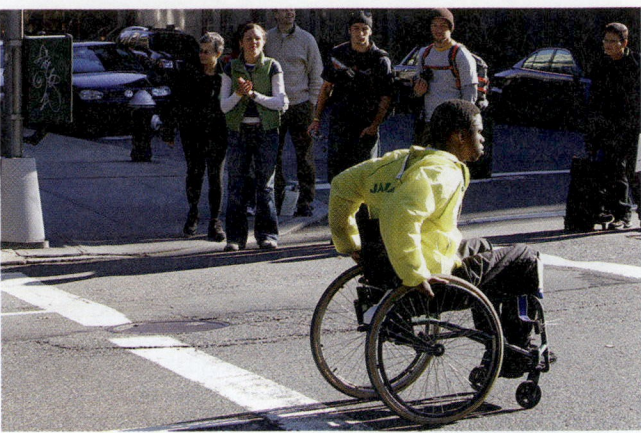

Wellness means striving to be the best you can be regardless of life's situations or circumstances.

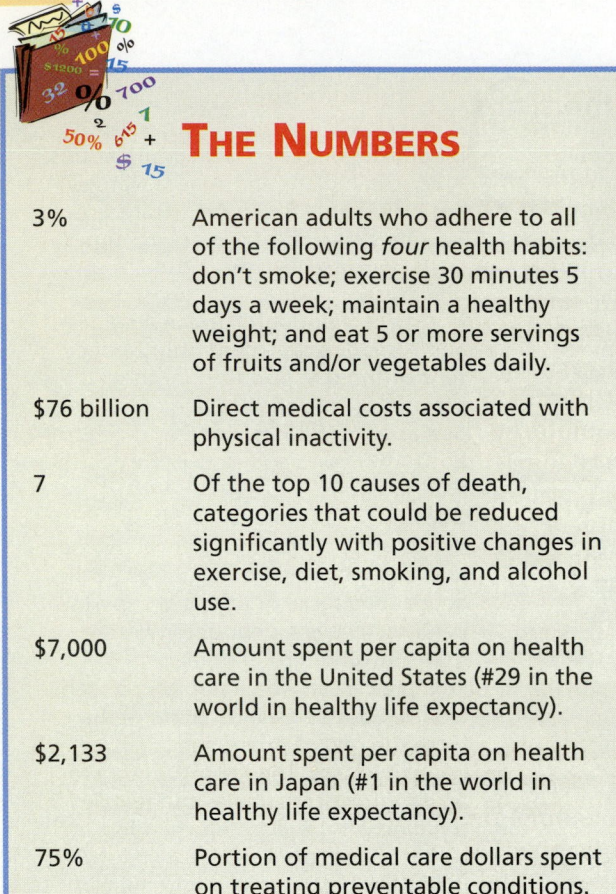

THE NUMBERS

3%	American adults who adhere to all of the following *four* health habits: don't smoke; exercise 30 minutes 5 days a week; maintain a healthy weight; and eat 5 or more servings of fruits and/or vegetables daily.
$76 billion	Direct medical costs associated with physical inactivity.
7	Of the top 10 causes of death, categories that could be reduced significantly with positive changes in exercise, diet, smoking, and alcohol use.
$7,000	Amount spent per capita on health care in the United States (#29 in the world in healthy life expectancy).
$2,133	Amount spent per capita on health care in Japan (#1 in the world in healthy life expectancy).
75%	Portion of medical care dollars spent on treating preventable conditions.

began writing about the upper limits of health—the *ultimate* in health. He was the first to use the word *wellness* in his writings in reference to the pursuit of optimal well-being. Dunn viewed "health" as a relatively passive and neutral state of existence—in contrast to "wellness," which he described as an ever-changing process of growth toward an *elevated* state of superb well-being, and where one is actively working to reach it. Today, **wellness** is defined as *an integrated and dynamic level of functioning oriented toward maximizing potential, dependent on self-responsibility.* Wellness involves not only preventive health behaviors but also a shift in *thinking* and *attitude.* Wellness is a mind-set of lifelong growth and achievement in the emotional, spiritual, physical, occupational, intellectual, environmental, and social dimensions. It means a lifetime of striving toward ever higher levels of functioning where complacency and passivity are not tolerated.

High-level wellness is achievable by people of all ages, all socioeconomic groups, and all types. It involves working toward becoming the best you can be without accepting "traditional" limitations (i.e., age, race, gender, heredity). Wellness is a way of living in which growth and improvement are sought in all areas. It involves a lifestyle of deliberate choices and self-responsibility, requiring conscien-

tious management and planning. Living a wellness lifestyle does not come about by accident or luck. It also involves much more than curing sickness, counting fat grams, jogging, and measuring body fat. It is a *mind-set* of personal empowerment. It means approaching life with optimism, confidence, and energy. Unlike sickness care, which involves treatment, wellness is a lifelong quest toward optimal functioning in which *you* take charge. Individuals who strive for wellness have an exceptional openness to experience. Rather than fearing new experiences and life's changes, they welcome them as a way to grow. They do not allow prejudices or stereotypes to distort their perceptions. They take control of life and face it with creativity and freshness. Living a wellness lifestyle has good potential for increasing longevity. However, this is not the sole purpose of wellness living. Wellness author and advocate Donald Ardell agrees. He states, "Wellness is not a goal to be attained but a process to be maintained." Simply put, wellness is the idea of being aware of and actively working toward better health. When you think of wellness, think of the phrase, "Make the *rest* of your life the *best* of your life." No matter where you are starting from or what you've done in the past, you have the capacity to take steps to improve your personal well-being.

Figure 1-2 shows a wellness continuum. You do not attain a "state of wellness" and then stop. Your personal choices dictate whether you are moving upward toward high-level wellness or downward away from your wellness potential. In what direction are you traveling on the wellness continuum?

The Dimensions of Wellness

The wellness lifestyle is a coordinated and integrated living pattern that involves seven dimensions: physical, intellectual, emotional, social, spiritual,

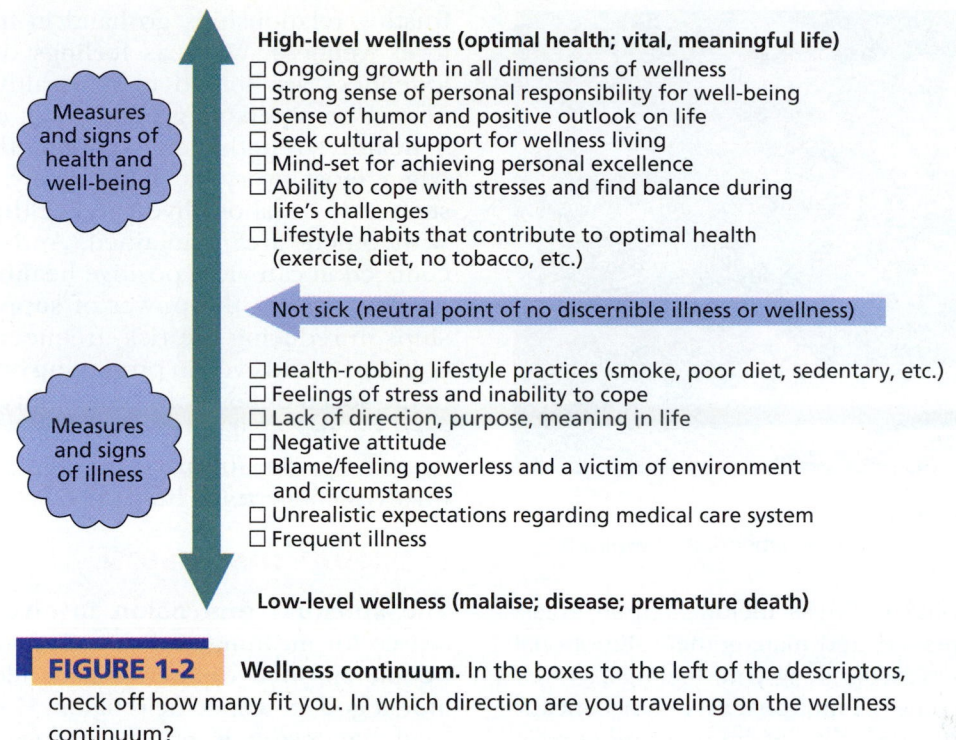

High-level wellness (optimal health; vital, meaningful life)
☐ Ongoing growth in all dimensions of wellness
☐ Strong sense of personal responsibility for well-being
☐ Sense of humor and positive outlook on life
☐ Seek cultural support for wellness living
☐ Mind-set for achieving personal excellence
☐ Ability to cope with stresses and find balance during
    life's challenges
☐ Lifestyle habits that contribute to optimal health
    (exercise, diet, no tobacco, etc.)

Measures and signs of health and well-being

Not sick (neutral point of no discernible illness or wellness)

Measures and signs of illness

☐ Health-robbing lifestyle practices (smoke, poor diet, sedentary, etc.)
☐ Feelings of stress and inability to cope
☐ Lack of direction, purpose, meaning in life
☐ Negative attitude
☐ Blame/feeling powerless and a victim of environment
    and circumstances
☐ Unrealistic expectations regarding medical care system
☐ Frequent illness

Low-level wellness (malaise; disease; premature death)

FIGURE 1-2   **Wellness continuum.** In the boxes to the left of the descriptors, check off how many fit you. In which direction are you traveling on the wellness continuum?

environmental, and occupational. There is a strong interconnection among these dimensions. For example, joining an exercise class in your community most notably enhances your physical well-being, but it can also be socially enriching and intellectually stimulating as you learn more about the functional capacity of the human body. It can also help relieve emotional stress. Attending the class with coworkers after work may improve your occupational wellness. In each dimension there is opportunity for personal growth, and due to the dimensions' interrelationships, growth in one area often sparks interest in another. *Balancing* these dimensions, however, is important in pursuing wellness. For example, being an avid reader yet not being able to get along with anyone is not an example of balanced wellness.

PHYSICAL DIMENSION

The **physical dimension** deals with the functional operation of the body. It involves the health-related components of physical fitness—muscular strength, muscular endurance, cardiorespiratory endurance, flexibility, and body composition. Dietary habits have a significant effect on physical well-being. Your sexual, drinking, and drug behaviors also play a role in physical health. Do you smoke? Do you get enough sleep? Are you overweight? Do you catch many colds? These questions deal with your physical dimension.

The physical dimension also includes medical self-care—regular self-tests, medical and dental checkups, proper use of medications, taking

necessary steps when you are ill, and appropriate use of the medical system. Managing your environment also affects physical well-being. For example, do you try to minimize your exposure to tobacco smoke and harmful pollutants? Your body is the vehicle in which you travel throughout life; treat it like the precious entity it is.

INTELLECTUAL DIMENSION

The **intellectual dimension** involves the use of your mind. Maintaining an active mind contributes to total well-being. Intellectual growth is not restricted to formal education—that is, school learning. It involves a continuous acquisition of knowledge throughout life, engaging your mind in creative and stimulating mental activities, and opening your mind to new ideas. Curiosity and learning should never stop. Reading, writing, and keeping abreast of current events are intellectual pursuits. Being able to think critically and analyze, evaluate, and apply knowledge is also associated with this dimension. Do you visit museums or attend cultural events? Do you watch educational programs on television? The link between intellectual stimulation and healthy living is undeniable.

EMOTIONAL DIMENSION

The abilities to laugh, enjoy life, adjust to change, cope with stress, and maintain intimate relationships are examples of the **emotional dimension** of

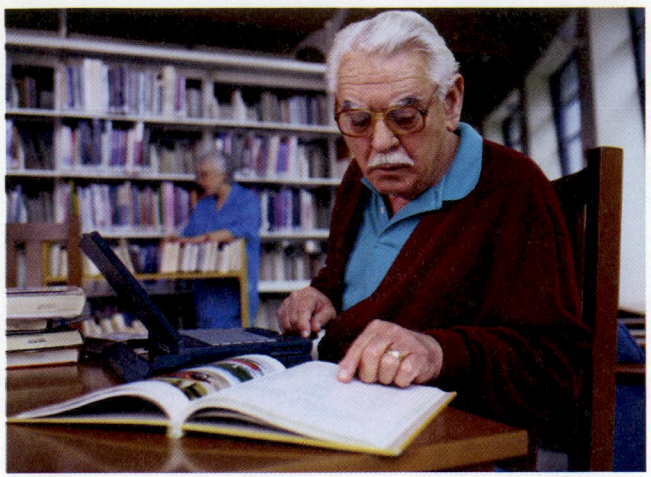

Having a strong desire to continue learning throughout life shows strength in the intellectual dimension of wellness.

wellness. Emotional wellness includes three areas: awareness, acceptance, and management. Emotional awareness involves recognizing your feelings, as well as the feelings of others. Emotional acceptance means understanding the normality of human emotion, in addition to assessing your personal abilities and limitations realistically. Emotional management is the ability to control or cope with personal feelings and knowing how to seek support when necessary. It involves having adequate stress-coping mechanisms.

At one time the mind was considered a separate entity from the physical body. Now, however, there is much research linking emotions to physical well-being. A complex system of chemical messengers connects the mind and body. The production of these chemicals can be turned on and off based on thoughts and emotions. Therefore, being stuck in a negative emotional state (anger, loss, depression, fear, anxiety, or hostility) can affect this chemical system, thereby reducing immune function and increasing illness. Conversely, emotions such as happiness, contentment, and joy can positively affect health and vitality.

Research shows that optimistic and positive-thinking people live longer. They become masters of their own fate not just because they *believe* good things will happen but also because they believe they can *make* good things happen. Having a positive mental state is directly linked to wellness.

SOCIAL DIMENSION

Everyone must interact with people. The **social dimension** of wellness involves the ability to get along with others, appreciate the uniqueness of others, and feel connected to others. You achieve social wellness when you feel a genuine sense of belonging to a social unit. Good friends, close family ties, volunteerism, community involvement, and trusting relationships go hand in hand with high-level wellness. Whereas feelings of isolation and loneliness are linked to ill health, feeling "connected" to a person, group, cause, or even a pet is a health strengthener. Granted, there are times when most everyone feels lonely. However, this state can be short lived if healthy relationships with others are maintained. And this feeling of connection can yield positive health benefits. Studies have shown the power of supportive relationships in reducing the risk, frequency, and severity of illness—and even in promoting healing. Included in the social dimension is the ability to exhibit concern for the welfare of your community and fairness and justice toward others. Social wellness also involves concern for humanity as a whole.

SPIRITUAL DIMENSION

The **spiritual dimension** involves the personal search for meaning and direction in life. For many people spiritual wellness means identifying a creator, a god, or a specific religion. However, the spiritual dimension is not always synonymous with religion. In its purest sense, spiritual wellness involves cultivating beliefs, principles, and values that provide guidance and strength throughout all of life's experiences. Why am I here? What path will lead to fulfillment in my life? What is life about? What are my values? These questions are most often answered within the context of a larger reality beyond the physical and material aspects of existence. Selflessness; compassion; honesty; joy for living; forgiveness; charity; and the development of a clear, comfortable sense of right and wrong are components of spiritual wellness. The Top 10 "Components of Spirituality" can help you gain an understanding of the components of a spiritual life.

There is a strong connection between spirituality and self-esteem because of the internal feelings of self-worth that occur when a sense of hope, purpose, and morality is developed. Attempts to achieve long-term self-esteem through external constructs of power, socioeconomic status, or physical appearance fail. Like all dimensions of wellness, spirituality does not "happen." It is a process of growth requiring time and attention. Medicine has begun to recognize the strong influence of spirituality on health and illness. Studies of cancer patients have shown that those who continuously pursue goals related to living a meaningful life boost the natural killer cell activity in their immune systems.

ENVIRONMENTAL DIMENSION

The **environmental dimension** of wellness deals with the preservation of natural resources as well as

TOP 10 LIST

Components of Spirituality

Spirituality and religion are related but not always synonymous. However, the practice of religion may deepen spirituality for some. One cannot discount the importance of organized religion to the spirituality of millions. Nevertheless, it is inappropriate to suggest that one must practice a specific religion to develop spiritual wellness. This list includes components that are typically seen in a spiritual life. Those who develop spiritual wellness see spirituality as a journey or process, not a destination. How many of these 10 components do you possess?

1. Belief in a higher power, being, or energy force greater than oneself that provides strength in coping with the demands and challenges of life.
2. Feelings of hope about the future.
3. Feelings of purpose, meaning, and direction in life.
4. Feelings of optimism; ability to see the best side of a situation.
5. Regular worship, prayer, meditation, or spiritual study/reflection.
6. Universal love and devotion to the welfare of others.
7. Possession of moral and ethical principles that reflect one's spiritual beliefs.
8. Possession of a clear set of values and ability to live according to those values.
9. Ability to share spiritual values with others and tolerance of others whose beliefs are different from yours.
10. Feeling a sense of unity with nature and the universe; inner peace.

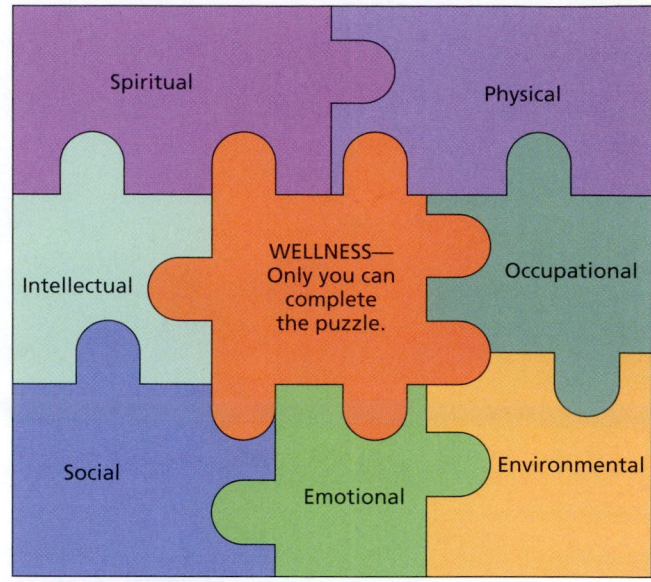

FIGURE 1-3 Wellness involves an interconnectedness of all seven dimensions.

the protection of plants and wildlife. We have basic biological needs that include safe air, water, and food. Our dependence on the automobile and the general industrialization of our world have created worldwide pollution and changes in the atmosphere. Habits such as recycling, limiting the use of pesticides, carpooling, and conserving electricity show positive involvement in the environmental dimension of wellness. Demonstrating a commitment to the protection of wildlife and plants is also a component of environmental wellness. We must *all* take part in sustaining and improving the quality of the environment for current and future generations.

OCCUPATIONAL DIMENSION

The **occupational dimension** involves deriving personal satisfaction from your vocation. Much of your life will be spent at work. Therefore, it is important that your chosen career provide the internal and external rewards you value. Do you want a job that allows for creativity, interaction with others, daily challenge, or autonomy? Do you prefer opportunities for advancement, personal entrepreneurship, leadership, or helping others? How do you feel about mobility? Is salary your major motivation? Answering these questions may help you with career selection. Occupational wellness also involves maintaining a satisfying balance between work time and leisure time. It involves a work environment that minimizes stress and exposure to physical health hazards. A majority of your college life is spent analyzing your skills and interests and integrating them with career choices. It is vital that your vocational choice be personally enriching and stimulating. If you are not happy with your occupation, you will find that your entire well-being suffers.

As depicted in Figure 1-3, wellness is an interlocking combination of all seven dimensions. It means striving for growth in each dimension and appreciating the interconnectedness among all of them. Is there one dimension in which you are strongest? Which dimension is your weakest? Neglecting any dimension destroys the balance critical to high-level wellness. Certain dimensions may take on a greater importance at different times throughout your life. Nevertheless, striving for balance contributes to your wholeness. To evaluate your wellness in the seven dimensions, you are encouraged to do Lab Activity 1-2, *Assessing Your Wellness*. Doing this assessment will also help you understand the broad array of choices within each dimension.

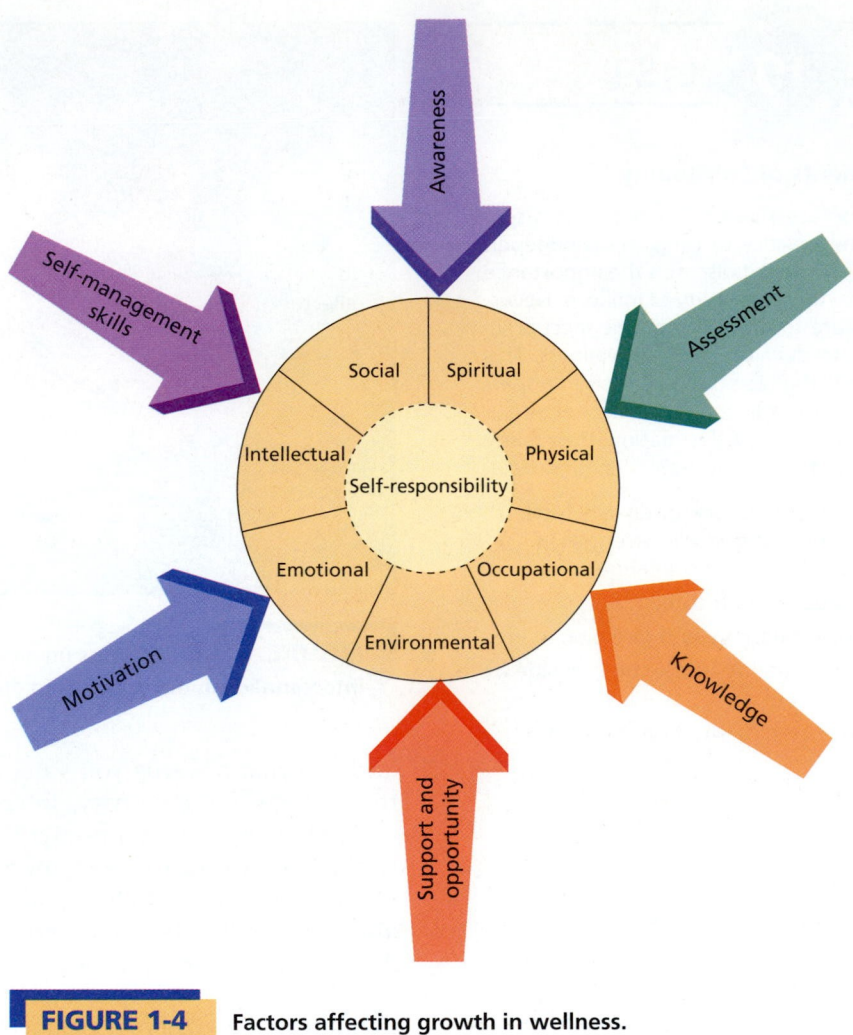

FIGURE 1-4   Factors affecting growth in wellness.

Growth in Wellness

We have described wellness as a dynamic course of action based on self-responsibility. The goal is to assume greater responsibility for your quality of life by making positive lifestyle decisions. How do you begin making positive lifestyle choices? How do you know the options available to you? How do you grow in wellness? As Figure 1-4 shows, growth in wellness is influenced by many factors. Wellness living is an *active* process, and so understanding how each of the factors contributes to your growth in each dimension is important.

AWARENESS

Before you can grow in wellness you must have an awareness of wellness options. You are now aware that your health, happiness, and quality of life are strongly affected by your willingness to make wellness choices. Your well-being is not solely the responsibility of the medical care system. You have

choices. The increasing general interest in wellness has made it easier for an individual to adopt a wellness lifestyle, because wellness choices now are not only available but valued.

Wellness is . . . .

wellness	is a continuous, active process—an ongoing, lifelong effort oriented toward maximizing one's potential.
wellness	is commitment—a determined choice to move toward optimal well-being.
wellness	is proactive—an approach to living, loving, working, and playing based on your values.
wellness	is a way of life—a lifestyle you design to achieve optimal health.
wellness	is an integration—an appreciation that everything you do, think, feel, and believe has an impact on your well-being.

ASSESSMENT

Once you are aware of the wellness option, you should assess your lifestyle. Assessment allows you to see how you are conducting your life and identify where changes should occur. An assessment can be anything from medical tests (cholesterol profile, blood pressure, bone density, etc.) to physical fitness tests. They can be stress inventories, health-risk appraisals, dietary logs, or even attitude questionnaires. Personality assessments can help you understand your social and professional relationships. Assessment offers an opportunity to begin the process of self-observation as you confront a wellness issue. You will find a wide variety of assessments throughout this book.

KNOWLEDGE

Having knowledge in the lifestyle areas helps you make decisions. For example, suppose from an assessment you learn your blood cholesterol level. What level constitutes high blood cholesterol? How do you go about reducing your cholesterol? What dietary changes can make an impact? Will exercise help? Having accurate knowledge about nutrition, fitness, stress, and other areas of health can help you understand your risks and become a foundation for you to build upon. However, knowledge is not enough. You must have self-management skills and motivation to put that knowledge to good use.

SELF-MANAGEMENT SKILLS

Self-management skills help you try some of the options. Skills in goal setting, behavior modification, and personal strategy building enable you to make the necessary lifestyle changes. How do I go about managing stress? Eating nutritiously in the residence hall or on a tight budget? Fitting regular exercise into my busy schedule? Self-management skills help you incorporate strategies of self-change into your life so that daily lifestyle choices are habitually "wellness choices." Realize that it takes time and practice to develop these skills into lifetime habits.

MOTIVATION

Motivation is the desire to do something—a stimulus to action. Motivation gets you started and keeps you going as you strive for continued wellness growth. It is also very personal and complex. It changes throughout life and is specific to each person. For example, a 19-year-old may be motivated to lose weight to look better. A 55-year-old may want to lose weight to help reduce high blood pressure.

Motivation is strongly influenced by locus of control. **Locus of control** is an individual's belief about how much power he or she has in regard to what happens to him or her. If you believe that personal actions can make a difference in your life, you have an *internal* locus of control. If you feel, however, that factors beyond your control—environment, heredity, chance, friends, luck—play a greater role, you have an *external* locus of control. Because those with an external locus of control do not relate their personal behavior to outcomes, they are less likely to be motivated to take charge of their lives. Having an internal locus of control makes it easier to be motivated and committed to a wellness lifestyle. Whether the goal is to lose weight, manage stress, or get along better with a roommate, a variety of complex factors affect a person's ability to change the behavior and sustain motivation. More detailed information relating to behavior-change techniques and motivation is given in Chapter 2.

SUPPORT AND OPPORTUNITY

Maintaining positive lifestyle choices is best achieved when there is support and encouragement from the organizations and environments surrounding you. For example, suppose you join a smoking cessation class. You are starting your climb toward permanent behavior change. If you face returning every day to a roommate who smokes or to a workplace where coworkers smoke, your chances of maintaining your new behavior are considerably lower. Your family, friends, and group affiliations have a strong influence on your behavior. It has been found that there are significant correlations among self-esteem, social support, and a healthy lifestyle. Choices are not made in a vacuum, and so the aim should be to establish a health-promoting environment in which persons like you can easily make health-significant decisions. Choosing a living or working environment where others strive for wellness can assist you in wellness growth. That is why it is important for schools, communities, and government agencies to provide wellness support to cultivate lifestyle changes. When people have an opportunity to practice healthy behaviors, they are more likely to do them. Making healthy choices is easier when one has access to healthy foods, safe and inviting places to exercise, and stress-reducing activities. Having a supportive environment may be the most powerful factor of all. Do you feel your roommates, friends, and family are supportive of wellness? How about your campus? Why or why not?

SELF-RESPONSIBILITY

At the center of wellness growth is self-responsibility. The goal is to assume greater responsibility for your quality of life by making positive lifestyle decisions.

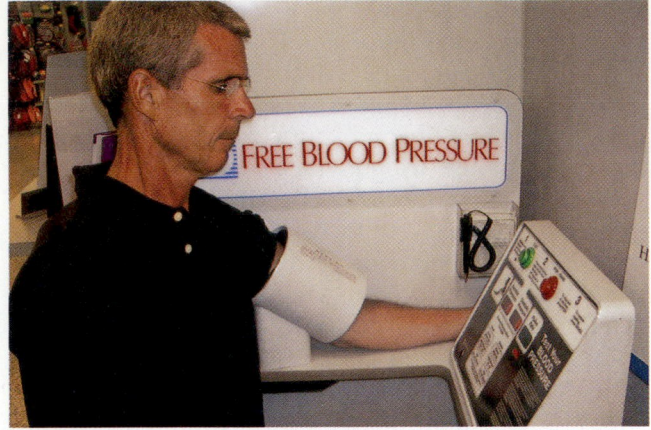

Checking your blood pressure is an example of a wellness assessment that you can do at many pharmacies and grocery stores.

Understandably, for every decision to be made there are alternatives and consequences. Your challenge is to make thoughtful decisions that direct you toward high-level wellness. You know what you can and cannot control. Part of self-responsibility is recognizing this. Heredity is an example of something you cannot control. You had no voice in selecting your genetic tendencies. A physical disability is another uncontrollable life situation. Self-responsibility in wellness is making the best of the "hand you are dealt" regardless of your stage in life or circumstances.

Self-responsibility in wellness also means active involvement. Having realistic expectations, a sense of personal accountability, and a sense of humor will help you see wellness living as a joyful experience. Self-responsibility involves self-control as opposed to going along with the crowd or merely reacting to what seems to happen. Because everyone else is eating a triple order of french fries, that does not mean you must. When everyone else is grumbling about the weather, why not find something positive about it? Wellness is about personal empowerment—having a sense of ownership and control of the decision-making process.

As you travel this wellness path, you will probably become more aware of how society can help and hinder your trip. Societal or environmental support has a powerful influence on promoting and maintaining a wellness lifestyle. Therefore, it is important to understand the power of societal norms.

◆ SOCIETAL NORMS

We are influenced by what we encounter every day. We are constantly bombarded by subtle yet extremely powerful messages that are sometimes obstacles to

TABLE 1-2   Societal Norms That Promote "Unwellness"

- The idea that everyone must be extremely thin (especially women)
- The assumption that alcohol abuse is an acceptable rite of passage into college
- The media's portrayal of sex as being glamorous, without commitment or consequences
- Social events, parties, celebrations where alcohol and food abuse is expected (New Year's Eve, wedding receptions, Super Bowl parties, tailgating, etc.)
- The number of high-sugar and high-fat gifts associated with holidays such as Valentine's Day, Easter, Halloween, and Christmas
- The habit of driving a car to go short distances
- Equating tanned skin with beauty, wealth, power, and sex appeal (thus, the emergence of thousands of tanning salons)
- Vending machines at offices and schools loaded with candy bars, chips, cookies, and doughnuts
- Fast-food restaurants that offer burgers and fries (with few healthy alternatives)
- Miles and miles of roads built *without* sidewalks or bike lanes
- The elimination of daily physical education in the schools coupled with the parental push for private sports lessons and competitive Little League football, baseball, soccer, etc. (often serving only the best athletes and emphasizing "winning" rather than lifetime participation)
- Access to television 24 hours a day, with a choice of hundreds of cable stations—all changed by remote control
- The notion that as you grow older it is OK to be inactive and fat
- Consistently driving 5–15 mph over the speed limit
- Extra large portions or an "all you can eat" emphasis at restaurants

wellness. Our behavioral choices are strongly affected by unwritten codes that permeate our daily lives and can contradict and sabotage a wellness lifestyle. **Societal norms** are behaviors or practices that are expected in a culture and that are accepted and supported by its members. Our society often makes it easy to do things we know are not good for us.

These unwritten rules are carried on from generation to generation. Table 1-2 lists circumstances and norms you have probably grown up with. As you look at them, consider the messages they give. Do they promote wellness as you know it? You can probably think of more examples.

Many of our norms encourage a sedentary lifestyle. Somehow we've absorbed the notion that minimal exertion is better. Heaven forbid if, when operating your car, you have to roll down your own windows, walk around the car to unlock the doors, or keep constant pressure on the accelerator while driving on the interstate. We push buttons to open

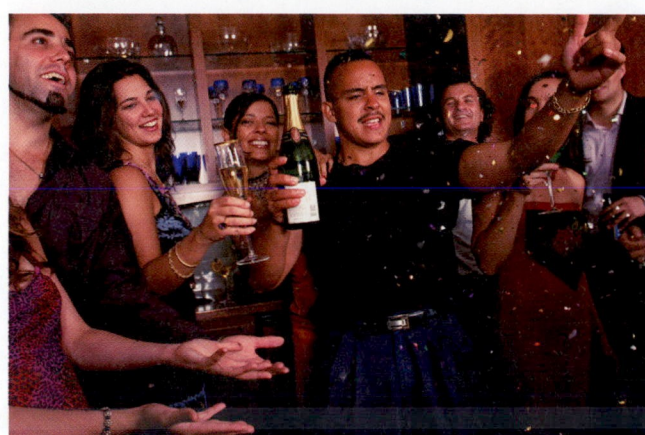

The alcohol abuse often associated with New Year's Eve parties is an example of an unhealthy social norm.

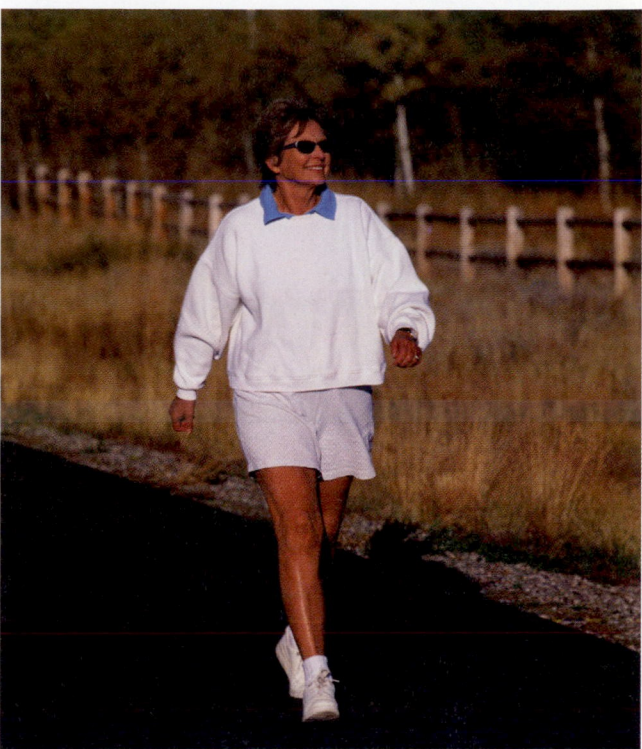

Many communities are converting old railroad tracks to paved exercise trails—an example of a commitment to wellness.

garage doors, change television channels, and order food delivery. You can go to the bank, a fast-food restaurant, a dry cleaner, and a drug store without ever leaving the comfort of your car. What kind of message is this sending?

The advertising industry is especially effective at influencing us with messages. We see former star athletes guzzling beer that is "less filling." Every Saturday morning high-sugar snacks are displayed on television. If thin, attractive movie stars enjoy smoking, perhaps you will, too. Lab Activity 1-3 allows you to explore the norms in your community or campus.

In traveling the road to optimum well-being, be aware of these pitfalls and obstacles in our society. Remember, it is you who will make the daily choices as to how to live your life. You are the one who must assess the traps that may impede your pursuit of wellness. Self-responsibility is the key.

Changing Times: Making Wellness the Norm

Now that the wellness concept has begun to invade the health care profession and society as a whole, we can see some norms changing. Thirty years ago the only people jogging were athletes in training or fitness "nuts." Now no one takes a second look even at senior citizens fitness walking along roads. Businesspeople pack their workout gear next to their business reports. Hotels provide workout facilities and hand out jogging maps to guests. Stress management, parenting, addictive behavior management, smoking cessation, and a multitude of other wellness topics are offered in community classes and workshops. As wellness permeates our society, there are more resources that support this lifestyle. There are positive choices available in grocery stores—more whole-wheat breads and cereals, low-sugar and low-salt products, low-fat dairy items, even take-out salad and fruit bars. Restaurants are also responding to consumer demand for more nutritious food selections. These are a few of the positive changes that reflect wellness awareness. Only by drawing together all available resources (individual, community, media, school, corporate, government) will we fix current health problems. This multilevel approach is necessary to bring about changes in societal norms.

For example, a study by the RAND Corporation found that as communities become more spread out and less walkable, chronic disease rates go up. Therefore, suburban design may be an important new avenue for health promotion. Our choices are shaped by our surroundings. If you live in a subdivision or work in an office park where you can't buy a stamp without getting on the interstate, you are going to rely on a car more than your own legs. Health messages and advice go only so far. The real secret to wellness is making the healthy choice the *easy* choice! City planners are now looking at ways to improve people's options. Bike lanes, walking paths, neighborhoods with sidewalks; shops, healthy restaurants, and office structures connected by walking bridges; and other improvements encourage more activity. This is a positive change from past cultural norms that engineered physical activity out of our daily lives.

Beyond the physical, health-related factors of wellness, it is important to change people's attitudes. It should not be considered bizarre for people to arrive at work or at a class full of enthusiasm rather than full of complaints. It is also not weird to take a few moments to stretch or close your eyes to relax during the day, congratulate another person for doing well on an exam, adhere to the speed limit, have a fruit juice rather than a beer at a party, give someone a hug, or have fun in life. These are behaviors that reflect wellness and are brought about by awareness, education, and growth in wellness. Perhaps wellness advocate Don Ardell says it best: "I urge people not to be 'normal.' A 'normal' lifestyle is hazardous to your health. Most 'normal' people are overstressed, overweight, underfit, and have given in to poor diets. In addition, most 'normal' people aren't having all that much fun living. Most normals aren't seeking added meaning and purpose in their lives."

It will take time for everyone to respond to this trend of positive lifestyle choices. You can do your part by encouraging those around you to make wellness a lifetime pursuit. Pass these attitudes and behaviors on to your children. Support changes in

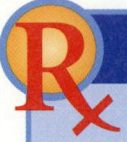

PRESCRIPTION FOR ACTION

You've read the chapter, now go do one or more of these.

✓ Schedule into your planner an exercise "appointment" with yourself.

✓ Read the entire front page of a major newspaper.

✓ Write down three positive wellness behaviors you can do today. Then do them!

✓ Do two anonymous good deeds for someone.

✓ Get 7 to 9 hours of sleep tonight.

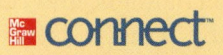

Go online to Connect to complete this activity.
http://connect.mcgraw-hill.com

society that make it easier for everyone to stay healthy. In doing so, you will help make wellness and self-responsibility society's norm.

Frequently Asked Questions

Q. I am 20 years old. I realize I don't have the best health habits. Like many college students, I eat a lot of fast foods at the food courts and am too busy to exercise. I smoke to relieve stress, and I drink alcohol. What's the point of adopting all these "healthy habits" at my age when I feel fine and have no symptoms of disease?

A. It is normal for young adults to feel healthy and invulnerable to future disease despite poor lifestyle choices. Nevertheless, these poor habits often become *lifetime habits!* Chronic diseases such as cancer, heart disease, type 2 diabetes, and osteoporosis take years to develop. Damage accumulates over time. Look at older friends and relatives who have practiced these habits for 30 years. Do you like what you see? Knowing this, you may find it easier to make gradual moderate lifestyle changes now rather than having to change "cold turkey" once a health scare has occurred. Those things you cannot feel (cells, artery walls, bones, organ tissues, etc.) will thank you in the long run. Also, there may be an immediate payoff. Do you feel as energized as you possibly could? Do you like what you see when you look in the mirror? If you begin now to change some of these habits, you'll reap the benefits immediately—and for

years. Remember, healthy living is not just an exercise in abstinence. It's about feeling better and looking better every day of your life.

Q. My father had a heart attack at age 50, and my mom has cancer. What impact does genetics have on my future health and longevity?

A. For some, familial tendencies constitute a psychological trap. If your father has heart disease and your mother has cancer, your chances of following in their footsteps are greater than those of someone whose parents are healthy at age 75. However, this is the case only if your parents' health problems were a result of genetics rather than environment or lifestyle abuse. If you inherited a genetic liability, this knowledge should give you additional motivation to live in such a way as to fight it—controlling your blood pressure and cholesterol, exercising regularly, not smoking, eating healthy foods, and so on. Heredity is only one factor in the link to health and well-being. Although our biological inheritance predisposes us to certain illnesses and protects us from others, it is the interaction of genetics, culture, environment, and habits that counts. Your environment and personal health habits can either magnify or inhibit the tendencies with which you were born.

Q. **Considering the health disparities and challenging diversity issues surrounding the health status of Americans, what can I do to make it better?**

A. *Healthy People 2020* defines the nation's health agenda through overarching goals. By identifying specific objectives within these goals, national, state, and local organizations and agencies can work together to disseminate preventive health information. Through school programs, Internet and media communications, and community programming a lot can be accomplished. However, change occurs one person at a time. As you assimilate the knowledge and practices that surround a wellness lifestyle and attitude, you are setting an example for those around you. You can communicate to others the benefits and advantages of taking personal responsibility for one's health destiny. You can become an advocate for wellness alternatives in your school and workplace. It can start with you!

Q. **I do well on a majority of health habits. However, I never seem to get enough sleep. Is it really that important to get 7 to 9 hours of sleep every night?**

A. You are not alone. Sleep has become a dwindling American resource, with only 33 percent of adults getting the recommended 7 to 9 hours a night. We are spending more hours working, watching television, socializing, and interacting with a computer at the expense of quality sleep. Chronic sleep deprivation can contribute to a weakened immune system, diabetes, high blood pressure, heart disease, mood disturbances, work inefficiency, traffic accidents, and even obesity. Shift workers who routinely get little sleep because of their irregular work hours live on average 10 years less than do those who work standard hours. Take heed and make an effort to turn off the TV and the computer and get to bed!

Q. **Why are U.S. health care costs so much higher per capita than other similar industrialized countries, and yet our healthy life expectancy is nowhere near the top?**

A. There is not a simple answer to this question. A multitude of factors are driving up the health care costs in the United States. Many feel that overtreatment is the cause (i.e., expensive medical tests and procedures ordered that may be unnecessary). Physicians fearing malpractice lawsuits fuel some of these ordered tests. Research shows that billions are spent each year on treatments, tests, and hospitalizations that do nothing to improve health. Others feel that drug development and the extensive advertising by pharmaceutical companies are contributors. Also, there are more specialists in the medical field, and they command higher salaries. Add into this mix the administrative paperwork of health insurance companies, which ties up almost one-third of overall health care costs.

Whatever the cause, 20 percent of patients account for 80 percent of the spending, and that 20 percent is made up mostly of the chronically ill. Diabetes, heart disease, high blood pressure, and obesity are chronic conditions that are driving up costs. Only when lifestyle and prevention strategies are embraced by society to prevent the early onset of chronic diseases will health care costs begin to fall. These preventive strategies can begin with *you*.

Summary

Many adults in the United States die prematurely from chronic diseases that are primarily a result of lifestyle abuse. Many others suffer from major limitations due to these chronic illnesses. Health promoters stress the importance of healthy behaviors in deterring the ravaging effects of such "diseases of choice," especially since the economic impact is so huge. With the cost of health care increasing so rapidly, we cannot effectively address these escalating health care costs without addressing the problem of chronic diseases. *Healthy People 2020* was published by the federal government in an effort to spark a national commitment to self-responsibility for well-being and acknowledge the need for community-based support systems to help those pursuing wellness lifestyles. There is a need for a nationwide, coordinated preventive approach that promotes healthy lifestyles, supports people of every age, and eliminates health disparities.

High-level wellness is a dynamic level of functioning that is oriented toward maximizing a person's potential. It is an integrated living pattern involving seven dimensions—physical, intellectual, emotional, social, spiritual, environmental, and occupational. It is a lifelong journey that involves a conscientious effort to reach one's full potential. The cornerstone of wellness living is self-responsibility. Wellness growth involves a multifaceted approach of awareness, assessment, motivation, knowledge, support, and self-management skills. It includes intelligent deciphering of societal norms, recognizing your power, making choices, interpreting risks, and understanding personal limitations.

The objective of wellness is a richer, more satisfying life. Wellness is an attitude of living so meaningfully and deliberately that in the end you will have lived a full life, no matter how long it is.

Terms

- chronic diseases
- emotional dimension
- environmental dimension
- health
- health promotion
- healthy life expectancy
- intellectual dimension
- locus of control
- occupational dimension
- physical dimension
- social dimension
- societal norms
- spiritual dimension
- wellness

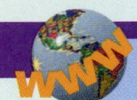

Internet Resources

Aetna Intelihealth

www.intelihealth.com

Provides consumer-oriented information on a variety of health topics, including lifestyle choices, disease conditions, and an array of interactive tools and assessments.

Centers for Disease Control and Prevention (CDC)

www.cdc.gov

Offers a vast amount of information on a variety of wellness topics on its site.

Columbia University Health Service

www.goaskalice.columbia.edu

This interactive site provides answers to college students' questions about relationships, sex, emotional health, fitness, nutrition, alcohol, and general health. Anyone can ask questions anonymously.

Healthfinder

www.healthfinder.gov

A guide to reliable health information, including diseases, Web sites of health organizations, recent health news, and online self-assessments and quizzes.

HealthierUS

www.healthierus.gov

As part of a nationwide initiative, this site encourages and emphasizes physical fitness, prevention, nutrition, and healthy choices. Included are links to many sources.

Healthy People 2020

www.healthypeople.gov

Provides information on the goals, objectives, leading health indicators, and priority areas in the federal government's publication *Healthy People 2020*.

Mayo Clinic

www.mayoclinic.com

Contains reliable health and wellness information on a variety of topics, including diseases and conditions, lifestyle choices, nutrition, aging, stress, fitness, and occupational and gender issues.

National Institutes of Health (NIH)

www.nih.gov

Provides extensive health information and scientific resources covering disease prevention, treatment, and a wide variety of wellness topics.

Real Age

www.realage.com

Provides unique personal health management tools that educate, empower, and support healthy behaviors. The interactive assessments provide individualized lifestyle information.

Trust for America's Health

http://healthyamericans.org

A nonprofit organization dedicated to protecting America's health and preventing disease. This site covers a wide variety of health topics, including statistics and health indicators on every state.

U.S. Department of Health and Human Services

www.dhhs.gov

Addresses all aspects of disease, health promotion, and wellness issues affecting people of all ages and sexes as well as specific populations.

U.S. National Library of Medicine

www.nlm.nih.gov

Links to a number of databases and electronic information such as Medline and other medical libraries.

Web MD

www.webmd.com

Provides valuable and up-to-date health information, tools for managing your health, and support for those who seek information.

Yahoo Health Directory

http://health.yahoo.com

Contains hundreds of health-related Web sites covering a wide range of topics and a search engine to help you go directly to the sites of interest.

Your Disease Risk

www.yourdiseaserisk.wustl.edu

Allows you to assess your risk of developing cancer, diabetes, heart disease, osteoporosis, and stroke. Also gives prevention tips.

LAB Activity 1-1

Healthy Lifestyle: A Self-Assessment

Everyone wants good health. However, many people do not have habits that contribute to health, well-being, and vitality. Health professionals now describe *lifestyle* as one of the most important factors affecting health. This lifestyle assessment, adapted from one created by the U.S. Public Health Service, will help you evaluate how well you are doing at managing the factors that strongly affect your present and future health. For each statement choose the answer that best describes your behavior. Then add up your scores for each section.

	Almost Always	Sometimes	Never
Tobacco **(If you never use tobacco, enter a score of 10 for this section and go to the next sections.)**			
1. I put limits on my tobacco use.	2	1	0
2. I smoke only low tar/nicotine cigarettes *or* I smoke a pipe or cigars *or* I use smokeless tobacco.	2	1	0
Tobacco Score _____			
Exercise/Fitness			
1. I engage in vigorous exercise (examples include jogging, swimming, brisk walking, cycling) for 20–60 minutes, 3–5 days a week.	4	1	0
2. I do exercises to develop muscular strength and endurance (examples include weight lifting, using exercise bands, pushups, abdominal curls) at least twice a week.	2	1	0
3. I spend some of my leisure time participating in physical activities such as golf, tennis, softball, bowling, or gardening.	2	1	0
4. I maintain a healthy weight, avoiding overweight and underweight.	2	1	0
Exercise/Fitness Score _____			
Nutrition			
1. I eat a variety of foods each day, including five or more servings of fruits and/or vegetables	3	1	0
2. I limit the amount of total fat, cholesterol, saturated fat, and trans fats in my diet.	3	1	0
3. I limit the amount of salt and sugar I eat.	2	1	0
4. I intentionally include whole grains and dairy/calcium products in my diet every day.	2	1	0
Nutrition Score _____			
Stress			
1. I enjoy being a student, and do other work that I enjoy.	2	1	0
2. I find it easy to relax and express my feelings freely.	2	1	0
3. I use healthy coping skills for managing the stress in my life.	2	1	0

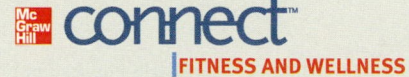

http://connect.mcgraw-hill.com

LAB Activity ■ **CHAPTER 1**

	Almost Always	Sometimes	Never
4. I have close friends, relatives, or others I can talk to about personal matters and call on for help when needed.	2	1	0
5. I participate in group activities (such as community, school, church organizations) and/or hobbies that I enjoy.	2	1	0

Stress Score _____

Alcohol and Drugs

	Almost Always	Sometimes	Never
1. I avoid alcohol *or* I drink no more than 1 (women) or 2 (men) drinks a day.	4	1	0
2. I avoid using alcohol or other drugs as a way of handling stressful situations or problems in my life.	2	1	0
3. I am careful not to drink alcohol when taking medications (such as for colds, allergies, pain) or when pregnant.	2	1	0
4. I read and follow the label directions when using prescribed and over-the-counter drugs.	2	1	0

Alcohol and Drugs Score _____

Safety

	Almost Always	Sometimes	Never
1. I wear a seat belt while driving or riding in a car.	2	1	0
2. I avoid driving while under the influence of alcohol or other drugs.	2	1	0
3. I obey traffic rules and the speed limit when driving.	2	1	0
4. I make sure I am fully alert when driving (not drowsy, not talking on a cell phone, not reading, not putting on makeup, etc.).	2	1	0
5. I am careful when using potentially hazardous products or substances such as chemicals, poisons, household cleaners, and electrical appliances.	2	1	0

Safety Score _____

Disease Prevention

	Almost Always	Sometimes	Never
1. I know the warning signs of cancer, heart attack, and stroke.	2	1	0
2. I avoid overexposure to the sun and use sunscreen.	2	1	0
3. I get recommended age-appropriate medical screening tests (examples include blood pressure and cholesterol checks, Pap tests, mammograms, dental exams), immunizations, and booster shots.	2	1	0
4. I practice monthly breast/testicular exams.	2	1	0
5. I am not sexually active *or* I have sex with only one mutually faithful partner *or* I use condoms, *and* I do not share needles to inject drugs.	2	1	0

Disease Prevention Score _____

WHAT YOUR SCORES MEAN

Scores of 9 and 10.
Excellent! Your answers show that you are aware of the importance of this area to your health. More important, you are putting your knowledge to work.

Scores of 6 to 8.
Good, but there is room for improvement. Look again at the items you answered with a "Sometimes" or "Never." What changes can you make to improve your score? Even a small change can help you achieve better health.

Scores of 3 to 5.
Your health risks are showing! Plan your strategies now for making changes.

Scores of 0 to 2.
Your present habits may seriously jeopardize your future health. Perhaps you were not aware of the risks. Change is within your grasp, and you are worth it!

SOURCE: Adapted from *Healthstyle: A Self-Test,* U.S. Department of Health and Human Services Public Health Service, DHHS Publication No. (PHS) 81-50155. (The behaviors covered in this assessment may not apply to people with certain chronic diseases or disabilities or to pregnant women, who may require special advice from their physician.)

EVALUATION

In which areas did you score the lowest or would you like to improve?

Identify three of your risky behaviors and then identify a strategy for making a change.

Examples: *Risky behavior:* Never obeying speed limits.

 Strategy: Put a sticky note on the dashboard reminding me to continually monitor my speed limit.

 Risky behavior: Rarely eating fruit.

 Strategy: Put a banana and an apple in my backpack every day before I leave for classes. Eat them between classes.

Risky Behavior	*Strategy*
1.	
2.	
3.	

LAB Activity 1-2

Assessing Your Wellness

Read each statement carefully and respond honestly by using the following scoring:

Almost always = 2 points
Sometimes/occasionally = 1 point
Very seldom = 0 points

Physical Dimension

_____ 1. I engage in vigorous exercise (examples include jogging, brisk walking, swimming, cycling) for 20–60 minutes at least four times per week.

_____ 2. I eat fruits, vegetables, and whole grains every day.

_____ 3. I avoid tobacco products.

_____ 4. I wear a seat belt while riding in and driving a car.

_____ 5. I deliberately minimize my intake of cholesterol, dietary fats, and trans fats.

_____ 6. I avoid drinking alcoholic beverages *or* I consume no more than one (women) or two (men) drinks per day.

_____ 7. I get 7–9 hours of sleep most nights.

_____ 8. I have adequate coping mechanisms for dealing with stress.

_____ 9. I maintain a regular schedule of immunizations, physical and dental checkups (including Pap tests, and blood pressure and cholesterol checks), and monthly self-exams of breasts/testicles.

_____ 10. I maintain a healthy weight, avoiding extremes of overweight and underweight.

_____ **Physical total**

Intellectual Dimension

_____ 1. I seek opportunities to learn new things.

_____ 2. I try to keep abreast of current affairs—local, national, and international.

_____ 3. I enjoy attending special lectures, plays, musical performances, museums, galleries, and/or libraries.

_____ 4. I enjoy watching educational programs on TV.

_____ 5. I enjoy creative and stimulating mental activities/games.

_____ 6. I am happy with the amount and variety that I read.

_____ 7. I make an effort to improve my verbal, writing, and expression skills.

_____ 8. A continuing education program is/will be important to me in my career.

_____ 9. I am able to analyze, synthesize, and see more than one side of an issue.

_____ 10. I enjoy engaging in intellectual discussions.

_____ **Intellectual total**

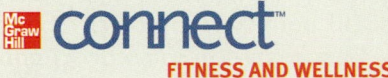

http://connect.mcgraw-hill.com

Emotional Dimension

_____ 1. I am able to develop and maintain close relationships.

_____ 2. I accept responsibility for my actions.

_____ 3. I see challenges and change as opportunities for growth.

_____ 4. I feel I have considerable control over my life.

_____ 5. I am able to laugh at life and myself.

_____ 6. I feel good about myself.

_____ 7. I am able to cope appropriately with stress and tension.

_____ 8. I am able to recognize my personal shortcomings and learn from my mistakes.

_____ 9. I am able to recognize and appropriately express my feelings.

_____ 10. I relax and enjoy life without the use of alcohol or drugs.

_____ **Emotional total**

Social Dimension

_____ 1. I contribute time and/or money to social and community projects.

_____ 2. I am committed to a lifetime of volunteerism.

_____ 3. I exhibit fairness and justice in dealing with people.

_____ 4. I have a network of close friends and/or family.

_____ 5. I am interested in others, including those with backgrounds different from my own.

_____ 6. I am able to balance my needs with the needs of others.

_____ 7. I am able to communicate with and get along with a wide variety of people.

_____ 8. I obey the laws and rules of our society.

_____ 9. I am a compassionate person and try to help others when I can.

_____ 10. I support and help with family, neighborhood, school, and work social gatherings.

_____ **Social total**

Spiritual Dimension

_____ 1. I feel comfortable and at ease with my spiritual life.

_____ 2. There is a direct relationship between my personal values and my daily actions.

_____ 3. When I get depressed or frustrated by problems, my spiritual beliefs and values give me direction.

_____ 4. Prayer, meditation, and/or quiet personal reflection is/are important in my life.

_____ 5. Life is meaningful for me, and I feel a purpose in life.

_____ 6. I am able to speak comfortably about my personal values and beliefs.

_____ 7. I am consistently striving to grow spiritually, and I see that as a lifelong process.

_____ 8. I am tolerant of and try to learn about others' beliefs and values.

_____ 9. I have a strong sense of hope and optimism in my life and use my thoughts and attitudes in life-affirming ways.

_____ 10. I appreciate the natural forces that exist in the universe.

_____ **Spiritual total**

Environmental Dimension

_____ 1. I consciously conserve energy (electricity, heat, light, water, etc.) in my place of residence and work.

_____ 2. I practice recycling (glass, paper, plastic, etc.).

_____ 3. I am committed to cleaning up the environment (air, soil, water, etc.).

_____ 4. I consciously carpool, ride a bicycle, walk, or use a gas-efficient vehicle to conserve fuel energy and lessen the pollution in the atmosphere.

_____ 5. I limit the use of fertilizers and chemicals when managing my yard/lawn/outdoor living space.

_____ 6. I limit my use of aerosol sprays.

_____ 7. I do not litter.

_____ 8. I volunteer my time for environmental conservation projects.

_____ 9. I purchase recycled items when possible, even if they cost more.

_____ 10. I feel strongly about doing *my* part to preserve the environment.

_____ **Environmental total**

Occupational Dimension

_____ 1. I am happy with my career choice.

_____ 2. I look forward to working in my career area.

_____ 3. The job responsibilities/duties of my career choice are consistent with my values.

_____ 4. The payoffs/advantages in my career choice are consistent with my values.

_____ 5. I am happy with the balance between my work/career choice time commitment and leisure time.

_____ 6. I am happy with the amount of control I have in my work/career choice.

_____ 7. My work/career choice gives me personal satisfaction and stimulation.

_____ 8. I am happy with the professional/personal growth provided by my job/career choice.

_____ 9. I feel my job/career choice allows me to make a difference in the world.

_____ 10. My job/career choice contributes positively to my overall well-being.

_____ **Occupational total**

SCORING

Add your total score for each dimension of wellness.

Scores of 15–20 Points
Excellent strength in this dimension.

Scores of 9–14 Points
There is room for improvement. Look again at the items in which you scored 1 or 0. What changes can you make to improve your score?

Scores of 0–8 Points
This dimension needs a lot of work. Look again at this dimension and challenge yourself to begin taking small steps toward growth. Remember, the goal is balanced wellness.

Take your score in each dimension of wellness and shade it in on the accompanying figure. How smoothly will your wellness wheel roll? A smooth ride indicates *balanced* wellness, and the *larger* the wheel, the better!

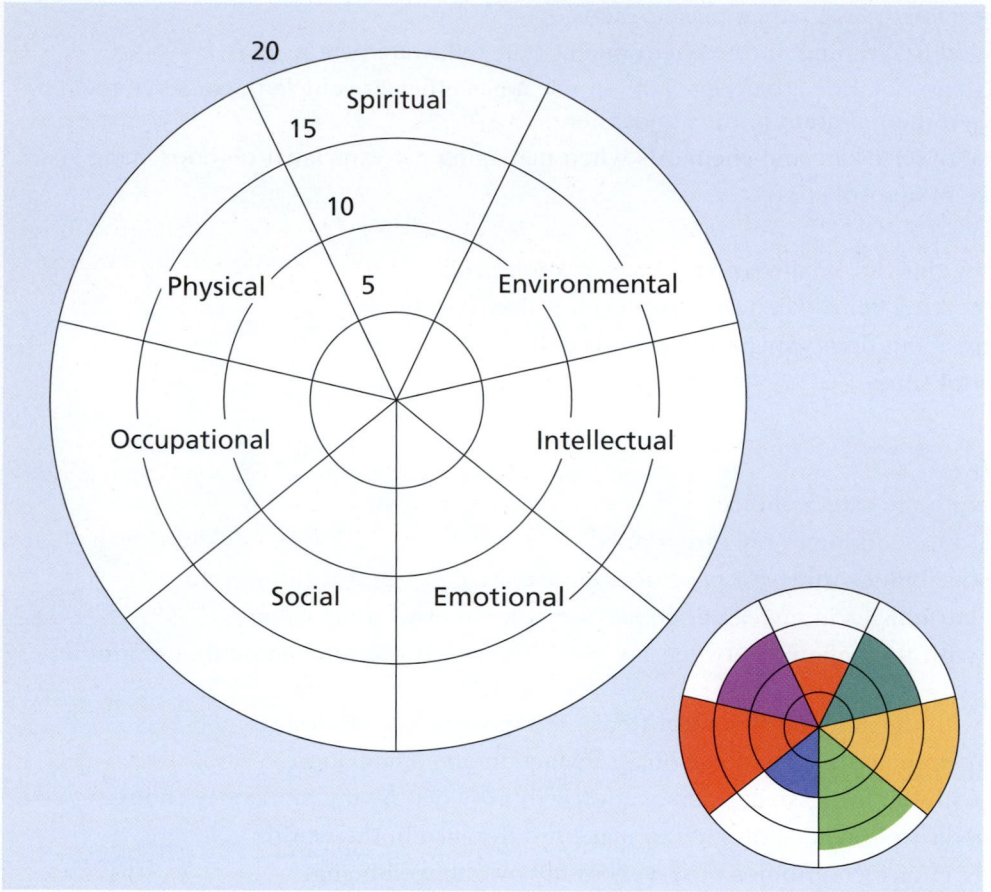

Wellness wheel

EVALUATION

Finish the following statements:

After completing "Assessing Your Wellness,"

1. I discovered I am strong in:

2. I discovered I am weak in:

3. I feel I can change:

LAB Activity 1-3

Name _____ Class/Activity Section _____ Date _____

Societal Norms: The Unwritten Codes

Societal norms that promote unhealthy habits permeate our daily lives. However, they don't have to be practiced and accepted by everyone. List three unhealthy societal norms that are prevalent in your community or around your campus. Then, list countering strategies, behaviors, choices, or policies that could help change these norms to be more positive. You may want to refer to Table 1-2 for ideas.

Example

1. *Unhealthy norm:* Residence hall student lounges have vending machines that offer only candy, cookies, and chips.
2. *Strategies:* (1) Meet with hall council and advocate for healthier items: apples, granola bars, pretzels, popcorn, etc. (2) Keep healthy snacks in the room so you don't have to use the vending machine. (3) Consider increasing the prices for the unhealthy choices. (4) Post on the vending machine the fat grams and calories of each item, as well as the number of minutes of exercise it would take to burn off each.

1. *Unhealthy norm:*	1. *Strategies:*
2. *Unhealthy norm:*	2. *Strategies:*

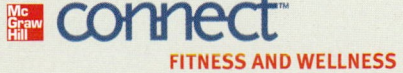

http://connect.mcgraw-hill.com

3. *Unhealthy norm:*

3. *Strategies:*

List two unhealthy societal norms that you have already observed to be in the process of changing to be more positive.

CHAPTER 2

Changing Behavior

STUDY QUESTIONS

You will have successfully mastered this chapter if you can answer the following:

1. What is self-efficacy and how does it affect behavior change?
2. Why is willpower alone not enough to change behavior permanently?
3. Can you identify and describe the five stages of change in the transtheoretical model of behavior change?
4. What are the nine processes of change and how do they relate to the stages of change in the transtheoretical model?
5. What are the elements of a well-designed behavior-change plan/contract?
6. What are the components of S.M.A.R.T. goal setting?
7. Can you name the two components of motivation and give ideas for sustaining motivation?
8. What are the three contributions to relapses during attempted behavior changes?
9. Can you list ways to prevent or recover from a relapse during behavior change?

You will find the answers as you read this chapter.

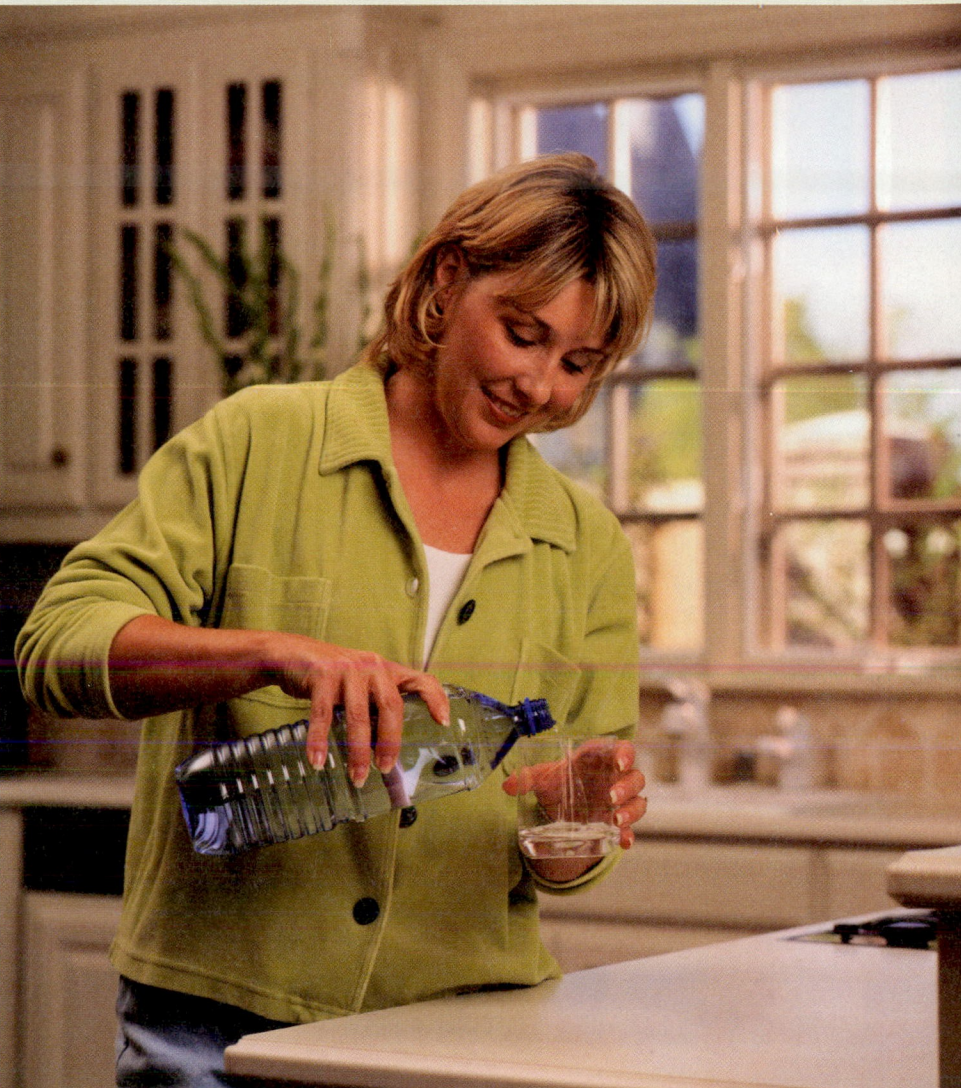

"*There are three kinds of people in this world: those who make things happen; those who see things happen; and far too many who say—"what happened?"*"

—Anonymous

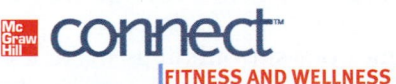

FITNESS AND WELLNESS

http://connect.mcgraw-hill.com

Megan is feeling overwhelmed because she needs to lose about 30 pounds. She doesn't know where to begin, so that frustration has prevented her from changing her diet.

Steve knows that he spends too much time on Facebook rather than studying. As a result, his grades are plummeting. He can't seem to get motivated to stop.

Jessica exercises for 30 minutes twice a week in her fitness class but doesn't feel that exercise is part of her normal daily routine. She wants to make exercise an everyday habit.

These scenarios are very common. Many people have a behavior that they would like to change—perhaps stopping a habit that is harming their health (like smoking or eating a lot of junk food) or beginning a wellness-promoting habit (like eating more vegetables or managing stress). Despite the strong evidence linking lifestyle abuse and lack of well-being, many people remain inactive, smoke cigarettes, drink excessive amounts of alcohol, burn out due to stress, and eat too much of the wrong foods. It is intriguing that knowledge is not always linked to action. Knowledge is not power; rather, knowledge is only potential power! Information is necessary but not sufficient for creating meaningful change. Traditional educational messages devised to arouse fear (antismoking brochures showing blackened lungs, seat belt campaigns showing crumpled cars, video clips of people having heart attacks) have eliminated high-risk behaviors in some people, but not in the majority of the population. Fear of a heart attack or cancer has not kept many Americans involved in ongoing programs of exercise and dietary change. Even when the information is positive or inspirational, many still have difficulty making lifestyle behavior changes. Our everyday behaviors are learned responses. They occur as we respond to a variety of societal influences—parents, friends, role models, media, and our environment. Many of our choices are

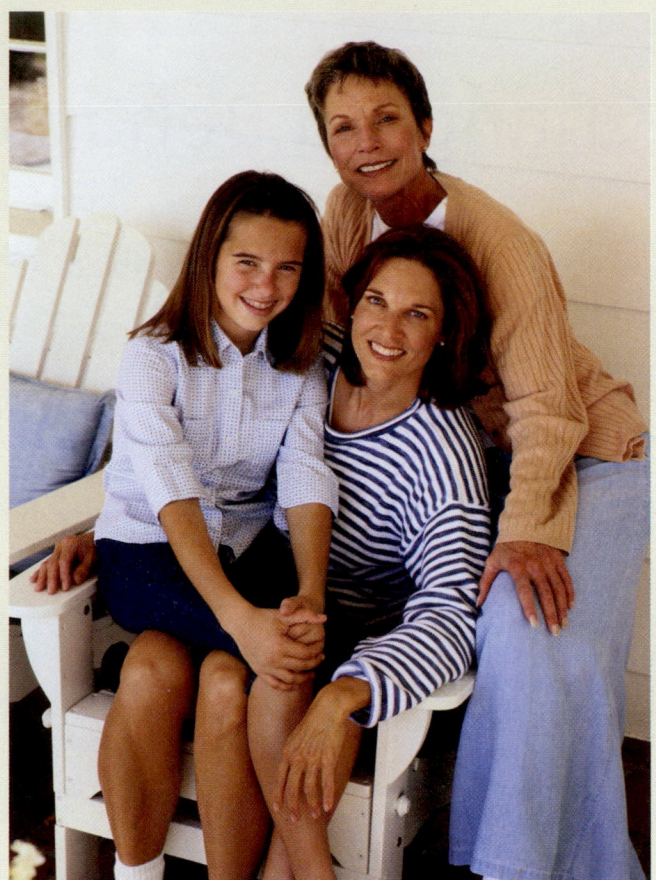

Daily choices affect health and vitality throughout the entire life span.

shaped by our surroundings. Called habits, these learned behaviors can also be unlearned. What is missing in the link between knowledge and action is a systematic strategy or plan.

◆ MORE THAN WILLPOWER

Change is difficult. All of us who have tried to give up old habits and start new ones know how hard it is. Attempts to change can sometimes leave us feeling overwhelmed and demoralized. We may want to give up, feeling it's easier to hang on to old habits. Change can be especially difficult when someone else tells us to do it—a physician, friend, parent, or spouse. For many of us who face imposed change, the first reaction is to get angry and defensive. We do not like feeling forced to do something even when the change may appear to be in our best interest.

Sometimes our surroundings make it easier *not* to change. For example, if your only lunch option is a food court loaded with high-fat, high-calorie foods,

it becomes the daily norm. Packing your own lunch with healthy fruits, vegetables, and yogurt may seem like a lot of trouble. In the same way, not having an accessible, safe place to jog, walk, or cycle makes exercising a more difficult task. Whatever the circumstances, behavior change starts in the mind. A new mind-set is needed to navigate this challenging path. *We* are the ones who initiate change; not someone else who nags us to do so.

Psychologists use the term **self-efficacy** in relation to behavior change. Self-efficacy is the amount of confidence an individual has in his or her own ability to carry out a desired behavior. You have a high level of self-efficacy if you feel confident in your ability to progress even amid tempting situations. Self-efficacy is also behavior-specific, which means you may have high self-efficacy regarding exercise but low self-efficacy with dietary changes. If you lack self-efficacy, you might not be able (or willing) to put in the sustained effort required to change. When you have self-efficacy, you are able to view little setbacks and bad days as interesting challenges to overcome. And, more important, you are able to transfer these experiences into opportunities to be more skillful—instead of feeling helpless. Having a high level of self-efficacy is one of the strongest factors in making positive wellness choices.

But what about good old willpower? Isn't that all it takes to change? No! Willpower is an ambiguous, nonspecific entity. Certainly desire for change is important, but the "just do it" approach has no strategy to follow. It isn't as simple as making a New Year's resolution either, and having changes miraculously occur the next day.

For many it is easier to make excuses for not changing. Excuses are rationalizations for avoiding personal accountability. In fact, most of us can relate to the Top 10 "Excuses for Not Changing a Behavior." How many of these excuses have you used?

Changing a behavior or breaking an unhealthy habit involves *learning new behavior*. Just as in learning anything else, you must understand and practice the basic skills and techniques of behavior change. The key to permanent change is having a plan. Merely being "motivated" is not enough. A tennis player may be motivated to win but neglect working on the skills necessary to be successful. Successful behavior change involves choosing specific goals and designing strategies to meet them. It is a learned skill that involves conscious decisions, including how to deal with setbacks, temptations, and the environment around you. Successful change occurs when *knowledge* and *action* are linked for the purpose of controlling behavior.

THE TRANSTHEORETICAL MODEL OF BEHAVIOR CHANGE

Changing a behavior is a complex process. It has puzzled behavioral scientists for years that some people can successfully self-initiate and maintain major lifestyle changes (stop smoking, lose weight, stick with exercise, cut fat in their diet, etc.) while others fail to make even moderate changes, even after participating in professional group programs (exercise groups, smoking cessation classes, low-fat cooking seminars, etc.). After spending years studying individuals who successfully changed health-related behaviors by themselves, James Prochaska, John Norcross, and Carlo DiClemente revolutionized

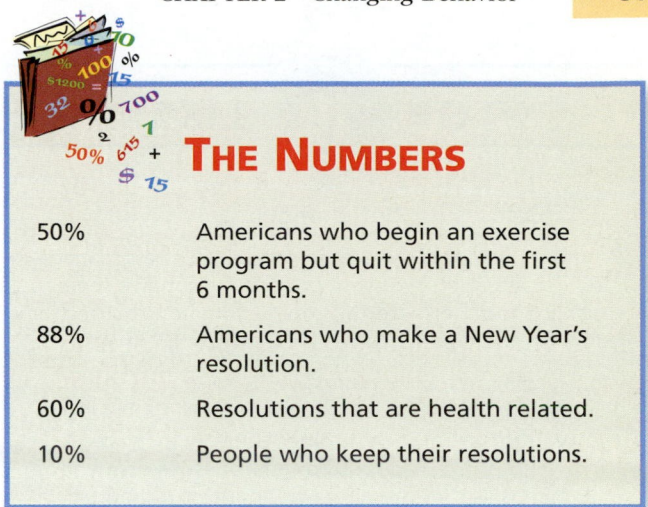

THE NUMBERS

50%	Americans who begin an exercise program but quit within the first 6 months.
88%	Americans who make a New Year's resolution.
60%	Resolutions that are health related.
10%	People who keep their resolutions.

behavior-change theory. They concluded that individuals engaging in a new behavior move through five distinct stages of change. This is called the **transtheoretical model of behavior change.** Rather than viewing behavior change as a single *event,* such as quitting overeating or becoming an exerciser, the transtheoretical model identifies change as a *progression* through five stages. These stages are identified as precontemplation, contemplation, preparation, action, and maintenance. This is a self-directed approach in which the person is fully involved in the process of change. Rather than focusing on social influences or biological reasons, the transtheoretical model focuses on *personal decision making*. It is a model of intentional change that unfolds gradually over time.

The following is a brief description of each stage, along with typical statements spoken by people in each stage:

Stage 1: **Precontemplation** ("I don't want to change.")

Precontemplation is the stage in which people are not even considering a change in their behavior. People may be in this stage because they are uninformed or underinformed about the consequences of their behavior. They are often in denial about their habit. For example, an obese woman might think she is simply "big-boned" and not at risk for any health problems. A sedentary middle-aged man may think that exercise is only for young people, and since he was an athlete back in high school, he doesn't need to exercise. Or the precontemplator may have tried unsuccessfully to change and become discouraged about his ability to change. In this stage the barriers to and cons of changing outweigh the pros or

TOP 10 LIST

Excuses for Not Changing a Behavior

Whether it involves our activity level, diet, stress management, or a tendency toward procrastination, we seem to resist change. Here are the top 10 common excuses for not changing.

1. *"It can't happen to me."*
   Denial is the first psychological barrier. Denial prevents us from seeing things the way they are. A wellness lifestyle requires an honest assessment of things as they are and a willingness to change.

2. *"I have no time to devote to this. I'll do it later."*
   Change is achieved in little steps, and the time to start is now. The rest of your life starts *today*, not "after the holidays" or "when this tough semester is over." Don't wait for *someday* to roll around.

3. *"I'll have to give up and lose the things I love."*
   Instead of focusing on the benefits of change, most people have a tendency to focus on what they're losing. Instead of mourning the loss of your chocolate cake, cigarettes, or TV time, focus on the gains: money saved, a leaner body, more self-respect, better breathing, etc.

4. *"It's someone else's fault that I am the way I am."*
   Wellness and lifestyle changes begin with self-responsibility and taking ownership of your problem. Blaming others or society in general is a trap, a way of avoiding self-responsibility.

5. *"The task is too overwhelming. It'll take too much work."*
   When you were a 1-year-old, the task of running around the block was also overwhelming! You started with baby steps (and some falls along the way).

6. *"It's too late to change now."*
   Nonsense! No matter what your age or how long you've been avoiding change, you will benefit from any positive lifestyle change.

7. *"If I fail, I'll look silly."*
   There is no such thing as failure; there are only learning experiences. Thomas Edison, for example, learned hundreds of ways *not* to make a lightbulb. All of us have setbacks from time to time.

8. *"I don't deserve to succeed."*
   One way to break through the barrier of negative self-dialogue is by affirming the positive. An affirmation is a conscious, positive statement or image that channels your energy into action. When you catch yourself feeling "that you don't deserve success," try visualizing that positive image or repeating a positive self-talk statement such as "I deserve success" or "I've worked hard for success."

9. *"My family/friends aren't particularly supportive."*
   This is a tough one. Have you discussed your plan with them? You may be surprised at how supportive (and proud) of you they are once you tell them how important it is to you.

10. *"I don't know how to begin."*
    Behavior change is a complex process that doesn't happen overnight. As you study the transtheoretical model in this chapter, you'll identify your current stage and the behavior processes that will help you move along. Formulate your plan and act on it.

benefits of changing. Precontemplators are often viewed as unmotivated, uncooperative, and defensive. They tend to avoid reading, talking, or thinking about their behavior. They have often constructed defenses that aid in the denial of the problem.

Typical statements made by precontemplators: "I think my diet is fine." "Smoking doesn't cause heart disease." "I'm too out of shape to exercise." "Individual recycling won't really make a difference." "My weight is not a problem."

Stage 2: **Contemplation** ("Is change worth it?") Contemplators have a sense of awareness about their problem behavior but are ambivalent about changing. In this stage, they may intend to take action, or are seriously thinking about it, but have not yet made a commitment to take action. They have to be convinced that the trip is worth the effort. They consider the barriers (e.g., time, expense, hassle, fear) as well as the benefits (e.g., feeling better, looking better, lower blood pressure). For them, however, the barriers and cons are still more overriding than the perceived pros or benefits. People may remain stuck in this stage for years as they contemplate the pros and cons of changing.

Typical statements made by contemplators: "I really should eat more fruits and vegetables, but I'm not ready." "I know drinking is bad, and maybe someday I'll quit." "Exercise would be good for me, but I don't want to do it." "I really get stressed out, but I don't have the time to work on stress management skills."

Stage 3: **Preparation** ("Count me in!") In this stage, the individual is on the verge of making a specific change. He or she is investigating the options available and may even experiment with small changes as the determination to change increases. This is a key stage where a transition is occurring from cognitive "thinking about it" to beginning to take action. These individuals are putting together a plan of action, having resolved that the pros of changing outweigh the cons. They are making a commitment to the change effort and taking small steps to facilitate the change.

Typical statements made by someone in the preparation stage: "Monday I start my diet." "I signed up for a Bible study class." "I purchased a treadmill and am going to start a walking program." "I bought a low-fat cookbook and have already tried a few of the recipes."

Stage 4: **Action** ("I'm doing it!")
In this stage the individual overtly takes definitive action, requiring a considerable commitment of time and energy. This stage is most visible to others who see the new behaviors taking place. This is a busy stage of change in which the person uses strategies to resist temptations, cope with everyday challenges, and prevent a relapse. Having a strong belief and confidence in the ability to change is a key element in this stage. That's why working toward small, attainable goals is important during the action stage. Most experts agree that one must be in the action stage for 6 months before moving to the maintenance stage.

Typical statements made by someone in the action stage: "I now walk for 20 minutes during my lunch hour." "My roommate and I now go to the library to study three nights a week from 8:00 to 10:00 P.M." "I've switched from doughnuts to a whole-grain cereal for breakfast and have a lot more energy throughout the morning as a result." "When I feel the urge to smoke, a sugar-free mint satisfies my urge."

Stage 5: **Maintenance** ("It's hard to imagine how it used to be.")
Maintenance is the stage in which a person is sustaining his or her new behavior, usually for 6 months to 5 years. Patterns are becoming more automatic. Maintainers are experiencing the benefits of their change and are increasingly confident in their ability to sustain this new lifestyle. The main goal in maintenance is relapse prevention. For this reason, maintenance is a long, ongoing process.

Typical statements made by maintainers: "I do my breast self-exam on the same day every month." "I haven't had a cigarette for 2 years and really don't miss them." "I prefer skim milk over 2% milk." "My day isn't complete without my evening workout."

Take a look at the flowchart in Figure 2-1. By answering each question you can identify your current stage of change.

The transtheoretical model acknowledges that each stage is equally important in the change process. To apply this model, you should understand the following principles:

✓ Movement through the five stages does not always occur in a distinct, linear manner. Some people spiral back and forth between stages and may be stuck in one stage for many years before the goal is reached (e.g., slip back from the "action" stage to the "contemplation" stage).

✓ Successful behavior change is a process that unfolds over time; it doesn't happen all at once. There is no "magic moment."

✓ You may be at different stages of change for different behaviors (e.g., be in maintenance for an exercise program but in contemplation for kicking your fast-food habit).

✓ Self-efficacy increases as one progresses through the five stages.

✓ Specific processes must be applied at the specific stages if progress through the stages is to occur.

✓ The key to successful behavior change is *identifying what stage of change you are in and then applying the processes of change that fit that particular stage* to move on to the next stage.

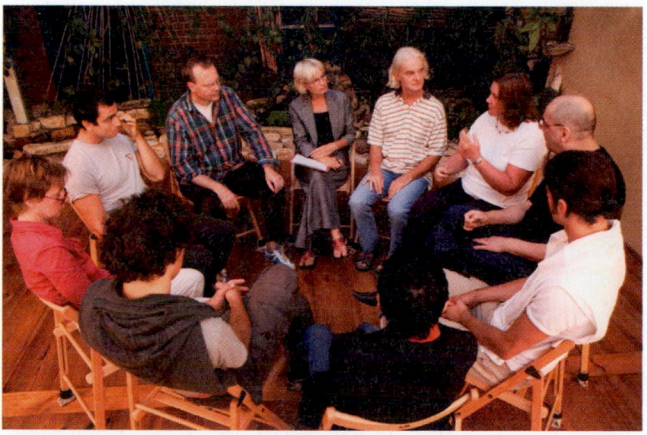

Joining a support group is especially helpful to someone in the *action* stage of change.

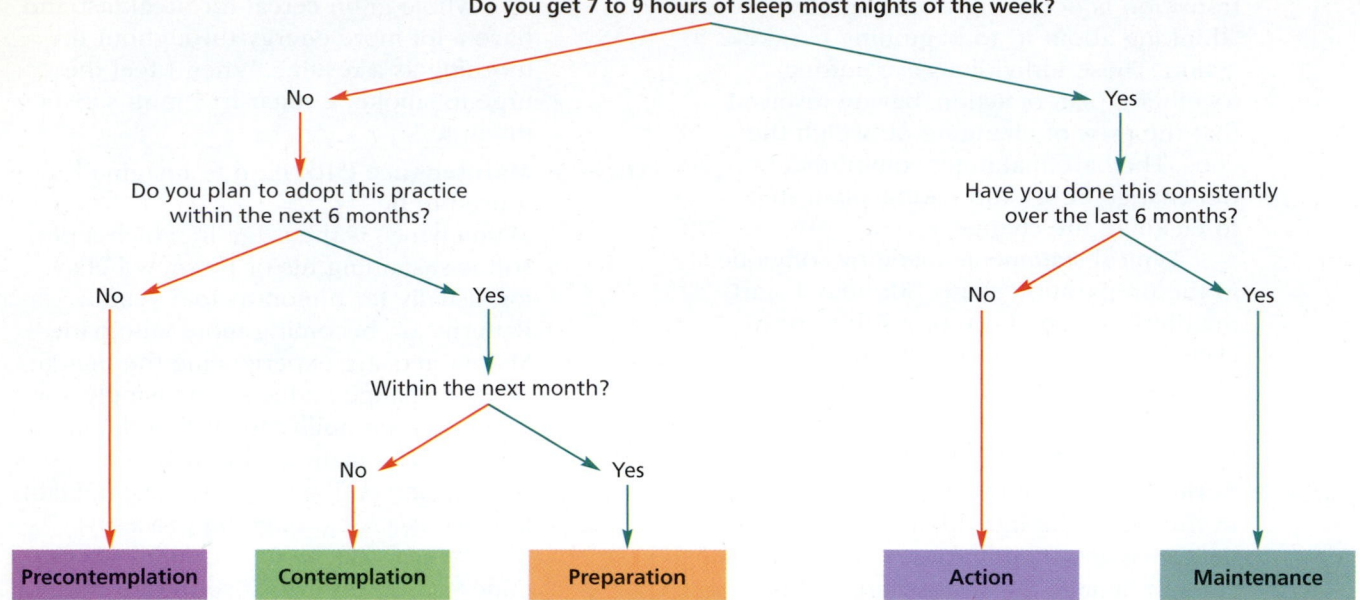

Do you get 7 to 9 hours of sleep most nights of the week?

No → **Do you plan to adopt this practice within the next 6 months?**

Yes → **Have you done this consistently over the last 6 months?**

No ← → Yes

No ← → Yes

Within the next month?

No ← → Yes

| Precontemplation | Contemplation | Preparation | Action | Maintenance |

You can substitute a variety of lifestyle questions for the initial question in this flowchart:
Try substituting: Do you recycle used newspapers, glass bottles, and aluminum cans?
Do you wear sunscreen when you know you'll be out in the sun for an hour or more?
Do you consistently limit the fat in your diet to under 70 grams per day?
Do you do aerobic exercise at least three to five times per week?
Do you regularly volunteer for community projects?

Can you think of other questions?

FIGURE 2-1   **A flowchart for determining your stage of change.**

The Processes of Change

Prochaska and his colleagues discovered that to help people progress through the stages toward maintenance, distinct behavioral strategies known as **processes of change** need to be practiced at different stages. These processes are covert and overt activities and experiences that individuals engage in when they attempt to modify problem behaviors. These nine processes and the behavioral change strategies they incorporate have been shown to be the *best* predictors of permanent lifestyle change because they incorporate personal decision making, feelings of self-involvement, and individual confidence. The degree of confidence individuals have that they can practice healthful behaviors across a broad range of daily situations has been shown to be critically important in progressing through behavior change. Table 2-1 explains the nine processes of change that Prochaska, Norcross, and DiClemente have

identified. Examples of behavioral strategies are listed for each process.

After looking over these strategies, you may say, "But I tried many of these techniques and *still* went back to my old habits!" The most dramatic implication of this behavior-change research is that efficient self-change depends on implementing the right behavioral strategies (processes) at the right time (stages). In this way, the key to successful change is *identifying* what stage you are in and matching the change process to maximize the problem-solving efforts. Figure 2-2 identifies the five stages of change and the nine processes that work best within each stage.

Suppose Rick, for example, has been a nonexerciser for more than 3 years. He competed in sports while in high school but stopped when he started college. He has gained 20 pounds and feels tired and sluggish. He knows he should exercise but feels overwhelmed with school and a part-time job at the video store. How can the transtheoretical model help Rick?

TABLE 2-1	The Processes of Change	
Process	**Description**	**Example Behavioral Strategies**
Consciousness-raising *Learn about it.*	Getting information about the nature and risk of unsafe behaviors; gaining awareness and feedback about a problem behavior; learning about the benefits of changing a problem behavior.	• Learning, "What are the long-term effects of inactivity?" • Assessing, "What foods in my diet are high in fat?" • Asking, "How many calories will I burn if I jog 3 miles?" • Investigating, "What actually triggers my smoking?" • Keep a log of available time for exercise, calories consumed, etc. • Thinking, "What would be the benefits of losing weight?" • Using lifestyle and health assessments to pinpoint problem areas
Social liberation *Is there help out there?*	Understanding and changing the contingencies that control or maintain the problem behavior; accepting and using new alternatives provided by the external environment; seeking social opportunities that support change.	• Investigating alternative environments (alcohol-free parties, smoke-free buildings, healthy lunch selections, walking clubs, etc.) • Identifying self-help groups and support groups • Utilizing low-fat menu choices in restaurants, campus workout facilities, recycling bins • Empowering policy changes (quiet hours, smoke-free lounges, healthier food court selections, etc.)
Emotional arousal *I don't want that to happen to me!*	Experiencing emotions related to the problem behavior.	• Watching a dramatization pertaining to the situation or problem • Using mental imagery to envision future health profile, weight, cholesterol, etc., if old habits do not change • Blowing cigarette smoke into a handkerchief to see the yellow stain; visiting a hospital cancer floor, emergency room, or drug rehab center • Reflecting about the illness or death of someone with heart disease or lung cancer, or who was in a DWI accident, etc.
Self-reevaluation *Is change really worth it?*	Determining consequences and impact on personal life with and without a particular habit; reevaluating values, sacrifices, level of commitment; weighing pros and cons.	• Listing pros and cons (benefits and barriers) of changing • Asking, "Is having a fit body worth the sacrifice?" • Reflecting, "Is tanning that important to me?" • Considering, "Will my friends respect me if I stop drinking?" • Asking, "Will studying at the library three nights per week diminish my social life?"
Self-liberation *I can do it!*	Accepting personal responsibility for changing, especially the belief that it *can* be done; committing and recommitting to act on that belief.	• Publicly announcing your intentions; making a New Year's resolution; setting a specific date • Creating a plan of action and taking small steps • Writing and signing a behavior-change contract • Posting motivational signs, pictures, affirmations • Keeping a log, chart, diary of progress
Reward *How can I reward myself along the way?*	Rewarding oneself or receiving rewards and reinforcement from others for positive changes.	• Using positive self-talk ("I'm looking better." "It feels good to be in control." "I like the compliments I'm receiving.") • Making bets, pacts with others; using money, gifts as goals are reached • Incorporating a step-by-step approach with rewards at each step
Countering *What can I do instead?*	Substituting alternative behaviors for problem behaviors.	• Walking with your spouse or partner rather than watching TV • Practicing relaxation rather than arguing/retaliating • Thinking positive, self-supporting thoughts • Drinking soda instead of beer • Chewing gum rather than smoking • Going to the gym rather than to "happy hour" • Reading a magazine rather than snacking

(continued)

TABLE 2-1   *The Processes of Change (continued)*

Process	Description	Example Behavioral Strategies
Environment control *My surroundings must make it convenient and easy.*	Restructuring the environment to reduce temptations; avoiding or controlling the situations that trigger the problem behavior.	• Having exercise clothes/gym locker conveniently ready or exercise equipment readily available • Removing ashtrays/cigarettes from the apartment • Never shopping at the grocery store when hungry and tempted to buy high-fat, high-calorie foods • Posting positive signs and reminders • Planning ahead by visualizing your action when confronted with a temptation/trigger
Helping relationships *Will you help me stick with this?*	Trusting, accepting, and using the support of others during attempts to change the problem behavior.	• Sharing your plans with others; asking for their support • Writing a partner contract with goals and partner's commitments • Enlisting someone else to "buddy up" and change with you; having someone to talk to • Joining support groups; being with others who are doing the same things

Identified Stage of Change: Contemplation (i.e., he knows he should but feels he has no time.)
Processes That Will Help Rick:

✓ Consciousness-raising behavioral strategies:

 • Read/learn/investigate the benefits of exercise throughout the life span.

• Keep a daily time log to see when a workout could possibly fit into his schedule.
• Investigate how many calories could be burned during a workout.

✓ Social liberation behavioral strategies:

 • Find out the open hours at the campus recreation center.

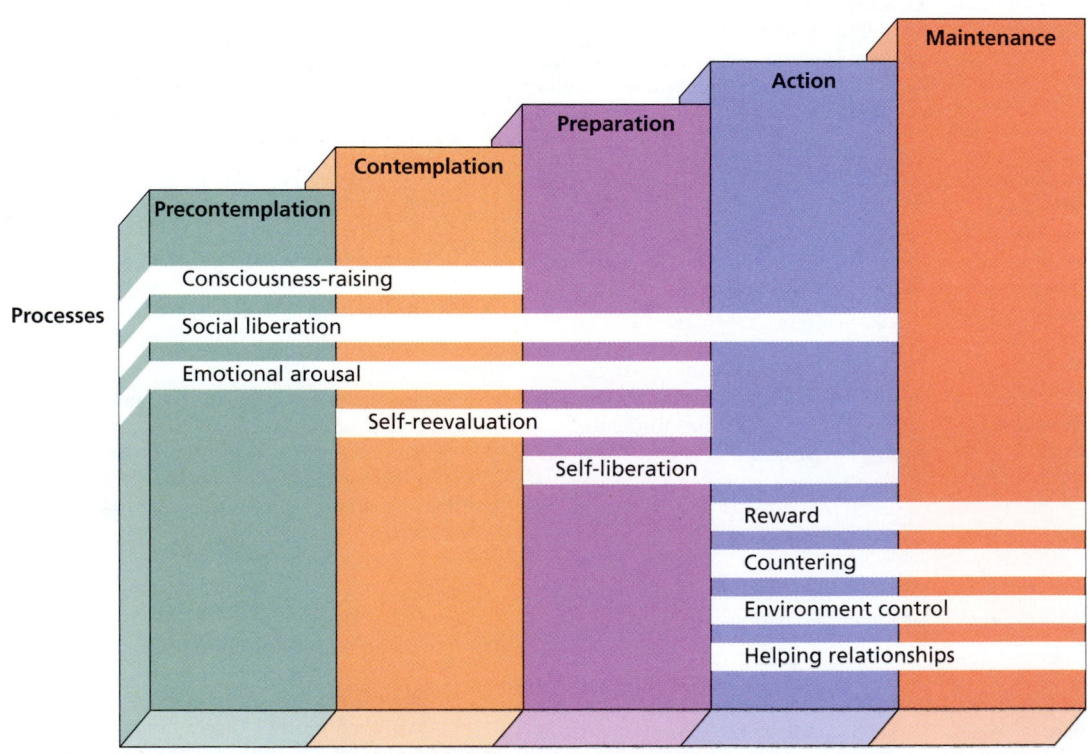

Stages of Change

FIGURE 2-2   **Stages of change and the processes found to be most useful in each stage.**

Source: James O. Prochaska, Cancer Prevention Research Center, University of Rhode Island.

- Map out a safe cycling/walking/jogging route from his apartment with various mileages.
- Investigate the cycling/jogging/swimming clubs on campus.

✓ Emotional arousal behavioral strategies:

- Reflect on father's heart attack at age 52.
- Look at high school pictures—a leaner, fit body.
- Look at latest blood/fitness profile—high body fat, high cholesterol, pre-hypertension.

✓ Self-reevaluation behavioral strategies:

- List pros and cons of daily exercise sessions.
- Imagine what his health profile will be in 5 years if he continues same inactive lifestyle.
- Analyze whether the sacrifice of time to exercise would be worth it.

By using these processes Rick has a good chance of transitioning successfully from the contemplative stage to the preparation stage. In contrast, starting Rick out by nagging him to join you in your 6:00 A.M. swim or buying him a YMCA membership for his birthday would be futile because Rick is not initially ready for "action." However, exposure to the processes that affect him as a contemplator can help him move on to the next stage where additional behavior strategies can then help him. Plus, Rick has taken some ownership and self-involvement in the change rather than being forced or cajoled by others.

Unfortunately, many health promotion programs address only the needs of people in the "action" stage of change (e.g., aerobics classes, low-fat cooking classes, stress management seminars). Yet a large proportion of individuals are precontemplators and contemplators who need other strategies. For these individuals, joining an action-oriented program often results in failure, guilt, or blame for the lack of willpower or motivation.

Prochaska's stages-of-change model is a self-directed model that you can use as you begin applying the correct *processes* according to the stage of change you are in.

Why is understanding the transtheoretical model important as you attempt to make a behavior change?

✓ Having a realistic view of the work involved may better prepare you for the effort and commitment needed to be successful.

✓ Even in the absence of pure action, you can make progress by gaining awareness about the problem behavior, experiencing emotions relative to the problem behavior, and changing your beliefs and attitudes about the problem behavior.

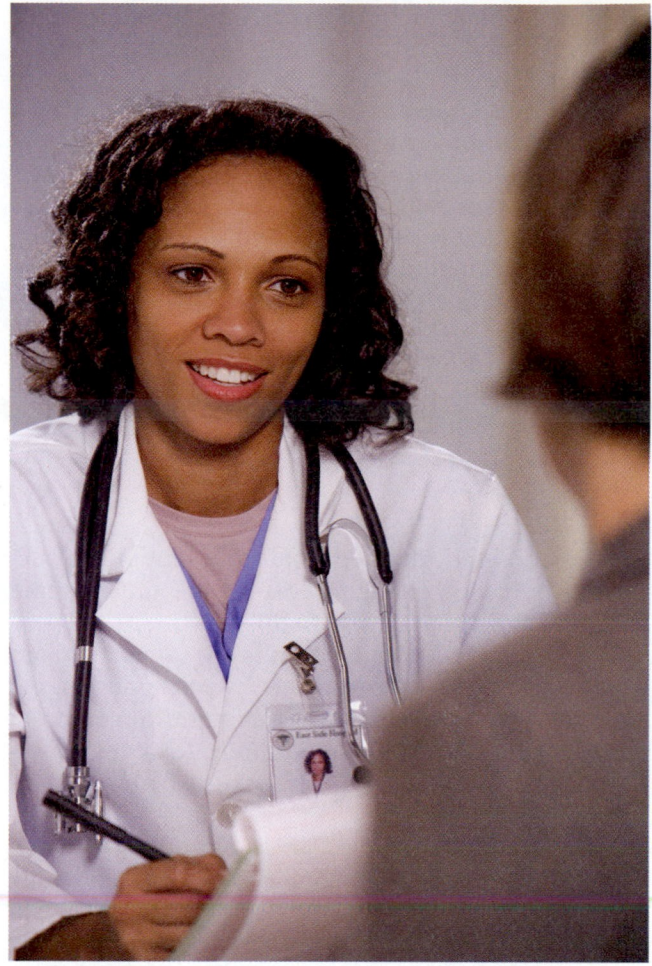

Learning about health risks is a strategy in the consciousness-raising process of change. This is helpful to someone in the precontemplation or contemplation stage of change.

✓ Knowing the factors that could cause a setback may help you prepare for success rather than fall into a relapse.

Remember . . . behavior change is a marathon, not a sprint.

◆ MAKING A PLAN

According to the *American Heritage Dictionary* a "plan" is a "detailed scheme, program, or method worked out beforehand to accomplish an objective." Too often people will say that they "plan" to eat healthier, stop smoking, or exercise. However, they fail to work out or think through the necessary details in advance.

One specific way to initiate a lifestyle change is to write a personal behavior-change contract or action plan incorporating the processes for the change. Writing it out makes you think through your plan in its entirety rather than letting things happen as they may. It specifies the *details* for carrying out your plan. Figure 2-3 shows a sample behavior-change contract. The changes you choose to make can pertain to any dimension of wellness—anything from improving study skills, to losing weight, to reducing stress, to controlling anger. The most important outcomes of writing a contract are the self-evaluating and planning involved. Having a *plan* is what differentiates a successful change from a fleeting New Year's resolution. A plan can turn a resolution into a reality. A blank contract and a behavior-change log are provided in the lab activities at the end of the chapter for your use. Remember, failing to plan is planning to fail!

Identifying Your Goal

Having a clearly defined goal is essential for successful behavior change. Most of the time people select a vague goal or one that is too broad. Or they try to change too many things at once. You are doomed to failure if you try to lose 40 pounds, get A's in all your classes, train for a marathon, and eat spinach every day—all at one time! However, developing one succinct, well-defined goal can get you headed toward success.

Self-change strategies are most effective when goals are stated in behavioral terms and quantified. ("I am going to walk 10,000 steps every day." "I am going to lose 10 pounds by spring break." "I am going to meditate for 15 minutes every morning before class.") In the business world successful leaders emphasize putting goals in writing. Therefore, as you develop your behavior-change goal, write it down and post it in a prominent place (bulletin board, day planner, bathroom mirror, car dashboard, refrigerator, etc.) where you will see it every day. Think of it this way: You would never attempt to drive from Boston to Chicago without a map. Just taking off and wandering probably would not get you there. Goal setting is like downloading a road map from Map Quest!

Many success coaches and business consultants use the acronym S.M.A.R.T. to explain goal setting. S.M.A.R.T. refers to **S**pecific, **M**easurable, **A**chievable, **R**eward, and **T**ime-defined.

S = **S**pecific
Goals need to be specific, not vague. *Not* "try to do better in history class" *but* "study my history class notes and chapter assignments every day after class." *Not* "try to eat better" *but* "add a serving of fruit and a serving of vegetables to every meal." *Not* "become more environmentally involved" *but* "recycle all of my aluminum cans." These are specific actions that contribute to the outcome.

M = **M**easurable
Goals should have concrete criteria for measuring progress (How much? How many? How will I know when it is accomplished?). *Not* "start exercising" *but* "go to the gym M, W, F, S at 5:30 P.M." *Not* "handle stress better" *but* "get up 15 minutes earlier in the morning to meditate." *Not* "lose some weight" *but* "lose 10 pounds." *Not* "save some money" *but* "set aside $50 per paycheck."

A = **A**chievable
Goals should be challenging but also within your capabilities—something you know you can achieve! *Not* "win Wimbledon" *but* "learn to play tennis at an intermediate level." *Not* "make straight A's all 4 years" *but* "maintain a 3.5 GPA." *Not* "run a marathon next month" *but* "run a 5K race next month."

R = **R**eward
You need to reward yourself along the way as you reach certain milestones (new shoes, a pedometer, a massage, a new CD, concert tickets, etc.).

T = **T**ime-defined
Establish some time frames for your goal—either when you'll *do* it or when you'll *accomplish* it. ("I'll study between 8 and 10 P.M. Sundays through Thursdays." "I'll lose 8 pounds by summer break." "I'll cycle the Hilly Hundred by October 15.")

Get started today by establishing your S.M.A.R.T. goal (see Lab Activity 2-1).

Listing Pros and Cons

The decision to move from one stage to the next is based largely on the weight given to the pros and cons of changing behavior. The pros represent

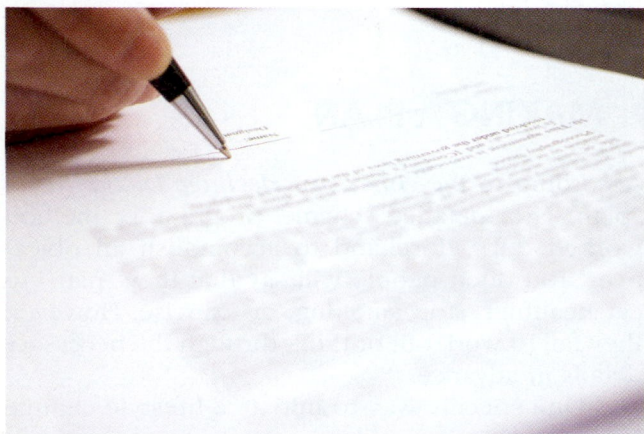

Putting your behavior-change plan into a written contract can help you think through all of your strategies.

Behavior-Change Contract (using the transtheoretical model)

Name _Kate Christopher_

Date _January 1_

Goal (Specific and
Measurable):   To be able to jog 4 miles nonstop by March 5
Pros/Benefits of Changing: Enhance my cardiorespiratory system; reduce my risk for chronic
diseases; lose weight; feel better; build better bones; relieve stress
Cons/Barriers of Changing: Hard to find the time; cold, snowy weather; sometimes feel too
tired to exercise; roommates are not exercisers

Identify stage of change currently in:

_____ Precontemplation   _____ Contemplation   _X_ Preparation
_____ Action   _____ Maintenance

Processes (with accompanying behavioral strategies)

1.   Consciousness-raising
a. Research the long-term benefits of
exercising
b. Keep a time-managment log to find
days/time when I could fit in a jog
c. Talk to other busy students who make
time for exercise and see how they do it

2.   Social liberation
a. Find out the winter hours for the indoor
track at the recreation center
b. Map out a safe 4-mile route starting from
my residence hall
c. Find out which residence halls have
treadmills available for student use

3.   Emotional arousal
a. Visualize my coronary arteries becoming
clogged
b. Think about my ill, overweight aunt with
a 320 cholesterol
c. Visit a hospital coronary care unit

4.   Self-reevaluation
a. List the pros and cons of daily exercise
b. Imagine how much *more* I'll be out of shape
in 5 years if I don't exercise regularly
c. Reflect on how important it is to me to be
more fit and feel better about myself

5.   Self-liberation
a. Make a chart to log miles with a specific
destination—the Grand Canyon
b. Post pictures on my bulletin board from a
running magazine
c. Write a daily training schedule with
specific mileages per day; put it on my
Outlook calendar

6.   Reward
a. Put a quarter in a jar for every nonstop
mile jogged . . . eventually buy a new CD
b. Use positive self-talk ("If Janet can do this,
so can I." "I've jogged 10 days in a row
and don't want to blow it now.")
c. Every Sunday morning jog to the coffee
shop and treat myself to a hazelnut
cappuccino

7.   Countering
a. Rather than driving, jog to the corner
pantry for my daily newspaper
b. Rather than taking the elevator, jog up
the stairs to my computer science class
c. When I go to the post office, jog rather
than drive

8.   Environment control
a. Get a locker at the recreation center and
keep a towel and extra workout clothes
there
b. Pack my workout bag each night before
bed so it is ready
c. Keep an extra pair of running shoes and
workout clothes in the car so I have them
when I go out of town to visit my
boyfriend

9.   Helping relationships
a. Invite my roommates to jog with me
b. Tell my boyfriend about my plan
c. Discuss my goal and plan with my
exercise physiology professor

FIGURE 2-3   **Behavior-Change Contract** (Note: This sample contract gives suggested
strategies for *each* process even though Kate, having identified herself as being in the
"preparation" stage, is best influenced by only four of the processes. Can you identify those four?
See below for answers.)

Social liberation, Emotional arousal, Self-reevaluation, Self-liberation

TOP 10 LIST

"S's" for Success in Changing a Behavior

1. **Self-monitoring:** Accurately observe your behavior by keeping a log or record of your habit. This increases self-awareness of cues, triggers, consequences, and challenges and gives you an honest accounting of your behavior.

2. **Self-efficacy:** The belief that you can do what is required of you to achieve an objective. If past failures have created low self-efficacy, you can build it up by breaking a large goal into positive, specific, realistic short-term goals.

3. **Set reasonable expectations:** Be realistic, but also challenge yourself.

4. **Start small:** Divide large tasks into a number of smaller steps. With each successful step, you gain confidence and skills that will help you continue.

5. **Self-talk:** You control your inner voice. Keep those silent words to yourself positive and encouraging.

6. **Social support:** Surround yourself with others who share your mission. These could be family members, friends, coworkers, a support group, or even strangers on an Internet message board.

7. **Surround yourself with positives:** Utilize positive and inspirational images, pictures, quotes, books, and music to keep you inspired and your spirits high.

8. **Setbacks:** There will be bad days or moments of weakness. Don't expect perfection and don't beat yourself up. Learn from it and move forward.

9. **Stress management:** Stress can trigger a major relapse. Make sure that you practice stress-management strategies daily.

10. **See your goal:** Put it in front of yourself over and over and over again!

positive aspects or benefits of changing. The cons represent negative aspects of changing behavior and may be thought of as barriers to change. It's helpful to make a list of the pros and cons as you contemplate a change. Seriously ask yourself how your life will be affected by your changed behavior. Realize that changing behavior brings consequences to you and, most likely, others. (By quitting drinking I will have better health and less likelihood of suffering from an alcohol-related accident. However, I may lose some social friends who like to party a lot.")

In the precontemplation stage of the transtheoretical model, the cons of changing outweigh the pros. In the contemplation stage, the pros may begin to match the cons. However, because they are so close to being equal, the resulting indecision and lack of commitment cause many individuals to become stuck in the contemplation stage. These individuals substitute *thinking* for *action* while continually weighing the costs and benefits of changing. As individuals move into preparation and through the final two stages, the positive aspects (pros) of changing progressively outweigh the negative aspects (cons).

Honestly assessing the costs of changing will help you face yourself and your true motivations. This will help you anticipate the obstacles ahead of you.

◆ STAYING MOTIVATED THROUGHOUT BEHAVIOR CHANGE

Many people think that "being motivated" means having no struggles. Not so. To look at people who manage their lives making positive wellness decisions, you would think that they live in a different world than you do. How do they stay motivated to exercise daily, manage their stress, study when they need to, refuse a beer at a party, apply sunscreen before going to the beach, or choose broccoli instead of french fries? Answer: They have developed coping and motivational strategies in our less-than-perfect world.

It is human nature to pursue gratification—both sensory and psychological. An immediate sensory gratification might be eating a piece of rich cheesecake. A psychological gratification might be

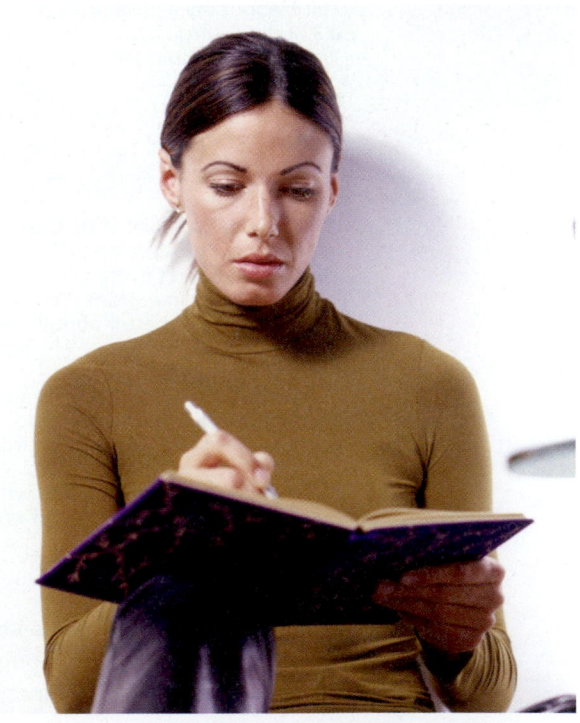

Keeping a log or diary of your behavior allows you to see your progress and can be a great motivator. It could be calories consumed, minutes of exercise, pounds lost, cookies eaten, hours studied, or any measurable behavior.

achieving a goal weight. Cheesecake + Weight Loss = Conflict. Viewing motivation as simply the ability to resist "bad" foods can lead to frustration. In reality, motivation involves two components: (1) the ability to give yourself the opportunity to make *conscious decisions* and *take responsibility* for these choices, and (2) *strategies* for keeping these conscious decisions ongoing. In the cheesecake example, perhaps a cup of creamy vanilla yogurt sprinkled with a tablespoon of granola will satisfy both the sensory gratification and the long-term psychological gratification of trying to lose weight. Motivation remains strong and continues.

Read the Top 10 "S's for Success in Changing Behavior" for tips to help you build your motivation reservoir. In this way you are in control rather than seeing yourself as a helpless victim of forces (or urges) over which you have no control. Lab 2-4 at the end of the chapter encourages you to brainstorm and apply these 10 "S's" to your personal behavior change circumstance.

Preventing Relapse

In the first line of his best-selling book *The Road Less Traveled,* Dr. M. Scott Peck writes, "Life is difficult." He further adds that "life is always difficult and is full of pain as well as joy." Changing a habit takes *effort,* but the joy in the growth and self-empowerment is the wellness journey. In our society we have become accustomed to the quick fix: instant cash at the ATM machine, fast food, credit cards, 24-hour Internet shopping, fax machines. Changing a behavior takes *time,* and setbacks are not uncommon. Instead of giving up forever, try to learn from your experiences.

New behaviors are fragile, so maintaining your plan will require flexibility, particularly if the plan is not working properly, if unexpected obstacles arise, or if a support system is failing. Reevaluation is a necessary component in making a permanent lifestyle change. A lapse or setback should be viewed as a mere "bump in the road" where learning and growth can occur. One problem many people have is believing that a setback is a *failure* rather than a temporary obstacle. How you respond to a temporary lapse determines what you will do after it occurs. Often the first line of defense against relapse is *planning.* If chocolate chip cookies are your downfall, don't buy any. (They'll keep calling your name from the cupboard.) If you've tried and can't get up 45 minutes earlier in the mornings to exercise, what about using your lunch hour to exercise? Take your walking shoes to work with you and invite a colleague to exercise with you. If you are trying to control your weight, you'll likely do better ordering from a menu than choosing the all-you-can-eat buffet. Plan so you'll *succeed.* It is important to recognize "high-risk" situations and have specific coping skills for those situations. Successfully managing high-risk situations can lead to increased feelings of self-efficacy. This means you've increased your behavior-changing skills, which in turn leads to decreased chances of relapse.

As you become the *cause* rather than the *effect* of actions, your confidence and self-esteem are enhanced. Emphasize the positive. Value your successes and your worth as a human being. Most of us do not realize that the majority of our supportive messages come from our internal thought processes rather than from external sources. We carry on a continuous dialogue with ourselves each day. Called *self-talk,* our inner voice can be a positive source of motivation. Mental health experts recognize self-talk

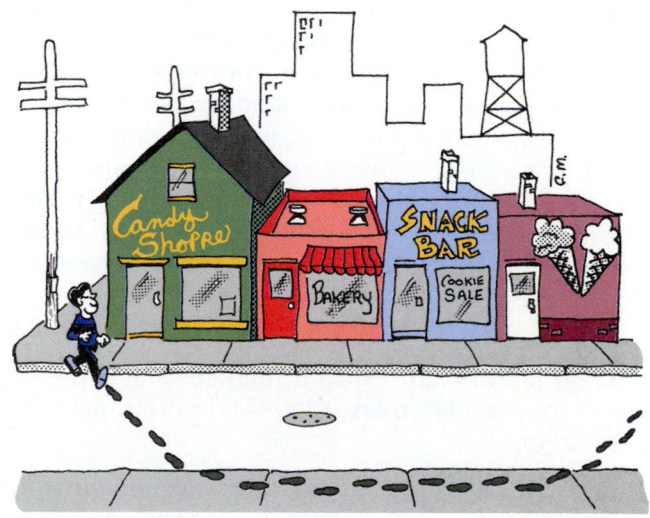

There are many ways to avoid temptations.

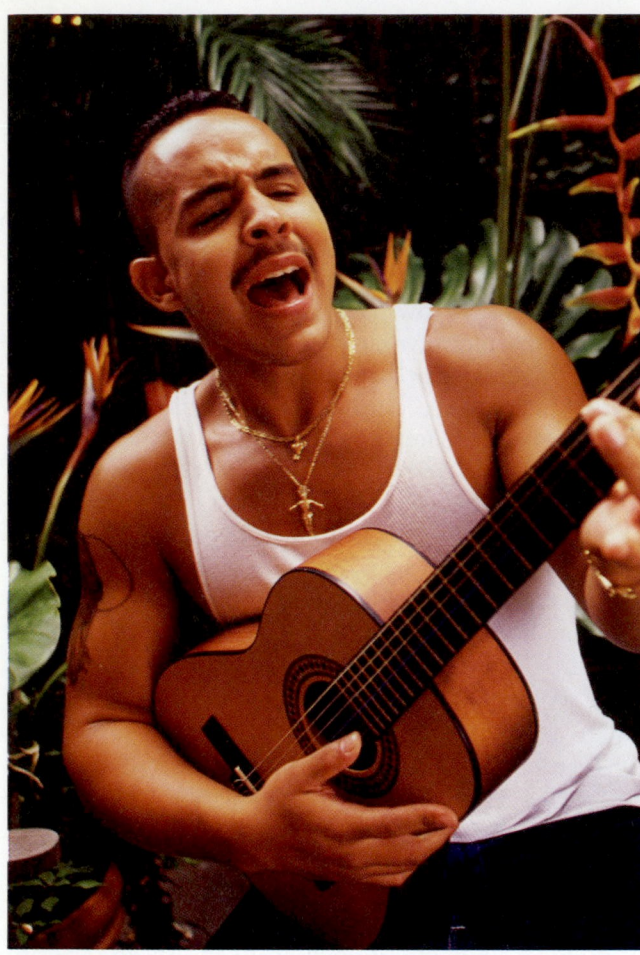

By playing the guitar to distract himself from the urge to smoke, this young man is utilizing the *countering* process of change.

as a powerful force for changing the way we think and behave. "We have a choice about how we think," states Martin Seligman, author of *Learned Optimism*. Self-talk that encourages us and reminds us of our achievements helps increase our self-esteem and motivation. Self-talk can also be negative and, as a result, a source of discouragement. For example, when confronted with tempting desserts at a holiday party, a positive self-talk statement would be "I'll have just a small amount because I am looking forward to wearing my new clothes." A negative self-talk statement would be "I'm already overweight, so it doesn't matter if I eat a lot." Remember . . . *you* control your thoughts, and they can be very powerful.

FACTORS THAT CONTRIBUTE TO RELAPSES

Several factors can cause a relapse. The top contributors are (1) stress, (2) social situations, and (3) cravings.

✓ Stress has a tendency to drain our energy and blur our focus. For example, suppose you have been exercising every Monday, Wednesday, and Thursday evening at the recreation center. Then you suffer a breakup with your partner. Feeling stressed, you suddenly find yourself skipping workouts and immersing yourself in television. These are times when it is important to have healthy stress-coping strategies. We all face life's stresses at times, and it is important not to give up during these times. See Chapter 10 for information on stress-management techniques.

✓ Social situations often present a challenge when trying to change a behavior. Other people may be ambivalent about your change and can consciously or unconsciously tempt you to revert to old habits. For example, suppose you have been cutting back on eating candy, limiting yourself to one small treat a week. Then, at a campus party you find yourself eating handfuls of chocolate peanuts from a big bowl. A remedy for social situations is to plan ahead for such high-risk situations—chew gum, position yourself away from the candy bowl, eat before the party, and so on.

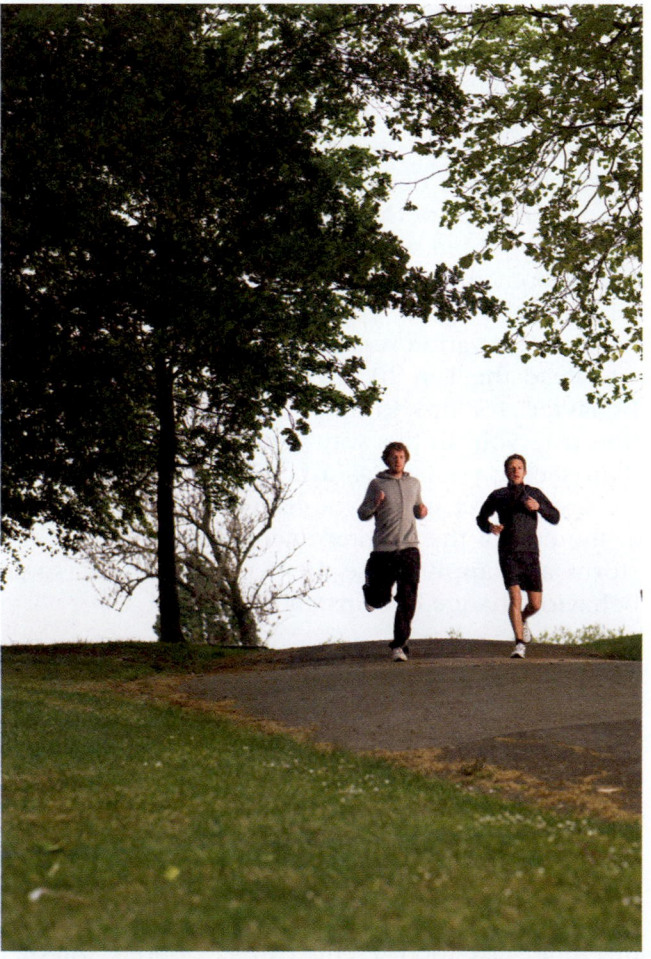

It is much easier to stick with a program when you have someone doing it with you. This is a strategy in the *helping relationships* process of change.

✓ Cravings are intense urges that involve emotional and physiological wants and needs. For example, suppose you haven't smoked a cigarette for 3 weeks. Then you attend your high school reunion and find yourself smoking again with old classmates. By using positive self-talk, mental imagery, and countering strategies, you can control cravings.

Regardless of the cause, if a relapse does occur, analyze what happened. Learn what you could do better in the next similar situation. Check out Table 2-2 for more specific tips.

Remember that changing a behavior is a process involving growth. It is a process of assessing and reassessing goals, monitoring behavior, reviewing strategies, learning from setbacks, and acknowledging the joy in the effort to be the best you can be. Successful behavior change requires time, attention, and effort. But you'll find it is well worth it!

Paul J. Meyer, an international self-empowerment author, acknowledges such effort by saying, "Ninety percent of all those who fail are not actually defeated. They simply quit."

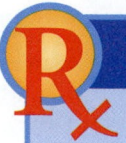

PRESCRIPTION FOR ACTION

You've read the chapter. Now go do one or more of these:

✓ Keep a log/journal of a habit you are thinking about changing.

✓ Write a specific, measurable behavior-change goal and post it in a prominent place.

✓ Identify two specific things you can and will do today to help you reach your goal.

✓ State one source of support (campus, community, friends, family, etc.) that could assist you in changing a habit.

✓ Identify one way you can modify your environment to help contribute to a successful behavior change.

Go online to Connect to complete this activity.
http://connect.mcgraw-hill.com

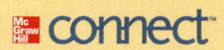

TABLE 2-2	*Tips for Getting Back on Track After a Setback*

1. Cut yourself some slack.
   Accept that you are human and that no one is perfect. If you slipped today, tomorrow is another day. More important, what have you learned from this setback? Remember that success does not hinge on 1 or 2 bad days. Therefore, praise yourself for the successes you *have* experienced. In this way you shift your focus from failures to successes. ("I did this successfully for 5 days; what made it work?")

2. Review your goal and plan.
   Make sure it is realistic and achievable. Don't set yourself up for failure. If you have never been an early riser, perhaps a 6:00 A.M. workout is not the best time for you. November, just before the holidays, may not be the best time to start a new weight-loss program. Readjust your plan: i.e., exercise at 3:00 P.M.; set a goal to *not gain* extra weight over the holidays.

3. Review your pros for changing.
   You must have had strong reasons for wanting to change. Was it to fit into that new swimsuit? Was it to lower your blood pressure? Was it to develop muscle definition? Go over your motivations again. Write them down and post them in a prominent place.

4. Anticipate obstacles.
   What do you think triggered this setback? Try to anticipate future triggers and roadblocks and find ways around them, or at least prepare for them. For example, your exercise routine may run afoul during holidays, travel, vacations, or bad weather. Look for hotels with fitness centers; pack a jump rope and an exercise band; investigate indoor facilities during bad weather; ask the concierge about jogging routes, facilities, etc.; organize a family walk after Thanksgiving dinner.

5. Look for role models.
   Do you know someone who has reached the goal you are striving for? If you do, chat with them about how they overcame obstacles and setbacks. Gain strength from their experiences. Perhaps you can pair up with a friend or join a group with similar goals. Even reading stories about strangers or celebrities who have succeeded can provide inspiration and hope. Also, look for ways to restructure your environment or personal living situation to make it easier to succeed.

6. For cravings, use the three **D'S.**
   Delay at least 10 minutes so that your actions are conscious, not impulsive.
   Distract yourself by engaging in an activity that requires concentration (e.g., play the piano, surf the Internet, do a crossword puzzle).
   Distance yourself from the temptation (e.g., stand away from the buffet table; don't walk past the donut shop; sit in the nonsmoking area).
   Substitute a fun-size candy bar for a king-size; a low-fat fudgesicle for a super premium turtle sundae; a mint rather than a cigarette; chew on a toothpick rather than fingernails; etc.

Frequently Asked Questions

Q. One of the processes of change in the transtheoretical model is called "countering." What are some of the specific strategies of this process?

A. Countering behaviors replace the problem behavior. This strategy is useful when one faces a craving or a social pressure. Try reading a magazine article; abdominal breathing; calling a friend; surfing the Internet; playing a musical instrument; putting on a CD and dancing or singing; going for a walk; watching a television program; playing a game of solitaire; practicing positive self-talk; doing sit-ups/push-ups; cross-stitching; watching a movie; reading scriptures; chewing gum; closing your eyes and practicing imagery; shooting baskets; practicing a new skill; drinking a diet soda; e-mailing a friend/family member. There are many more. The intention is to divert your attention for 10 to 15 minutes while you refocus on your goals.

Q. My behavior-change needs involve time management—specifically, making myself go to the library 4 nights per week from 7:00 to 10:00 P.M. to do homework. I wrote a contract and did well for 4 weeks; then I missed several nights. Now I feel like a failure and am having a hard time getting back on track. Help!

A. The problem of relapse is an important challenge in changing behavior. When individuals experience a *lapse* (a few days of not complying with a new behavior), they need to avoid the feeling that they are doomed. For dieters, it is the belief that one cookie terminates a diet. For exercisers, it is the belief that one missed exercise class means they are no longer "exercisers." Remember that a lapse is a slip, a *relapse* is a string of lapses, and a *collapse* is when the person gives up and returns to past behaviors. Everyone has lapses. Analyze what influenced your lapse. Did you have some other commitments? An invitation to go shopping? A birthday party

to attend? Maybe you'd be better off scheduling your 3 hours at the library from 2:00 to 5:00 P.M. Readjust, refocus, recommit, and don't let a mere lapse turn into a major relapse or collapse.

Q. Is there a way to increase my self-efficacy?

A. Yes. Since self-efficacy deals with your perception of your ability to perform a task or engage in a behavior, you can improve your confidence by using four methods: (1) hands-on practice (give it a try!), (2) observing others like you who are doing it successfully (modeling), (3) internalizing the benefits you'll be getting (positive expectations), and (4) beginning to feel or see results (positive feedback/reinforcement).

Q. My best friend is very inactive, and I am an avid exerciser. She makes fun of me sometimes! Even though she is trim, I worry about her future health. I have begged her to go to the gym with me, but she just laughs and says she doesn't need to exercise since she is slim. What can I do to change her mind?

A. Like millions of others, your friend is in the precontemplation stage. She doesn't see the need for exercise or is in denial about the benefits of exercise for her. The three processes that will have the most impact on her are consciousness-raising, social liberation, and emotional arousal. Therefore, find opportunities to casually bring up the benefits of exercise. Verbalize how good you feel after your workout and how it reduces your stress. Talk about how nice the campus recreation center is, or how you've met some great new friends there. Mention the awesome aerobics class that you are taking, or how excited you are about the bike club trip next weekend. Making comments like these in a nonthreatening manner raises your friend's awareness. Letting her know about available campus resources may also help. As time goes by, she may consider giving it a try—or at least move on to the contemplation stage.

Summary

Following a great musician's performance, an admirer said to him, "I'd give my life to play like that." The brilliant performer hesitated for a moment and then replied, "I did." We often view a performance by an athlete or artist with envy. Accomplishment is often deceptive, because we don't see the perseverance that produces it. We don't see the good times and bad, the setbacks and the obstacles. Changing behavior also

involves a certain amount of perseverance and discipline. Many desire the benefits of a healthy lifestyle but fail to commit to its precepts.

It takes more than willpower to change a behavior. Permanent behavior change involves passing through five distinct transitional stages, while using the corresponding problem-solving processes and strategies within each stage. Just as special tools are needed in building a house, having skills in the various processes of change will help you "build your new self." Making a plan, S.M.A.R.T. goal setting, listing pros and cons, and understanding relapses are important skills. Writing a contract helps you construct a plan in its entirety, and keeping a behavior-change log helps you monitor daily activity. Though setbacks may occur, a mind-set of commitment and self-empowerment can help you continue the journey.

Think about a business that places this sign in its window: "UNDER NEW MANAGEMENT." Imagine that your body/life is your "business" and you're the new manager who's been brought in to turn this business around. It's going to be challenging, and you're going to have to make some tough decisions. It'll take effort and commitment, but it is your job! And think of the benefits! So declare it now: "MY LIFE IS UNDER NEW MANAGEMENT!"

Terms

- action stage
- contemplation stage
- maintenance stage
- precontemplation stage
- preparation stage
- processes of change
- self-efficacy
- transtheoretical model of behavior change

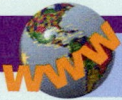

Internet Resources

American Academy of Health Behavior
www.ajhb.org

Offers current and archived abstracts of articles from the *American Journal of Health Behavior* with an emphasis on health behavior research.

Health Behavior News Service
www.cfah.org/hbns

Has recent scientific research and news stories pertaining to how people can change their behavior to improve and manage existing illnesses.

Home of the Transtheoretical Model
www.uri.edu/research/cprc

Offers detailed information about the transtheoretical model of behavior change. Included are assessment inventories for various behaviors and habits.

Psychology Today
www.psychologytoday.com

Accesses thousands of articles related to a variety of psychological topics: anxiety, behavior, depression, family, personality, relationships, stress, and addictions.

Spark People
www.sparkpeople.com/resource/motivation.asp

A public site with information and articles on motivation for exercise, weight loss, and other healthy habits. Also includes message boards involving people who have positively changed their habits.

LAB Activity 2-1

Identify Your S.M.A.R.T. Goal

By using the information in this chapter on goal setting, identify your **S.M.A.R.T.** goal.

S (Specific):
(Examples: Poor = "I want to look better."; Good = "I am going to increase the muscle definition in my arms.")

M (Measurable):
(Examples: Poor = "I want to try to eat more fruit."; Good = "I will eat 4 servings of fruit every day.")

A (Achievable):
(Examples: Poor = "I will lose 120 pounds."; Good = "I will lose 10 pounds.")

R (Reward):
(Examples: Poor = "For every pound that I lose, I am going to treat myself to a hot fudge sundae."; Good = "For every pound that I lose, I am going to put $2 in a jar toward the purchase of a new outfit.")

T (Time-defined):
(Examples: Poor = "I want to stop biting my nails." Good = "I will stop biting my nails by spring break.")

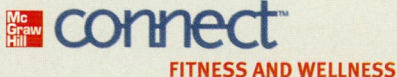

http://connect.mcgraw-hill.com

Now . . . state your *final, completed goal statement* using all S.M.A.R.T. factors:
(Example: "I will get up at 7:30 A.M. on MWF to do 20 minutes of spiritual reading and journaling, and my reward for sticking with it for a whole month will be to treat myself to a massage.")

_____

_____

_____

_____

_____

Anticipated obstacles, barriers, or high-risk situations:

Strategies for overcoming obstacles, barriers, or high-risk situations:

Name _____ **Class/Activity Section** _____ **Date** _____

Behavior-Change Contract (Using the Transtheoretical Model)

Writing a contract makes you think through your plan in its entirety. It specifies the *details* for carrying out your plan.

STEP 1: Turn your personal goal into a question (see Figure 2-1), and write it on the line below. Then trace a path along the flowchart to find your current stage of change.

Do you _____?

(Example: Do you consume at least 1,000 mg of calcium every day?)

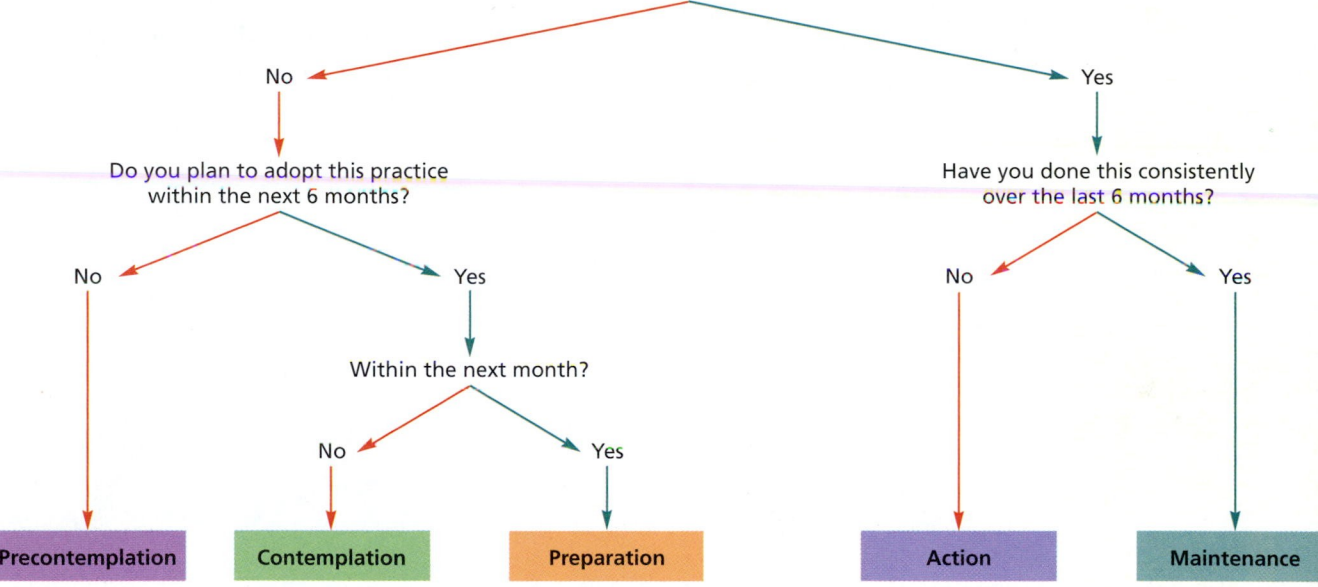

STEP 2: Write your contract, using your behavioral strategies. (See Figure 2-3 for a sample contract.)
Goal (specific and measurable):

Pros/Benefits of changing:

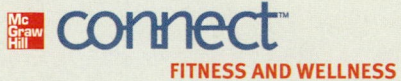
FITNESS AND WELLNESS

http://connect.mcgraw-hill.com

Cons/Barriers of changing:

State your current stage of change (as identified by the flowchart):

_____

Now identify three *processes* of change that correspond to your personal stage of change (see Figure 2-2), and list two specific behavioral strategies you will use for each process. (See Table 2-1 and Figure 2-3 for several examples of behavioral strategies.)

Example:

1. Process: _____

    Strategies: (1)

    Process: <u>Consciousness-raising</u>

    Strategies: (1) Find out amount of calcium I need for my age.

        (2)

        (2) Keep track of my daily calcium intake to see what I currently get.

2. Process: _____

    Strategies: (1)

        (2)

3. Process: _____

    Strategies: (1)

        (2)

    Witness (optional) _____

Name _____ **Class/Activity Section** _____ **Date** _____

Using the "S's for Success" in Changing Your Behavior

Staying engaged and motivated throughout your behavior change means using strategies and attitudes that help keep you going. Using the Top 10 List in Chapter 2 ("S's for Success in Changing a Behavior"), write your ideas on how you can utilize each of the "S's" to help you reach your goal.

GOAL (specific and measurable):

1. Self-monitoring:

2. Self-efficacy:

3. Set reasonable expectations:

4. Start small:

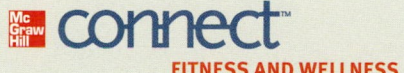

http://connect.mcgraw-hill.com

5. Self-talk:

6. Social support:

7. Surround yourself with positives:

8. Setbacks:

9. Stress management:

10. See your goal:

Developing and Assessing Physical Fitness

STUDY QUESTIONS

You will have successfully mastered this chapter if you can answer the following:

1. What are the benefits of physical fitness?
2. What are the five health-related fitness components?
3. What are the purpose, content, and time of the three parts of a workout?
4. What are the principles of fitness development?
5. What is cross training? Give one example.
6. What are one or more tests for each component of health-related fitness?

You will find the answers as you read this chapter.

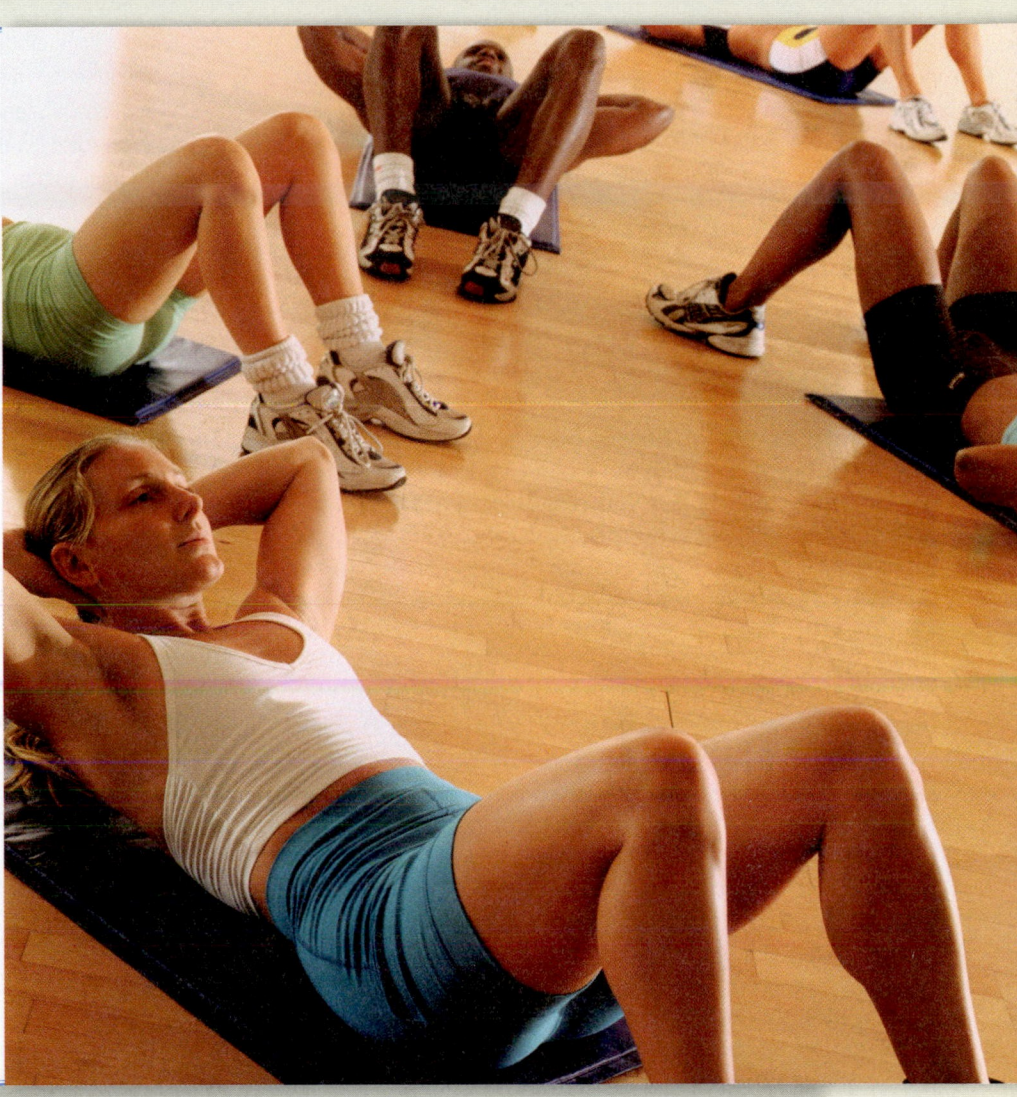

> " *Our medicines are no further away than the shelves of the grocery and the sidewalks that we can use for a brisk walk.* "
> —Tommy Thompson, former Secretary of Health and Human Services

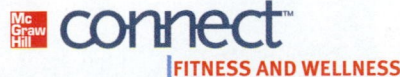

connect™
FITNESS AND WELLNESS

http://connect.mcgraw-hill.com

If there was a magic potion that you could take to increase your energy and help you manage weight, decrease stress, feel better, and decrease the risk of heart disease, cancer, and diabetes, would you be interested? The benefits of regular physical activity include these and many more. It is perhaps our cheapest preventive medicine. Since 1993 we have known that three behaviors account for 78 percent of the risk of chronic disease: tobacco use, diet, and physical activity. Exercise alone cuts the risk of premature death in half. To live a wellness lifestyle, you must be physically active. While moderate levels of activity produce improvements in health, physical fitness requires higher-intensity activity and produces greater benefits. Physical fitness is an important component of wellness because what affects the body ultimately affects the mind. Physical fitness enables you to function at the peak of your capacity physically and mentally—to enjoy life more fully—to be all that you can be.

You want to become more physically fit. How do you begin? This chapter discusses the benefits of physical activity and how much activity is needed to maintain health. It reviews basic principles of developing physical fitness, gives guidelines for health benefits, and details methods of assessing the health-related physical fitness components. This enables you to measure your current fitness levels, set goals, and develop a plan for working toward those goals. It will provide you with the information you need to begin a fitness program so that you can reap the benefits for life!

◆ IMPORTANCE OF EXERCISE

The natural peak of fitness occurs at physiological maturity, in the late teens to early twenties. After this, life becomes a slide down the aging curve for sedentary individuals, who gradually lose 1 to 3 percent per year of their cardiorespiratory endurance, muscle mass, flexibility, and so on. If you have observed friends who are older, you have seen that many of them are beginning to show physical deterioration due to lack of exercise: decreasing energy levels, increasing body fat, loss of muscle tone. Our bodies were designed for physical activity, but few occupations provide enough to maintain health or fitness. Homemakers, office workers, and students have busy, stressful lives and may feel tired at the end of the day, but they often lack the physical activity vital to tone muscles, stimulate the heart and lungs, or produce a training effect. This has resulted in an epidemic of **hypokinetic diseases** related to an inactive lifestyle, such as obesity, coronary heart disease, cancer, osteoporosis, and diabetes. Older adults are sometimes erroneously told to "slow down" and "take it easy," resulting in increasing weakness and accelerated physical decline. Unfortunately, too many people feel that they don't have time for exercise and are satisfied with minimal exertion in their lives. Approximately 250,000 premature deaths per year in the United States can be attributed to lack of exercise. According to Dr. Steven Blair, epidemiologist for the Cooper Institute for Aerobics Research, a sedentary lifestyle is as much a risk factor for disease as are smoking, obesity, and high blood pressure, but inactivity is more prevalent.

Inactivity also contributes to the problem of obesity in our country. Nearly 73 percent of American adults are overweight, and a third are obese. The average American gains 1 to 2 pounds per year throughout adulthood. Our nation's children are fatter too, and about half are not physically active enough for aerobic benefit; this increases their risk of heart disease. Consuming too many calories and not getting enough exercise are to blame. The problem is compounded by the abundance of labor-saving devices, such as remote controls, computers, and riding lawn mowers. Americans spend more than half their time sitting, from working at desks to sitting in cars. Children's playtime often consists of watching television; surfing the Internet; or sports lessons where sitting, standing, or watching consumes a major portion of the time. To make matters worse, although childhood is the best time to develop a lifelong habit of physical activity, many physical education programs face elimination because they are considered a frill when educational budgets are crunched. In a world filled with labor-saving devices, it is more important than ever to build exercise into our lives for optimal health and well-being.

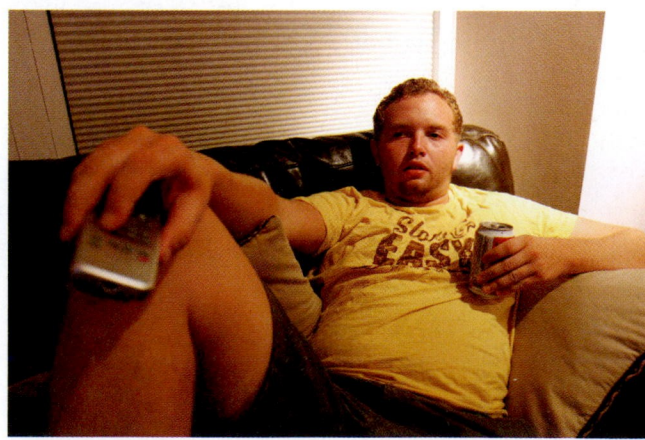

We have become a nation of spectators. The average American spends 5 hours per day watching TV or online.

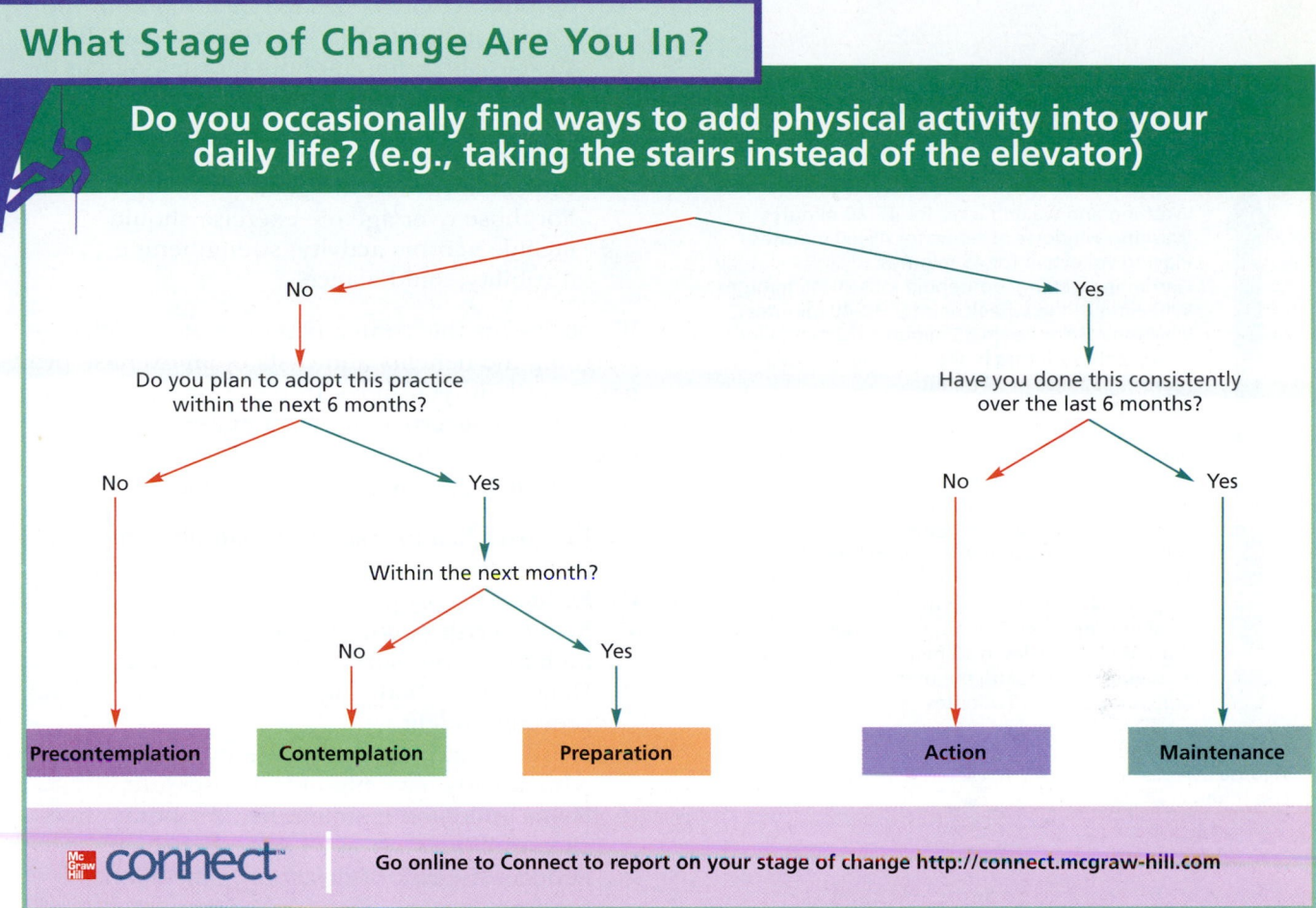

What Stage of Change Are You In?

Do you occasionally find ways to add physical activity into your daily life? (e.g., taking the stairs instead of the elevator)

No — Do you plan to adopt this practice within the next 6 months? — No → **Precontemplation** ; Yes → Within the next month? — No → **Contemplation** ; Yes → **Preparation**

Yes — Have you done this consistently over the last 6 months? — No → **Action** ; Yes → **Maintenance**

Go online to Connect to report on your stage of change http://connect.mcgraw-hill.com

For young people, levels of physical activity decline sharply through adolescence. Many college students show early signs of hypokinetic disease. If you are concerned about slowly gaining weight from pizza, shakes, and fries, a good fitness program can reverse the trend. If normal daily activities leave you feeling worn out, you can boost your energy with regular exercise 3 to 5 days a week. Because routine activities such as sitting in class, watching TV, and walking across campus seldom require the physical effort needed to develop fitness, we must plan for daily vigorous exercise. The old saying "Use it or lose it" has never been more true.

◆ PHYSICAL ACTIVITY AND HEALTH

We know that many people can improve their health and the quality of their lives with lifelong physical activity, yet about 60 percent of adult Americans are not regularly active and nearly 90 percent need more physical activity to improve their health. Almost half our young people are not vigorously active.

Healthy People 2020 (see Chapter 1) contains exercise objectives, which include the following:

✓ To reduce the proportion of adults who engage in no leisure-time physical activity.
✓ To increase the proportion of adults that meet current federal physical activity guidelines for aerobic physical activity and for muscle strength training.

Unfortunately, Americans have not made progress toward these goals in the past 20 years.

To encourage Americans to get moving and reverse the increasing toll of health care costs related to chronic diseases, the American College of Sports Medicine and the American Heart Association issued a joint recommendation for the quantity of physical activity needed by healthy adults to improve and maintain health:

1. To promote and maintain health, all healthy adults ages 18 to 65 should maintain an active lifestyle.
2. Include moderately intense aerobic exercise 30 minutes a day, 5 days a week, or vigorously

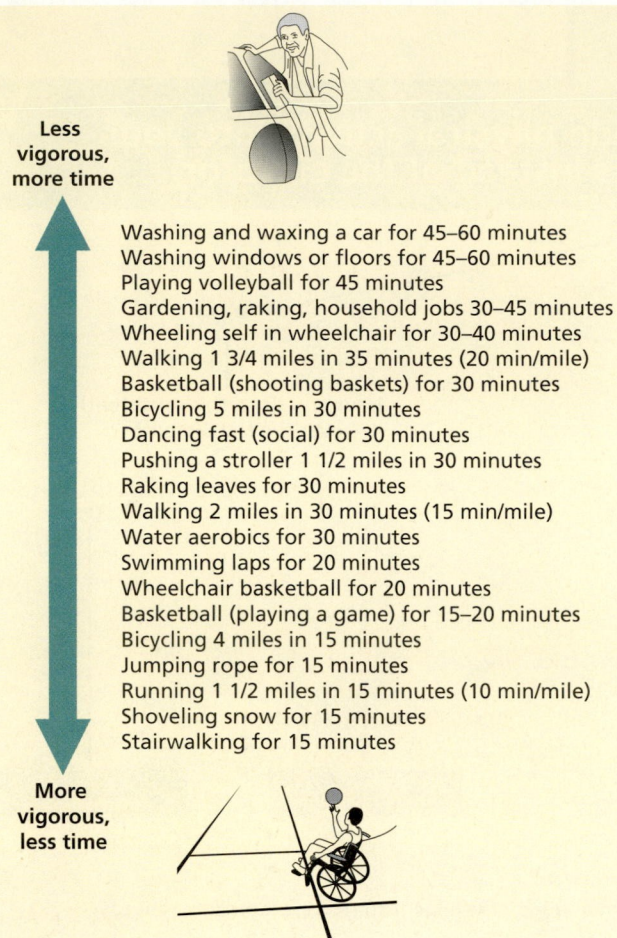

Less vigorous, more time

Washing and waxing a car for 45–60 minutes
Washing windows or floors for 45–60 minutes
Playing volleyball for 45 minutes
Gardening, raking, household jobs 30–45 minutes
Wheeling self in wheelchair for 30–40 minutes
Walking 1 3/4 miles in 35 minutes (20 min/mile)
Basketball (shooting baskets) for 30 minutes
Bicycling 5 miles in 30 minutes
Dancing fast (social) for 30 minutes
Pushing a stroller 1 1/2 miles in 30 minutes
Raking leaves for 30 minutes
Walking 2 miles in 30 minutes (15 min/mile)
Water aerobics for 30 minutes
Swimming laps for 20 minutes
Wheelchair basketball for 20 minutes
Basketball (playing a game) for 15–20 minutes
Bicycling 4 miles in 15 minutes
Jumping rope for 15 minutes
Running 1 1/2 miles in 15 minutes (10 min/mile)
Shoveling snow for 15 minutes
Stairwalking for 15 minutes

More vigorous, less time

FIGURE 3-1   Moderate amounts of physical activity.

intense aerobic exercise 20 minutes a day, 3 days a week.

3. The 30 minutes of moderate-intensity exercise can be accumulated in bouts of 10 minutes or more. Examples of moderate-intensity exercise are given in Figure 3-1. Combinations of moderate- and vigorous-intensity exercise can be done, such as 30 minutes of brisk walking 2 days during the week and 20 minutes of jogging another 2 days.

4. Also do 8–10 strength-training exercises, 8–12 repetitions of each, twice a week on nonconsecutive days. This can include lifting weights, calisthenics, elastic bands, etc., using major muscle groups.

5. "More is better." Because greater amounts of physical activity (longer duration or greater intensity) can provide additional health benefits, people who wish to further improve their fitness, reduce risk for chronic disease, or prevent weight gain may benefit by exceeding the minimum recommended amounts of exercise.

6. Aerobic activity is needed in addition to the routine light-intensity activities of daily life, such as shopping, mopping, or taking out the trash. However, moderate to vigorous activities performed for more than 10 minutes, such as shoveling snow or walking to work, can count toward the goal.

7. For those over age 65, exercise should include aerobic activity, strengthening, flexibility, and balance.

If you are in the contemplation stage of change, weighing the benefits and costs of an exercise program can help you move to the next stage. If lack of time is a concern, note that a minimum of 1 hour of exercise (20 minutes × 3 days) out of 168 hours in your week pays big health dividends:

✓ Increases health span, the span of your healthy life.
✓ Reduces risk of premature death.
✓ Reduces risk of coronary heart disease, stroke, high blood pressure, cancer, and diabetes.
✓ Helps reduce body fat, abdominal obesity, and prevents weight gain.
✓ Helps reduce blood pressure in some people who already have high blood pressure.
✓ Helps build and maintain healthy bones, muscles, and joints.
✓ Reduces the risk of developing metabolic syndrome.
✓ Improves sleep quality.
✓ May improve sexual function.
✓ Reduces risk of low back pain.
✓ Prevents cognitive decline in older individuals and improves cognitive performance in people of all ages.
✓ Reduces stress, anger, and depression and improves mood.
✓ Promotes psychological well-being, increases self-esteem, and improves life satisfaction.

A landmark study conducted at the Institute for Aerobics Research in Dallas by Steven Blair et al. provides evidence that physical fitness is associated with longevity (Figure 3-2). In this 8-year study, physical fitness was quantified by using an exercise tolerance test on a treadmill. The subjects were categorized into physical fitness levels based on the treadmill test. The greatest reduction in risk of death occurred between the low and medium levels of fitness. A similar study of 4,300 people tracked for 20 years showed that the mortality rate for the least fit was twice that of the medium fit and four times that of the highest fitness group. Therefore, a modest improvement in fitness among the most unfit can bring about substantial health benefits.

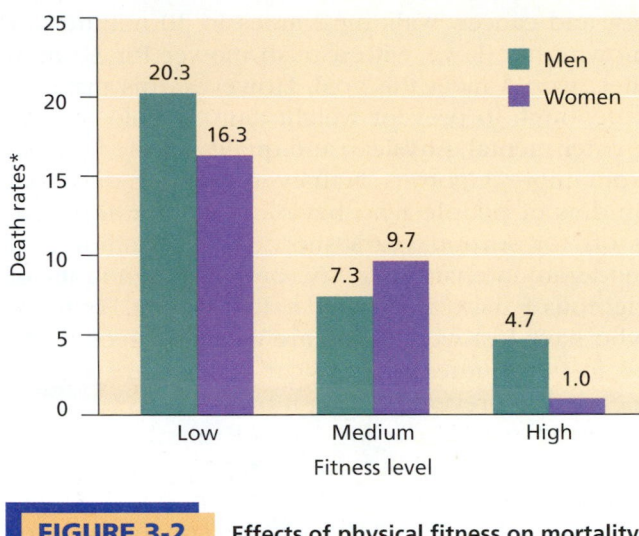

FIGURE 3-2   **Effects of physical fitness on mortality rates.**

*Age-adjusted per 10,000 person-years at follow-up.

Physical Activity Guidelines for Americans

To encourage Americans to improve health through physical activity, the U.S. Department of Health and Human Services issued the first-ever *Physical Activity Guidelines for Americans.* Noting that the current level of inactivity puts Americans at unnecessary health risk, they divided physical activity into two types: baseline and health enhancing. Baseline activity refers to normal lifestyle activity that occurs throughout the day such as standing, walking slowly, and lifting light objects. It can also include short bouts of vigorous activities like climbing a few flights of stairs, but these short episodes don't meet the guidelines. People who do only baseline activity are considered inactive and are in the highest health-risk category. Health-enhancing physical activity, such as brisk walking and lifting weights, when added to baseline, produces health benefits. This report recommended that adults should accumulate at least 2 1/2 hours a week of moderate intensity or 75 minutes of vigorous intensity aerobic physical activity, or equivalent combination. This can be done in segments of at least 10 minutes, preferably distributed throughout the week. Additional health benefits occur by accumulating up to 5 hours of moderate- or 2 1/2 hours of vigorous-intensity physical activity or a combination of both. Also, adults should do muscle strengthening activities 2 or more days per week. These guidelines support and are similar to the ASCM recommendations but are intentionally more general in allowing accumulation of exercise time across the week in various ways.

Moderate Physical Activity for Health Promotion

There are differences in the intensity and duration of physical activity needed for health, for physical fitness, and for performance, such as in athletics. What is involved in adopting a moderately active lifestyle?

First, realize that physical activity does not have to be punishing to be beneficial. The emphasis should be on activity of *moderate* intensity. This would be equivalent to walking approximately 2 miles at a pace of 15 minutes per mile for improvements in health to occur.

Second, exercise does not have to be done all at one time. We know that 20 minutes or more of vigorous exercise is recommended for high-level fitness (full cardiorespiratory benefit), but all activity is beneficial to our health. Something is better than nothing. Incorporate bits of activity every day whenever and wherever you can. For example: Ride your bike to mail a letter; play racquetball, walk, swim, or run at noon; take a walk after dinner;

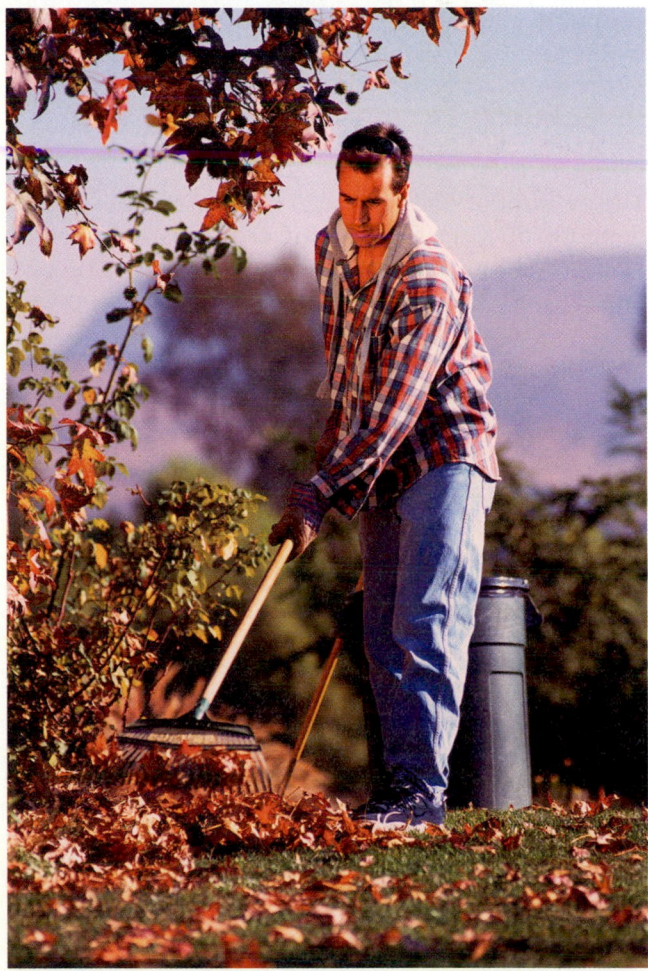

Just 30 minutes of moderate activity can provide many health benefits.

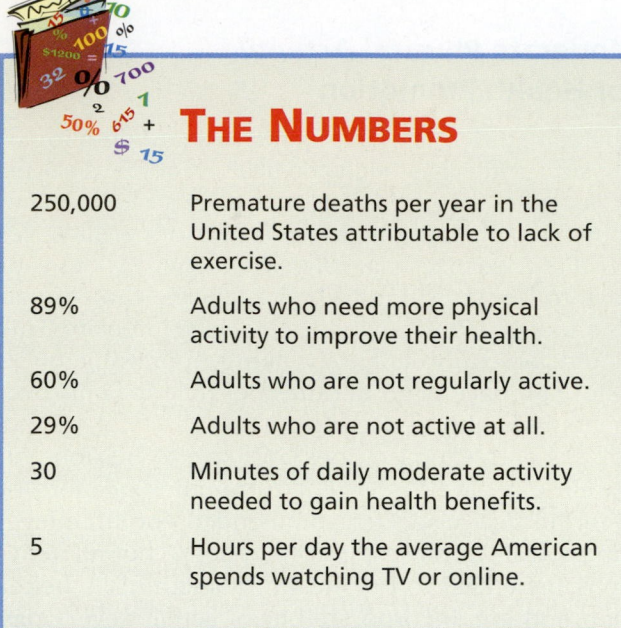

THE NUMBERS

250,000	Premature deaths per year in the United States attributable to lack of exercise.
89%	Adults who need more physical activity to improve their health.
60%	Adults who are not regularly active.
29%	Adults who are not active at all.
30	Minutes of daily moderate activity needed to gain health benefits.
5	Hours per day the average American spends watching TV or online.

wash the car; rake the leaves; walk to the grocery when you need only a few items. *Look* for opportunities to add daily activity—get up earlier, use TV commercial time, when working out a problem, when visiting a friend, and so on.

HOW MUCH EXERCISE IS NEEDED FOR HEALTH—30, 60, OR 90 MINUTES?

The amount of daily physical activity recommended depends on your goal. To lower the risk of chronic diseases, 30 minutes of moderate activity is recommended on 5 days of the week. This is important for reducing risk of coronary heart disease, diabe-

Tips for Behavior Change

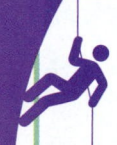

- Take your dog for a walk, and if you don't have one, borrow a friend's
- Wash and wax your car by hand
- Switch from a self-propelled to a push mower
- Pack a healthy lunch and walk to a nearby park to enjoy it
- If your destination is within 1/2 mile, walk instead of driving (i.e. post office, library, etc.)
- Put something you use frequently on a high shelf so that you will need to stretch to reach it
- Start a garden

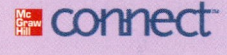 **Go online to Connect to complete this activity. http://connect.mcgraw-hill.com**

tes, and cancer. Walking 2 miles in 30 minutes, or mowing the lawn with a push mower for 30 minutes, would meet the goal. However, this may not be enough to prevent weight gain. People can get greater mental, physical, and quality of life benefits from more vigorous activity or longer duration. Studies of people who have lost weight and kept it off for several years show that 60 minutes of moderate-intensity activity, or lesser amounts of vigorous activity, are needed to lose weight. For those who have lost weight and are trying to keep it off, 60 to 90 minutes of physical activity are recommended to prevent gaining it back.

Most people declare lack of time as a reason for not exercising, but the average person spends 5 hours per day watching television. For the time-crunched, Figure 3-1 has some suggestions for working exercise into your day.

THE ACTIVITY PYRAMID

The Activity Pyramid (Figure 3-3), like the Food Guide Pyramid (see Chapter 11), is a guide to help you choose activities to improve your health and fitness level. The activities at the base of the pyramid, such as walking the dog and using the stairs more often, can be built into your everyday life. If you are currently sedentary, this is the place to start. If you are already moderately active, begin a formal exercise program (the second level of the pyramid) at least three times per week. Aerobic exercise is the most beneficial in promoting health benefits and cardiorespiratory fitness. Vigorous recreational sports also promote cardiorespiratory fitness. Extra healthful benefits can be achieved at the third level, which recommends strength exercises at least twice per week to build balanced fitness, especially if you already do aerobic exercise regularly. The fourth level adds flexibility and leisure activities two or three times per week. The top of the pyramid suggests what to do *least*, including sitting and watching TV.

You are faced with a tremendous challenge. Because you are our nation's future homemakers, parents, and leaders, the responsibility for the health and well-being of the next generation rests in your hands. You can make an enormous impact on the activity patterns of your children, family, friends, and neighbors by setting a good example. So go to it: Get up off the sofa, turn off the TV, and accept the challenge to enjoy exercise daily.

Encourage your friends and neighbors to get out and work in the garden, walk around the block, mow the lawn, walk the dog, participate in recreational sports (bowling, tennis, golf, softball), and go dancing. Anyone can begin the journey toward wellness with a single step and begin reaping health benefits immediately.

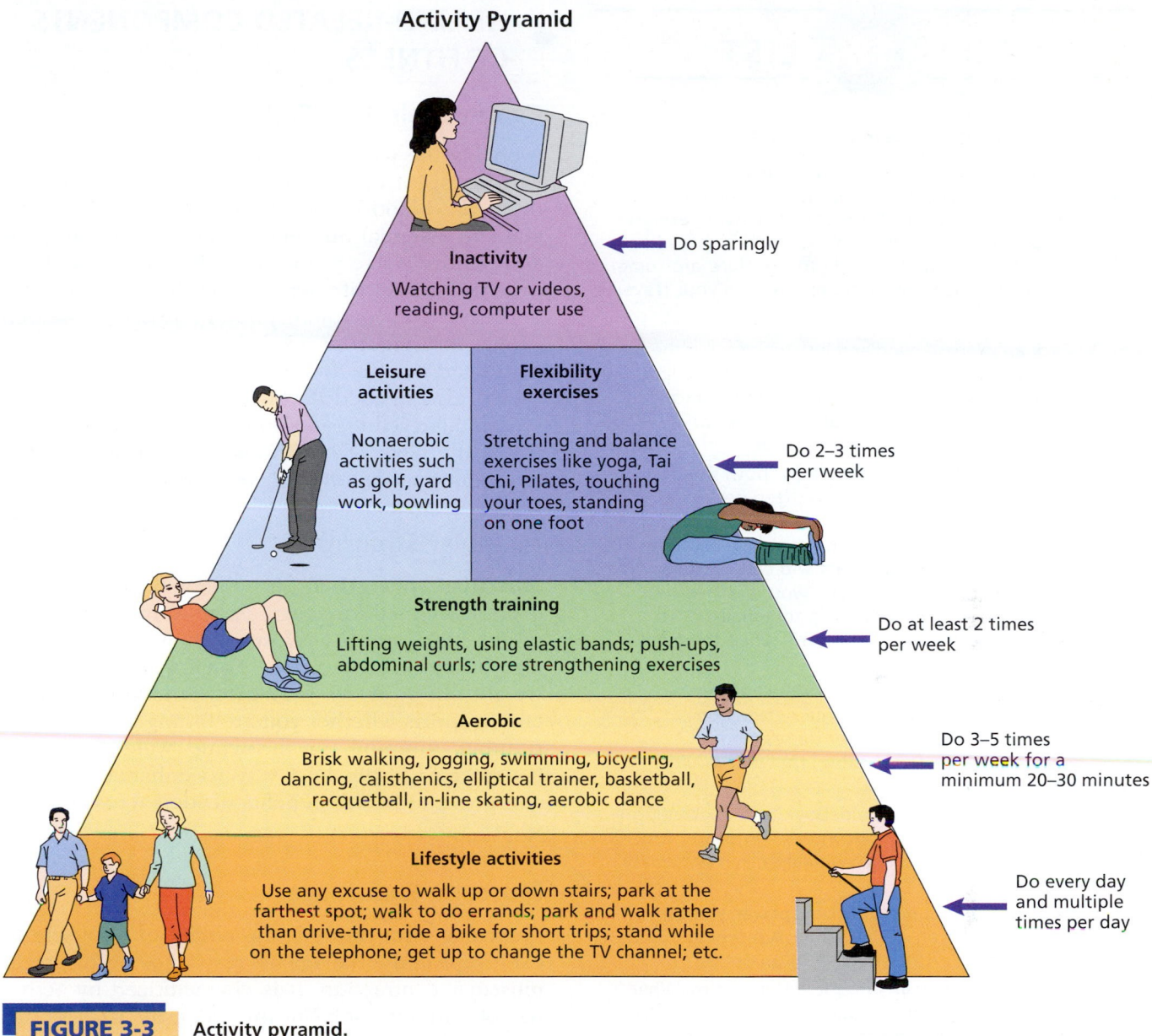

FIGURE 3-3   Activity pyramid.

While moderate activity can improve health, physical fitness requires more vigorous exercise to cause long-term beneficial physiological changes. Specific activity examples are given in Figure 3-1. Next, we look at the components of physical fitness and basic principles of fitness development.

◆ WHAT IS PHYSICAL FITNESS?

Physical fitness is the ability of the body to function at optimal efficiency. The fit individual is able to complete the normal routine for the day and still have ample reserve energy to meet the other demands of daily life—recreational sports and other leisure activities—and to handle life's emergency

situations. Physical fitness involves performance-related and health-related components, which are listed below. The *performance-related* components of fitness are important to athletic success and are not crucial for health. The five *health-related* components of fitness are important for health and performance of daily functional activities.

Performance-Related	**Health-Related**
✓ Speed	✓ Cardiorespiratory endurance
✓ Power	
✓ Agility	✓ Muscular strength
✓ Balance	✓ Muscular endurance
✓ Reaction time	✓ Flexibility
✓ Coordination	✓ Body composition

TOP 10 LIST

Ways to Exercise on the Go

When you travel for business or pleasure, fitting in exercise presents a special challenge. As much as possible, plan ahead when/where you will fit in exercise during your trip. Pack your exercise clothes and a small towel so that you will be ready to go. Here are some suggestions for incorporating exercise into your travel plans.

1. Pack an exercise band and instructions (see the back cover of this book). Exercise bands are lightweight and take very little space in the suitcase. They are inexpensive and allow a wide variety of exercises for different muscle groups.

2. Lace up your shoes and walk for both sightseeing and exercise. You can often get route directions and maps from hotel personnel or a city guidebook. Walk wherever and whenever possible, avoiding cars and cabs. If the weather is extreme and you would rather walk indoors, combine a trip to a mall with a 30-minute walk. Try to go early when the mall is least crowded.

3. Before you leave home, check the Internet for a list of gyms close to your destination and call or check online for classes (yoga, spinning, Pilates, kickboxing) that you would like to try.

4. Use the Internet or a guidebook to check out local activities that you can incorporate into your trip like kayaking, climbing, swimming, and horseback riding.

5. With a laptop or portable DVD player, you can work out with an exercise DVD. A morning exercise program on TV may also be an option.

6. Pack two large empty plastic water bottles. When at your destination, fill the bottles with water to use as hand weights for upper-body exercises.

7. An inexpensive exercise mat is easy to pack and can be used for stretching and calisthenics as shown in Chapters 5 and 6.

8. If you have a few hours between flights, use them to walk the airport, stretch, or do a few exercises with your exercise band. Some airports have a fitness facility that you can use for a small fee. You can also stretch and use the exercise band for sitting exercises while on the plane.

9. If you would rather exercise indoors, take a jump rope. It can provide you with a way to do an aerobic workout in a small area.

10. If you are spending time on the beach, take a Frisbee and plan to be active rather than lying in the sand all day.

HEALTH-RELATED COMPONENTS OF FITNESS

Cardiorespiratory Endurance

Probably the most important fitness component is **cardiorespiratory endurance (CRE),** the ability of the heart, blood vessels, and lungs to deliver oxygen and essential nutrients to the working muscles and remove waste products during vigorous physical activity. Your life depends on the efficient functioning of your cardiorespiratory system. Research shows that vigorous exercise is needed to keep your heart healthy and prevent heart disease. Good CRE is also needed if you want to enjoy running, swimming, cycling, and other vigorous activities to live at the peak of health and enjoy a full life. For more information on CRE, see Chapter 4.

Muscular Strength

Muscular strength is the ability of a muscle to exert a maximal force against resistance. Short-duration, high-intensity efforts such as moving furniture, lifting a heavy suitcase, and lifting a 100-pound weight one time are examples. Strength is important in sports whether you are hitting a tennis ball, running, jumping, or throwing. Weight training (Chapter 6) is the best way to enhance strength and provides health benefits needed across the life span.

Muscular Endurance

Muscular endurance is the ability of a muscle to exert repeated force against resistance or to sustain muscular contraction. It is characterized by activities of long duration but low intensity, such as doing repetitions of push-ups or sit-ups. Muscular endurance is essential in everyday activities such as housework, yard work, and recreational sports. Muscular strength and endurance tend to decline with age along with activity levels, making it difficult to perform daily activities such as getting in and out of a car and standing up from the floor. This loss can be delayed and muscular fitness can be maintained by participating in a resistance training program.

Flexibility

Flexibility is movement of a joint through a full range of motion. Flexibility is essential to smooth, efficient movement and may help prevent muscle strains. It is specific to each joint; you may have flexible shoulders but tight hip flexors or vice versa.

Can you sit and touch your toes without bending your knees? This requires hamstring flexibility. You need arm and shoulder flexibility to scratch your back. Women usually have more joint flexibility than men because men have bulkier skeletal muscles. Older adults may have trouble performing routine tasks such as turning to watch traffic while driving and dressing when clothes fasten at the back because flexibility diminishes with age. This loss can be countered if stretching is part of your lifetime exercise program. Chapter 5 has more information about flexibility.

Body Composition

Body composition is the amount of body fat in proportion to fat-free weight. The ratio between body fat and fat-free weight is a better gauge of fatness than is body weight alone. There are various ways to measure body composition, and all are superior to the height/weight chart method. For instance, a height/weight chart may label a 6-foot, 210-pound football player as overweight, when in reality he has only 10 percent body fat, as measured with skinfold calipers. On the other hand, a sedentary person may look okay, but when body composition is analyzed, it is calculated to be 30 percent body fat. Have your body composition analyzed by a professional. Obesity is both unhealthy and uncomfortable and is associated with increased risk for heart disease, diabetes, high blood pressure, cancer, and joint and lower back problems.

THINK ABOUT IT

There is a variety of exercise equipment advertised by models and celebrities who state that their device is the fast, easy solution to total fitness. Do you feel that a celebrity endorsement makes it more likely that the equipment will produce results advertised? Why or why not? What are guidelines to follow to help a person differentiate useful exercise equipment from overhyped junk?

McGraw Hill connect™
Go online to Connect to complete this activity.
http://connect.mcgraw-hill.com

TABLE 3-1	*Benefits of Physical Fitness on Wellness Dimensions*
Physical	Slows the aging process; increases energy; improves posture and physical appearance; helps control weight; improves flexibility; improves muscular strength and endurance; strengthens bones and reduces osteoporosis; reduces risk for coronary heart disease.
Emotional	Relieves tension; aids in stress management; improves self-image; evens emotional swings; provides time for adult play; promotes psychological well-being.
Social	Enhances relationships with family and friends; increases opportunity for social contacts.
Intellectual	Develops concepts of mind and body oneness; increases alertness; enhances concentration; motivates toward improved personal habits (smoking cessation, reducing drug and alcohol use, better nutrition); stimulates creative thoughts.
Occupational	Decreases absenteeism; increases productivity; decreases disability days; lowers medical care costs; lowers job turnover rate; increases networking possibilities.
Spritual	Develops appreciation of body–mind connection; enhances appreciation for healthy environment; builds compassion for those less able.
Environmental	Develops appreciation for healthy air and water; increases concern for recycling and preservation of natural resources; increases interest in eliminating toxins and chemicals from food chain.

PHYSICAL FITNESS AND WELLNESS

Becoming physically fit is a positive health habit that has a major impact on all dimensions of wellness (Table 3-1). It is one area where you can assume control of your lifestyle. See the Prescription for Action box at the end of this chapter for suggestions on getting started today.

THREE-PART WORKOUT

An exercise session includes three parts: a warm-up, a conditioning bout, and a cool-down.

Warm-Up

The **warm-up** is an important beginning to an exercise session. Two important physiological changes occur during the warm-up. The internal temperature of the muscles increases, enhancing their elasticity. Heart rate and respiration increase, thus providing greater blood flow to the exercising muscles. The warm-up prepares the body physically and mentally for the conditioning bout and may reduce the chance of injury while exercising. There is no set length of time for the warm-up, although 5 to 15 minutes is adequate. On cold days or when you feel sluggish, the warm-up may take longer. When you're feeling energetic or when the temperature is warm, the warm-up period may be shorter. A good method of gauging whether you have had an adequate warm-up is to pay attention to how you feel. Do you feel ready to exercise vigorously? If you still feel stiff and sluggish, you need a longer warm-up. A slight sweat, reflecting an increase in deep muscle temperature, is another indication of an adequate warm-up.

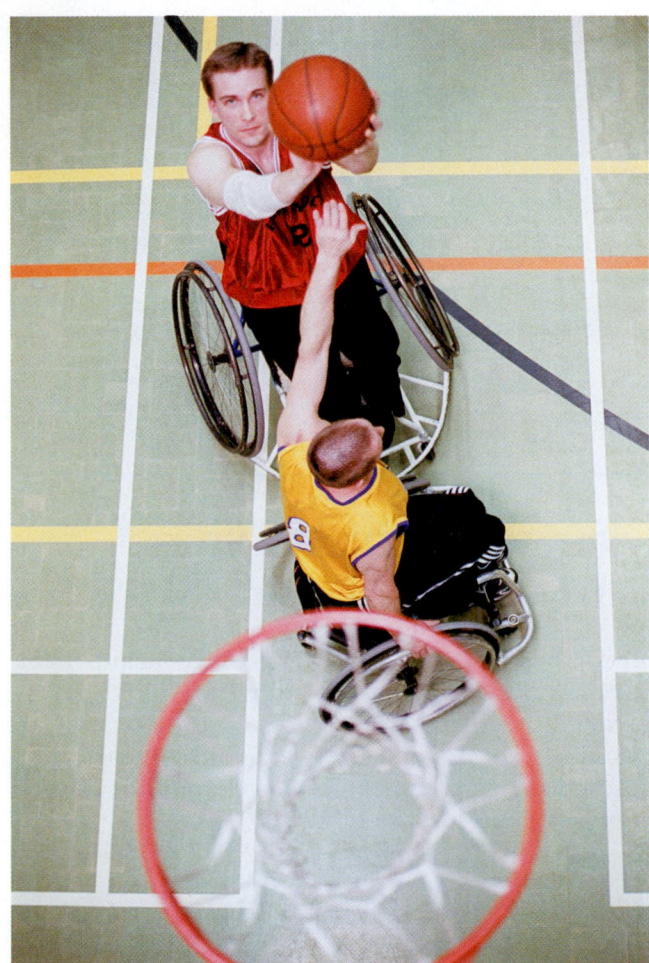

Everybody benefits from physical activity.

Three activities may be included in the warm-up: walking briskly, mild stretching exercises, and a short period of task-specific activity. Stretching during a warm-up is mainly preparation for the activity, not for flexibility. Gentle **static stretching,** in which a stretch is held for 10 to 30 seconds at the point of tightness, is best. **Ballistic stretching,** with jerking and bouncing movements, should not be used because it can strain cold muscles. See Figures 5-1 and 5-2 for more information on types of stretching and specific exercises. Most experts agree that the best time to stretch for flexibility is during the cool-down phase because the muscles are warmer and more elastic.

The **task-specific activity** is an exercise using the same muscles that will be used in the conditioning bout but at a lowered intensity level (lower heart rate). For example, joggers should include a short period of brisk walking or slow jogging before increasing to normal intensity.

Conditioning Bout

The **conditioning bout** is the main part of the workout: 20 to 30 minutes or more. It may include a variety of activities for building cardiorespiratory endurance, muscular strength and endurance, or flexibility, depending on your goals. Gradually increase the frequency, time, and intensity of your exercise sessions until you reach a maintenance level. Progress slowly and listen to your body. If the exercise is at an appropriate level, you should recover within an hour. If you are too tired afterward or if the fatigue lingers until the next day, ease back on the workout time, intensity, or frequency to find an appropriate level. Your goal is a lifetime of exercise. Select one or more activities you will enjoy. Depending on your age, current fitness level, and physical abilities, enjoy walking, cycling, weight training, or any other vigorous activity you prefer.

Cool-Down

The **cool-down** is the final segment of the exercise session. The purpose of the cool-down is to ease your body back to its resting state. It will usually take 5 to 15 minutes to reduce the intensity of exercise. It should begin with the same activity performed in the conditioning bout, but at a lowered intensity. For example, if you jog, reduce the pace and end with a period of walking. Failure to cool down may allow the muscles to tighten further, potentially causing soreness and stiffness. Another problem with an inadequate cool-down is the possibility of venous blood pooling in the lower extremities, resulting in faintness and dizziness. The cool-down should continue until the heart rate is approximately 100 to 110 beats per minute or less. In the cool-down, spend a few minutes stretching while the muscles are thoroughly warm and elastic. Use the stretching exercises illustrated in Figures 5-1 and 5-2. Greater flexibility is achieved when stretching occurs in the cool-down segment of the workout.

PRINCIPLES OF FITNESS DEVELOPMENT

When a person begins an exercise program, the body adapts over time to the demands placed on it. The beneficial long-term changes that occur with regular exercise depend on several factors. To put together an effective exercise program, it is important to understand several principles of fitness development, including overload, specificity, reversibility, and individual differences.

Progressive Overload

Progressive overload is a gradual increase in physical activity, working a muscle group or body system beyond accustomed levels. Overload is perhaps the most important factor in developing physical fitness. When the amount of exercise is gradually increased, the muscle group or system, such as the cardiorespiratory system, gradually adapts, resulting in improved physiological functioning. In addition, a decrease in the severity and a delay in the onset of fatigue occur. If there is insufficient overload, there is no fitness improvement, but too much overload can cause injury. The key to gradual overload is to increase slowly.

To progress in cardiorespiratory exercise, gradually increase the frequency of workouts, starting with three and progressing to five workouts per week, adding one workout each week. Second, increase time. Start with workouts of 20 minutes (or less, if your fitness is very low), and lengthen the workouts by no more than 10 percent per week. For example, if the conditioning bout is 20 minutes, the next week's workout can be 22 minutes. Third, increase the workout intensity by no more than 10 percent per week. See Chapter 4 for further information on developing cardiorespiratory fitness.

The old saying "No pain, no gain!" is inappropriate advice for fitness exercisers. To increase your level of fitness and minimize the risk of overuse injury, follow the prescription factors in the correct order and listen to your body. Don't rush to get into shape in a few weeks. Exercise is for a lifetime.

Specificity

The **principle of specificity** means that only the muscles or body systems being exercised will show beneficial changes. To improve the cardiorespiratory system, exercise the heart and lungs through aerobic activities; to improve flexibility, do stretching exercises; and to improve muscular strength, lift weights. You cannot strengthen the muscles of the arms by jogging or increase cardiorespiratory fitness by doing yoga. This principle also helps explain why you are "wiped out" after swimming 10 minutes even though you can run for 30 minutes.

Reversibility

The **principle of reversibility** states that changes occurring with exercise are reversible and that if a person stops exercising, the body will decondition and adapt to the decreased activity level. Rate of fitness loss varies, but if a person stops exercising, a gradual loss of fitness begins within 48 hours. All fitness improvements can be lost within 2 to 4 months. If a person must decrease activity, the greatest benefits can be retained by maintaining intensity while decreasing the frequency or time of exercise. For example, if a person is traveling for 2 weeks and doesn't have time for the regular 30-minute run, 5 days a week, dropping to 20 minutes or 3 days a week at the usual target heart rate (THR) will help maintain training effect benefits.

Individual Differences

The **principle of individual differences** states that people vary in their ability to develop fitness components. Some people find that it is relatively easy to build strength, but they have to work hard to maintain their desired body composition. Others find that it is easier to increase their cardiorespiratory endurance than their flexibility. We differ in our genetic endowment, and there are limits on our ability to improve any particular fitness component. Some have estimated that maximal oxygen uptake can be improved by only about 15 to 30 percent with aerobic exercise. Even that amount of increase can make a tremendous difference in quality of life. Within our genetic endowment, we have potential for improvement. You don't have to be an Olympic athlete to gain the health benefits of physical activity.

TABLE 3-2   *Activities for Cross Training*

Exercise Goal	Activity
Cardiorespiratory endurance	Running, fitness walking, aerobic dance, bench and stair stepping, rope jumping, cross-country skiing, swimming, cycling, water exercise, in-line skating, ice skating, full-court basketball, ultimate Frisbee, soccer
Flexibility	Stretching, yoga, Tai Chi, Pilates
Muscular strength	Resistance training with weight machines, free weights, elastic bands, gymnastics
Muscular endurance	Calisthenics (push-ups, pull-ups, abdominal curls), weight training with light weights and high repetitions
Body composition	Cardiorespiratory endurance exercises burn calories at the highest rate per minute. Resistance training builds muscle, which increases metabolic rate for a greater calorie burn 24 hours a day.

Cross Training

Cross training involves participating in two or more types of exercise in one session or in alternate sessions for balanced fitness. An easy way to start is to vary activities; for example, you could add one swimming session and two weight training days to a three-times-per-week jogging program and stretch daily. Or within one exercise bout you may spend a few minutes warming up on a treadmill, lift weights, do stationary cycling for 20 minutes, and finish with stretching. See Table 3-2 for cross-training activities. Cross training provides several advantages for the health/fitness exerciser:

✓ It adds variety to your exercise sessions and makes them more interesting, preventing boredom and making it easier to stick to an exercise program.

✓ It provides a greater variety of fitness benefits than does any single activity alone. For example, weight training improves muscular strength and endurance but does little for cardiorespiratory endurance or flexibility. Running increases cardiorespiratory endurance but does little for upper-body strength. Cross training can be used to develop all five fitness components.

✓ It reduces the risk of injury because the bones, joints, and muscles are not subjected to the same repetitive stresses of one activity, which leads to overuse injuries (e.g., shin splints from excessive impact).

✓ Changing activities utilizes muscles differently, promoting muscle symmetry, a balance of strength, and flexibility in opposing muscle groups. Using only one activity tends to cause some muscles to grow strong and their opposing muscles to grow disproportionately weak.

✓ You may continue to train while allowing an injury to heal by using activities that do not stress the injured area.

✓ It develops balanced fitness, because optimal performance in any activity usually requires more than one fitness component. For example, a distance runner may benefit from greater strength and anaerobic fitness to run uphill or sprint to the finish line.

◆ ASSESSING PHYSICAL FITNESS

Physical fitness tests are often divided into two categories: health-related and skill-related. Skill-related tests, such as a vertical jump or shuttle run, are performance-based and are related to athletic ability. Health-related tests are related to functional well-being in the areas of cardiorespiratory endurance, muscular strength and endurance, flexibility, and body composition. These areas of physiological functioning can be improved or maintained through regular exercise and offer protection against the negative effects of a sedentary lifestyle.

Do you know how fit you are? We seem to have a natural curiosity about how we compare to others. The purpose of fitness testing is to help you identify your current fitness levels in several health-related categories. Such an evaluation should tell you whether your current lifestyle is effective in developing and maintaining a level of fitness conducive to optimal wellness. Your results can be used as a basis for setting personal fitness goals; for developing an appropriate individualized exercise prescription; and finally, for measuring the effectiveness of your fitness program in reaching your goals.

The remainder of this chapter gives norms that enable you to compare your fitness levels with those of other students. Norms reflect achievements of thousands of people who have completed a 12- to 15-week fitness course. When evaluating your fitness and setting goals, keep in mind that scoring in the "low" category does not reflect negatively on you. People often score in this category if they have not previously been exercising. While "superior" is an attainable goal for some, relatively few people achieve this level in one or more areas of fitness. *Health-related fitness benefits can be experienced at the "average" fitness level.* Bodies are different. Your current fitness level does not indicate your potential. Physical capacity to achieve any particular level of fitness is partially genetically determined. You may find that you gain strength easily but must constantly work on flexibility or vice versa.

Also keep in mind that all tests are subject to some measurement variability. Results of tests of aerobic capacity and muscular fitness are influenced by a person's level of motivation. If you don't try hard, your fitness will be underestimated. Use these norms as guidelines. Finally, testing should not dominate your program but help you measure its effectiveness. You may wish to measure at the beginning of your program and remeasure 8 to 12 weeks into the program to see how you are progressing.

A *Personal Fitness Profile* is located in Lab Activity 3-3. When completed, it will indicate areas of fitness you can maintain and areas needing improvement. It will help you decide where to begin in your fitness program. Norms for fitness tests are given in Table 3-3 and detailed instructions are given in Labs 3-4 through 3-10 at the end of this chapter.

Note: **Many different tests are provided as options. Select tests appropriate for your condition and goals. Do one or more, but do not feel that you must do all of them!**

◆ GUIDELINES FOR MEDICAL CLEARANCE

According to American College of Sports Medicine guidelines, it is generally safe for men under age 40 and women under 50 to begin a vigorous exercise program if they are healthy and have had a satisfactory medical checkup in the last 2 years. Also, if you have been exercising regularly, it is probably safe to continue progressing gradually from your current activity level. Prior to participation, you should complete the *Student Precourse Health Assessment* form found in Lab Activity 3-1 to identify any potential health concerns.

If you are over these age guidelines or if, regardless of age, you have had health concerns noted on the *Student Precourse Health Assessment* form, it is important to check with your physician before taking a cardiorespiratory fitness test or participating in vigorous exercise. The *Physician-Approved Exercise Clearance Form* in Lab Activity 3-2 is designed for individuals with special health concerns to assist your instructor in individualizing your fitness program according to your physician's recommendations. You may need to have a medical checkup and a diagnostic exercise test. If you smoke cigarettes, have been sedentary over the last several months, are pregnant, have diabetes, are 20 or more pounds overweight, or have family members who have positive risk factors for heart disease, it is particularly important that you see your physician and ask him or her to fill out the *Physician-Approved Exercise Clearance Form*. Also, check with your physician if you are unsure or have concerns about your health.

◆ CARDIORESPIRATORY ENDURANCE TESTS

High-level wellness is inextricably tied to a physically active lifestyle. If you want to be an active participant in life—not just a spectator—cardiorespiratory fitness is essential. A person with a high level of cardiorespiratory fitness can do more work with less fatigue than can a person with low cardiorespiratory fitness. Increased cardiorespiratory fitness can enhance quality of life by increasing the rate of energy production during physical activity. Low levels of cardiorespiratory fitness may result in a limited lifestyle due to low energy reserves, quick exhaustion after moderate exertion, and resulting inability to participate in vigorous, oxygen-demanding activities. The ability of your heart and lungs to supply oxygen during activity is one of the best indicators of overall physical fitness. There are several ways to measure your body's ability to use oxygen. The most accurate method is an **exercise tolerance test** on a treadmill or on a bicycle ergometer in a laboratory (see Figure 3-4). In an exercise tolerance test, a person exercises strenuously while heart rate and oxygen consumption are measured. This, however, is complex, expensive, and time-consuming and requires elaborate equipment and trained personnel. It is impractical for testing large numbers of people.

Cardiorespiratory fitness can also be measured in field tests conducted out of the laboratory setting. What these tests lose in accuracy they make up in the practicality of self-testing or testing many people at the same time. Field tests of cardiorespiratory endurance are generally based on physiological performance (distance or time tests) or a parameter such as pulse rate (step test).

TABLE 3-3	*Fitness Test Norms*

1.5-Mile Run

Age	18–29		30–39		40–49		50–59	
	F	M	F	M	F	M	F	M
Superior	<12:34	<8:26	<13:34	<9:10	<14:34	<9:55	<15:34	<10:40
Good	12:34–13:40	8:26–10:24	13:34–14:40	9:10–11:10	14:34–15:40	9:55–12:00	15:34–16:40	10:40–12:50
Average	13:41–14:45	10:25–12:31	14:41–15:45	11:11–13:45	15:41–16:45	12:01–14:55	16:41–17:45	12:51–16:05
Fair	14:46–16:00	12:32–14:49	15:46–17:00	13:46–16:00	16:46–18:00	14:56–17:15	17:46–19:00	16:06–18:30
Low	>16:00	>14:49	>17:00	>16:00	>18:00	>17:15	>19:00	>18:30

1.0-Mile Walk

Age	18–29		30–39		40–49		50–59	
	F	M	F	M	F	M	F	M
Superior	<12:34	<11:39	<13:34	<12:40	<14:34	<13:40	<15:34	<14:10
Good	12:34–13:40	11:39–12:59	13:34–14:40	12:40–14:00	14:34–15:40	13:40–14:40	15:34–16:40	14:10–15:20
Average	13:41–14:45	13:00–14:21	14:41–15:45	14:01–15:20	15:41–16:45	14:41–15:55	16:41–17:45	15:21–16:25
Fair	14:46–16:00	14:22–15:43	15:46–17:00	15:21–16:15	16:46–18:00	15:56–16:45	17:46–19:00	16:26–17:25
Low	>16:00	>15:43	>17:00	>16:15	>18:00	>16:45	>19:00	>17:25

3.0-Mile Bicycle Ride

Age	18–29		30–39		40–49		50–59	
	F	M	F	M	F	M	F	M
Superior	<9:18	<8:24	<9:54	<9:00	<10:30	<9:36	<11:06	<10:12
Good	9:18–10:06	8:24–9:12	9:54–10:42	9:00–9:42	10:30–11:06	9:36–10:12	11:06–11:36	10:12–10:42
Average	10:07–11:06	9:13–10:12	10:43–11:42	9:43–10:48	11:07–12:18	10:13–11:24	11:37–12:54	10:43–12:00
Fair	11:07–12:00	10:13–11:06	11:43–12:30	10:49–11:35	12:19–13:00	11:25–12:06	12:55–13:30	12:01–12:48
Low	>12:00	>11:06	>12:30	>11:35	>13:00	>12:06	>13:30	>12:48

500-Yard Swim

Age	18–29		30–39		40–49		50–59	
	F	M	F	M	F	M	F	M
Superior	<7:05	<6:12	<7:35	<6:30	<8:05	<7:00	<8:35	<7:30
Good	7:05–8:49	6:12–7:44	7:35–9:19	6:30–8:14	8:05–9:49	7:00–8:44	8:35–10:19	7:30–9:14
Average	8:50–10:34	7:45–9:19	9:20–11:04	8:15–9:49	9:50–11:34	8:45–10:19	10:20–12:04	9:15–10:49
Fair	10:35–12:19	9:20–10:51	11:05–12:49	9:50–11:22	11:35–13:19	10:20–11:52	12:05–13:49	10:50–11:22
Low	>12:19	>10:52	>12:49	>11:22	>13:19	>11:52	>13:49	>11:22

500-Yard Water Run

Age	18–29		30–39		40–49		50–59	
	F	M	F	M	F	M	F	M
Superior	<7:59	<6:53	<8:30	<7:20	<9:00	<7:50	<9:30	<8:20
Good	7:59–8:38	6:53–7:44	8:30–9:08	7:20–8:15	9:00–9:38	7:50–8:45	9:30–10:08	8:20–9:15
Average	8:39–9:18	7:45–8:38	9:09–9:48	8:16–9:05	9:39–10:18	8:46–9:35	10:09–10:48	9:16–10:05
Fair	9:19–9:58	8:39–9:32	9:49–10:28	9:06–10:00	10:19–10:58	9:36–10:30	10:49–11:28	10:06–11:00
Low	>9:58	>9:32	>10:28	>10:00	>10:58	>10:30	>11:28	>11:00

*Norms reflect the achievements of thousands of people who have completed a 12- to 15-week fitness course. Norms are revised yearly.

(continued)

A field test used to estimate oxygen consumption measures the time it takes you to jog 1.5 miles. Studies have shown that time on the 1.5-mile run correlates well with your maximal ability to utilize oxygen. The faster you cover the distance, the more efficient your heart and lungs are at their job of supplying oxygenated blood and nutrients to the working muscles. Field tests make it easy for you to measure your fitness and detect progress as you train. Keep in mind that if you retest within a few weeks, early improvements may be due to a "learning effect" rather than true cardiovascular changes.

TABLE 3-3   *Fitness Test Norms*   (continued)

1-Minute Abdominal Curls

Age	18–29		30–39		40–49		50–59	
	F	M	F	M	F	M	F	M
Superior	>88	>93	>70	>78	>56	>65	>45	>49
Good	75–88	79–93	60–70	62–78	48–56	53–65	38–45	42–49
Average	60–74	64–78	47–59	51–61	37–47	42–52	29–37	35–41
Fair	45–59	50–63	35–46	40–50	27–36	36–41	21–28	28–34
Low	<45	<50	<35	<40	<27	<36	<21	<28

1-Minute Push-Ups

Age	18–29		30–39		40–49		50–59	
	F	M	F	M	F	M	F	M
Superior	>54	>64	>43	>54	>33	>43	>23	>33
Good	44–54	51–64	32–43	41–54	26–33	32–43	18–23	26–33
Average	32–43	37–50	22–31	27–40	17–25	22–31	11–17	17–25
Fair	20–31	23–36	13–21	18–26	8–16	13–21	6–10	8–16
Low	<20	<23	<13	<18	<8	<13	<6	<8

Sit and Reach (inches)

Age	18–29		30–39		40–49		50–59	
	F	M	F	M	F	M	F	M
Superior	>8.5	>7.0	>8	>6	>7	>5	>6	>4
Good	6.5–8.5	4.0–7.0	5–8	3–6	4–7	2–5	3–6	1–4
Average	4.0–6.4	1.0–3.9	3–4.9	0–2.9	2–3.9	−1–1.9	1–2.9	−3–0
Fair	1.0–3.9	−2.0–0.9	0–2.9	−3−−0.1	−1–1.9	−4−−1.1	−2–0.9	−5−−3.1
Low	<1.0	<−2.0	<0	<−3	<−1	<−4	<−2	<−5

Leg Press (max/body weight)

Age	18–29		30–39		40–49		50–59	
	F	M	F	M	F	M	F	M
Superior	>1.97	>2.39	>1.67	>2.19	>1.56	>2.01	>1.42	>1.89
Good	1.68–1.97	2.13–2.39	1.47–1.67	1.93–2.19	1.37–1.56	1.82–2.01	1.25–1.42	1.71–1.89
Average	1.50–1.67	1.97–2.12	1.33–1.46	1.77–1.92	1.23–1.36	1.68–1.81	1.10–1.24	1.58–1.70
Fair	1.37–1.49	1.83–1.96	1.21–1.32	1.65–1.76	1.13–1.22	1.57–1.67	.99–1.09	1.46–1.57
Low	<1.37	<1.83	<1.21	<1.65	<1.13	<1.57	<0.99	<1.46

Bench Press (max/body weight)

Age	18–29		30–39		40–49		50–59	
	F	M	F	M	F	M	F	M
Superior	>1.00	>1.62	>.79	>1.34	>.76	>1.19	>.67	>1.04
Good	.80–1.00	1.32–1.62	.70–.79	1.12–1.34	.62–.76	1.00–1.19	.55–.67	.90–1.04
Average	.70–.79	1.14–1.31	.60–.69	.98–1.11	.54–.61	.88–.99	.48–.54	.79–.89
Fair	.59–.69	.99–1.13	.53–.59	.88–.97	.50–.53	.80–.87	.44–.47	.71–.78
Low	<.59	<.99	<.53	<.88	<.50	<.80	<.44	<.71

SOURCES: For norms in 1.5-mile run, 1.0-mile walk, 3.0-mile bicycle ride, 500-yard swim, 500-yard water run, 1-minute abdominal curls, 1-minute push-ups, and sit and reach: E. Keener et al. "Undergraduate Student Physical Fitness Assessment," Muncie, IN: Ball State University (originally published Spring 1989; latest compiled data shown here); source for norms in leg press and bench press: based on norms from the Cooper Institute for Aerobics Research, Dallas, TX, revised 2000, used with permission.

That is, you will learn to pace yourself better throughout the distance. It will take 8 to 12 weeks for significant cardiovascular improvement to occur. You should take the *1.5-Mile Run Test* only if you are conditioned for it. It is best if you have been building up to the distance gradually for several weeks prior to taking the test. Other field tests that measure cardiorespiratory endurance are the *1-Mile Walk Test*, the *3-Mile Bicycling Test*, the *500-Yard Swim Test*, the *500-Yard Water Run Test*, and

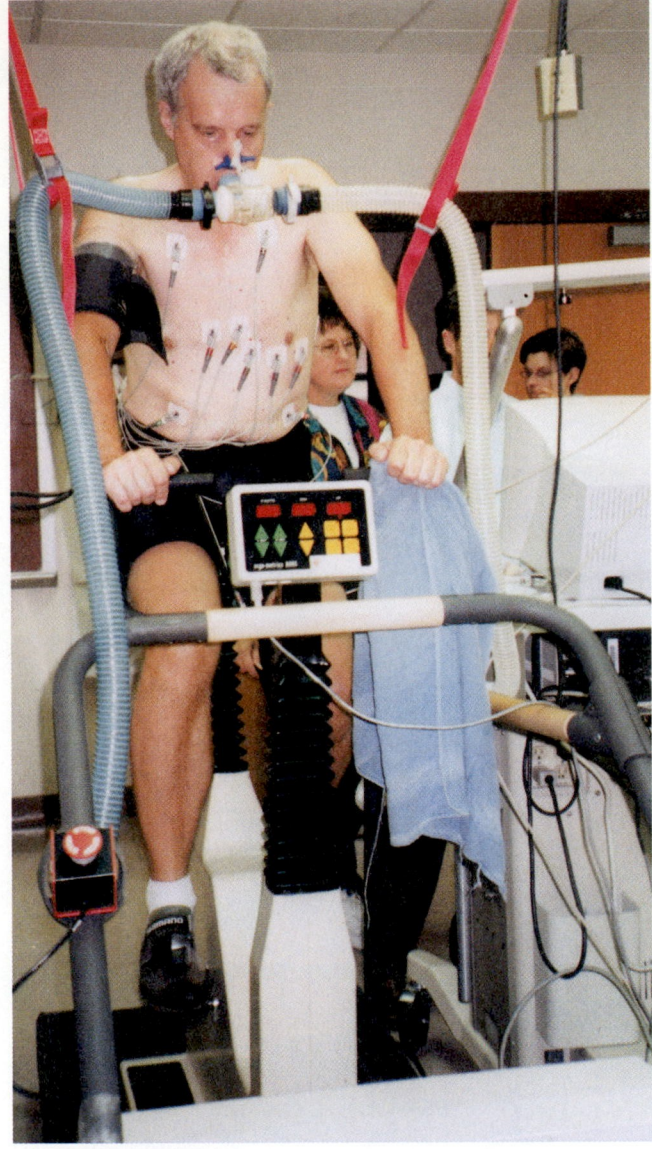

FIGURE 3-4   Exercise tolerance test on a bicycle ergometer.

the *3-Minute Step Test*. You can choose the test most appropriate for your chosen physical conditioning activity. Detailed instructions for these tests are in Labs 3-4 through 3-6.

Pretest Instructions

For any of the cardiorespiratory endurance tests, you will need comfortable clothes appropriate for the activity and a stopwatch or a watch with a second hand.

✓ If possible, avoid taking the test under conditions of extreme heat or cold, particularly if you are not accustomed to exercising under those conditions.

✓ Do not eat a heavy meal, consume alcohol, take caffeine, or smoke for up to 3 hours prior to the test.
✓ Drink plenty of fluids the day before testing.
✓ Rest from vigorous exercise at least 1 day prior to taking the test.
✓ Get adequate sleep (7 to 9 hours) the night before testing.
✓ Warm up and stretch before taking the test and then cool down and restretch afterward.
✓ If at any point during the test you begin to feel ill, dizzy, faint, or extremely short of breath, stop! Your body is telling you that you are not ready for this level of exertion.

Do not be ashamed of stopping before completing the test, especially if you are unfit. Test performance may be limited by local muscular endurance or by aerobic capacity. You may record the amount of time in the test you were able to complete and work toward a fitness level that will enable you to complete the test.

1.5-Mile Run Test

The *1.5-Mile Run Test* requires six laps around a standard quarter-mile track, or it can be done on a measured section of road that has few stoplights. Consider taking this test only if you have been exercising previously. The *1-Mile Walk Test* may be more appropriate for you if you are over 35 years of age or 20 or more pounds overweight or if you have been out of shape for some time but are otherwise in good health. See Lab 3-4 for detailed instructions.

1-Mile Walk Test

For those who are starting a walking program or for whom the *1.5-Mile Run Test* may be too vigorous, the *1-Mile Walk Test* is an option. You will need a 1-mile measured course (four laps of a quarter-mile track), your walking shoes, and a watch with a second hand. See Lab 3-4 for detailed instructions.

3-Mile Bicycling Test

If your main fitness activity is bicycling, you can test your cardiorespiratory fitness with a timed 3-mile bicycle ride. This test can be done on a bike track or on a measured section of road with few stoplights or stop signs. See Lab 3-4 for detailed instructions.

500-Yard Swim Test

If your fitness program consists primarily of swimming, you will find a swimming endurance test useful. A regulation 25-yard pool is recommended, and you will need a friend to time you. You may swim any stroke, although best results will be obtained with the front crawl. See Lab 3-5 for detailed instructions.

500-Yard Water Run Test

The *500-Yard Water Run Test* was designed for those involved in aerobic water exercise programs in which swimming skills are not required. It can be done lengthwise in a pool of constant depth or widthwise across the shallow end of a pool of variable depth. It helps to work in pairs, with one partner on deck counting completed laps for the other. For the most accurate results, runners should carve their own paths through the water and avoid drafting in the wake of other runners. Runners should use their arms to pull as they run but must maintain a vertical body position. No swimming is allowed. See Lab 3-5 for detailed instructions.

3-Minute Step Test

A variety of step tests are useful for testing cardiorespiratory fitness indoors. They involve stepping on and off a bench for a 3- to 5-minute period and measuring the heart rate recovery. The step test is based on the fact that the heart rate of a person who is physically fit is lower at any workload and recovers faster than does the heart rate of a person who is unfit. Although it is not the best measure of cardiorespiratory fitness, it is a quick and simple way to evaluate the heart's response to exercise. It is easy to administer to an individual or to large groups, requires no special skill to perform, and requires little equipment. See Lab 3-6 for detailed instructions.

◆ MUSCULAR STRENGTH AND ENDURANCE TESTS

Muscular strength and endurance are assets in the ability to perform daily activities—lifting, carrying, pushing, pulling—without strain or undue fatigue. Strength and endurance of the abdominal muscles are particularly important for good posture and lower back health. Muscular fitness activities add shape and firmness to muscles, resulting in a trim, well-toned appearance.

Muscular strength and muscular endurance tests have been used as a measure of physical fitness for years. Physical conditioning activities require and can develop both components. Strength is best developed by weight training and is often measured by one maximal lift with weights. Muscular endurance can be measured without special equipment by using the tests provided in Lab 3-7.

Muscular strength and muscular endurance are measured by different tests. You can assess the strength of major muscle groups by taking the *Leg Press Strength Test* and the *Bench Press Strength Test* using the guidelines provided in Lab 3-8. Alternatively, you may use a one-rep max calculator listed under Internet resources at the end of this chapter. Muscular strength is not often tested as part of a general fitness assessment unless prior training and special equipment are provided.

Abdominal Curls and Push-Ups

Abdominal curls are perhaps the best way to assess the endurance of the abdominal muscles. The traditional *Bent-Knee Sit-Up Test* requires use of the thighs and hip flexors as well as abdominals and may put the back at risk. Abdominal curls isolate and test only abdominal muscles, decreasing risk to the lower back. Push-ups test the muscular endurance of the arms and upper-body muscles. Directions and norms for abdominal curls and push-ups are given in Lab 3-7.

Leg Press Strength Test

The "Gold standard" of strength measurements is one single maximal lift (one-rep max). This should be attempted only after several weeks of weight training, emphasizing proper lifting form for safety, as the risk of injury is high for an inexperienced lifter. If you have knee, ankle, or lower back problems, check with your physician before attempting a maximal lift. As there is no industry standard for resistance levels on weight machines, "70 pounds" will give a slightly different resistance level on a Universal, Cybex, or Nautilus. Strength testing using a machine is encouraged as it is safer than using free weights. You will need a leg press machine and a weight scale. Detailed instructions are given in Lab 3-8. If you prefer to estimate your one-rep max from a submax effort, an online calculator is listed under Internet resources.

Bench Press Strength Test

If you have shoulder problems, check with your physician before attempting a maximal lift. While free weights may be used, strength testing using a machine is encouraged because it is safer than using free weights. You will need a bench press machine and a weight scale. See Lab 3-8 for detailed instructions.

 ## FLEXIBILITY TESTS

Flexibility is a valuable asset in daily activities or in any type of vigorous exercise program. The ability to move joints through a full range of motion without stiffness or tightness makes exercise more comfortable and may decrease the risk of injury. The tests included in this section will indicate whether you have a normal range of motion in the lower back and other important areas.

Quick Checks for Flexibility

The quick checks for flexibility in Lab 3-9 are easy ways of measuring the flexibility of major muscle groups often shortened and tightened in daily activities. Each quick check is also a stretch, so if your range of motion is limited or if you feel excessive tightness in a joint or muscle group, use the same position to improve flexibility in that area (see Chapter 5 for basic fitness flexibility guidelines). Note that the hamstring flexibility test (Lab 3-9) eliminates the problem of arm-leg length discrepancy found in the traditional sit and reach test.

Sit and Reach Test

The *Sit and Reach Test* (Lab 3-9), which measures back and hamstring flexibility, can be done with a flex box. If you do not have a flex box, the test can be performed with a ruler on a bench or on the ground with feet flexed. Norms are given using the soles of the feet as the 0 inches mark.

Sit and Reach Wall Test

The *Sit and Reach Wall Test* is a self-check for flexibility and can quickly be performed by a large number of people. All you need is a wall. See Lab 3-9 for detailed instructions.

 ## BODY COMPOSITION TESTS

A certain amount of body fat is essential to good health. Fat acts as an insulator, conserving body heat. It pads bones and cushions internal organs, and it stores and supplies energy for later use.

In a diet-obsessed society in which both obesity and eating disorders abound, few people realize that excessive leanness can be as unhealthy as excessive fatness. For young adults, an average range of body fat for women is 21 to 24 percent, and for men it is 14 to 17 percent (Table 3-4). Keep in mind that each of us has inherited a certain body build and fat distribution; it is natural for some bodies to carry more fat than others do. It is also natural to increase body fat slightly as we age.

While weight scales can tell you how much you weigh, they cannot tell you how much of your body is composed of fat or lean tissue. A sedentary individual may maintain a normal weight for height but increase fat and lose **lean body mass** (muscle tissue) over time. A body builder may be "overweight" according to height-weight charts, but this is due to the development of muscle and bone rather than fat. Being overweight due to having a substantial amount of lean muscle tissue is not the same as being overweight due to excess fat tissue. People who have a muscular build may think they are too heavy when the weight is mainly lean tissue. They could jeopardize their health trying to lose weight unnecessarily. On the other hand, sedentary people who are satisfied with their weight may be shocked to discover that their body fat percentage is over 30 percent, high enough to pose a health risk. In the early stages of a fitness program, excess fat will often be lost and lean muscle weight will increase as fitness improves. Even if no significant weight change occurs, the exerciser is leaner and appears trimmer because a pound of muscle is denser than a pound of fat.

Body fat is measured by using several different techniques. Laboratory tests include DEXA and hydrostatic weighing. Nonlaboratory tests that use indirect techniques to estimate body composition include bioelectrical impedance, skinfold assessment, and measurements of circumference. A Body Mass Index (BMI) calculator is available in Chapter 12. While these tests are not 100 percent accurate, they are useful for assessing change in body composition.

Dual energy X-ray absorptiometry (DEXA) is a laboratory test that uses very low-dose X-ray energy to measure body fat, muscle, and bone mineral. It is considered to be more accurate and valid than underwater weighing. When having the scan done, a person lies still on the DEXA table for about 12 minutes as the computer produces an estimate of body fat, muscle, and bone mineral. Two drawbacks are that it is an expensive test and is not readily available to fitness participants.

Underwater (hydrostatic) weighing is based on Archimedes' principle, which states that when a body is submerged in water, there is a buoyant counterforce equal to the weight of the water that is displaced. A person's weight on land and weight in water are compared. Because bone and muscle are denser than water, a person with a larger percentage of **fat-free tissue** is heavier in the water and records a lower percentage of body fat. However, fat floats, and so a large amount of fat mass will weigh less in the water. This technique reports an accuracy of ±2 percent and has been used by research laboratories to assess body composition for decades. The drawbacks are that it requires elaborate equipment, trained personnel, and about 30 minutes to test each person. Also, emptying the lungs of air (since air makes the body float) and repeatedly submerging underwater may be difficult for some individuals.

Bioelectrical impedance analysis (BIA) is based on the principle that an electrical current travels through fat-free tissue (all parts of the body except fat) with its high water and electrolyte content more readily than it does through fat. By measuring resistance to the current (which is too mild to be felt), the machine estimates body fat. Machines are inexpensive, are easy to use, and include handheld devices and weight scales with built-in electrodes (see Figure 3-5). However, the results vary with differences in hydration, placement of electrodes, and type of machine. BIA tends to overestimate lean individuals and underestimate those who are obese. Hydration plays an important role in BIA and can cause inaccurate results. Dehydration, which can be caused by exercising before testing, not drinking enough fluids, diuretics, illness, and drinking alcohol or caffeine, will cause overestimation of fat percentage. If these variables are controlled, BIA gives a fairly good estimate of body fat, with accuracy reported as ±2 to 5 percent.

Another technique for measuring body composition involves the use of **skinfold calipers.** A caliper is a device that compresses the skin at a pressure determined by a spring. Skinfold measurements can be used to assess your proportion of fat to lean tissue because about 50 percent of your fat is **subcutaneous fat**—located directly under the skin between the skin and the underlying muscle. The amount of subcutaneous fat you have correlates highly with total body fat. An experienced measurer can assess body fat with skinfold calipers to within a range of ±2 to 5 percent. An inexperienced tester may be less accurate. Two or more body sites may be measured, and accuracy increases with the number of sites sampled. Accuracy diminishes at the ends of the scale—for the very obese and the very lean—but for the average individual, skinfolds are reliable.

A self-test of body composition, though considerably less accurate than skinfold caliper measurements, involves body girth measures of body fat. Keep in mind that greater fitness is not guaranteed by low body fat, and what constitutes a healthy fat percentage for you is an individual matter.

Body Composition Assessment Using Skinfold Calipers

Goal: To measure subcutaneous body fat accurately.

Directions: Have a person trained in the use of skinfold calipers perform the following steps.

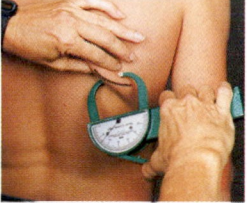

Skinfold measuring technique.

1. Measure skinfolds on the right side of the body by using a skinfold caliper.
2. Grasp a fold of skin between thumb and forefinger, pulling it away from the underlying muscle.
3. Apply the calipers about 0.25 inch below the fingers holding the skinfold.
4. For men, take triceps and thigh measurements on a vertical skinfold. For women, take subscapular and suprailiac measures on a slight lateral slant along the natural fold of the skin.
5. Measure twice. Take readings to the nearest half millimeter. If the readings do not match, take a third measurement and average the closest two measurements.

FIGURE 3-5   **Bioelectrical impedance devices estimate body fat percentage.**

6. Skinfold sites for women are the following:

   a. **Triceps.** Measure a vertical skinfold on the back of the arm midway between the shoulder and the elbow.

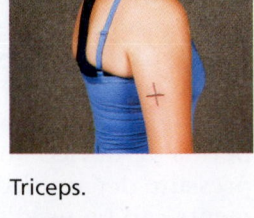

Triceps.

   b. **Suprailiac.** Measure a slightly lateral fold at the middle of the side of the body just above the hip bone (iliac crest).

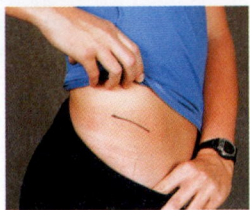

Suprailiac.

7. Skinfold sites for men are the following:

   a. **Subscapular.** Measure a diagonal fold just under the right shoulder blade (scapula).

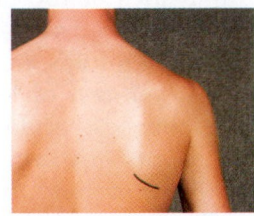

Subscapular.

   b. **Thigh.** Measure a vertical fold on the front of the thigh midway between the inguinal fold (where the hip bends in front) and the top of the patella (knee cap).

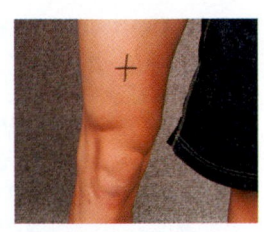

Thigh.

8. Mark your two skinfold measurements on the *Percent Body Fat Nomogram* (Figure 3-7) and connect the marks with a straight line. Read your percent of fat on the center scale. See Table 3-4 for your body composition evaluation. If your body fat is not on the nomogram, use the following formula (Sloan-Weir):

Female (percent body fat formula)

% Body fat = [(4.57 ÷ (1.0764 − (0.00081 × suprailiac skinfold, mm) − (0.00088 × triceps skinfold, mm))) − 4.142] × 100

Male (percent body fat formula)

Percent body fat = [(4.57 ÷ (1.1043 − (0.00133 × thigh skinfold, mm) − (0.00131 × subscapula skinfold, mm))) − 4.142] × 100

Example: A male with thigh skinfold = **10 mm** and subscapular skinfold = **10 mm**

Percent body fat = [(4.57 ÷ (1.1043 − (0.00133 × 10 mm) − (0.00131 × 10 mm))) − 4.142] × 100
= [(4.57 ÷ (1.1043 − 0.0133 − 0.0131)) − 4.142] × 100
= [(4.57 ÷ 1.0779) − 4.142] × 100
= .0977 × 100
= 9.77% body fat

If you prefer to use the 3- or 7-site skinfold tests, online instructions are listed under Internet resources at the end of this chapter.

Body Girth Measures

Many people begin a fitness program because they are concerned about their physical appearance. Basic body build is an inherited characteristic, and less than 5 percent of the population can aspire to the current cultural "ideal" of model-like proportions. Take a look at your parents and grandparents to get an idea of your genetic endowment and what is realistic for you. While your basic structure cannot be altered, as fitness improves, fat may be lost from deposit areas and muscles will become firmer, enhancing body contours. You may notice a loss of unwanted inches from the waist, hips, or thighs or a desirable reshaping of body contours before noticing any weight change. Body girth measures will help you set goals to work for a trim, healthy body shape.

Goal: To measure body girths.

Directions: Recruit a partner to measure you. You will need a measuring tape. For each measurement, pull the tape snugly, but do not indent the flesh. Take the measurements at the following sites (Figure 3-6):

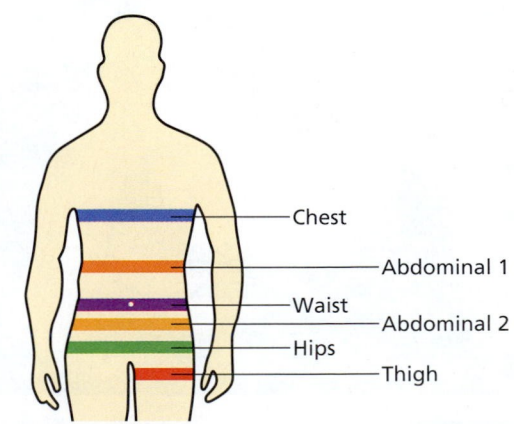

FIGURE 3-6   Body girth measurement sites.

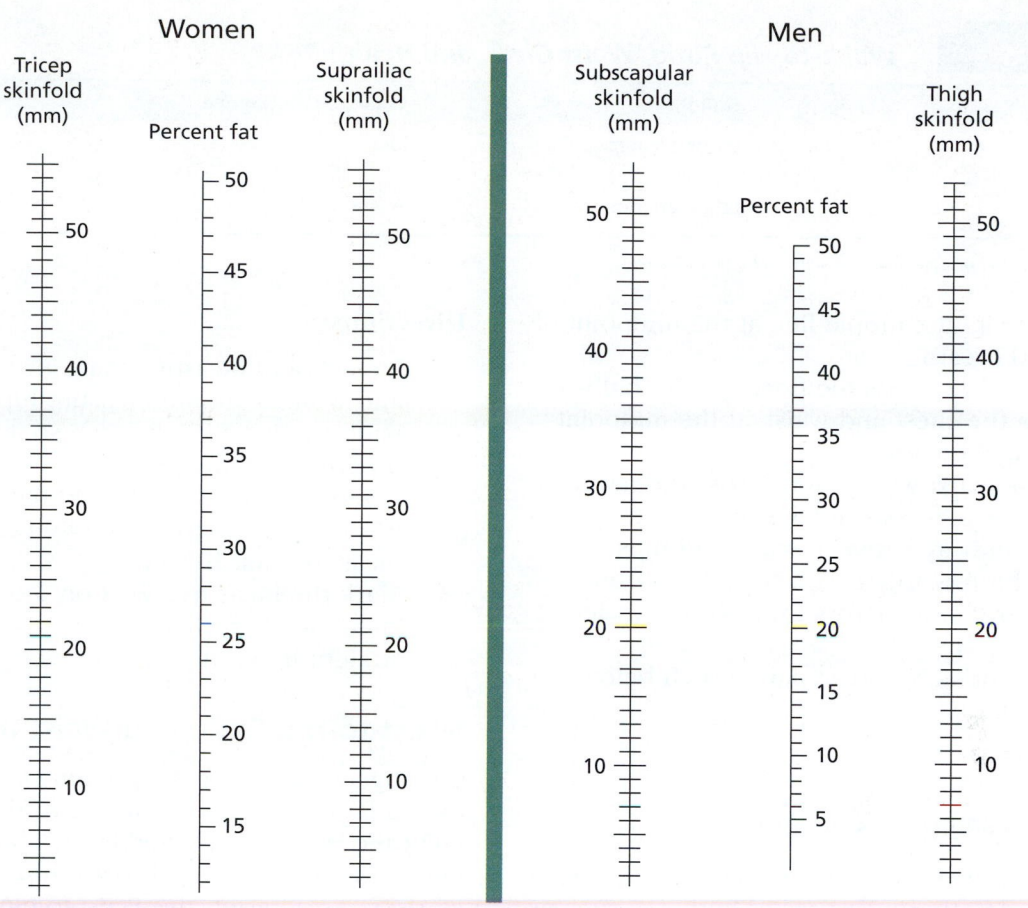

FIGURE 3-7   **Percent body fat nomogram.**

SOURCE: A. W. Sloan and J. Weir, "Nomograms for Prediction of Body Density and Total Body Fat from Skinfold Measurements." *Journal of Applied Physiology* 28:2 (1970): 221–222. Reprinted by permission of the American Physiological Society.

TABLE 3-4   *Body Fat Norm Percentages*

Ages	18–29		30–39		40–49		50+	
	F	M	F	M	F	M	F	M
Very low fat	<17	<10	<18	<11	<19	<13	<20	<15
Low fat (trim)	17–20	10–13	18–20	11–16	19–21	13–18	20–22	15–19
Average	21–24	14–17	21–24	17–19	22–24	19–21	23–25	20–22
Above average (fat)	25–27	18–20	25–27	20–22	25–27	22–23	26–28	23–24
High fat	28–30	21–25	28–30	23–25	28–30	24–25	29–31	25–26
Obese	>30	>25	>30	>25	>30	>25	>31	>26

SOURCE: E. Keener et al. "Undergraduate Student Physical Fitness Assessment." Muncie, IN: Ball State University (originally published Spring 1997; latest compiled data shown here).

TABLE 3-5	Waist-to-Hip Ratio, Waist Girth, and Health Risk*		
Waist-to-Hip Ratio	**High Risk**	**Waist Circumference**	**High Risk**
Men	.95 or greater	Men	over 40 inches
Women	.80 or greater	Women	over 35 inches

*Risk of cardiovascular disease, hypertension, and type 2 diabetes

✓ *Chest:* across the nipple line at the midpoint of a normal breath
✓ *Abdominal 1:* across the floating ribs, halfway between the chest and waist, at the midpoint of a normal breath
✓ *Waist:* the narrowest point, across the navel
✓ *Abdominal 2:* across the iliac crest (hip bones), midway between waist and hips
✓ *Hips:* with feet together, across the pubic bone in front and across the widest part in back
✓ *Thigh:* right side, widest part, 1 inch below the crotch

Body Girth Measures of Body Fat

Body girth measures of fatness have greater variability than do other measures of body fat, such as skinfolds. However, their advantage is that they do not require special equipment or training and can be done with a measuring tape at home.

Directions:

1. Men should measure waist girth at the navel, and women should measure hips at the widest point. Pull the tape so it is snug but does not indent the skin.
2. Remove shoes. Men should measure their weight without clothing. Women should measure their height.
3. Mark the measurements on the appropriate circumference chart and connect them with a straight line (Figure 3-8).

Waist-to-Hip Ratio and Waist Girth

Investigations have begun pointing to the location of excess fat as a risk factor for heart disease and certain cancers. Fat distributed in the abdominal area is linked to increased health risks; hip/thigh fat is not as risky. As a result, the waist-to-hip ratio has become a common assessment for health-risk identification (see Table 3-5). To compute this ratio, divide the waist measurement by the hip measurement.

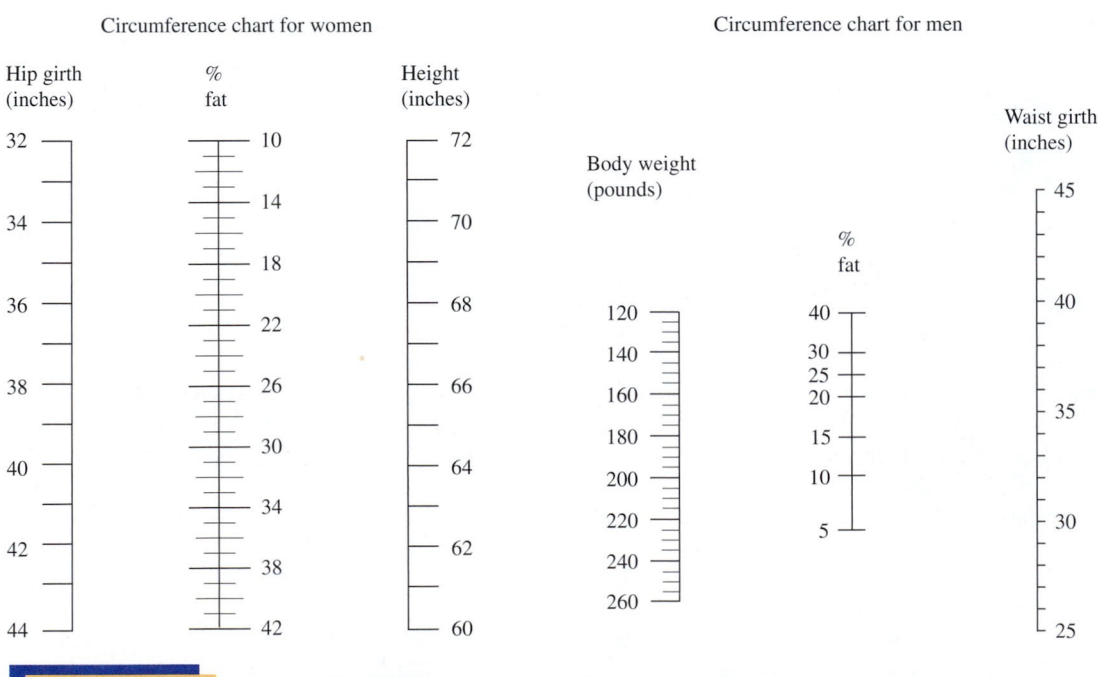

FIGURE 3-8   Circumference charts.

SOURCE: Nomograms developed by Jack Wilmore, University of Texas. Used by permission.

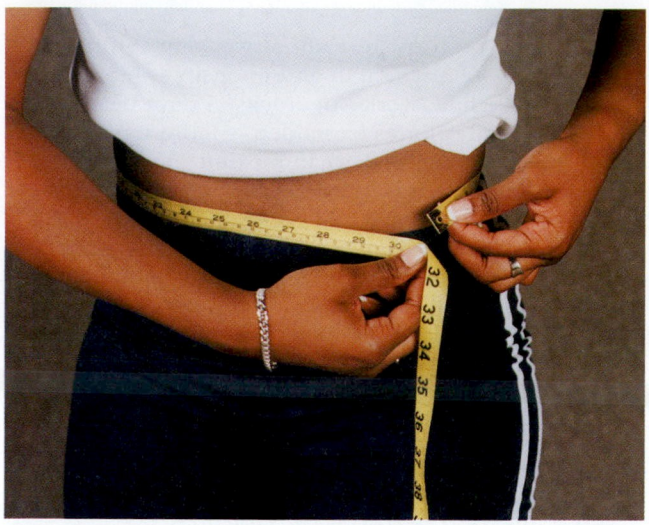

Waist-to-hip ratio or waist girth alone can identify health risk.

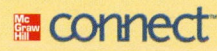

$$\frac{29 \text{ in. waist}}{38 \text{ in. hip}} = 0.76 \qquad \frac{42 \text{ in. waist}}{36 \text{ in. hip}} = 1.17$$

Studies indicate that health problems are increased for women whose ratio is 0.80 or higher and for men whose ratio is 0.95 or higher. You may also use waist girth alone. Health risks are higher for women with a waist measurement over 35 inches, and for men with one over 40 inches. (See Chapter 12 for more information on waist-to-hip ratio as a health-risk factor.)

PRESCRIPTION FOR ACTION

You've read the chapter. Now go do one or more of these.

✔ Write down three reasons your last exercise program did not work and a solution for each.

✔ Schedule exercise on your calendar for a specific time 3 to 5 days this week.

✔ Take a 15-minute study break and go for a walk or do some gentle stretching.

✔ Get to your job 30 minutes earlier and walk before starting work.

✔ Pack a sack lunch and take a 30-minute walk on your lunch break.

✔ Call a friend and make a date to bicycle, play tennis, or walk after dinner.

✔ Jump rope or use a stationary cycle while watching the news.

✔ Trade your desk chair for a fitness ball.

✔ Keep on exercise band at your desk and do an exercise between tasks.

connect Go online to Connect to complete this activity. http://connect.mcgraw-hill.com

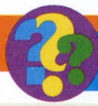

Frequently Asked Questions

Q. I have bad knees/bad ankles/shin splints . . . what kind of physical activity can I do?
A. Low-impact or nonimpact activities will be least likely to make your legs ache. Try swimming, water running, bicycling, Precor, yoga, Pilates, and strength training using upper body exercises.

Q. I heard that stair stepping will make your rear end bigger . . . is this true?
A. No, stair stepping is a good aerobic activity that strengthens quadriceps and glutes, as well as burning calories and improving aerobic fitness. Firmer, toned muscles will look more shapely, regardless of size.

Q. What is the best way to reduce my belly fat/lose the gut?
A. Exercise alone or diet alone will not guarantee a flat abdomen. Combine a healthy diet with regular exercise, and give this prescription time to work. If you are overweight, reducing excess calories is the first step (see Chapter 12). Combine this with 30 minutes of aerobic exercise 5 days per week and abdominal toning exercises 3 days per week (see Chapter 6, Figure 6-5). Give yourself at least 8 weeks to see results.

Q. What is Zumba?
A. Zumba is an exercise program based on Latin dance. Check out Zumba.com for details.

Q. I sweat a lot during exercise, is this a problem?
A. Not at all. It is normal for your body temperature to increase during exercise, and evaporation of sweat is the way your body prevents overheating. You will notice sweat more when the humidity is high, because that slows evaporation. Turning a fan on in an indoor exercise area

Q. I want to exercise, but after a full day of work and classes I feel too tired, plus exercise makes me more tired. What should I do?

A. Schedule a time that works for you. Some people have more energy in the morning and get up a half hour early for a brisk walk. Others take time during their lunch hour. Still others schedule a class (like aerobics or spinning) at the end of the day. Whatever time you choose, schedule it in like an appointment. Some days you will start with more energy, and other days less, but generally, if the intensity is appropriate, you will find yourself invigorated rather than exhausted at the end of the workout. Use the "talk test" to judge if you are exercising at the correct intensity. It may also help if you exercise with a friend; that way it will seem more like fun and less like work. Review the Top 10 "Ways to Stick with Exercise" in Chapter 4 for more tips on maintaining your exercise program.

Q. How many calories do I burn while walking or jogging a mile?

A. Caloric expenditure is based on body weight. You burn about 62 calories per 100 pounds per mile whether walking or jogging. It's a principle of physics. It takes a certain amount of energy to move weight a certain distance. If you weigh 150 pounds, you burn $62 \times 1.50 = 93$ calories per mile.

Q. I want to lose weight. Is it better to exercise for a longer time at a lower intensity or for a shorter time at a higher intensity?

A. If your main goal is weight control, the most important factor, besides a low-calorie, nutritious diet, is to be consistent about working aerobic exercise—of any length and intensity—into your daily schedule. Work out at least 5 days per week. Total calories expended is more important than intensity of activity in maximizing weight loss. One or two weight-training sessions per week also lead to weight control. Moderate-intensity exercise is recommended because it allows you to exercise longer, accumulate more total work, and thus burn more calories, and it is less likely to cause discomfort or injury. Moderate-intensity activity can also help you keep off lost weight. If your goal is high-level fitness, exercise at a higher intensity is necessary.

Q. I swim/cycle regularly and feel like I'm in pretty good shape. Why did I score only "average" on the 1.5-mile walk/run?

A. It's the rule of specificity. Your aerobic fitness will show best if you use the test specific to your activity. Swimmers should use the 500-yard swim, cyclists the 3-mile ride, for results that better reflect their aerobic fitness level. Likewise, someone who usually runs for exercise would find a cycling or swimming test more difficult.

Q. I had my body fat tested by skinfold calipers and bioelectrical impedance. They gave different results. Which is more accurate?

A. Both are reasonably accurate when used by an experienced tester, with average errors of 2 to 5 percent. Skinfold calipers are more accurate if multiple sites are measured to get a better picture of total fat distribution. Bioelectrical impedance can overestimate fat percentage if you are dehydrated, and results vary depending on where the electrodes are placed and the type of machine used.

Summary

The sedentary lifestyle of most Americans is seriously undermining the health and welfare of our nation. We are fast becoming overfat and underfit, resulting in reduced levels of well-being. From the information you have acquired in this chapter, you now have the necessary tools to develop a personalized physical fitness program, based on sound scientific principles and using your age, resting heart rate, interests, and abilities. You have also gained a better understanding of the health benefits that can be achieved by incorporating moderate levels of physical activity into your daily life. By applying the concept of a three-segment workout and finding ways to increase daily activity, you can be on your way to a lifetime of improved health, fitness, and wellness.

Assessment is a critical tool in developing any dimension of wellness. It helps you understand your strengths and weaknesses and decide whether your current levels of cardiorespiratory endurance, muscular endurance, flexibility, and body fat are conducive to optimal wellness. With this knowledge, you can set reasonable fitness goals, establish a starting point for a fitness program, and develop a plan of action. Specific workout programs for different aerobic activities can be found in Chapter 4. A *Student*

Precourse Health Assessment form and a *Personal Fitness Profile* are also available in the Lab Activities section of this chapter.

As you progress in your fitness program, it may be useful to retest occasionally. While testing should not dominate your program, it will allow you to monitor your progress and can give you additional motivation to continue regular exercise.

Terms

- ballistic stretching
- body composition
- cardiorespiratory endurance (CRE)
- conditioning bout
- cool-down
- cross training
- exercise tolerance test
- fat-free tissue
- flexibility
- hypokinetic disease
- lean body mass
- muscular endurance
- muscular strength
- physical fitness
- principle of individual differences
- principle of reversibility
- principle of specificity
- progressive overload
- skinfold calipers
- static stretching
- subcutaneous fat
- task-specific activity
- warm-up

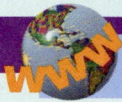

Internet Resources

American Academy of Family Physicians

www.familydoctor.org

Promotes healthy behaviors with fact sheets on many health topics, including exercise and fitness.

American College of Sports Medicine

www.acsm.org

Information on sports research, health and fitness, and aerobic exercise guidelines, along with a quarterly fitness newsletter. "News Releases" give information on a variety of exercise topics of recent interest.

American Council on Exercise

www.acefitness.org/fitfacts/

Features 100 fitness fact sheets, free e-newsletters, and a variety of different fitness activities from bicycling to swimming.

American Heart Association

www.heart.org

Health tools include an exercise diary and body mass calculator. Information includes exercise and fitness promotion for women, children, seniors; information on how exercise affects heart health; exercise tips; and a healthy heart workout quiz.

Centers for Disease Control and Prevention

www.cdc.gov/chronicdisease/index.htm

Information on getting started in physical activity, exercise tips, links to other fitness resources, and health promotion for increasing physical activity in your school or community.

Fitness Fundamentals

www.Hoptechno.com/book11.htm

Developed by the President's Council on Physical Fitness and Sports, contains guidelines for developing a personal exercise program, checking your health, developing workout schedules, and controlling your weight.

Fitness Partner

http://primusweb.com/fitnesspartner/

Includes an activity calorie calculator, articles on how to get and stay active, and weight management tips.

Healthfinder

http://healthfinder.gov/

Reliable health information resources related to the 28 focus areas of *Healthy People 2020,* including physical activity.

Livestrong.com

http://www.livestrong.com/loops/

Map your local running, cycling, walking, and hiking routes or find one created for your area and track your calorie burn.

Mayo Clinic

http://tinyurl.com/ch3mayo

Fitness basics including aerobic exercise, strengthening, stretching, nutrition, and motivation.

Medline Plus

www.nlm.nih.gov/medlineplus

Consumer site with comprehensive information on many health topics, including physical fitness benefits, health, weight management, and fitness at any age.

National Center for Chronic Disease Prevention and Health Promotion

www.cdc.gov/nccdphp/dnpao/index.html

Information on nutrition, physical fitness, and preventing chronic diseases such as diabetes and cancer.

National Heart, Lung, and Blood Institute

www.nhlbisupport.com/bmi

Calculate your body mass index, assess your risk, and find information and recipes for weight control.

President's Council on Physical Fitness and Sports

www.fitness.gov

Information on fitness and health, weight control, exercise for kids and seniors, videos, and sports and fitness awards, along with fact sheets on fitness and health.

Shape Up America!

www.shapeup.org

Information and guidance on fitness, the 10,000 step program, weight management, plus a body fat lab.

Fitness Calculators Online

BMI calculator: **http://tinyurl.com/ch3bmicalc**

Body fat test:
http://tinyurl.com/ch3bdfattest

Home step test:
www.brianmac.co.uk/homestep.htm

One-rep max calculator:
www.exrx.net/Calculators/OneRepMax.html

RealAge estimator:
http://www.realage.com/

Three- and Seven-site skinfold measurements:
www.exrx.net/Testing/SkinfoldProcedures.html

Videos

ACSM Exercise is Medicine series:
http://www.exerciseismedicine.org/keys.htm

How sitting too much affects health:
http://tinyurl.com/ch3sitting

Stay active and feel better, stay active to be healthy:
http://www.healthyroadsmedia.org/english/index/htm

How exercise can protect against diseases of aging:
http://tinyurl.com/ch3exaging

Fitness basics:
http://tinyurl.com/ch3sportfitness

LAB Activity 3-1

Student Precourse Health Assessment

Student ID# _____ Age _____ Date of last medical checkup _____

Please answer all of the questions completely and honestly. This document is confidential between the student, instructor, and administration. This form is used to help you stay safe in courses that have physical activities. If at any time you do not feel well or experience an injury, please tell your instructor immediately. If you must leave the activity area to get water or use the restroom take a classmate with you. While your participation in this course may enhance your health and well-being, you are advised that participation in some activities may be extremely vigorous and have potential risks. Some sports have inherent risks associated with them. If you have any questions about the course or activities, please talk to your instructor. If you are over age 40 (for men) or 50 (for women), it is highly recommended that you see your personal physician before you begin this class. The presence of some of the following conditions may affect your performance. Please check any conditions listed that pertain to you.

___ Cardiac/respiratory problems ___ Asthma (any)   ___ High blood pressure (140/90 or above)

___ Chest pain or discomfort   ___ Epilepsy (seizures/grand ___ Pregnancy
                                   mal, 3+ min.)

___ Severe allergic reactions   ___ Diabetes   ___ Severe headaches

___ Fainting spells/sudden unconsciousness   ___ Family history of heart disease

___ Other life-threatening conditions (please list): _____

_____

___ Knee injuries   ___ Epilepsy (seizures/petit mal) ___ Smoker   ___ Foot injuries

___ Back injuries   ___ Shoulder injuries   ___ Ankle injuries   ___ Allergies

___ Scoliosis   ___ Neck/spinal injuries   ___ Other, please list below

Please list any other medical conditions or information you think should be brought to the attention of your instructor.

_____

Please list all medications that you take regularly.

_____

If during this class/course your physical health changes in regard to any of the listed or other conditions, please notify your instructor immediately. If you have concerns about your health, are sedentary, diabetic, pregnant, 20 or more pounds overweight, smoke, or have a family history of heart disease, it is important that you complete the *Physician-Approved Exercise Clearance Form.*

   By signing this form I understand my responsibility toward staying safe in this course and informing my instructor that I am not withholding any information regarding my health status. (Please sign, date, and return this form to your instructor.)

Student Signature _____ Date _____ Student Phone Number _____

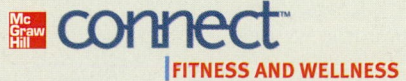

http://connect.mcgraw-hill.com

Name _____ Class/Activity Section _____ Date _____

Physician-Approved Exercise Clearance Form

Student ID# _____ Age_____ Date of last medical checkup_____

This form is designed for individuals with special health concerns to assist your instructor in individualizing your fitness program according to your physician's recommendations.

This section is to be completed by the Lab Instructor:

(Name of student) _____ is presently enrolled in (name of course) _____ and he/she has identified the following health problems on the Student Precourse Health Assessment Form that may affect participation in the activities of this course.

_____

_____

This class/course will include the following activities:

_____

The above information was provided by **(instructor's name)** _____ Date _____

This section is to be completed by the Physician:

NOTE TO PHYSICIAN: **PLEASE REVIEW THE STUDENT PRECOURSE HEALTH ASSESSMENT FORM.**

After reviewing the form, I recommend the following level of participation:

_____ Full participation   _____ Modified participation as indicated   _____ No participation*
                                  (Please indicate below):

_____

_____

*If the student may not participate in this class, list the activities in which the student may participate:

_____

_____

_____   _____   _____
Signature of Physician   **Date (mm/dd/yy)**   **Physician's Printed Name**

_____   _____
Physician's Fax Number   **Physician's Phone Number**

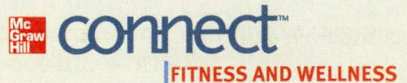

http://connect.mcgraw-hill.com

LAB Activity 3-3

Personal Fitness Profile

Note: Do not feel that you must do all of these tests.
Select tests appropriate for your condition and goals.

	Pretest Date: _____	Posttest Date: _____
1. **Resting heart rate**	_____	_____
2. **Cardiorespiratory endurance** (Labs 3-4, 3-5, 3-6)		
1.5-mile run	_____	_____
1.0-mile walk	_____	_____
500-yard swim or water run	_____	_____
Other_____	_____	_____
Exercise pulse	_____	_____
3. **Muscular endurance** (Lab 3-7)		
Abdominal curls	_____	_____
Push-ups	_____	_____
4. **Muscular strength** (Lab 3-8)		
Leg press	_____	_____
Bench press	_____	_____
5. **Flexibility** (Lab 3-9)		
Sit and reach	_____	_____
6. **Body girth measurements** (Figure 3-6)		
Hips—biggest part	_____	_____
Thigh—1 inch below crotch	_____	_____
Chest—nipple line	_____	_____
Waist—smallest part	_____	_____
Abdominal 1—halfway between chest and navel	_____	_____
Abdominal 2—halfway between navel and pubic bone	_____	_____
7. **Waist-to-hip ratio** (Lab 3-10)	_____	_____
8. **Body mass index** (Table 12-1)	_____	_____
9. **Body composition**		
Female *Male*		
Triceps Subscapula	_____	_____
Iliac Thigh	_____	_____
Percent body fat (see nomogram in Figure 3-7)	_____	_____
10. **Weight**	_____	_____
11. **Height**	_____	_____
12. **Quick checks (pass or fail)** (Lab 3-9, Figures 3-15 to 3-19)	P/F	P/F
a. Erector spinae	_____	_____
b. Iliopsoas	_____	_____
c. Quadriceps	_____	_____
d. Hamstrings	_____	_____
e. Gastrocnemius	_____	_____

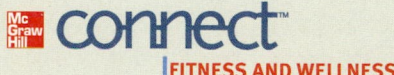

connect

FITNESS AND WELLNESS

http://connect.mcgraw-hill.com

Name _____ Class/Activity Section _____ Date _____

Evaluating Your Cardiorespiratory Fitness: 1.5-Mile Run Test, 1.0-Mile Walk Test, and 3.0-Mile Bicycling Test

1.5-MILE RUN TEST

EQUIPMENT NEEDED:

A track or premeasured course of 1.5 miles
Stopwatch or a watch with a second hand

PROCEDURE

1. Before taking the test, warm up with walking, stretching, and a slow jog.
2. This is a test of maximum capacity, so push yourself to cover the distance as quickly as possible without overdoing it. Try to maintain a continuous, even pace. Run as long as you can and then walk if necessary. When you complete the 1.5-mile distance, record your time.

   Running time: _____
3. Cool down by walking slowly for several minutes and stretching.
4. Check the table below for your fitness rating.

   Cardiorespiratory fitness rating: _____

1.5-Mile Run

Age	18–29		30–39		40–49		50–59	
	F	M	F	M	F	M	F	M
Superior	<12:34	<8:26	<13:34	<9:10	<14:34	<9:55	<15:34	<10:40
Good	12:34–13:40	8:26–10:24	13:34–14:40	9:10–11:10	14:34–15:40	9:55–12:00	15:34–16:40	10:40–12:50
Average	13:41–14:45	10:25–12:31	14:41–15:45	11:11–13:45	15:41–16:45	12:01–14:55	16:41–17:45	12:51–16:05
Fair	14:46–16:00	12:32–14:49	15:46–17:00	13:46–16:00	16:46–18:00	14:56–17:15	17:46–19:00	16:06–18:30
Low	>16:00	>14:49	>17:00	>16:00	>18:00	>17:15	>19:00	>18:30

1.0-MILE WALK TEST

EQUIPMENT NEEDED:

A track or premeasured course of 1.0 miles
Stopwatch

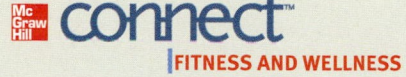

http://connect.mcgraw-hill.com

FITNESS AND WELLNESS

PROCEDURE

1. Before taking the test, warm up with walking and stretching.
2. This is a test of maximum capacity, so push yourself to walk the mile as quickly as possible without overdoing it. Try to maintain a continuous, even pace. When you complete the 1-mile distance, record your time.

   Walking time: _____
3. Cool down by walking slowly for several minutes and stretching.
4. Check the table below for your fitness rating.

   Cardiorespiratory fitness rating: _____

1.0-Mile Walk

Age	18–29		30–39		40–49		50–59	
	F	M	F	M	F	M	F	M
Superior	<12:34	<11:39	<13:34	<12:40	<14:34	<13:40	<15:34	<14:10
Good	12:34–13:40	11:39–12:59	13:34–14:40	12:40–14:00	14:34–15:40	13:40–14:40	15:34–16:40	14:10–15:20
Average	13:41–14:45	13:00–14:21	14:41–15:45	14:01–15:20	15:41–16:45	14:41–15:55	16:41–17:45	15:21–16:25
Fair	14:46–16:00	14:22–15:43	15:46–17:00	15:21–16:15	16:46–18:00	15:56–16:45	17:46–19:00	16:26–17:25
Low	>16:00	>15:43	>17:00	>16:15	>18:00	>16:45	>19:00	>17:25

3.0-MILE BICYCLING TEST

If your main fitness activity is bicycling, you can test your cardiorespiratory fitness with a timed 3-mile bicycle ride.

EQUIPMENT NEEDED:

Bicycle
Stopwatch
A measured section of road with few stoplights or stop signs

PROCEDURE

1. Warm up by riding for a few minutes and stretching.
2. Cycle 3 miles as quickly as you can. If you are doing this on the road, be careful to obey traffic rules.
3. Try to pace evenly. Time the ride with a stopwatch or a watch with a second hand. Record the time. Record your exercise pulse.
4. Cool down and stretch.
5. Check the table below for your fitness rating.

   Cardiorespiratory fitness rating: _____

3.0-Mile Bicycle Ride

Age	18–29		30–39		40–49		50–59	
	F	M	F	M	F	M	F	M
Superior	<9:18	<8:24	<9:54	<9:00	<10:30	<9:36	<11:06	<10:12
Good	9:18–10:06	8:24–9:12	9:54–10:42	9:00–9:42	10:30–11:06	9:36–10:12	11:06–11:36	10:12–10:42
Average	10:07–11:06	9:13–10:12	10:43–11:42	9:43–10:48	11:07–12:18	10:13–11:24	11:37–12:54	10:43–12:00
Fair	11:07–12:00	10:13–11:06	11:43–12:30	10:49–11:35	12:19–13:00	11:25–12:06	12:55–13:30	12:01–12:48
Low	>12:00	>11:06	>12:30	>11:35	>13:00	>12:06	>13:30	>12:48

Name _____ Class/Activity Section _____ Date _____

Evaluating Your Cardiorespiratory Fitness: 500-Yard Water Run Test and 500-Yard Swim Test

500-YARD WATER RUN TEST

EQUIPMENT NEEDED:

A regulation 25-yard pool
Stopwatch
Partner to time you
Measuring tape to measure width of pool

PROCEDURE

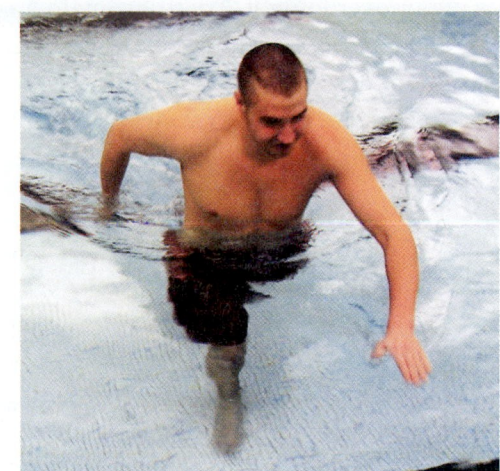

1. Measure pool width and calculate the number of widths required to cover 500 yards.
2. Have a partner on the deck to count laps and keep the time.
3. Before taking the test, warm up with a couple minutes of easy jogging in the water.
4. Select a starting point along the wall where the water level is at a midpoint between the runner's navel and nipple (Figure 3-9). Shorter runners will start in shallower water, taller runners in deeper water.

FIGURE 3-9 Water run test.

5. This is a test of maximum capacity, so push yourself to cover the distance as quickly as possible without overdoing it. Try to maintain a continuous, even pace. Run the necessary number of widths and record your time to the nearest second.

   500-yard water run time: _____

6. Cool down by walking in the water for several minutes and stretching.
7. Check the table for your fitness rating.

   Cardiorespiratory fitness rating: _____

500-Yard Water Run

Age	18–29		30–39		40–49		50–59	
	F	M	F	M	F	M	F	M
Superior	<7:59	<6:53	<8:30	<7:20	<9:00	<7:50	<9:30	<8:20
Good	7:59–8:38	6:53–7:44	8:30–9:08	7:20–8:15	9:00–9:38	7:50–8:45	9:30–10:08	8:20–9:15
Average	8:39–9:18	7:45–8:38	9:09–9:48	8:16–9:05	9:39–10:18	8:46–9:35	10:09–10:48	9:16–10:05
Fair	9:19–9:58	8:39–9:32	9:49–10:28	9:06–10:00	10:19–10:58	9:36–10:30	10:49–11:28	10:06–11:00
Low	>9:58	>9:32	>10:28	>10:00	>10:58	>10:30	>11:28	>11:00

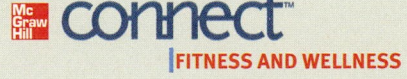

http://connect.mcgraw-hill.com

500-YARD SWIM TEST

EQUIPMENT NEEDED:

A regulation 25-yard pool
Stopwatch
Partner to time you

PROCEDURE

1. Have a partner on the deck to count laps and keep the time. In a 25-yard pool, 500 yards is 20 lengths.
2. Before taking the test, warm up with a couple of easy laps.
3. This is a test of maximum capacity, so push yourself to cover the distance as quickly as possible without overdoing it. Try to maintain a continuous, even pace. Record your time to the nearest second.

   500-yard swim time: _____
4. Cool down and stretch.
5. Check the table for your fitness rating.

   Cardiorespiratory fitness rating: _____

500-Yard Swim

Age	18–29		30–39		40–49		50–59	
	F	M	F	M	F	M	F	M
Superior	<7:05	<6:12	<7:35	<6:30	<8:05	<7:00	<8:35	<7:30
Good	7:05–8:49	6:12–7:44	7:35–9:19	6:30–8:14	8:05–9:49	7:00–8:44	8:35–10:19	7:30–9:14
Average	8:50–10:34	7:45–9:19	9:20–11:04	8:15–9:49	9:50–11:34	8:45–10:19	10:20–12:04	9:15–10:49
Fair	10:35–12:19	9:20–10:51	11:05–12:49	9:50–11:22	11:35–13:19	10:20–11:52	12:05–13:49	10:50–11:22
Low	>12:19	>10:52	>12:49	>11:22	>13:19	>11:52	>13:49	>11:22

LAB Activity 3-6

Evaluating Your Cardiorespiratory Fitness: 3-Minute Step Test

EQUIPMENT NEEDED:

A 12-inch bench or 16-inch roll-out bleacher step
Stopwatch
Metronome or recorded music at a tempo of 96 beats per minute

PROCEDURE

1. Before taking the test, warm up with easy stepping and stretching.

2. You will need to step up and down at a tempo of 96 counts per minute (24 cycles of up-up-down-down). Step up with your right foot, and then your left foot, and then step down with your right and then your left (Figure 3-10). Continue for 3 minutes. Straighten your knees as you step up on the bench. To prevent leg soreness, you may want to switch lead legs about halfway through the test.

   Pulse rate: _____

3. Stop at the end of 3 minutes and sit down. Five seconds after completing the test, the tester should count the partner's pulse for 15 seconds. The tester can check the partner's carotid pulse by lightly pressing against the neck under the jawbone. The partner being tested can double-check his or her own pulse at the radial artery, located on the thumb side of the wrist. The partners' pulse counts should not vary more than one or two beats if counting is accurate.

4. Record the pulse.

5. Cool down by walking slowly for several minutes and stretching.

6. Check the table below for your fitness rating.

   Cardiorespiratory fitness rating: _____

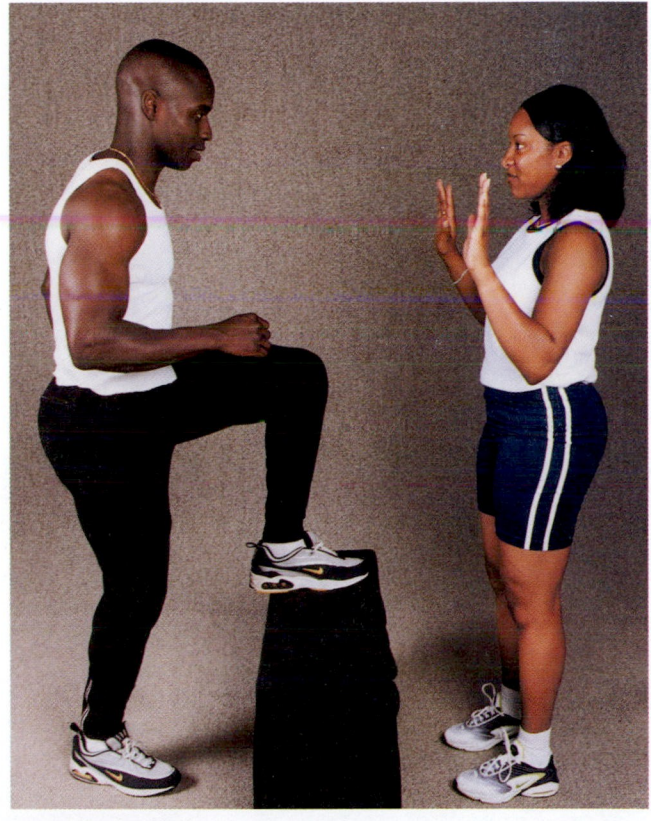

FIGURE 3-10 Step test.

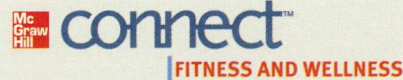

http://connect.mcgraw-hill.com

3-Minute Step Test Norms

Bench Height	Men		Women	
	12-inch	16-inch	12-inch	16-inch
Superior	<20	<31	<21	<37
Good	20–24	31–37	21–25	37–41
Average	25–28	38–41	26–30	42–44
Fair	29–32	42–45	31–35	45–49
Low	>32	>45	>35	>49

SOURCE: F. W. Kasch and J. L. Boyer. *Adult Fitness: Principles and Practices*. Mountain View, CA: Mayfield, 1968. Used by permission.

LAB Activity 3-7

Evaluating Your Muscular Endurance: The Abdominal Curls Test and Push-Ups Test

THE ABDOMINAL CURLS TEST

EQUIPMENT NEEDED:

Ruler
Adhesive tape
Mat
Stopwatch or watch with a second hand

PROCEDURE

1. Tape a 3-inch-wide strip on a mat or the floor and lie on your back with your fingertips at the edge of the strip (Figure 3-11). Bend your knees, and bring your heels as close as possible to your buttocks.

FIGURE 3-11 Abdominal curls test.

2. Curl forward until your fingertips have moved forward across the 3-inch strip and then curl back until your shoulder blades touch the floor. Your shoulders should lift from the floor with each curl, but the lower back should stay on the ground.

3. Complete as many curls as possible in 1 minute, then check the results in the table below.

   Number of abdominal curls: _____

   Muscular endurance rating: _____

1-Minute Abdominal Curls

Age	18–29		30–39		40–49		50–59	
	F	M	F	M	F	M	F	M
Superior	>88	>93	>70	>78	>56	>65	>45	>49
Good	75–88	79–93	60–70	62–78	48–56	53–65	38–45	42–49
Average	60–74	64–78	47–59	51–61	37–47	42–52	29–37	35–41
Fair	45–59	50–63	35–46	40–50	27–36	36–41	21–28	28–34
Low	<45	<50	<35	<40	<27	<36	<21	<28

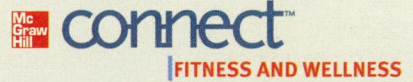

http://connect.mcgraw-hill.com

CHAPTER 3 ■ **LAB Activity**

THE PUSH-UPS TEST

EQUIPMENT NEEDED:

Mat
Stopwatch or watch with a second hand

PROCEDURE

1. Start in an "up" position with your weight on your hands and toes (men) (Figure 3-12) or knees (women) (Figure 3-13).

2. Lower yourself until your elbows form a right angle and your upper arms are parallel to the floor. Be sure to keep your abdominals tight, hips slightly piked, and your back straight to protect your lower back.

3. Complete as many push-ups as possible in 1 minute; record, then check the results in the table below.

Number of push-ups: _____

Muscular endurance rating: _____

1-Minute Push-Ups

Age	18–29		30–39		40–49		50–59	
	F	M	F	M	F	M	F	M
Superior	>54	>64	>43	>54	>33	>43	>23	>33
Good	44–54	51–64	32–43	41–54	26–33	32–43	18–23	26–33
Average	32–43	37–50	22–31	27–40	17–25	22–31	11–17	17–25
Fair	20–31	23–36	13–21	18–26	8–16	13–21	6–10	8–16
Low	<20	<23	<13	<18	<8	<13	<6	<8

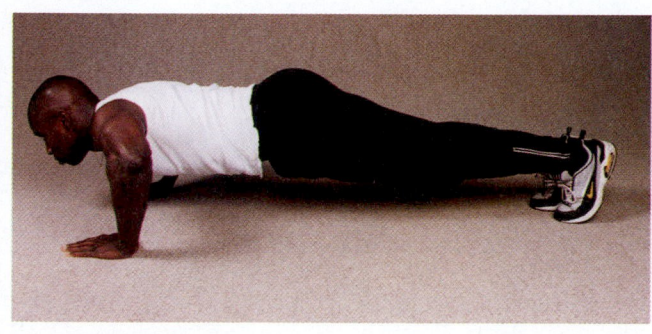

FIGURE 3-12 Push-up—standard position. (Note the 90-degree elbow angle.)

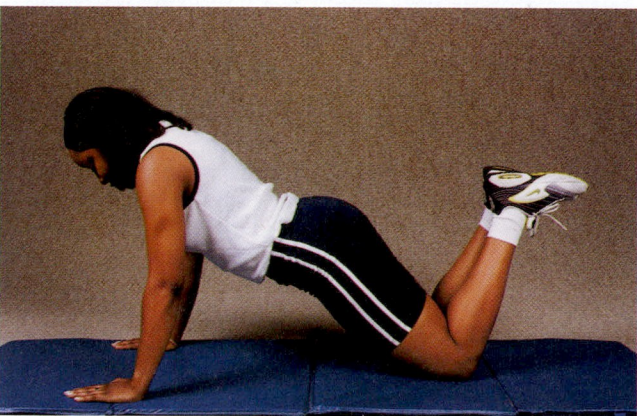

FIGURE 3-13 Push-up—modified position.

Name _____ **Class/Activity Section** _____ **Date** _____

Evaluating Your Muscular Strength: Leg Press Strength Test and Bench Press Strength Test

LEG PRESS STRENGTH TEST

EQUIPMENT NEEDED:

Leg press machine If free weights are used, the following equipment is needed:
Weight scale   Weight scale   Barbell
                 Squat rack   Assorted weight plates
                 One or two spotters

PROCEDURE

1. If you have a history of ankle, knee, hip, or lower back injuries, check with your physician before doing this test.
2. Before taking the test, warm up with several light lifts and stretching.
3. Set the leg press machine for a weight that is lighter than the amount you think you can press one time. Press to full extension. If you can press the weight to extension, add more weight and try again. Rest a few minutes between attempts. It may take several attempts to find your maximum lift.
4. Stop when you reach a weight that you cannot move through a full range of motion. The heaviest weight that you can move through a full range of motion is your max.
5. Divide your max by your body weight.

   Max: _____ Body weight: _____

   Max / Body weight = _____

   Check the table below for your fitness rating.

   Muscular strength rating: _____

Leg Press (max/body weight)

Age	18–29		30–39		40–49		50–59	
	F	M	F	M	F	M	F	M
Superior	>1.97	>2.39	>1.67	>2.19	>1.56	>2.01	>1.42	>1.89
Good	1.68–1.97	2.13–2.39	1.47–1.67	1.93–2.19	1.37–1.56	1.82–2.01	1.25–1.42	1.71–1.89
Average	1.50–1.67	1.97–2.12	1.33–1.46	1.77–1.92	1.23–1.36	1.68–1.81	1.10–1.24	1.58–1.70
Fair	1.37–1.49	1.83–1.96	1.21–1.32	1.65–1.76	1.13–1.22	1.57–1.67	0.99–1.09	1.46–1.57
Low	<1.37	<1.83	<1.21	<1.65	<1.13	<1.57	<0.99	<1.46

SOURCE: Based on norms from the Cooper Institute for Aerobics Research, Dallas, Texas, revised 2000, used with permission.

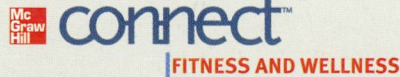

http://connect.mcgraw-hill.com

BENCH PRESS STRENGTH TEST

EQUIPMENT NEEDED:

Bench press machine   If free weights are used, the following equipment is needed:
Weight scale

Weight scale	Barbell
Flat bench	Assorted weight plates
One or two spotters	Weight scale

PROCEDURE

1. If you have a history of shoulder, wrist, or lower back injuries, check with your physician before doing this test.

2. Before taking the test, warm up with several light lifts and stretching.

3. Set the bench press machine for a weight that is lighter than the amount you think you can press one time. Press to full extension. If you can press the weight to extension, add more weight and try again. Rest a few minutes between attempts. It may take several attempts to find your maximum lift.

4. Stop when you reach a weight that you cannot move through a full range of motion. The heaviest weight that you can move through a full range of motion is your max.

5. Divide your max by your body weight.

    Max: _____ Body weight: _____

    Max / Body weight = _____

    Check the table below for your fitness rating.

    Muscular strength rating: _____

	Bench Press (max/body weight)							
Age	20–29		30–39		40–49		50–59	
	F	M	F	M	F	M	F	M
Superior	>1.00	>1.62	>.79	>1.34	>.76	>1.19	>.67	>1.04
Good	.80–1.00	1.32–1.62	.70–.79	1.12–1.34	.62–.76	1.00–1.19	.55–.67	.90–1.04
Average	.70–.79	1.14–1.31	.60–.69	.98–1.11	.54–.61	.88–.99	.48–.54	.79–.89
Fair	.59–.69	.99–1.13	.53–.59	.88–.97	.50–.53	.80–.87	.44–.47	.71–.78
Low	<.59	<.99	<.53	<.88	<.50	<.80	<.44	<.71

Source: Based on norms from the Cooper Institute for Aerobics Research, Dallas, Texas, revised 2000, used with permission.

If you prefer to estimate your one-rep max from a submax effort, an online calculator is listed under Internet Resources.

LAB Activity 3-9

Evaluating Your Flexibility: Sit and Reach, Sit and Reach Wall Test, and Flexibility Quick Checks

SIT AND REACH

EQUIPMENT NEEDED:

Flex box
Mat

PROCEDURE

1. Warm up with walking or light calisthenics.
2. Sit with your feet flat against the flex box about 5 inches apart.
3. Place your hands together. Without bending your knees, reach as far forward as possible, extending fingertips along the box (Figure 3-14). Hold the position for 3 seconds.
   Sit and reach score: _____ inches
4. Check the table below for your flexibility rating.   Flexibility rating: _____

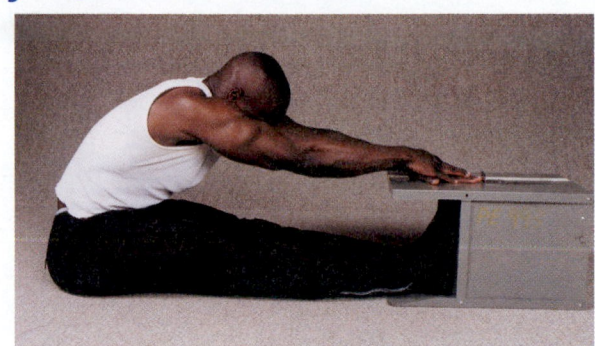

FIGURE 3-14 Sit and reach test.

Sit and Reach (inches)

Age	18–29		30–39		40–49		50–59	
	F	M	F	M	F	M	F	M
Superior	>8.5	>7.0	>8	>6	>7	>5	>6	>4
Good	6.5–8.5	4.0–7.0	5–8	3–6	4–7	2–5	3–6	1–4
Average	4.0–6.4	1.0–3.9	3–4.9	0–2.9	2–3.9	−1–1.9	1–2.9	−3–0
Fair	1.0–3.9	−2.0–0.9	0–2.9	−3––0.1	−1–1.9	−4––1.1	−2–0.9	−5––3.1
Low	<1.0	<−2.0	<0	<−3	<−1	<−4	<−2	<−5

SIT AND REACH WALL TEST

EQUIPMENT NEEDED:

Wall
Mat

PROCEDURE

1. Warm up by walking and static stretching.
2. Remove shoes, sit facing a wall, and keep your feet flat against the wall and your knees straight.
3. Reach forward as far as possible to touch your fingertips, knuckles, or palms to the wall and hold the position for 3 seconds.   Result: _____
4. Check your flexibility evaluation in the accompanying table.

SIT AND REACH WALL TEST SCORES

Result	Flexibility
Cannot touch wall	Low
Fingertips touch wall	Average
Knuckles touch wall	Good
Palms touch wall	Superior

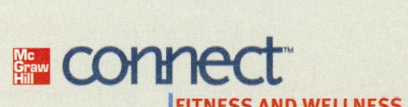

LAB Activity ■ CHAPTER 3

FLEXIBILITY QUICK CHECKS

EQUIPMENT NEEDED:

Mat

PROCEDURE

1. Warm up with walking or light calisthenics.
2. Complete the flexibility quick checks shown in Figures 3-15 through 3-19.
   Record the results (*pass* or *fail*).

	Pass	Fail
Low back flexibility test	_____	_____
Hip flexor flexibility test	_____	_____
Quadriceps flexibility test	_____	_____
Hamstring flexibility test	_____	_____
Calf flexibility test	_____	_____

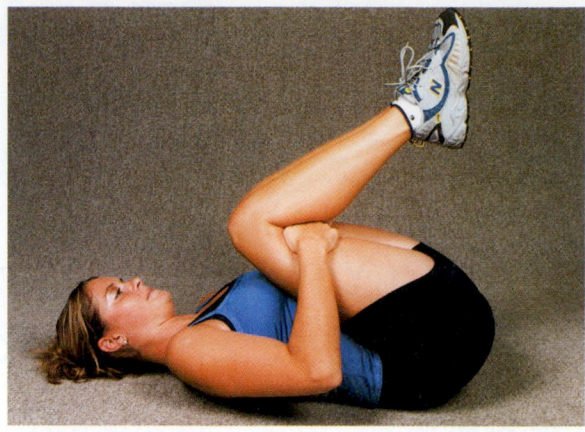

FIGURE 3-15 Low back flexibility test.
Muscle: Erector spinae (lower back)
Test: Lying on your back, pull thighs to chest.
Passing: Thighs should touch chest.

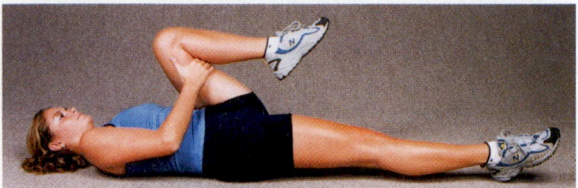

FIGURE 3-16 Hip flexor flexibility test.
Muscle: Iliopsoas (hip flexor)
Test: Lying on your back, pull one knee to chest, keeping other leg fully extended on the floor.
Passing: Calf of extended leg must remain on the floor; knee must not bend.

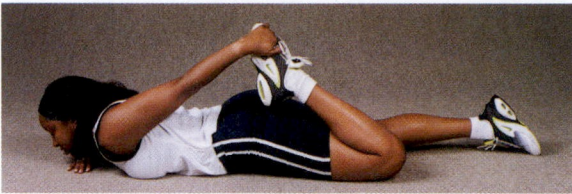

FIGURE 3-17 Quadriceps flexibility test. Caution: Avoid if you have or experience knee problems.
Muscle: Quadriceps (front of thigh)
Test: Lying face down with knees together, pull heel toward buttocks.
Passing: Heel should comfortably touch buttocks.

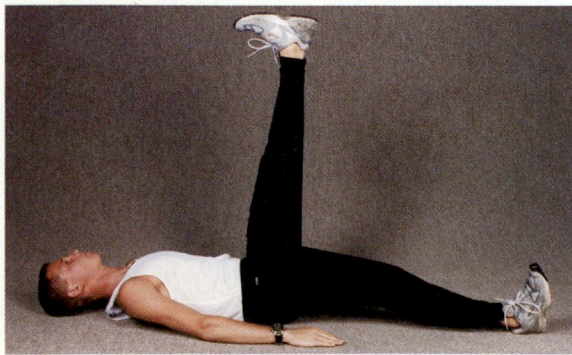

FIGURE 3-18 Hamstring flexibility test.
Muscle: Hamstring (back of thigh)
Test: Lying on your back, lift one leg, keeping other leg straight on the floor without bending either knee.
Passing: The raised leg must be vertical (90 degrees).

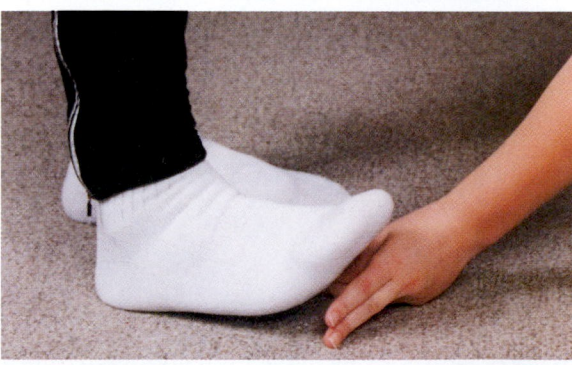

FIGURE 3-19 Calf flexibility test.
Muscle: Gastrocnemius (calf)
Test: Standing without shoes, raise one forefoot off floor, keeping knees relaxed and heels down.
Passing: Ball of foot should clear floor by height equal to width of two fingers.

LAB Activity 3-10

Body Composition Assessment

EQUIPMENT NEEDED:

Measuring tape
Skinfold calipers
Height/weight scales

Read about body composition tests in Chapter 3 for more information about these assessments.

WAIST-TO-HIP RATIO

1. Measure your waist at the smallest circumference and hips at the greatest circumference. Record the results.

   Hips: _____ inches   Waist: _____ inches

2. Divide your waist measurement by your hip measurement and check your rating.

   Waist/Hip = _____   Rating: _____

Waist-to-Hip Ratio	High Risk
Men	.95 or higher
Women	.80 or higher

WAIST GIRTH

Measure your waist at the smallest circumference and record the results.

Waist: _____ inches   Rating: _____

Waist Circumference	High Risk
Men	over 40 inches
Women	over 35 inches

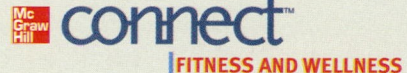

http://connect.mcgraw-hill.com

BODY MASS INDEX

1. Measure your height and weight and record the results.

    Height: _____ feet _____ inches   Weight: _____ pounds

2. Check your BMI using Table 12-1 on page 408.

    BMI: _____   Rating: _____

BODY FAT PERCENTAGE

1. Read the section in Chapter 3 on body composition assessment using skinfold calipers.
2. Measure skinfolds on the right side of the body using a skinfold caliper and record the results.
3. Check the results on the nomogram in Figure 3-7 and Table 3-4.

    Female: Triceps   _____
                  Suprailiac   _____
                  Percent body fat   _____

    Male: Subscapula   _____
                  Thigh   _____
                  Percent body fat   _____

DESIRABLE WEIGHT

1. Percent body fat × weight (lbs) = Fat weight (lbs)

    _____ × _____ = _____ lbs

2. Weight (lbs) − fat weight = lean body weight (lbs)

    _____ − _____ = _____ lbs

3. Desirable weight for females (at 18%):
    lean body weight /.82 = desirable weight
    _____ /.82 = _____ lbs

4. Desirable weight for males (at 12%):
    lean body weight /.88 = desirable weight
    _____ /.88 = _____ lbs

Maximizing Cardiorespiratory Fitness

STUDY QUESTIONS

You will have successfully mastered this chapter if you can answer the following:

1. Why is exercise called "medicine"?
2. What are the benefits of cardiorespiratory fitness?
3. How are the FITT prescription factors for developing physical fitness defined and applied?
4. How is training heart rate calculated using the Karvonen formula?
5. How is the Rate of Perceived Exertion Scale used to measure workout intensity?
6. How is the progressive overload principle applied to a cardiorespiratory exercise program?
7. What are specific goals for the FITT and the U.S. Department of Health and Human Services (USDHHS) exercise guidelines?
8. Which aerobic exercise activity (of the eight found in this chapter) would you be most interested in to develop cardiorespiratory endurance (CRE)? (The eight activities include aerobic dance, bicycling, fitness swimming, fitness walking, indoor exercise equipment, in-line skating, jogging, and water exercise/aqua aerobics.)
9. What are the guidelines for beginning the aerobic activity (of the eight in the chapter) you selected?
10. How would you describe the 10,000 steps per day wellness goal? How would you initiate it?

You will find the answers as you read this chapter.

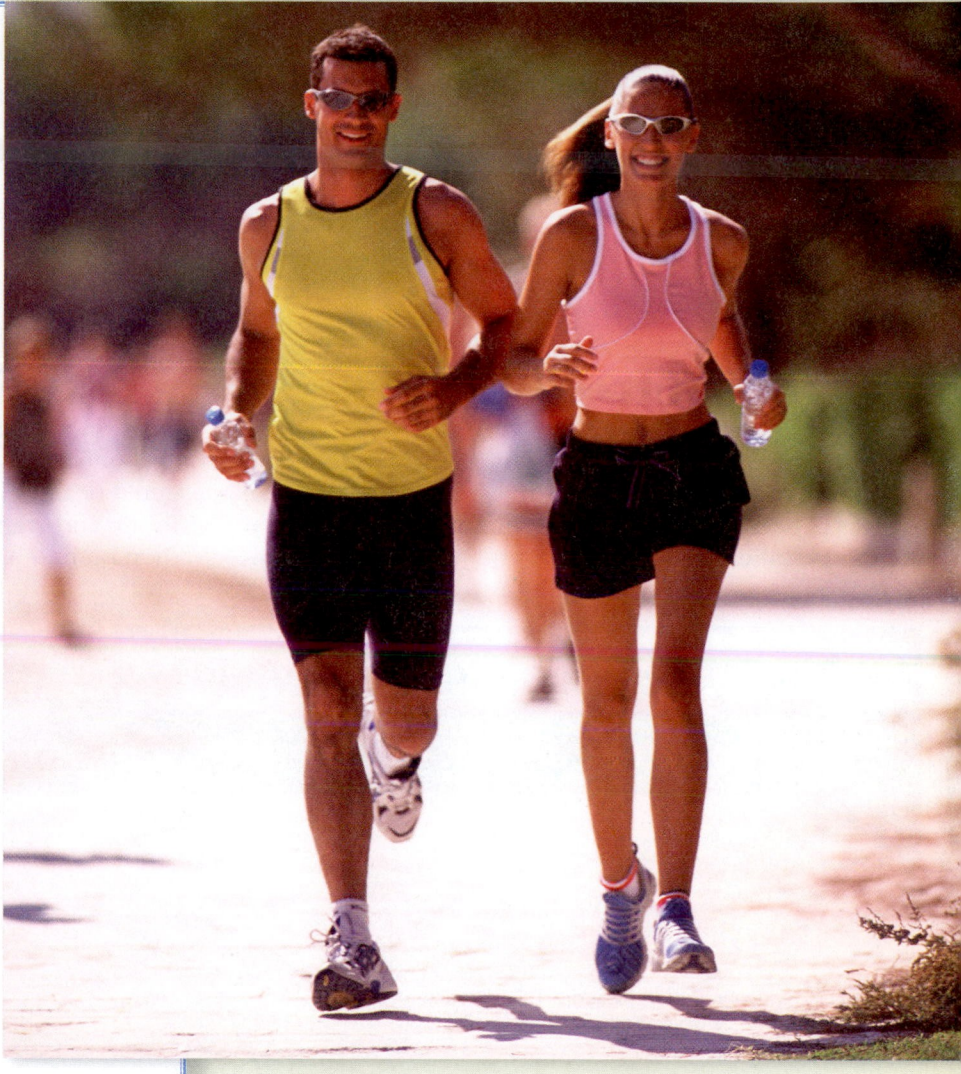

> *A journey of a thousand miles starts with a single step.*
> —Lao Tse

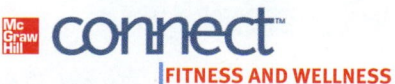

FITNESS AND WELLNESS

http://connect.mcgraw-hill.com

The number one reason people begin exercising is to improve their physical appearance—to decrease body fat and develop firm, well-toned muscles. They find that these benefits are only the beginning.

Would you be interested in a prescription for a medicine that does all of the following: lowers blood pressure, blood sugar, and weight; improves cholesterol, sleep, and bone and heart health; decreases the risk of cancer; wards off type 2 diabetes; improves memory and academic performance; increases length of life; and increases fitness? Imagine one prescription that could do all these things and more. Well, that prescription really exists. There's just one catch: You'll need 20–60 minutes each day to take it. The "medicine" is *exercise.* Cardiorespiratory endurance plays an important role in developing physical fitness and wellness. A number of physiological (cardiorespiratory, body composition, and metabolic) and psychological (mental and emotional) health benefits are yours in return for a small investment of time and effort.

A variety of exercise programs and recreational activities can enhance health and fitness. Nearly everyone can find one or two activities that are satisfying and enjoyable. This chapter focuses on the many benefits that can be gained from cardiorespiratory endurance, the prescription factors for fitness, and information about a variety of lifetime exercise activities to get you started on the path to a vigorous and vibrant life.

◆ CARDIORESPIRATORY ENDURANCE AND MAXIMAL OXYGEN UPTAKE

Cardiorespiratory endurance is often expressed in terms of **maximal oxygen uptake** (VO_{2max} or **aerobic capacity**), the greatest amount of oxygen that can be taken in and used by the body during high-intensity exercise. You can live several days without water, several weeks without food, but only minutes without oxygen. Most fitness experts agree that VO_{2max} is the best measure of cardiorespiratory fitness. Energy for physical activity and body processes is produced by burning fuel in the presence of oxygen. For muscles to use oxygen, the lungs must take in air and transfer it to the blood. The blood must then be pumped to the muscles. Finally, the muscles

What Stage of Change Are You In?

Do you do aerobic exercise at least three to five times a week?

- **No**
  - Do you plan to adopt this practice within the next 6 months?
    - **No** → **Precontemplation**
    - **Yes**
      - Within the next month?
        - **No** → **Contemplation**
        - **Yes** → **Preparation**
- **Yes**
  - Have you done this consistently over the last 6 months?
    - **No** → **Action**
    - **Yes** → **Maintenance**

Go online to Connect to report on your stage of change http://connect.mcgraw-hill.com

must take the oxygen from the blood and use it. During exercise, the ability of the body to utilize oxygen and remove waste products depends on the efficient functioning of the cardiorespiratory system, which includes the heart, blood vessels, lungs, and muscles. When a person exercises, the working muscles demand more oxygen and nutrients and the heart must work harder to keep up with the demand. The demand for oxygen increases in direct proportion to the intensity of exercise.

VO_{2max} is determined partly by genetics and partly by training. As fitness improves, many factors contribute to greater VO_{2max}. The heart is a muscle and, like any muscle, grows stronger with training. A fit, trained heart can pump more oxygenated blood to exercising muscles than an unfit heart can. Cardiorespiratory training increases both stroke volume, the volume of blood pumped per heartbeat, and **cardiac output,** the volume of blood pumped per minute. Similarly, trained skeletal muscles can utilize oxygen and nutrients delivered by the blood to produce energy more efficiently than untrained muscles can. Ventilation and blood flow to the lungs improve. Blood flow of the muscles improves. Muscle cells become more efficient at extracting oxygen and producing energy for muscular contraction. Waste products are removed more efficiently. VO_{2max} determines how intensely and how long you can perform aerobic exercise and is considered one of the best overall indicators of physiological well-being.

While natural cardiorespiratory endowment may vary among individuals, with training, maximal oxygen uptake can improve 20 to 30 percent, depending on pretraining status and the frequency, intensity, and duration of training. Beneficial physiological changes persist as long as aerobic training continues, but inactivity produces physical decline. If training stops, VO_{2max} returns to pretraining levels within a few months. With aging, aerobic capacity decreases about 1 percent per year after age 25. This decline is related closely to decreasing levels of activity rather than to growing older. Declines in VO_{2max} may be slowed dramatically by those who exercise across the lifetime. See the section on aging in Chapter 7 for more information on the effects of exercise on aging.

The ability to utilize oxygen during exercise can be measured in a laboratory on a treadmill or in a field test. Several tests in Chapter 3 can be used to assess your cardiorespiratory endurance. They include the 1.5-mile run, the 1-mile walk, the 500-yard water run, the 500-yard swim, the 3-mile bicycling test, and the 3-minute step test. *Norms were developed by testing thousands of college students at the end of 12 to 15 weeks of aerobic fitness classes,* so you can compare your results with the standards for your selected activity.

Benefits of Aerobic Exercise

Aerobic exercise has both short- and long-term effects. The immediate effects of vigorous exercise, regardless of fitness level, are an increase in the respiration rate, an increase in the heart rate, and an increase in body temperature. After a few weeks of regular, vigorous exercise, the body begins to adapt to meeting the demands. These physiological adaptations to exercise (the total beneficial changes) are called the **training effect** and are detailed in the following lists. The benefits of flexibility and muscular fitness are discussed in Chapters 5 and 6.

Cardiorespiratory Benefits

1. Lower resting heart rate
2. Increased stroke volume (the amount of blood pumped out of the heart with each beat), improving heart efficiency
3. Increased rest for the heart between beats due to slower resting heart rate and increased stroke volume
4. Increased oxygen-carrying capacity of the blood due to the greater supply of red blood cells and hemoglobin; greater endurance in exercising muscles due to increased energy and improved elimination of waste products
5. Improved exercise performance on timed tests due to more efficient use of oxygen
6. Reduced blood pressure
7. Improved blood lipid profile by increasing the number of protective high-density lipoproteins (HDLs)
8. Quicker recovery to resting heart rate after vigorous exercise due to improved cardiac efficiency
9. Possible regression of atherosclerosis
10. Fewer illnesses and deaths due to coronary heart disease

Body Composition/Physical Appearance Benefits

1. Reduced body fat percentage
2. Increased lean body mass
3. Firmer, more toned muscles
4. More positive body image

Psychological, Mental, and Emotional Benefits

1. Enhanced sense of well-being and self-esteem, resulting in increased energy, alertness, and vitality
2. Increased sense of self-discipline due to the determination needed to stick to an exercise program
3. Reduced state of anxiety and mental tension, thereby increasing stress-coping ability

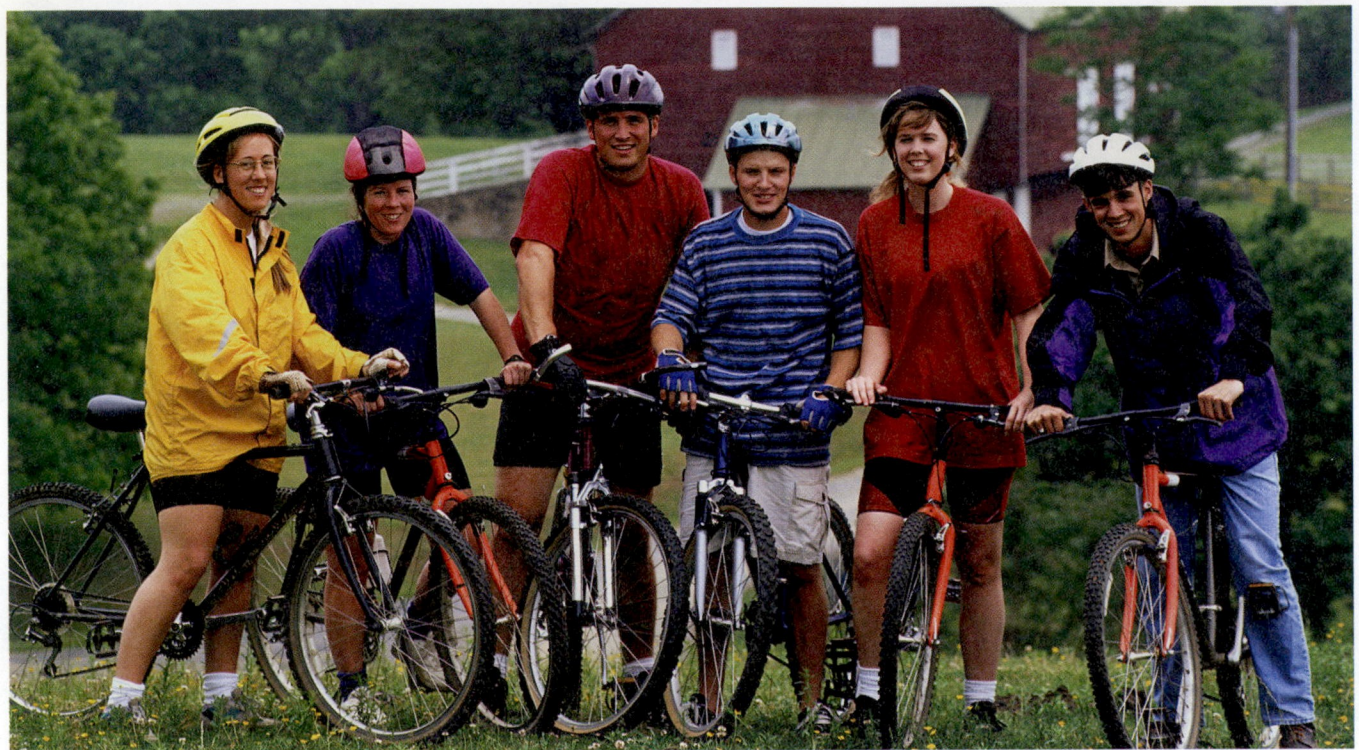

The U.S. Department of Health and Human Services is urging doctors to prescribe the medicine that aids more ills than any other. Exercise! The Rx is . . . move at least 2½ hours each week.

4. Improved quality of sleep; sleep soundly and wake up refreshed
5. Decreased level of mild to moderate depression
6. Improved mental acuity, learning, memory, and other higher thought processes
7. Feeling of relaxation
8. Improved mood
9. Reduced cognitive decline and dementia

The psychological benefits are very rewarding and are often the main reason people keep exercising. More detail on these and other benefits of cardiorespiratory fitness follows.

IMPROVED MENTAL HEALTH

People who exercise regularly report improved mood, higher self-confidence and self-esteem, and less stress compared with nonexercisers. Research indicates that aerobic exercise can also enhance psychological well-being by reducing depression and anxiety. The best results were obtained after several weeks of regular exercise, with more vigorous exercise, and in those who were high in anxiety or depression to begin with. During aerobic exercise, some people experience the effects of **endorphins.** This is sometimes called "a runner's high." Endorphins are opiate-like chemicals released by the brain that work like "natural pain-relievers." Recent studies report that the feelings of well-being endorphins provide last about half a day, 12 times longer than previously thought. While it may not work for everyone and we can't say exactly how much exercise is needed, for many individuals being able to say "exercise makes me feel better" is a significant benefit.

IMPROVED COGNITIVE FUNCTION

Recent research reveals that exercise also makes us smarter! For children, even a few games of kickball can boost the brain in widespread, long-lasting ways. This is why many teachers are lobbying for more time in physical education class.

It has been confirmed that aerobic exercise helps the heart pump more blood to the brain, as well as to the rest of the body. More blood means more oxygen and better-nourished brain cells. Science has now demonstrated a link between exercise and cognition, or neurogenesis, the scientific term for the process by which new brain cells are generated. The mental effects of exercise are far more profound than once thought. Exercised muscles send out chemicals that travel through the bloodstream and into the brain itself. There, these chemicals ramp up production of several brain chemicals that fuel almost all the activities that lead to higher thought. With regular exercise, the body builds up its levels of chemicals, and the brain's nerve cells start to branch out, join together, and communicate with each other in new ways. This is the process that underlies learning. Brains with more of these specific chemicals have a greater capacity for knowledge. On the other hand, a brain that is low on these chemicals shuts itself off to new information. These new findings have a profound impact on learning, memory, and many other processes of higher thought for the young, the college student, and the elderly.

The human brain gradually loses tissue from age 30 onward, and this is reflected in gradual declines in cognitive function. Cardiorespiratory fitness has been associated with preservation of cognitive function in healthy adults. One study that followed subjects for 10 years indicated that middle-aged aerobic exercisers compared with sedentary individuals have a significantly slower rate of memory decline and better memory performance. In subjects over 55, the positive effect of exercise was greatest on the "executive control" functions of judgment, planning, and the coordination of actions to achieve a goal. In elderly subjects age 60 to 76, 2 months of aerobic training significantly improved cognitive test scores, and the effect was equal to 2 months of mental training.

IMPROVED SLEEP

Many studies support the positive effects of exercise on sleep. In studies of individuals who exercised aerobically, exercisers went to sleep more quickly, slept longer, and had a more restful sleep than did those who did not exercise.

IMMUNE SYSTEM FUNCTION

Those who participate in regular moderate exercise enjoy enhanced levels of well-being, including fewer colds and minor respiratory infections compared with sedentary peers. Moderate workouts temporarily strengthen your defenses by boosting the circulation of white blood cells throughout the body, which allows them to detect invading and infected cells earlier. Exercise also may enhance immunity by flushing bacteria from the lungs through increased output of urine and sweat. Avoid overtraining, however, as exercising to exhaustion can weaken immune system function.

IMPROVED BODY COMPOSITION AND WEIGHT MANAGEMENT

Regular endurance exercise burns excess calories and can help maintain muscle mass and reduce excess body fat. Increasing levels of overweight and obesity in the United States at all age levels may be due as much to decreased physical activity as to increased caloric intake. For this reason, at least 60 minutes of vigorous physical activity daily is recommended for weight management. Even if exercise does not reduce body fat significantly, research indicates that those who exercise regularly significantly reduce the risk of chronic diseases compared with sedentary individuals.

REDUCED RISK OF CHRONIC DISEASES

Cardiorespiratory fitness can reduce the risk of developing several chronic diseases. For those who already have one of these diseases, a carefully monitored aerobic program is often recommended as a part of treatment to improve health and physiological resilience.

Cardiovascular Disease Cardiorespiratory exercise reduces the risk of having cardiovascular disease and the risk of dying from it. Cardiovascular disease does not develop suddenly in middle age. It begins much earlier, in childhood and the teens and twenties, and continues to progress silently for many years. Young adults can reduce the risk of cardiovascular disease by developing a habit of regular exercise and managing the other risk factors described in Chapter 9.

High Blood Pressure Exercise prevents or delays the development of high blood pressure. High blood pressure is associated with the risk of stroke, kidney failure, and coronary heart disease. People with high blood pressure can reduce it by improving cardiorespiratory fitness, particularly if they lose weight as a result of exercise.

Type 2 Diabetes Regular aerobic exercise is associated with a lower risk of developing type 2 diabetes. Type 2 diabetes is associated with the risk of several chronic diseases that can make one's life miserable and shorten one's life span. Exercise helps prevent obesity, which is related to the onset of diabetes. It burns excess blood sugar and increases cells' sensitivity to insulin, which helps regulate blood sugar. For those with diabetes, exercise is an important adjunct to other treatments. Additionally, regular exercise dramatically reduces the risk of metabolic syndrome, a dangerous group of risk factors that have been shown to raise the risk of diabetes and heart disease. See Chapter 9.

Cancer One-third of cancer deaths in the United States each year are attributed to some combination of physical inactivity, poor diet, and obesity. The strongest evidence for an exercise–cancer link is with breast cancer and colorectal cancer. Part of the protection provided by exercise may be through weight control, but other independent effects (altering hormones, improving immune system function, speeding movement of foods through the digestive tract, etc.) are also important. Exercise also may improve survival rates for individuals battling cancer. The evidence is particularly strong for women fighting breast cancer. (See Chapter 13 for more information.)

Osteoarthritis   Regular exercise may prevent or delay osteoarthritis. Osteoarthritis is most common at weight-bearing joints such as the hips, knees, and ankles and is exacerbated by increased weight on those joints. Exercise maintains the strength of the muscles that surround and support the joints and helps maintain normal joint function. For those who have osteoarthritis, regular exercise such as walking is recommended for maintenance of normal joint function and reduction of excess body fat.

Osteoporosis   Osteoporosis is another disease that has its beginning in the teens and twenties with inadequate exercise and eating habits. Weight-bearing exercise such as running, walking, and aerobics can decrease the risk of osteoporosis by building optimal bone mass in young adults and in slowing its loss with age (see Chapter 7).

The benefits of aerobic fitness can enhance health and well-being across the life span. They can be gained by following the FITT prescription for cardiorespiratory fitness.

◆ THE FITT PRESCRIPTION FOR CARDIORESPIRATORY FITNESS

Cardiorespiratory fitness development involves four **FITT factors:** **F**requency, **I**ntensity, **T**ime, and **T**ype of exercise. The prescription for cardiorespiratory fitness for healthy adults is given in Figure 4-1. The prescription may be adjusted for older and sedentary individuals, who can begin with shorter times and lower intensity. While athletes may use this prescription to maintain fitness in the off-season, a greater investment of time and effort may be needed for in-season training.

"F" Equals Frequency

How often should you exercise? Exercise three to five times per week with no more than 48 hours between workouts. After 48 hours, the body starts

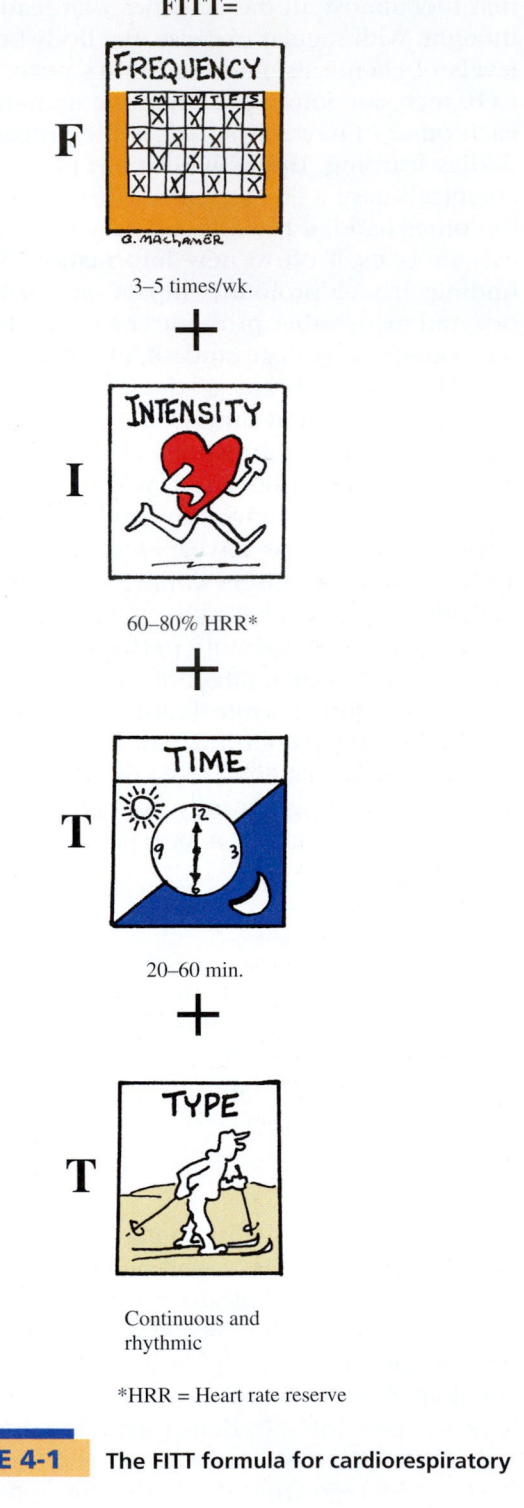

FITT=

F   FREQUENCY   ©. MACHAMER
3–5 times/wk.

+

I   INTENSITY
60–80% HRR*

+

T   TIME
20–60 min.

+

T   TYPE
Continuous and rhythmic

*HRR = Heart rate reserve

FIGURE 4-1   **The FITT formula for cardiorespiratory fitness.**

to decondition and lose some of the benefits gained in the last workout. It is not necessary to exercise every day to develop fitness, although 5-day-a-week programs produce greater improvements than do 3-day-a-week programs. Working out three times per week is the *minimum* and appropriate only for beginners or those recovering from an injury or illness. If your goal is to lose weight or reduce stress, at least 5 days of exercise a week is recommended. However, time for recovery is important, especially if you are just beginning a fitness program. The body needs time to adapt, so start slowly, working out every other day, gradually increasing the frequency as your fitness improves.

"I" Equals Intensity

How hard should you exercise? In athletics, a coach may ask you to give 100 percent effort, but this level of intensity is not needed to develop health-related fitness. Depending on the initial fitness level, about half to over three-quarters effort allows adequate stimulation of the cardiorespiratory system to produce training effect benefits. The American College of Sports Medicine (ACSM) recommends a workout intensity of 60 to 80 percent of your heart rate reserve for healthy, active individuals. For low fit, deconditioned, or older adults, intensities as low as 40 to 50 percent may be adequate for cardiorespiratory improvement. While this intensity will not produce excellent cardiorespiratory fitness, it does provide health benefits and reduces the risk for chronic diseases. Intensity of effort is directly reflected by exercise pulse rate and is perhaps the most important factor in gaining training effect benefits from your exercise program. You must put in enough effort to force the body to adapt and produce fitness improvements. If intensity is too low, there will still be health benefits but no increase in physical fitness. There are three ways to judge intensity: target heart rate, rate of perceived exertion, and the talk test.

TARGET HEART RATE: KARVONEN EQUATION

To determine your **target heart rate (THR)** range for cardiorespiratory exercise, we will use the **Karvonen equation,** which takes into account your age and resting heart rate (RHR). Karvonen, a Finnish researcher, discovered that the heart rate during exercise must be raised by at least 60 percent of the difference between resting and maximal heart rates (called the **heart rate reserve, HRR**) to gain cardiorespiratory fitness. An adequate upper intensity is 80 percent of HRR.

It is necessary to know your **maximal heart rate (HR$_{max}$)** to calculate your target heart rate range. The HR$_{max}$ is your highest possible heart rate. It can be directly determined during a treadmill exercise tolerance test in a laboratory or can be predicted based on your age. The maximal heart rate ranges from 180 to 200 beats per minute (bpm)

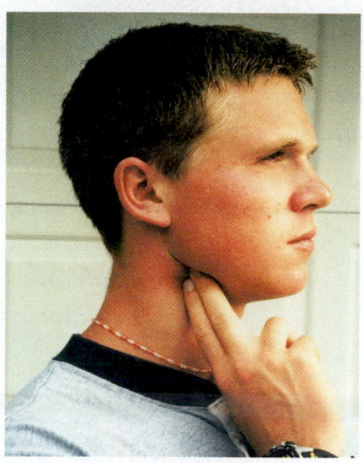

FIGURE 4-2   **Pulse at carotid artery.**

in young people and decreases with age. Most people can estimate their HR$_{max}$ by subtracting their age from 220. For example, if you are 23 years old, your estimated HR$_{max}$ is $220 - 23 = 197$.

Next, you will need to know your RHR for 1 minute. Check it by using a stopwatch or a watch with a second hand. The best time to check it is in the morning before you get out of bed. You also may check it after you have been sitting quietly for 20 minutes or more. Ideally, you should check it several times over a few days. You can find the pulse with your fingertips (not the thumb) at the carotid artery in the neck or on the thumb side of the wrist (Figures 4-2 and 4-3). Be careful not to apply too much pressure at the carotid artery site because the body's natural response is to suppress the heart rate when this occurs. Count the number of beats for 30 seconds and multiply by two to calculate your 1-minute pulse. By using your age and your RHR, you can calculate your target heart rate

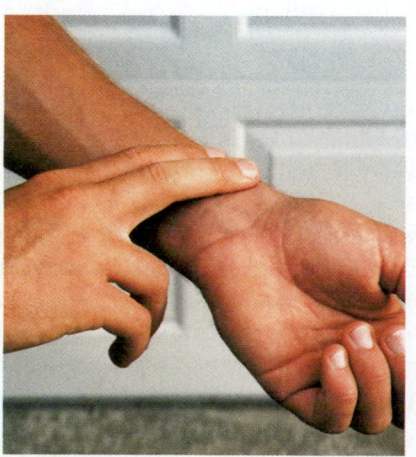

FIGURE 4-3   **Pulse at the thumb side of wrist.**

TABLE 4-1	*Calculating Target Heart Rate Range Using the Karvonen Formula*

This example shows a 23-year-old with a resting heart rate (HR$_{rest}$) of 72 bpm:

- Estimation of HR$_{max}$ = 220 − 23 = 197
- HR$_{rest}$ = pulse at complete rest for 1 minute
- Intensity = range of 60% to 80%

THR = (HR$_{max}$ − HR$_{rest}$) × intensity + HR$_{rest}$

a.   220   −   23   =   197

(HR$_{max}$)   (age)   (estimated maximal heart rate [MHR])

b.   197   −   72   =   125

(MHR)   (resting HR)   (heart rate reserve)

c.   125   ×   .60   =   75 + 72 = 147

(HR reserve)   (lower intensity)   (resting HR)   (lower target heart rate)

d.   125   ×   .80   =   100 + 72 = 172

(HR reserve)   (higher intensity)   (resting HR)   (higher target heart rate)

Target heart rate is **147** to **172** beats per minute.

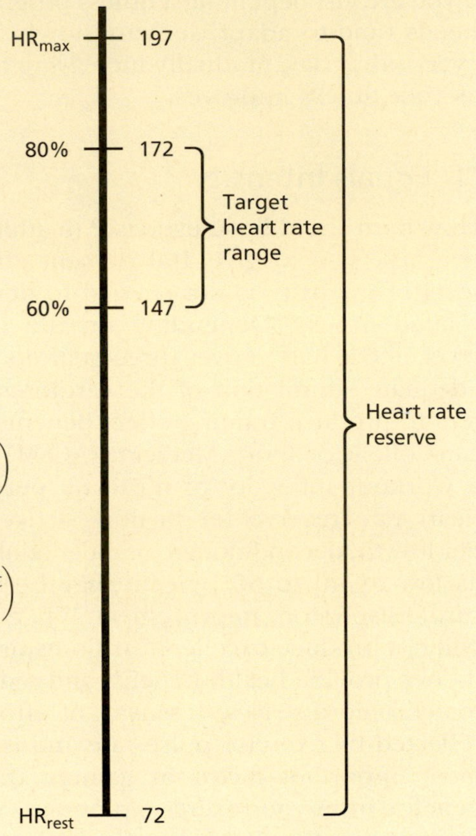

HR$_{max}$ — 197
80% — 172
60% — 147
HR$_{rest}$ — 72

Target heart rate range

Heart rate reserve

SOURCE: Adapted from Karvonen, M., Kentala, K., and Mustala, O. "The Effects of Training on Heart Rate: A Longitudinal Study." *Annals of Medicine and Experimental Biology* 35 (1957): 307–315.

range (Table 4-1). There is also a target heart rate worksheet in Lab Activity 4-1.

Now that you know your target heart rate range, you will be able to measure the intensity of every exercise session. Count your pulse during exercise and immediately after a conditioning bout. Because your pulse drops rapidly when you stop exercising, rather than counting your pulse for a full minute, you may find it easier to count for 6 seconds (e.g., if you count 15 beats in 6 seconds, your pulse is 150). It will take some practice, but in time you will become accurate at checking your heart rate.

Exercise heart rates differ by age (Figure 4-4). For most young adults, a THR is in the range of 140 to 170 beats per minute, but for older adults, a rate of 120 to 140 beats per minute may be adequate. Exercising at a heart rate above your THR is not necessary for fitness, does not increase health benefits, but may increase the risk of injury. Keep in mind that because the maximal heart rate is estimated, any error in that estimate is carried over into the THR calculation. Actual THR can vary plus or

minus 10 beats. A general rule is to apply the talk test and/or the rate of perceived exertion (RPE).

TALK TEST

The **talk test** is another way to gauge the intensity of exercise. You should be able to carry on a

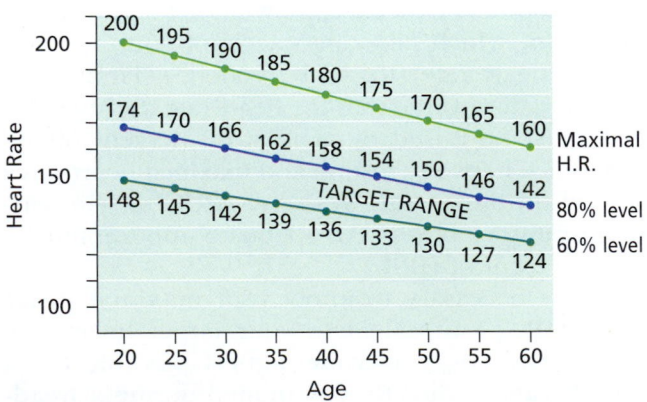

FIGURE 4-4	**Estimated target heart rate range (based on RHR of 70 bpm).**

conversation with a companion while exercising. If you are too breathless to talk, you are exercising too hard. Research has confirmed that at the point where speech is just becoming difficult, the exercise intensity is almost exactly equivalent to the target heart rate. When speech is not comfortable, exercise intensity is consistently above target heart rate. Listen to your body and adjust exercise intensity accordingly.

RATE OF PERCEIVED EXERTION (RPE)

Many people do not check their heart rate during exercise and judge intensity of exercise by **rate of perceived exertion (RPE),** sensing how hard or easy a workout feels. This method uses a scale developed by Gunnar Borg (an easy way to use an adaptation of Borg's scale is found in Table 4-2). Borg discovered that exercisers are able to "sense" their exercise intensity levels and that the RPE scale correlated with heart rate. Borg found that the descriptive words in the right column closely paralleled the heart rate of the exerciser, which is illustrated by the numbers in the left column. To receive cardiorespiratory benefit from the exercise and improve fitness, you should feel the effort is "Moderate" to "Hard," or 4–6 on the RPE chart. This exertion intensity approximates an intensity of 60 to 80 percent of the heart rate reserve method discussed earlier. It is helpful to cross-check your heart rate with your perceived rating when you first begin to use this method. Experienced exercisers can use RPE to determine if they are in their target HR zone and adjust the exercise intensity accordingly. Younger, more fit exercisers, competitive athletes,

or those doing interval training may workout up to an RPE of 7 and beyond for a more vigorous exercise bout. This is a safe and accurate way to monitor exercise intensity anywhere, anytime without using a stopwatch.

THR During Non-Weight-Bearing Activities

When you swim, bike, or water run, an adequate target pulse rate is lower than it is when you are running. Weight-bearing activities, such as running and walking, use more oxygen and make your heart beat faster than it does when you exercise by cycling or swimming—at the same perceived level of effort. As a general rule, reduce cycling THR by 5 percent and swimming THR by 10 percent. In any case, you should be able to pass the talk test. For example, if your THR for running/walking is 150–170 bpm, your swimming THR will be

1. $150 \times .10 = 15$; $170 \times .10 = 17$
2. $150 - 15 = 135$; $170 - 17 = 153$
3. THR $= 135 - 153$ bpm

Also remember to set different goals for cross training. A good way to achieve an effective workout is to monitor your rate of perceived exertion (RPE).

TARGET HEART RATE: PERCENTAGE OF MAXIMAL HEART RATE

An old method of determining the target heart rate used a straight percentage of the maximal heart rate. The ACSM recommends using 70 to 90 percent of an individual's maximal heart rate to set exercise intensity. For example, if a person's estimated maximal pulse was 200, the target heart rate range would be 140 ($200 \times .7$) to 180 ($200 \times .90$) beats per minute. The advantage of this method is that it is simple to compute. Its drawback is that it does not take resting pulse into account.

"T" Equals Time

How long should each workout be? The ACSM recommends a conditioning bout of 20 to 60 minutes at an intensity of 60 to 80 percent, not including warm-up and cool-down. The 20 to 60 minutes does not have to be completed in one workout. It is acceptable to accumulate the time in 10-minute bouts of exercise throughout the day—for example, 10 minutes in the morning, 10 more minutes at lunchtime, and 10 minutes (or more) after work or school.

Duration is inversely related to the intensity of the activity. A similar exercise volume may be obtained at a low intensity and a longer time (60 percent intensity, 30 to 60 minutes) or a higher intensity and a shorter time (80 percent intensity, 20 minutes). See Figure 3-1 in Chapter 3 for a comparison of

TABLE 4-2	Rate of Perceived Exertion (RPE)
RPE Chart	
0 No exertion (resting)	
1 Extremely easy	Warm-up/Cool-down zone
2 Very easy	
3 Easy	
4 Moderate	
5 Somewhat hard	Target zone
6 Hard (heavy)	
7 Very hard	
8 Extremely hard	Working too hard zone
9 Near maximal exertion	
10 Maximal exertion	

SOURCE: Adapted from G. Borg's Perceived Rate of Exertion.

exercise intensities and times. However, risk of injury does increase at higher intensities. Because many traditional-aged college students (18 to 24 years) have difficulty reaching their THR during some fitness activities (such as fitness walking), or find it is always at the low end of the THR range, they may wish to extend the time of the workout to 60 minutes or more. If time permits and the exercise session is enjoyable, if weight management is a goal, or if you are training for a long-distance event (e.g., mini-marathon), exercising for longer than 60 minutes is fine, but it is not necessary for cardiorespiratory fitness benefits. A typical exercise session would be as follows:

Warm-up 5–15 min.	+	Conditioning bout 20–60 min. or more	+	Cool-down 5–15 min.

When beginning a fitness program, it is best to limit your conditioning periods to 20 minutes or less (e.g., four 5-minute bouts with a rest in between if needed), then progress slowly until you can comfortably work out for 20 to 60 minutes or more in your target heart rate range. If you wish to progress beyond a basic level, you should apply the progressive overload principle discussed in Chapter 3.

THINK ABOUT IT

One of the latest fitness machines advertised on the Internet is the ROM QuickGym. ("ROM" stands for Range of Motion.) You can evaluate some of its claims online at www.quickgym.com. For example, this Cross Trainer promises to deliver 45–90 minutes of exercise in just FOUR MINUTES, uses 12-times more muscles than used in walking or running, and stretches and lengthens muscles. All this can be yours for a mere $14,614! Compare the cost and benefits promised by this machine with those of other fitness machines on the market today. Are there other, less expensive ways, to achieve the same results? What factors such as convenience, efficiency, and promised results might influence someone's decision to purchase a fitness machine? What do you think fitness experts world say about the ROM QuickGym?

Go online to Connect to complete this activity.
http://connect.mcgraw-hill.com

Many people think they don't have time to exercise, but if you do the minimum 20 minutes, 3 days per week, it takes only 1 hour in your week—a small investment that pays big dividends. Complete Lab activity 4-4 to help you overcome any obstacles that are keeping you from exercising on a regular basis.

"T" Equals Type

What type of exercise promotes aerobic fitness? The term **aerobic** means "with oxygen." Aerobic activities are ones that demand large amounts of oxygen and improve cardiorespiratory endurance. They are vigorous, continuous, and rhythmic. Aerobic dancing, swimming, cycling, and jogging are all good, as are other vigorous activities that sustain a target heart rate. Rope jumping, playing a game of basketball, or stair climbing, even going through a circuit in the weight room rapidly can be an aerobic activity as long as the FITT prescription factors are met. However, riding a bike a short distance across campus is not adequate

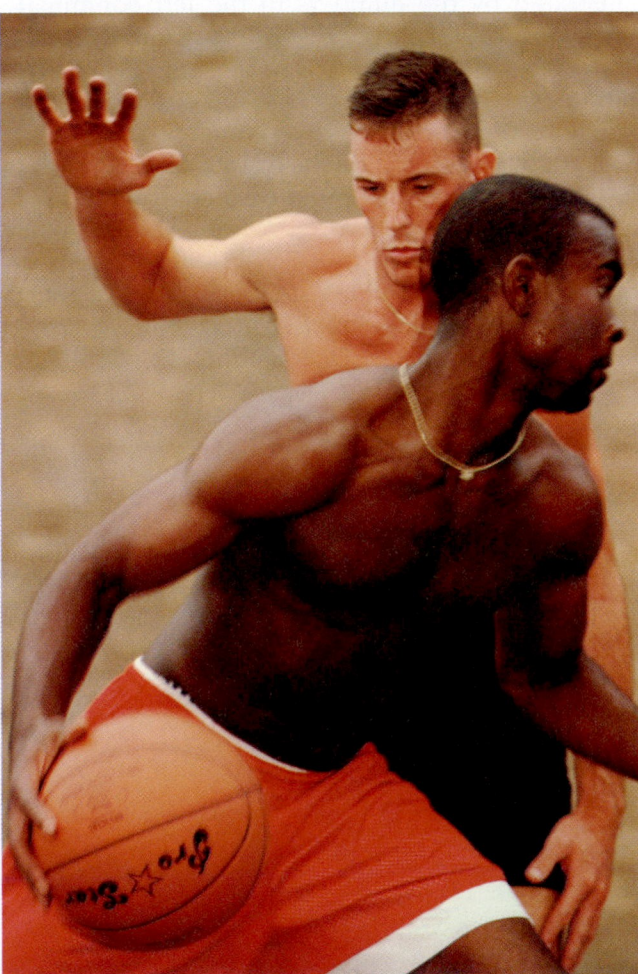

Enjoy playing a game of basketball. It can be aerobic if the FITT prescription factors are met.

in intensity or time to develop fitness. Ask, "Did I keep my heart rate in the target heart range for 20 to 60 minutes or more?" Bowling, golf, and softball, although enjoyable recreational activities, are not aerobic. What other activities meet the FITT prescription?

Anaerobic exercise means "without oxygen." Anaerobic activities are of high intensity and short duration, such as sprinting. This type of activity demands more oxygen than the body can supply while exercising, causing an oxygen debt. Anaerobic exercise causes waste products (lactic acid) to accumulate in muscles, which, along with the depletion of stored energy, leads to exhaustion. Many activities—tennis, volleyball, and weight training—are anaerobic. They aid in the development of agility, eye-hand coordination, and muscular strength and endurance, as well as flexibility, but they are not aerobic and are not an efficient way to increase cardiorespiratory fitness unless they follow the FITT formula.

How Long Before Results Become Apparent?

This varies with the individual. Within the first few exercise sessions, many people report that they feel better. Measurable differences such as decreased heart rate and improved aerobic fitness can occur within 8 to 12 weeks. The key is staying with the exercise program. Studies indicate that over 50 percent of adults who start an exercise program quit within the first 3 to 6 months. Regular exercisers focus on the positive benefits of exercise, reminding themselves how good they feel after exercise, and pat themselves on the back for making progress. So how do you stay with an exercise program long enough to experience the benefits of the training effect? See the Top 10 "Ways to Stick with Exercise" on page 111 for examples of ways to keep a commitment to a healthy lifestyle.

FITT vs. Department of Health and Human Services (DHHS) Physical Activity Guidelines for Americans

You have learned that to develop aerobic fitness you should follow the FITT prescription. Does this conflict with the recently released Department of Health and Human Services (DHHS) Physical Activity Guidelines? Not really. The new guidelines parallel the FITT prescription; they are a health recommendation designed to improve health by warding off chronic diseases (diabetes, heart disease, etc.) and are backed by solid scientific evidence. The goal is health. The FITT prescription is designed to improve health by reducing risk of chronic disease and is also backed

Exercise Guidelines	
FITT (for CRE fitness)	• 20 to 60 minutes (minimum of 20–30 minutes) • Moderate to vigorous intensity: 60–80% HRR (Example: walking 4.0–4.5 mph, jogging 5 mph, biking 10 mph) • 3 to 5 days per week
DHHS Guidelines for Americans (for health)	**Per Week** • All adults should avoid inactivity • At least 2½ hrs (150 minutes) of moderate-intensity aerobic activity: 40–60% HRR (Example: brisk walking @ 3.5 mph) **Or** • 1¼ hrs (75 minutes) of vigorous-intensity aerobic activity (Example: jogging, swimming laps) • Activity should be done in at least 10-minute bouts and can be spread throughout the week **For More Health Benefits** • 5 hours (300 minutes) of moderate-intensity aerobic activity **Or** • 2½ hours (150 minutes) of vigorous-intensity aerobic activity **And** • Muscle-strengthening activities (moderate or high-intensity, all muscle groups) 2 or more days per week
For weight loss or weight loss maintenance (for FITT/DHHS Guidelines)	• 1 hour per day at least five times per week (300 minutes per week at least) • Moderate aerobic activity • May require more activity than base amount needed for health benefits • Try to accumulate 450 minutes or more per week to keep weight off

by science. However, the FITT prescription's primary goal is cardiorespiratory endurance, or aerobic fitness, which is the most important component of fitness. As you recall, there are five components of health-related fitness, and a balance among the five is important for complete health and fitness. See Chapter 3.

Look at the *Exercise Guidelines box* to see how the FITT and the DHHS Physical Activity guidelines compare. The government's recommendations here are for healthy adults age 18 to 64. Also, examine the *Sample Physical Activity Workouts to meet the DHHS Guidelines box.* There are numerous ways fitness activities can be combined to meet the guidelines. Note: If you follow the FITT prescription, you will

Sample Physical Activity Workouts to meet DHHS Guidelines	
Workout	**Total Weekly Minutes**
• 30 minutes fitness walking (moderate)/ 5 days; resistance bands/2 days	150
• 20 minutes jogging (vigorous)/5 days; calisthentics (push-ups, ab curls)/5 days	100
• 30 minutes indoor cycling class (vigorous)/1 day; 60 minutes aerobics class (vigorous)/1 day; 30 minutes fitness walking (moderate)/1 day; resistance bands/2 days	120
• 20 minutes jogging (vigorous)/2 days; 30 minutes fitness walking (moderate)/ 2 days; 60 minutes basketball (moderate to vigorous)/1 day; free weight workout/2 days	160
• 60 minutes fitness walking (moderate)/ 5 days; resistance bands and free weights/ 2 days	300

most likely exceed the DHHS Physical Activity Guidelines and in turn reap even greater health and fitness benefits. Have you noticed both stress and longer duration of exercise if the goal is weight loss or weight loss maintenance? What is the recommendation for duration and intensity of exercise if you wish to lose weight? For a more thorough look at the Physical Activity Guidelines for Americans go to www.health.gov/paguidelines. You will find physical activity guidelines for all ages and special population groups.

10,000 STEPS: A DAILY LIFESTYLE GOAL

Many fitness experts believe that we could manage weight control and enhance fitness if we would accumulate 10,000 steps in our activity each day. The goal of this new recommendation is to increase the activity levels of the American public by encouraging more people to move about at least 10,000 steps per day—the equivalent of about 5 miles. A mile can be anywhere from 1,800 to 2,000 steps, depending on stride length and pace. Sedentary individuals typically move about (or walk) less than 5,000 steps in a day, moderately active people take 5,000 to 7,500 steps per day, and active people take at least 10,000 steps per day. The goal of 10,000 steps per day is applicable regardless of how much a person weighs or what his or her cardiorespiratory endurance fitness level is. A young person could accumulate steps through jogging, playing basketball, or other activities, while an older person could meet the recommendation by walking. Some fitness experts believe that people who regularly

work out at a high intensity level may not need to achieve the daily 10,000 step count. However, the jury is still out on this concept.

How do you measure the number of steps taken per day? A basic pedometer, by detecting vertical movement of the hips, is an inexpensive and simple way to monitor the total volume of physical activity performed on a daily basis. See the Internet Resources section for information on pedometers. Pedometers are motivational, fitness experts contend. By keeping track of how many steps have been taken, one can check quickly to see how many more steps must be taken to reach the goal of 10,000 steps that day. You will probably discover that it is nearly impossible to take 10,000 steps in a day without intentionally adding some type of fitness workout such as a jog, a walk, or a game of tennis or basketball.

Pedometers accurately measure any form of physical activity that involves the vertical movement at the hip, such as walking, jogging, tennis, basketball, some cardio-machines, and even climbing stairs, shoveling, gardening, and raking. It is

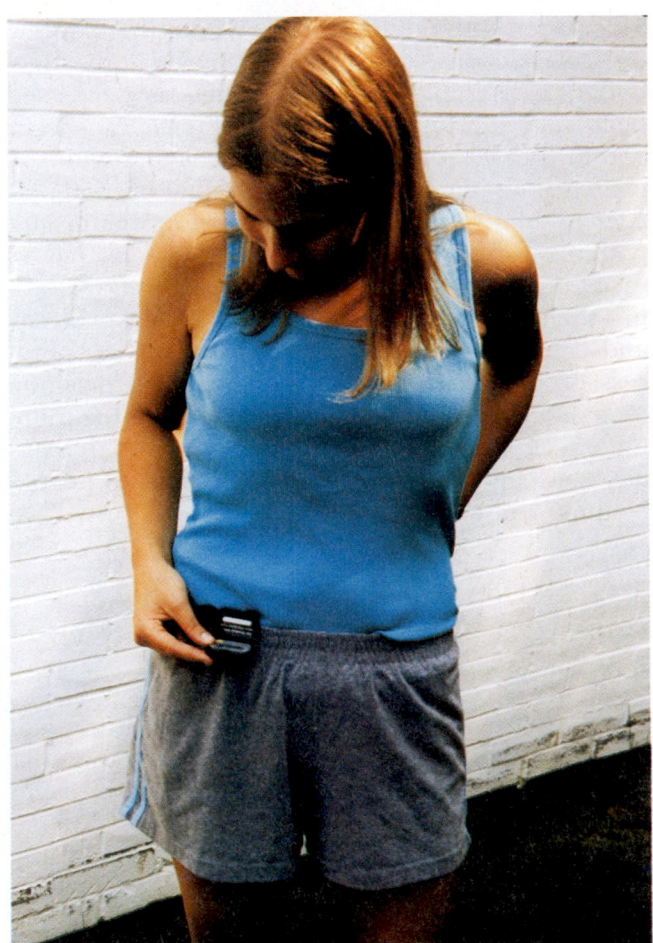

Use a pedometer to motivate you to get more activity every day. People who wear a pedometer walk about 2,500 steps more—or about another mile—than those who don't. How many steps are you getting each day?

important to note that there are some activities and factors in which the pedometer will not accurately register movement counts at the hip:

✓ cross-country skiing
✓ activities on wheels (e.g., bicycling, skateboarding, and in-line skating)
✓ swimming activity (most pedometers are not waterproof)
✓ moving slowly (less than 2.5 miles per hour)
✓ walking with an uneven gait or scuffing the feet
✓ walking on thick carpet
✓ wearing the pedometer on a flimsy waistband (this forces it out of the vertical position)

A good pedometer need not be expensive or have multiple functions in order to be reliable and valid. Pedometers requiring the calculation of the step-stride distance are not necessary either. Keep it simple but do get one with a safety strap. This protects against loss or damage if it should fall off the waistband.

Here are guidelines for using pedometers correctly:

✓ Pedometers can be worn on either the right or the left side of the body.
✓ Place the pedometer on the waistband (or belt) in line with the midpoint of the thigh and kneecap. Reset it to zero. The pedometer will register counts only when the lid is closed (if the brand you have has a lid).
✓ Perform the 20-Step Accuracy Check before use to ensure the pedometer is in the correct spot on the waistband.

  • Begin walking at a normal cadence while counting the number of steps taken. Stop immediately when 20 steps are reached. Check the pedometer's step count reading. If the step count reads 19–21, the placement is accurate.
  • If the step count is not accurate; move the pedometer slightly to the right or left. Reset, take 20 steps, and recheck for accuracy as previously described. Continue with the Accuracy Check until proper placement is reached.

✓ Attach a safety strap to clip the pedometer to your waistband, or simply use a safety pin to keep it from falling off.
✓ Pedometers *must remain in the upright vertical position to measure steps accurately.* Undercounting errors may occur for individuals who are overweight because the pedometer may be turned away from the vertical plane and moved toward the horizontal plane by the excess body fat around the waist. Wearing loose-fitting clothing may also affect the

accuracy of the pedometer because it absorbs slight vertical force that occurs with each step. In these cases, placement at waist level behind the hip on the back is often accurate. Check the accuracy as described previously.

The 10,000-step goal may be too high for some people at first. Follow the five steps outlined in Table 4-3 for guidelines to safely reach your 10,000-step goal and for tips on how to incorporate more physical activity, fun, and variety into your daily life. Also see Lab Activity 4-2 for help reaching 10,000 steps per day.

Use the 1-Mile Equivalent Chart in Lab Activity 4-3 for additional ideas on how to add more steps to your lifestyle. Do you realize that ancient people took approximately 30,000 steps per day to survive and hunt for food? How many steps are you getting on most days of the week? Check "The Numbers" to see how modern society compares to the Amish lifestyle.

THE NUMBERS

2½	Minimum number of hours of physical activity per week needed to meet the government's physical activity guidelines—most Americans *watch more hours of TV a day* than this!
3,000	Number of steps in 30 minutes, 5 days a week, that will help you meet the government's recommended fitness goals. (That's 1,000 steps per 10 minutes.)
3 in 4	Adults do not engage in sufficent exercise despite the common knowledge that inactivity is related to specific chronic diseases (such as heart disease, and diabetes, obesity, etc.)
18,000	Average number of steps that men in an Old Order Amish community in Ontario, Canada, took per day. On average, women in the same community took 14,000 steps per day. (Data from a University of Tennesee study.)
2,000–4,000	Number of steps the average American takes per day.
100–125	Number of steps per minute that meet the ACSM fitness guidelines for moderate-intensity exercise. This equals approximately 3,000 steps in 30 minutes.

TABLE 4-3   *Five Steps to Reach 10,000 Steps a Day*

To avoid injury, you need to work up to 10,000 steps slowly. If you have any concerns about your joints (ankles, knees, hips), discuss your exercise plans with your physician. Check with your physician if you experience any pain or discomfort that concerns you. The goal is to be active for the rest of your life. Don't go overboard at the beginning and develop an injury that will prevent you from having an active lifestyle.

Step Conversion		
1 step	=	2.64 feet
1 mile	=	2,000 steps
5 miles	=	10,000 steps
10 miles	=	20,000 steps
25 miles	=	50,000 steps

1. Week 1: Start by wearing the pedometer for one full "normal" or typical week. Record the number of steps taken each day. Use the log sheet in Lab Activity 4-2. Calculate a daily average for 1 week. This is your Baseline Activity Level and a reference point for setting a personal, realistic, and progressive goal.

2. Weeks 2 and 3: Establish your personal goal by taking the Baseline Activity Level and adding 10 percent more steps to that level.

   For example: If your baseline is 6,000 steps per day, your personal goal would be 6,000 steps plus 600 (10 percent) more steps for a total of 6,600 steps. This will be your personal goal for the next 2 weeks. If the goal is reached for a majority of days during this period, another 10 percent (600 steps) is added to the baseline and the process is repeated each 2-week period thereafter until you reach the goal of 10,000 steps a day. (Example: Weeks 4–5 your goal will be 7,200 steps; weeks 6–7 your goal will be 7,800 steps, and so on.)

   Alternate Method: After the baseline is determined, establish progressive step goals based on the premise that approximately 100 steps are taken every minute. If you wish to increase your activity level by 5 minutes a day, then 500 steps should be added as a goal. One thousand steps should be added for an additional 10 minutes, and so on. Continue adding 500 steps per day (or 1,000 steps per day) to your daily goal until you reach the 10,000-step goal. (Example: If your Baseline Activity Level is 6,000 steps per day, your step goal for weeks 2–3 will be 6,500 steps; for weeks 4–5 your step goal will be 7,000 steps per day; and for weeks 6–7 your step goal will be 7,500 steps per day, and so on.)

3. Decrease your goal or stay at the same goal for longer if you wish or if you are not ready to increase.

4. Pedometers are accurate for walking, running, tennis, and so on, but not for bicycling, swimming, activities on wheels, and some cardio equipment in the fitness center. Use the 1-Mile Equivalent Chart in Lab Activity 4-3 to estimate your steps if you enjoy those activities. They can count toward the 10,000-step goal.

5. Use "Exercise Across the U.S.A." to have fun adding activity to your daily life. Pick a state and exercise/walk across it (see Lab Activity 4-3). At 10,000 steps per day, how many days would it take you to travel the length of the Mississippi River, the Grand Canyon, the circumference of Earth, or go to the moon, or cross the state of Illinois? Or, use the "Activity Step Equivalents" below if you enjoy these activities.

Activity Step Equivalents	
Activity	**Steps per Minute**
Aerobic dance	150–200
Basketball	200–220
Bicycling (6 mph)	70–100
Bicycling (10 mph)	130–140
Gardening	100–130
Housework	80–100
Jumping rope	230–250
In-line skating	135–200
Rowing machine	170–200
Snow shoveling	140–180
Stair climbing	200–230
Swimming	200–300
Tennis (doubles)	100–150
Tennis (singles)	160–200
Weight training	100–130
Yoga	70–100

Example: A 30-minute aerobic dance workout would equate to 4,500–6,000 steps (or between 2.25 miles and 3 miles).

◆ LIFETIME EXERCISE ACTIVITIES

Physical activity is touted as the single most effective lifestyle behavior for promoting better health. See "The Numbers" for the number of Americans who don't engage in sufficient exercise. What impact does this have on our nation's health?

You can do your part to help improve the health of our nation by selecting and participating in one of the eight exercise activities in this chapter. Select the activity you wish to pursue to reach your fitness goals and then follow the FITT prescription factors. Next, thoroughly read the activity unit of your choice. This will provide you with the helpful guidelines necessary to assist you in reaching these goals. *Take time now to read the Top 10 list "Ways to Stick with Exercise."*

As you begin your exercise program, let the thoughtful words of the Reverend Jesse Jackson inspire you: "Both tears and sweat are salty, but they render a different result. Tears will get you sympathy, sweat will get you change."

◆ AEROBIC FITNESS CLASSES

(Including Aerobic Dance, Step Aerobics, and Spinning)

ADVANTAGES/DISADVANTAGES

Aerobic dancing is a popular fitness activity. Usually performed under the leadership of an instructor, it combines the cardiovascular benefits of jogging with the joy of dancing. The variety of movements not only strengthens the cardiorespiratory system but also increases flexibility, tones muscles, and enhances body composition. It is a total body workout. The upbeat music tempo creates an atmosphere of excitement; exercising in a group is fun and emotionally stimulating. The popular music and group camaraderie help prevent boredom and can keep you motivated. Aerobic dancing can be so much fun, you often forget you are exercising. Because the participants focus on the instructor, aerobic dance classes are good for the beginning or self-conscious exerciser. Aerobic dance allows for individualization of a workout. The same movement sequence or exercise can be done by a well-conditioned participant and a beginning exerciser with variation in the intensity or the number of repetitions. Because aerobic dance is done indoors, the environment provides security and comfort.

Aerobic dance has excellent potential for developing all components of physical fitness, but it can have some drawbacks. Although participants are urged by instructors to work at their own pace, some exercisers overdo it. These exercisers try to keep up with the group or work as hard as the instructor even though they may not be ready for this intensity. Many times the result is excessive soreness or fatigue. Performing aerobic dance on a hard, unyielding surface (such as cement) or while wearing inappropriate shoes also increases the risk of injury. Some overzealous aerobics participants attend classes one or more times a day, leading to overuse. Excessive impact may cause leg and foot problems. Also, not all aerobic dance instructors have had training in exercise instruction and safety and may teach improper technique. Unless good body mechanics and reasonable progressions are emphasized in a class, the result can be discomfort rather than exhilaration and a desire to continue exercising. Having to join or travel to a fitness facility to take an aerobics class may be viewed as a disadvantage by some exercisers. Others find it motivating to have a set time, to have made a financial investment, and to have a group of friends to exercise with. Aerobic dance videotapes are available for the home exerciser. They allow exercising in private but lack the spontaneity, instruction, and enthusiasm available in a live class.

TOP 10 LIST

Ways to Stick with Exercise

1. *Pick an activity you enjoy.* Exercise should be fun, not merely work. Try different activities until you find one or two you like.

2. *Make exercise social.* Exercising with a partner or a group of friends is more fun than working out alone. Friends rely on each other for moral support and help each other stay committed to the fitness program. An "exercise date" once or twice a week can keep you going.

3. *Take lessons.* Join an aerobic dance class or a health club. Start slowly and progress gradually to avoid injuries. If exercise is too difficult or too intense, you are not likely to want to stay on the program.

4. *Make it convenient.* Develop a home gym or purchase a couple of exercise videos. Keep your exercise gear available so that you can squeeze in a quick workout.

5. *Treat exercise like an appointment.* Schedule a time that works best for you, whether morning, noon, or evening.

6. *Keep a chart to monitor your progress.* It's rewarding to see how much you have progressed.

7. *Add variety.* To keep your program fresh, walk or jog different routes or exercise in a park or around a golf course. Alternate swimming, walking, and bicycling. While pedaling a stationary bike, read, listen to music, or watch TV. (But don't wear headphones when exercising outside near traffic.)

8. *Have a backup plan in case of bad weather or conflicts.*

9. *Be patient with yourself.* Expect ups and downs. Some days you will be more energetic, some days less. If you're not feeling like a workout, tell yourself you will do a little and you may find that after a few minutes you perk up. If you have been doing too much, a rest may do you more good than another workout.

10. *Finally, don't stop!* It's difficult to get going again. Remember to plan for changes in your schedule (for example, pack your exercise equipment when you travel). However, don't feel guilty if you miss an exercise session. Taking a few days off due to illness or injury isn't a disaster. Consider this a lifetime commitment and resume exercising as soon as possible.

TECHNIQUES AND SAFETY TIPS

Many injuries and much discomfort can be avoided in aerobic dance with proper shoes, gradual progression, and exercising on a resilient surface. Chapter 8 provides several general suggestions for preventing injury in fitness activities. In aerobic dance, careful attention to technique and body mechanics further eliminates chance for injury and heightens the enjoyment of the activity.

1. *Always warm up with low-intensity, whole-body movements.* Your warm-up should include slow, full-range-of-motion joint movements. Static stretching should also be included in the warm-up.
2. *Keep abdominals pulled in and buttocks tucked under.*
3. *Avoid twisting the spinal column excessively* (windmill toe touches, elbow-to-knee lunges, etc.).
4. *Limit the hopping on one foot* to a maximum of four consecutive times.
5. *Soften your jumps and bounces by maintaining a slightly bent-knee landing position.*
6. *Try to make your heels go all the way to the floor when landing from jumps.*
7. *Never fling or throw your arms or legs.* Maintain control of limbs throughout movements.
8. *Avoid hyperextending your elbows, knees, or lower back.*
9. *Listen to your body.* If a stretch, exercise, or position causes pain or a burning sensation, do not do it.
10. *Wear supportive shoes designed for the impact of aerobic dance.* The shoe should allow for lateral movement and not have the wide heel flare found on a jogging shoe.

The amount of concern for technique and safety in the class depends on your instructor. A wise wellness consumer chooses a knowledgeable, trained instructor. The popularity of aerobic dance has skyrocketed, and the number of qualified instructors has not kept pace. While standards and certification programs have been established, it is up to you to select a class. Do not be shy. Check the instructor's qualifications. Is she or he

✓ Certified by a national fitness organization?
✓ Knowledgeable in anatomy, exercise physiology, kinesiology, and first aid?
✓ Currently certified in CPR (cardiopulmonary resuscitation)?
✓ Doing some health screening or fitness assessment of students?
✓ Supervising the class effectively?
✓ Monitoring the intensity of the workout with periodic heart-rate checks?
✓ Beginning with a good warm-up and ending with a cool-down period?
✓ Giving corrective cues and technique suggestions throughout the workout?

✓ Considering the variances in fitness levels in the class by showing how to modify the intensity of the workout?
✓ Easy to follow?
✓ Educating the participants on injury prevention and signs of fatigue?

Looking good in a leotard and being a fluid dancer are not requirements for being a quality aerobic dance instructor. Most important is the ability to conduct a safe yet invigorating workout from which all participants can benefit.

HOW TO BEGIN AND PROGRESS

As with any other fitness activity, begin slowly. Attend no more than three classes per week for several weeks. Start with 5 to 10 minutes of the aerobic phase and progress gradually. If the aerobic portion of the class is 30 minutes, do low-impact moves or walk in place while the experienced exercisers continue. Monitor your pulse and stay within your target heart-rate range. You should be able to talk or sing with the music throughout the entire workout. Gradually add a few minutes weekly to the aerobic phase until you can exercise aerobically for 20 to 60 minutes. Use Lab Activity 4-5 to record your progress.

Some exercisers prefer low-impact aerobics to high-impact aerobics. Low-impact aerobics reduces the strain on knees and ankles by minimizing jumping and bouncing movements. In low-impact aerobics, one foot is in contact with the ground at all times. *Low impact* does not necessarily mean *low intensity*. To maintain a training heart rate, move your arms vigorously and travel along the floor by wide-stride walking, sliding, and sidestepping. Beginners and well-trained exercisers with joint problems can benefit from low-impact aerobics. You may want to combine low-impact and high-impact

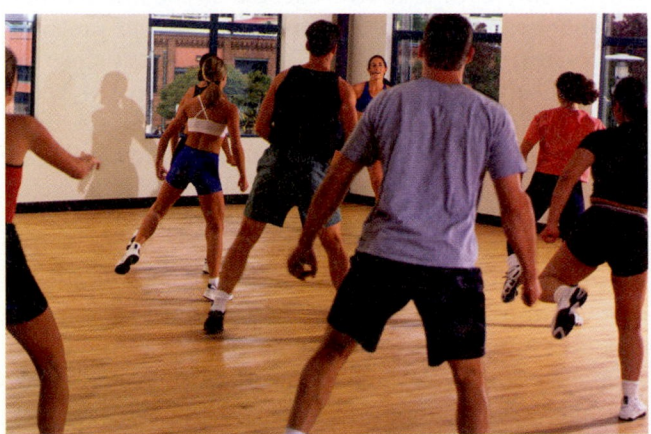

Working out in a class setting is social and fun.

moves. Most jumps and steps can be modified to become low-impact steps.

Most aerobic dance classes incorporate in the workout a body toning segment. Once again, use common sense. Do not try to do as many repetitions as the teacher unless you are equally fit. Stop and stretch if you feel pain or a burning sensation in the muscle. Aerobic dance participants often tend to compare themselves or compete with others in the class. Avoid falling into this trap. Work to be the best you can be without shame or guilt.

VARIETY

It is easy to add variety to aerobic dance. Vary the music. Use pop, jazz, country, or classical music. Try some holiday or theme music when appropriate. Vary the routines or steps. Aerobics can be taught by using set routines (repetitive movements in a programmed format) or in a freestyle format (participants mimic the instructor and change accordingly). Varying between learned routines and a freestyle approach helps keep interest high. Try circuit aerobic dance. Set up exercise stations around the room. Do different aerobic movements for 1 to 2 minutes per station and then jog to the next station to sustain your training heart rate. There are many other ways to add variety to aerobic dance. One- to two-pound hand weights can be used during aerobic routines to increase upper-body endurance and maintain a training heart rate. Heavier hand weights are often used during stationary power moves to tone arms and legs. To prevent knee injuries, do not wear ankle weights while doing aerobic dance steps. Weights are, however, an effective way to add resistance while doing floor toning. Thick rubber bands and elastic tubing can also be used to increase the efficiency of body toning exercises.

Step Aerobics

Also known as *bench/step training,* step aerobics is an innovative activity that involves stepping up and down on a 4- to 12-inch platform. Combining a variety of stepping patterns with kicks, turns, and upper-body movements results in a brisk workout. Step aerobics appeals to a wide range of exercisers for several reasons: It can be a high-intensity workout with low-impact force; it is adaptable to different fitness levels by adjusting the bench height, adding jumps, varying arm gestures, and adding light hand weights; and it is easy to do. Step aerobics has become especially popular with men, who may be put off by "dancelike" aerobics classes. As with all aerobic exercise activities, proper form and technique are necessary to prevent injury.

To prevent injury while stepping:

1. As much as possible, keep your shoulders aligned over your hips.
2. Step up lightly, making sure the whole foot lands on the platform.
3. Keep your knees aligned over your feet when they're pulling your body weight onto the platform.
4. At the top, straighten your legs but don't lock your knees.
5. Do not pivot a bent, supporting knee.
6. As you step down, stay close to the platform.

If you are a beginner at step aerobics, start with the lowest bench and keep your eyes on the bench until you adjust to the activity. Once you learn the stepping patterns, you can add arm movements and light hand weights or challenge yourself by raising the height of the bench. (However, never use a height that flexes your knees to an angle less than 90 degrees.)

Step aerobics is a great workout for the lower body and, when combined with a variety of arm movements, an exciting variation in aerobic exercise.

Indoor Cycling Classes (Spinning or Fit Ride)

Indoor cycling class is a stationary cycling workout that uses motivational techniques. The instructor leads a group of riders on a scenic stationary trail ride by using visualization techniques, motivational strategies, and videotapes and music. The instructor prompts you on when to crank up or loosen the tension and when to pedal faster. The indoor cycling class allows people of all ages and fitness levels to take a stationary bike and transform it into a powerful workout. Participants vary the workout by making changes in the speed and resistance of the bike. Indoor cycling classes allow participants to experience road cycling without the associated dangers. The program is also a great choice for the cyclist who wants to take his or her outdoor program inside during inclement weather.

A drawback to this excellent aerobic exercise program is the necessity to join a class that provides the certified trained instructor and appropriate bikes. Access to a health/fitness club or university fitness class is usually required for this activity.

For added comfort and enjoyment while Spinning, follow these guidelines:

1. Adjust the seat high enough so that the leg fully extends at the bottom of each pedal stroke with a slight bend in the knee.

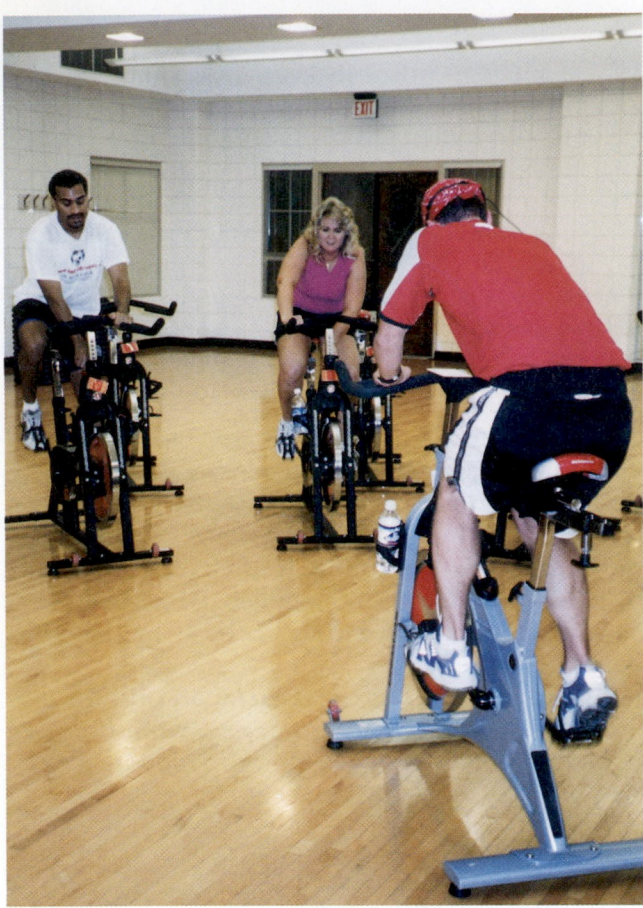

Indoor cycling class is a popular indoor fitness activity and can be quite challenging. The optimal pace is 60 to 80 rpm. A racer's pace is 80 to 100 rpm or more.

2. If possible, move the seat forward or back so that the bent knee, at the top of the stroke, rests just above midfoot.
3. Use toe clips or clipless pedals to help prevent foot fatigue.
4. Tilt the seat slightly downward to avoid crotch numbness.
5. For added comfort, buy a cover to pad the seat (or a gel cover) and invest in cycling shorts.
6. Adjust handlebar height to reduce hand/wrist pressure.
7. Add resistance when pedals (instead of your thigh muscles) are propelling your foot or the instructor advises you to do so.
8. Always warm up and cool down properly. Don't try to compete with class members; ride at your fitness level. Use your THR or RPE as a guide.
9. Listen to your body and stop before you feel fatigued.

Common Discomforts

As in most fitness activities, mild soreness can be anticipated by the beginning exerciser. Some discomfort may be avoided by emphasizing stretching and toning the first 3 to 4 weeks to condition muscles and connective tissue for the stress of impact and the new movements. Veteran exercisers can suffer pain or injury by increasing frequency, time, or intensity too rapidly. Most aerobic dance discomfort is found in the legs, so be sure to warm up and stretch this area. Exercise fatigue can also occur due to dehydration or lack of sleep/rest. Refer to Chapter 8 for further information about prevention and treatment of injuries. If you use hand weights, elbow and shoulder strain can be avoided by not flinging the weights. Always move the weights with control. Having a towel or exercise mat with you provides additional comfort and padding for floor exercises.

◆ BICYCLING

ADVANTAGES/DISADVANTAGES

Cycling is a popular choice for people of all ages. You can fit in a cycling workout while running errands, while going to work, or at home in front of the TV (on rollers or a stationary bike). You can cycle alone, with family, or with friends. If you have a small child, you can take him or her along in a bike seat instead of having to hire a sitter while you get a workout. It is nonimpact exercise, minimizing stress to the back, shins, and ankles.

There are a few drawbacks, though. You must have a bicycle, keep it in good working condition, and store it securely to prevent theft. Cycling in traffic requires alertness and the use of defensive driving skills to prevent accidents. Cycling in rain, snow, or icy conditions is uncomfortable and hazardous. Also, bicycles are so efficient that they can do most of the work for you. Cycling to class or for short distances is fine for transportation, but if you want to get in shape, you will need to put in more effort. Nevertheless, cycling produces cardiorespiratory benefits without impact, making it the third most popular activity in the United States. It can be enjoyed throughout a lifetime.

EQUIPMENT

There are plenty of bike–pedestrian and bike–car accidents, and the bicyclist is usually at fault. Always wear a helmet even if you're going only a short distance. The sidewalk is a hard surface. You may lose some skin in a slide or break some bones,

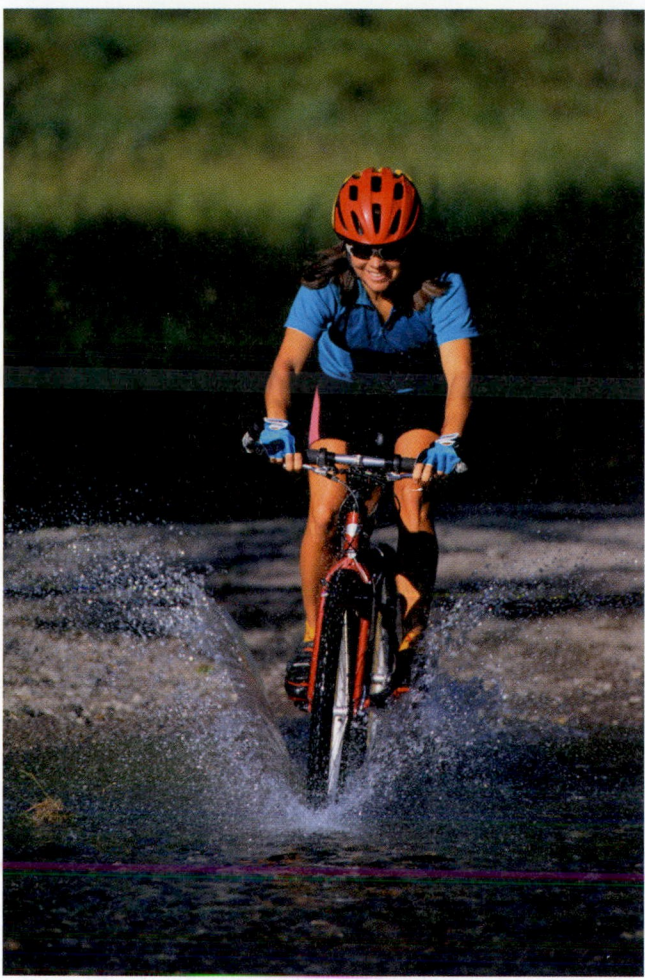

Bicycling is a great fitness activity across the life span. Always wear a helmet.

but they will heal. Your brain won't. Head injuries account for over 75 percent of deaths and permanent disabilities in cycling crashes. Only 18% of cyclists wear a helmet all or most of the time. If you hit something and go flying headfirst, wearing a good helmet is the best way to prevent serious injury.

When you are choosing a helmet, make sure that it has the following characteristics:

- ✓ Outer shell or cover that is brightly colored (i.e., yellow, white, or red) so that you are easily visible to drivers
- ✓ Hard shell lined with polystyrene or polystyrene alone
- ✓ Secure chin strap
- ✓ Label indicating that the helmet is Consumer Product Safety Commission, American Society of Testing and Materials (ASTM), or Snell Memorial Foundation approved

Helmets are single-use devices designed to crush and absorb shock upon impact. You should replace a helmet that has been in a significant crash.

A water bottle is essential for workouts, particularly in the heat. Because sweat evaporates so quickly while you are riding, you may not realize how quickly water is lost. Dehydration, leading to heat illness, can easily occur. Drinking regularly from a water bottle to maintain an adequate level of hydration during a workout is a necessity, not a luxury.

Recumbent bicycles have recently become popular, especially for riders with back problems. Because they are low to the ground, they are not as visible to motorists. Be sure to use a warning flag on the bike.

It doesn't matter what type of bike you ride, but it does matter that you keep it in good working order. If you are not mechanically inclined, your local bicycle shop can help. Most people ride with the bike seat too low, which is inefficient and can make the knees hurt. The bike seat should be high enough that when you sit centered on the seat with your heel on the pedal at its lowest point, your knee is only slightly bent. That way, when you move the ball of your foot to its proper position on the pedal, your knee will be almost fully extended at the bottom of the stroke. If the seat is too high, you'll tend to rock from side to side with each footstroke and may develop a sore crotch. A sore crotch also can be caused by improper seat tilt. Start with the nose of the seat level. If it bothers you, tilt it down slightly. Pedals, wheels, and steering should turn or spin freely with no binding, catch, or click. The derailleur should shift smoothly. Brakes should close and release easily. Brake shoes should be ⅛ inch or less from and level with the rim of the bike. If they are badly worn, replace them. The air in the tires usually needs to be topped off weekly to keep them hard and rolling smoothly, but use caution when filling them. The air pumps at service stations are designed for cars, and it's easy to explode a bicycle tire by overfilling it. If a bike wheel is badly out of true and wobbles, it may hit the brake shoe with each revolution. A bike shop can true a wheel; lubricate sticky brake cables; adjust the derailleur; and show you how to keep your machine running smoothly, which makes riding safe and enjoyable.

TECHNIQUE AND SAFETY TIPS

Shifting On multispeeds, the gears overlap slightly and you have to shift by feel. To shift, continue pedaling but ease up on the pedal pressure. Shifting without pedaling can cause a bent or broken chain or gear teeth. As you shift, you should not hear a loud clunk or a constant rubbing sound if you are shifting smoothly and getting it into gear correctly.

Most beginners gear too high and pedal too slowly. They feel like they're not getting any exercise unless they're pushing against resistance. This is inefficient and can increase fatigue and cause knees to ache. It is better to pedal quickly against light resistance. An optimal pedal rate is 60 to 80 rpm, with a range of 80 to 100 rpm. Racers and experienced tourists often cycle at 90 to 110 rpm.

If your bike has several gears, practice using them. Gearing is a matter of maintaining an even cadence regardless of terrain, weather, or wind conditions. If you're going uphill, shift before you have to slow your cadence so that you can go up smoothly. Also practice down-shifting before stop signs so that you don't have to stand on the pedals to get going again.

Pedaling Ride with the ball of your foot on the pedal. If you have toe clips or clipless pedals, you can try ankling—pulling up as well as pushing down on the pedal with each stroke—which doubles your efficiency.

Braking Look ahead, signal, slow down, and learn to anticipate problems instead of simply reacting to them. Be careful not to jam on the brakes too suddenly or you can pitch headfirst over the handlebars. The front brake is the most powerful because as you decelerate, your weight shifts forward, lessening the weight over the back tire. For the most efficient stop, keep your body weight back, gradually increase pressure on the front brake, and hold pressure on the back brake just below the point where the wheel will skid. In wet conditions, brakes lose up to 90 percent of their braking ability. It is good to frequently apply the brakes lightly to wipe water off the rims and allow extra stopping distance. When going downhill, pump the brakes to avoid overheating the wheel rims or brake shoes. When in doubt, favor the rear brake.

Bumps When you come up to bumps, holes, and railroad tracks, shift your weight to pedals and handlebars to absorb the shock. It's better for you and for your bike.

SAFETY TIPS

1. Wear bright colors or reflective clothing so drivers can see you; wear a helmet, and carry water.
2. Keep to the right side of the road and ride in a straight line. Always ride in single file with traffic.
3. Do not make sudden turns or swerves. Signal turns and stops. Try to make eye contact with drivers when you are turning so you know they have seen you.

4. Stay alert. Look out for cars pulling out into traffic or turning. Listen constantly for traffic approaching out of your line of vision.
5. Observe traffic regulations as if you were driving a car—red and green lights, one-way streets, stop signs. Slow down at all street intersections and look right and left before crossing.
6. Be sure the brakes are operating efficiently and keep your bicycle in perfect running condition. Keep your hands on or near the brakes at all times.
7. Keep speed under control, especially on long downhill runs. Speed should be low enough that you can stop quickly.
8. In rainy weather, allow much more distance for stopping and don't take corners too fast.
9. Watch for sudden door openings from parked cars. Ride at least 3 feet away from them.
10. Avoid sewer grates that parallel your direction.
11. If railroad tracks are rough, walk your bike across them (to prevent a blowout or other damage to the bicycle). If you choose to ride over the tracks, cross them at a 90-degree angle.
12. Make sure you are at least 3 feet off the traveled portion of the road when you stop or park.
13. Hug the right-hand shoulder of the road on all curves.
14. Give pedestrians the right-of-way. Avoid sidewalks.
15. Watch out for child cyclists. Children on bicycles usually weave from side to side and turn unpredictably without signaling and can run into you when you are passing them.
16. Dogs are potential adversaries. If a dog is far enough away, you can probably outrun it. Water from your bottle or a bike pump may scare the dog off. If you stop, keep the bike between you and the dog. Walk slowly away. Usually a dog will leave you alone, but watch the dog carefully before you get under way again. You can also buy a small can of "dog repellent," which will shoot a thin stream of chemical about 10 feet. Although the effects are potent, no permanent damage is done to the animal. Don't try to run down or kick at a dog—this can cause a crash. If you are scared, you can yell "Out" at the dog, mimicking a noise made by mother dogs when disciplining their puppies. This will usually startle a dog enough to give you a chance to escape.
17. Don't wear headphones—they block out street sounds that enable you to anticipate traffic.

18. Don't wear a heavy backpack. It can throw off your balance. Carry packages in baskets or bags attached to the cycle.
19. Learn to shift gears while keeping your eyes on the road.
20. If you use toe clips or clipless pedals, practice getting in and out of them in a safe area.
21. Tuck in your shoelaces.
22. Don't drink and cycle.
23. Avoid loose-fitting garments, which can get caught in the chain or wheels, and sandals, which can slip off the pedals. Use clips to keep pant cuffs from getting caught.
24. A pair of bicycling shorts makes long rides more comfortable.

HOW TO BEGIN AND PROGRESS

First, measure your fitness level by using the 3-mile timed ride test in Chapter 3. Remember that your *current* fitness level does not indicate your potential. Allow yourself several weeks to show significant improvement. Begin at the step indicated by your current fitness level in the *Bicycling Program box*. If you cannot complete the test, begin at level 1. Exercise 3 to 5 days a week at your training pulse. (An appropriate pulse for bicycling appears to be about 5 percent lower than that for other exercise, so subtract 5 percent to adjust for this difference.) It is also appropriate to use the RPE. You may work at one level until you can comfortably handle the recommended distance and intensity; then move to the next step. To develop balanced fitness, add 25 to 30 push-ups, a minute of abdominal curls, and 5 to 15 minutes of stretching to each workout. Use Lab Activity 4-5 to record your progress.

Bicycling Program

Fitness Category	Starting Level
Low	1 or 2
Fair	3
Average	4
Good	5
Superior	6

Level	Cycling	Total Distance
1	20–30 min. (8–10 mph)	3–5 miles
2	20–30 min. (10–12 mph)	4–6 miles
3	30–45 min. (10–12 mph)	4–8 miles
4	30–60 min. (10–15 mph)	7–15 miles
5	40–75 min. (10–15 mph)	10–18 miles
6	40–90 min. (10–15 mph)	10–22 miles

VARIETY

Part of the appeal of bicycling is being able to explore an area and see things you normally wouldn't notice as you whizzed past in a car. Try cycling to a park, a lake, or a scenic spot or just go exploring on a bicycle. Plan an outing with a picnic or refreshment break halfway. Ride to a nearby small town and back. Plan a bike rally, similar to a car rally with checkpoints, or a bike scavenger hunt in which you gather bits of information from locations (e.g., what is the name of the store at 21 Oak Street?). If you are interested in more alternatives, consult your local bicycle shop for bicycling organizations in your area and find out what rides and tours are planned.

COMMON DISCOMFORTS

Bicyclists beginning a conditioning program often experience a sore crotch the first week or two. As you and your saddle adjust to each other, the syndrome should disappear. Check to see that the seat is not too high. An overly high seat causes you to rock from side to side with each pedal stroke, and the constant rubbing will prolong soreness. It may help to tilt the nose of the saddle down a bit (not so much that you slide off!), to try a different saddle, one with padding under the "sit bones," or to consider padded cycling shorts. See the section "Males and Exercise" in Chapter 7.

Sore knees? A seat that is too low so that your knees are excessively bent throughout the pedal stroke is one cause. Riding with excessive resistance at too low a cadence increases pressure on the knees and is another easily remedied cause. A relatively high cadence against light resistance reduces the frequency of overuse injuries.

If your fingers feel numb after cycling, you need to change hand position more frequently and ride with the elbows slightly bent, not locked. The ulnar nerve runs across the palm, and constant pressure on the hands can temporarily cut off sensation to the area. Wearing padded cycling gloves or cushioning your handlebars with foam grips may also help.

Neck or back soreness usually disappears in a week or so once you grow accustomed to riding. If it does not, try changing hand positions frequently, riding with the elbows slightly bent, moving the seat forward a little, or perhaps switching to upright handlebars.

Do your toes tend to go numb on long rides? If you are using toe clips or clipless pedals, it may be that pedaling tends to push your foot forward into your shoes until your toes touch the end, reducing blood flow to the area. Try lacing your shoes snugly enough so that they hold your foot back in the heel of the shoe but not so tightly that circulation is hindered. Also, try loosening your toe clips or repositioning the cleats on your cycling shoes.

FITNESS SWIMMING

ADVANTAGES/DISADVANTAGES

Swimming is a superb form of exercise. It is a total body workout that uses the major muscle groups of both the upper and lower body. Other forms of aerobic exercise, jogging, for example, use mainly large muscles of the lower body. In addition, water exercise is a natural form of strength training. Resistance of the water against the body's movements enhances muscle strength. Swimmers are also subject to fewer injuries than are participants in many other activities. Joint and muscle injuries are not common among swimmers because of water buoyancy. Water supports the body, alleviating the jarring effects of weight-bearing exercise such as aerobics or jogging. Swimming is ideal for the overweight, the arthritic, the injured, the elderly, and those prone to joint problems.

Another advantage of swimming is that participants rarely experience heat exhaustion and heat stroke. This can be a concern when exercising in hot, humid weather. If you don't like to sweat, you will probably prefer to exercise in water.

Swimming does have drawbacks. You must have some swimming ability and have access to a pool at a time convenient for you. That first plunge into the water may be difficult for some, but after a brief warm-up period, the cool water temperature will be invigorating. Warm water quickly becomes uncomfortable during a vigorous workout.

Although the injury rate is low, you may experience some minor annoyances as you train in water. Eye irritations and "swimmer's ear" are the most common.

The inconvenience of having to redo makeup and hair is minor when you measure the positive outcomes of aquatic exercise. After the workout, an efficient hair and makeup routine develops quickly.

TECHNIQUE AND SAFETY TIPS

Learn to swim the following five basic strokes efficiently: sidestroke, elementary backstroke, breaststroke, back crawl, and front crawl. Incorporate stroke mechanics sessions on these strokes into each workout. The butterfly stroke is too strenuous for most fitness swimmers.

Learn and practice the front crawl and back crawl turns. These will make lap swimming more enjoyable. Construct your daily training program to include a water warm-up, conditioning bout, and water cool-down. Monitor your heart rate (or use the RPE) and do not allow it to exceed your swimming target zone. Use hand paddles, kickboards, pull buoys, and swim fins to increase muscular strength and stroke efficiency. Hyperextension of the lower back (arching) is natural in water exercise. It is important to strengthen the abdominal muscles and always stretch the lower back area to counteract this tendency.

Here are other safety tips:

1. *Never swim alone.* A lifeguard should be present. Safety equipment, such as a ring buoy and a reaching pole, should also be available.
2. *Do not dive into the pool at the shallow end.* The risk is too great. Even experienced swimmers have misjudged the depth of the water and hit the bottom, resulting in serious injuries.
3. *Stay to the right of the lane and make your turns counterclockwise.*
4. *If resting at the pool edge, keep to one side of the lane to allow other swimmers to turn easily.*
5. *Be careful with electrical equipment around the pool* (radios, pace clocks, etc.). Make sure electrical outlets are grounded.
6. *Keep telephone and emergency rescue numbers in the pool area.*
7. *Keep all doors going into the pool area locked unless there is a lifeguard on duty.*

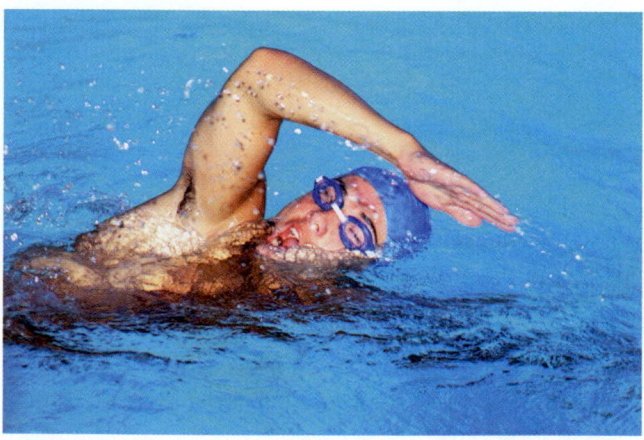

Swimming is one of the best whole-body workouts. It builds heart and lung capacity, tones all major muscles (arms, shoulders, waist, hips, and legs), improves flexibility, and reduces stress.

HOW TO BEGIN AND PROGRESS

Assess your aerobic swimming fitness on the 500-yard swim test as described in Chapter 3. Based on your fitness category, begin at the appropriate starting level in the fitness *S.W.I.M. Program box.* Progress through each level, one step at a time. Do not skip steps and stay on each one as long as necessary to adapt to that workload. Remember to monitor your pulse and do not exceed your swimming target heart rate range. When you have completed level M, you may want to swim continuously for distance or time or continue with the routine of four lengths and a brief rest for the measured distance or time. Keep in mind the THR for swimming is 10 percent less than for weight-bearing activities. You may also use the RPE.

In this program, swim the number of lengths suggested, but if the workout feels too hard, rest a few seconds by climbing out of the pool and walking back to the starting point or rest at the end of the pool for a few seconds before continuing the workout. Swim the front crawl, if possible, or any stroke that allows you to reach the prescribed swimming target heart rate. Consult the pool distance table. Use Lab Activity 4-5 to record your progress.

VARIETY

To add variety to your swimming workouts, practice stroke mechanics on the five basic strokes. This will allow you to use a variety of strokes in your workouts instead of being limited to one or two. Swim for time instead of distance for a change or vice versa. Use equipment: a kickboard is good for practicing kicks and for strengthening your legs; swim fins help you develop leg and abdominal muscles and increase ankle flexibility; hand paddles give your shoulders, chest, arms, and back an extra workout. Webbed gloves or a tethering system add interest to your workouts and improve strength and stroke efficiency. Use a waterproof CD player or digital music player if you find swimming monotonous. For a complete change of pace, try an aquacircuiting or water running session in shallow water or a deep-water jogging workout using some type of flotation device. See the section on water exercise/aqua aerobics later in this chapter.

COMMON DISCOMFORTS

While swimmers are less susceptible to injuries, they may experience a few minor discomforts. Eye irritations are caused by an imbalance in the pH of the water (balance of acidity and alkalinity) or excessive amounts of chlorine. Wear goggles and you will have no problem. Swimmer's ear refers to a

Pool Distance
Most standard pools are 25 yards in length.
One length = 25 yards
One lap = two lengths (50 yards)

18 lengths = 1/4 mile	(approx. 450 yds.)
35 lengths = 1/2 mile	(approx. 875 yds.)
53 lengths = 3/4 mile	(approx. 1325 yds.)
70 lengths = 1 mile	(approx. 1750 yds.)

25 Meter Pools
16 lengths = 1/4 mile (approx. 402.25 m)
32 lengths = 1/2 mile (approx. 804.50 m)
48 lengths = 3/4 mile (approx. 1206.75 m)
64 lengths = 1 mile (approx. 1609 m)

Fitness S.W.I.M. Program

Fitness Category	Starting Level
Low	S
Fair	S
Average	W
Good	I
Superior	M

S.W.I.M. Program

Level S				Level W		
Lengths	Repeats	Distance		Lengths	Repeats	Distance
1	× 4	= 100 yds./m		2	× 4	= 200 yds./m
1	× 6	= 150 yds./m		2	× 5	= 250 yds./m
1	× 8	= 200 yds./m		2	× 6	= 300 yds./m
1	× 10	= 250 yds./m		2	× 7	= 350 yds./m
				2	× 8	= 400 yds./m
				2	× 9	= 450 yds./m
				2	× 10	= 500 yds./m
				2	× 11	= 550 yds./m

Level I				Level M		
Lengths	Repeats	Distance		Lengths	Repeats	Distance
3	× 7	= 525 yds./m		4	× 7	= 700 yds./m
3	× 8	= 600 yds./m		4	× 8	= 800 yds./m
3	× 9	= 675 yds./m		4	× 9	= 900 yds./m
3	× 10	= 750 yds./m		4	× 10	= 1000 yds./m
3	× 11	= 825 yds./m		4	× 11	= 1100 yds./m
3	× 12	= 900 yds./m		4	× 12	= 1200 yds./m
3	× 13	= 975 yds./m				
3	× 14	= 1050 yds./m				

rashlike inflammation of the ear canal that is caused by frequent exposure to moisture. Dry your ears thoroughly with a towel to prevent this nuisance. If you have frequent ear infections, it would be wise to purchase a pair of ear plugs. See a specialist to get a good fit; those purchased over the counter do not fit well enough to keep water out of the ear canal. A few swimmers complain of sore shoulders. A certain amount of soreness is normal during the first weeks of training. But if pain persists, you may be developing tendinitis. Shoulder tendinitis may be caused by an inherent structural shoulder problem, the use of hand paddles, or improper stroke mechanics. See an orthopedic specialist if shoulder pain persists, and use strokes with an underwater recovery (i.e., breaststroke, sidestroke, and elementary backstroke). Some swimmers experience knee pain, especially along the inner borders of the knees, when swimming the breaststroke and elementary backstroke. This is caused by the kick used in these strokes. Do not swim the breaststroke or elementary backstroke until the pain subsides, or avoid them altogether. It is a common myth that you are more susceptible to colds if you participate in aquatic activities, especially during the winter. Colds and respiratory infections are caused by viruses and are spread by contact with infected individuals. You are more likely to catch a cold in a warm, dry, crowded room than in a swimming pool. Another myth is that swimming during menstruation is prohibited. Minor discomfort during this time may be alleviated by exercise. If cramps are severe, use your judgment.

 ## FITNESS WALKING

ADVANTAGES/DISADVANTAGES

Walking is simple, enjoyable, and probably the safest form of aerobic exercise known. It is inexpensive and can be done by almost anyone, anyplace, anytime. There is no need to join a club or find partners or opponents. It is a wise exercise choice for the overweight, the older adult, the very out of shape, the postsurgical patient, and the individual in a cardiac rehabilitation program. Appropriate shoes and comfortable clothes are the only equipment you need.

Studies show that walking generates a downward force of about one and one-half times your body weight, so wearing appropriate shoes is important in helping you progress smoothly and injury-free. A good pair of shoes will help protect your feet, legs, and back. When purchasing new shoes, go to a reputable store and ask for a trained salesperson. Look for shoes with a cushioned heel, a flexible sole, firm heel support, and arch supports that fit your feet. The toe box must provide room for the toes to work to prevent blisters. Try a walking shoe or one made for cross training or jogging, but be sure it fits your foot. The shoe should never feel like it needs to be broken in.

Do you replace your worn-out shoes soon enough? A study at Tulane University found that all shoes, regardless of brand, price, or type of construction, lose most of their shock absorbency after

500 miles of use. This is a good reason for keeping records of your mileage. See Lab Activity 4-5. Take your old shoes with you when shopping for a new pair so that a knowledgeable salesperson can

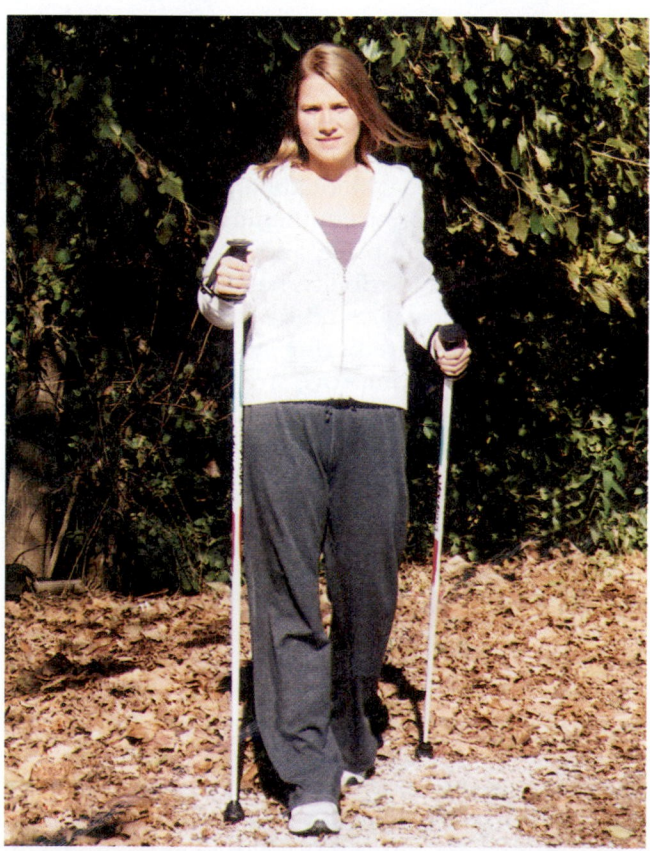

Walking poles safely increase the intensity of a fitness walking workout.

Correct Walking Form

To check your form, have a friend watch you walk, or walk on a treadmill in front of a mirror. Here are the key points for good walking posture.

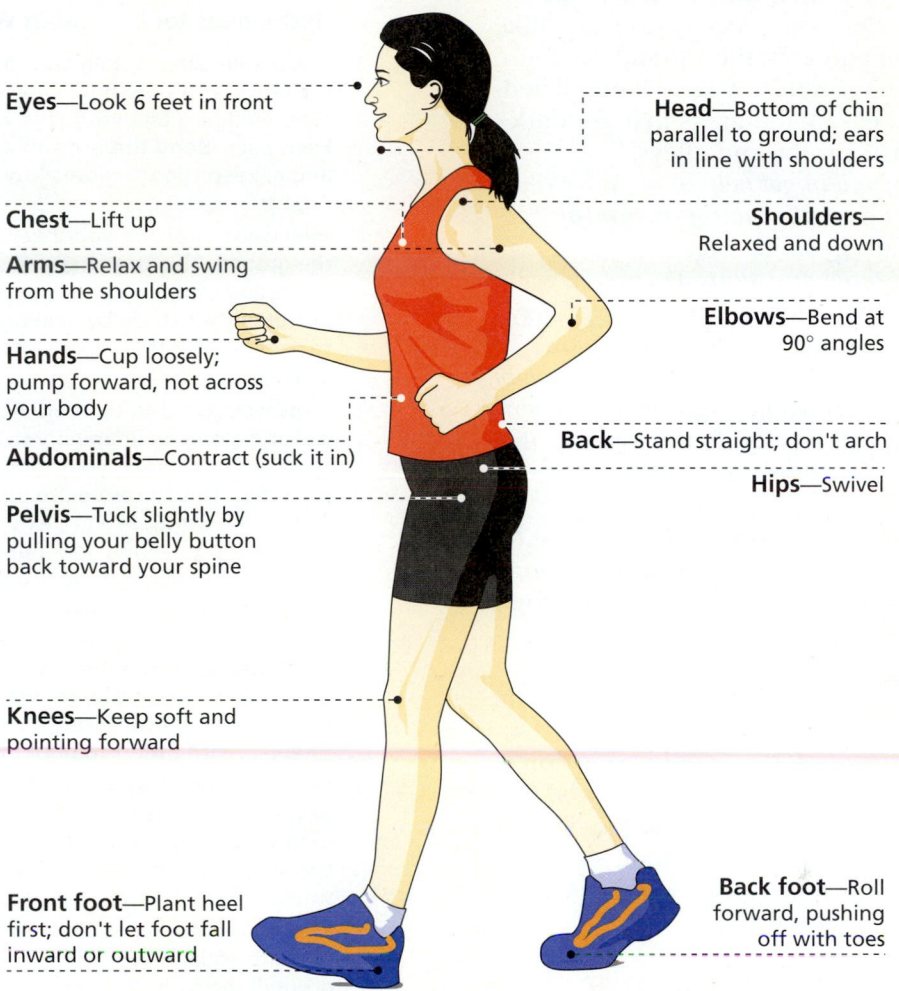

Eyes—Look 6 feet in front

Head—Bottom of chin parallel to ground; ears in line with shoulders

Chest—Lift up

Shoulders—Relaxed and down

Arms—Relax and swing from the shoulders

Elbows—Bend at 90° angles

Hands—Cup loosely; pump forward, not across your body

Abdominals—Contract (suck it in)

Back—Stand straight; don't arch

Hips—Swivel

Pelvis—Tuck slightly by pulling your belly button back toward your spine

Knees—Keep soft and pointing forward

Front foot—Plant heel first; don't let foot fall inward or outward

Back foot—Roll forward, pushing off with toes

Feet—Point toes forward, keeping feet parallel

evaluate the wear pattern to help you choose a suitable shoe.

Walking is excellent for weight control. You use as many calories walking a mile as you would jogging the same distance. The difference is that walking takes longer. Even though the injury rate is low, some walkers who try to increase distance and pace too quickly may experience sore muscles and knees or other types of discomfort. Another disadvantage to walking is that the already physically fit may not be able to elevate the heart rate into the target zone. In this case, try one of the advanced forms of fitness walking, such as power walking (with hand weights or walking poles) or race walking. Dogs and inclement weather present other problems to the walker. Many shopping malls have opened their doors for early morning walking and also to provide a safe, weather-controlled environment year-round.

TECHNIQUE AND SAFETY TIPS

Walking posture is erect but relaxed (see Correct Walking Form). To alleviate tension, the abdomen should be pulled in, the rib cage lifted, and the shoulders pulled down. This will help you keep relaxed and increase your endurance. Your arms should be bent at about a 90-degree angle, and your hands (loose fist) should swing slightly above your waist. Your arms counterbalance your leg motion. You may discover during your walk that your arms have dropped, resulting in a slower pace. Do you ever see joggers with their arms at their sides? Visualize that you are walking in a straight line. Hold your head up with the eyes focused ahead, watching the ground but not your feet. Your foot contact should be a heel roll to the ball of the foot and toes for pushing off. Resist the tendency to lean forward at the waist.

While you are walking, keep in mind these tips for a safe workout:

1. *Always carry some form of identification* (include pertinent medical information).
2. *Choose a safe time and place to exercise.* Take keys with you, and lock the car and/or house.
3. *Plan your route carefully.* Use well-populated, well-lighted areas. Avoid areas that are dark and have dense shrubs and alleys.
4. *Know where you can get help along your route.*
5. *Use sidewalks or walk facing oncoming traffic* and walk in single file.
6. *Obey traffic signals and signs.* Do not jaywalk.
7. *Keep alert at all times.* Give the right-of-way to cars. Don't assume the driver sees you.
8. *Wear bright, reflective clothing at dusk or night.*
9. *Tell someone where you are going and when you think you will return.* Better yet, use the buddy system. It's more fun to walk with someone.
10. *Avoid dogs by selecting routes that are free of them.* The best advice is to ignore a barking dog and never walk between a barking dog and its human, especially if the human is a child.
11. *For the cleanest air, walk in the morning.* The air is more polluted at midday or later.
12. *Don't wear a headset;* you would be losing one of your most valuable sensory aids. If you wear a headset, keep volume low so that you can hear traffic or approaching strangers.
13. *Avoid peak traffic hours* unless you can use a jogging path or a sidewalk.

TIPS FOR INCREASING WALKING PACE

What is your current walking pace? If you do not know, here is how you can measure your effort. Go to a quarter-mile track or measure 1 mile on a road with your car odometer. Time yourself walking for 1 mile. If it takes you 20 minutes, you are walking at 3 mph; if it takes you 17 minutes, you are walking at 3.5 mph; if it takes you 15 minutes, you are walking a 4 mph pace; if it takes you about 13 minutes, you are walking at a 4.5 mph pace; if you do it in 12 minutes, you have reached a 5 mph pace. You can also calculate your speed by counting how many steps you take in 1 minute:

✓ 115 steps = 2.5–3.5 mph
✓ 125 steps = 3.0–4.0 mph
✓ 135 steps = 3.5–4.5 mph
✓ 150 steps = 5.0 mph

If you would like to increase your fitness walking pace, try the Top 10 "Techniques for Increasing Walking Pace."

TOP 10 LIST

Techniques for Increasing Walking Pace

1. *Pump your arms.* When your arms drag, the tendency is to slow down. Resist this. Keep your arms pumping and your legs will be forced to keep pace. Bend the arms to a full 90-degree angle; keep the shoulders low and relaxed (not raised).

2. *Heel walks.* Walk on your heels, with your toes off the ground. This stretches and strengthens your calves and especially your shins, training that puts power in your stride by helping you develop a stronger push-off and prevents the development of shin splints.

3. *Crossovers.* On a track, road, or sidewalk, practice walking along an imaginary straight line. Engage your hips by crossing your foot across the line with each step. This forces you to adopt the signature race-walking wiggle. Plus, extending your legs from your hips allows your pelvis to rotate forward so you can cover more ground with each step without overstriding.

4. *Use interval training.* Walk as fast as you can for 1 minute, then slow the pace for 4 minutes. Gradually increase the intervals by 1 minute every 2 weeks until you can do intense 4-minute intervals with only 1 minute at the slower pace.

5. *Simultaneously begin using the hard/easy system of training.* Go hard one day—either by taking a long walk or by doing intervals or hills—and easy the next. Practice at least 2 training days per week.

6. *Streamline your form.* Alter your strike to a straight-leg landing. When your heel touches the ground, the front leg should be straight. Your forefoot is flexed momentarily to land on the heel rather than the sole of the foot.

7. *Set "walk-to" targets.* Set a "walk-to" target a short distance in front of you (about 30 yards). Walk quickly to the target, reset the target, and walk fast to the new target. Keep resetting the walk-to targets throughout the route. Use mailboxes, driveways, road signs, and trees for targets. This technique helps keep you mentally involved in your fitness walking workout and helps you resist the tendency to stroll.

8. *Add bends and straightaways.* On a track, warm up for 10 minutes and then go your fastest on the straightaways, using the curves for slow recovery walks. Start with 6 to 8 laps, building to 15.

9. *Count steps.* Accelerate 100 steps five times in 30 minutes. This will teach your legs to move faster.

10. *Don't overdo it.* Limit speed workouts to twice a week so that sore muscles won't sideline you for the next day's walk.

Carrying hand weights and using walking poles, Powerbelts, and the like while fitness walking will increase the intensity of your workouts. Pumping your arms will accomplish the same effects. While the majority of healthy men and women can achieve a training heart rate with unaided walking, there are some people who may be too fit to achieve this threshold (e.g., young college students). Research shows that adding external weight to the body or involving the upper extremities during exercise can increase the intensity of walking.

For people who want to increase the overall intensity of their workout or make walking more of a total body workout, there are a variety of reasonably priced adjuncts to consider, such as weighted belts, gloves, vests, and walking poles (a.k.a. Nordic walking). They are safe and effective and can increase CRE and weight control benefits of a regular walking program. See Table 4-4.

When using the walking equipment described in Table 4-5, be aware that 50 to 70 percent of the increase in oxygen consumption and caloric expenditure comes from swinging the arms to a greater degree. In one study, for example, participants walked on a treadmill at 3.0 mph, VO_{2max} was 15.9 ml/kg/min. Walking at the same speed while swinging the arms to chin height required 17.8 ml/kg/min. The addition of 2-pound weights further increased the oxygen cost to 18.9 ml/kg/min. Thus 63 percent of the increase above normal walking was attributed to the exaggerated arm swing. Swinging the arms may serve as a good intermediate step for increasing walking intensity without being encumbered with extra equipment.

TABLE 4-4   *Pros and Cons of Walking Equipment*

Walking Equipment	Pros	Cons
Weighted Vests	• Form-fitting • Comfortable	• Minimal aerobic benefit • Expensive (compared with other equipment)
Wrist/Hand Weights	• Inexpensive • Easy to use • Moderate increase in intensity	• May elicit exaggerated blood pressure responses • No place to put the weight if you get tired • May increase incidence of overuse injuries
Walking Poles	• Excellent increases in intensity/caloric expenditure/VO_2 • Upper-body muscular endurance increases • Puts less stress on knees	• May elicit a pressor response due to gripping poles • Not adjustable; different height people need different poles • No place to put poles if you get tired
Powerbelts	• Excellent potential aerobic benefit • May increase muscular strength • Good for interval training • Resistance cords retract when not in use	• Higher levels may be too difficult to maintain • May elicit exaggerated blood pressure responses due to high degree of muscular effort

TABLE 4-5   *Heart Rate Increase, Oxygen Consumption, and Calorie Expenditures of Various Walking Equipment*

Walking Equipment	Heart Rate Increases (bpm)	Oxygen Consumption (ml/kg/min)	Calorie Expenditures (% of increase)
Weighted Vests (5–10% of Body Wt)	3–7	1.3–2.5	3–10
Hand Weights/Weighted Gloves (1–3 lb.)	6–13	1.5–4.0	5–15
Walking Poles	10–15	4.5–5.5	20–25
Powerbelts			
Base unit	25–30	6.3–6.7	40–45
Powerpack 1	30–35	6.7–7.0	45–50
Powerpack 2	35–40	7.0–8.0	50–60
Powerpack 3	40–45	8.0–9.5	60–65

W.A.L.K.S. Program

Fitness Category	Starting Program
Low	W Level
Fair	A Level
Average	L Level
Good	K Level
Superior	S Level

W Level

Week	1–2	3–4	5–6	7–8	9–10	11–12	13–14
Warm-up (min.)	5–10	5–10	5–10	5–10	5–10	5–10	5–10
Conditioning bout (mileage)	1.00	1.25	1.50	1.75	2.00	2.25	2.50
Intensity % (target heart rate)	60–80	60–80	60–80	60–80	60–80	60–80	60–80
Cool-down (min.)	5–10	5–10	5–10	5–10	5–10	5–10	5–10
Frequency	3	3	3	3	4	4	4

A Level

Week	1–2	3–4	5–6	7–8	9–10	11–12	13–14
Warm-up (min.)	5–10	5–10	5–10	5–10	5–10	5–10	5–10
Conditioning bout (mileage)	2.00	2.25	2.50	2.75	3.00	3.25	3.50
Intensity % (target heart rate)	60–80	60–80	60–80	60–80	60–80	60–80	60–80
Cool-down (min.)	5–10	5–10	5–10	5–10	5–10	5–10	5–10
Frequency	3	3	3	4	4	4	4

L Level

Week	1–2	3–4	5–6	7–8	9–10	11–12	13–14
Warm-up (min.)	5–10	5–10	5–10	5–10	5–10	5–10	5–10
Conditioning bout (mileage)	3.00	3.25	3.50	3.70	3.75	4.00	
Intensity % (target heart rate)	60–80	60–80	60–80	60–80	60–80	60–80	60–80
Cool-down (min.)	5–10	5–10	5–10	5–10	5–10	5–10	5–10
Frequency	3	3	4	4	4	4	4

K Level

Week	1–2	3–4	5–6	7–8	9–10	11–12	13–14
Warm-up (min.)	5–10	5–10	5–10	5–10	5–10	5–10	5–10
Conditioning bout (mileage)	3.50	3.75	3.75	4.00	4.00	4.00	4.00
Intensity % (target heart rate)	60–80	60–80	60–80	60–80	60–80	60–80	60–80
Cool-down (min.)	5–10	5–10	5–10	5–10	5–10	5–10	5–10
Frequency	4	4	4	4	5	5	5

S Level

Week	1–2	3–4	5–6	7–8	9–10	11–12	13–14
Warm-up (min.)	5–10	5–10	5–10	5–10	5–10	5–10	5–10
Conditioning bout (mileage)	4.00	4.00	4.00	4.25	4.25	4.50	4.50
Intensity % (target heart rate)	60–80	60–80	60–80	60–80	60–80	60–80	60–80
Cool-down (min.)	5–10	5–10	5–10	5–10	5–10	5–10	5–10
Frequency	5	5	5	5	5	5	5

W.A.L.K.S. Maintenance Program (for a lifetime of fitness)

Warm-up:	5–10 min.
Conditioning bout:	3–5 miles per workout
Intensity %:	60–80
Cool-down:	5–10 min.
Frequency:	3–5 times per week
Weekly mileage:	9–25 miles

HOW TO BEGIN AND PROGRESS

Test your fitness using the 1-mile walk test described in Chapter 3. Then follow the appropriate level on the *W.A.L.K.S. Program box*. After completing the "S" level, continue on the W.A.L.K.S. Maintenance Program for a lifetime of fitness.

Warm up for 5 to 10 minutes before starting the conditioning segment of your workout. The warm-up should be activity-specific, so for fitness walking begin gradually increasing the pace to that at your conditioning level. During the conditioning bout, always check your heart rate to be sure it stays within the target zone. Also use the RPE or talk test. Listen to your body, and progress slowly for optimal results.

Cool down for 5 to 10 minutes after the conditioning bout. As in the warm-up, the cool-down should be activity-specific. Thus, reduce your pace, finishing with 5 to 10 minutes of slow walking.

For total fitness, stretch for flexibility. Improved flexibility is best achieved if it occurs at the end of the cool-down, when the muscles and joints are thoroughly warmed and pliable. Use flexibility exercises for your stretching routine.

Take each step on the chart and don't skip ahead. If the increase is too difficult, go back to the preceding level for a while. You should feel energized after your workout, not exhausted. Use Lab Activity 4-5 to record your progress.

VARIETY

Adding variety to your walking workouts can keep you enthused about the activity for many years.

Varying your walking routes gives you a change of scenery. Drive the car to a new area, park, and explore the surroundings during your workout. Mailing a letter, walking an errand, taking window shopping walks, and doing shopping mall workouts can be fun. Walk with a friend, in a group, or by yourself for a change. Dogs are excellent walking companions. For a challenge, try an advanced exercise walking technique such as race walking, power walking, hill walking, or walking a fitness trail. Participate in a volksmarch, a competitive walking event, or join a Hashing Club (described in the Jogging section). Water walking (walking in waist-deep water) is popular in many areas; give it a try. Some people enjoy listening to music while exercising in a traffic-free area. Schedule walking meetings with coworkers. Train for a half-marathon (mini); see sample training program in the Jogging section. Try "Exercise Across the U.S.A." (Lab Activity 4-3) for added incentives to keep walking. You won't become stale or bored with exercise if you vary your workouts.

COMMON DISCOMFORTS

As in running, most aches, pains, and injuries from walking occur from overuse. Listen to your body. Don't attempt to work through an injury. It will only aggravate the condition. The two most common walking complaints are shin splints and back-of-the-knee soreness. Refer to Chapter 8 for information about shin splints. Cut back on pace and distance until soreness subsides. Comfortable, well-fitting shoes will help prevent blisters. Consult a sports podiatrist if you suffer from foot problems such as calluses, bunions, heel spurs, ingrown toenails, high arches, flat feet, and an overly pronated foot. These conditions can be remedied, but if not corrected, they may prevent you from fully enjoying your walking program.

INDOOR EXERCISE EQUIPMENT

(Including Stationary Bikes, Steppers, Treadmills, Rowing Machines, and Elliptical Trainers)

ADVANTAGES/DISADVANTAGES

When winter's plummeting temperatures, ice, snow, and chilly winds make outdoor exercise difficult, indoor exercise equipment may be for you. If it is too rainy, too hot, too dark, or unsafe to exercise outside, you can work out in the relative comfort and safety of a health club or your home. Indoor exercise equipment allows you to alternate indoor and outdoor workouts according to the weather, your schedule, and your mood. Be aware: The "calories expended" feature on most cardioexercise machines is not accurate.

Indoor workouts can be done on either your equipment at home or equipment in a health club. If you like working out with others, don't want to deal with equipment maintenance, and enjoy a variety of different types of exercise, a health club is a good place to start. At a club, you can try different types of equipment—bicycles, steppers, treadmills, rowers, and elliptical trainers—and see what you like best. If you can't seem to make time to get to the health club, with exercise equipment at home you don't have to go anywhere. You can exercise before or after work, be with your family, and read or watch TV at the same time. If you have children, you can keep an eye on them and won't have to hire a sitter while you work out. The main advantage to working out at home is the convenience.

Disadvantages of home exercise equipment are that you have to decide what type of equipment and features you want, purchase it, make room for it in your house, perform your own maintenance, and find someone to repair it (or fix it yourself) if it breaks. You will probably be working out alone and may get bored with the same workout day after day. Also, if your enthusiasm wanes, the equipment may become a constant reminder of failed resolutions. However, working out in private is very appealing to many people. You know who used the equipment last, and for what you pay for a 1-year club membership, you can have your own equipment at home.

Advantages of working out at a health club include that you can switch from one type of equipment to another to avoid boredom or work different muscle groups; you can meet a lot of people; professionals are readily available to answer your questions; you don't have to buy, maintain, and repair the equipment; and you don't have to make space at home for it year-round.

Disadvantages of working out at a health club include that you will have to pay membership fees, schedule it in your day, have transportation, and at popular workout times possibly wait to get on some equipment.

EQUIPMENT

Equipment comes in two main types: aerobic and strength machines. Strength training information is covered in Chapter 6. This section focuses on aerobic equipment. Indoor exercise equipment need not be expensive. A jump rope, an exercise mat, elastic resistance bands, a step or a slide mat, and an aerobics video are low-budget. More costly exercise machines include steppers, climbers, treadmills, exercise bicycles, rowers, and elliptical trainers.

If you would like to work out at home and are not familiar with the variety of equipment available, join a health club for a 1- to 3-month trial period to try out and compare the different types. Then you will know what type of equipment you want to purchase and will be more familiar with the features available. Shop informed. Ask friends and family about equipment and features they like.

Be choosy. Avoid cheap equipment, which may be flimsy, noisy, unstable, or jerky and can make the whole workout experience so unpleasant that you'll soon use the machine as a coat rack. Shop for well-designed exercise equipment from a specialty retailer rather than from a TV infomercial or chain department store. The quality and durability will be worth the cost in terms of ease of use and maintenance. Think compact. Unless you have a lot of space, you probably will not want equipment that takes up a whole room. Steppers and exercise bicycles have the smallest "footprint" and are easily moved to the side when not being used. Think simple. Not much can go wrong with a jump rope, but plenty can go wrong with a flimsy treadmill. The more complicated a piece of equipment is to use and adjust, the more maintenance it needs.

Before you invest in home exercise equipment, try out several models and ask these questions:

1. How much will I use this? Do I enjoy this type of exercise?
2. Does the sales staff ask about my needs and fitness goals before helping me select equipment, or do they automatically recommend the most expensive machine?
3. Does it have the features I want?
4. Is it easy to assemble?
5. If it breaks, how will I get it repaired? Can it be fixed locally?
6. What kind of warranty comes with it? What is the store's return policy?
7. Is it well constructed of steel or alloy to last 10 or more years?
8. What kind of maintenance is needed, according to the manual?
9. Are the seats and grips comfortable, durable, and easily adjustable?
10. Does it work smoothly? How stable is it? Is it relatively quiet? Is it safe?
11. Where will I put it? How much space does it require?
12. Does the manual show how to use the equipment correctly and how to reach my target heart rate?
13. Do I need all the fancy gadgets, or will a more simple model do?
14. Can I get a workout with this machine that is intense enough for my current and future fitness levels?

Stationary Bikes

ADVANTAGES/DISADVANTAGES

Most models work the lower body—primarily legs, hips, and buttocks—but some models have handlebars for exercising arms and shoulders. Some of the more expensive electronic models have programmed workouts such as interval training or hills to add variety. Upright models make efficient use of space, and you can read or watch TV as you exercise. They give you a good nonimpact workout that is easier on the joints than treadmills are. They are particularly good for overweight people who need to avoid extra stress on the back, knees, and ankles. Both upright and recumbent models are effective. Recumbent bikes, in which you sit back on a seat and pedal in front of the body, tend to be more expensive and need at least 6 to 7 feet of space but are easier on the back. Bicycle trainers, which put your regular bicycle on a stand with resistance to the rear wheel, require balance but are less expensive than stationary bicycles.

HOW TO SELECT

A good machine is easy to adjust, moves smoothly, and feels stable. The seat should be comfortable and should adjust to your height. In many models, handlebars are also adjustable. The controls should be within easy reach, and the workload should adjust smoothly and easily. Look for a smooth, quiet ride; a sturdy frame; a wide, comfortable, adjustable seat; and an easy-to-read instrument panel. Cheaper models are made of flimsier metal; the resistance mechanism may be grabby, the seat less comfortable, and the whole device more "tippy."

TECHNIQUE AND SAFETY TIPS

Proper seat height and pedaling cadence are the keys to avoiding knee problems. Seat height should be adjusted so that when you sit on the seat, your knee is almost fully extended on the downstroke. Also, keep the resistance moderate so that you maintain a cadence of about 60 to 100 rpm. Racers cycle at 80 to 100 rpm.

Steppers

ADVANTAGES/DISADVANTAGES

Steppers primarily work the legs, hips, and buttocks and do not work the upper body. They take relatively little space and allow you to read or watch TV as you exercise. They may aggravate some knee problems. They tend to work the calves more than other types of equipment do.

HOW TO SELECT

Steppers come with either dependent or independent pedals. With dependent pedals, as one goes down, the other goes up. The machine does some of the work for you because you are exercising one foot at a time. Independent pedal models, in which both feet have to be working at the same time, take a little more work to get the rhythm and coordination but give you a better workout. Hydraulic resistance mechanisms provide a fluid feel at an affordable price. High-end models have computerized interval resistance programs that can increase and decrease the workload through the exercise bout. Self-leveling pedals are a nice feature. Make sure pedals are big enough for you to balance on them comfortably. Some also come with poles for working the arms. Less expensive models are manually adjustable, so if you want to change resistance in the middle of a workout, you will have to get off and turn knobs or slide levers. They still give you a good workout, however, and so the lower price may be worth the minor inconvenience.

TECHNIQUE AND SAFETY TIPS

Rest your hands lightly on the handlebars or railings for balance and take small steps at first. Stand tall and gradually begin to take deeper steps after you warm up. Do not lean on the railings because you will decrease the effectiveness of the workout.

Treadmills

ADVANTAGES/DISADVANTAGES

Treadmills are popular and easy to use, giving you a good cardiovascular and lower-body workout. They also tend to be used more than other types of equipment. However, they are noisy and more prone to breakdowns than other types of equipment. They also require a large space, about 6 by 4 feet, though you can purchase models that fold for storage. See Lab Activity 4-6 on the book's Web site for sample workouts.

HOW TO SELECT

✓ A motorized treadmill should have at least a 1.5-horsepower continuous-duty motor to be strong enough to maintain even speed. Two horsepower is even better.

✓ It should have a running belt that is at least 20 to 24 inches wide and a length of at least 48 inches.

✓ Look for a machine that will reach a top speed of at least 9 miles per hour. Even if you don't walk/run at this speed, higher speeds are useful for interval training.

✓ Ability to simulate at least a 10 percent incline is important for you to always be able to reach your target pulse.

✓ Look for a safety lock so a child cannot accidentally start the treadmill and an emergency shut-off button to cut power immediately.

✓ You need at least one handrail, preferably two for balance, and wide footrails. Also look for a wide 2-ply rubber belt for durability on the running surface and some flexibility so that it gives a little with each stride.

Decide if you want a motorized or hand-crank incline and what other computerized features you desire, such as heart rate or calorie counting. Less expensive machines tend to have a shorter, narrower bed, lower horsepower, a faster starting speed, a lower top speed, a less durable 1-ply belt, and fewer computerized features. They are also noisier, wear out faster, and may not keep the belt speed as consistent as the higher-end models do.

Nonmotorized treadmills are cheaper but move only with the pull of your feet on the belt, and they slow down if you do. They are better for walking than for running and may be harder on the joints than motorized treadmills, which move continuously at a preset speed.

Investigate the warranty. Ask what's covered in the agreement, including parts and labor; who will service the treadmill; and length of coverage (average is 3 years).

TECHNIQUE AND SAFETY TIPS

Start the machine at a slow pace. Straddle the belt, step with one foot a few times to get a feel for the speed, and then begin. Increase to normal speed as you warm up. Keep near the front of the belt at all times.

Rowing Machines

ADVANTAGES/DISADVANTAGES

Rowers provide an excellent upper- as well as lower-body workout, toning the shoulders, back, arms, and legs. They do, however, require a lot of space, up to 8 feet by 3 feet. They can also be noisy, and you cannot read while working out.

HOW TO SELECT

They come in piston and flywheel models. The piston models are cheaper and more compact, but flywheel models have smoother action. Some models give strokes per minute, total distance, time, and power output per stroke.

TECHNIQUE AND SAFETY TIPS

Correct rowing technique takes practice to master and is important to avoid back injury. Do not lean into the pull but keep upright throughout the range of motion. Your legs, arms, and shoulders, not your back, should do much of the work, and your arms should move forward before you bend your knees. With a flywheel model, pull the bar into your abdomen, not your chin. The workout can be intense.

Elliptical Trainers

ADVANTAGES/DISADVANTAGES

This machine simulates a combination of walking, running, and stair climbing in one motion. The workout is weight-bearing, but there is none of the jarring impact that occurs when you are exercising on pavement, a track, or a treadmill. The motion is even smoother than that of step machines. Physical therapists and athletic trainers love these machines because they allow athletes to continue their training regimen even while rehabilitating an overuse injury, such as Achilles tendinitis, runner's knee, shin splints, and even a stress fracture. Elliptical trainers offer the cardiorespiratory endurance and muscular benefits of running as well as a refuge from nature's wrath and the dangers of dodging traffic.

Like all exercise machines, elliptical trainers have some drawbacks, though they are minimal. Because the muscles do not have to adjust for landing on the ground with each stride as they do with actual running, the overall muscle action (and thus, the overall workout) is not quite as intense on an elliptical trainer. The estimated overall workout benefit on an elliptical trainer is anywhere from 75 to 90 percent of that of a running workout. Ellipticals require minimal use of the arms and shoulders, and so they do not offer a total body workout. Elliptical trainers with arm-pole attachments reduce this drawback.

Ellipticals tend to be rather large machines, so they do not offer the mobility and ease of storage offered by some other indoor exercise machines.

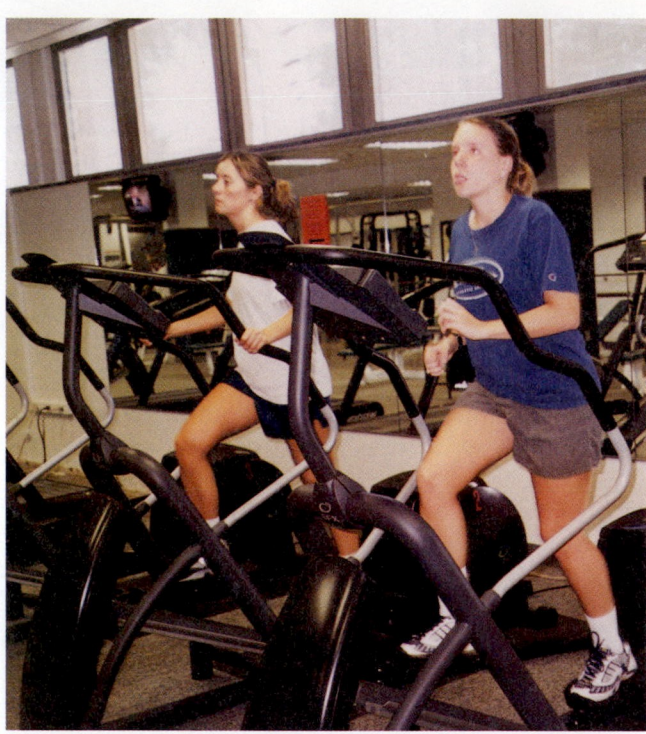

You will burn more calories if you let go of the handrails of treadmills and elliptical trainers and swing your arms.

Cost may be a drawback unless you can comfortably afford the $300 to $3,000 (health club model) price tag. Keep in mind that you get what you pay for.

HOW TO SELECT

The elliptical trainer you select should have tension control that allows you to adjust and vary the resistance against the running ramps. The ramp elevation option on some machines is nice but not essential. You can get the same effect by running faster and/or adjusting the ramp resistance control to a higher tension setting. You may select a machine with arm poles similar to those on cross-country ski machines, thus allowing you to use them for an upper-body workout. These are nice but not essential.

Experts recommend selecting a machine that has a readout screen that shows information such as calories burned, time and distance run, and strides per minute.

A final piece of advice if you plan on buying an elliptical trainer: Try out a number of models before making a final decision.

TECHNIQUE AND SAFETY TIPS

When you exercise on an elliptical trainer, you stand on two platforms, or ramps, "suspended" between wheel-gear and roller mechanisms. When you move your legs in a running motion, one ramp moves forward and slightly upward while the other ramp moves backward and slightly downward. You will leave your arms free (as in running) or hold on to the handrails on the side of the machine.

Stand upright. Elliptical trainers can put pressure on the lower back if you lean forward or lean on the handrails while exercising. If you feel low back discomfort during or after the workout, check your posture. Feet that are too far apart can cause the hips to shift excessively, putting strain on the lumbar region. To stabilize, bring your feet closer together on the pedals.

HOW TO BEGIN AND PROGRESS

Consult your owner's manual for guidelines on how to begin and progress. In general, treadmills and stationary bikes have the quickest learning curves, and steppers run third. Rowers require more balance and skill. But, for the time invested in the rower, you can get a better upper-body workout along with aerobic fitness, and so the time is well spent. Also, the rule of specificity applies, so if you are in great running shape but begin working out on a stepper or cycle, give yourself some time to build up to the same level of intensity and duration. If you are a beginner, start with 5 to 10 minutes, low intensity, 3 days the first week to get a feel for correct mechanics and how to use the equipment. Increase the workout by a couple of minutes each week. Pace your progress according to how you feel during and after the workout. If you feel tired and washed out, you are trying to progress too quickly and need to move back or maintain the same level until your endurance increases. If you feel good, you can continue to add a couple of minutes a week to each workout until you reach 20 to 30 minutes of continuous activity. To increase frequency, add an additional day each month until you are exercising up to 5 days a week at your target pulse. Use Lab Activity 4-5 to record your progress. A suggested workout schedule follows:

Sample Beginning Program

Week	1–2	3–4	5–6	7–8	9–10	11–15
Warm-up (min.)	5–10	5–10	5–10	5–10	5–10	5–10
Conditioning bout (min.)	5–10	8–14	12–18	17–22	21–26	25–30
Intensity (target heart rate)	50–60	60–80	60–80	60–80	60–80	60–80
Cool-down (min.)	5–10	5–10	5–10	5–10	5–10	5–10
Frequency	3	3	3	3–4	3–4	3–5

IN-LINE SKATING

ADVANTAGES/DISADVANTAGES

Modern skating has gone in-line. Instead of four wheels situated in box formation under the skate, the new skating gear has four urethane wheels positioned down the center of a supportive boot complete with brake pads. Skaters also need protective pads and a helmet to lower injury risk, which can be substantial.

Ice hockey players in Minnesota designed the first prototype for today's in-line skates. They enjoyed their dryland workouts so much that they began skating out of season for fun! The popularity of in-line skating exploded in the 1990s primarily because it is so easy to learn and convenient. People are no longer intimidated by the misconception that only the super-coordinated can skate on a single row of wheels.

In-line skating can be a competitive sport involving speed or fancy tricks, known as freestyle skating. Other sports, such as basketball and hockey, can be played on in-line skates, and skiers may cross train on in-line skates in the off-season. But the majority of in-line skaters do it primarily for fitness, recreational, social, or transportation purposes. Thirty-five percent of in-line skaters report using skates as a mode of transportation.

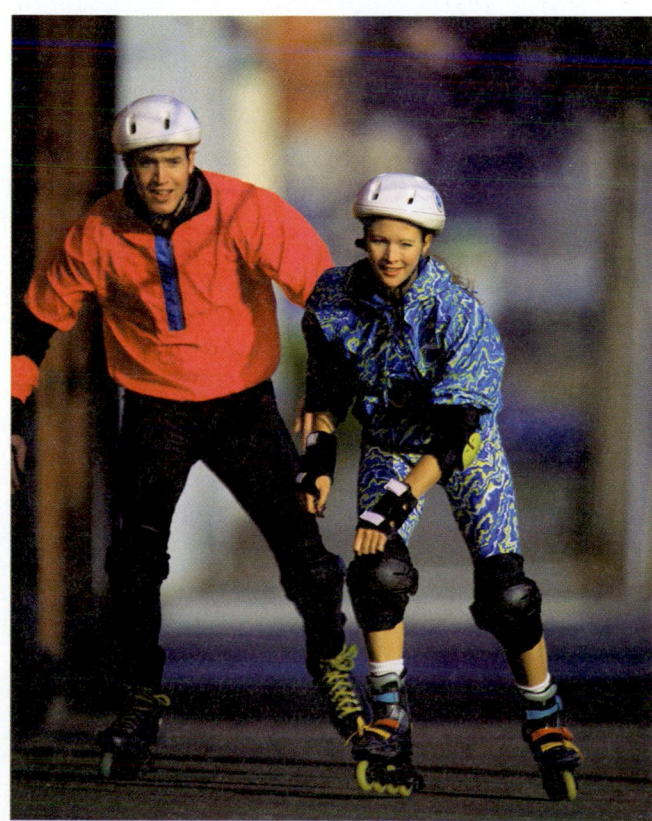

Wear protective gear every time you skate.

In-line skating has excellent potential for developing physical fitness, especially cardiorespiratory endurance and muscular endurance, plus it is invigoratingly fun. Vigorous and continuous striding can burn as many calories as jogging or cycling does. Skating is one of the best activities for improving balance and is ideal for cross training for any fitness activity. Serious skating increases muscular strength and endurance. It strengthens the musculature in the entire upper leg, including the hamstrings and quadriceps as well as the buttocks, hips, and lower back muscles. If you swing and pump the arms vigorously during skating, the biceps, triceps, and shoulder muscles can be strengthened and toned.

In-line skaters reap all the benefits of other forms of exercise: improved physical fitness; increased energy levels; lower blood pressure; weight control; relaxation; and a reduced risk of cancer, heart disease, and stroke. Physiological responses measured during in-line skating indicate that individuals with average fitness levels can achieve appropriate exercise training effect on flat terrain, although the highly fit may need to skate uphill or skate fast to achieve the same benefit.

In-line skating does have a few drawbacks. This fun, aerobic, low-impact sport can be dangerous to skaters who don't wear helmets and protective pads or who do not learn safe starting and stopping techniques. If you have a fear of falling, suffer from osteoporosis, or have balance problems, in-line skating is not a good exercise choice. Another disadvantage with in-line skating is cost. In-line skates and the necessary safety gear can be expensive.

NECESSARY GEAR

✓ *Skates:* Good in-line skates are not cheap. Expect to pay $100 to $400. The rule to follow is to buy the best possible skates you can afford. Originally, the skate boot was made from molded polyurethane, a lightweight but extremely sturdy material. But since 1994, the soft-boot in-line design skate boot has been the industry standard. The new boot fits like a hiking boot instead of a plastic ski boot. The fit should not be too tight or too loose. It should be flexible from the ankle up. It should allow some room for the toes (about one-fourth inch from the end of the longest toe to the end of the boot). In-line boots use laces, buckles, Velcro straps, or a combination of laces and buckles to tighten and secure the boot. The most effective and popular style is a boot that laces on the lower part and buckles on the ankle for maximum support. Boots with vents

to allow liberal air circulation are recommended. A foam liner, either built into the skate or an insert purchased separately, provides added comfort and helps prevent blisters. Look for liners with vents to aid breathability.

✓ *Helmet:* Select a helmet that provides a snug, comfortable fit. Look for approval by the two national helmet testing bodies, SNELL and ANSI.

✓ *Wrist Guards:* This is a fingerless glove with a hard plastic splint running down the front. The plastic is curved slightly—not enough to hinder wrist and hand movement but enough to act as a shock absorber in the event of a fall.

✓ *Knee and Elbow Pads:* These are designed to prevent scrapes and bruises. Use only the style that has a hard plastic shield over the pad. Do not use cloth-covered pads from other sports, such as volleyball.

TECHNIQUES AND SAFETY TIPS

Taking a few in-line skating lessons and studying an instructional video are the recommended methods for learning this sport. It is imperative to practice the following basic skills before you take to the street or trails: ready position, forward fall, forward stride and glide, basic turning, braking, and making emergency stops. Find a conveniently located paved area where you can go often to practice. It must be smooth and level with enough room to move about unobstructed. Empty parking lots and unused ball courts are ideal if they are free of pedestrians, debris, and bike traffic. Avoid hills until your skills are proficient. Table 4-6 lists some safety guidelines you need to follow.

TABLE 4–6 *Safety Guidelines for In-Line Skating*
1. Always wear full protective gear.
2. Achieve a basic skating level before taking to the road. Practice basic skills on a smooth, flat surface away from traffic.
3. Stay alert and courteous at all times.
4. Always skate under control.
5. Skate on the right side of paths, trails, and sidewalks.
6. Overtake pedestrians, cyclists, and other skaters on the left. Announce your intentions by saying, "Passing on your left."
7. Avoid water, oil, or debris on the trail and uneven, broken pavement.
8. Obey all traffic regulations.
9. Avoid areas with heavy automotive traffic.
10. Always yield to pedestrians.
11. Keep your gear in proper working order.

SKATE MAINTENANCE

In-line skates are relatively low-maintenance; that is one of the inviting aspects of the sport. You can put on your skates and get a good workout without much setup or cleanup time. However, your skates will need occasional attention.

Tools It's a good idea to put together a skate repair kit that can be carried in your skate bag. Be sure to choose components and tools that fit your particular model of skate. Your local skate shop can help you with the selection of components and tools.

Wheel Rotation or Replacement The most common maintenance activity is rotation of the wheels. Wheels wear down while skating; therefore, to get maximum mileage proper rotation is necessary. Rotation is changing the position of the wheels on the frame and turning the wheels over so the inside edges become the outside edges. To rotate your wheels, follow these directions:

Wheel in Position	Move to Position
1	3
2	4
3	1
4	2

Bearing Replacement Bearings allow the wheels to spin smoothly and have the greatest effect on the performance of the skate. Buy the best bearings you can afford. Each skate has two sets of bearings, one on each side of the wheel. ABEC bearings range from 1 to 7, with 1 creating the least amount of speed and 7 the greatest amount of speed. Fitness/recreation skaters usually use ABEC 3 bearings.

Brake Replacement Brakes should be replaced when you have to lift your toe too high to be stable when stopping or when the bolt holding the brake in place begins to rub the ground. Loosen the bolt, remove the brake, and attach the new brake.

HOW TO BEGIN AND PROGRESS

First, assess your fitness level by using the 1.5-mile timed run test described in Chapter 3. Remember that your current fitness level does not indicate your potential. Based on your fitness category, begin at the appropriate starting level in *In-Line Skating Program box*. Progress through each level, one step at a time. Do not skip steps, and stay on each as long as necessary to adapt to that workload. Remember to monitor your pulse, and do not exceed your target heart rate range. Or, if you prefer, use the RPE to monitor your intensity level during the workout. Keep in mind the FITT prescription factors.

Don't forget to warm up and cool down during each workout. To develop balanced fitness add 25 to 30 push-ups, 1 minute of abdominal curls, and 5 to 15 minutes of stretching per workout. Use Lab Activity 4-5 to record your progress.

In-Line Skating Program

Fitness Category	Starting Level
Low	1 or 2
Fair	3
Average	4
Good	5
Superior	6

Level	Skating
1	10–15 min.
2	10–20 min.
3	15–25 min.
4	20–40 min.
5	30–45 min.
6	45–75 min.

VARIETY

Adding variety to your skating workouts can keep you enthused about the sport for many years. Varying your skating routes gives you a change of scenery. Drive the car to a new area, park, and explore the area. Find new trails, paths, sidewalks, and parking lots on which to skate. Use your skates for transportation to and from school or work several days a week. Keep your skates in the trunk of the car and strap them on for a spontaneous workout when you see an opportunity (e.g., at lunchtime). Be sociable; skate with a friend or join a skating club. Pack a backpack with a water bottle and a snack for a longer than usual workout. Try speed skating, amateur racing, or freestyle or artistic skating, which is similar to ice figure skating. Extreme skating involves tricks, jumps, and ramps that might appeal to you. You won't become bored with exercise if you vary your workouts.

COMMON DISCOMFORTS

Each year more than 100,000 people are treated in hospital emergency rooms for in-line skating injuries. In-line skaters can reach speeds of 50 miles per hour or more, yet two-thirds do not wear protective clothing. Spontaneous loss of balance; falling due to debris or an irregularity on the skating surface; colliding with a fellow skater; and striking a stationary hazard, such as a tree, are the most common causes of falls by in-line skaters. Blisters, strains, sprains, and many other general complaints are addressed in Chapter 8.

Falling is the biggest concern when skating, so you won't be surprised to learn that the number one injury site is the wrist. One-fourth of all skating injuries are injuries to the wrist, and over 40 percent of all these injuries result in fractures. "Skitching" can be deadly and should never be attempted. This is a popular activity in which a skater hooks onto a motor vehicle and attempts to hang on while coasting behind or beside the vehicle. The U.S. Consumer Product Safety Commission (CPSC) and the International In-line Skating Association (IISA) recommend that a helmet, elbow and knee pads, and wrist guards with fingerless gloves be worn while skating to reduce the risk and severity of injuries, especially those involving the wrist.

 ## JOGGING

ADVANTAGES/DISADVANTAGES

Running is a simple way to develop cardiorespiratory endurance. You can do it alone, with a partner, or with a group. A good pair of running shoes is the only equipment you need. Finding a place to run is as simple as walking out your front door. Getting a full workout through running takes less time than do many other aerobic activities. It can be done in most types of weather, on vacation, or during a lunch break. As a weight-bearing exercise, jogging provides stress to the long bones, which aids in the maintenance of bone mineralization and decreases the risk of osteoporosis. Like other aerobic activities, jogging has positive benefits in terms of reducing obesity, stress, type 2 diabetes, and several heart disease risk factors.

Drawbacks to running include traffic, uneven pavement, and, occasionally, an aggressive dog. Trying to progress too quickly may cause impact problems such as shin splints and sore knees. Jogging is not for everyone. For individuals prone to musculoskeletal problems, low- or nonimpact activities such as bicycling and water exercise are less likely to precipitate injury. If you are overweight or out of shape, it may be best to start with a less intense activity, such as walking. Nonetheless, a carefully planned program of progressive activity enables many people to enjoy running as part of a fitness program.

Keep in mind that when you are running you generate a great deal of body heat. When you are warmed up, it will feel about 20 degrees warmer than the actual temperature. A hot day would be 70 degrees or higher, a warm day 50 to 60 degrees, a cool day 30 to 40 degrees, and a cold day below freezing. High humidity on hot days and the

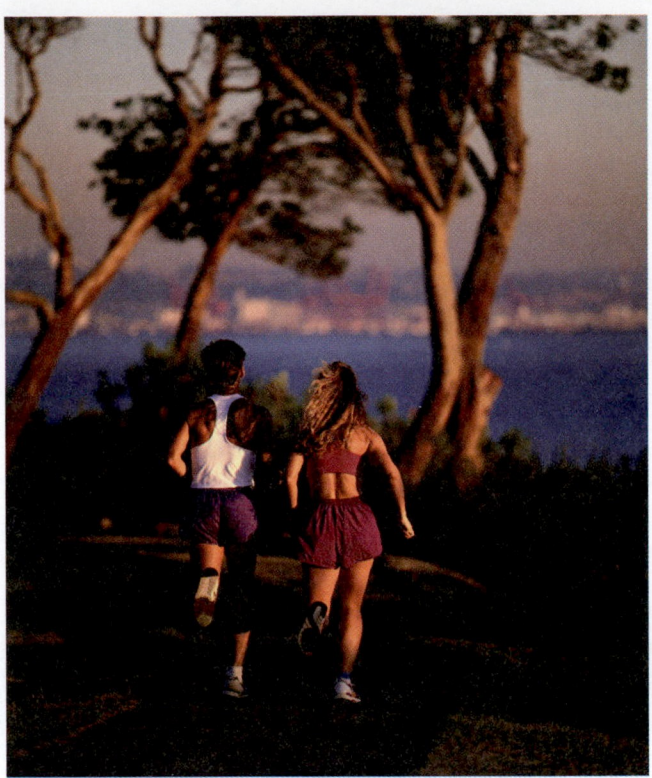

Vary your jogging workouts to avoid becoming bored and stale.

wind-chill factor on cold days should also be considered (see Chapter 7).

A good pair of properly fitted running shoes is important in preventing injuries. When running, your foot strikes the ground with *an impact of approximately three times your body weight*. A well-made running shoe fitted by a trained salesperson can absorb shock and support the foot. A cheap pair of poor-quality shoes is no bargain if it leaves you with blisters or shin splints.

You can run in almost any kind of weather if you dress appropriately. On hot days, wear as little as decently possible—shoes, socks, shirt, and shorts. For cooler weather, add layers: a long-sleeved T-shirt and tights or long pants. In cold weather, add a jacket or a turtleneck sweater and, to protect the ears and hands, a stocking cap and mittens. In wet weather, wear a cap with a brim to keep rain out of your eyes and rain-repellent clothing, if desired.

TECHNIQUE AND SAFETY TIPS

Good running form is relaxed and mechanically efficient. Your energy goes into moving yourself forward and is not dissipated in extraneous movements. Maintain a relaxed, erect posture, head up, eyes looking ahead. Keep your shoulders relaxed and level, arms swinging freely from the shoulder, and hands unclenched, traveling between the hips and lower chest. Avoid hunching forward, your eyes watching your feet, your arms held stiffly or swinging across the midline of your body. Knees and feet should aim ahead, not to the center or side. Foot contact should be heel to ball or midfoot, not on the toes like a sprinter. Keep your stride length comfortable and effortless, with your foot landing under your center of gravity. Be careful not to overstride or bounce when you run. Stride length is a product of speed and leg strength. Unless you increase one of these elements, attempts to increase your stride length will waste energy. Breathe through your mouth and nose. It is hard to get enough air breathing through the nose alone.

While you are working on your running form, there are some safety guidelines you need to keep in mind:

1. *Before leaving home, let someone know your route* and when you expect to return. Carry identification.
2. *If you wear a headset, keep the volume low* enough so that you can hear approaching traffic.
3. *Keep alert.*
4. *If there is a sidewalk, jog on it.*
5. *If there is no sidewalk, run facing traffic on the extreme left edge or shoulder of the road.*
6. *Respect private property.* Do not run across lawns.
7. *Obey traffic signs and signals.* When crossing a street at the light, cross with the green light only.
8. *Maintain eye contact with motorists* whenever you cross in front of them.
9. *Give the right-of-way to cars.* Don't antagonize drivers even if they try your patience.
10. *If you run at night, wear light-colored clothing with reflective strips.*
11. *At night, do not run in unfamiliar areas.*
12. *Do not wear a vinyl sweat suit* while exercising, ever!

HOW TO BEGIN AND PROGRESS

Begin at the level indicated by your cardiorespiratory fitness assessment (Chapter 3) and progress slowly. See the *Run Walk Program box.* If you cannot complete a mile in 15 minutes, begin with walking briskly 15 to 30 minutes until your heart rate stays within the target range. When you can comfortably handle 2 miles in 30 minutes, you may begin the jog/walk program. As in all activities, follow the FITT guidelines.

Run/Walk Program

Fitness Category		Starting Level
Low		1, 2, or 3
Fair		4
Average		5 or 6
Good		7 or 8
Superior		9 or 10

Level	Run	Walk	Repeats
1	–	15–20 min.	1
2	–	20–30 min.	1
3	30 sec.	30 sec.	8–12 plus 10- to 15-min. walk
4	1 min.	30 sec.	6–10 plus 10-min. walk
5	2 min.	30 sec.	4–10 plus 5- to 10-min. walk
6	4 min.	1 min.	4–6
7	6 min.	1 min.	4–5
8	8 min.	1–2 min.	3–4
9	12 min.	2 min.	2
10	20–30 min.	5 min.	1
11	up to 60 min.	–	1

Start at the level appropriate for your fitness category. Remember that your starting level does not indicate your potential. For each run-walk interval, begin with the lowest number of repeats indicated, and with each successive workout, add one repeat. When you can do the maximum number of intervals at one level, move to the next level. A 5-minute warm-up and 5-minute cool-down should accompany each workout. You may stay at one level as long as you need to or even move back a step if the beginning level is too difficult. If the workout has been appropriate, you should feel refreshed and relaxed, not exhausted, after exercise. Use Lab Activity 4-5 to record your progress.

VARIETY

Much of the variety in running comes from running different routes and observing the changing scenery and seasons. If you run alone, you may wish to run occasionally with a partner or a group. Instead of taking a long run at a continuous pace, you might try *fartlek,* a Swedish term for *speed-play.* Fartlek mixes fast-paced runs, brief all-out sprints, and slow-paced recovery intervals. It is best done on uneven or hilly terrain such as a park or golf course. Interval training done once or no more than twice a week can add a change of pace. This alternates a fast-paced run over a predetermined distance with walking or a slow recovery jog. An example might be running 220 yards four to six times in 40 to 50 seconds with a 220-yard walk after each run. With interval training, you may vary the distance run, recovery interval, number of repetitions, and time or pace of the run. These workouts are usually done on the track but can be done on the road by running and then walking a set amount of time, running a certain number of telephone pole intervals, or selecting a long hill on your route and running up it several times. A fitness trail, or parcour, with exercise stations linked by a running trail, may be available at a local park or university or you can make your own. To simulate a parcour on a regular running route, stop every 2 to 4 minutes to do a stretching or toning exercise (e.g., hamstring stretch, run 2 minutes, calf stretch, run 3 minutes, push-ups, run 3 minutes, abdominal curls, . . .).

Some activities are suitable for a small group. You can take a tennis or foam ball along to toss among some friends. You'll get quite a workout because this mixes sprinting and upper-body exercise into the run. This is safer if your route has little traffic. Hashing is a popular club sport in the southern United States, Europe, and Russia. The idea is for a group to follow a marked course through an unfamiliar area. Elected group members meet at an earlier time to mark the route, usually with flour. Orienteering is popular in some areas. This is a cross-country type of activity in which participants navigate from point to point, using a map and compass, covering distances from 2 to 10 miles. Local fun-runs give you a chance to run with and meet other runners in a noncompetitive atmosphere. If you like competition, you can get information on road races from your local running club or athletic shoe store.

COMMON DISCOMFORTS

Most aches and pains in running do not occur suddenly. They are often from overuse—a long steady erosion that wears down the body. Many general complaints are addressed in Chapter 8. Specific to running, two additional discomforts, easily avoided, occasionally occur. If you run with shoes that are too short or don't fit well, in addition to developing blisters you could injure a toe. The toenail may turn black and possibly fall off. While painful, the condition is not permanent. The nail will grow back. If your thighs rub together when you run, you may suffer an abrasion. The solution is to apply petroleum jelly to the area and wear tights or shorts that cover your thighs.

◆ WATER EXERCISE/AQUA AEROBICS

ADVANTAGES/DISADVANTAGES

You don't have to know how to swim to get a vigorous workout in the water. You don't even have to get your head wet! As more people are discover-

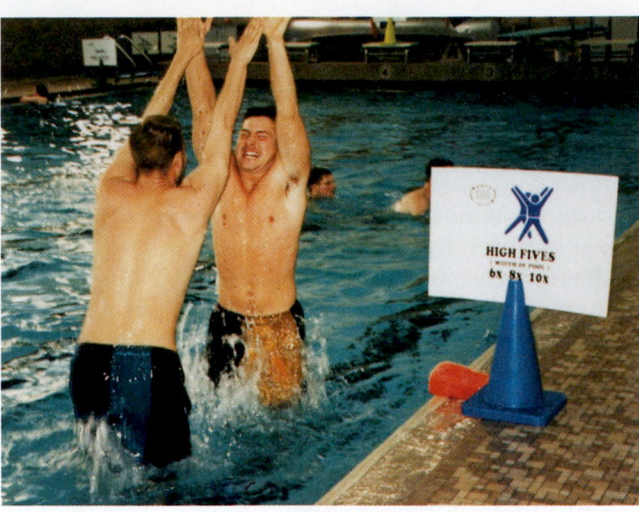

Nonswimming water workouts are one of the best forms of exercise because they build muscular strength and endurance as well as cardiorespiratory endurance. The faster you move, the harder your muscles work.

ing, exercising against water resistance in shallow water is a fine workout and great fun, especially with a group. Water exercise can be a social activity because you can carry on a conversation while working out. It is low-impact, so joint problems are rare. The supportive effect of water buoyancy makes water exercise enjoyable and relaxing for individuals who have concerns about other forms of exercise. In chest-deep water, a person weighs only about a tenth of what he or she does on land. People who have arthritis or joint problems find that this buoyancy decreases stress to the joints, allowing a fuller range of motion than is possible on land. It is easy to individualize intensity levels so that you get a good workout, whatever your level of fitness.

Water has at least 12 times the resistance of air, and that number increases as movement speed increases. Thus, muscular conditioning improves, and in a time-efficient program as well. For example, biceps and triceps can be overloaded concentrically during the same exercise.

Hydrostatic (water) pressure pushes against the chest and body. This helps strengthen the breathing system and makes breathing on land easier. Hydrostatic pressure aids venous circulation and contributes to reduction in edema (swelling), which is especially helpful for expectant moms.

Water currents constantly challenge the trunk core muscles to maintain proper alignment when starting, stopping, and changing direction in the water. The abs have to work the entire time—a great plus.

Inclement weather is not a problem. Water exercise is cool even on the hottest summer days, so heat stress is eliminated. It is also a comfortable indoor workout for rainy or cold winter days. If you are overweight and sensitive about exercising in public, the water covers you up so that you don't feel so self-conscious. Water exercise is also beneficial during pregnancy because of both decreased joint stress and decreased heat stress compared with other forms of exercise.

The drawbacks are few. You need access to a pool at a time when you can have a lane separate from lap swimmers. It is probably best to first join a class to learn the exercises and activities. Then you can work out on your own.

TECHNIQUE AND SAFETY TIPS

Workouts may have a muscle toning emphasis or an aerobic emphasis or a combination of the two. In constructing workouts, maintain muscle balance by exercising all major muscle groups. Particularly emphasize stretching tight muscle groups (e.g., lower back, hamstrings, calves) and toning weak areas (e.g., abdominals, upper body). To overload, keep in mind that as in weight training, water adds resistance. The harder you push and pull, the more resistance you create and the more benefit you receive. In any activity, limit back hyperextension by keeping the abdominals firm while exercises are being performed. In the water, as on land, workouts must maintain a training heart rate for 20 to 30 minutes to produce aerobic benefit. Training heart rates for swimmers appear to be about 10 percent lower than those for land exercisers. This may also be true for other cardiorespiratory water exercise. To calculate an appropriate exercise intensity for water exercise, subtract 10 percent from your training pulse on land. Jogging in the water, aqua aerobics, and other vigorous activities can provide aerobic benefit if an adequate overload occurs. Several books that give examples of water exercises are available and are listed at the end of this chapter.

Whenever you exercise in the water, a few safety guidelines must be followed:

1. *Never work out in the water alone.* A lifeguard or workout partner, preferably one who can swim, should be present. Safety equipment, such as a life ring or a reaching pole, should also be available.
2. *Shower before entering the pool.*
3. *Do not go into the deep water unless you can swim.*
4. *Don't mix water and electricity.* If you like to exercise to music, keep electrical equipment away from the water and make sure that all electric outlets have ground-fault circuit interrupters that shut off the electricity if it contacts water. Better yet, use battery-powered equipment.
5. *Do not enter the pool if you have an open sore, infection, or rash.*
6. *Do all exercises through a full range of motion with slow, controlled movements.* Swinging or flinging movements can injure joints.
7. *Maintain good body alignment in walking and jogging.* Keep abdominals tight and hips tucked under and avoid excessive forward lean.

HOW TO BEGIN AND PROGRESS

Water exercise workouts, like other aerobic programs, should incorporate a warm-up, conditioning period, and cool-down. The warm-up may be started on deck or in the water. A cardiorespiratory warm-up transitions the heart, lungs, and muscles gradually to an increased intensity level. Water exercise may involve many different activities—aerobic, muscle toning, and stretching. Recommendations on how to progress are given for the aerobic portion of the workout (e.g., water running) in terms of length of time at a training heart rate. Test your fitness by using the 500-yard water run test described in Chapter 3. Then follow the appropriate level in the *Water Exercise Program box*. Stay on each level as long as necessary; don't skip levels. Go back a level if the next feels too strenuous. Progress slowly, listen to your body, and follow the FITT factors. Monitor your THR or use the RPE.

Water Exercise Program

Fitness Category	Starting Level
Low	1
Fair	2
Average	3
Good	4
Superior	5 or 6

Level	Vigorous	Easy	Sets	Total Time
1	1 min.	30 secs.	8–12	10–18 mins.
2	2 mins.	30 secs.	6–8	15–20 mins.
3	4 mins.	30 secs.	4–6	18–27 mins.
4	6 mins.	30 secs.	3–4	19–26 mins.
5	8–10 mins.	1 min.	3	26–32 mins.
6	Continuous		1	30 mins. or more

Follow the conditioning bout with a 5- to 10-minute cool-down combining a period of gradually decreasing intensity exercise with stretching for flexibility.

VARIETY

Exercise with friends or with music. After mastering the exercises with only water resistance, you may wish to add kickboards, pull buoys, or other water exercise equipment to increase resistance. Vary the exercises and activities so that you don't do the same workout 2 days in a row. For example, an aerobic workout may involve, on different days, running or walking widths, aqua aerobics, step aerobics, water games, deepwater running, treading and kicking drills, or circuit training. There are so many different things to do in the water that it is easy to add variety. Some examples of different types of workouts follow.

Muscular strength and endurance are built by performing repeats of exercises against resistance: side leg swings to tone inner thigh and outer hip, straight arm raises to tone deltoids, back leg swings to strengthen hamstrings and gluteus. A series of 8 to 12 exercises covering all major muscle groups can be performed for 1 minute each and repeated two to three times for a thorough muscular workout.

Water walking involves walking in waist- to chest-deep water fast enough to produce a target heart rate. Good body alignment during walking and jogging is important. Walk tall with abdominals pulled in and buttocks tucked in to avoid leaning forward. It is also essential, for muscle balance, to vary the walking movements. Variations include walking forward, backward, or sideways and adding different arm variations, such as forward pulls, breaststroke, and backstroke.

Shallow water jogging is similar to water walking but is more intense, using a faster, bounding stride. A common error is running too much on the balls of the feet, which causes calf tightness. Try to press your heel to the pool bottom before pushing off on your toes.

Deepwater jogging is a nonimpact workout. Exercisers may wear a flotation vest or belt and run, varying directions and arm movements. Deepwater jogging without a flotation belt is strenuous. See the Guidelines for Deepwater Jogging below.

Interval training alternates high- and low-intensity workout segments. This can allow even the most athletic exerciser to get a vigorous workout. For example, you might alternate four laps of shallow water running with two laps of water walking.

GUIDELINES FOR DEEPWATER JOGGING

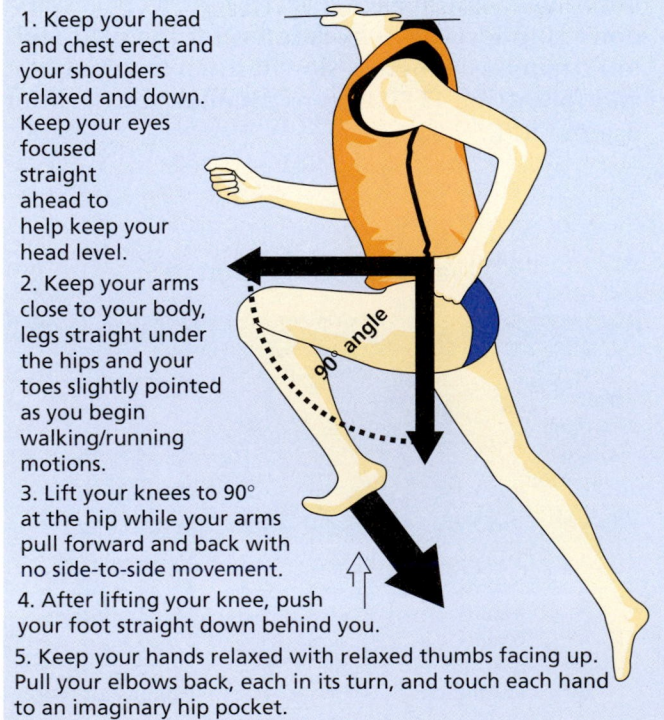

1. Keep your head and chest erect and your shoulders relaxed and down. Keep your eyes focused straight ahead to help keep your head level.

2. Keep your arms close to your body, legs straight under the hips and your toes slightly pointed as you begin walking/running motions.

3. Lift your knees to 90° at the hip while your arms pull forward and back with no side-to-side movement.

4. After lifting your knee, push your foot straight down behind you.

5. Keep your hands relaxed with relaxed thumbs facing up. Pull your elbows back, each in its turn, and touch each hand to an imaginary hip pocket.

90° angle

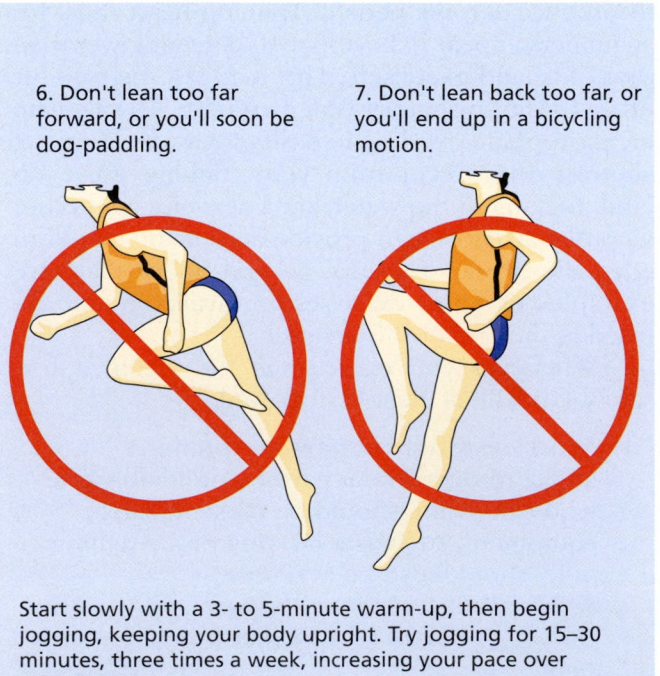

6. Don't lean too far forward, or you'll soon be dog-paddling.

7. Don't lean back too far, or you'll end up in a bicycling motion.

Start slowly with a 3- to 5-minute warm-up, then begin jogging, keeping your body upright. Try jogging for 15–30 minutes, three times a week, increasing your pace over a few weeks.

Water aerobics, like land aerobics, puts exercise to music. Workouts may be choreographed or freestyle. Bench step workouts have also made the transition into the aquatic environment, with benefits similar to those in land workouts.

Plyometrics are vigorous jumping and bounding exercises that increase muscle strength and power. They are also aerobic. Examples include high jumps in place, bounding across the pool, and a series of high 2-foot hops. Because these are impact exercises, they can cause injury, are only for well-conditioned exercisers, and should be avoided if you have ankle, knee, or back problems. Water buoyancy lessens the risk of injury.

In *circuit training*, a series of exercises are performed for a certain number of repetitions or a given amount of time (e.g., 1 minute each of side leg circles, jumping jacks, push-ups, forward kicks). Exercises may be written on numbered cards placed around the pool edge, and as each exercise is completed, participants move quickly to the next exercise station. Exercises may stress one fitness component or several. A set of 8 to 12 exercises can be repeated, or time at each station can be increased to produce overload.

Flexibility exercises are often used as a part of a water exercise program. A static stretch is held 20 to 30 seconds or more for each major muscle group to increase range of motion.

Occasionally, it is fun to try a water game for variety. Examples include shallow water polo, inner-tube water polo, water baseball, freeze tag, sharks and minnows, water basketball, and volleyball.

COMMON DISCOMFORTS

The most common discomforts water exercisers encounter are tight calves and blisters from running barefoot on the pool bottom. Blisters can be avoided by starting with only a few minutes of running in the pool and giving the feet time to toughen as you gradually progress in workouts. You could also wear pool shoes or clean sneakers during workouts. Calves tend to get tight because, due to buoyancy, most running and walking in the pool is done on the ball of the foot. Take care to stretch calves before and after the workout.

PRESCRIPTION FOR ACTION

You've read the chapter. Now go do one or more of these:

✓ Walk an extra 2,000 steps. Wear a pedometer all day today. (Hints: Pace around as you talk on the phone; take a walk as you return phone calls; take a marching-in-place minute once an hour; meet with a friend for a walk instead of a soda or coffee; walk around [even in place] during TV commercials.)

✓ Try a new cardio machine in the fitness gym.

✓ Enroll in a fitness class.

✓ Add hand weights to your walking workout.

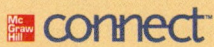 Go online to Connect to complete this activity.
http://connect.mcgraw-hill.com

Tips for Behavior Change

Refer to the Stage of Change flowchart on page 98. What is your stage of change after answering the questions and tracing the flowchart?

To see which processes of change are most effective for facilitating your transition from your current stage to the next stage (or *maintaining* your behavior if you are already in the maintenance stage), refer to Figure 2-2 on page 36. Here are some behavioral examples for selected processes of change:

Consciousness-raising: Keep a log of how often you exercise aerobically now. Evaluate your cardiovascular fitness level with one of the CRE fitness tests.

Social liberation: Find out the open hours at the campus recreation center. Map out safe fitness trails with various mileages in your area.

Emotional arousal: Imagine what your health profile will be in 10 years (weight, waist size, cholesterol, blood pressure, etc.) if old habits don't change.

Environment control: Have exercise clothes ready at all times . . . in your room, car, or locker at the gym.

Helping relationships: Join a fitness class at the campus recreation center.

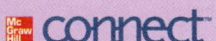 Go online to Connect to complete this activity.
http://connect.mcgraw-hill.com

Frequently Asked Questions

Q. During the winter and at other times when the weather is bad I work out in the fitness gym. How can I avoid picking up a cold, flu, staph infections, and other germs from the equipment?

A. These six simple tips can help you stay healthy at the gym all year long:

- Wipe down equipment with the alcohol spray that most gyms provide.
- Keep your hands clean. After touching weights and machine handrails, keep your hands away from your eyes, nose, ears, and mouth until you can wash them. Shower right after you exercise.
- Take two towels. One for yourself and one to wipe down the machines and mats before you use them. Don't share towels with others.
- Cover up. The less skin-to-equipment contact you have, the better. Keep cuts clean and bandaged. Wear flip-flops in the shower.
- Use your own mat in classes like yoga, etc.
- Launder workout clothes after every workout.

Q. What happens to your body when you quit exercising?

A. The initial changes can be as subtle as tiring easily during everyday activities like climbing the stairs. Over the course of 10 weeks, however, you will end up losing much of the gains made from regular workouts (i.e., drop in muscle strength, flexibility, and heart health). Plus, you will probably experience weight gain as well as an increase in blood pressure, cholesterol, and resting heart rate. Your psychological well-being is likely to suffer, too (i.e., increased mood swings, poor self-image, and even mild depression). It takes effort to keep up your present level of fitness. Don't be discouraged if you miss several days or weeks of exercise. Do what you can and get back into your regular routine as soon as you can.

Q. What is the difference between physical activity and exercise?

A. The terms are sometimes used interchangeably even though they represent different things. Physical activity refers to any movement produced by muscular contractions that burns extra calories. Examples include raking leaves, pushing a stroller, and washing a car.

Exercise is a specific type of physical activity that includes any planned, structured, and repetitive bodily movement done specifically to improve or maintain one or more components of physical fitness. Brisk walking, swimming, and lifting weights are examples.

Q. What is the Pilates Method of body conditioning?

A. The Pilates (pronounced puh-LAH-teez) Method was developed in the 1920s by physical trainer Joseph H. Pilates for rehabilitation for dancers. It is an exercise system that isolates and strengthens muscles without joint stress and without building bulk. It is a system of controlled exercises aimed at stretching and strengthening muscles of the back, buttocks, and abdomen for improved posture, better balance, relief of aches/pains, and increased flexibility. Pilates movements generate from the "powerhouse" or the "core" (the abdomen, lower back, and buttocks). Today's Pilates classes primarily use mat work, but classes featuring Pilates machines, which magnify resistance by using springs and pulleys, are also available.

Q. Is balance training beneficial?

A. Yes! Balance training improves posture, enhances movement skills for sports and daily living, is good for fall prevention, and improves mental focus. Balance exercises can be done with or without equipment.

Q. My hands swell when I'm fitness walking. Is this a problem? It feels funny and I don't like it.

A. Swelling in your hands is normal. When you swing your arms, the blood rushes down into your hands. It isn't harmful but it can be uncomfortable, especially if you wear rings. It's a good idea to take them off before you walk. To improve venous blood flow back to the heart and minimize swelling, keep your elbows bent at a 90-degree angle as you swing your arms. See "Correct Walking Form" in this chapter. You can also try squeezing your hands into fists from time to time as you walk. This helps push blood back from the fingers to the heart.

Q. Are yoga and Tai Chi really considered exercise?

A. Absolutely. In addition to enhancing balance, flexibility, and strength, these ancient disciplines can improve mood and provide some cardiovascular benefit. For example, an Australian study found that Tai Chi reduces heart rate, blood pressure, and stress hormones as effectively as brisk walking does. Yoga can decrease blood pressure; although traditional versions typically do not supply much aerobic benefit, newer "power yoga" classes incorporate standard yoga poses into a strenuous session that works both the heart and the lungs.

Q. How much benefit do I get from a sport like golf?

A. To get much benefit from golf, you will have to abandon the cart because the major exercise is in the walking. In a Finnish study, middle-aged former golfers resumed their game, without carts, two to three times per week. After 5 months, they had increased their aerobic performance and endurance, raised their "good" HDL-cholesterol level, and lost an average of 3 pounds and nearly an inch from their waistlines.

Q. My fitness level has plateaued. What can I do to jump-start it?

A. To keep improving, change a variable in the FITT prescription every 4 to 6 weeks.

- **Frequency:** If you exercise three times a week and aren't seeing improvement, try adding another day.
- **Intensity:** Slowly increase your speed or incline when using cardio machines.
- **Time:** Add 10 percent to each workout, or add 5 minutes to each workout, or make one weekly workout twice as long.
- **Type:** Try a different cardio machine or take a class to add interest to your continuous, rhythmic exercise; add resistance training to your exercise program.

Q. What are the most common mistakes made by individuals who engage in aerobic exercise?

A. Here are the top 10 common mistakes made by individuals who engage in aerobic exercise:

1. Relying on "muscle burn" as an accurate indicator of exercise intensity. Your heart's response to the demands of exercise is not related to how much your muscles "burn" during physical activity. For a training effect to occur, individuals must exercise within their training heart rate zone. It is okay to use your perception of effort (i.e., rating of perceived exertion, or RPE).
2. Mistaking neuromuscular difficulty as a meaningful barometer of training intensity. Even though individuals may find it relatively difficult to perform whatever combination of limb and trunk movements are involved in a particular activity (e.g., exercising on a cross-country skiing machine), it does not necessarily mean that they are achieving the desired training effect.
3. Working out at an inappropriate level of intensity. Getting the most out of your aerobic exercise efforts requires that you exercise within the appropriate training zone.
4. Engaging in activities that place too much stress on the lower extremities. Some aerobic activities involve a greater degree of impact forces on the lower body of the exerciser than do others. Also, some individuals can withstand greater loads on their lower extremities than can others. It is critical that you select your aerobic exercise modality wisely.
5. Worrying more about the exercise clothes on their body than the footwear on their feet.
6. Leaning on the exercise machine while working out. Many individuals compromise the safety and quality of their aerobic workouts by excessively leaning on the handrails of whatever aerobic equipment they are using while exercising (e.g., treadmills, ellipticals, cross trainers, or stair climbers).
7. Failing to warm up before exercising.
8. Failing to cool down after exercising.
9. Failing to get enough rest. Even though you may feel passionate about exercising, you need to give your body adequate rest from working out to provide it with the opportunity to recover from the physical demands you have placed on it.
10. Relying on aerobic exercise gimmicks marketed on television and the Internet. Geared to individuals who are wishfully looking for a quick, easy, and painless way to achieve the innumerable benefits of proper exercise, most of these items look too good to be true, and they are.

Q. My friends and I want to join a health club. What are some tips so we don't get ripped off?

A. Follow these 7 tips on how to select a health club:

- Ask friends and family about local clubs, equipment, and advantages and disadvantages.
- Visit several clubs at times you would be going, such as after work, to see how crowded they are. Check out the bathrooms, locker room, pool, and weight room. All should be clean and well maintained. Equipment should be in good repair. Talk to the regulars to see how they judge it. See that it has the features and types of equipment you want to use.
- Professionals should be available to show you how to use the equipment correctly for the most effective workout and to avoid injury. Ask about instructor qualifications. Certification by a professional group demonstrates a commitment to quality instruction. Many national certifying organizations certify instructors in different activities. Some of these are the American College of Sports Medicine, YMCA, YWCA, International Dance-Exercise Association, Aerobics and Fitness Association of America, and National Strength and Conditioning Association.
- Look for a health club with at least 3 years of continuous operation. Call the local Better Business Bureau or your state or local consumer protection agency to check if any negative reports have been filed. Ask to see evidence of bonding from the club (this protects you if the club goes out of business).
- Membership fees are negotiable, so no matter what is printed on the brochure, negotiate!
- Start with a short-term membership. Only 10 percent of members are still working out after 3 months, so either pay on a monthly basis or sign up for a 3-month trial membership.
- Read the contract carefully before signing, making sure it covers everything you have discussed with the club employees. If you change your mind, most states have a 3-day cooling-off period during which you can void the contract and get a full refund.

Summary

Cardiorespiratory endurance is perhaps the most important component of health-related fitness. It is measured by VO_{2max}, your body's maximal ability to transport and utilize oxygen during exercise. VO_{2max} can be increased by training, and decreases with inactivity or aging. It is often measured in field tests such as the 1.5-mile run or 1-mile walk. Benefits of long-term cardiorespiratory fitness training include improvements in exercise capacity, exercise recovery, muscular fitness, weight management, cognitive function, and psychological well-being. Regular exercise also reduces risk of chronic diseases such as cardiovascular disease, high blood pressure, type 2 diabetes, and certain types of cancer. The FITT prescription factors for cardiorespiratory fitness can be applied to many different activities to produce high-level fitness. Intensity of exercise, measured by heart rate, is a key factor in developing cardiorespiratory endurance. The Karvonen equation can be used to determine an adequate target heart rate range to produce cardiorespiratory benefits in many fitness activities. The Perceived Rate of Exertion can also be used.

The DHHS 2008 Physical Activity Guidelines for Americans are outlined in this chapter. How to use a pedometer to accumulate 10,000 steps is discussed.

The eight fitness activities in this chapter are aerobic dance, bicycling, fitness swimming, fitness walking, indoor exercise equipment, in-line skating, jogging, and water exercise/aqua aerobics. Each activity unit gave you valuable information concerning taking part in the activity. Now you have the necessary tools to begin a program of aerobic activity—one you will enjoy and pursue for a lifetime. You will also have the satisfaction of knowing you are nurturing the most important habit you can adopt to safeguard your health. The ball is in your court. Select an activity and go to it. We wish you well.

Terms

- aerobic
- aerobic capacity
- anaerobic
- cardiac output
- endorphins
- FITT factors
- heart rate reserve (HRR)
- Karvonen equation
- maximal heart rate (HR_{max})
- maximal oxygen uptake (VO_{2max})
- rate of perceived exertion (RPE)
- talk test
- target heart rate (THR)
- training effect

General Resources

Dynamix Music Service, 733 W. 40th St., Suite 10, Baltimore, MD 21211, (800) 843–6499.

Muscle Mixes, P.O. Box 533967, Orlando, FL 32853, (800) 52–MIXES or (407) 872–7576.

Power Productions, P.O. Box 550, Gaithersburg, MD 20884–0550, (301) 926–0707 or (800) 777–BEAT (call for a free catalogue).

Collage Video Specialists, 5390 Main St. N.E. Dept. 1, Minneapolis, MN 55421, (800) 433–6769. (Pilates, yoga, Tai Chi)

Creative Instructors Aerobics Educational Videos, 2314 Naudain Street, Philadelphia, PA 19146, (215) 790–9767 or (800) 435–0055.

IDEA Resource Library: Aqua Exercise, IDEA: The Association for Fitness Professionals, 6190 Cornerstone Court E., Suite 204, San Diego, CA 92121–3773.

Resources for Walking Equipment: Wrist/hand/ankle Weights: any large department and sporting equipment stores.

Weighted Vests: Smart Vest, Training Zone Concepts, Inc. Flint, MI (888) 797–8378.

Walking Poles: Exerstrider, Exerstrider Products Inc., Madison, WI (800) 554–0989.

Powerbelts: Inergi Fitness, Norcross, GA (800) 797–2358.

Pedometers: Digi-Walker, www.digiwalker.com (888) 748–5377.

Accusplit Eagle, (800) 935–1996.

Internet Resources

Aerobics Fitness Association of America

www.afaa.com

Includes "Exercise Gets Personal," an interactive site where you can design a customized exercise program.

America on the Move

www.americaonthemove.org

Inspirational hints to help increase walking.

American College of Sports Medicine

www.acsm.org/

Information on sports research, health and fitness, and aerobic exercise guidelines, along with a quarterly fitness newsletter. News releases give information on a variety of exercise topics of recent interest.

American Council on Exercise

www.acefitness.org/

Features 100 fitness fact sheets, free e-newsletters, and a variety of different fitness activities from bicycling to swimming.

American Heart Association

www.heart.org

Health tools include an exercise diary and a body mass calculator. Information includes exercise and fitness promotion for women, children, and seniors; information on how exercise affects heart health; exercise tips; and a health heart workout quiz.

American Volkssport Association

www.ava.org (800–830–9255)

Walking and hiking events sponsored by chapters throughout the United States.

Centers for Disease Control and Prevention

www.cdc.gov/

Information on getting started in physical activity, exercise tips, links to other fitness resources, and health promotion for increasing physical activity in your school or community.

The Cooper Institute for Aerobics Research

www.cooperinst.org

Discover the latest fitness news, from aerobics to weight loss.

Department of Health and Human Services Physical Activity Guidelines for Americans

www.health.gov/paguidelines

Summarizes the latest physical activity guidelines for Americans—all age groups and virtually all populations.

Digiwalker pedometers

www.thepedometercompany.com/

Information on programs and how to purchase this pedometer.

Exercise Calorie Expenditure

www.nutribase.com/exercala:htm

Calculates how many calories are expended for 30 minutes for specific body weights.

International Dance-Exercise Association (IDEA)

http://www.ideafit.com

Information about certification and equipment.

The President's Council on Physical Fitness and Sports

www.fitness.gov/

Information on award programs such as Presidential Active Lifestyle Award (PALA). Site explains how to count steps using a pedometer.

Shape Up America

www.shapeup.org

Provides information, programs, and tips on weight management.

Small Step

www.smallstep.gov

A U.S. Department of Health and Human Services Web site; helps people get started toward a more active and healthy lifestyle. Gives tips to eat healthier and get more activity.

Marathoning: Listings of marathons, training logs, charts, race results, and other helpful links.

Marathon Guide

www.marathonguide.com

Chicago Marathon Program (designed by Hal Higdon)

http://www.halhigdon.com/marathon/Mar00index.htm

Galloway Program (designed by Jeff Galloway)

www.jeffgalloway.com

National President's Challenge

www.presidentschallenge.org

Contains a personal activity log, allows you to choose a program, encourages participation in advanced exercise programs.

LAB Activity 4-1

Calculate Your Target Heart Rate (THR) Range

The target heart rate represents the intensity level at which you should exercise to produce cardiorespiratory benefits. This amount of exercise (overload) is enough to condition the heart, lungs, and muscles but is not overly strenuous. Monitoring intensity during a workout is done by measuring the heart rate. For fitness to occur, your heart rate must be raised to approximately 60 percent of the difference between the resting and maximal heart rates. An increase in heart rate equal to 80 percent of the difference between resting and maximal rates is a reasonable upper intensity level for most exercises. This is the target heart rate range (or training heart range). The Karvonen formula for calculating your target heart rate is as follows:

THR = (maximal HR* − resting HR**) × Intensity % + Resting HR

   *Maximal HR = 220 minus age
   **Resting HR = count your pulse at rest for 60 seconds

When estimating your target heart rate range, two factors are involved:

- Your age: _____.
- Your resting heart rate (RHR): _____.

Use these numbers in the formula that follows:

1. 220 − _____ = _____
         your age   (estimated maximal heart rate [MHR])

2. _____ − _____ = _____
   MHR   (resting HR)   HR reserve

3. _____ × 0.60 + _____ = _____
   (HR reserve)   (lower intensity)   (resting HR)   (lower target heart rate)
   _____ × 0.80 + _____ = _____
   (HR reserve)   (higher intensity)   (resting HR)   (higher target heart rate)

4. Target heart rate range is _____ to _____ beats per minute.

5. For a quick pulse check during exercise, my THR ÷ 10 is _____ to _____ beats.

Example: Jeff is 23 years old and has a resting heart rate of 72 beats per minute.

1. 220 − 23 = 197 MHR
2. 197 − 72 = 125 heart rate reserve
3. 125 × .60 = 75 + 72 = 147
   125 × .80 = 100 + 72 = 172
4. THR range is 147 to 172 beats per minute.
5. THR ÷ 10 is 15 to 17 beats.

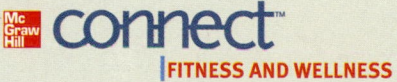

http://connect.mcgraw-hill.com

Name _____ **Class/Activity Section** _____ **Date** _____

Using a Pedometer: "How Many Steps Do I Take?"

Wear your pedometer for one full "normal" or "typical" week. Put it on first thing in the morning and wear it until you go to bed at night. Before you go to bed, record your steps for that day. Read the section in this chapter about pedometer use, and see Table 4-3, "Five Steps to Reach 10,000 Steps a Day." See the "1-Mile Equivalent" section in Lab Activity 4-3 for additional activities that can count toward your step goal.

1. Week 1: Steps I accumulated each day.

   Day/date _____   Steps = _____

   Day/date _____   Steps = _____

   Day/date _____   Steps = _____

   Day/date _____   Steps = _____

   Day/date _____   Steps = _____

   Day/date _____   Steps = _____

   Day/date _____   Steps = _____

   Total number of steps for Week 1 is _____

2. Divide by 7. This is your 7-day step average, also known as your **baseline activity level.**

What is your **7-day step average or baseline activity level?** _____

Any surprises? _____

_____

3. Weeks 2 and 3:

   - Calculate your **step count goal** using the 10% method. This is the number of steps you wish to add each day beyond your baseline activity level. Example: If your baseline activity level is 6,000 steps, an increase of 10% will be 600 steps $(6,000 \times .10 = 600)$. During Weeks 2–3 you would accumulate 6,600 steps per day. To progress, you would plan to add 600 steps every 2 weeks thereafter. (Example: Weeks 3–4 your goal would be to increase to 7,200 steps; Weeks 5–6 your goal would be to increase to 7,800 steps; Weeks 7–8 your goal would be to increase to 8,400 steps, and so on until you reach your ultimate goal of 10,000 steps or more.)

     What is your personal DAILY STEP COUNT GOAL for Week 2 and Week 3?

     _____ steps. (Your 7-DAY AVERAGE/BASELINE ACTIVITY $\times .10$)

     OR

   - ALTERNATIVE METHOD: Calculate your personal 7-DAY AVERAGE or BASELINE ACTIVITY LEVEL using the 500-Step Method. Increase your 7-Day Average by 500 steps instead of using the 10% Method. (Example: If your baseline is 6,000 steps, add 500 steps to set the goal for Weeks 2–3. This would be $6,000 + 500 = 6,500$; Weeks 4–5 would be 7,000 steps; Weeks 6–7 would be 7,500, and so on until you reach your ultimate goal of 10,000 steps or more.)

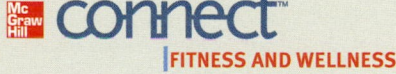

http://connect.mcgraw-hill.com

CHAPTER 4 ■ **LAB** Activity

What is your personal DAILY STEP COUNT GOAL for Week 2 and Week 3?

_____ steps. (Your 7-DAY AVERAGE/BASELINE + 500)

4. Calculate your personal activity goals using the 10% Method or the 500-Step Method for the next 12 weeks. Your instructor may prefer one method over the other. Use the pedometer log to record your daily activity.

Weeks 2–3: _____ steps per day

Weeks 4–5: _____ steps per day

Weeks 6–7: _____ steps per day

Weeks 8–9: _____ steps per day

Weeks 10–11: _____ steps per day

Weeks 12+: _____ steps per day

5. List specific strategies you plan to use in order to work toward your step goals.

PEDOMETER LOG

Name _____   Class/Activity Section _____

	Sunday	Monday	Tuesday	Wednesday	Thursday	Friday	Saturday	Weekly Average
Week of: Goal: _____ Steps = Miles =	_____ _____ _____ _____	_____ _____ _____ _____	_____ _____ _____ _____	_____ _____ _____ _____	_____ _____ _____ _____	_____ _____ _____ _____	_____ _____ _____ _____	_____ _____ _____ _____
Week of: Goal: _____ Steps = Miles =	_____ _____ _____ _____	_____ _____ _____ _____	_____ _____ _____ _____	_____ _____ _____ _____	_____ _____ _____ _____	_____ _____ _____ _____	_____ _____ _____ _____	_____ _____ _____ _____
Week of: Goal: _____ Steps = Miles =	_____ _____ _____ _____	_____ _____ _____ _____	_____ _____ _____ _____	_____ _____ _____ _____	_____ _____ _____ _____	_____ _____ _____ _____	_____ _____ _____ _____	_____ _____ _____ _____
Week of: Goal: _____ Steps = Miles =	_____ _____ _____ _____	_____ _____ _____ _____	_____ _____ _____ _____	_____ _____ _____ _____	_____ _____ _____ _____	_____ _____ _____ _____	_____ _____ _____ _____	_____ _____ _____ _____
Week of: Goal: _____ Steps = Miles =	_____ _____ _____ _____	_____ _____ _____ _____	_____ _____ _____ _____	_____ _____ _____ _____	_____ _____ _____ _____	_____ _____ _____ _____	_____ _____ _____ _____	_____ _____ _____ _____

NOTE: Approximately 2,000 Steps = 1 Mile
List the specific strategies you use to work toward your step goals:
(make copies as needed)

Name _____

Class/Activity Section _____

Date _____

Exercise Across the U.S.A. Log (make copies as needed)

Activity(s) _____　　　Start date _____　　　End date _____

State/distance _____

Month: ___		Month: ___		Month: ___		Month: ___		Month: ___		Month: ___	
1	17	1	17	1	17	1	17	1	17	1	17
2	18	2	18	2	18	2	18	2	18	2	18
3	19	3	19	3	19	3	19	3	19	3	19
4	20	4	20	4	20	4	20	4	20	4	20
5	21	5	21	5	21	5	21	5	21	5	21
6	22	6	22	6	22	6	22	6	22	6	22
7	23	7	23	7	23	7	23	7	23	7	23
8	24	8	24	8	24	8	24	8	24	8	24
9	25	9	25	9	25	9	25	9	25	9	25
10	26	10	26	10	26	10	26	10	26	10	26
11	27	11	27	11	27	11	27	11	27	11	27
12	28	12	28	12	28	12	28	12	28	12	28
13	29	13	29	13	29	13	29	13	29	13	29
14	30	14	30	14	30	14	30	14	30	14	30
15	31	15	31	15	31	15	31	15	31	15	31
16	Total	16	Total	16	Total	16	Total	16	Total	16	Total

Name _____ Class/Activity Section _____ Date _____

Exercise Across the U.S.A.

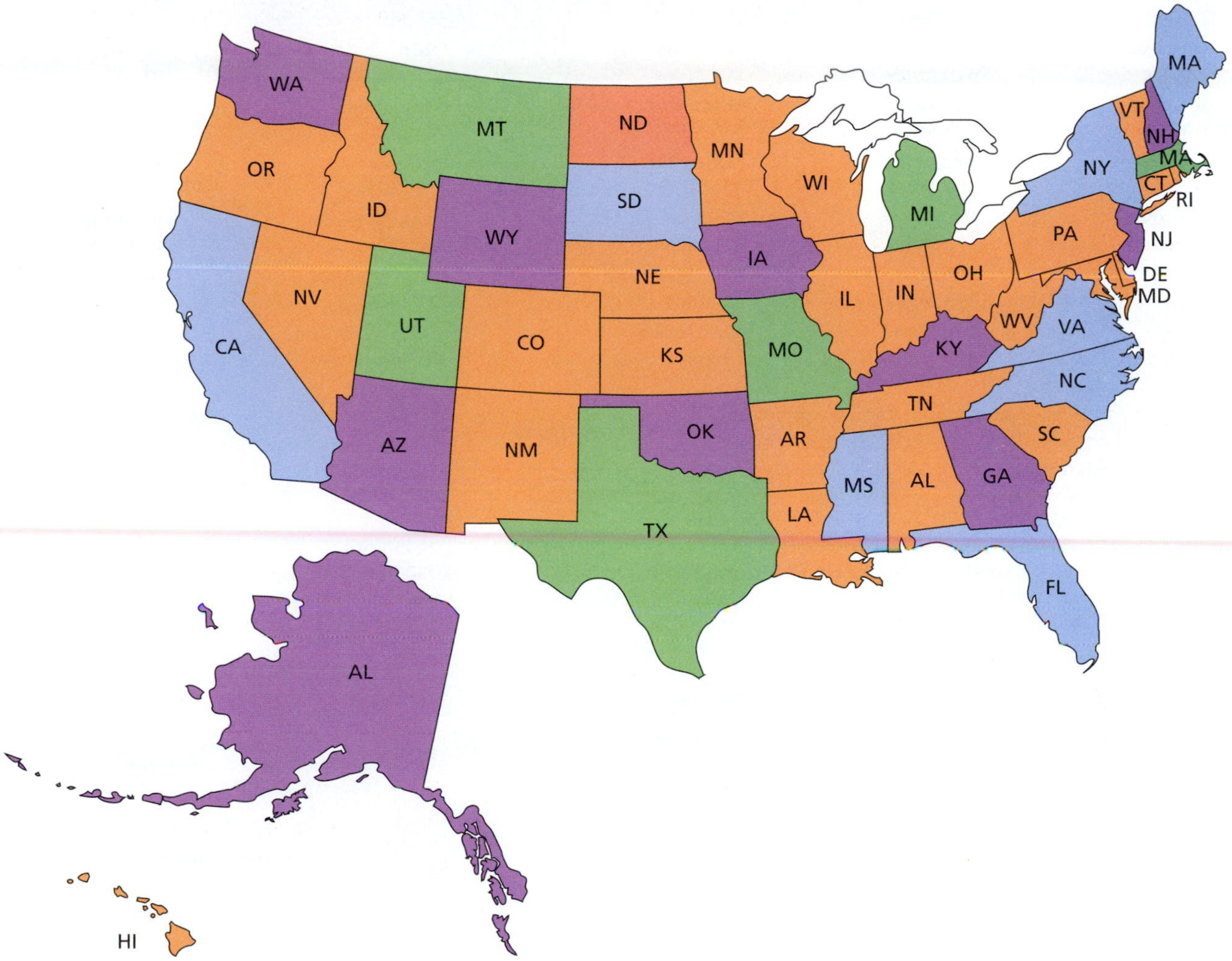

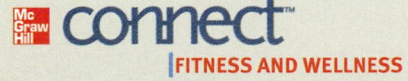

DIRECTIONS: (NOTE: ALL MILEAGE IS APPROXIMATE.)

1. Select a state to exercise across or go for the coast-to-coast challenge and a grand total of 2,755 miles.
2. Record your exercise miles on the Exercise Across the U.S.A. log form.
3. If you wish, you may make the trip interesting by incorporating different activities to reach your total mileage goal. Many sports are easy to measure in miles, but if you prefer a different activity, see the 1-Mile Equivalents chart, which is measured in minutes (estimated for a 143-pound person).

McGraw Hill **connect** | FITNESS AND WELLNESS

http://connect.mcgraw-hill.com

Exercise Across the U.S.A
(Grand Total: 2,775 Miles)

Pick a State

Alabama 195 Miles	**Hawaii** 75 Miles	**Massachusetts** 25 Miles	**New Mexico** 340 Miles	**South Dakota** 379 Miles
Alaska 858 Miles	**Idaho** 302 Miles	**Michigan** 185 Miles	**New York** 285 Miles	**Tennessee** 439 Miles
Arizona 315 Miles	**Illinois** 212 Miles	**Minnesota** 273 Miles	**North Carolina** 396 Miles	**Texas** 661 Miles
Arkansas 227 Miles	**Indiana** 139 Miles	**Mississippi** 273 Miles	**North Dakota** 355 Miles	**Utah** 267 Miles
California 247 Miles	**Iowa** 310 Miles	**Missouri** 295 Miles	**Ohio** 225 Miles	**Vermont** 81 Miles
Colorado 371 Miles	**Kansas** 390 Miles	**Montana** 546 Miles	**Oklahoma** 305 Miles	**Virginia** 340 Miles
Connecticut 80 Miles	**Kentucky** 351 Miles	**Nebraska** 400 Miles	**Oregon** 358 Miles	**Washington** 335 Miles
Delaware 36 Miles	**Louisiana** 177 Miles	**Nevada** 317 Miles	**Pennsylvania** 286 Miles	**West Virginia** 149 Miles
Florida 138 Miles	**Maine** 198 Miles	**New Hampshire** 76 Miles	**Rhode Island** 27 Miles	**Wisconsin** 254 Miles
Georgia 227 Miles	**Maryland** 215 Miles	**New Jersey** 72 Miles	**South Carolina** 207 Miles	**Wyoming** 348 Miles

Other Destinations

Length of Mississippi River	740 miles
Circumference of Earth	24,901 miles
Length of Grand Canyon	277 miles
To the moon	238,330 miles
The Lewis and Clark Expedition (from St. Louis to the Pacific Ocean)	4,000 miles
The Pony Express Trail (from St. Joseph, MO, to Sacramento, CA)	1,966 miles
The Great Wall of China	3,517 miles

1-Mile Equivalents (Approximately 2,000 Steps)

Activity	Minutes	Activity	Minutes	Activity	Minutes
Aerobic dance	18	Gardening		Rowing	12
Basketball	13	Digging	15	Skiing	
		Mowing	16	Cross country	13
Biking		Raking	32	Downhill	16
Leisure	29	Golf (without cart)	21		
Moderate	19			Softball (fielder)	32
Racing	11	In-line skating		Stair climbing	9
Calisthenics		(use actual distance covered)	16	Swimming	12
(Sit-ups, push-ups, etc.)	25	Jumping rope	11	Tennis	16
Canoeing (leisure pace)	40	Karate	9	Weight training	15

LAB Activity 4-4

"I Have No Time..." Overcoming Obstacles to Exercise

Many people have reasons, excuses, or obstacles that keep them from exercising on a regular basis. Some of these reasons are perceived; others are legitimate. With varied social, environmental, and motivational challenges, it is important to find ways to overcome these barriers. Reread the Top 10 lists "Ways to Stick with Exercise" and "Reasons to Pursue Lifetime Exercise" now for help in making exercise a priority in your life.

Listed below are the most common reasons for not exercising. Under each reason, list two or more ways one might overcome each challenge.

1. Lack of time

2. Lack of willpower/motivation

3. Lack of resources (money, facilities, equipment, etc.)

4. Lack of social support (friends, family, coworkers, etc.)

5. Weather issues (too hot, too cold, rainy, snowy, etc.)

6. Family/child care obligations

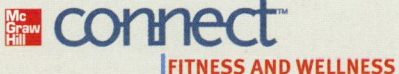

http://connect.mcgraw-hill.com

7. Injuries/disabilities

8. Fear of failure (too old, too out of shape, too fat, too much to overcome, etc.)

What are **your** three biggest personal challenges/obstacles in maintaining a regular exercise program?

1.

2.

3.

List two or more ways you could overcome each of these challenges/obstacles.

Obstacle 1

Obstacle 2

Obstacle 3

LAB Activity 4-5

Cardiorespiratory Exercise Log Sheet

(Note: Record only the information you find necessary.)

(Make Copies of this Form as Needed)

	Week	Sun	Mon	Tues	Wed	Thurs	Fri	Sat	Total
1	Date: RHR: Distance/time/steps: Type of activity: EHR: Location:								
2	Date: RHR: Distance/time/steps: Type of activity: EHR: Location:								
3	Date: RHR: Distance/time/steps: Type of activity: EHR: Location:								
4	Date: RHR: Distance/time/steps: Type of activity: EHR: Location:								

Comments/Goals: _____

_____

_____

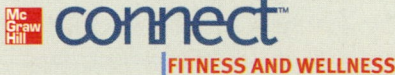

http://connect.mcgraw-hill.com

LAB Activity ■ **CHAPTER 4**

153

(Make Copies of this Form as Needed)

Name _____

Week _____   RHR _____   THR _____

Goals: _____

Date	RHR	Distance/time/steps	HR (at end of workout)	Location	Comments
Sun					
Mon					
Tues					
Wed					
Thur					
Fri					
Sat					

Total _____

CHAPTER 5

Developing Flexibility

STUDY QUESTIONS

You will have successfully mastered this chapter if you can answer the following:

1. What are the benefits of and five cautions for stretching?
2. What factors affect flexibility?
3. What are the two types of flexibility?
4. What are the four types of stretching?
5. What are some basic guidelines for flexibility development?
6. What are the five principles of flexibility development?
7. What are five flexibility exercises for basic fitness?
8. Can you differentiate between the safe and contraindicated exercises illustrated in the chapter?
9. What are the general guidelines for identifying exercises that increase risk of injury?
10. How do flexibility and muscular fitness contribute to wellness?

You will find the answers as you read this chapter.

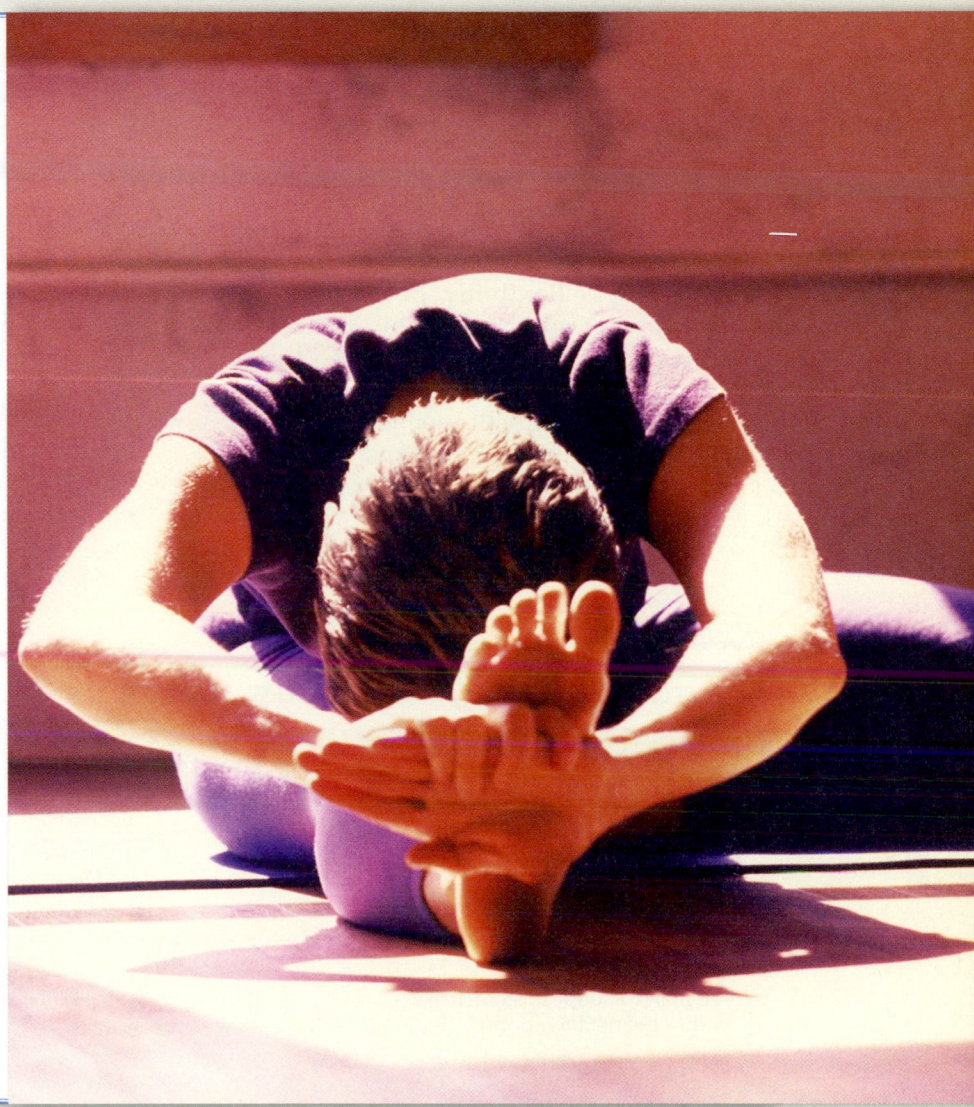

"Blessed are the flexible for they shall not be bent out of shape."
—Author unknown

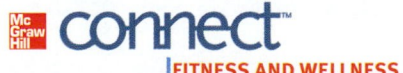

FITNESS AND WELLNESS

http://connect.mcgraw-hill.com

Flexibility, the ability to move the joints through their full range of motion, is an important factor in achieving wellness throughout the life span. It enables us to reach, bend, twist, and perform movements without excessive tightness or stiffness. As children, we are naturally flexible, but as we age, flexibility tends to decrease.

Disuse, injury, scar tissue, excessive body fat, and muscle imbalances are common factors associated with loss of range of motion. This chapter covers many aspects of flexibility—its benefits, types, cautions, principles, and guidelines. In addition, it highlights illustrated programs for developing this important component of fitness.

◆ FLEXIBILITY

You can maintain youthful flexibility by incorporating stretching into your regular workouts. The flexibility exercises in this section are grouped as follows: a basic fitness flexibility program with exercises for joggers, walkers, aerobic dancers, cyclists, swimmers, and water exercisers and examples of PNF partner-assisted stretches. Contraindicated exercises, safer substitutes, and general rules for identifying common exercises that put back and joints at increased risk of injury are also discussed.

Benefits of Flexibility

Several benefits can be gained from flexibility development:

✓ *Decreased aches and pains.* Tight, inflexible muscles pull unevenly across joints, causing skeletal misalignment, poor posture, unnecessary fatigue, and muscle and joint pain. Stretching can alleviate these problems.

✓ *Enhanced ability to move freely and easily* and to perform activities such as bending down to tie your shoes, scratching your back, and turning to look back as you are driving.

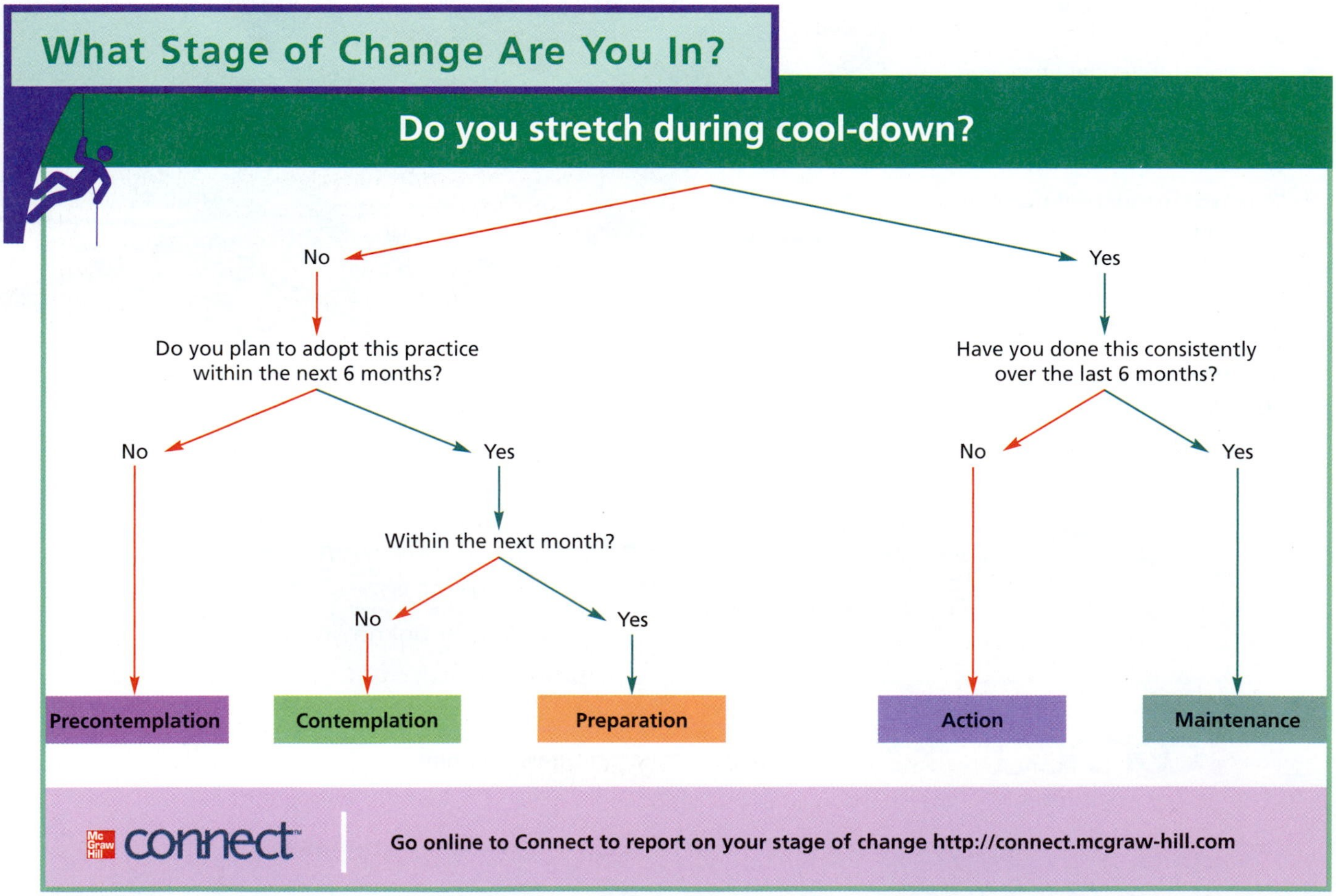

What Stage of Change Are You In?

Do you stretch during cool-down?

No → Do you plan to adopt this practice within the next 6 months?

- No → **Precontemplation**
- Yes → Within the next month?
  - No → **Contemplation**
  - Yes → **Preparation**

Yes → Have you done this consistently over the last 6 months?

- No → **Action**
- Yes → **Maintenance**

connect™ | Go online to Connect to report on your stage of change http://connect.mcgraw-hill.com

✓ *Possible decreased risk of injury.* When tight muscles restrict the natural range of motion of a joint, the slightest unusual twist can cause a strain or pull, such as a strained hamstring. Inflexibility also is a precipitating factor in overuse injuries such as tendinitis, because inelastic muscles transfer excessive stress to even less pliable connective tissue.

Some research indicates that the importance of stretching in injury prevention may vary depending on the type of activity to follow. It may be more important in activities involving vigorous jumping and bouncing (like soccer or basketball) in which the muscle-tendon unit undergoes high-intensity stretch-shortening cycles. It may be less important in activities with limited demands for stretch-shortening cycles (e.g., jogging, walking). While the effects of stretching in injury prevention are controversial and research has generally not shown that stretching before exercise decreases risk of injury, a long-term flexibility program designed to alleviate muscle tightness and imbalance can offer benefits. Excessively tight areas, identified by flexibility assessment, can be corrected and adequate flexibility restored for sports and daily activities. Many rehabilitation professionals would agree that injury resistance is best enhanced by including in your weekly workouts exercises designed to enhance both flexibility and strength as part of a balanced muscular fitness program.

✓ *Recovery from injury.* Athletic trainers and physical therapists commonly utilize stretching in injury rehabilitation programs. Research has shown that gentle stretching in a pain-free range of motion is important in shortening the rehabilitation period after injury. This enables a person to more quickly regain normal range of motion and return to activity.

✓ *Enhanced athletic performance.* In racquetball, golf, tennis, volleyball, and swimming, greater range of motion and ability to apply force through that range of motion can confer a winning edge. However, research indicates that stretching routines preceding strength-dependent activities appear to decrease subsequent performance. Therefore, it may be best to minimize stretching prior to competitive events and to delay stretching for flexibility until after strength-building exercise sessions.

✓ *Reversal of age-related flexibility declines.* We tend to lose flexibility as we age, partly due to age-related changes in connective tissue and muscle, partly due to decreasing levels of activity. A regular stretching program can improve flexibility at any age.

✓ *Improved posture, appearance.* We look and feel better when we carry ourselves tall with shoulders back, chest high, and back straight. Unfortunately, over time, we may tend to "sag into gravity" and develop a "hunched over" appearance with rounded shoulders, forward head, and sagging abdominals. Muscle tightness across the chest, hamstrings, and lower back coupled with weakness of opposing muscles can contribute to and perpetuate poor postural habits. Over time, poor posture tends to worsen and becomes harder to self-correct as muscle imbalances increase. Stretching to correct shortened muscles, along with strengthening the weak opposing muscles, can enhance posture and help a person "stand tall" naturally without continual conscious effort.

✓ *Decreased muscle soreness after exercise.* Research has shown that delayed onset muscle soreness and stiffness that occurs 1–2 days after exercise can be decreased by stretching the affected muscles.

✓ *It feels good.* Stretching reduces muscular tension, promoting relaxation.

CAUTIONS

If carelessly done, stretching may cause injury. You must be careful not to overstretch, particularly when muscles are cold and tight. Stretch just to the point of tightness and hold. Stretching is not a competitive activity, so don't try to imitate the most flexible person in your class. Injured areas should be stretched with great care and not into pain, which risks reinjury. If you feel pain during stretching, particularly joint pain, stop!

While less flexible individuals may envy those who can do splits with ease, keep in mind that more flexibility is better only up to a point. There is concern that excessive flexibility, unless accompanied by muscular strength, may overstretch ligaments and tendons and increase joint laxity and susceptibility to injury. For this reason, it is wise to strengthen muscles that you stretch and to stretch muscles that you strengthen for optimal fitness benefits.

Be aware that some studies show that static stretching immediately preceding activities requiring high levels of strength or power decreases performance approximately 10 percent. Studies also show decreased vertical jump performance immediately following some types of stretching. Therefore, delaying stretching until after competitive or strength-dependent activities would enable

all. Little difference was seen among the groups in leg strength, but power measures for both stretching groups were reduced, prompting the researchers to recommend a dynamic warm-up before, and stretching after competition.

Duration of stretching can also affect subsequent performance. Researchers had athletes perform 2, 4, or 6 repetitions of a stretch for 15 seconds. There was no difference in performance with the 2 and 4 repetition groups, but the 6 repetition group (total 90 seconds of stretching) experienced a decrease in muscle power as shown by vertical jump height. Therefore, researchers recommended that athletes perform a whole-body warm-up activity, followed by stretching for flexibility, after—not before—an athletic performance that requires maximum power, such as football or sprinting.

In sports that require above-average flexibility (gymnasts, dancers), static stretching enhances performance. A study of different durations of static stretching on dynamic balance showed improved balance with 3 repetitions of a 15-second stretch, but no improvement when the stretch duration was increased to 45 seconds. Two other studies have shown greater improvements in flexibility from static stretching as compared to dynamic stretching.

Dynamic stretching has not been encouraged in personal fitness programs due to concerns over possible increased risk of injury and muscle soreness. Guidelines for the fitness exerciser and the recreational athlete are as follows:

1. Always warm up first.
2. The small decrease in muscle power after stretching may not warrant a change in warm-up routine, especially for activities such as fitness walking or jogging that do not require high levels of muscular power.
3. Static stretching after your workout to maintain or improve flexibility is beneficial.
4. For health-related fitness, 2 to 4 repetitions of a static stretch is sufficient and can improve dynamic balance and flexibility.
5. Before athletic activities requiring high muscular forces, dynamic exercises can increase blood flow, deep-muscle temperature, and metabolic activity.

Do you want to add a few dynamic exercises to your warm-up? Realize that they are most effective when sport specific. For recreational runners and walkers, try incorporating 5 to 10 minutes of exercises such as leg swings forward and back, lunges, squats, and butt-kicks (walking or jogging while trying to kick your buttocks with your heels).

For activities with rapid directional changes such as tennis and soccer, try arm swings, shoulder rolls, hip circles, high-knee skipping or bounding, and carioca (grapevine). Other commonly used dynamic flexibility exercises include walking with exaggerated knee lift, lunging to front or side, and toe walks or heel walks. Videos of these dynamic flexibility exercises are listed in the Internet Resources at the and of the chapter.

Static and dynamic stretching can be performed actively or passively. With **active stretching,** you use your own muscle forces to stretch yourself. For example, you can actively stretch calves by sitting and flexing your ankles to pull the toes back. With **passive stretching,** someone or something else assists with a stretch. The assist could be gravity, body weight, a strap, or leverage: for example, using gravity or a slant board to assist with a calf stretch. You relax the muscle you are trying to stretch and use the external assist to apply force. Both active and passive stretching improve flexibility, but passive stretching is more commonly used.

Guidelines for Flexibility Development

Flexibility exercises are part of a balanced fitness program. The goal is to develop and maintain an adequate range of joint motion for ease of movement in your daily activities. Flexibility gains are proportional to the overload applied: to the frequency, intensity, and time (duration) of stretching.

Depending on the number of stretches and length of repetitions, a flexibility session can last 10 to 30 minutes. See the Top 10 list for "Tips for Developing Flexibility."

Prescription for Flexibility	
Frequency	• Stretch at least 2 to 3 days a week, daily if possible. Greater flexibility is produced by more frequent stretching.
Intensity	• Low-intensity stretching is best. Progress at your speed. Stretching is not competitive. Flexibility changes from day to day, and on some days you might not be able to stretch as far as you did the day before. Stretch slightly beyond the normal range of motion, to the point of tension, and hold. Do not force a stretch.
Time	• The ACSM recommends a 10- to 30-second stretch during cool-down for optimal benefit.
Repetitions	• At least four 10- to 30-second sustained stretches for each muscle group are recommended.

Tips for Behavior Change

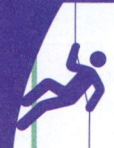

- Check this chapter and the Internet Resources for stretches recommended for your chosen fitness activity.
- Consider the benefits of enhanced flexibility in your daily activities.
- Make a checklist of your stretches and record each day you do them.
- Retest your flexibility after 6 weeks using the tests in Chapter 3 to measure your progress.

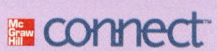 **connect**

Go online to Connect to complete this activity.
http://connect.mcgraw-hill.com

TOP 10 LIST

Tips for Developing Flexibility

Everyone can benefit from flexibility. To maximize the results from the time invested, implement the following guidelines in your next stretching session:

1. *Warm up before stretching.* An increase in muscle temperature produced by fast walking, slow jogging, or other large-muscle exercises will make stretching safer and more productive. You are sufficiently warmed up when you begin to feel warmer or when you begin to sweat.

2. *After warm-up, use stretching as preparation for activity.* While some believe that stretching during warm-up decreases the risk of injury in the activity that follows, there is no evidence that this is true. Warm-up stretching is different from a planned program of stretching for general flexibility. Warm-up stretching can be limited to what is essential, avoiding overstretching. Stretch the muscle groups used in the activity with static or dynamic exercises, and do not push for flexibility increases. Any gains will be minimal due to the tightening effect of the workout that follows.

3. *Stretch for flexibility during cool-down.* Muscles are warmest and most elastic at this point. Stretching is easier. More permanent changes in muscle lengthening occur with low-force, long-duration stretching if muscles are allowed to cool in a stretched position. Cooling muscles before releasing tension apparently causes muscle collagen (connective tissue), like stretched taffy, to stabilize toward its new stretched length.

4. *Stop at the point of tension, not pain.* Stretching to the point of pain, or until muscles quiver, can risk overstretching injury.

5. *Stretch slowly and evenly,* hold 10 to 30 seconds, and release slowly.

6. *Try to consciously relax* the target muscle as you stretch. Stretching should be felt in the muscle, not the joint.

7. *Maintain a regular breathing pattern* as you stretch.

8. *Don't bounce.* A slow sustained stretch is more effective.

9. *Incorporate 8 to 12 stretches into your program.* Flexibility is specific to a joint, so a well-planned program for general flexibility will contain one stretch for each major muscle group. Warm-up or cool-down stretching may contain fewer exercises because such stretching is activity specific and has different goals. Pay particular attention to body areas that are least flexible and stretch them more often.

10. *Strive for muscle balance.* When stretching muscles on one side of a joint, stretch those on the other side as well; for example, if you stretch hamstrings, stretch quadriceps too.

Principles of Flexibility Development

Over time, a program of regular stretching can produce beneficial changes in muscle and joint range of motion. To develop an effective stretching program, several principles affecting flexibility development must be considered. These principles include progressive overload, specificity, reversibility, individual differences, and balance.

PROGRESSIVE OVERLOAD

Improvement in joint range of motion can occur when sustained stretching produces elastic and plastic elongation. **Elastic elongation,** the temporary lengthening of soft tissue, occurs when muscle is stretched and returns to its resting length. Connective tissue within and surrounding muscle has both elastic and plastic properties. Longer or more intense stretching can produce **plastic elongation,** a semi-permanent lengthening of tissues. After a

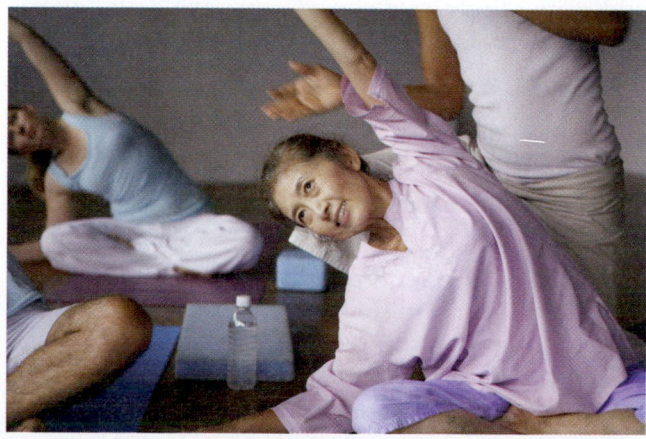

Flexibility can be improved at any age.

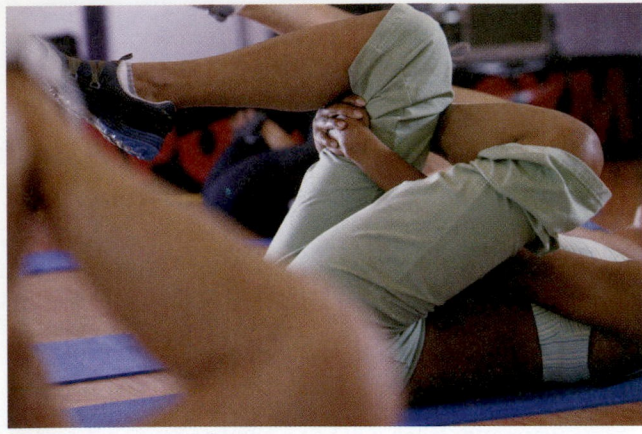

Flexibility gains are greatest during cool-down stretching.

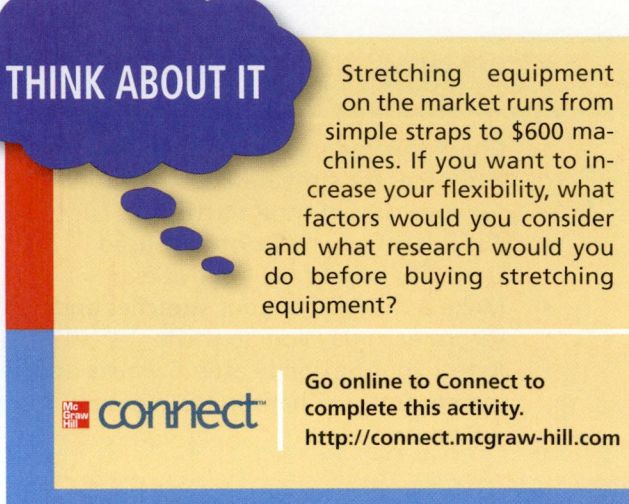

THINK ABOUT IT

Stretching equipment on the market runs from simple straps to $600 machines. If you want to increase your flexibility, what factors would you consider and what research would you do before buying stretching equipment?

connect Go online to Connect to complete this activity. http://connect.mcgraw-hill.com

stretch is removed, elastic elongation reverses and plastic elongation remains. Plastic elongation is the goal of stretching programs. It is best obtained through static or slow, sustained stretching. The amount of plastic elongation is considered time-dependent and is proportional to the amount of force applied. If tissue is stretched to the point of tension but not pain (which may activate the stretch reflex) and held, the tissue will gradually relax and elongate, and require less force to maintain the new length. A prolonged stretch is needed to achieve plastic elongation.

SPECIFICITY

Flexibility is specific to a joint; that is, flexibility in one leg does not guarantee flexibility in the other leg, and flexibility in the shoulders does not ensure flexibility in the lower back. It is also specific to joint angles—a person who can do front splits may be less flexible in side splits.

REVERSIBILITY

Like any other fitness component, flexibility changes are reversible. If a person stops stretching, over time, range of motion will decrease back to levels sustained by daily activities. Gains from flexibility can be lost in as little as 3 to 4 weeks without stretching. On the other hand, flexibility can be maintained with stretching as few as 2 to 3 days per week.

INDIVIDUAL DIFFERENCES

People vary in their ability to develop flexibility. Variations in proportions of collagen and elastin in muscle tissue, joint structure, length of muscles, and attachment points of tendons on bones may contribute to differences in joint range of motion as well as ability to increase that range. Within your genetic endowment, you do have potential for improvement. A regular stretching program can help you enhance and maintain your flexibility within your genetically determined range.

BALANCE

We often have muscles that are tighter on one side of the body (right-left or front-back). Pay attention to flexibility differences and work to improve them. Your hamstrings may be tighter on one side than the other. It is common for chest muscles to be tighter than the opposing upper back muscles, and lower back muscles are often tighter than abdominals. Spend more time stretching the tighter areas to alleviate the imbalance.

Flexibility Exercises for Basic Fitness

After a good general warm-up or as part of a cool-down, exercises A through F in Figure 5-1 are important for runners, walkers, and aerobic dancers. Cyclists, swimmers, and water exercisers should add upper-body stretches G through I. If time is limited, save stretching for the cool-down. For basic fitness flexibility, perform the full program of exercises in Figure 5-1. Hold each one 10 to 30 seconds and repeat at least four times. Lab Activity 5-1 gives an introductory flexibility session that you can incorporate into your routine.

A. Hamstring stretch
    Sit and extend one leg in front, with the other bent and tucked as shown in diagram (a). Keeping shoulders erect, press abdomen forward. Hold. Repeat with other leg.
B. Lower back/hip flexor stretch
    Lie on your back with one leg straight and one bent. With hands behind thigh,

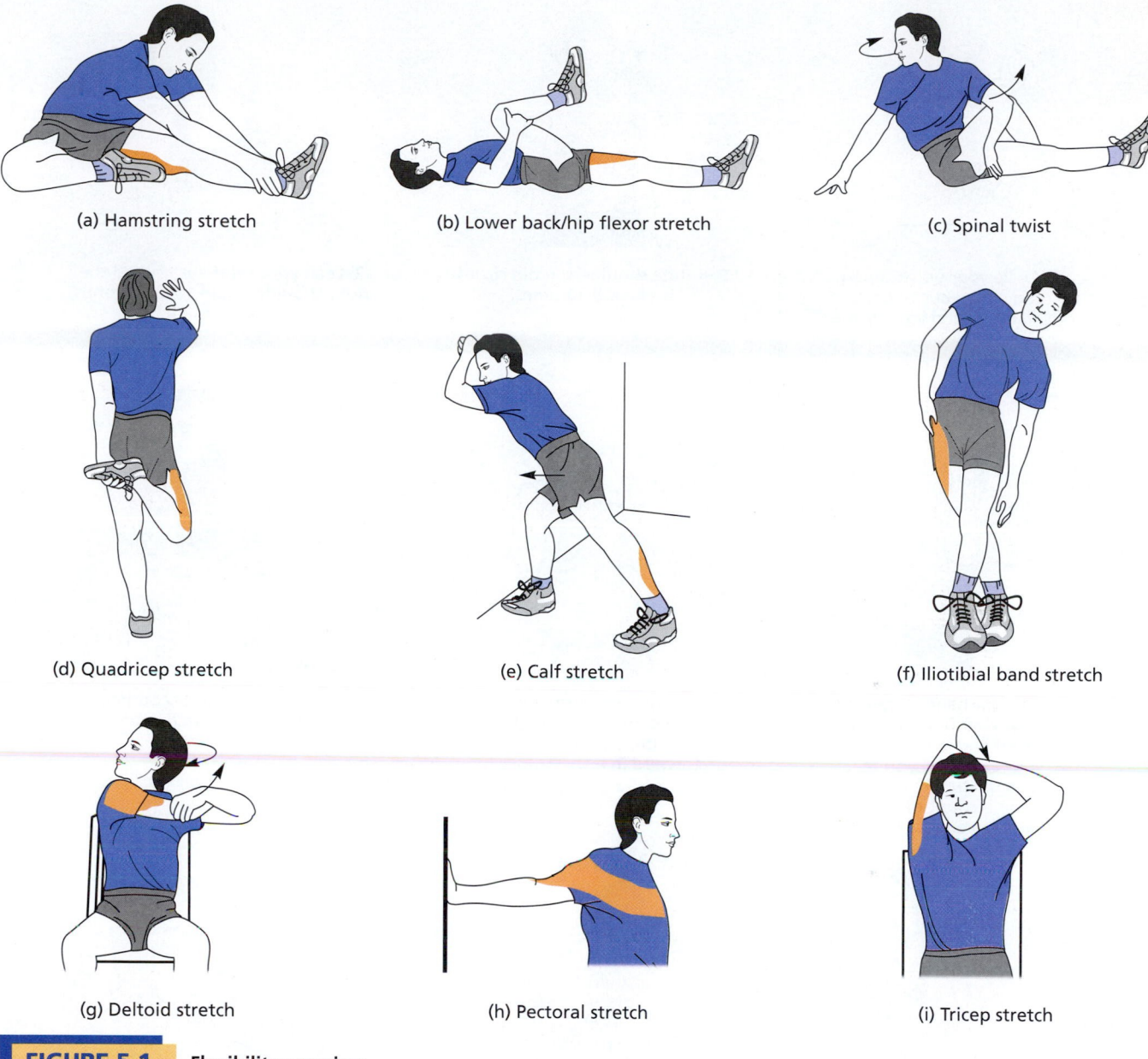

(a) Hamstring stretch   (b) Lower back/hip flexor stretch   (c) Spinal twist

(d) Quadricep stretch   (e) Calf stretch   (f) Iliotibial band stretch

(g) Deltoid stretch   (h) Pectoral stretch   (i) Tricep stretch

FIGURE 5-1   **Flexibility exercises.**

press thigh toward chest. Keep extended leg straight. Repeat left.

C.   Spinal twist (lower back and hip abductors)
Sit with right leg extended, step left leg over right, and turn upper body toward left. Repeat on other side.

D.   Quadriceps stretch
Stand with right leg bent at the knee. With left hand, pull right heel toward buttocks. Keep shoulders up, abdominals tight, and hips tucked under to prevent back hyperextension. Omit if you have knee problems.

E.   Calf/achilles stretch
Standing in forward lunge position, toes pointing forward, press heel toward floor.

Repeat with other leg. Bend back knee to stretch soleus.

F.   Iliotibial band stretch
Cross left foot over right, press hips to right. Repeat with other side.

G.   Deltoid stretch
Cross right arm in front of body and pull it in toward midline with left hand. Repeat on other side.

H.   Pectoral stretch
Place right hand on wall, with elbow extended but not locked. Twist shoulders left. Repeat with left arm.

I.   Triceps stretch
Pull left elbow behind head. Repeat right.

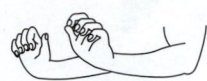
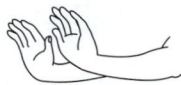

1. Circle your wrists, open and close your fingers, flex and extend your wrists

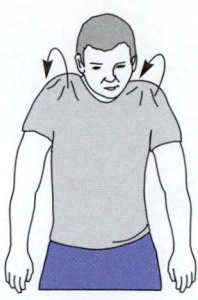

2. Rotate shoulders in big circles backward 10 times.

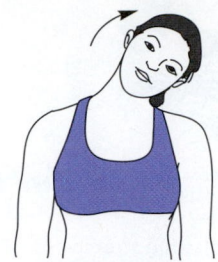

3. Lean your right ear toward the right shoulder, hold 10–20 seconds, repeat to the left.

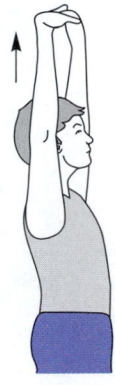

4. Place your hands together in front of your body, raise your arms overhead and back toward your ears until you feel a chest stretch. Inhale, hold for a count of 5, exhale and lower your arms.

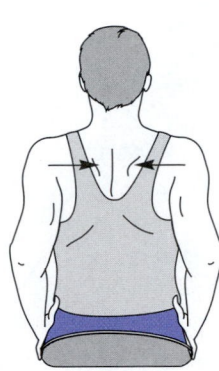

5. Put your hands on your hips. Pull your shoulder blades back and press your chest forward in a chest stretch.

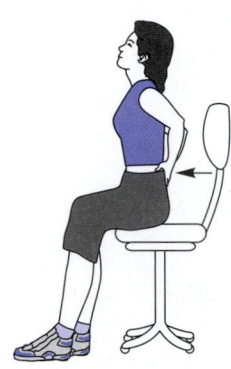

6. Gently press your abdomen forward and arch your lower back.

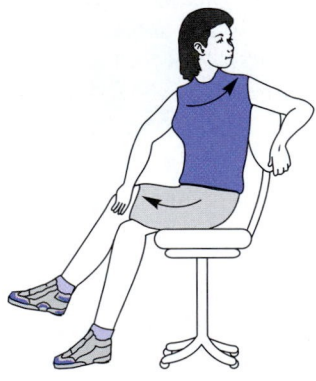

7. Cross left knee over right. Place hands on your knee and hip. Rotate your trunk to look back over your left shoulder. Repeat to the other side.

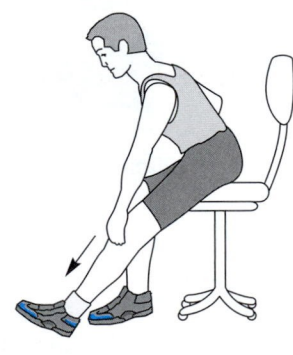

8. Extend one knee, lean toward it trying to bring your belly button toward your thigh until you feel a gentle stretch in your hamstring. Hold. Repeat to the other side.

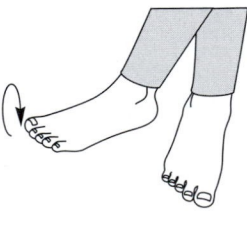

9. Point and flex your ankles several times, circle your ankles

FIGURE 5-2   **Seated stretches**

Seated Stretches

Do you find yourself doing a lot of desk work and needing to relax tight muscles? Do you feel you don't have much of an opportunity to stretch? Figure 5-2 illustrates some stretches you can do without leaving your desk, while at the computer, or when watching television. Choose those that you find most beneficial and do them a few times throughout the day to feel refreshed. (Also see Lab Activity 5-2.)

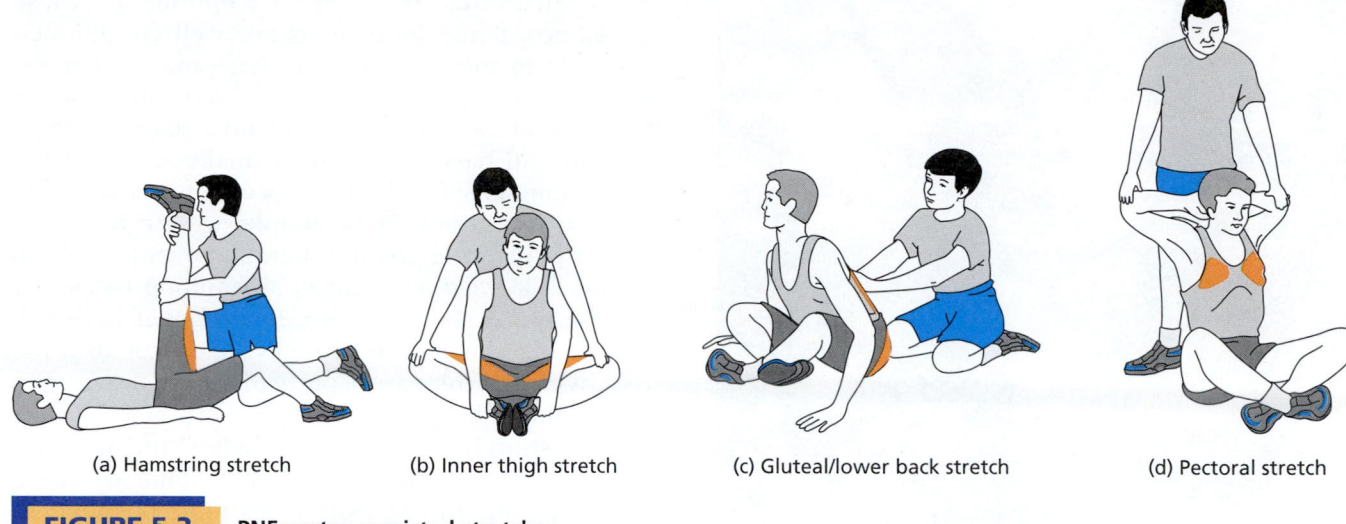

(a) Hamstring stretch   (b) Inner thigh stretch   (c) Gluteal/lower back stretch   (d) Pectoral stretch

FIGURE 5-3   PNF partner-assisted stretches.

PNF Partner-Assisted Stretches

A type of static stretching called **proprioceptive neuromuscular facilitation (PNF),** a partner-assisted stretch often used by athletic trainers, is highly effective for increasing flexibility. It utilizes the nervous and muscular systems to facilitate stretching. It was developed by Herman Kabat, MD, and two physical therapists in the 1940s for use on paralysis patients to improve flexibility and strength. PNF utilizes the inverse stretch reflex produced by golgi tendon organs to relax the target muscle and allow a greater stretch. It is thought that when the muscle is first stretched, then contracted, the GTO reflexes are stimulated, relaxing the muscle. To perform a PNF contract-relax stretch, you first perform a 10- to 30-second static stretch, then contract the muscle for 6 seconds to produce fatigue, and then relax while a partner stretches your limb for 10 to 30 seconds. The forced contraction fatigues the muscle and increases the muscle's ability to relax while being stretched.

Another type of PNF stretching called the *contract-relax-agonist contract* inserts a contraction of the opposing muscle group before the final stretch; for example, in the hamstring stretch, after contracting hamstrings, the person would contract quadriceps, pulling the leg back as far as possible for about 10 seconds. If the quadriceps is contracted, through reciprocal innervation, the hamstring relaxes even more and can be passively stretched to a greater range of motion. Some research indicates that the contract-relax-agonist contract method is the most effective PNF technique.

For safety, be sensitive to your partner's needs and flexibility levels. Be sure to communicate when more or less resistance or pressure is needed throughout each exercise. Work with the same partner throughout the series. Switching partners can lead to injury because of unfamiliarity with the flexibility limits of the person being stretched. Some examples of PNF stretches are illustrated in Figure 5-3.

A. Hamstring stretch
    Lie on your back and lift one leg into the air. Partner supports ankle and knee in a static stretch. Keeping knee extended but not locked, push against your partner as he or she resists. Stretch and then relax as partner eases leg into a new stretch.

B. Inner thigh stretch
    Sit with knees out and bottoms of feet together. Press down on knees in a static stretch. Partner kneels behind and resists on knees as you press them upward. Finally, relax as partner gently presses knees toward the floor in a stretch.

C. Gluteal/lower back stretch
    Sit cross-legged and stretch forward. Partner kneels behind you with hands on your upper back. Next, resist back against partner. Then stretch forward as partner assists.

D. Pectoral stretch
    Sit cross-legged with fingers interlaced behind your head and back, supported by partner's thigh. Partner gently pulls your elbows back for 10 seconds and then resists as you attempt to pull them forward. Next, relax as partner gently stretches them back.

Other Programs for Enhancing Flexibility

Tai Chi and yoga are very old yet newly popular activities that can enhance flexibility and balance as well as reduce stress.

Tai Chi is an ancient Chinese exercise known for its slow, graceful movements. It originated as a self-

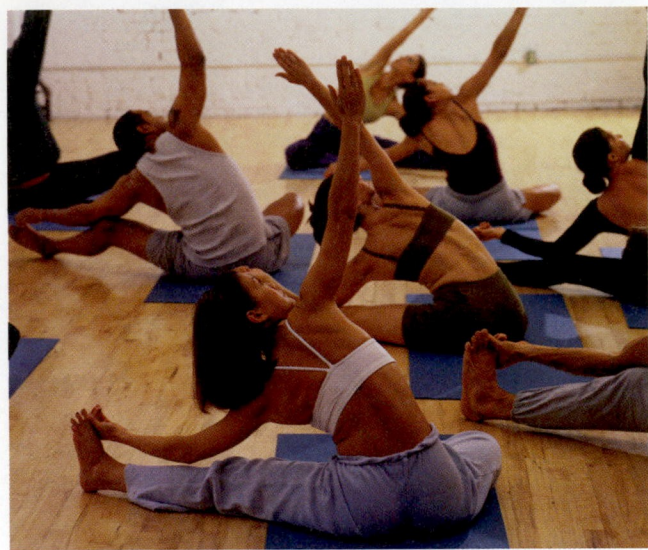

Yoga can improve flexibility and balance.

defense activity but now is used to enhance standing balance, flexibility, lower-body strength, and neuromuscular control. It is a good exercise for people of all ages and can be enjoyed throughout the lifetime.

Yoga, which means to yoke or unite, is another ancient art with several branches, each with its own style. Hatha yoga is the most widely practiced in the United States. It involves using mental focus and coordinated breathing while assuming a series of physical postures. Some people do yoga to reduce stress, others to improve flexibility and balance. Some forms of yoga are more vigorous than others; some are more relaxing. If one type doesn't appeal to you, investigate others.

One way to get started in yoga or Tai Chi is to enroll in a class. Either can be learned at a beginning level in a few weeks of instruction, though mastery may take years. Instructional DVDs are available for home use and can be obtained at a video store or library. The Yoga Sun Salutation, a series of yoga poses, is pictured and described in Lab Activity 5-3 for you to experience.

Other activities with a notable flexibility component include Pilates (Chapter 6) and water exercise (Chapter 4).

◆ CONTRAINDICATED EXERCISES

A few stretching and toning exercises added to an aerobic program can promote balanced fitness by increasing flexibility in tight muscles and strengthening weak ones. However, not all conditioning exercises commonly done in classes or seen on videotapes are good for everyone. These potentially harmful exercises are labeled *contraindicated exercises*.

Realize that there are exceptions to these guidelines. Some individuals are well conditioned and able to minimize risk in these moves. For example, a competitive hurdler needs to practice hurdle stretches for the sport, and a dance or yoga student will have an instructor make sure that the positioning is safe. The body is able to move safely in many directions. For example, we are rarely injured by squatting down or bending over to pick up a shoe. Likewise an occasional standing toe touch will be harmless for most people, but if high-risk moves are practiced repeatedly, day after day, the risk of injury increases, particularly in those with preexisting joint problems.

By studying people with aches and injuries, fitness experts have learned that some common stretching and toning exercises should be avoided. Others should be modified for safety and effectiveness. Be aware of which commonly done high-risk movements you should avoid and which high-benefit, low-risk exercises you should do instead. Figure 5-4 shows some examples of each.

Your body is meant to move in many ways—to bend, twist, and stretch. Some people can do high-risk exercises for years with no ill effects. For others, after only a few repetitions, injury occurs. You may not know into which category you fit until it is too late. The problem is that some movements increase risks to muscles, joints, and connective tissue. While you may need to do deep squats if you are a competitive weightlifter or a yoga plow if you are in a yoga class, these moves don't offer any special benefit for the fitness exerciser. Low-benefit, high-risk exercises should be minimized in programs designed to emphasize personal fitness. Follow these general rules when exercising:

1. Do not hyperflex the knee.
2. Do not hyperextend the knee, neck, or lower back.
3. Do not apply a twisting or lateral force to the knee.
4. Avoid holding your breath during exercise.
5. Avoid stretching long/weak muscles (e.g., abdominals) and avoid shortening already short/strong muscles (e.g., hip flexors). See common muscle imbalances in Table 8-2.
   a. Most people should avoid aggravating common postural faults: forward head, dorsal kyphosis (rounded upper back), medial rotations of the thigh, and pronation of the foot.
   b. Most people need to stretch the chest muscles, hip flexors, calves, hamstrings, lower back, and medial thigh rotators.

Don't	**Do**	**Explanation**

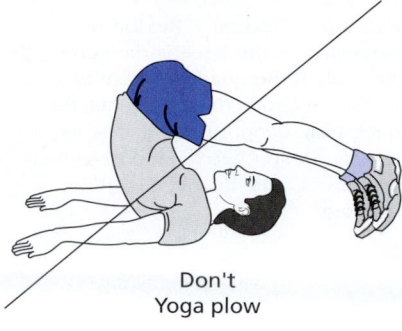 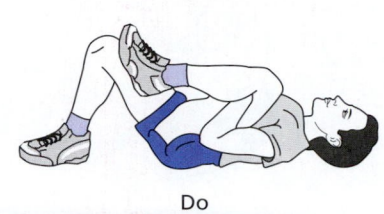

Don't
Yoga plow

Do
Single-knee tuck to chest

1. *Yoga plow:* Sometimes done as a back stretch, this exercise can injure discs, ligaments, and nerves in the neck and back. A better back stretch is a single-or double-knee tuck to the chest.

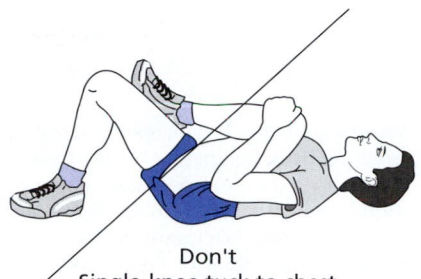 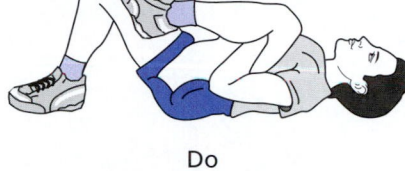

Don't
Single-knee tuck to chest

Do
Single-knee tuck to chest
Note: Hug the **thigh**, not the knee.

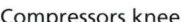
Compressors knee

2. *Knee tuck to chest:* Hyperflexing the knee by pulling it to the body with the arms or hands placed on top of the tibia places undue stress on the knee joint. Note: The hand position should be *changed to hug the thigh rather than the shin.*

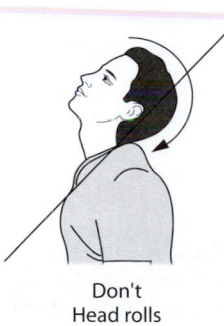 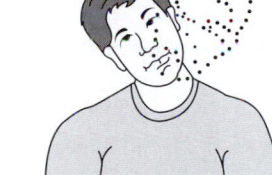

Don't
Head rolls

Do
Half-head rolls

3. *Head roll:* Hyperextension can injure discs in the neck. Safer neck stretches include half-head rolls to the front, turning the head side to side so that the chin touches the right and left shoulders, and touching an ear to each shoulder.

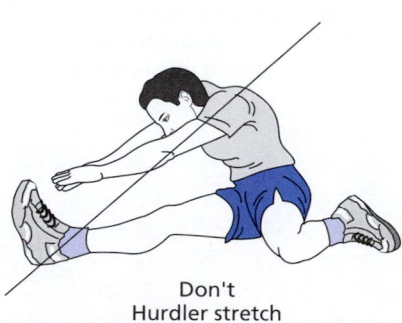 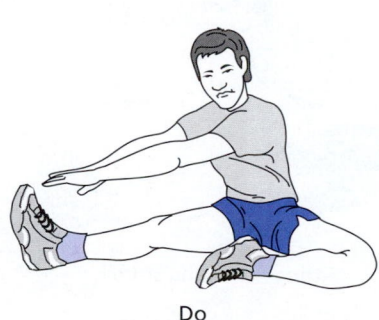

Don't
Hurdler stretch

Do
Alternative hurdler stretch

4. *Hurdler stretch:* This stretch can cause groin pull, injure knee cartilage, and overstretch the medial collateral ligament—the one that helps stabilize the knee. It may also cause hip joint discomfort because the femur of the leg that is tucked behind is in a position of extreme rotation in the joint capsule. The alternative hurdler stretch safely stretches hamstrings.

FIGURE 5-4   **Contraindicated exercises.**

Don't	Do	Explanation

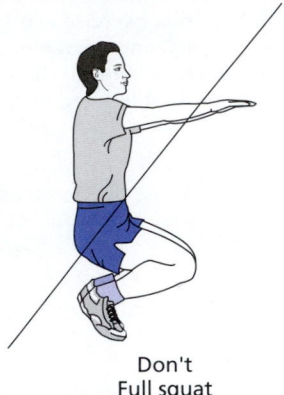

Don't
Full squat

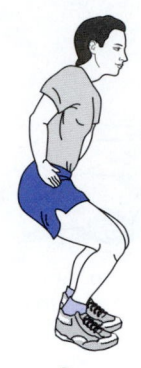

Do
Half-knee bend

5. *Full squat:* Excessive flexion or extension of the knee is dangerous. To strengthen the quadriceps, substitute half-knee bends for full squats, the duckwalk, deep lunges, and squat thrusts. Deep knee flexion exercises overstress knee ligaments and cartilage.

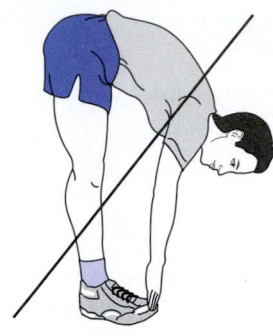

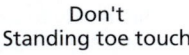

Don't
Standing toe touch

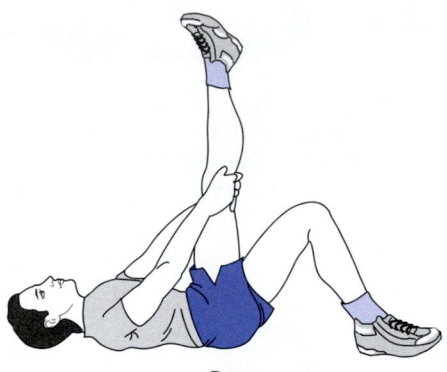

Do
Lying hamstring stretch

6. *Standing toe touch:* This exercise risks straining back ligaments. Limit forward flexion in a standing position. As your trunk dips below a 25- to 45-degree angle, the lower back muscles cease to work and the posterior ligaments joining bone to bone must support the load.

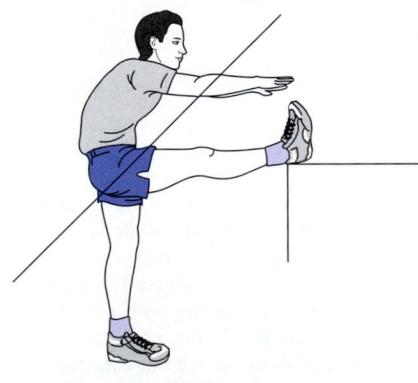

Don't
Ballet bar leg stretch

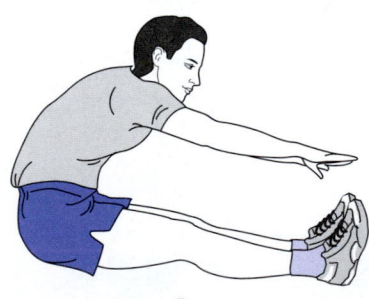

Do
Sitting hamstring stretch

7. *Leg stretches at a ballet bar (or other high object):* These may be potentially harmful. When the extended leg is raised 90 degrees or more and the trunk is bent over the leg, it may lead to sciatica problems, especially when the exerciser has limited flexibility. Substitute the back and hamstring stretches suggested in 1,4, and 6.

FIGURE 5-4   **Contraindicated exercises. (*continued*)**

Don't   **Do**   **Explanation**

8. *Leaning forward and twisting the trunk to the side:* These moves are particularly hazardous to the lower back, adding a shearing force to the stress on back ligaments. Avoid swinging hands and the trunk through the knees, windmill toe touches, waist circles, and elbow-knee lunges. There is no exercise you can do standing to tone your waist. The most effective exercise for reducing the waist is aerobic exercise and sensible nutrition. To tone oblique abdominals, the muscles that underlie the waist area, use twisting bent-knee abdominal curls. Lying on your back with heels close to your buttocks and crossing your arms across your chest (or with a hand touching each shoulder), curl the shoulders first toward the right knee and then toward the left knee.

Don't
Windmill toe touches

Do
Oblique abdominal curls

9. *Double-leg lifts, straight-leg sit-ups, and low leg scissors:* These do little or nothing to tone the abdominals. They tighten hip flexors, which in most people are too tight already, causing lordosis (swayback). They may also cause lower back strain. The most effective exercise for toning abdominals is bent-knee abdominal curls in which the lower back stays on the ground while the shoulders curl forward about 3 inches. To avoid jerking on the head or neck, cross your arms across your chest or behind your head with a hand touching each shoulder.

Don't
Straight-leg sit-ups

Do
Bent-knee abdominal curls

Don't
Double-leg lifts

10. *The swan arch, prone double-leg raises, and yoga cobra:* These produce excessive back hyperextension and possible back strain. In a prone position, raise your right arm and the opposite leg a few inches off the ground and then switch; this will strengthen the back safely.

Right arm needs to be raised.

Don't
Swan arch

Do
Single arm/leg raises

11. *Donkey kicks or fire hydrants:* Done on hands and knees with the back hyperextended, these may strain the lower back. To protect the back, hold your abdominals tight, round your back, and raise your leg no higher than 6 to 12 inches.

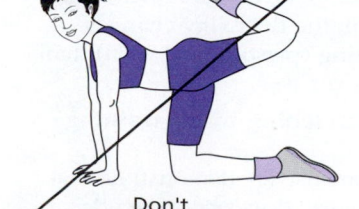

Don't
Donkey kicks

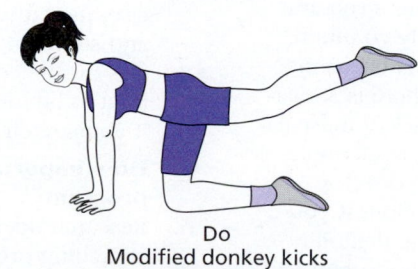

Do
Modified donkey kicks
(can be done with forearms on floor)

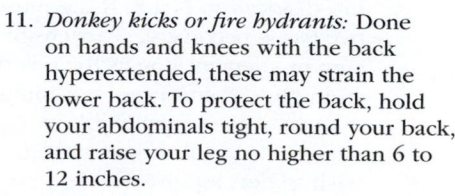

FIGURE 5-4   **Contraindicated exercises. (*continued*)**

6. Avoid stretching any joint to the point of pain.

7. Be especially careful when using passive stretches with another person (unless the person is a physical therapist).

8. Avoid movements that place acute compressional forces on spinal discs, such as extending and rotating the spine simultaneously (e.g., trunk and neck circling and double-leg lifts).

9. Avoid movements that cause joint impingements or cartilage damage, such as arm circles in the palm-down position.

10. If the nature of your sport regularly requires the violation of good mechanics (baseball catcher assuming a deep squat position or gymnast performing double-leg lifts), make certain the muscles are as strong as possible to endure the stress.

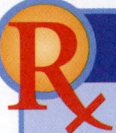

PRESCRIPTION FOR ACTION

You've read the chapter. Now go do one or more of these.

✓ While studying or reading the morning paper, sit on the floor and stretch hamstrings.

✓ While on the phone, do calf and quadriceps stretches.

✓ If you have a desk job, take a 5-minute stretch break every hour—do ankle circles, half head rolls, and shoulder stretches.

✓ After every hour of computer use, stretch wrists, back, and shoulders.

✓ While watching TV, stretch during commercials.

McGraw Hill **connect**™

Go online to Connect to complete this activity.
http://connect.mcgraw-hill.com

Frequently Asked Questions

Q. Is it possible to become too flexible? Is that a problem?

A. It is possible for the muscles and connective tissue surrounding a joint to become too flexible. Joints are constructed to move within a certain range of motion. Excessive motion can damage tendons and ligaments and tear the joint capsule. Once a muscle has been stretched to its maximum length, further stretching will only loosen tendons and ligaments (which you do not want to stretch), which can cause joint instability and increase the risk of injury. There is a trade-off between flexibility and stability. The greater the joint's range of motion, the less stable the joint is structurally and the more it must rely on the muscles supporting it to control the range of motion. For example, the shoulder has relatively high flexibility compared with the hip, which has greater structural stability. Shoulder dislocation is fairly common; hip dislocation is not. If the muscles and connective tissue become very extensible, there is a measure of safety as long as there is sufficient muscular strength to control the movement. For example, gymnasts are very flexible but also develop strength to control that range of motion. If you wish to develop greater than average flexibility for a sport or physical activity, it is important to strengthen the muscles that you stretch (and vice versa) for balanced fitness.

Q. What are the advantages and disadvantages of stretching with a partner?

A. On the plus side, stretching with a partner adds a social element that makes it more fun. It's a good way to get to know your classmates if you stretch with different people. You can relax while your partner stretches you, so you may get a better stretch. On the minus side, you and your partner must communicate well to minimize the risk of overstretching, and stretching with a partner takes longer than stretching alone. A good compromise is to do a few partner stretches along with individual stretches.

Q. If I am short on time, is it better to stretch before or after exercise?

A. When you stretch before exercise, the muscles tighten up again during the workout. After exercise, the muscles are warmer, more extensible, and stretching is easier. Also, if you stretch muscles during cool-down, the flexibility changes tend to be longer lasting (plastic elongation) than if you stretch before exercise.

Q. How important is stretching in my training program?

A. Research does not conclusively demonstrate that stretching prevents injury. However, we tend to lose flexibility and move more stiffly as we age, and regular stretching prevents this loss.

Maintaining youthful flexibility can enhance your ability to perform daily activities, such as turning to look as you are backing up your car. It also enhances performance of athletic activities—making it easier to get a full stride as you run or a full reach in swimming. Being able to apply forces through a full range of motion gives more power to athletic skills.

Summary

Flexibility is an important asset in fitness and daily activities. It enhances the ability to move freely and easily, aids with posture and appearance, helps with recovery from injury, and can reverse joint stiffness and tightness that creeps up over time. Factors that affect flexibility include joint structure, soft tissues, inactivity, muscle temperature, age, genetics, gender, obesity or excessive muscle hypertrophy, injury and scar tissue, as well as neural factors. Flexibility gains are proportional to the overload applied, to the frequency, intensity, and time of stretching. While static stretching is recommended for most fitness activities, dynamic stretches may better for certain athletic activities, and both types may be done either passively or actively. Principles of flexibility development include progressive overload, specificity, reversibility, and balance. A series of stretches for basic fitness was given, as well as PNF partner-assisted stretches. Some potentially harmful or contraindicated exercises that put joints at increased risk of injury, and guidelines for identifying them, were also discussed.

Terms

- active stretching
- collagen
- dynamic flexibility
- dynamic stretching
- elastic elongation
- elastin

- golgi tendon organ (GTO)
- inverse stretch reflex
- muscle spindle
- passive stretching
- plastic elongation

- proprioceptive neuromuscular facilitation (PNF)
- reciprocal inhibition
- static flexibility
- static stretching
- stretch reflex

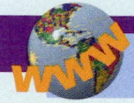 Internet Resources

About.com

http://tinyurl.com/ch5stretchex

Stretching exercises described and illustrated for various joints, muscles and activities

American College of Sports Medicine

www.acsm.org

Information on sports research, health and fitness, aerobic exercise guidelines, and a quarterly fitness newsletter. The "Fit Society Page" and "Current Comments" give information on a variety of exercise topics of recent interest.

International Fitness Association

www.ifafitness.com

Provides information about physical fitness, strength training, types of stretching, and the physiology of stretching.

Mayo Clinic

www.mayoclinic.com

Videos on stretching for the office and slide shows showing stretching exercises.

Mayo Clinic

Information on stretching
http://tinyurl.com/ch5stretching

Information on Tai Chi to improve balance and reduce stress
http://mayoclinic.com/health/tai-chi/SA00087

Slide show on how to stretch your muscle groups
http://tinyurl.com/ch5mgroups

Slide show on stretches you can do in your office
http://tinyurl.com/ch5office

The Stretching Institute
http://www.thestretchinghandbook.com/
Information on stretches for different activities and to alleviate specific injuries.

The Ultimate handbook
http://tinyurl.com/ch5handbook
Information on warmup, basic stretches, active isolated and PNF stretching, improving mobility and Yoga.

Videos

American College of Sports Medicine
Exercise Is Medicine—Keys to Exercise—Flexibility
http://tinyurl.com/ch5flexible

Mayo Clinic.com
Back exercises in 15 minutes a day
http://tinyurl.com/ch5backex
Forearm stretches for the office
http://tinyurl.com/ch5forearm
Neck stretches for the office
http://tinyurl.com/ch5neck
Seated stretches for the office
http://tinyurl.com/ch5seated
Standing stretches for the office
http://tinyurl.com/ch5standing

Upper body stretches for the office
http://tinyurl.com/ch5upbody
Yoga for Stress Management
http://tinyurl.com/ch5yoga

NY Times.com
Stretching: The Truth. Explains the benefits of dynamic stretching.
http://tinyurl.com/ch5nytstretch

Youtube.com
Dynamic Flexibility Exercises
http://tinyurl.com/ch5dynamic1
http://tinyurl.com/ch5dynamic2
http://tinyurl.com/ch5dynamic3
Basic Tai Chi Exercises
http://tinyurl.com/ch5tcbasic
28 Form Tai Chi for Beginners
http://tinyurl.com/ch5begintc
Yang Tai Chi 24 Form (in Chinese)
http://tinyurl.com/ch5yang
Hatha Yoga Workout: Sun Salutation
http://tinyurl.com/ch5hatha1
http://tinyurl.com/ch5hatha2

LAB Activity 5-1

Name _____ Class/Activity Section _____ Date _____

Introductory Flexibility Session

Equipment Needed:

Mat

Procedure

Read Chapter 5, warm up, and then complete these exercises as illustrated in Figure 5-1. Hold each stretch 10 to 30 seconds and repeat two to four times. You can tear out this lab and follow the exercise descriptions on the back of this page.

FLEXIBILITY EXERCISES

Exercise	Time/ Repetitions	Exercise	Time/ Repetitions	Exercise	Time/ Repetitions
A. Hamstring stretch	_____	D. Quadriceps stretch	_____	G. Deltoid stretch	_____
B. Lower back/hip flexor stretch	_____	E. Calf/Achilles stretch	_____	H. Pectoral stretch	_____
C. Spinal twist	_____	F. Iliotibial band stretch	_____	I. Triceps stretch	_____

See back of page for instructions.

Results

1. What stretches were the most challenging due to muscle or joint tightness?

2. What stretches were easiest for you? You will want to maintain this flexibility.

3. Considering your own tight or flexible areas, as well as the rule of specificity, which are the most important stretches for you to incorporate into your exercise program?

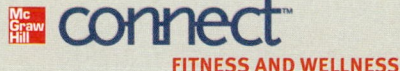

http://connect.mcgraw-hill.com

FITNESS AND WELLNESS

A. Hamstring stretch

   Sit and extend one leg in front, with the other bent and tucked. Keeping shoulders erect, press abdomen forward. Hold. Repeat with other leg.

B. Lower back/hip flexor stretch

   Lie on your back with one leg straight and one bent. With hands behind thigh, press thigh toward chest. Keep extended leg straight. Repeat with other leg.

C. Spinal twist (lower back and hip abductors)

   Sit with right leg extended, step left leg over right, and turn upper body toward left. Repeat on other side.

D. Quadriceps stretch

   Stand with right leg bent at the knee. With left hand, pull right heel toward buttocks. Keep shoulders up, abdominals tight, and hips tucked under to prevent back hyperextension. Omit if you have knee problems.

E. Calf/achilles stretch

   Standing in forward lunge position, toes pointing forward, press heel toward floor. Repeat with other leg. Bend back knee to stretch soleus.

F. Iliotibial band stretch

   Cross left foot over right, press hips to right. Repeat with other side.

G. Deltoid stretch

   Cross right arm in front of body and pull it in toward midline with left hand. Repeat with left arm.

H. Pectoral stretch

   Place right hand on wall, with elbow extended but not locked. Twist shoulders left. Repeat with left arm.

I. Triceps stretch

   Pull left elbow behind head. Repeat with right arm.

LAB Activity 5-2

Seated Stretching Session

Equipment Needed:

Chair

Procedure:

Here is a set of stretches that can be done during the day while sitting at your desk to relieve muscle tension and tightness. After remaining seated for an hour or more at your desk, complete these exercises as illustrated, then answer the questions below. This is a tear-out sheet that may be used anywhere.

SEATED STRETCHES

Results

1. Which stretches revealed muscle or joint tightness?

2. Considering your own tight or flexible areas, which are the most beneficial stretches for you to use when you find yourself doing a lot of seated work?

connect
FITNESS AND WELLNESS

http://connect.mcgraw-hill.com

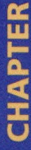

LAB Activity ■ CHAPTER 5

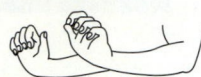
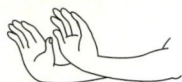

1. Circle your wrists, open and close your fingers, flex and extend your wrists

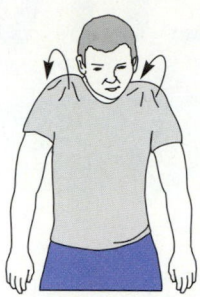

2. Rotate shoulders in big circles backward 10 times.

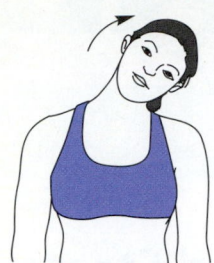

3. Lean your right ear toward the right shoulder, hold 10–20 seconds, repeat to the left.

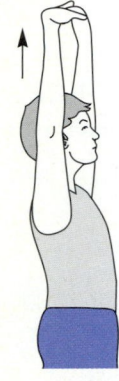

4. Place your hands together in front of your body, raise your arms overhead and back toward your ears until you feel a chest stretch. Inhale, hold for a count of 5, exhale and lower your arms.

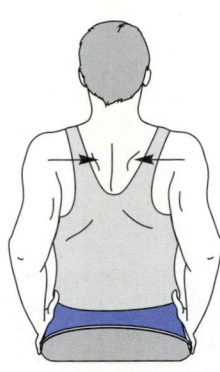

5. Put your hands on your hips. Pull your shoulder blades back and press your chest forward in a chest stretch.

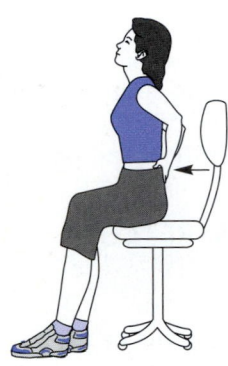

6. Gently press your abdomen forward and arch your lower back.

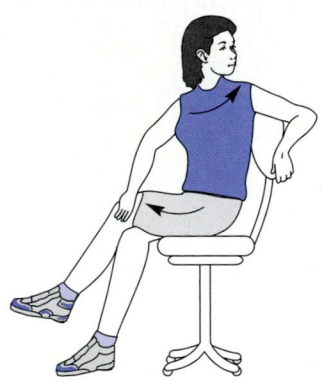

7. Cross left knee over right. Place hands on your knee and hip. Rotate your trunk to look back over your left shoulder. Repeat to the other side.

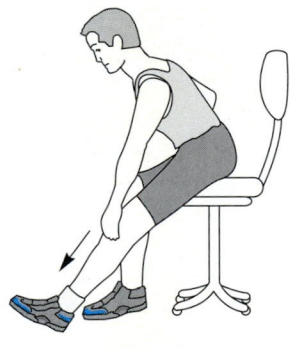

8. Extend one knee, lean toward it trying to bring your belly button toward your thigh until you feel a gentle stretch in your hamstring. Hold. Repeat to the other side.

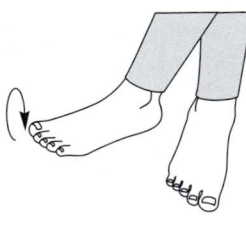

9. Point and flex your ankles several times, circle your ankles

LAB Activity 5-3

Name _____ Class/Activity Section _____ Date _____

Hatha Yoga Workout: Sun Salutation (or Salute to the Sun)

Introduction: The Sun Salutation, one of the most popular yoga routines, is a series of 12 postures (poses) performed in a single, graceful flow. Each movement is coordinated with the breath. Inhale as you extend or stretch, and exhale as you fold or contract. Complete the instructions below and answer the questions. The Sun Salutation is on the back of this page. This is a tear-out exercise that may be used anywhere.

1. Go through the Sun Salutation routine slowly several times. One complete routine consists of two sequences: one for the right side of the body, and one for the left. Concentrate on the proper order of the poses during this initial practice session.

2. Now practice the routine concentrating on inhaling and exhaling at the correct time.

3. Describe how the arms and shoulders feel after going through this yoga workout.

4. Were you able to step each leg up between the hands in one movement on the Lunge pose? Yes/No Discuss:

5. Were you able to press the heels of the feet down to the floor on the Downward Dog pose? Yes/No Discuss:

6. What is your evaluation of the Sun Salutation as a strength and flexibility exercise routine?

7. Is there any way to make this routine aerobic? If so, how?

8. How could this routine help with stress management?

_____

Video illustrating the Hatha Yoga Sun Salutation can be found at http://tinyurl.com/ch5hatha1 and http://tinyurl.com/ch5hatha2

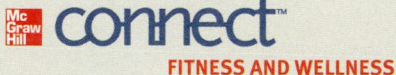

http://connect.mcgraw-hill.com

FITNESS AND WELLNESS

LAB Activity ■ CHAPTER 5

Sun Salutations

1
Mountain

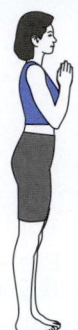

Stand with feet together, slightly pigeon-toed (big toes touching, heels apart), with your hands together, palm to palm, at heart level. Take several deep breaths. **Exhale.**

2
Slight Arch

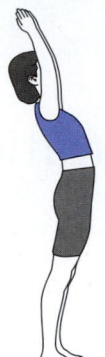

Inhale. Tighten buttocks, stretch arms upward, gently arching your back as far as feels comfortable and safe.

3
Standing
Forward Bend

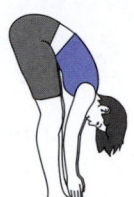

Exhale, while bending forward and downward, bringing your hands flat to the floor beside your feet, bending the knees if necessary. Touch head to knees, if possible.

4
Lunge

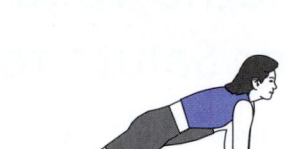

Inhale and step the right leg back in a wide backward lunge. Keep left foot between hands.

5
Plank

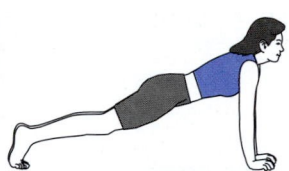

Exhale and step left leg back into plank. **Inhale.** Hold the position and breathe. Tighten abs.

6
Knees and Chest

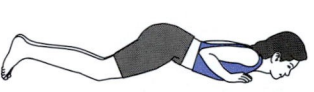

Hold your breath and lower the body in one unit, close to the floor. **Exhale** as you touch knees, chest, and chin to the floor. Lower hips, point feet and toes.

7
Cobra

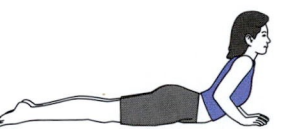

Inhale, lifting your chest toward the sky, with elbows slightly bent and pressed into your ribs. Straighten arms as much as feels comfortable.

8
Downward Dog

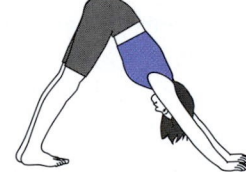

Exhale, tuck toes under lifting hips up and bringing the body into inverted V. Align head with arms. Press heels down.

9
Lunge

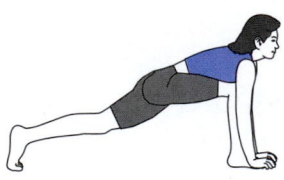

Inhale. Lift head and step the right foot up between hands.

10
Standing Forward
Bend

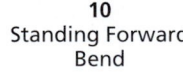
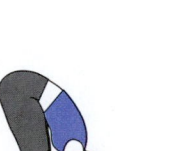

Exhale. Bring the left foot up and go into standing forward bend.

11
Slight Arch

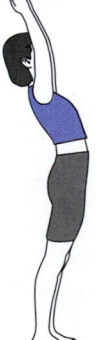

Inhale. Rise slowly. Tighten buttocks, lift arms overhead, and arch back.

12
Mountain

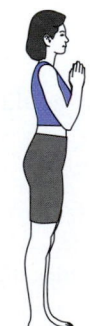

Exhale. Return to position number 1. Repeat the sequence, stepping with the left leg.

CHAPTER 6

Developing Muscular Fitness

STUDY QUESTIONS

You will have successfully mastered this chapter if you can answer the following:

1. What are the five benefits of and five cautions for resistance training?
2. What are the differences between training programs for strength and programs for muscular endurance?
3. What are the two basic types of muscular exercise? Give an example of each.
4. What are the three principles of resistance training?
5. What are the correct safety guidelines for weight training?
6. What are the four types of resistance training programs?
7. How does muscular fitness contribute to wellness?

You will find the answers as you read this chapter.

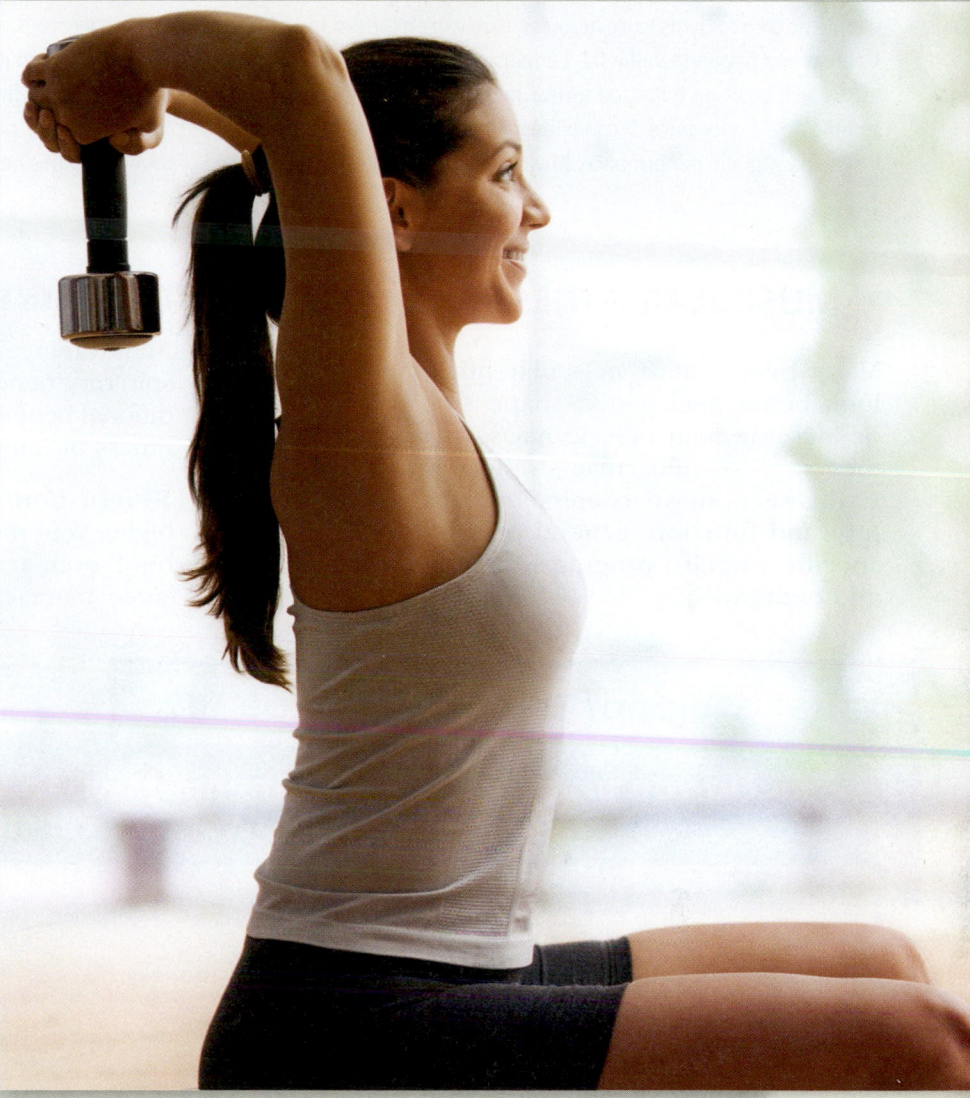

" *Exercise is a gift you give yourself.* "

—Anonymous

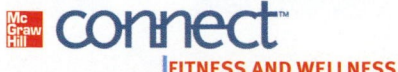

http://connect.mcgraw-hill.com

FITNESS AND WELLNESS

At one time physical fitness programs consisted almost entirely of strength and flexibility exercises. Then, in the 1970s, aerobic activities rose to prominence. As a result, strength and flexibility exercises were swept into the role of supplemental activities and added to the main workout only if time permitted. As people flocked to gyms to do aerobics, they were exposed to weight training and began to value the benefits of muscular fitness. Today, as the emphasis on balanced fitness grows, muscular fitness is assuming new importance. It can enhance the ability to perform daily tasks and athletic performance. Muscular fitness makes it easier to perform routine activities such as carrying groceries upstairs, lifting a child, and moving the couch. It is perhaps the most important fitness component for older adults because muscular fitness is essential for carrying out activities of daily living that help maintain functional independence. Enhanced muscular fitness allows us to perform vigorous activities with less risk of straining muscles or connective tissue, so it is important in the prevention and rehabilitation of injuries. This chapter covers muscular fitness benefits, cautions, principles, and guidelines, along with illustrated programs for developing this important fitness component.

◆ MUSCULAR FITNESS

Many people start muscular fitness programs to look better, feel better, shape and tone muscles, or increase lean muscle mass. At the same time, they increase muscular strength and endurance. In this section, we examine benefits, muscle structure and function, general principles, safety, and specific exercise programs for muscular strength and endurance.

Resistance Training: Benefits and Cautions

An advantage of aerobic activities is their cardiorespiratory benefits. Resistance training can offer additional benefits whether your goal is health-related fitness or improved athletic performance.

Weight Control The more muscle you have, the higher your metabolism is and the more calories you burn, even at rest. This is one reason men can consume more calories without gaining weight than

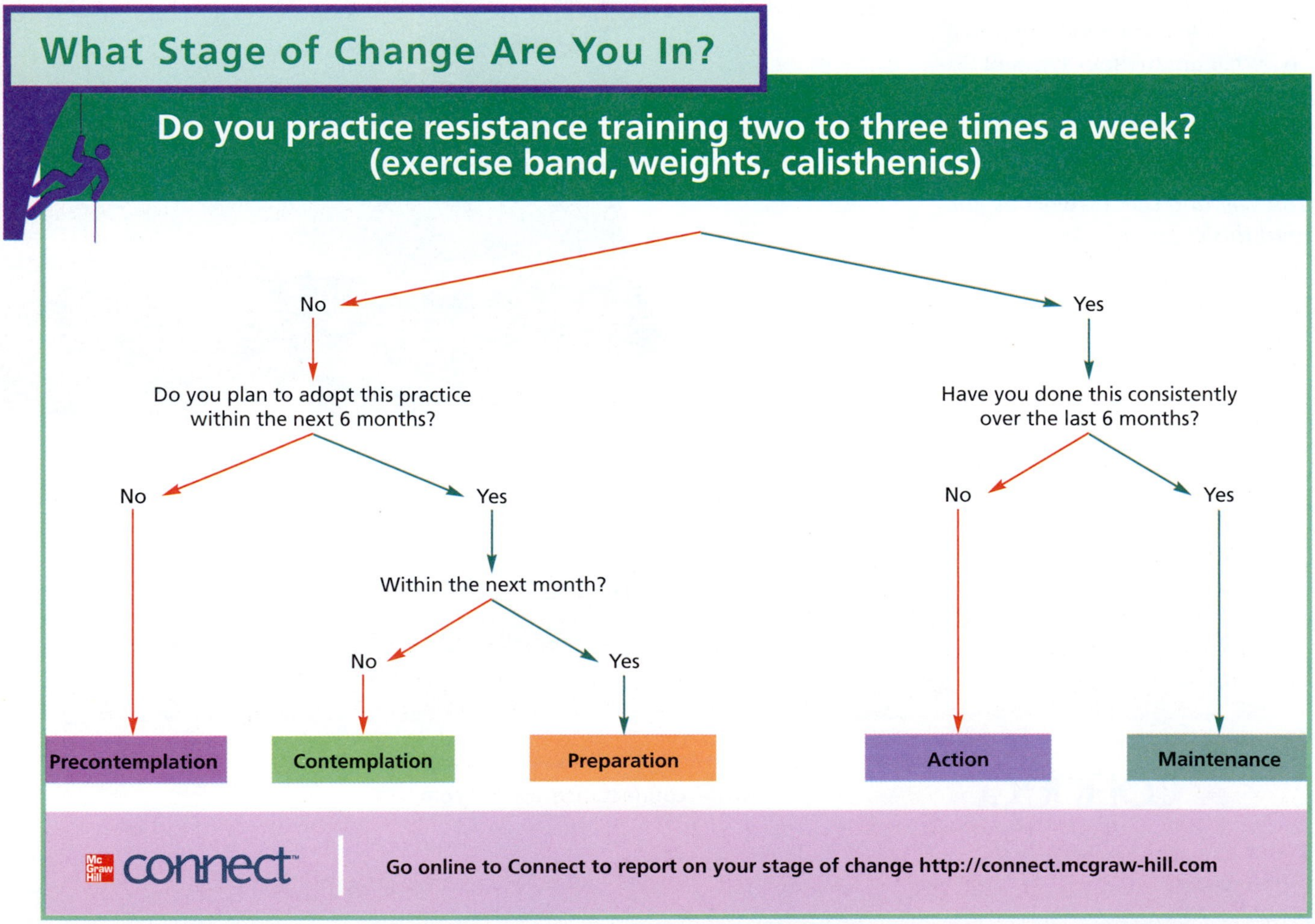

What Stage of Change Are You In?

Do you practice resistance training two to three times a week?
(exercise band, weights, calisthenics)

No → Do you plan to adopt this practice within the next 6 months?

    No → **Precontemplation**

    Yes → Within the next month?

        No → **Contemplation**

        Yes → **Preparation**

Yes → Have you done this consistently over the last 6 months?

    No → **Action**

    Yes → **Maintenance**

 connect™ | Go online to Connect to report on your stage of change http://connect.mcgraw-hill.com

can women of equal size—the average male has roughly twice the muscle mass of the average female. Muscle is active, high-metabolic tissue; fat is storage tissue. Resistance training increases muscle mass, which increases the rate at which you burn calories 24 hours a day, not just during the workout. This makes weight control easier. While women do not appear to gain as much muscle as men do from weight training, when differences in body size are taken into account, gains are comparable. Over a 4- to 6-month period, a man may gain 4 to 6 pounds of muscle, and a woman 2 to 3 pounds. Muscle is denser than fat and pound for pound takes up less space, so as muscle is gained, if fat is lost, the result is a loss of unwanted inches. Aerobic exercise and a nutritious low-fat diet are the quickest ways to reduce body fat, but weight training offers advantages for long-term weight control.

Weight Gain   For those who wish to gain weight, increasing lean muscle mass, not fat, is a desirable goal, and there is no better way to do this than weight training. However, rate and quantity of muscle tissue gains vary from person to person because they are partially genetically determined. Those with a naturally tall, lean build tend to gain muscle more slowly than do those with a stockier build, and men gain faster than women do. A bodybuilding program is outlined in the weight-training section for those who wish to increase lean weight.

Appearance   Developing a lean, well-toned body is the main reason many people exercise. If you think that you need to lose weight, but your body fat percentage is in the average range, reevaluate. Weight loss alone does not give a firm, well-toned appearance to flabby thighs or abdominals. Resistance training is the most effective way to shape and tone muscles, resulting in a trimmer appearance. Posture improves when agonist and antagonist muscles are in balance. Strengthening weak muscles and stretching tight, inflexible muscles help develop good body alignment so that you move more fluidly and feel and look better.

Time Economy   Instead of doing 50 leg lifts without weights, you can cut your workout time by adding resistance. Lift a weight heavy enough to produce fatigue in 8 to 12 repetitions, and you will get more benefit in fewer lifts. For basic muscular fitness, a balanced resistance-training workout of 10 to 12 exercises takes approximately 30 minutes to complete. Despite what you may observe in the gym, more is not necessary. While body builders, competitive weightlifters, and other strength-event athletes work out much more than this, keep in mind that

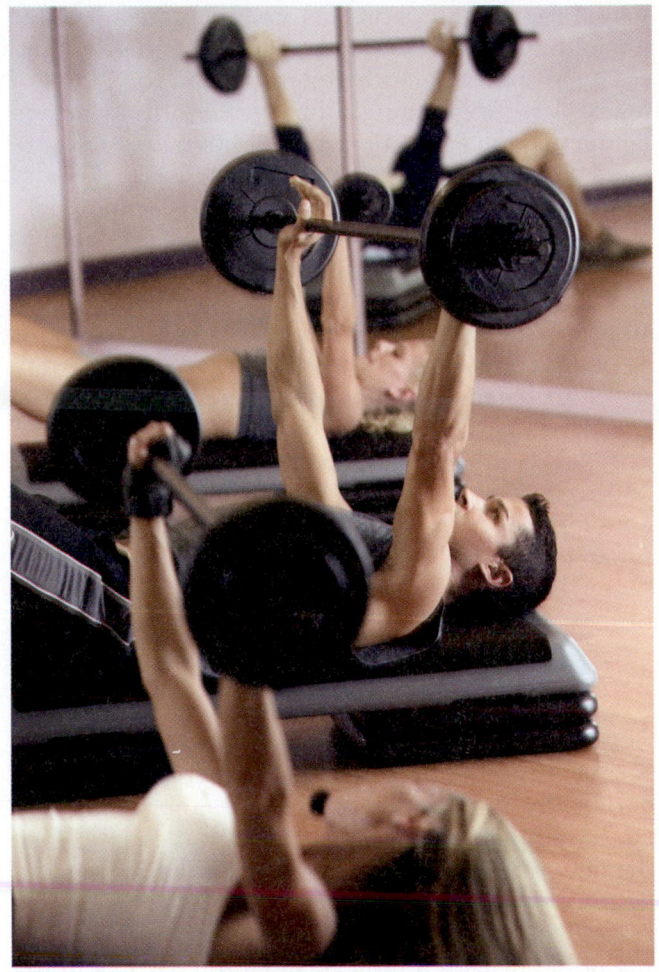

Resistance training is the most effective way to shape and tone muscles and is an important part of a balanced fitness program.

they have different goals. Health-related fitness levels can be developed and maintained in much less training time than is needed for competition.

Energy   Performance and efficiency improve with resistance training—more work can be done with less effort as muscular strength and endurance increase.

Athletic Performance   Stronger muscles enable you to better control the forces of movement—self-generated and external—as well as your body position during activity. Improved muscular fitness contributes to skill-related components of balance, speed, power, coordination, and agility. All other things being equal, a strong person can run faster, jump higher, and throw a ball farther than can a weaker individual.

Injury Prevention   Aerobic exercises such as jogging and aerobic dance have the potential to cause injury through repetitive, forceful impact against unyielding surfaces. Strong, flexible muscles and connective tissue can better withstand the stress of many forceful landings during a workout. When ligaments, tendons, muscle, and bone are strengthened through muscular exercise, the risk of injury is decreased. Many aerobic activities tend to develop strength in only a few groups of muscles, leaving others weak. For example, jogging strengthens the quadriceps but leaves the hamstrings weak. Weak muscle groups are more susceptible to strains or pulls. A well-designed resistance-training program develops balanced, proportional strength in agonists (prime movers) and antagonists (opposing muscle groups). If injury does occur, it may be less severe and may heal more quickly if the muscle is well conditioned. A carefully designed program can also rehabilitate injuries to help you regain normal (or better) strength levels. For more detailed information on injury prevention, see Chapter 8.

Bone Strength Resistance exercises decrease the risk of osteoporosis. This is important not only for the elderly but for young people as well. Osteoporosis may cause a fracture at age 60, but it starts much earlier—in the teens and twenties. You need good exercise and eating habits to build adequate bone density. The pull of muscles on bone in weight-bearing exercise stimulates development of increased bone density and bone quality and preserves existing bone. Research indicates that intensity of lifting is clearly related to bone mineralization. Lifting relatively heavy weights in a few repetitions may be more effective in increasing bone mass than lifting a light weight many times.

Flexibility Moving weights through a full range of motion, from full extension to full contraction, stretches and tones muscles. This is an important training technique to master to maintain flexibility. Muscles become short and tight if exercises are performed repeatedly through only a partial range of motion.

Balance Strong, fatigue-resistant muscles mean better balance during static and dynamic activities not only in athletics but in functional activities for people of all ages. Studies show improvements in balance for elderly people participating in strength training. This may translate into improved gait stability, decreased risk of falls, and reduced frequency of hip fractures—even for people in their eighties.

Cardiovascular Health Resistance training may enhance cardiovascular health by reducing several risk factors associated with cardiovascular disease. Studies show a decrease in resting diastolic blood

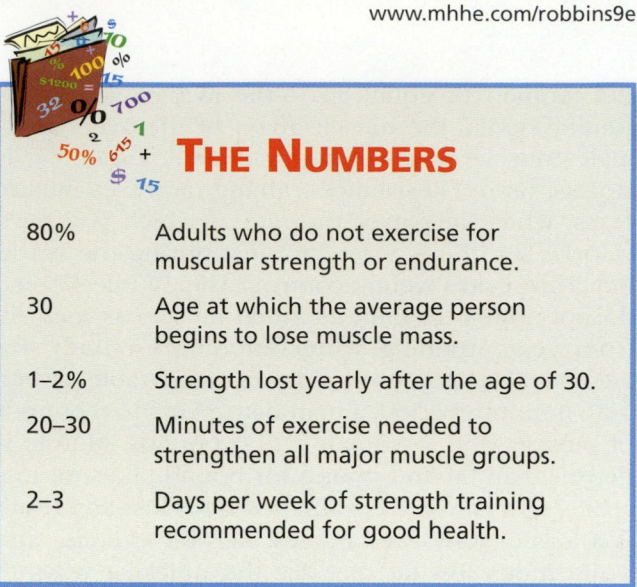

THE NUMBERS

80%	Adults who do not exercise for muscular strength or endurance.
30	Age at which the average person begins to lose muscle mass.
1–2%	Strength lost yearly after the age of 30.
20–30	Minutes of exercise needed to strengthen all major muscle groups.
2–3	Days per week of strength training recommended for good health.

pressure that is most significant in individuals with previously elevated blood pressure; decreases in exercise heart rate and exercise blood pressure; increased exercise tolerance; and modest improvements in blood lipid profile. Resistance training has also been shown to increase insulin sensitivity and decrease glucose intolerance in diabetic exercisers. Although little change in VO_{2max} occurs with traditional weight training, if a circuit weight-training program consisting of 10 exercises, 15 repetitions each, with a short (15 to 30 seconds) rest between is followed, modest improvements in VO_{2max} of 5 to 8 percent have been recorded.

Psychological Benefits Although many people begin an exercise program to improve appearance, many other less visible but equally important ef-

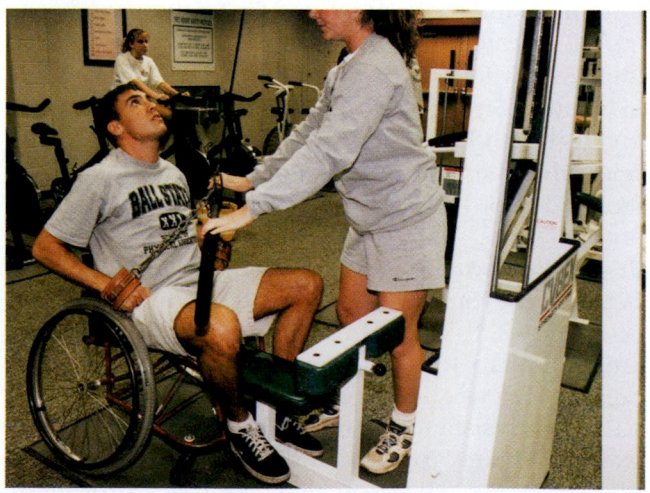

Resistance training benefits everyone. Greater muscular fitness improves performance of everyday activities and recreational and competitive sports.

fects may result. Benefits in the emotional dimension of wellness from regular exercise include feeling better, decreased stress, decreased depression, and enhanced self-esteem and self-confidence.

Social Benefits In addition to offering physical and psychological benefits, lifting with a partner or friend offers social benefits. There are many more opportunities for conversation and interaction when you work out with someone than when you watch a movie.

Benefits at Any Age Regardless of your age, you can benefit from resistance training. It is untrue that loss of strength is inevitable with age or that older people cannot gain strength. While the typical sedentary individual can lose up to 30 percent of his or her muscle mass between the ages of 20 and 70, this loss is more from atrophy due to disuse than from aging alone. Adequate levels of muscular strength are particularly important to older adults to maintain their functional independence and quality of life. Several studies including people in their seventies, eighties, and nineties participating in resistance training show that they increased muscle mass, decreased fat, more than doubled their strength, and improved their functional mobility and ability to perform daily living activities.

Disadvantages and Cautions Although resistance training has many benefits, it does have disadvantages. Resistance training is not a complete exercise program because it does not develop cardiorespiratory endurance. As in any physical activity, injury is possible if you are careless or ignore safety procedures. You may have trouble accessing equipment. Also, you can expect some mild muscle soreness during the first week of the program.

Individuals with cardiovascular problems or high blood pressure should seek medical guidance due to the tendency of blood pressure to increase during strength training. Those who have hernias, arthritis, or lower back problems should also seek medical clearance. Individuals with these health concerns may benefit from resistance training but should be aware that they may need special exercise modifications.

Avoid use of hand and ankle weights during jogging, high-impact aerobic dance workouts, and other activities involving running and jumping. Ankle weights may distort proper form, increase stress to legs and feet, and increase the risk of strains and sprains. While small increases in oxygen consumption and caloric expenditure result from using light weights, the same effect can be produced with less risk by exercising longer or harder.

When used with controlled form and rhythm in a muscle toning or walking program, however, light weights are beneficial for increasing heart rate and muscular fitness in the upper body. All in all, resistance training offers few drawbacks and many major advantages for the time invested.

Muscle Function

Muscles are made of individual muscle fibers bound together and sheathed in connective tissue. They end in a tendon that connects the muscle to a bone. An example is the Achilles tendon, which you can feel above your heel, connecting your calf to your foot. Muscle fibers can contract to shorten the muscle or relax and return to their resting length. They are also elastic. They can be stretched and will spring back to their resting length.

Muscle fibers are classified into types based on their endurance, speed of contraction, and ability to exert force. **Slow-twitch** (ST) **muscle fibers** have high aerobic capacity but low power and are recruited primarily for endurance-type activities such as jogging. **Fast-twitch** (FT) **muscle fibers** are able to contract more quickly and generate more force but fatigue relatively quickly. They are important for short-burst, powerful activities such as sprinting and jumping. ST fibers are recruited initially during muscular contraction, and FT fibers are recruited when weight training becomes more intense and requires greater speed or force. The ratio of ST to FT muscle fibers is genetically determined and varies from one person to another. Resistance training increases the size and strength of both fiber types as well as their ability to exert force.

Muscles cannot expand and push. Movement is produced as muscle contracts, shortens, and pulls on bones across a joint. As a muscle on one side of a bone contracts, muscles on the other side must relax to allow movement to occur. The contracting muscle that initiates movement is called the **agonist.** The opposing muscle is called the **antagonist.** In a biceps curl (Figure 6-1), the agonist is the biceps and the antagonist is the triceps. In a triceps extension, the roles reverse. What is the agonist in a hamstring curl? What is the antagonist?

Determinants of Muscular Fitness Gains

Gains in muscular fitness result from neurological and muscular adaptations. Dramatic strength gains early in a program are often due to a "learning effect"—that is, you learn how to lift weights more efficiently. Your body represses its self-protective reflexes and increases its ability to recruit muscle fibers fully when needed.

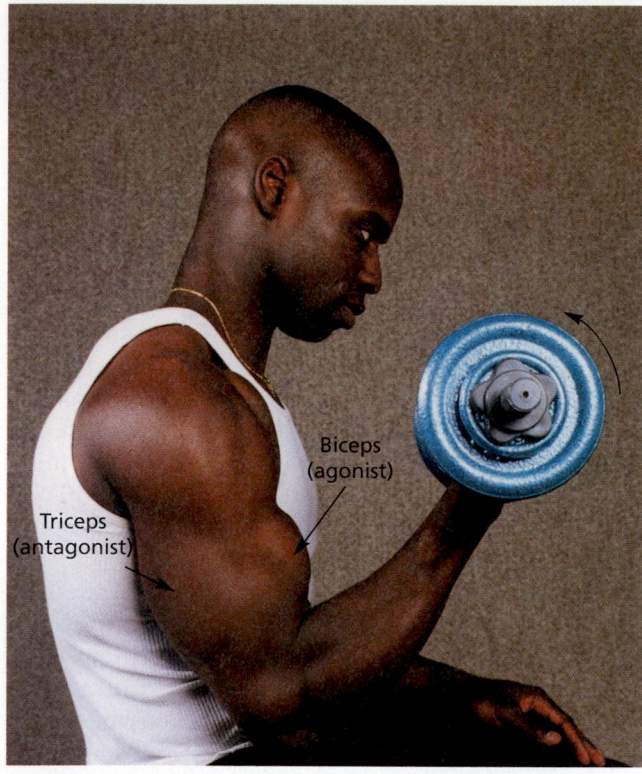

FIGURE 6-1   A biceps curl demonstrating muscle function.

Your overall potential for the development of muscular fitness is determined by many factors, including the types, number, and size of muscle fibers you possess and how well your muscular system can recruit them during muscular effort. The more muscle fibers you have, the larger they are, and the better your system is at activating them during muscular effort, the greater your strength is. While the types and number of muscle fibers you possess are genetically determined, size and muscle fiber recruitment are a product of training.

MUSCLE FIBER RECRUITMENT

When a muscle contracts, only the number of muscle fibers required for that momentary effort will shorten. Individual muscle fibers cannot contract partially. They are working as hard as possible or not at all. This is called the *all-or-nothing principle.* For example, when a biceps curl calls for a 50 percent effort, all fibers in the muscle do not contract at 50 percent effort; rather, a portion of the muscle's fibers contract fully while the remainder rest. After these first muscle fibers contract, fatigue slightly decreases their ability to apply force. On each subsequent contraction, more fibers must be recruited to continue to lift the same weight. After several muscle contractions, enough fibers are fatigued

that the muscle temporarily can no longer generate the same effort in what is called *temporary muscular failure.* Muscle fibers increase strength only if they are stimulated by intensity of effort. If your goal is to develop maximal muscular strength, try to recruit, or activate, as many muscle fibers as possible by working a muscle to a state of temporary muscular failure. If you are working for health-related fitness levels, a less intense effort is adequate.

MUSCLE ATROPHY AND HYPERTROPHY

Muscles adapt to the load placed on them. When the load increases over time, muscular strength and endurance improve. When muscles are not used, they grow weaker, stiffen, and **atrophy,** or shrink in size. A dramatic example of muscle atrophy occurs when a person has an injured limb in a cast for several weeks. When the cast is removed, the muscles of the affected limb are noticeably smaller. Increasing amounts of exercise over time are necessary to rebuild muscle strength, size, and flexibility.

When muscles are stimulated by an increased workload, they grow stronger and muscle fibers experience **hypertrophy,** or increase in size. This increase occurs in both men and women and is proportional to muscle mass. The average man has about twice the muscle mass of the average woman, so hypertrophy in men is more pronounced.

GENDER DIFFERENCES

Some women worry that they will develop big shoulders or massive, masculine musculature because of weight training. This myth is reinforced by televised images of women's bodybuilding competitions. Be assured that shoulder width, like hip width, is

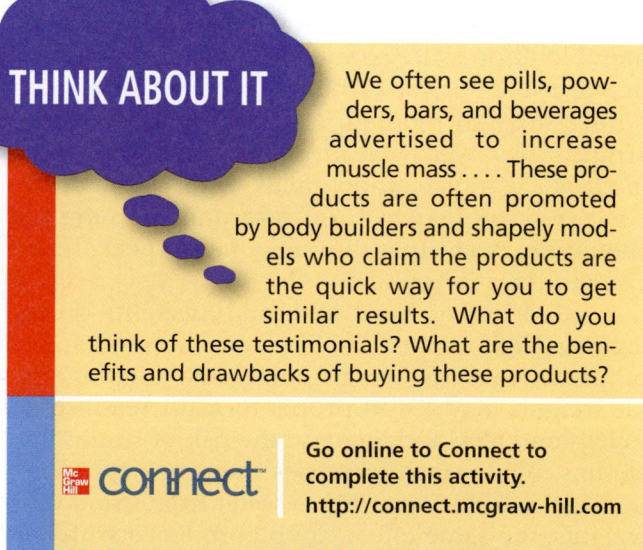

THINK ABOUT IT   We often see pills, powders, bars, and beverages advertised to increase muscle mass . . . . These products are often promoted by body builders and shapely models who claim the products are the quick way for you to get similar results. What do you think of these testimonials? What are the benefits and drawbacks of buying these products?

Go online to Connect to complete this activity. http://connect.mcgraw-hill.com

influenced by genetics and that significant muscle gains require hours of strenuous weight lifting for many months. Dramatic muscle hypertrophy and masculinization can also occur with anabolic steroid abuse (see Chapter 14). Men have a greater potential for muscle hypertrophy than women do because men have higher levels of the sex hormone testosterone, which promotes muscle growth. Some of the strongest women athletes are gymnasts, who have very feminine physiques. Weight training is also popular with TV and movie stars who exercise to maintain a fit, toned appearance and help control weight. Be assured that massive muscles don't occur by accident or with a 20- to 30-minute muscle-toning workout twice a week.

Types of Resistance Training

Two basic types of muscular exercise are static (isometric) and dynamic (isotonic). Different resistance programs have been developed using each type of exercise.

STATIC (ISOMETRIC) EXERCISE

Static (isometric) exercise is exercise in which the muscle contracts but does not change length and little or no movement occurs. If you pushed your palms together hard, your pectoral muscles would contract and try to shorten, but your arms would not move. An advantage of static exercise is that it requires little or no equipment and can be done almost anywhere—for instance, while sitting at a desk. However, these exercises are not widely used because resistance is applied at only one point in your range of motion, and thus strength development is limited. Also, it is difficult to know how much force is being exerted, and so strength gains are not as easy to observe as they are when equipment is being used. However, static exercises can be useful in strengthening muscles after an injury, when dynamic movement would be painful or even increase injury.

DYNAMIC (ISOTONIC) EXERCISE

Dynamic (isotonic) exercise is exercise in which the muscle contracts and shortens and movement occurs. Most daily activities, such as pushing, pulling, and lifting, are dynamic. Dynamic exercise programs can be done with free weights, exercise machines, elastic resistance, or calisthenics such as crunches and push-ups. Dynamic exercise involves two types of muscle contractions: concentric and eccentric.

In a **concentric contraction,** a muscle shortens as it overcomes resistance. For example, a weight is lifted as the biceps contract during the lifting phase

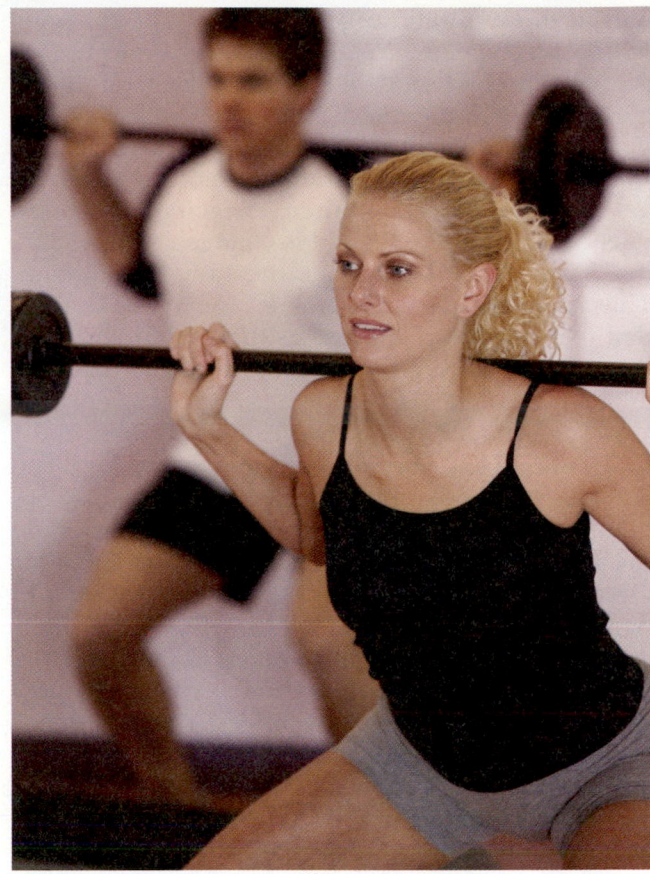

Weight training can help maintain a fit, toned appearance and control weight.

of a biceps curl. **Eccentric contraction** occurs when a muscle lengthens and contracts at the same time, gradually allowing a force to overcome muscular resistance; for example, the biceps contract eccentrically during the lowering phase of a biceps curl. Eccentric contraction is a beneficial component of strength development because it makes up half of the muscular effort. The same muscles are involved in eccentric and concentric contractions, so lowering should be done in a smooth, controlled manner for maximal benefit and to prevent potential injury from dropping the weight.

Advantages of dynamic exercise are that it strengthens through a full range of motion, the load is measurable, and a variety of isotonic programs are available. Calisthenics, free weights, and machines such as Universal or Nautilus use dynamic exercise.

Two common types of dynamic exercises involve constant resistance or variable resistance. In **constant resistance exercise,** a constant resistance (weight) is used throughout the range of motion. However, the force needed to move the weight varies with leverage determined by the angle of the joint; that is, it increases or decreases as the load is moved through the range of motion. For example, with a biceps curl, it is easier to move the weight through the first and last thirds of the motion and harder through the middle third. The ability to lift a weight is limited by the amount of strength required to move it through this "sticking point."

In **variable resistance exercise,** the force needed to move the weight is changed to provide a maximum load throughout the range of motion. This requires special machines, such as Nautilus, that increase the resistance as the weight is moved through the ends of the range of motion where you are able to exert greater force.

Another type of dynamic exercise is **isokinetic,** in which the speed of movement is controlled. The advantage of isokinetic work is that the load applied mirrors the force exerted by the user while the speed remains constant. Isokinetic machinery is often used in rehabilitation and is not common in most fitness centers.

Both constant resistance exercise and variable resistance exercise are effective in developing muscular fitness. Different types of exercises and equipment have advantages and disadvantages, but the most important factor in fitness gains is a person's motivation and effort rather than the type of equipment used.

Principles of Resistance Training

Strength gains are proportional to the load applied and the frequency and intensity of effort. Basic principles of resistance training include progressive overload, specificity, and recovery.

PROGRESSIVE OVERLOAD

Progressive overload is the most important principle of resistance training. To stimulate a muscle to increase strength or endurance, it must gradually be overloaded or forced to work at a higher than normal effort. Either the number of lifts **(repetitions)** performed or the amount of weight (load or resistance) must gradually be increased or recovery time between exercises must be decreased. Increasing the number of repetitions or decreasing rest increases muscular endurance. Increasing the weight lifted increases strength. General programs increase load and repetitions until a desired maintenance goal is reached.

You must exercise two to three times a week to improve muscular fitness. Significant strength gains require at least 8 consecutive weeks of training. To maintain strength, one intense workout is adequate for health fitness. Athletes need to train at least twice a week to maintain fitness in the off-season.

SPECIFICITY

The speed of contraction, range of motion, amount and type of resistance, and number and type of exercise are a few of the variables that determine the results of strength training. If you desire a specific result, such as an increase in muscle mass, your program must be designed and executed to produce that result.

RECOVERY

Exercise stimulates a muscle to take in more protein and nutrients and undergo changes that increase its ability to contract forcefully. After a workout, you will be weaker, not stronger, due to fatigue. Improvement occurs during recovery, which gives the muscle fibers time to repair and grow. This requires more recovery time than for the cardiorespiratory system. Strength workouts are best done with 2 to 3 days of rest between sessions to allow recovery and improvement to occur. Lifting may be done more frequently, using a split routine with the upper body one day and the lower body the next.

Guidelines for Developing Muscular Fitness

In increasing muscular strength, endurance, or power, the key variables are resistance, repetitions, and speed. The purest example of strength is one maximal lift, and the closer a program comes to this, the greater the strength gains are. However, risk of injury is high when working at or near maximal levels. Athletes working to develop strength often exercise at 80 to 90 percent or higher effort a few (five to eight) times. Muscular endurance is enhanced by contracting repeatedly (e.g., one to two sets of 15 to 20 reps) with moderate (50 to 60 percent) effort.

There is some crossover effect between muscular strength and muscular endurance. Development of muscular strength also produces an increase in muscular endurance; for example, if you can lift a 100-pound weight 5 times, you can probably lift a 5-pound weight 20 times. However, muscular endurance does not enhance strength. If you can lift a 5-pound weight 20 times, you may not be able to lift a 100-pound weight even once. If you want to develop both muscular strength and endurance, a muscular strength program can provide double benefits.

Muscular power, a function of strength and speed, is the ability to apply force rapidly. Power is increased by performing a muscle contraction quickly, as in the plyometric exercises often used in athletics. While muscular power is not necessary for health-related physical fitness, it is an asset in many sports.

TABLE 6-1	Guidelines for Resistance Training Programs			
	Muscular Endurance	Health Fitness	Bodybuilding (Muscle hypertrophy)	Muscular Strength
Frequency (workouts per week)	3–5	2–3	4–10	2–3
Resistance (% of 1 RM)	50–60%	70–75%	70–80%	80–90%
Repetitions	15–20	8–12	5–10	5–8
Sets	1–2	1–2	3–5	1–3
Rest between sets*	1/2–1 min.	1–2 min.	1–3 min.	2–4 min.

*Rest between sets may be decreased by alternating lifts using different body parts.

TABLE 6-2	Safety Guidelines for Resistance Training

1. Warm up before each workout and stretch afterward. Stretching before lifting impairs muscle performance.
2. Use good technique—keep your abdominals tight, back straight, hips tucked under, knees relaxed.
3. Work each exercise through a full range of motion from full extension without lockout to full contraction.
4. Perform each exercise smoothly, with control. Do not swing the limbs or use momentum. Faster is not better.
5. Before you lift, inhale. Exhale on the exertion. Do not hold your breath.

Guidelines for resistance training programs are summarized in Table 6-1. Optimal results can be obtained from any resistance training program, and risk of injury can be minimized if you follow the guidelines in Table 6-2.

SEQUENCE

Ideally, first work large muscle groups and complex multiple joint exercises, ending with small muscle groups and isolated single joint exercises. It is difficult to exercise large muscle groups adequately if you have already fatigued the smaller supporting muscles. The suggested order of exercises is hips/legs, torso, arms, abdominals (see the sample weight-training program).

FORM

✓ Never sacrifice form for weight. After progressive overload, correct exercise form is the most important (and most neglected) factor in maximizing strength gains and minimizing the risk of injury. Improvement is more rapid if correct technique, not only quantity of weight, is emphasized.

✓ Always work through a complete range of motion for flexibility and maximum strength gains. Move from full extension without lockout to full flexion.
✓ Keep your back straight and abdominals tight to protect your lower back.
✓ When doing standing exercises, keep the knees slightly bent and the hips tucked under to support your back.
✓ Avoid "cheating," a breakdown in exercise form that occurs when extra muscles are used to complete the exercise, decreasing the load to the prime mover. Cheating occurs when the load is too heavy or you are fatigued. Remember: Quality of work is more important than the number of repetitions or amount of weight lifted.

REST BETWEEN SETS

A **set** is a group of lifts followed by a rest period. For example, a person doing eight biceps curls has done one set of eight repetitions. A rest period between sets of an exercise should allow sufficient recovery so that good form can be maintained. This time will vary, depending on the intensity of lifting with 1 to 2 minutes of rest recommended between sets of a health fitness program and 2 to 4 minutes between sets of a strength program. To make efficient use of time, you may alternate exercises on different body parts—for example, legs, then arms—so that one muscle group is recovering while you are working another.

MUSCLE BALANCE

Muscles work in pairs, so it is important to strengthen muscles on both sides of a bone so that they pull evenly across joints and maintain body alignment. For example, if pectorals are stronger than upper back muscles, rounded shoulders result. When upper back muscles are strengthened, shoulders are naturally held erect. Tight lower

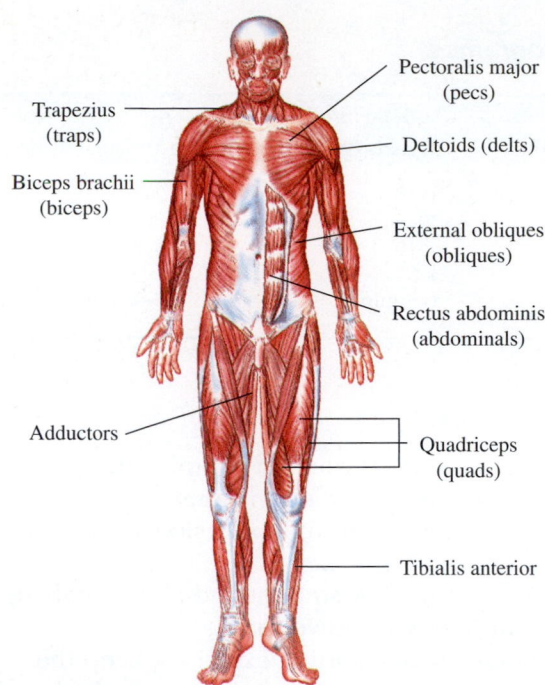

FIGURE 6-2A Major muscles of the body. Front.

Source: From John W. Hole Jr., *Human Anatomy and Physiology,*
4th ed. Copyright © 1987 Wm. C. Brown Publishers, Dubuque, Iowa.
All Rights Reserved. Reprinted by permission.

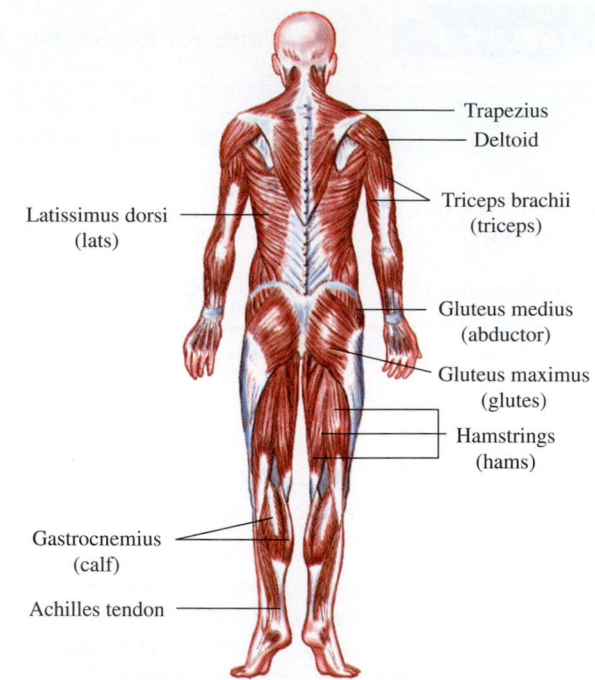

FIGURE 6-2B Major muscles of the body. Back.

Source: From John W. Hole Jr., *Human Anatomy and Physiology,*
4th ed. Copyright © 1987 Wm. C. Brown Publishers, Dubuque, Iowa.
All Rights Reserved. Reprinted by permission.

back muscles opposed by weak, sagging abdominals pull the back into an exaggerated curve. This stresses lumbar vertebrae, increasing back fatigue and the risk of lower back pain. Well-toned abdominals support the back, improve appearance, and prevent back problems. Resistance programs must be planned to develop proportional strength in the following muscle pairs: biceps/triceps, pectorals/trapezius-rhomboids, abdominals/lower back, hamstrings/quadriceps, gastrocnemius/anterior tibialis, and deltoids/latissimus dorsi (Figure 6-2a and 6-2b).

BREATHING

Exhale as you push or pull; inhale as you lower the weight. For example, on a biceps curl, exhale as you lift the weight and inhale as you lower it to the starting position. *Do not hold your breath.* Holding your breath while you strain against a closed epiglottis is called the **Valsalva maneuver.** This can elevate blood pressure dangerously and cause dizziness or fainting.

SPEED OF MOVEMENT

Exercising in a smooth, controlled manner maximizes strength gains and reduces injuries. Take 2 seconds to lift (concentric or shortening contraction) and 2 to 4 seconds to lower (eccentric or lengthening

contraction). Control the movement; do not fling, swing, or kick. Jerky movements will cause excessive wear and tear on your joints. Also, when you use momentum to perform an exercise, you apply force and develop strength only through the first part of the movement. Lower a limb with the same control used to lift it. Do not drop weights with a crash. You are stronger lowering a weight than lifting it.

Tips for Behavior Change

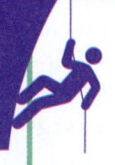

- Think about which benefits of strength training are most important to you.
- Decide where (home, gym) you would like to strength train and when (days, time).
- Test your strength and muscular endurance using the tests in Chapter 3 now and again in 6 weeks to check your progress.
- Use Online Lab Activity 6-6 (www. mhhe.com/robbins9e) to keep track of your workouts.

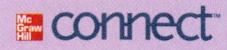

Go online to Connect to
complete this activity.
http://connect.mcgraw-hill.com

Resistance Training Programs

There are many types of resistance training programs. The type of program you select will depend on your goals and the type of equipment (if any) you plan to use. Four basic resistance training programs are shown in Table 6-3. Regardless of the type of program you select, you can keep track of your progress with the Resistance Training Log in Online Lab Activity 6-6 at www.mhhe.com/robbins9e.

WEIGHT TRAINING

Weight training is a noncompetitive exercise program used to develop several health-related physical fitness components: muscular strength, muscular endurance, flexibility, and body composition. It differs significantly in its goals from the competitive sports of weight lifting and bodybuilding. Male, female, young, old, athlete, and fitness exerciser—all benefit from weight training. Beginners with low levels of muscular fitness benefit the most and will notice results more quickly than will experienced lifters. Weight training can build muscular fitness levels so that recreational, competitive, and daily activities are accomplished more easily, with less strain and fatigue.

FREE WEIGHTS VERSUS MACHINES

For beginners, it really doesn't matter what type of equipment is used. A beginner will improve on almost any type of program as long as an adequate overload is provided. Two major types of equipment used in weight training are free weights and machines. Both have advantages and disadvantages:

✓ Free weights are far less expensive than machines, so you can have your own set at home. Free weights cost about $100 on sale, double that if you add a padded bench and rack. Machines can cost upward of $500 to $5,000.

✓ You have more variety of exercises on free weights than on machines because you have the freedom to lift in so many different positions.

✓ Lifting with proper technique is crucial. A wrong move can cause injury with any lifting but particularly with free weights.

✓ To lift free weights safely, you must have a skilled spotting partner who can handle the weight in case you start to lose control.

✓ For muscular fitness development, free weights have an advantage over machines because they not only develop strength in the prime movers, but also develop balance and coordination by

TABLE 6-3	**Basic Resistance Training Programs**			
	Machines	**Free Weights**	**Elastic Band**	**No Weights**
Legs	Leg press Leg extension Hamstring curl	Squats Lunges	Squats Leg extension Hamstring curl Side leg lift Inner thigh lift Three-way leg pointer	Wall sit Lunges Partner leg extension Partner hamstring curl Partner inner/outer thigh press
Ankles, Calves	Toe press	Calf raise	Toe press Toe lifts	Calf raise Partner foot flexion
Chest	Bench press	Bench press	Push-ups	Push-ups Dips Partner elbow press forward
Shoulders	Military press	Military press	Deltoid raise	Partner overhead press
Back	Lat pull Rowing Back extension	Bent-over rowing Back extension	Lat pull Rowing	Partner lat pull Partner elbow press backward Core exercises
Abdominals	Abdominal curls	Abdominal curls	Abdominal curls	Core exercises
Arms	Triceps press Biceps curl	Triceps press Biceps curl	Tricep press Biceps curl	Push-ups Pull-ups Partner biceps curl

TABLE 6-4   *Preventing Injuries*

1. Never attempt to lift more than you know you can handle. Work out—don't show off.
2. Always make sure that the weight pins, bars, and collars are secure.
3. Don't lift weights alone. Always work with someone else.
4. Keep sweat wiped off your hands; it makes weights slippery.
5. When using free weights, work with a trained spotter.
6. Return all equipment to the proper place. Don't leave it lying around for someone to trip over.

strengthening other muscles required to balance and control the weight.

✓ Machines such as Nautilus and Universal are easy to use and safer than free weights because they guide your movements and control the weights. An advantage of Nautilus equipment is that it provides variable resistance, adjusting the load for strength variations throughout a lift.

✓ Because of the cost of machines, it is best to start your machine-workout program at a health club or gym.

✓ Proper lifting technique is easier to learn on machines, and you won't need a spotting partner.

✓ Loads can be changed quickly, so the workout may take less time than with free weights.

For safety, convenience, and time, machines have the edge. Whether you use free weights or machines, always follow the safety guidelines in Table 6-4 to minimize risk of injury.

WEIGHT ROOM ETIQUETTE

Be aware of and follow common weight room etiquette guidelines while working out:

✓ Wipe sweat off benches after use.
✓ Rerack weights when you are done.
✓ Let others work in between sets while you are resting. Don't lie around on the equipment chatting between sets if people are waiting to use the machine.
✓ Don't drop or bang the weights together. This can damage the equipment and increases the noise level unnecessarily.
✓ If you want to listen to music, wear a headset; don't play your music loudly.
✓ Exhale, don't grunt, while lifting.

PROGRAM FOR HEALTH FITNESS

A conditioning program should develop balanced strength. Many muscle strains occur because of weakness in the pulled muscle or its opposing muscle. A

TOP 10 LIST

Resistance Training Mistakes to Avoid

Resistance training is a great way to shape and tone muscles. If done wrong, however, it can elevate blood pressure and cause back strain, sore knees, or ankle sprain. Also, training mistakes slow your progress. Here are the most common errors to avoid:

1. *Holding your breath during lifting.* This can cause a dangerous increase in blood pressure. Exhale on exertion, inhale on release.
2. *Lifting too heavy a weight.* If you can't lift it with full range of motion with good form, lighten the load. Train, don't strain.
3. *Arching the back.* During the bench press or military press, this can strain back ligaments. Tighten abdominals and keep the back straight.
4. *Using momentum.* "Kicking" the weight up in the quadriceps extension or hamstring curl decreases the load through the full range of motion and slows progress. Bouncing or jerking a lift strains ligaments and indicates the weight is too heavy or you are getting too tired to lift smoothly.
5. *Doing reps too quickly.* Length of time a force is applied is a factor in muscle fitness. Lift for two to four counts and lower slowly for two to four counts for best results. Yes, it is harder than lifting fast. It takes fewer reps to get the same result compared to lifting fast.
6. *Not using full range of motion.* Strength is built only in the range of motion used. If you stop before the "sticking point," you are building muscle imbalances.
7. *Not wiping off sweat.* Sweat makes your grip slippery.
8. *Going too deep in squats or leg press.* This strains knee ligaments. Don't go below 90 degrees.
9. *Letting ankles roll out when legs are loaded.* This can cause ankle sprain. Keep ankles straight in squats or toe presses.
10. *Working only "problem" areas.* Or working the agonist but not its opposing antagonist. In other words, working biceps but not triceps or abdominals but not the back. This causes muscle imbalances, increasing risk of injury.

well-planned strength program prevents strength imbalances. If you exercised only problem areas, you would increase imbalances. Prime muscle movers, the muscle(s) mainly responsible for the joint movement, are listed and can be found in Figures 6-2a and 6-2b. The following exercises, listed in the order of large muscle groups and complex multiple joint exercises to isolated single joint exercises and small muscle groups, may be done on machines (Figure 6-3). Free weight exercises are also described and illustrated (Figure 6-4). If you plan to use machines, your first workouts should include learning how to adjust and efficiently use the equipment. Videos illustrating these exercises are listed under Internet Resources at the end of this chapter.

Weight Training Exercises

1. Leg press
   Prime movers: quadriceps, hamstrings, and gluteus maximus
   On leg press, sit on seat, adjust position to last slot or to a 90-degree knee angle.
   Place feet squarely on pedals, press out smoothly (do not lock knees), and return to starting position.

2. Leg extension
   Prime movers: quadriceps
   Sit on bench with both feet under the rollers. Toe in slightly. Do not lie back.
   Extend your legs, hold 1 second, and return to starting position.

3. Hamstring curl
   Prime movers: hamstrings and gluteus maximus
   Lie face down on the bench, hook both heels under the rollers. Position knees at the pivot point where the rollers attach to the bench. Pull up to 90 degrees, hold for 1 second, and return to starting position.

4. Toe press
   Prime mover: gastrocnemius
   On leg press station, place feet squarely on pedals, press out to full leg extension without knee lockout. Press with toes from flat-footed position to foot extension and return.

5. Bench press
   Prime movers: pectorals and triceps
   Lie on bench, head next to the machine. The grips should be lined up approximately with the shoulders. Place your feet flat on the bench with knees bent and back flat. Press to extension and return. If you tend to have shoulder problems, lower the bar to only 4 inches above your chest, then extend.

6. Military press
   Prime movers: deltoids and triceps
   Sit on the stool or stand with abdominals tight, back flat, and knees slightly bent. With shoulders close to handles, extend upward with arms until they are straight but not locked and return.

7. Lat pull
   Prime movers: latissimus dorsi
   Grip bar directly above shoulders or at handles. Pull down until you are kneeling or sitting. From this position, pull down to chest and return.

8. Rowing
   Prime movers: rhomboids, latissimus dorsi, and biceps
   Sit on the machine with arms almost fully extended. Pull back as far as possible, drawing shoulder blades together. Return to starting position.

9. Back extension
   Prime movers: erector spinae, gluteus maximus, and quadratus lumborum
   Sit on the machine with back against upper back pad and feet under ankle rollers. Fasten hip belt if one is available to keep hips from lifting or sliding out of position. Slowly extend trunk back fully and slowly return to starting position.

10. Abdominal curls
    Prime movers: abdominals and hip flexors
    Sit with pad on upper chest, knees flexed, and feet on footpad. Use seat belt if provided to keep hips from lifting off seat. Flex trunk as far forward as possible. Return slowly to starting position.

11. Triceps press
    Prime movers: triceps
    Stand facing lat bar. With palms facing down, grasp the bar so that hands are shoulder width apart. Keep elbows at waist. Press down to extension and return.

12. Biceps curl
    Prime movers: biceps
    Stand facing the weights, hold bar with both hands, palms up. Flex arms until the bar meets shoulders. Return to starting position. Keep back straight, abdominals firm.

Free Weight Exercises   These exercises (Figure 6-4) may be done with a set of barbells or hand weights. Practice each move without weights before attempting weighted sets. Free weights provide additional challenge over machines because balance and coordination are developed in addition to strength. Strict attention to lifting form is critical because with free weights, a moment's carelessness can cause an injury. Always work with an experienced spotter in case you have difficulty. When possible, use power/squat racks with adjustable supports for added safety. To protect the back, you need to keep abdominals firm, back straight. Breathe continuously; do not hold your breath.

1. Squats
   Prime movers: gluteus maximus, quadriceps, and hamstrings
   Start standing upright with the bar resting on your shoulders. Keep the head up, abdominals tight, back flat, feet a bit wider than your

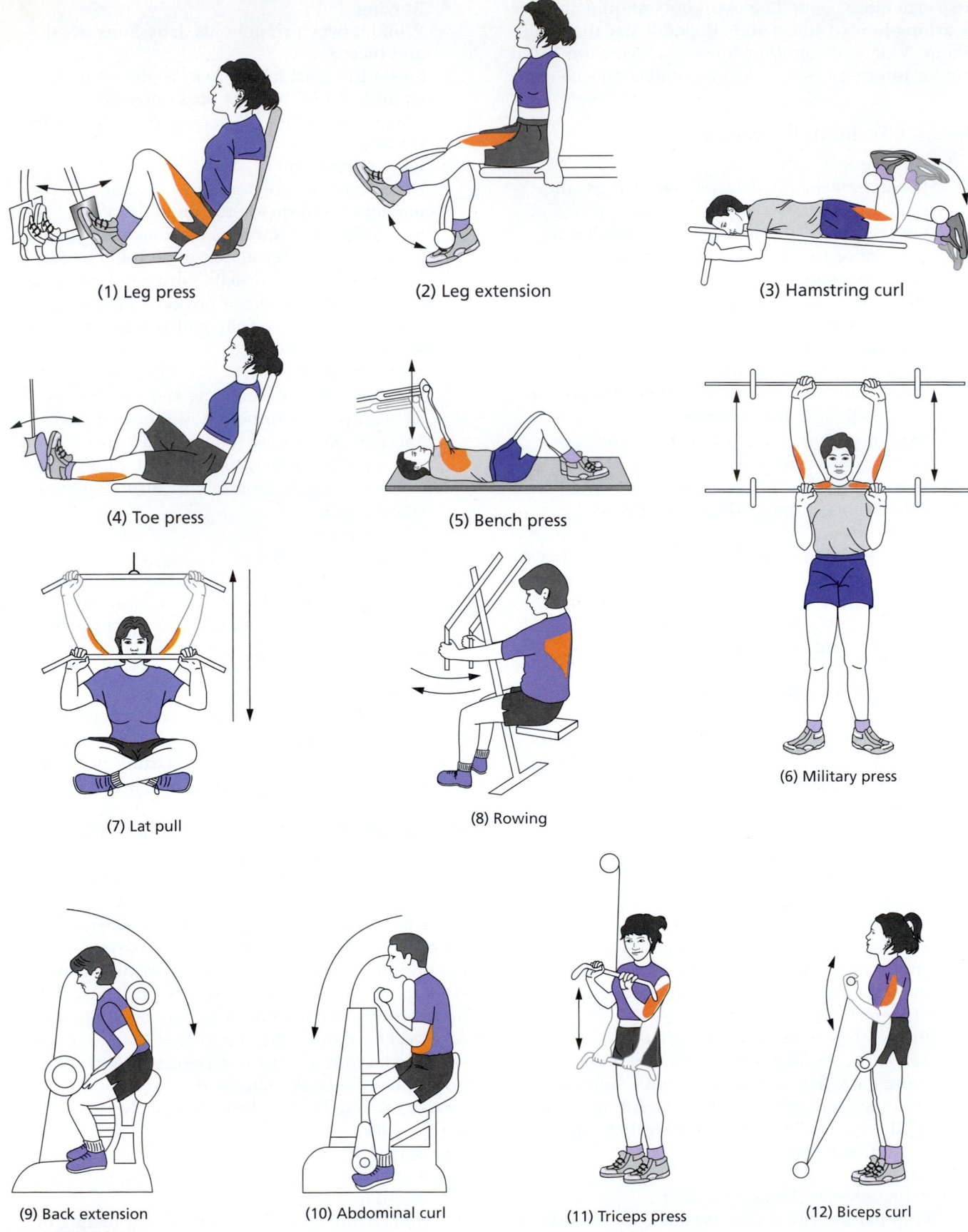

(1) Leg press (2) Leg extension (3) Hamstring curl

(4) Toe press (5) Bench press (6) Military press

(7) Lat pull (8) Rowing

(9) Back extension (10) Abdominal curl (11) Triceps press (12) Biceps curl

FIGURE 6-3   **Weight training exercises.**

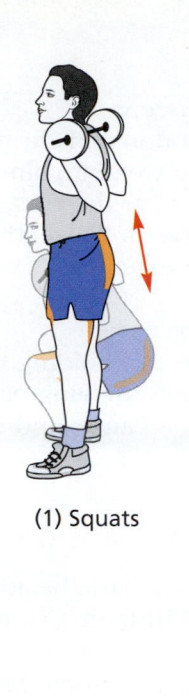

(1) Squats

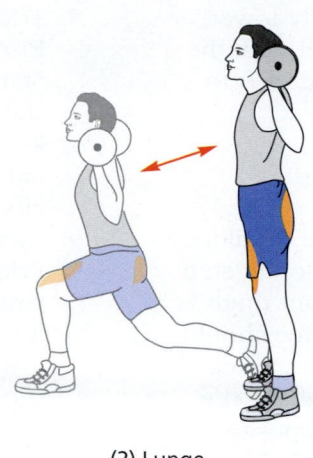

(2) Lunge

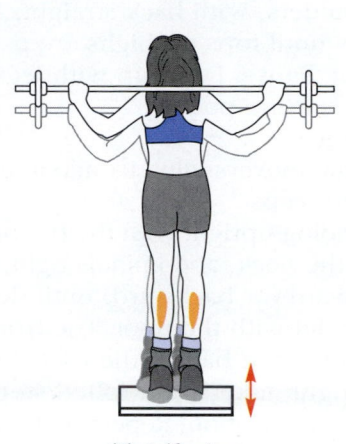

(3) Calf raise

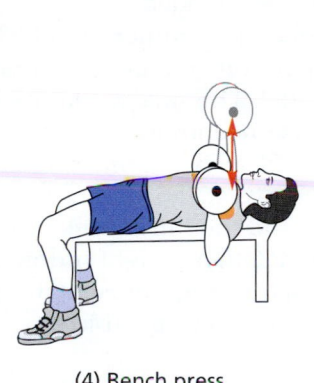

(4) Bench press

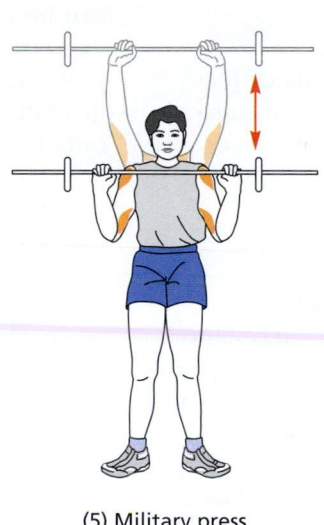

(5) Military press

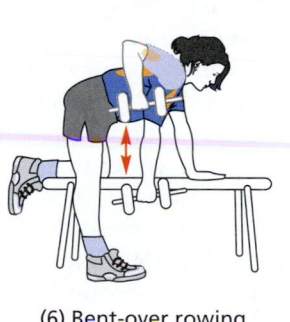

(6) Bent-over rowing

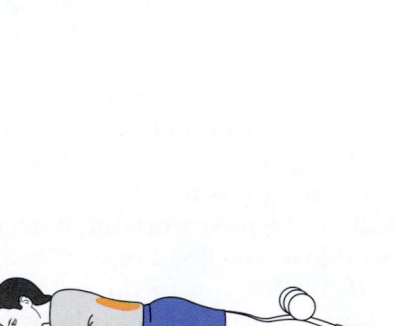

(7) Back extension

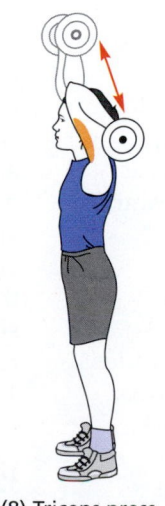

(8) Triceps press

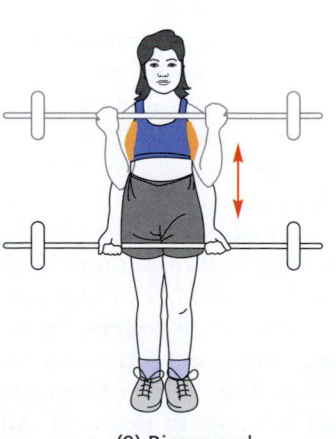

(9) Biceps curl

FIGURE 6-4 Free weight exercises.

shoulders. With back straight, slowly lower hips until tops of thighs are parallel with the floor. Pause. Drive up with legs and hips to the starting position.

2. Lunge
Prime movers: gluteus maximus and quadriceps
Standing upright with the bar on the shoulders off the neck, abdominals tight, back flat, step forward (or backward) until the front thigh is parallel with the floor. The front knee should be over the ball of the foot. Keeping back straight, take a controlled step back to the starting position. Repeat with the opposite leg. This exercise requires considerable balance. You may wish to start first with dumbbells and progress slowly to use of a barbell.

3. Calf raise
Prime mover: gastrocnemius/soleus
Place bar on shoulders, position balls of feet on board and heels off board. Press up onto balls of feet, then lower with control. Knees straight tones gastrocnemius, knees bent tones soleus.

4. Bench press
Prime movers: pectorals and triceps
Lie with head and buttocks on bench, feet stabilized on ground for balance and safety. Grip about 4 inches wider than shoulders, palms under bar (pronated). Lower bar to chest. Focus eyes up to the sky; do not watch bar. Elbows should be directly under bar and forearms perpendicular to ground. Do not let bar slide to the neck. Press to extension and return.

5. Military press
Prime movers: deltoids and triceps
Sit on bench or stand. With barbell on chest, press upward with arms until they are straight overhead but not locked, and return.

6. Bent-over rowing
Prime movers: rhomboids and latissimus dorsi
Stabilize one knee and hand on a bench; opposite hand holds the weight, and foot is flat on the floor. Pull elbow up and in toward the spine.

7. Back extension
Prime movers: erector spinae, gluteus maximus, and quadratus lumborum
Lie with your hips on the seat pad and ankles under the ankle rollers, arms crossed across chest. Slowly extend trunk to a horizontal position, hold 3 to 5 seconds, and slowly lower to starting position. After you can easily do 15–20 repetitions, you may increase resistance by holding light hand weights to your chest.

8. Triceps press
Prime movers: triceps
Standing with abdominals firm, feet apart for stability, grip the weight, palms up, and keeping elbows near the ears, slowly lower bar behind the head. Pause, then press until elbows are fully extended.

9. Biceps curl
Prime movers: biceps
Grasp bar, palms up, holding bar about thigh level. Bend elbows, moving bar in an arc toward shoulders. Pause, and slowly return to starting position.

HOW TO BEGIN AND PROGRESS

According to the ACSM, basic health fitness benefits can be obtained by lifting in a single set of 8 to 12 exercises. If time permits, you may choose to do multiple sets for optimal muscle fitness and muscle growth. A minimum of two to three intense workouts a week is recommended.

The first week, a beginner should lift for one set of 8 to 12 repetitions under the supervision of a trained professional. The first workouts should use light weights and concentrate on form, rhythm, and breathing. This will also minimize muscular soreness. The second week, an additional set can be added if desired, and the third week, a starting load can be established. Other weight training programs for goals of increasing muscular endurance, strength, or size are given in Table 6-3.

ESTABLISHING YOUR WORKLOAD

After several weeks of conditioning and working on lifting form, you may establish an appropriate workload. For each exercise find the maximum amount of weight you can lift once with good form (one **repetition maximum** or **1 RM**). In a general conditioning program, 75 percent of that weight will be your workload. In the workout, lift to fatigue at each station. If you can do fewer than 6 reps, the weight is too heavy. If you can do 12 or more reps at that load, the weight is too light. Increase or decrease the load in the next workout, if necessary. At the correct workload, the last 2 reps of each exercise should be difficult for you to do, and you should reach temporary muscular failure between 8 and 12 reps.

INCREASING YOUR WORKLOAD

When you can do 12 reps, increase the amount of weight. If you can do at least 6 reps at the new weight, stay with that weight until you can do

12 reps. If, when you increase the weight, you cannot do at least 6 reps, drop back to your old weight and increase the number of reps each time until you can do 15. You should then be able to increase the weight and do at least 6 reps. In general,

✓ Increase only one variable at a time (reps, sets, resistance).
✓ Increase reps or sets first, then resistance.
✓ When increasing resistance, decrease reps.
✓ To increase muscular endurance, increase the number of reps or sets or decrease rest between sets.
✓ Increase the workload by no more than 5 to 10 percent each time.

VARIETY

You can incorporate variety into your workout by changing the workload, recovery period, number of sets, reps, rhythm, and number or order of lifts. Here are a few examples of different programs, and see Internet Resources at the end of this chapter for further ideas.

1. *Health fitness:* One to two sets of 8 to 12 reps at 70 to 75 percent 1 RM. Rest 1 to 2 minutes between sets.
2. *Muscular strength:* One to three sets of 5 to 8 reps at 80 to 90 percent 1 RM. Rest 2 to 4 minutes between sets.
3. *Muscular endurance:* One to three sets of 20 reps at 50 to 60 percent 1 RM. Rest 30 to 60 seconds between sets.
4. *Bone strength:* Two to three sets of 8 to 12 reps at 70 to 85 percent 1 RM. Rest 2 minutes between sets. Do two to three times per week.
5. *Eccentric emphasis (negatives):* Lift for two counts, lower for eight. Some experts say that lowering the weight is more important to strength development than lifting it. This does tend to promote more muscle soreness. Strength increases occur with eccentric lifting alone, and because you can lower more weight than you can lift, you may need to increase resistance.
6. *Supersets:* Work opposite muscle groups immediately (triceps/biceps, hams/quads).
7. *Continuous set:* Lift to muscular exhaustion at your regular weight, lower one plate and lift to exhaustion, and continue to lower weight as you fatigue. This is a type of muscular endurance program. It is supposed to increase muscular definition. It can be done with machines but is difficult with free weights.

8. *Pyramid:* Lift 6 reps at 70 percent 1 RM, 4 reps at 80 percent 1 RM, 2 reps at 90 percent 1 RM, 1 rep at 100 percent 1 RM. This program emphasizes strength.
9. *Split routine:* Work upper body one day and lower body the next day or do pushers (e.g., quads, triceps) one day and pullers (e.g., hams, biceps) the next. You must work 4 to 6 days per week. This reduces total body fatigue but requires more time.
10. *Aerobic circuit:* A circuit is a group of exercises performed with little rest after each. Lighten weight to 40 to 60 percent of 1 RM. Lift quickly 30 seconds (15 to 20 lifts), recover for 15 to 30 seconds, while switching to the next station and setting the weight. Perform an upper body, lower body, and core exercise with no rest in between, then an aerobic exercise for 1 minute (cycle, jump rope, jumping jacks). Begin with one set of 10 to 12 exercises and work up to three sets, maintaining a target pulse. This is designed to strengthen the heart as well as develop muscular endurance. Be careful to maintain good form—it is easy to get sloppy and hurt yourself in this workout because the lifting rhythm is so quick.
11. *Muscle size (weight gain) program:* A bulk-up of three to five sets of 5, gradually increasing to 10 reps at 70 to 80 percent effort should be performed for several months to increase lean weight.

COMMON DISCOMFORTS AND TRAINING ERRORS

After lifting for a few weeks, you may notice a buildup of callus on your palms. If it bothers you, lifting gloves will offer some protection. If you experience nausea or light-headedness, stop and figure out the cause.

✓ Did you allow enough time since your last meal?
✓ Are you exhaling on the effort?
✓ Are you trying to progress too quickly?

If you experience pain, particularly joint pain, pay attention. It could be an early warning sign of injury. You may be lifting too heavy a weight or stressing your joints with poor form. Lifting too heavy a weight leads to poor form and increases the risk of injury. Jerking, straining, holding your breath, using momentum, bouncing, and arching the back are problems that need to be corrected. Have a professional check your form periodically to make sure you are not falling into bad habits.

TABLE 6-5   *Performance Aids Promoted to Weight Trainers*

Substance	Advertised Claim	Effects/Side Effects
Amino acid and protein supplements	Muscle growth	May cause unbalanced protein metabolism, dehydration, gout, liver and kidney disease, calcium excretion
Anabolic steroids	Increased muscle mass, strength	Increased muscle mass, strength, aggression, testicular atrophy, acne, impotence, masculinizes women (see Chapter 7, Exploring Special Exercise Considerations)
Caffeine	Increased endurance	Increased endurance, nervousness, tremors
Chromium	Muscle growth	No effect on body composition or strength
Clenbuterol and beta 2 agonists	Increased muscle mass, cuts fat	Rapid heart rate, tremor, anxiety, headache, no proven effect on strength or endurance
Creatine monohydrate	Increased energy, muscle growth	Increased power in short-term high-intensity exercise, weight gain, muscle cramps, increased risk of heat stroke, decreased endurance
Ephedrine and other stimulants	Increased energy	Anxiety, tremor, cardiac arrhythmia Increased risk of heat stroke due to cardiac and central nervous system effects
Growth hormone	Increased muscle size, strength	Slight increase in fat-free mass and water No increase in strength or endurance Acromegaly, diabetes, hypothyroidism
HNB (beta-hydroxy beta-methybutyrate)	Enhanced strength and body composition	No benefit for strength or body composition in trained individuals
Megadose vitamins	Increased energy, strength	No benefit (see Chapter 11, Eating for Wellness) Excess water-soluble excreted Excess fat-soluble can be toxic Excess of one vitamin may decrease absorption of others

PERFORMANCE AIDS

Many people take nutritional supplements or try other products that claim to increase strength, build muscle, or reduce fat. Unfortunately, most of these products do not live up to their advertised claims and are a waste of money, and some are even potentially dangerous. Table 6-5 lists several performance aids used by weight trainers and their effects and side effects. See "Drugs Affecting Physical Performance" in Chapter 7 for further information.

How to Shape and Tone Without Weights

There are many ways to develop muscular strength and endurance. While weight training is an excellent program, it is not always convenient. The programs described next can be done at home or while traveling. The abdominal and core strengthening, hip and thigh, and upper body programs require no special equipment. Partner exercises add a social dimension to a workout. Elastic resistance produces results without bulky equipment and is easy to take with you for exercise on a trip.

While weights add intensity to a workout, they are not always necessary when the goal is to shape and tone. Muscles develop firmness by working against a resistance, and that resistance can be your body weight. These programs emphasize muscular endurance rather than strength by increasing time in contraction or reps. Core trunk muscles in particular benefit from a muscular endurance routine because their function is one of endurance—sustained contraction. If you would like a total body program, combine this with the upper body routine that follows.

ABDOMINAL AND CORE STRENGTHENING EXERCISES

Core trunk stabilizers include all the trunk muscles—the abdominals and the hip and back muscles—which support the body, hold us upright, absorb and transmit forces, and enable us to twist, turn, and bend. Trunk strength is important because it provides a base of stability and power from which the arms and legs work. Most functional movements originate in or rely on trunk stability for efficient performance. Weakness in the trunk musculature increases stress on joints, ligaments, and tendons; impedes performance; and increases the risk of injury. Strong core stabilizers make the body more

Strength Training Myths and Facts

Many common misconceptions regarding strength training have arisen over time and stubbornly persist, passed from one exerciser to the next, despite research evidence to the contrary. Myths are persistent partly because we wish they were true and partly because it is easy to believe testimonials from models and athletes in advertisements and infomercials. Several common myths are discussed here along with the facts you need to debunk them.

Myth	Fact
You can reduce fat around the abdominals, waist, and thighs with specific exercises.	✓ If this were true, people who talk a lot would have thin faces. You can tone underlying muscles with area-specific exercises but many studies have shown that fat burns off all over. If you want to get rid of unsightly bulges, your best bet is a combination of calorie control and aerobic exercise to reduce body fat, with area-specific exercise to tighten the underlying muscles.
You can work upper and lower abdominals separately.	✓ Based on electromyographic studies of people doing various types of abdominal and core exercises, people cannot selectively recruit upper versus lower abdominal muscles. The rectus abdominis acts as a sheet, and contracts as a whole. During certain exercises, like leg lifts, a person may feel greater fatigue in the lower abdominal region because the iliopsoas "hip flexor" is being worked, and it originates below the lower abdominal region. A person can selectively train transverse abdominals, which connect hip-to-hip, by contracting the abdominals, trying to pull the navel toward the spine, holding for 5 seconds, and repeating four or five times.
When you stop exercising, muscle turns to fat.	✓ Muscle and fat (adipose tissue) are made up of different types of cells. Lack of exercise allows muscles to atrophy and turn flabby. Without exercise, a person burns fewer calories and may add pounds of fat. Muscle tissue can no more be turned into fat tissue than a cat can be turned into a dog!
Strength training gives women bulky muscles.	✓ The hormone testosterone is responsible for increases in muscle size seen in men who weight train. Women have only about one-tenth as much testosterone as men, not enough to build huge muscles. The myth persists, probably because of competitive women bodybuilders. To gain the muscle size seen in professional women bodybuilders requires spending hours lifting weights plus taking anabolic steroids. These females should not be confused with women who do not take anabolic drugs and who use resistance training to shape and tone in a fitness program. For additional information, see the section on "Gender Differences" in this chapter.
To tone muscles or to burn fat you should use light weights and high reps.	✓ Magazines and infomercials often suggest that women should lift this way to tone and burn fat without getting big muscles. Lifting light weights and high reps does build muscular endurance, which has its place in your program, but lifting a strength program of heavy weights and fewer reps also will enhance muscle tone, and takes less time than a program requiring multiple sets of reps. Whichever you do, to be effective, you should lift enough weight that you can complete *only* the desired reps with good form. Achieving a lean, toned look may require controlling body fat by creating a calorie deficit with aerobic exercise and a sensible diet as well.
You can get "too old" for strength training.	✓ Many studies show that even people in their seventies and eighties can benefit from exercise with improved strength, balance, and ability to perform activities of daily living. If you have any medical issues or conditions, you will need to get your doctor's clearance, but there is no age limit on health benefits from improving your strength. See the section on "Benefits at Any Age" in this chapter.
Strength training reduces flexibility.	✓ If you exercise without moving your joints through their full range of motion, you can lose flexibility, but that is poor technique. Strength training exercises correctly performed through a full range of motion enhance flexibility, especially if you stretch at the end of your workout.
If you lift weights, you need to eat a lot more protein.	✓ Lots of nutrition hype—most of it untrue—circulates around weight lifting and bodybuilding. Unfortunately, many weight lifters listen to testimonials that fuel the supplement market. The RDA protein requirement is 0.8 gm per kilogram of body weight for adults, which works out to about 46–50 gm of protein per day for women and 56–63 gm for men. For athletes, the protein need is only slightly higher, 1–1.2 gm per kilo of body weight (1 kilo = 2.2 lb), or about 10 to 15 percent of calories.

Research has shown that the primary fuel for muscle is carbohydrate, in the form of glycogen. The body is unable to store extra protein, and excess protein is converted to fat, not used to build muscle. The average American already consumes 1½ to 2 times the RDA of protein. Excess protein can also promote dehydration and loss of calcium, which can increase risk of osteoporosis. The American Dietetic Association (ADA) states that a balanced diet will supply all the protein a weight trainer needs. Exercise scientists and dieticians agree that if you want to build muscle, you should concentrate on a well-balanced diet combined with resistance training.

If you are interested in sports nutrition, try "Sports Nutrition" by Dan Benardot PhD, RD, or online at http://www.dietitian.com/sportnut.html. |

efficient and decrease the risk of back pain or injury. They also improve posture, appearance, breathing, and athletic performance.

A set of strengthening exercises for abdominals (1–9), gluteus (10, 11), and back muscles (12, 13) is shown in Figure 6-5. Also see Internet Resources at the end of this chapter for information about core and abdominal exercises. The exercises should be performed at a slow, steady pace with equal effort in both directions. Lift two counts and lower two counts—don't just lift and fall out of the contraction. The abdominal exercises chosen include those listed as most effective in a study by Peter Francis at San Diego State University. Core muscles can be worked 3 to 5 days a week because they are endurance muscles designed for sustained contraction. You will want a mat or carpeted surface to work on.

1. Bicycle exercise
   Lie on your back with hands behind your head. Raise knees to a 45-degree angle and slowly do a bicycle pedal motion. Touch right elbow to left knee and left elbow to right knee.
2. Abdominal curl "crunch" on stability ball
   Lie on stability ball with feet flat on floor, thighs and trunk parallel to floor. Cross arms behind shoulders or across chest; contract abdominals by raising trunk about 45 degrees. Spread feet apart for better balance. To work obliques more, bring feet closer together.
3. Vertical leg crunch
   Lie on your back with legs raised in the air, knees slightly bent and crossed at the ankles. Cross hands behind the shoulders to support the head. Keep chin lifted to prevent jerking the head. Lift the trunk and slowly lower.
4. Reverse crunch
   Lie on your back with ankles crossed, feet off the ground, and knees at about a 90-degree angle. Place arms on the floor beside your trunk. Press lower back to the ground, contract the abdominals, and rotate hips 1 to 2 inches. Your feet will lift slightly toward the ceiling with each contraction.
5. Plank
   Lie face down, propped with elbows under chest, palms down. Lift up on toes and tighten back and abdominals, keeping body straight and head and spine neutral. Hold 10 to 60 seconds, rest, repeat. If a straight-back position is too difficult, begin with hips hiked up or hold the contraction a shorter amount of time. Do not let the hips sag.

6. Side plank
   Lie on side with weight balanced between forearm, palm, and feet. Keep elbow directly under shoulder to avoid irritating the rotator cuff. Contract back and abdominals to hold body straight. Do not push hips out behind the body. Hold 10 to 30 seconds, rest, repeat on the other side. If a full-body position is too difficult, begin with the half-plank, balancing weight between knees and forearm. For an advanced version, try lifting the top foot in the air for 5 to 10 seconds.
7. Long arm crunch
   Lie on your back with knees bent and heels next to buttocks. Extend arms alongside your ears, chin raised, eyes focused on ceiling. Contract abdominals, keeping lower back to floor, lift shoulders as for a basic crunch, lower slowly.
8. Abdominal curl "crunch"
   Lie on your back with knees bent, heels next to buttocks. Place hands across chest or behind shoulders. Keep eyes focused on ceiling, chin up and about a fist distance from your chest. Contract your abdominals; do not jerk your head forward as you curl. Keeping lower back on the ground, curl shoulders up 3 inches and slowly lower.
9. Oblique abdominal curl
   Lie on the back as for the basic crunch but add a twist, bringing right elbow toward left knee, then left elbow toward right knee. Elbow does not have to touch knee.
10. Rear leg lift (gluteus)
    On hands and knees, hollow abdomen and round back to protect it. Extend right leg to the rear. Tense gluteus. Raise and lower leg slowly six to eight counts. Repeat left.
11. Glute squeeze
    Lying on back with knees bent, squeeze gluteus hard, raising hips no more than 3 inches from floor. Do not arch back. Hold for a count of five, relax, repeat.
12. Back extension
    Lie on your stomach with feet on the floor, head neutral, hands touching shoulders. Slowly lift head, shoulders, and chest. Hold 5 to 10 seconds, slowly lower. Variation: Squeeze shoulder blades in toward spine while holding trunk lift.
13. Alternate arm/leg lift
    Lie on your stomach with arms extended in front. Raise right arm while lifting left leg. Hold 5 to 10 seconds. Repeat on other side. Keep head neutral.

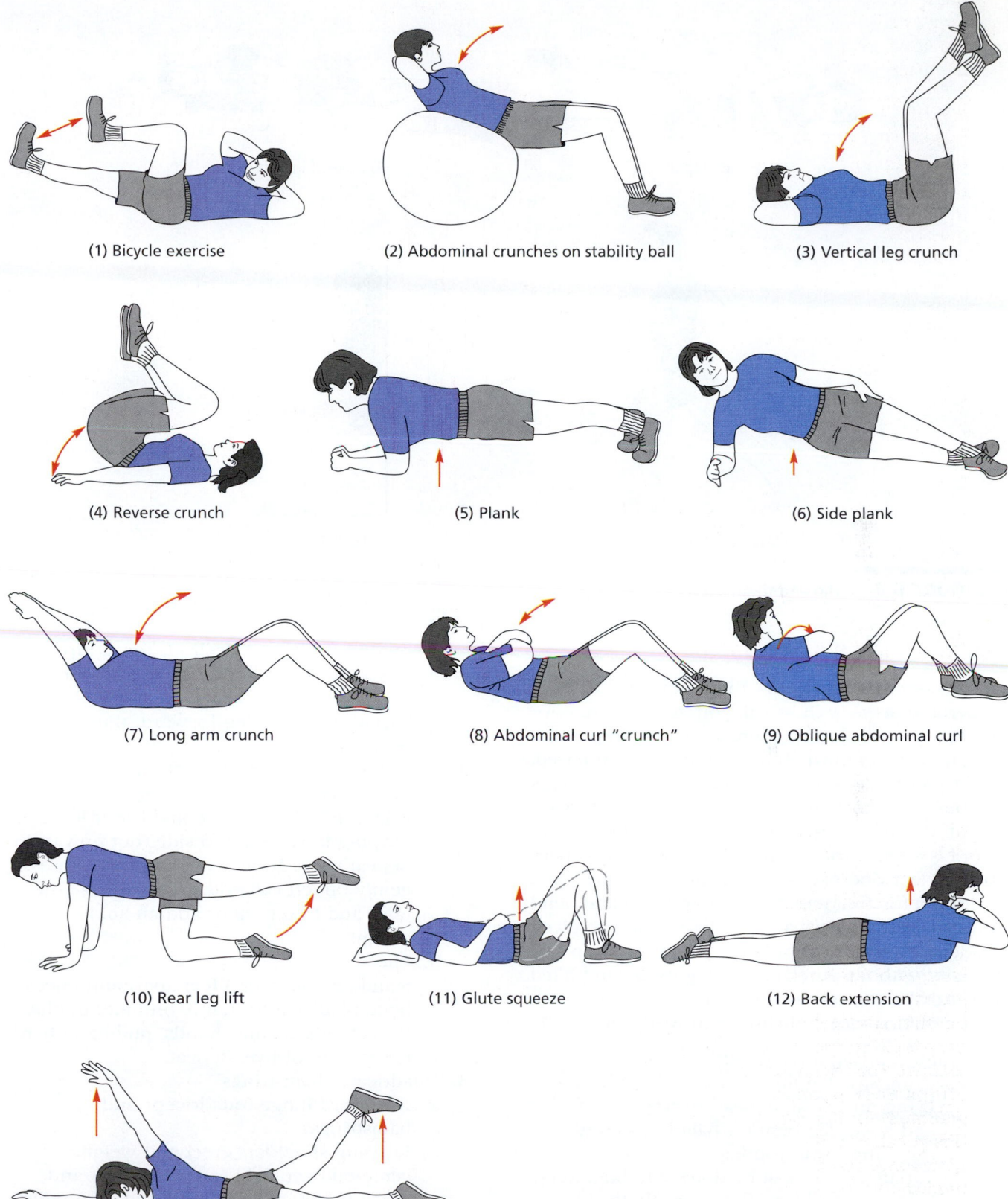

(1) Bicycle exercise

(2) Abdominal crunches on stability ball

(3) Vertical leg crunch

(4) Reverse crunch

(5) Plank

(6) Side plank

(7) Long arm crunch

(8) Abdominal curl "crunch"

(9) Oblique abdominal curl

(10) Rear leg lift

(11) Glute squeeze

(12) Back extension

(13) Alternate arm/leg lift

FIGURE 6-5   Abdominal and core strengthening exercises.

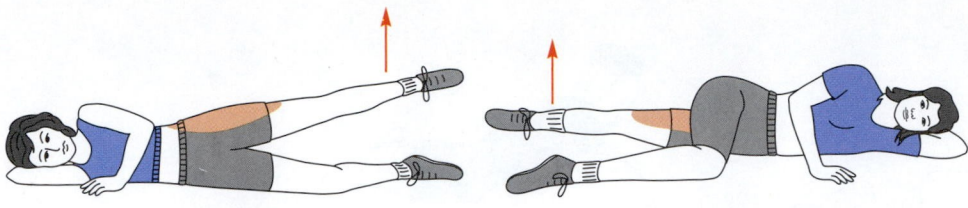

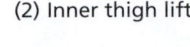

(1) Side leg lift   (2) Inner thigh lift

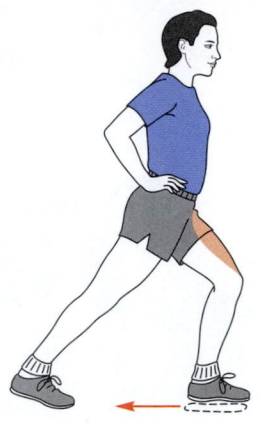

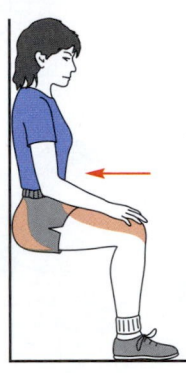

(3a) Backward lunge   (3b) Wall sit

FIGURE 6-6   Hip and thigh exercises.

HIP AND THIGH EXERCISES

These exercises (Figure 6-6) will not burn calories as aerobic work will, so if you want to remove inches, diet and aerobic exercise are still important. Also, fat will not burn off only in the area exercised. While you can't spot reduce fat, say, in the thighs by doing leg lifts, you can spot tone flabby muscles. Be patient and you may begin to see a difference in 8 to 12 weeks. You do not need to count repetitions. Select one exercise for each body area and perform it for 1 minute. Start with one set and build up to two sets, 3 days a week. Variations are given to add variety to your program. If you wish to add intensity without purchasing weights, a sand-filled sock can be tied on as an ankle weight. You will want a mat or carpeted surface to work on.

1. Outer hip (hip abductors)
   a. Lying side leg lift
      Lying on one side, head resting on arm and lower leg bent for balance, slowly raise and lower top leg.
      Variation: This can be done standing. Keep foot level and leg lifting directly to side, not toward front.
   b. Kneeling side leg lift
      Take a hands-and-knees position with one leg extended to side.
      Tighten abdominals, and round back to protect it. You may also support weight on one forearm if desired. Tense hip and raise and lower leg slowly no higher than 6 inches.
      Variation: Circle leg forward, then reverse.
2. Inner thigh (thigh adductors)
   a. Inner thigh lift
      Lying on left side, raise and lower left leg, keeping foot turned to side (not upward). Repeat right. To increase resistance, press gently on left calf with right foot as you raise and lower leg or add an ankle weight.
   b. Plié
      Standing with feet 3 feet apart and knees bent, place hands lightly on inner thighs. Press thighs against hands, pulling in hard for a count of five. Repeat.
3. Quadriceps, hamstrings
   a. Backward lunge (quadriceps and hamstrings)
      Keeping shoulders erect and weight centered over right foot, step back and touch lightly with left foot and then return to starting position. Repeat. Switch legs after 1 minute of reps.
   b. Wall sit (quads)
      Hold a sitting position with back against a wall for balance. Keep hips above knee level.

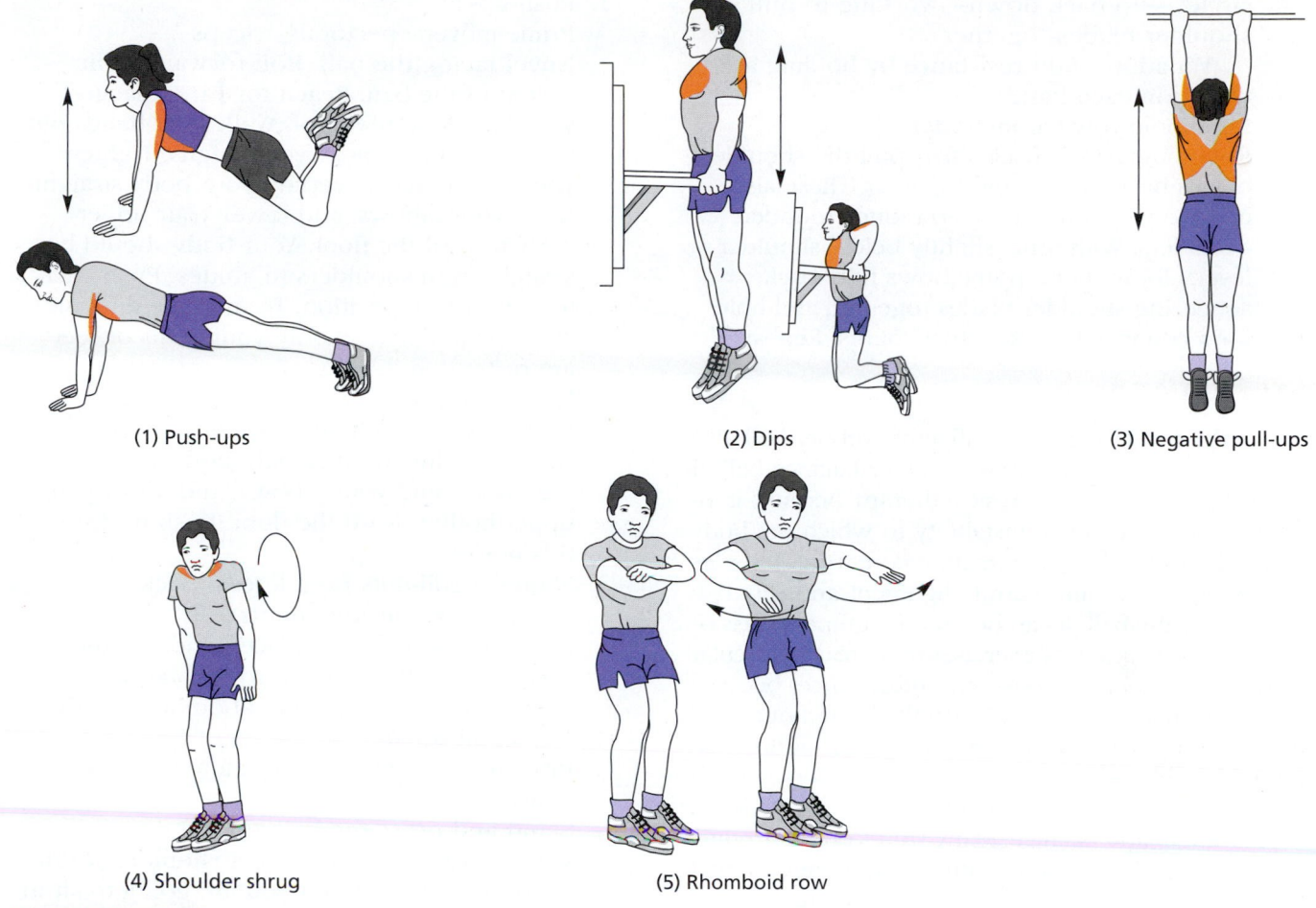

(1) Push-ups   (2) Dips   (3) Negative pull-ups

(4) Shoulder shrug   (5) Rhomboid row

FIGURE 6-7   **Upper body exercises.**

UPPER BODY EXERCISES

Upper body exercises can improve appearance by straightening rounded shoulders, firming upper arm muscles, and toning pectorals that underlie and support the breasts. You do not need to count repetitions. Select one exercise for each body area and repeat for 1 minute. If you wish to increase resistance, bricks, books, or cans of food can serve as hand weights. Upper body exercises are illustrated in Figure 6-7.

1. Push-ups (pectorals/triceps)
   These may be done standing, with hands against a wall and feet placed about 3 feet away from the wall (easiest), on the floor with knees bent (medium), or with weight supported on hands and feet (hardest). Keep abdominals firm and hips slightly flexed to support back. Lower to right angles of arms and then press back to arm extension.

   Variations: Keeping hands close emphasizes triceps. Keeping hands wide increases pectoral strengthening.

2. Dips (pectorals/triceps)
   Dips are an alternative way to tone the same muscle groups that push-ups tone. They may be done on a dip bar or using chairs. With weight evenly distributed between bars or two sturdy chairs, place a hand on each. Bend knees or extend legs so that weight is on arms, not feet. Bend arms to right angles and return to extension.

3. Negative pull-ups (latissimus dorsi/biceps)
   Negative pull-ups offer the same benefits as full pull-ups for upper back and arms. Stand on a chair if necessary to grasp a pull-up bar with arms flexed. SLOWLY lower yourself to a count of five. As you gain strength over several weeks, try to start with a few full pull-ups and finish with negatives.

4. Shoulder shrugs (trapezius)
   Shoulder shrugs can tighten upper back muscles to reduce rounded shoulders. Combine this with pectoral stretches for best results. Rotate shoulders in full

circles—up-back-down—working to pull shoulder blades together.
   Variations: Add resistance by holding a weight in each hand.

5. Rhomboid row (rhomboids)
   Rhomboids are muscles that pull the shoulder blades back, down, and together. These also need to be strengthened to reduce rounded shoulders. With arms slightly below shoulder level, elbows bent, pull elbows fully back, squeezing shoulder blades together, and hold for a count of five. Rest two counts. Repeat.

STABILITY BALLS

The stability ball is a large inflatable rubber ball also known as a Swiss ball, fitness ball, or balance ball. It has long been used in physical therapy because it introduces an element of instability to which the body naturally responds by contracting core trunk muscles to keep the spine in neutral alignment and stay balanced over the ball. It can be used in a fitness class or at home for a variety of exercises to increase muscular fitness, core strength, posture, and balance, because you must maintain a stable trunk throughout each exercise. To start, you can use it for abdominal crunches, obliques, and back extensions. You can also sit on the ball and exercise with hand weights to build core strength and balance. Many stores offer introductory videos or DVDs along with the equipment so that you can learn to use it in an effective manner.

Stability Ball Exercise Guidelines

✓ To choose a ball size—when you sit on the ball, your knees should be at a 90-degree angle and your thighs parallel to the floor.
✓ The ball should be inflated so that it is firm, but can still contour to your body. Do not inflate it until it is "hard."
✓ It is important to maintain good posture while working out. Keep your abdominals tight to protect your lower back. Avoid back and neck hyperextension.
✓ Do each exercise slowly.
✓ If you have never used a ball, start with sitting on the ball and rocking the hips, then try the easiest skills like back extension or bridging. Place the ball against a wall or keep your hands and/or feet on the floor for stability. Ball placement affects exercise difficulty.
✓ Attempt more difficult skills only after mastering the easier exercises.
✓ Strength exercises should be done for 8–12 repetitions.

Ten exercises that you can do with a stability ball are illustrated in Figure 6-8.

1. Push-ups
   Prime movers: pectorals, triceps
   Kneel facing the ball. Roll forward to lie on top of the ball. Reach forward, placing your hands on the floor. Walk your hands out until the ball is under your thighs. Tighten your abdominals, keeping your body straight. Bend your elbows, and lower your upper body toward the floor. Your body should be straight from shoulders to ankles. Push back to the starting position. To increase difficulty, roll the ball back so only your shins or feet are resting on it.

2. Knee tuck press
   Prime movers: deltoids, triceps
   Kneel on the stability ball, and hands on the floor. Bend your elbows, and lower your upper body toward the floor. Push up from this position.

3. Shoulder roll-outs from knees (back extensors, rectus abdominis)
   Kneeling on the floor, place hands on the stability ball. Roll it forward and back, keeping back straight and abdominals tight.

4. Back wall squat
   Prime movers: quadriceps, gluteus maximus, hamstrings
   Stand and press the ball against a wall with your back. Position feet shoulder width apart and forward as if you are going to sit in a chair. Bend your knees, rolling the ball down until your knees are at a 90-degree angle and your thighs are parallel to the floor. Keeping your back pressed against the ball, hold for 5 counts. Straighten your knees and return to the starting position.

5. Ball transfer
   Prime movers: rectus abdominis
   Lie on your back with hands resting on the floor and grip ball between your ankles. Curl the pelvis to lift the ball off the floor into the air, reach up, and transfer it to your hands, then back to your ankles.

6. Prone knee tucks
   Prime movers: rectus abdominis
   Place shins on the stability ball and hands on the floor. Roll the ball back away from your hands, keeping shoulders aligned with hands, abdominals tight, body straight. Extend legs, then bend knees in toward your chest and roll the ball forward until your knees are at your chest. To increase difficulty, try from a bent elbow position on the floor.

7. Oblique curls
   Prime movers: rectus abdominis, external and internal oblique abdominals

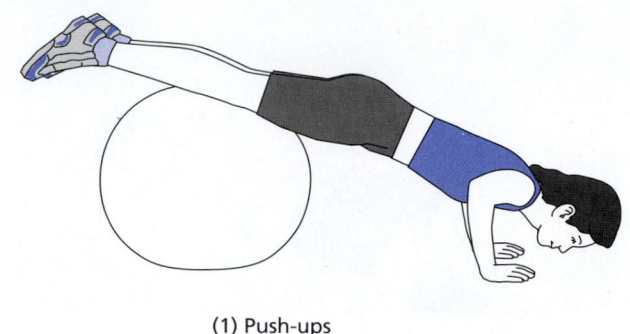

(1) Push-ups

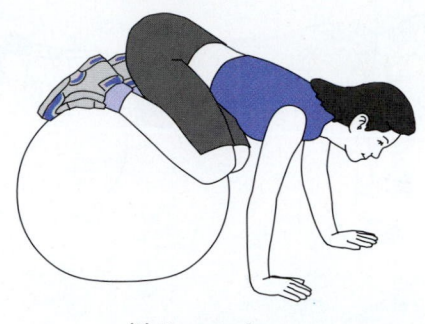

(2) Knee tuck press

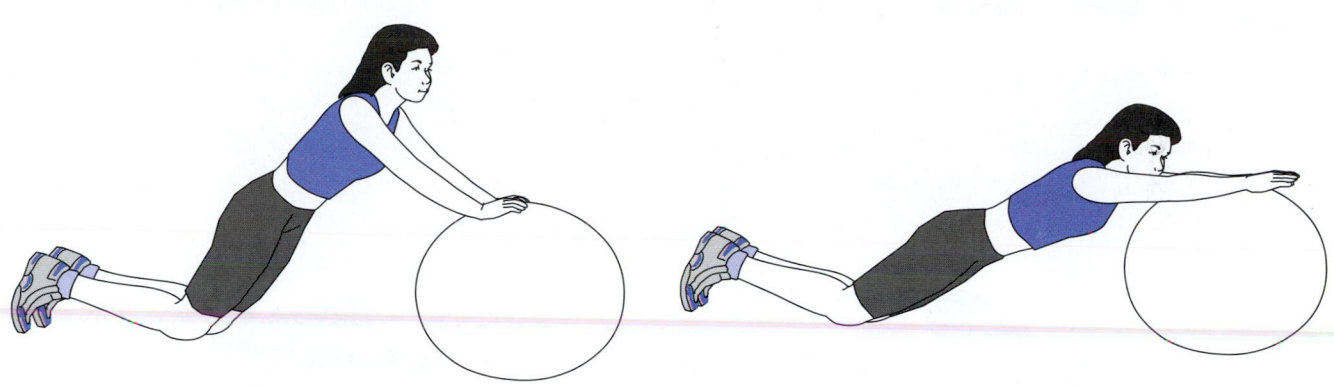

(3) Shoulder roll-outs

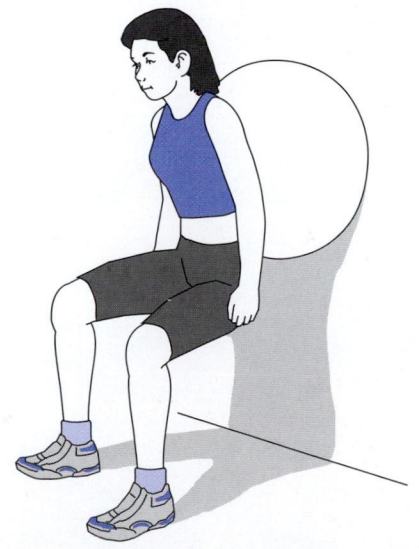

(4) Back wall squat

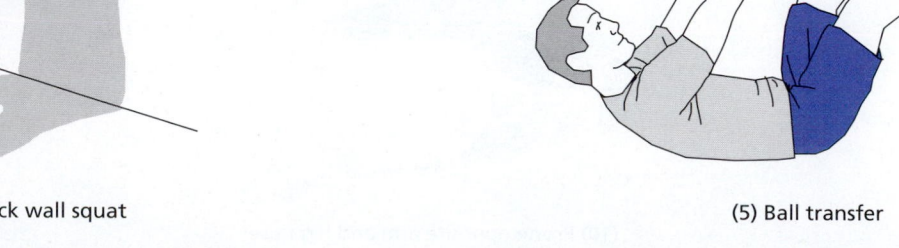

(5) Ball transfer

FIGURE 6-8   **Stability ball exercises.**

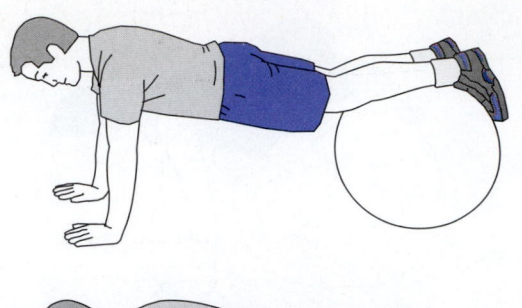

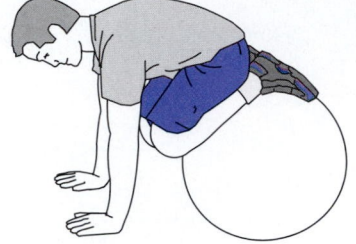

(6) Prone knee tucks

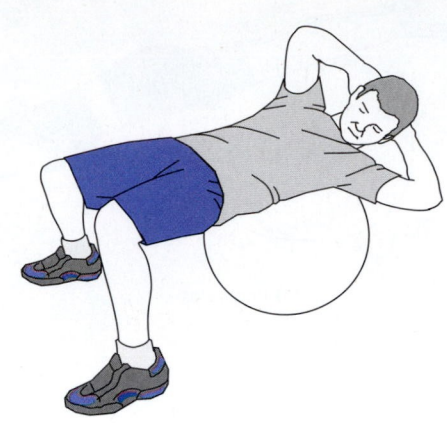

(7) Oblique curls

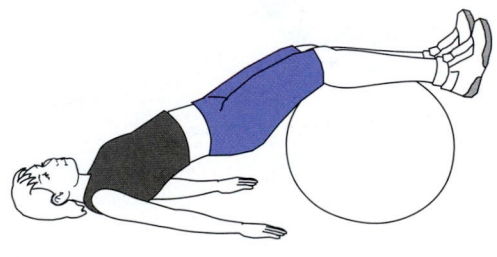

(8) Bridges

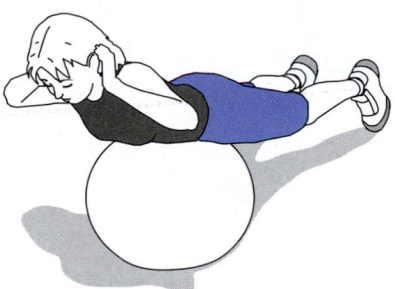

(9) Back extension

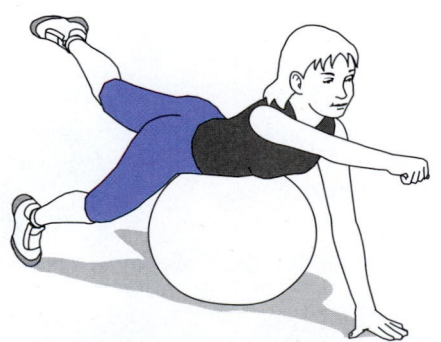

(10) Prone opposite arm and leg raise

FIGURE 6-8   Stability ball exercises. (*continued*)

Lie with the top of the ball beneath the center of your back, feet spread wide on the floor for stability. Rotate hips to one side, and slowly curl the right side of the upper body toward the left leg. Return to starting position; repeat, alternating sides.

8. Bridges

Prime movers: back extensors, gluteus maximus, hamstrings

Lie on your back with legs on the ball, hands resting beside you on the floor. Slowly lift hips until your back is straight and weight is on your upper back. Pause, then return slowly to the starting position. Avoid pressing the neck into the floor or arching the back. To make it easier, place ball under knees. To make it harder, place under heels.

9. Back extension

Prime movers: back extensors

Lie prone with hips on the ball, feet on the floor, and trunk slightly flexed. Arms may be at your side or behind shoulders. Tighten your upper back, slowly raising shoulders until the spine is straight or slightly extended. Keep head neutral to avoid neck hyperextension. Hold, relax slowly to starting position. Repeat.

10. Prone opposite arm/leg raise

Prime movers: back extensors, gluteus maximus, hamstrings, deltoids

Lying prone on the ball, extend right leg behind you, foot touching floor. Keep head neutral. Reach in front with the left arm, raising it close to your ear. Lift the arm and leg slowly at the same time, pause as you reach extension, then lower slowly. Repeat, alternating sides. To increase difficulty, lift the non-active arm a few inches off the floor instead of using it to balance.

PILATES

Pilates is a program that originally was used by dancers to improve core muscle strength, balance, muscle control, and flexibility. It now is being offered in fitness centers and is enjoyed by many exercisers for its health benefits. Development of strength and control in abdominal and back muscles is important for preventing back pain. Pilates emphasizes proper breathing, correct spinal and pelvic alignment, and concentration on smooth, flowing movement. It incorporates a series of group mat exercises and Pilates exercise equipment that uses springs to create resistance. If you are interested in trying Pilates, many fitness centers offer introductory sessions and many fitness retailers have DVDs available for home use.

TOP 10 LIST

Tips for Elastic Resistance Exercise

Exercising with elastic bands has its risks as well as its benefits. To maximize your results and minimize the risk of getting snapped by an elastic band, follow these tips:

1. *Check the band for tears before every workout.* Do not use it if it shows cracks or tears because it may break.
2. *Point the band away from your face.* Never point it toward another person.
3. *Keep a towel handy to wipe off sweat.* Sweat makes the band slippery.
4. *Leave slight tension on the band between reps.* This maximizes muscle toning. Do not let the band go slack.
5. *Wear socks.* This prevents the band from biting into the ankles in leg exercises.
6. *Men may want to wear exercise pants.* This will prevent the band from ripping out leg hair.
7. *Keep the wrist in line with the forearm.* Wrist hyperextension, a common mistake in lat pulls and bicep curls, stresses the carpal joints of the wrist.
8. *Stretch the band slowly and release slowly.* Use a controlled rhythm—pull 2 seconds, hold briefly, release 2 seconds. Begin with 30 seconds of repetitions and work up to 1 minute for each exercise. Completing 1 to 2 sets is a good goal.
9. *Progress to a stronger band.* Or add a second band to progress when the workout gets too easy (eventually it will).
10. *Powder the band lightly with cornstarch after use to keep it in good condition.*

Elastic Resistance

Elastic resistance exercise was developed in the 1950s. It was originally used by physical therapists who gave patients surgical rubber tubing to add resistance to rehabilitative exercise programs. Elastic bands and tubing are lightweight, portable, and readily available at fitness centers and medical supply companies. They are inexpensive but do not last forever and need to be replaced as they wear out. Safety tips are listed in the Top 10 "Tips for Elastic Resistance Exercise." They come in different strengths, based on the thickness of the elastic. Thin bands are best for beginners and for upper body work. Thicker bands are useful for lower body work. Two thin bands can be used in place of one thick band. The principles of form, rhythm, and breathing apply here as for any strength training program. Elastic resistance exercises are illustrated in Figure 6-9.

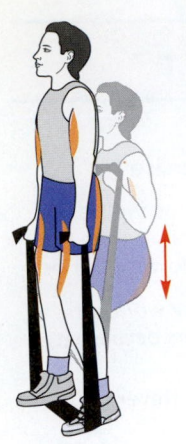

(1) Squats

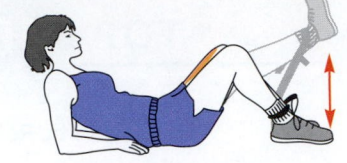

(2) Leg extension

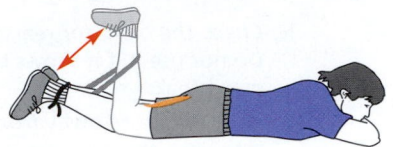

(3) Hamstring curl

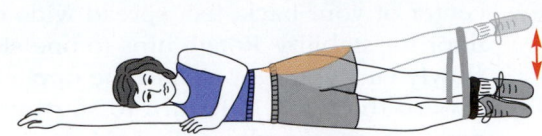

(4) Side leg lift

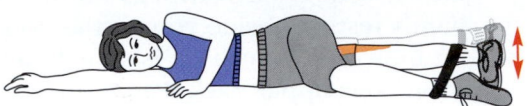

(5) Inner thigh lift

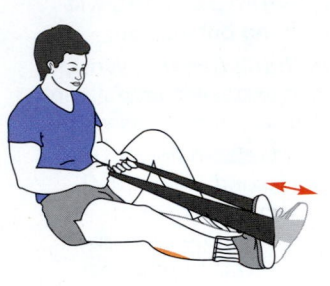

(6) Toe press

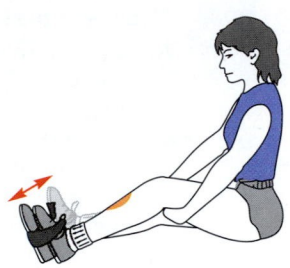

(7) Toe lifts

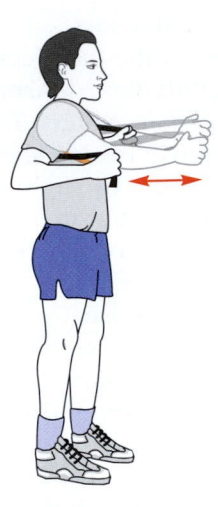

(8) Standing push-ups

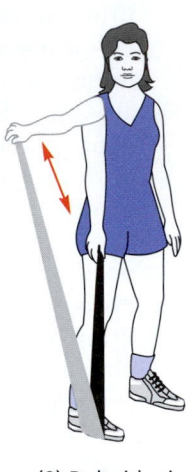

(9) Deltoid raise

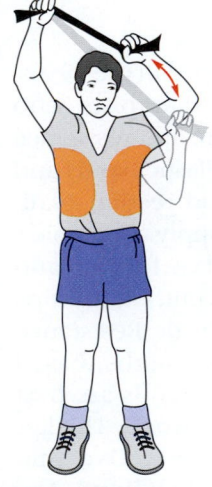

(10) Lat pull

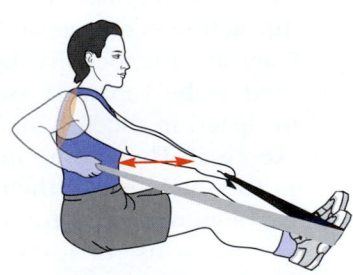

(11) Rowing

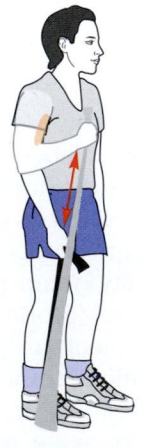

(12) Biceps curl

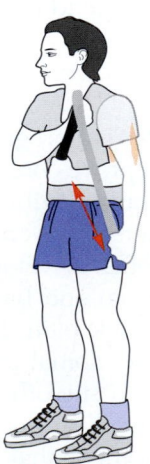

(13) Triceps extension

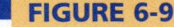

FIGURE 6-9   **Elastic resistance exercises.**

Elastic Resistance Exercises

1. Squats
   Prime movers: gluteus maximus, quadriceps, hamstrings, biceps
   Step on the band with feet about shoulder width apart and hold ends of the band low enough to feel moderate tension. Slowly squat until hips are just above knees, bending elbows to maintain tension in the band. Return to standing.

2. Leg extension
   Prime movers: quadriceps
   Tie band around ankles. Lie back, knees bent and feet on floor. Keeping knees and thighs together, straighten knee, lifting the foot as high as possible. Release slowly and repeat. Change legs.

3. Hamstring curl
   Prime movers: hamstrings, gluteus maximus
   Place the band around ankles. Lie face down with arms under the chin or hands under hips. Bending knee, slowly lift one foot. Release slowly, maintaining some tension in the band. Repeat. Change legs.

4. Side leg lift
   Prime movers: hip abductors
   Place the band around both legs—around ankles is hardest, around knees easiest. Lying on right side, torso supported by arms, slightly bend lower leg for support. Keep hips facing forward, lift upper leg. Lower, keeping tension on the band, and repeat. Change sides.

5. Inner thigh lift
   Prime movers: thigh adductors
   Place band around left arch and right ankle. Lie on right side with trunk supported by arms. Lift bottom leg slowly, hold briefly, lower slowly, repeat. Switch sides.

6. Toe press
   Prime movers: gastrocnemius, soleus
   Holding ends of band, place around ball of foot. With knee straight, slowly press through ball of foot from extension to flexion and back (gastrocnemius). To emphasize soleus, repeat with knee slightly bent.

7. Toe lifts
   Prime movers: tibialis anterior
   Tie band around arches. Place heels about 6 inches apart forward to back. Keeping one foot pointed, pull toes of the other foot back toward your face. Relax. Repeat on both feet.

8. Standing push-ups
   Prime movers: pectorals and biceps
   Wrap the band around your back and under your arms. Bend elbows and grasp ends of band. Extend arms forward, return slowly.

9. Deltoid raise
   Prime movers: deltoid and triceps
   Place one end of band under foot, hold the other end by your hip. Standing with good posture, lift arm to shoulder level, lower slowly.

10. Lat pull
    Prime mover: latissimus dorsi
    Hold band overhead, elbows extended but not locked. Pull arms apart to shoulder level. Be careful not to get hair caught in band.

11. Rowing
    Prime mover: rhomboids
    With band around arches and knees extended, grasp band about mid-shin. Pull elbows back and try to bring shoulder blades together. Release slowly.

12. Biceps curl
    Prime mover: biceps
    Place one end of band under foot, grasp other end low, and, keeping elbow at your side, curl right arm to shoulder. Slowly release.

13. Triceps extension
    Prime mover: triceps
    Standing with good posture, grasp ends of band. Press lower hand toward hip, pause, slowly release. Do both arms.

Partner Resistance Exercises

Exercising with a partner can be both challenging and enjoyable. Partner communication and sensitivity to your levels of strength and fatigue are important. The partner must vary resistance for different muscle groups and increase resistance during the eccentric part of each contraction. While many of these exercises can be done without equipment, to add variety, you may wish to try them using a towel to pull on (biceps curls) or a broomstick (overhead press). This is a balanced program of four lower-body and five upper-body exercises. You may either count reps or perform each exercise for a minute and work up to two to three sets (Figure 6-10).

1. Leg extension
   Prime mover: quadriceps
   Sit on a bench or chair. Move one leg from flexion to full extension and back as partner resists by pressing on front of lower leg.

2. Hamstring curl
   Prime movers: hamstrings, gluteus
   Lie face down while partner straddles your back and places a hand on each ankle. Bend knees and curl calves toward buttocks as

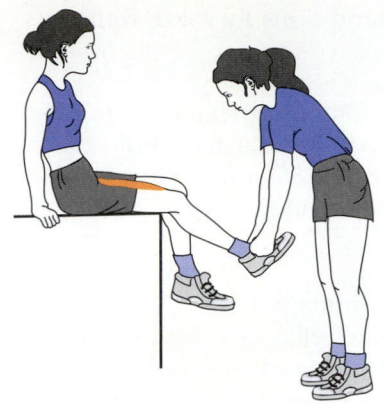

(1) Leg extension

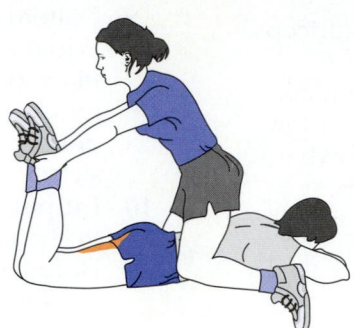

(2) Hamstring curl

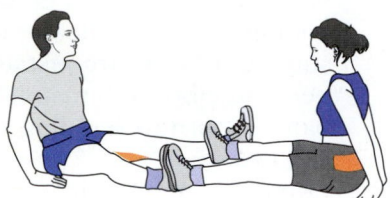

(3) Inner/outer thigh press

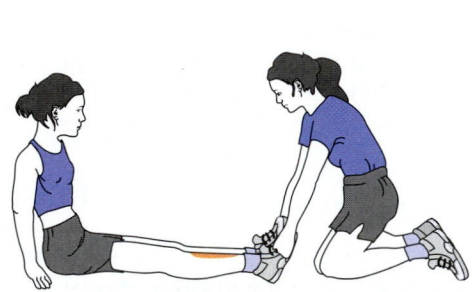

(4) Foot flexion

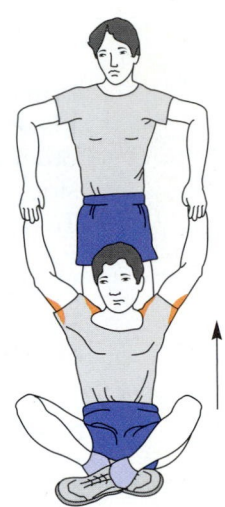

(5) Overhead press

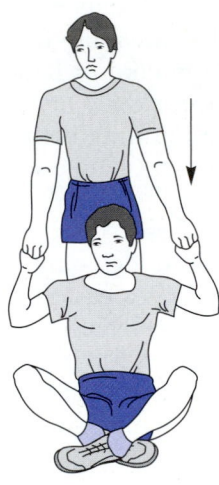

(6) Lat pull

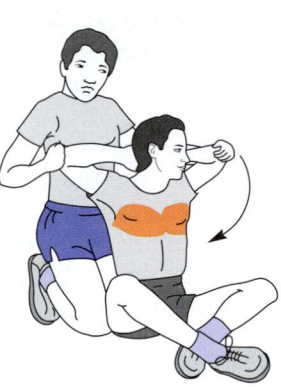

(7) Elbow press forward

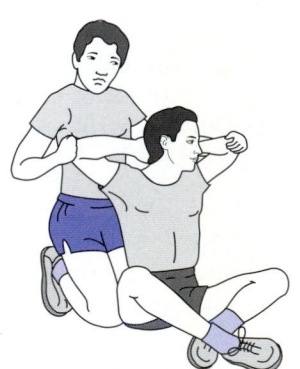

(8) Elbow press backward

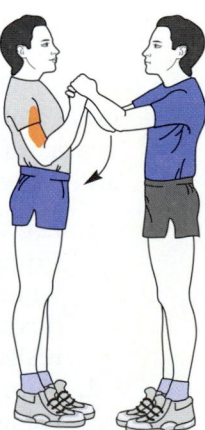

(9) Biceps curl

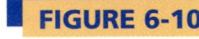

FIGURE 6-10 **Partner resistance exercises.**

your partner resists. Continue the resistance as you return to the starting position.

3. Inner/outer thigh press
Prime movers: thigh adductors and abductors
Sit, facing each other, legs forward, hands behind hips for balance. One partner places both feet inside the other's feet and presses outward as the other partner resists by pressing inward. Switch positions after six to eight reps.

4. Foot flexion
Prime mover: anterior tibialis
Sit with legs extended. Partner kneels and presses down on top of both feet as you flex them and then return to extension.

5. Overhead press
Prime movers: deltoids, triceps
Sit with hands at shoulder level, palms up. As partner resists, press up toward ceiling and then return to starting position.

6. Lat pull
Prime mover: latissimus dorsi
Sit and reach high overhead to grasp partner's hands. As partner resists, pull down to shoulder level and slowly return to starting position.

7. Elbow press forward
Prime mover: pectorals
Sit with elbows out and hands touchingshoulders. As partner resists at the elbows, pull them in toward your midline and return to starting position.

8. Elbow press backward
Prime mover: rhomboids
Sit with elbows out or with arms crossed. Partner sits behind, pressing on your elbows as you press back, pulling shoulder blades together. As partner continues resistance, return to starting position.

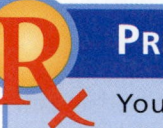

PRESCRIPTION FOR ACTION

You've read the chapter. Now go do one or more of these:

✔ While watching TV, use your exercise band during commercials.

✔ While sitting, do abdominal isometric contractions or press knees together hard for 6 seconds, 5–10 times, to tone inner thigh.

✔ Treat yourself with an exercise ball and video to add variety to your exercise program.

✔ Carry and load your own groceries; take the stairs instead of the elevator.

✔ If you usually use weight machines, make an appointment for instruction to enable you to try free weight exercises, and vice versa.

✔ Try a personal trainer for one session to check your lifting form and technique and make suggestions for improvement in your lifting program.

Mc Graw Hill connect™   **Go online to Connect to complete this activity.**
http://connect.mcgraw-hill.com

9. Biceps curl
Prime mover: biceps
Stand, palms facing upward. Partner resists on your palms as you curl arm from extension to flexion and back. This may also be done holding a towel in one hand in front of body. Partner sits or kneels facing you, resisting on other end of towel as you curl your arm.

Frequently Asked Questions

Q. I have been doing 100 abdominal crunches a day for 6 weeks, and still my abdominals aren't flat. Why? They feel really strong and tight.

A. A layer of fat often overlays the abdominals, giving them a rounded appearance. Crunches will strengthen the abdominals, making them feel firm. If you are overweight, diet will help reduce the fat layer to get the results you seek. If you are of normal weight, check your posture—habitually standing with an overarched lower back will make the abdominals protrude even if they are firm.

Q. Why should I add resistance exercises to my exercise program?

A. Strength training is an important part of a balanced fitness program. Stronger muscles help prevent injury, improve your ability to participate in sports, and prevent loss of muscle fibers that begins around age 25.

Q. Which is better, free weights or machines?

A. It depends on your goals. A beginner will improve with overload from either system. Machines are safer and you don't need a spotter, but they are expensive to buy or you need access to a gym. With free weights, you need a spotter for safety, but they are inexpensive, and so you can have a set at home. Free weights allow a greater variety of exercises than do machines and develop balance, timing, and muscular fitness, so many athletes prefer them. If you have access to both, start with machines, and as you gain strength, gradually work in a few free weight exercises to see which you like better.

Q. I just started a weight-training program. How long until I see results?

A. Rate of improvement varies with individuals—some gain quickly, others more slowly. If you are lifting 2 to 3 days a week using a general program of one to two sets of 8 to 12 reps at 75 percent 1 rep max, you may begin increasing reps or load within 3 to 4 weeks. The most rapid gains are seen in the first 6 months, but people can continue to improve for years. Other factors affecting rate of improvement include good nutrition, adequate recovery between workouts, and sufficient sleep.

Q. How good is the abdominal equipment on TV infomercials?

A. There is no piece of equipment that tones abdominals better than the abdominal exercises in Figure 6-5. Before you rush out to buy the newest advertised piece of abdominal gear, ask yourself if you will use it regularly. Be skeptical of any equipment that promises effortless results, spot reduction, burning more calories, or greater weight loss than other methods. While you can spot tone, you can't wear the fat off just one body area. Loss of abdominal fat requires regular exercise that works the whole body, as well as cutting back on calories. To help you decide, go to a gym or fitness center and try out various types of equipment to see what you like and what meets your needs.

Q. What do I do if I hit a plateau in weight training?

A. While initial progress may be rapid, after about 6 months of strength training, a plateau is common. If you have been doing the same program for months, it is time to vary the routine. You may benefit from changing the sequence of exercises so that muscles are fatigued in a different order. You can replace some of the exercises with ones that strengthen the same muscle group (e.g., fly instead of chest press or squats instead of leg press). If you have been lifting more than 12 repetitions of a weight, increasing the intensity and dropping the number of repetitions will make the muscles work harder. Also, make sure that you are giving your muscles sufficient recovery time, at least 48 hours between workouts.

Q. Does strength training decrease risk for osteoporosis?

A. Bones are living tissue, constantly remodeling to the stresses placed on them. Without weight-bearing exercise, bones demineralize. They require the regular stimulus of weight-bearing exercise to take up bone mineral. Walking and jogging using the resistance of body weight are excellent leg and hip-bone strengtheners. Weight training at an intensity of 70 to 85 percent of 1 RM, 2 to 3 sets of 8 to 12 repetitions, 2 to 3 days per week has been shown to produce gradual increases in bone density, which decreases risk of osteoporosis. Like muscle, the rule is "use it or lose it."

Summary

Muscular strength and muscular endurance exercises are a vital supplement to a regular program of aerobic exercise. They can enhance appearance by improving the shape, firmness, and tone of muscles. Enhanced posture, decreased risk of lower back pain, greater ease of movement, improved athletic performance, and more energy are benefits. While injury is possible in any exercise program if safety guidelines are ignored, sensible strengthening programs decrease the risk of injury for those who participate in health-related fitness programs or athletics.

Terms

- agonist
- antagonist
- atrophy
- concentric contraction
- constant resistance exercise
- dynamic (isotonic) exercise
- eccentric contraction
- fast-twitch muscle fiber
- hypertrophy
- isokinetic
- muscular power
- progressive overload
- repetition (rep)
- repetition maximum (1 RM)
- set
- slow-twitch muscle fiber
- static (isometric) exercise
- Valsalva maneuver
- variable resistance exercise

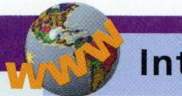

Internet Resources

American College of Sports Medicine

www.acsm.org/sportsmed

Provides information on sports research and health and fitness, aerobic exercise guidelines, and a quarterly fitness newsletter. "Current Comments" gives information on a variety of exercise topics of recent interest.

American Council on Exercise

www.acefitness.org

Has fitfacts information sheets on over 100 different health and fitness topics, health and fitness tips, fitness questions and answers, healthy recipes, and a free monthly e-newsletter on health and fitness topics.

ExRx.net

www.exrx.net

Exercise information including weight training, fitness testing, bodybuilding, anabolic steroids, and weight management.

International Fitness Association

www.ifafitness.com/wttrain/index.html

Illustrates 26 weight training exercises with moving diagrams and detailed information on lifting technique.

National Strength and Conditioning Association

www.nsca-lift.org

Provides research-based information on strength training and conditioning for improving fitness and athletic performance.

Additional Fitness Resources

Please note: All links were active at time of publication. If one is not working for you, try a search at the root Web site (mayoclinic.com or workoutz.com).

Mayo Clinic

www.mayoclinic.com

Under the fitness tab, provides information on stretching strength training, aerobic exercise, and sports nutrition. Includes videos and slide shows.

Fitness in Depth: Strength Training http://www.tinyurl.com/ch6strength

Strength training with resistance tubing http://tinyurl.com/ch6tubing

Slide show: Core exercises with a fitness ball http://tinyurl.com/ch6fitball

Abdominal Exercises—Best Abdominal Exercises and Core Workouts http://tinyurl.com/ch6bestabs

The Best and the Worst Ab Exercises http://tinyurl.com/ch6bestandworst

Top 10 questions about abdominal exercises http://tinyurl.com/ch6core

Podcast: Weight training tips for busy people—5 time-saving tips http://tinyurl.com/ch6timesaving

Exercise Video

ACSM Exercise Is Medicine—Keys to Exercise—Strength http://tinyurl.com/ch6ACSMstrength
ACSM Exercise Is Medicine—Keys to Exercise—Home Gym http://tinyurl.com/ch6homegym
Pilates Abs Workout http://tinyurl.com/ch6hpilatesabs

Videos for Figure 6-3 Weight training exercises with machines

1. Leg press — http://tinyurl.com/ch6hlegpress
2. Leg extension — http://tinyurl.com/ch6kextension
3. Hamstring curl — http://tinyurl.com/ch6hscurl
4. Toe press — http://tinyurl.com/ch6toepress
5. Bench press — http://tinyurl.com/ch6benchpress
6. Military press — http://tinyurl.com/ch6mpress
7. Lat pull — http://tinyurl.com/ch6latpulldown
8. Rowing — http://tinyurl.com/ch6rowing
9. Back extension — http://tinyurl.com/ch6backex
10. Abdominal curl — http://tinyurl.com/ch6abcurl
11. Triceps press — http://tinyurl.com/ch6tpress
12. Biceps curl — http://tinyurl.com/ch6bcurl

Videos for Figure 6–4 Free weight exercises

1. Squats — http://tinyurl.com/ch6squats
2. Lunge — http://tinyurl.com/ch6lunge
3. Calf raise — http://tinyurl.com/ch6calf
4. Bench press — http://tinyurl.com/ch6bpress
5. Military press — http://tinyurl.com/ch6milpress
6. Bent-over rowing — http://tinyurl.com/ch6borow
7. Back extension — http://tinyurl.com/ch6backex2
8. Triceps press — http://tinyurl.com/ch6tpress2
9. Biceps curl — http://tinyurl.com/ch6bcurl2

Videos for Figure 6-5 Abdominal and core strengthening exercises

1. Bicycle exercise — http://tinyurl.com/ch6bicycle
2. Abdominal crunches on stability ball — http://tinyurl.com/ch6stabcrunch
3. Vertical leg crunch — http://preview.tinyurl.com/ch6vert-leg
4. Reverse crunch — http://tinyurl.com/ch6reverunch
5. Plank — http://tinyurl.com/ch6plank
6. Side plank — http://tinyurl.com/ch6sideplank
7. Long arm crunch — http://tinyurl.com/ch6larmcrunch
8. Abdominal curl "crunch" — http://tinyurl.com/ch6abcurl2
9. Oblique abdominal curl — http://tinyurl.com/ch6oblique
10. Rear leg lift — http://tinyurl.com/ch6rleglift
11. Glute squeeze — http://tinyurl.com/ch6glutesqueez
12. Back extension — http://tinyurl.com/ch6backex3
13. Alternate arm/leg lift — http://tinyurl.com/ch6aall

Videos for Figure 6-6 Hip and thigh exercises

1a.	Side leg lift	http://www.workoutz.com/exercise/outer_thigh_lift
2a.	Inner thigh lift	http://www.workoutz.com/exercise/inner_thigh_lift
3a.	Backward lunge	http://www.workoutz.com/exercise/reverse_lunge
3b.	Wall sit	http://tinyurl.com/ch6wallsit

Videos for Figure 6-7 Upper body exercises

1.	Push-ups	http://tinyurl.com/ch6pushups
2.	Dips	http://tinyurl.com/ch6dips
3.	Negative pull-ups	N/A
4.	Shoulder shrug	http://tinyurl.com/ch6shrug

Videos for Figure 6-8 Stability ball exercises

1.	Push-ups	http://tinyurl.com/ch6sbpu
2.	Knee tuck press	http://tinyurl.com/ch6sbtuck
3.	Shoulder roll-outs	http://tinyurl.com/ch6sbrollout
4.	Back wall squat	http://tinyurl.com/ch6sbsquat
5.	Ball transfer	http://tinyurl.com/ch6sbtransfer
6.	Prone knee tucks	http://tinyurl.com/ch6sbtuck
7.	Oblique curls	http://tinyurl.com/ch6sboblique
8.	Bridges	http://tinyurl.com/ch6sbbridges
9.	Back extension	http://tinyurl.com/ch6sbbackex
10.	Prone opposite arm and leg raise	http://tinyurl.com/ch6sboalr

Videos for Figure 6-9 Elastic resistance exercises

1.	Squats	http://tinyurl.com/ch6ressquat
2.	Leg extension	N/A
3.	Hamstring curl	N/A
4.	Side leg lift	http://tinyurl.com/ch6ressideleg
5.	Inner thigh lift	N/A
6.	Toe press	N/A
7.	Toe lifts	N/A
8.	Standing push-ups	http://tinyurl.com/ch6respushup
9.	Deltoid raise	http://tinyurl.com/ch6resdeltoid
10.	Lat pull	http://tinyurl.com/ch6latpull
11.	Rowing	http://tinyurl.com/ch6resrowing
12.	Biceps curl	http://tinyurl.com/ch6resbcurl
13.	Triceps extension	http://tinyurl.com/ch6restriceps

LAB Activity 6-1

Name _____ Class/Activity Section _____ Date _____

Weight Training Experience

Equipment Needed:

Weight training machines or free weights

Purpose

To experience a weight training program

Procedure

Read about resistance training in this chapter and review Figures 6-3 and 6-4, then select one of the weight training programs listed on the next two pages. Perform the exercises using a weight that you can lift 8 to 12 repetitions for one to two sets. As this is an introductory session, use light weights and concentrate on correct form, rhythm, and breathing. If you want to perform and compare the two types of programs, rest 1 day between workouts for best results. If assigned by your instructor, track your weight training program on the Resistance Training Log Online Lab Activity 6-6. This is a stand-alone lab with complete instructions and illustrations of the free weight exercises. You can tear out this lab and use the exercise descriptions on the back of the page. If using free weights, use a spotter, and follow all safety recommendations with both programs.

WEIGHT TRAINING EXERCISES

(Choose one program)

Machines	Weight	Repetitions	Free Weight	Weight	Repetitions
1. Leg press	_____	_____	1. Squats	_____	_____
2. Leg extension	_____	_____	2. Lunge	_____	_____
3. Hamstring curl	_____	_____	3. Calf raise	_____	_____
4. Toe press	_____	_____	4. Bench press	_____	_____
5. Bench press	_____	_____	5. Military press	_____	_____
6. Military press	_____	_____	6. Bent-over rowing	_____	_____
7. Lat pull	_____	_____	7. Back extension	_____	_____
8. Rowing	_____	_____	8. Triceps press	_____	_____
9. Back extension	_____	_____	9. Biceps curl	_____	_____
10. Abdominal curl	_____	_____			
11. Triceps press	_____	_____			
12. Biceps curl	_____	_____			

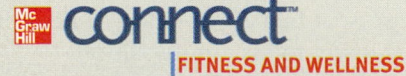

http://connect.mcgraw-hill.com

Results

1. What are three things you learned about weight training by doing this program?

2. If you tried both types of weight training, how did they compare? Which did you prefer and why?

3. What did you learn about your strength levels in different muscle groups?

Weight Training Exercises

1. Leg press
    Prime movers: quadriceps, hamstrings, and gluteus maximus
    On leg press, sit on seat, adjust position to last slot or to a 90-degree knee angle.
    Place feet squarely on pedals, press out smoothly (do not lock knees), and return to starting position.
2. Leg extension
    Prime movers: quadriceps
    Sit on bench with both feet under the rollers. Toe in slightly. Do not lie back.
    Extend your legs, hold 1 second, and return to starting position.
3. Hamstring curl
    Prime movers: hamstrings and gluteus maximus
    Lie face down on the bench, hook both heels under the rollers. Position knees at the pivot point where the rollers attach to the bench. Pull up to 90 degrees, hold for 1 second, and return to starting position.
4. Toe press
    Prime mover: gastrocnemius
    On leg press station, place feet squarely on pedals, press out to full leg extension without knee lockout. Press with toes from flat-footed position to foot extension and return.
5. Bench press
    Prime movers: pectorals and triceps
    Lie on bench, head next to the machine. The grips should be lined up approximately with the shoulders. Place your feet flat on the bench with knees bent and back flat. Press to extension and return. If you tend to have shoulder problems, lower the bar to only 4 inches above your chest, then extend.
6. Military press
    Prime movers: deltoids and triceps
    Sit on the stool or stand with abdominals tight, back flat, and knees slightly bent. With shoulders close to handles, extend upward with arms until they are straight but not locked and return.
7. Lat pull
    Prime movers: latissimus dorsi
    Grip bar directly above shoulders or at handles. Pull down until you are kneeling or sitting. From this position, pull down to chest and return.
8. Rowing
    Prime movers: rhomboids, latissimus dorsi, and biceps
    Sit on the machine with arms almost fully extended. Pull back as far as possible, drawing shoulder blades together. Return to starting position.
9. Back extension
    Prime movers: erector spinae, gluteus maximus, and quadratus lumborum
    Sit on the machine with back against upper back pad and feet under ankle rollers. Fasten hip belt if one is available to keep hips from lifting or sliding out of position. Slowly extend trunk back fully and slowly return to starting position.
10. Abdominal curl
    Prime movers: abdominals and hip flexors
    Sit with pad on upper chest, knees flexed, and feet on footpad. Use seat belt if provided to keep hips from lifting off seat. Flex trunk as far forward as possible. Return slowly to starting position.

11. Triceps press
     Prime movers: triceps
     Stand facing lat bar. With palms facing down, grasp the bar so that hands are shoulder width apart.
     Keep elbows at waist. Press down to extension and return.
12. Biceps curl
     Prime movers: biceps
     Stand facing the weights, hold bar with both hands, palms up. Flex arms until the bar meets shoulders.
     Return to starting position. Keep back straight, abdominals firm.

Free Weight Exercises

1. Squats
    Prime movers: gluteus maximus, quadriceps, and hamstrings
    Start standing upright with the bar resting on your shoulders. Keep the head up, abdominals tight, back
    flat, feet a bit wider than your shoulders. With back straight, slowly lower hips until tops of thighs are
    parallel with the floor. Pause. Drive up with legs and hips to the starting position.
2. Lunge
    Prime movers: gluteus maximus and quadriceps
    Standing upright with the bar on the shoulders off the neck, abdominals tight, back flat, step forward
    (or backward) until the front thigh is parallel with the floor. The front knee should be over the ball of
    the foot. Keeping back straight, take a controlled step back to the starting position. Repeat with the
    opposite leg. This exercise requires considerable balance. You may wish to start first with dumbbells
    and progress slowly to use of a barbell.
3. Calf raise
    Prime mover: gastrocnemius/soleus
    Place bar on shoulders, position balls of feet on board and heels off board. Press up onto balls of feet,
    then lower with control. Knees straight tones gastrocnemius, knees bent tones soleus.
4. Bench press
    Prime movers: pectorals and triceps
    Lie with head and buttocks on bench, feet stabilized on ground for balance and safety. Grip about 4
    inches wider than shoulders, palms under bar (pronated). Lower bar to chest. Focus eyes up to the sky;
    do not watch bar. Elbows should be directly under bar and forearms perpendicular to ground. Do not
    let bar slide to the neck. Press to extension, and return.
5. Military press
    Prime movers: deltoids and triceps
    Sit on bench or stand. With barbell on chest, press upward with arms until they are straight overhead
    but not locked, and return.
6. Bent-over rowing
    Prime movers: rhomboids and latissimus dorsi
    Stabilize one knee and hand on a bench; opposite hand holds the weight, and foot is flat on the floor.
    Pull elbow up and in toward the spine.
7. Back extension
    Prime movers: erector spinae, gluteus maximus, and quadratus lumborum
    Lie with your hips on the seat pad and ankles under the ankle rollers, arms crossed across chest.
    Slowly extend trunk to a horizontal position, hold 3 to 5 seconds, and slowly lower to starting
    position. After you can easily do 15–20 repititions, you may increase resistance by holding light hand
    weights to your chest.
8. Triceps press
    Prime movers: triceps
    Standing with abdominals firm, feet apart for stability, grip the weight, palms up, and keeping
    elbows near the ears, slowly lower bar behind the head. Pause, then press until elbows are fully
    extended.
9. Biceps curl
    Prime movers: biceps
    Grasp bar, palms up, holding bar about thigh level. Bend elbows, moving bar in an arc toward shoul-
    ders. Pause, and slowly return to starting position.

LAB Activity 6-2

Abdominal and Core Strengthening Workout

Equipment Needed:

Floor mat or carpeted surface
Stability ball

Procedure

These exercises are presented in Chapter 6, Figure 6-5. You can add or delete exercises depending on your goals. They should be performed at a slow, steady pace with equal effort in both directions. You can tear out this lab and use the exercise descriptions on the back of this page along with the illustrations in the back of the book.

ABDOMINAL AND CORE STRENGTHENING EXERCISES

Exercise	Repetitions
1. Bicycle exercise	_____
2. Abdominal crunch on stability ball	_____
3. Vertical leg crunch	_____
4. Reverse crunch	_____
5. Plank	_____
6. Side plank	_____
7. Long arm crunch	_____
8. Abdominal curl "crunch"	_____
9. Oblique abdominal curl	_____
10. Rear leg lift	_____
11. Glute squeeze	_____
12. Back extension	_____
13. Alternate arm/leg lift	_____

Results

1. What are three things you learned about abdominal and core strengthening by doing this program?

2. What did you learn about your muscular endurance levels in different muscle groups?

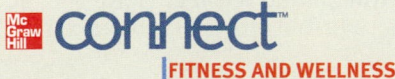

http://connect.mcgraw-hill.com

LAB Activity ■ **CHAPTER 6**

ABDOMINAL AND CORE STRENGTHENING EXERCISES

Exercise Instructions

1. Bicycle exercise
   Lie on your back with hands behind your head. Raise knees to a 45-degree angle and slowly do a bicycle pedal motion as in the figure. Touch right elbow to left knee, left elbow to right knee.
2. Abdominal curl "crunch" on stability ball
   Lie on stability ball with feet flat on floor, thighs and trunk parallel to floor. Cross arms behind shoulders or across chest, contract abdominals by raising trunk about 45 degrees. Spread feet apart for better balance. To work obliques more, bring feet closer together.
3. Vertical leg crunch
   Lie on your back with legs raised in the air, knees slightly bent and crossed at the ankles. Cross hands behind the shoulders to support the head. Keep chin lifted to prevent jerking the head. Lift the trunk and slowly lower.
4. Reverse crunch
   Lie on the back with ankles crossed, feet off the ground and knees about a 90-degree angle. Place arms on the floor beside your trunk. Press lower back to the ground, contract the abdominals, and rotate hips 1 to 2 inches. Your feet will lift slightly toward the ceiling each contraction.
5. Plank
   Lie face down propped with elbows under chest, palms down. Lift up on toes, tighten back and abdominals, keeping body straight, head and spine neutral. Hold 10–60 seconds, rest, repeat. If a straight-back position is too difficult, begin with hips hiked up, or hold the contraction a shorter amount of time. Do not let the hips sag.
6. Side plank
   Lie on side with weight balanced between forearm, flat palm, and feet. Contract back and abdominals to hold body straight. Do not push hips out behind the body. Hold 10–30 seconds, rest, repeat on the other side. If a full-body position is too difficult, begin with the half-plank balancing weight between knees and forearm. For an advanced version, try lifting the top foot in the air 5–10 seconds.
7. Long arm crunch
   Lie on your back with knees bent, heels next to buttocks. Extend arms alongside your ears, chin raised, eyes focused on ceiling. Contract abdominals, keeping lower back to floor, lift shoulders as for a basic crunch, lower slowly.
8. Abdominal curl "crunch"
   Lie on your back with knees bent, heels next to buttocks. Place hands across chest or behind shoulders. Keep eyes focused on ceiling, chin up and about a fist distance from your chest. Contract your abdominals, do not jerk your head forward as you curl. Keeping lower back on the ground, curl shoulders up 3 inches and slowly lower.
9. Oblique abdominal curls
   Lie on the back as for the basic crunch, but add a twist, bringing right elbow toward left knee, then left elbow toward right knee. Elbow does not have to touch knee.
10. Rear leg lift
    On hands and knees, hollow abdomen and round back to protect it. Extend right leg to the rear. Tense gluteus. Raise and lower leg slowly, six to eight counts. Repeat left.
11. Glute squeeze
    Lying on back with knees bent, squeeze gluteus hard, raising hips no more than 3 inches from floor. Do not arch back. Hold for a count of five, relax, repeat. This may also be done with legs extended, feet on stability ball, back on floor.
12. Back extension
    Lie on your stomach with feet on the floor, head neutral, hands touching shoulders. Slowly lift head, shoulders, and chest. Hold 5–10 seconds, slowly lower. Variation: Squeeze shoulder blades in toward spine while holding trunk lift.
13. Alternate arm/leg lift
    Lie on your stomach with arms extended in front. Raise right arm while lifting left leg. Hold 5–10 seconds. Repeat on other side. Keep head neutral.

Name _____ **Class/Activity Section** _____ **Date** _____

Stability Ball Workout

Equipment Needed:

Stability ball

Procedure

Read the stability ball section in Chapter 6 and review Figure 6-8. You can tear out this lab and use the exercise descriptions on the back of the page. Do these exercises slowly for best results.

STABILITY BALL EXERCISES

Exercise	Repetitions
1. Push-ups	_____
2. Knee tuck press	_____
3. Shoulder roll-outs from knees	_____
4. Back wall squat	_____
5. Ball transfer	_____
6. Prone knee tucks	_____
7. Oblique curls	_____
8. Bridges	_____
9. Back extension	_____
10. Prone opposite arm and leg raise	_____

Results

1. What are three things you learned about abdominal and core strengthening by doing this program?

2. What did you learn about your muscular endurance levels in different muscle groups?

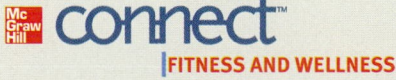

http://connect.mcgraw-hill.com

STABILITY BALL EXERCISES

Here are 10 exercises that you can do with a stability ball. They are illustrated in Figure 6-8.

1. Push-ups (pectorals, triceps)
    Kneel facing the ball. Roll forward to lie on top of the ball. Reach forward, placing your hands on the floor. Walk your hands out until the ball is under your thighs. Tighten your abdominals, keeping your body straight. Bend your elbows, and lower your upper body toward the floor. Your body should be straight from shoulders to ankles. Push back to the starting position. To increase difficulty, roll the ball back so only your shins or feet are resting on it.

2. Knee tuck press (deltoids, triceps)
    Kneel on the stability ball, and hands on the floor. Bend your elbows, and lower your upper body toward the floor. Push up from this position.

3. Shoulder roll-outs from knees (back extensors, rectus abdominis)
    Kneeling on the floor, place hands on the stability ball. Roll it forward and back, keeping back straight and abdominals tight.

4. Back wall squat (quadriceps, gluteus maximus, hamstrings)
    Stand and press the ball against a wall with your back. Position feet shoulder width apart and forward as if you are going to sit in a chair. Bend your knees, rolling the ball down until your knees are at a 90-degree angle and your thighs are parallel to the floor. Keeping your back pressed against the ball, hold for five counts. Straighten your knees and return to the starting position.

5. Ball transfer (rectus abdominis)
    Lie on your back with hands resting on the floor and grip ball between your ankles. Curl the pelvis to lift the ball off the floor into the air, reach up, and transfer it to your hands, then back to ankles. Return to starting position.

6. Prone knee tucks (rectus abdominis)
    Place shins on the stability ball and hands on the floor. Roll the ball back away from your hands, keeping shoulders aligned with hands, abdominals tight, body straight. Extend legs, then bend knees in toward your chest and roll the ball forward until your knees are at your chest. To increase difficulty, try from a bent elbow position on the floor.

7. Oblique curls (rectus abdominis, external and internal oblique abdominals)
    Lie with the top of the ball beneath the center of your back, feet spread wide on the floor for stability. Rotate hips to one side, and slowly curl the right side of the upper body toward the left leg. Return to starting position; repeat, alternating sides.

8. Bridges (back extensors, gluteus maximus, hamstrings)
    Lie on your back with legs on the ball, hands resting beside you on the floor. Slowly lift hips until your back is straight and weight is on your upper back. Pause, then return slowly to the starting position. Avoid pressing the neck into the floor or arching the back. To make it easier, place ball under knees. To make it harder, place under heels.

9. Back extension (back extensors)
    Lie prone with hips on the ball, feet on the floor, and trunk slightly flexed. Arms may be at your side or behind shoulders. Tighten your upper back, slowly raising shoulders until the spine is straight or slightly extended. Keep head neutral to avoid neck hyperextension. Hold, relax slowly to starting position. Repeat.

10. Prone opposite arm/leg raise (back extensors, gluteus maximus, hamstrings, deltoids)
    Lying prone on the ball, extend right leg behind you, foot touching floor. Keep head neutral. Reach in front with the left arm, raising it close to your ear. Lift the arm and leg slowly at the same time, pause as you reach extension, then lower slowly. Repeat, alternating sides.

Name _____ **Class/Activity Section** _____ **Date** _____

Elastic Band Workout

Equipment Needed:

Elastic bands

Purpose

To experience a strength-training workout with elastic bands

Procedure

Read the "Elastic Resistance" section and then perform the exercises shown in Figure 6-9 for 8 to 12 repetitions for one to two sets. As this is an introductory session, concentrate on correct form, rhythm, and breathing. You can tear out this lab and use the exercise descriptions on the back of the page. Also see the illustrations of these exercises on the back cover of this text. If assigned by your instructor, track your program on the Resistance Training Log.

ELASTIC BAND EXERCISES

Exercise	Repetitions	Exercise	Repetitions
1. Squats	_____	8. Standing push-ups	_____
2. Leg extension	_____	9. Deltoid raise	_____
3. Hamstring curl	_____	10. Lat pull	_____
4. Side leg lift	_____	11. Rowing	_____
5. Inner thigh lift	_____	12. Biceps curl	_____
6. Toe press	_____	13. Triceps extension	_____
7. Toe lifts	_____		

Results

1. What are three things you learned about resistance training with elastic bands by doing this program?

2. What did you learn about your strength levels in different muscle groups?

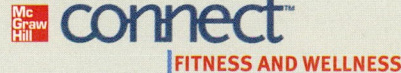

McGraw Hill **connect™** **FITNESS AND WELLNESS**   http://connect.mcgraw-hill.com

Elastic Resistance Exercises

1. Squats (gluteus maximus, quadriceps, hamstrings, biceps)
   Step on the band with feet about shoulder width apart and hold ends of the band low enough to feel moderate tension. Slowly squat until hips are just above knees, bending elbows to maintain tension in the band. Return to standing.

2. Leg extension (quadriceps)
   Tie band around ankles. Lie back, knees bent and feet on floor. Keeping knees and thighs together, straighten knee, lifting the foot as high as possible. Release slowly and repeat. Change legs.

3. Hamstring curl (hamstrings, gluteus maximus)
   Place the band around ankles. Lie face down with arms under the chin or hands under hips. Bending knee, slowly lift one foot. Release slowly, maintaining some tension in the band. Repeat. Change legs.

4. Side leg lift (hip abductors)
   Place the band around both legs—around ankles is hardest, around knees easiest. Lying on right side, torso supported by arms, slightly bend lower leg for support. Keep hips facing forward, lift upper leg. Lower, keeping tension on the band, and repeat. Change sides.

5. Inner thigh lift (thigh adductors)
   Place band around left arch and right ankle. Lie on right side with trunk supported by arms. Lift bottom leg slowly, hold briefly, lower slowly, repeat. Switch sides.

6. Toe press (gastrocnemius, soleus)
   Holding ends of band, place around ball of foot. With knee straight, slowly press through ball of foot from extension to flexion and back (gastrocnemius). To emphasize soleus, repeat with knee slightly bent. Change sides.

7. Toe lifts (tibialis anterior)
   Tie band around arches. Place heels about 6 inches apart forward to back. Keeping one foot pointed, pull toes of the other foot back toward your face. Relax. Repeat on both feet.

8. Standing push-ups
   Wrap the band around your back and under your arms. Bend elbows and grasp ends of band. Extend arms forward, return slowly.

9. Deltoid raise (deltoid and triceps)
   Place one end of band under foot, hold the other end by your hip. Standing with good posture, lift arm to shoulder level, lower slowly. Change sides.

10. Lat pull (latissimus dorsi)
    Hold band overhead with one arm, elbow extended but not locked. Pull other end of band to shoulder level bringing elbows to your side. Be careful not to get hair caught in band.

11. Rowing (rhomboids)
    With band around arches and knees extended, grasp band about mid-shin. Pull elbows back and try to bring shoulder blades together. Release slowly.

12. Biceps curl (biceps)
    Place one end of band under foot, grasp other end low, and, keeping elbow at your side, curl right arm to shoulder. Slowly release. Change sides.

13. Triceps extension (triceps)
    Standing with good posture, grasp ends of band. Press lower hand toward hip, pause, slowly release. Change sides.

LAB Activity 6-5

Partner Resistance Workout

Equipment Needed:

Floor mat or carpeted surface
Partner
Towel or broomstick

Procedure

These exercises are presented in Chapter 6, Figure 6-10. You can add or delete exercises depending on your goals. They should be performed at a slow, steady pace with equal effort in both directions. Perform 6–8 repetitions or about 1 minute of each exercise. You can tear out this lab and follow the exercise descriptions on the back of the page.

PARTNER RESISTANCE EXERCISES

Exercise	Repetitions or time
1. Leg extension	_____
2. Hamstring curl	_____
3. Inner/outer thigh press	_____
4. Foot flexion	_____
5. Overhead press	_____
6. Lat pull	_____
7. Elbow press forward	_____
8. Elbow press backward	_____
9. Biceps curl	_____

Results

1. What are three things you learned about abdominal and core strengthening by doing this program?

2. What did you learn about your muscular fitness levels in different muscle groups?

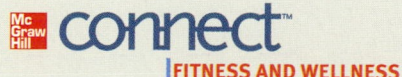

http://connect.mcgraw-hill.com

1. Leg extension (quadriceps)
    Sit on a bench or chair. Move one leg from flexion to full extension and back as partner resists by pressing on front of lower leg.

2. Hamstring curl (hamstrings, gluteus)
    Lie face down while partner straddles your back and places a hand on each ankle. Bend knees and curl calves toward buttocks as your partner resists. Continue the resistance as you return to the starting position.

3. Inner/outer thigh press (thigh adductors and abductors)
    Sit, facing each other, legs forward, hands behind hips for balance. One partner places both feet inside the other's feet and presses outward as the other partner resists by pressing inward. Switch positions after six to eight reps.

4. Foot flexion (anterior tibialis)
    Sit with legs extended. Partner kneels and presses down on top of both feet as you flex them and then return to extension.

5. Overhead press (deltoids, triceps)
    Sit with hands at shoulder level, palms up. As partner resists, press up toward ceiling and then return to starting position.

6. Lat pull (latissimus dorsi)
    Sit and reach high overhead to grasp partner's hands. As partner resists, pull down to shoulder level and slowly return to starting position.

7. Elbow press forward (pectorals)
    Sit with elbows out and hands touching shoulders. As partner resists at the elbows, pull them in toward your midline and return to starting position.

8. Elbow press backward (rhomboids)
    Sit with elbows out or with arms crossed. Partner sits behind, pressing on your elbows as you press back, pulling shoulder blades together. As partner continues resistance, return to starting position.

9. Biceps curl (biceps)
    Stand, palms facing upward. Partner resists on your palms as you curl arm from extension to flexion and back. This may also be done holding a towel in one hand in front of body. Partner sits or kneels facing you, resisting on other end of towel as you curl your arm.

CHAPTER 7

Exploring Special Exercise Considerations

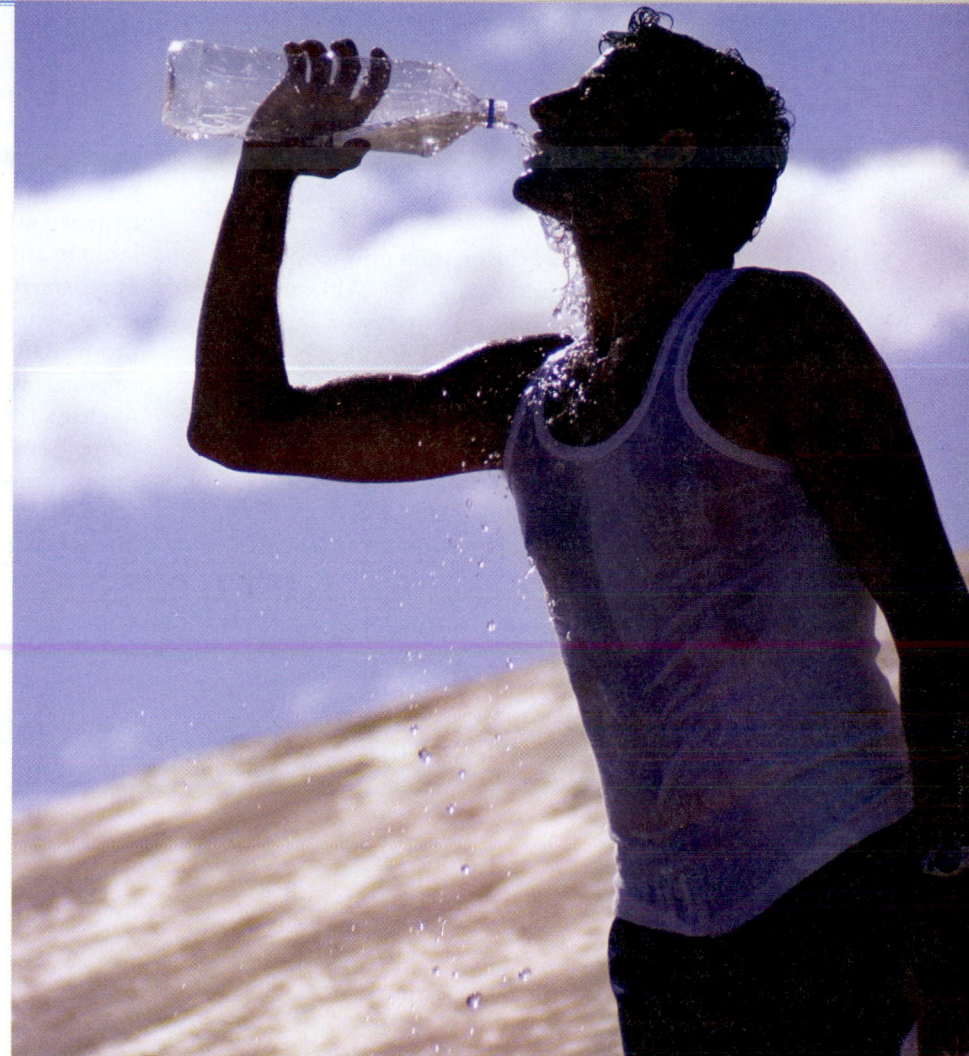

STUDY QUESTIONS

You will have successfully mastered this chapter if you can answer the following:

1. What are the physiological differences in men's and women's exercise performance levels?

2. What are the similarities in men's and women's responses to exercise?

3. What are the recommendations for exercise during pregnancy and postpartum?

4. What is exercise addiction?

5. How does exercise affect disease resistance?

6. What are the recommendations for exercising safely in hot and cold weather?

7. What are the best replacement fluids to prevent dehydration during exercise in hot weather?

8. What drugs affect physical performance? How do they do so?

9. What are the effects of a regular program of exercise on the aging process?

10. What are the recommendations for exercise for individuals with chronic health conditions such as arthritis, asthma, diabetes, hypertension, and osteoporosis?

You will find the answers as you read this chapter.

> " *Obstacles are those frightful things you see when you take your eye off the goal.* "
> —Hannah More, English author

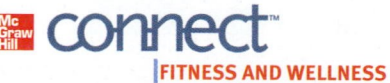

FITNESS AND WELLNESS

http://connect.mcgraw-hill.com

This chapter brings together several concerns related to exercise participation. Nine major areas are addressed: similarities and differences in men's and women's exercise performance, females and exercise, males and exercise, exercise addiction, exercise and disease resistance, environmental considerations, drugs that affect physical performance, aging and physical activity, and exercise and chronic health conditions. With increased knowledge of these special exercise considerations you will have a greater understanding of how to participate in and enjoy physical exercise throughout your life span. Be motivated to do so by these words: "Don't wait for your ship to come in. Row out to meet it."

◆ SIMILARITIES AND DIFFERENCES IN MEN'S AND WOMEN'S EXERCISE PERFORMANCE

While performance levels may differ, men and women respond to exercise in a similar manner. Although women have approximately 20 percent lower maximal oxygen uptake than men (due to smaller heart size), with exercise they show similar rates of improvement. Performance levels differ for several reasons.

✓ *Strength:* Due to hormonal changes during puberty, a woman adds fat because of estrogen, while a man's muscle mass doubles because of testosterone. In fact, women have half as much or more muscle to move their weight and more inactive fat weight to carry. Due to men's greater muscle mass, men are about 50 percent stronger than women. See "The Numbers" later in this chapter.

✓ *Performance and endurance:* Physically the male heart and lungs are larger than those of the female. The larger male heart and lungs produce higher stroke volumes and vital capacities than those of females. Men also have more **hemoglobin** (the oxygen-carrying component in red blood cells) in their arterial blood than do women. Both the larger heart size and more oxygen in the blood result in greater car-

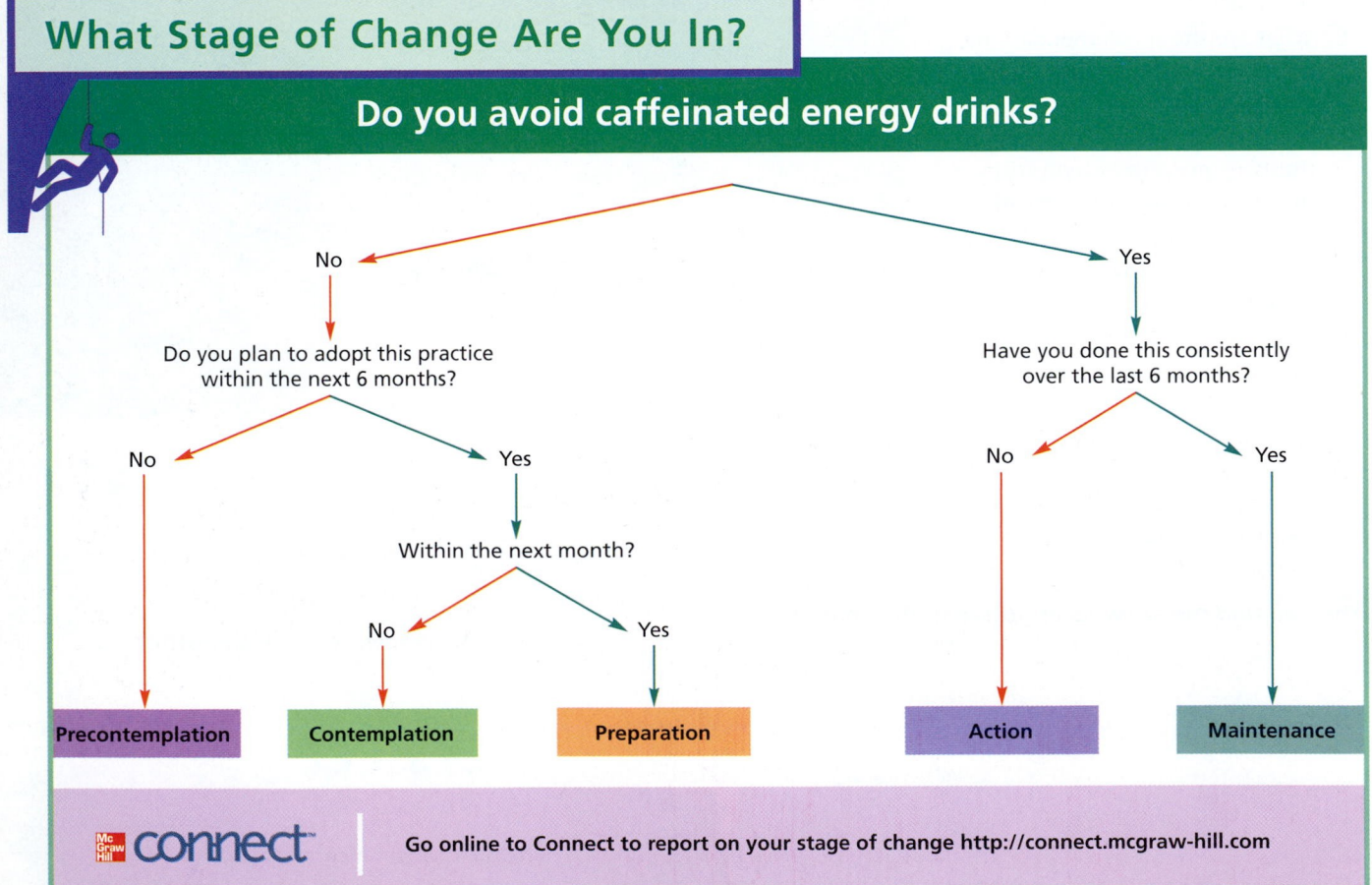

What Stage of Change Are You In?

Do you avoid caffeinated energy drinks?

- No
  - Do you plan to adopt this practice within the next 6 months?
    - No → **Precontemplation**
    - Yes
      - Within the next month?
        - No → **Contemplation**
        - Yes → **Preparation**
- Yes
  - Have you done this consistently over the last 6 months?
    - No → **Action**
    - Yes → **Maintenance**

Go online to Connect to report on your stage of change http://connect.mcgraw-hill.com

diac output and greater maximal oxygen uptake. Women have less bone mass than men, but their pelvic structure is wider. This gives men an advantage in running efficiency. In total, these factors give males advantages in terms of performance and endurance.

✓ *Heat tolerance:* Women have a higher body temperature at rest, fewer sweat glands, lower sweat production, and a propensity to start sweating at higher temperatures than do men. A woman's greater amount of adipose tissue (fat) serves as insulation and inhibits heat dissipation. The implication of these differences is that women have less tolerance to heat than do men, but women adapt to heat just as well as men. Regardless of gender, individuals with a greater level of fitness generally better tolerate and more readily adapt to heat stress than do those who are less fit.

Even though women are at a disadvantage in terms of physical performance, they benefit equally from aerobic exercise in terms of fitness improvement. Training effect benefits such as loss of fat from deposit areas, increased bone density, and decreased exercise heart rates are similar for men and women. When differences in body size are taken into account, fitness gains for men and women are *essentially* the same.

Some women fear that exercise will make them develop large or bulky muscles or a masculine appearance. This is not likely unless a woman is using anabolic steroids and spending many hours doing extremely strenuous weight training. A person's potential for muscular development is genetically determined by levels of the sex hormone testosterone, and women have only one-tenth as much of this hormone as men. While women, like men, vary in their potential for muscular size development, what most women want from exercise is exactly what they will gain: decreased fat, increased lean body tissue, and firmer, toned muscles.

◆ FEMALES AND EXERCISE

Once the sight of a female training on the road or competing in a race was sufficiently unusual that people would stop and stare. As late as 1965 women were threatened with banishment from international competition if they ran races longer than 1.5 miles, and it was 1984 before the first women's Olympic marathon took place. As the interest in fitness as a lifestyle has grown, so has the number of women participants in aerobic activities and athletics. Now that large numbers of females have adopted a physically active lifestyle, research has provided us with new information about topics of special interest to women.

Menstruation

Is it safe to exercise during menstruation? Yes. Menstruation is only one small part of the ongoing female reproductive cycle. In the past women sometimes used this as an excuse to avoid exercise, but now women are encouraged to follow a normal routine during all parts of the reproductive cycle. Research indicates that physical activity has little or no effect on the average woman's menstrual cycle. Accordingly, no restriction should be placed on the physical activity level of the average woman at any phase of her cycle. The way women experience menstruation varies greatly. Most feel no different than usual; some may experience abdominal and leg cramps, backache, or mood swings, particularly during the first 2 days of the menstrual flow.

Dysmenorrhea, or painful menstruation, is probably neither caused nor cured by exercise. However, there is some evidence that enhanced fitness leads to a reduction in menstrual complaints, although this is still being researched. Some studies indicate that exercise decreases mood swings and relieves depression, anxiety, and irritability. Excess

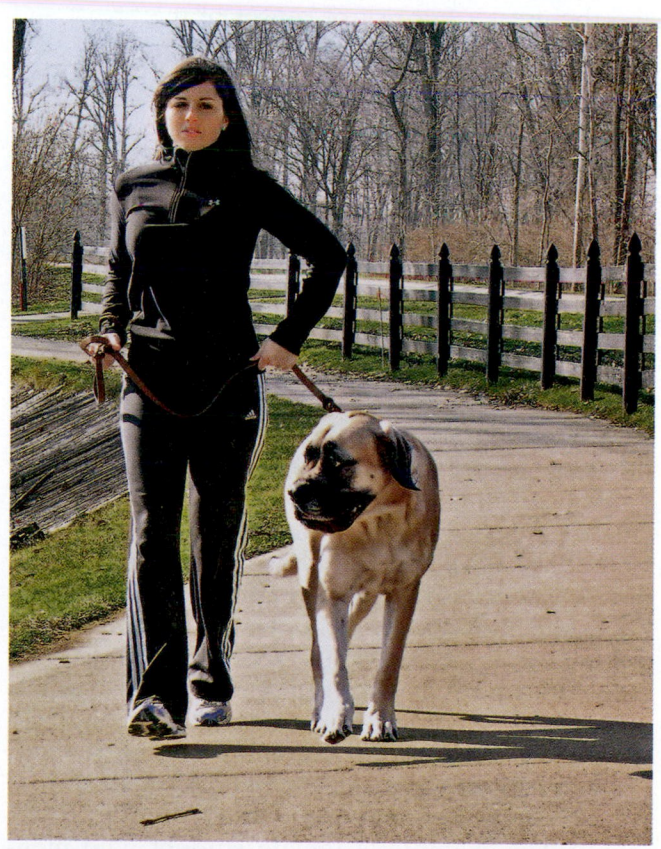

More women are discovering how enjoyable physical activity can be.

body water lost through perspiration can reduce weight gain due to water retention, relieving premenstrual bloating and edema. While no specific exercises cure severe cramps, participation in a program of regular exercise has been shown to decrease the frequency of minor menstrual cramps. This is perhaps due to increased abdominal tone, increased circulation to the uterus, or increased levels of natural pain-relieving endorphins.

Menstruation should be treated as a normal physiological function, not an illness. As long as she is comfortable, a woman should continue her regular exercise program. For women who want to look and feel their best, exercise is beneficial at any time of the month.

Studies indicate that young girls who exercise vigorously may experience a delay in **menarche,** the start of the menstrual cycle, decreasing their risk of cancer later in life. While the average American girl experiences menarche between ages 11 and 12, those who train vigorously experience the first menstrual cycle at an average age of 15½, the same as the average age for menarche 100 years ago. This delay may be natural and even desirable because it reduces the body's lifetime exposure to **estrogen,** a female sex hormone. The more menstrual cycles a woman has over her lifetime, the longer her exposure to estrogen and the greater her risk of cancer of the breast and reproductive organs. In addition, women who exercise tend to be leaner, thus producing less potent estrogen. In one study, women who had been athletic in high school and college compared with sedentary women had half the incidence of breast and reproductive cancer in later life. A sedentary lifestyle is considered a primary risk factor for cancer.

Menstrual abnormalities such as **oligomenorrhea** (infrequent or irregular menses) and **amenorrhea** (absent menses) occur in about 2 to 5 percent of the general population of women and in up to 28 percent of women athletes. In athletes, the prevalence appears high in sports that require greater intensity, frequency, and duration of training (e.g., distance running and swimming) or sports that emphasize low body weight or involve competition by weight class (e.g., dance, gymnastics, boxing, wrestling). Numerous factors, physiological and psychological, including change in diet or inadequate diet and physical and emotional stress, may affect menstruation abnormally (for example, stressors such as heavy athletic training and competition acting synergistically with other stressors in life). In athletes, the vast majority of cases of amenorrhea stem from an imbalance between activity level and nutritional intake. For example, a female student who menstruates during her off-season may lose her periods once preseason training begins because of increases in her activity level without corresponding increases

THINK ABOUT IT

Energy drinks (Monster Hitman, Energy Shooter, Full Throttle, 5-Hour Energy, Rockstar Energy Shot, etc.) have risen in popularity recently. Loaded with caffeine and guarana, they promise to boost energy, enhance performance, and keep you awake. Spend some time in your local supermarket reading the labels of several different energy drinks, and make a note of unfamiliar ingredients. Do these energy drinks seem likely to provide any benefits to your health or psychological well-being? Are there any potential dangers? What are arguments for and against consuming these drinks?

Go online to Connect to complete this activity. http://connect.mcgraw-hill.com

in her nutritional intake. Her body can't sustain all its functions without adequate calories and nutrition, and reproduction mechanisms are the first to shut down.

Exercise-induced oligomenorrhea and amenorrhea are rare in women doing moderate amounts of exercise as part of a fitness program. They are more common among those whose menstrual cycles started late, past age 15, or who had a history of irregularity before starting exercise programs. Although no specific body fat percentage has been associated with the development of exercise-induced amenorrhea, the evidence suggests that decreased fat levels may lead to decreased production of one form of estrogen. Thus, as fat percentages decrease, estrogen levels decline, and the evidence of amenorrhea increases. Some scientists have suggested that the critical body fat level may be as low as 13 percent or that there may be no such critical level. If such a critical fat percentage does exist, it probably varies widely from individual to individual.

The focus of research is on how all the factors mentioned here may affect the hypothalamus, thereby influencing the production of important regulatory hormones relative to menstruation and metabolism, including estrogen, epinephrine, and corticoids. Whatever the cause, exercise-induced amenorrhea is considered reversible. Normal menstrual cycles resume with as minor a change in lifestyle as a 10 percent decrease in exercise, improved nutrition, or a weight gain of 4 to 5 pounds. Also, exercise-induced amenorrhea does not seem to affect long-term fertility. While a woman with amenorrhea does not experience a regular menstrual cycle, she may still ovulate

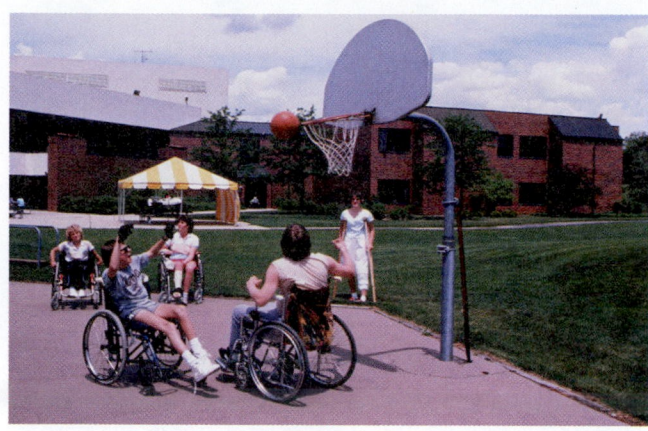

Everybody benefits from physical activity.

and become pregnant. She should not rely on this for birth control and should continue her regular birth control method if pregnancy is not desired. Any active woman should be aware of her normal menstrual cycle and should discuss any irregularities with her physician to rule out conditions such as thyroid disorders, ovarian cysts, brain tumors, and pregnancy.

Female Athlete Triad

Some female athletes and other physically active women who are underweight and nonmenstruating are being diagnosed as victims of the **female athlete triad.** This is a life-threatening syndrome marked by three disorders:

- ✓ Disordered eating habits (inadequate food, energy intake insufficient to meet metabolic demands)
- ✓ Amenorrhea (for more than 3 months)
- ✓ Osteoporosis

Sports can be a win-win activity for young women. Research shows that exercise builds strong bones, helps control weight, and improves mood. It also reduces the risk of developing serious illnesses such as heart disease and breast cancer. But it also comes with risks such as female athlete triad.

Societal pressure on females to have an unrealistically low body weight fuels this condition. Fitness professionals who work with physically active females should learn ways to prevent, recognize, treat, and reduce its risks.

The problem has caught the attention of the International Olympic Committee Medical Commission, which recently developed a consensus statement on the dangers and possible treatments, and the National Collegiate Athletic Association, which published a coach's handbook on the topic.

The female athlete triad is not limited to college or elite athletes. It occurs in high school and middle school girls as well as other women who are physically active. Any woman, even one in her forties, who has disordered eating and becomes amenorrheic will lose bone. A woman who has been amenorrheic for several years can have the bones of a 70- or 80-year-old woman.

Bone loss also can occur in men who have eating disorders. Those at risk are athletes in sports in which body weight is important, such as running, wrestling, and ski jumping. There is no triad for men at this time.

The problem begins when women do not consume enough calories for their activity levels; their energy deficits may disrupt their menstrual cycles. Estrogen, which is critical for preserving bone, drops to the level of postmenopausal women. At the same time, inadequate nutrition leads to other hormonal changes that inhibit the ability to build bone. With restrictive dieting, women often limit calcium-rich dairy products and other important nutrients for bone health. Such behaviors are especially harmful during the teen years up until about age 21 because women at those ages are still building bone.

No one knows how long women can go without menstruating before they experience bone loss, but going 3 months without a period is considered extremely dangerous. The exception is when the pause is recommended and supervised by a physician. The weakened skeletons of athletes (or other physically active women) can lead to fractures, especially in the legs, hips, and pelvis.

Amenorrhea can often be reversed with an increase in calories or a decrease in physical activity. Bone density does increase with a resumption in normal estrogen levels, but it does not appear to recover fully. Active young women who have not been menstruating regularly should have a bone-mineral density test, discuss low-dose estrogen replacement therapy with a physician, and consume a calcium intake of 1,500 mg/day (about 5 cups of milk). See the Top 10 list "Who's at Risk for Osteoporosis?"

Pregnancy

Is exercise advisable during pregnancy? How much? What are the benefits? Are there limitations or cautions to keep in mind? Are some exercises better than others?

Pregnancy is a natural and normal physiological function, not an illness. A pregnant woman is not fragile. Although she should always discuss her exercise plan with her physician, evidence keeps rolling in that exercise is more than just okay for a pregnant woman—it is good for both her and her baby and the benefits far outweigh the risks. In fact, a recent study revealed that most women (approximately two-thirds) are doing some sort of exercise during pregnancy. General advice for a healthy woman having an uncomplicated pregnancy is to perform some sort of physical activity most, if not all, days of the week,

TOP 10 LIST

Who's at Risk for Osteoporosis?

Although no one is immune to osteoporosis, the following factors increase one's risk:

1. Female
2. Postmenopausal
3. Amenorrheic
4. Small-boned
5. Eating a diet low in calcium and vitamin D
6. Alcohol, tobacco, and caffeine use
7. Eating a diet high in protein
8. A sedentary lifestyle and/or getting only low-impact exercise
9. Medications (including both oral and inhaled steroids for asthma)
10. A family history of osteoporosis

Note: Some vegetarian diets also increase the risk.

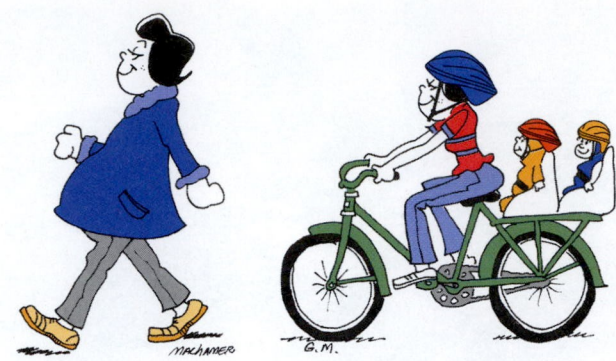

Exercise during and after pregnancy has many advantages.

or to continue her regular exercise program, unless symptoms indicate otherwise. The old recommendation from the American College of Obstetricians and Gynecologists (ACOG) that strenuous activities should not exceed 15 minutes in duration and the infamous advice that maternal heart rate should not exceed 140 bpm has been completely discredited by newer research. Now women are encouraged to limit their exercise routines based solely on *maternal symptoms* and *rate of perceived exertion*. However, if a pregnant woman notices any of the warning signs for discontinuing exercise (Table 7-2), she should contact her physician immediately.

Physical activity is encouraged, but precautions should be heeded. Pregnant women should be counseled not to undertake excessive physical activity in a hot climate to which they are not acclimated. A gradual weight gain, which is natural and desirable, is likely to increase stress to joints, ligaments, and muscles. Also, muscles and connective tissues become more lax as they gradually undergo hormonal changes. Increases in the pregnancy hormone relaxin help facilitate the baby's birth but make the pregnant woman more susceptible to strains and sprains. Therefore, during late pregnancy and the early postdelivery period, vigorous increases in flexibility should not be pursued.

Due to increasing weight and joint flexibility as the pregnancy progresses, impact activities may become uncomfortable. At this time, many women switch to low- or no-impact exercises such as walking, swimming, and stationary cycling. Some women continue their normal exercise program to the day of

delivery with no ill effects, but don't feel guilty if you feel a need to cut back. Toward the end of pregnancy, if you fatigue easily and exercise seems to require more effort, it is natural to decrease the activity level. After the first trimester it is not advised to do exercises that require lying on your back (i.e., supine position). This position can block the blood supply to the uterus (by compressing the aorta and/or the vena cava), resulting in depression of the fetal heart rate.

One of the most frequent questions pregnant women ask is, "Can I lift weights?" Experts do not recommend beginning a power-lifting routine during pregnancy, but there is no evidence that general resistance training causes any harm. Decreased resistance and shorter sets may be advised to reduce undue fatigue. Of most concern are breath-holding Valsalva maneuvers, which should be avoided, pregnant or not, and balancing issues, which may occur with heavy barbells. Resistance bands and weight machines should be used instead.

Throughout pregnancy, a woman needs to listen to her body and adjust her exercise level to maintain comfort. Specific pregnancy exercise guidelines from the American College of Obstetricians and Gynecologists are listed in Table 7-1. Also review Table 7-2.

Exercise is important during pregnancy for many reasons. The physiological changes of pregnancy place a great demand on the body. Labor and delivery are perhaps the most physically demanding events a woman will experience. Exercise can maintain optimal fitness, enabling a woman to control weight gain, improve muscle tone, improve posture, decrease backache, and decrease constipation. Exercise can also aid in increasing energy, increasing psychological well-being, managing stress, enhancing sleep at night, and regaining a prepregnancy figure.

While fitness is no guarantee of a quick labor or an easy delivery, endurance and increased capacity to deal with the physical stress of childbirth are assets that come from fitness. A fit mother can enjoy a quicker recovery from childbirth and can regain her normal fitness and activity levels in less time than can the unfit.

TABLE 7-1	*ACOG Guidelines for Exercise During Pregnancy and Postpartum*

1. Enjoy physical activity on most, if not all, days of the week.
2. No exercise should be performed while in a supine position after the first trimester. This slows blood flow back to the heart and decreases its output. Also, avoid *motionless standing,* which may decrease heart output.
3. Avoid activities with a high risk of falling because of a changing center of gravity (i.e., gymnastics, horseback riding, downhill skiing, high-impact sports, etc.) or those with a high potential for impact of abdominal trauma.
4. Previously inactive women or those with medical or obstetric complications should be evaluated before an exercise program begins.
5. Women with a history or risk for pre-term labor or fetal growth restriction should reduce physical activity in the second and third trimesters.
6. Take steps to avoid a heat injury. Avoid exercise in hot, humid weather or when you have a fever.
7. Avoid extremes of barometric pressure. Avoid scuba diving and exercising at altitudes of more than 6,000 feet.
8. Ballistic movements (jerky, bouncy motions) should be avoided. Exercise should be done on a wooden floor or a tightly carpeted surface to reduce shock and provide a sure footing.
9. Deep flexion or extension of joints should be avoided because of connective tissue laxity. Activities that require jumping, jarring motions, or rapid changes in direction should be performed with caution because of joint instability and high risk of injury.
10. Always warm up and cool down. This can be accomplished by slow walking or stationary cycling with low resistance.
11. Use the "talk test" or RPE to gauge exercise intensity. Slow down if you cannot comfortably maintain a conversation or if RPE is too extreme.
12. Care should be taken to rise gradually from the floor to avoid a sudden drop in blood pressure. Some form of activity involving the legs should be continued for a brief period.
13. Exercises that employ the Valsalva maneuver should be avoided.
14. Caloric intake should be adequate to meet not only the extra energy needs of pregnancy but also those of the exercise performed.
15. Liquids should be taken liberally before and after exercise to prevent dehydration. If necessary, activity should be interrupted to replenish fluids.
16. Women who have led sedentary lifestyles should begin with physical activity of low intensity and advance activity levels gradually.
17. Activity should be stopped and the physician consulted if any unusual symptoms appear. (See Table 7-2.)

TABLE 7-2	*Reasons to Discontinue Exercise and Seek Medical Advice During Pregnancy*

1. Vaginal bleeding.
2. Leakage of amniotic fluid.
3. Sudden swelling of the ankles, hands, or face.
4. Persistent, severe headaches and/or visual disturbance; unexplained spell of faintness or dizziness.
5. Swelling, pain, and redness in the calf of one leg (phlebitis).
6. Elevation of pulse rate or blood pressure that persists after exercise.
7. Excessive fatigue, palpitations, chest pain.
8. Persistent contractions (more than six to eight per hour) that may suggest onset of premature labor.
9. Unexplained abdominal pain.
10. Insufficient weight gain during the last two trimesters.
11. Decreased fetal movement.

STRESS INCONTINENCE

Stress incontinence, an involuntary leakage of urine when you laugh, cough, sneeze, or exercise, is a common problem, particularly in women over 30 who have given birth. During pregnancy and birth, these muscles become weakened and stretched. One solution is to wear a sanitary pad, but a better approach is to strengthen the perineal muscles that control this function. The pelvic floor is a hammocklike muscle layer attached at the front and back of the pelvis. It supports the pelvic organs, including the bladder, uterus, and rectum. Kegel exercises, named after the Los Angeles physician who developed them, strengthen the pelvic floor muscles and may prevent or cure stress incontinence. As a side benefit, many women report increased pleasure during intercourse.

KEGEL EXERCISE

Kegel exercises are done by contracting the perineal muscles, which surround the bladder neck and vagina. To learn the exercise, when urinating stop and start the flow. Hold the contraction for 3 to 4 seconds during the stop phase. The muscle action you take to do this when urinating is the action you must take when doing Kegel exercises. You can do these exercises anytime—contract hard and then release. Do 10 in a row, and work up to five sets of 10 daily. Do these exercises before, during, and after pregnancy.

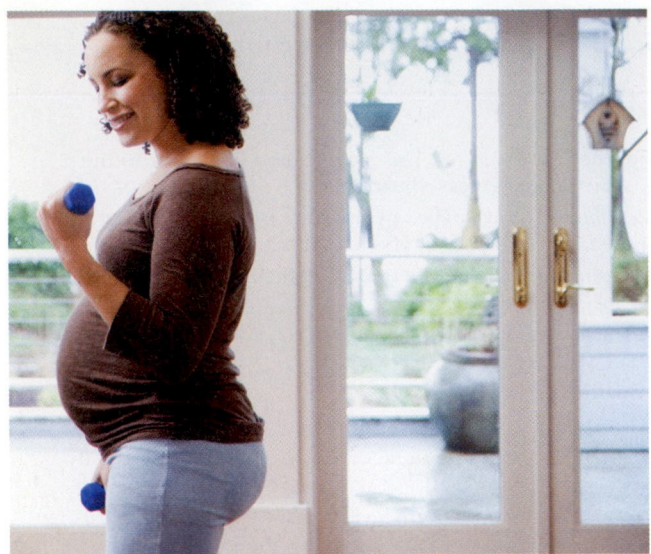

Exercise keeps both mother and baby healthy, but always get the workout approved by your health care provider. No exercise should be performed while lying on the back after the first trimester.

POSTPARTUM: GETTING BACK INTO SHAPE

Giving birth and coping with the demands of a new baby are both joyful and stressful for a new mother. The main problem in resuming exercise is not fatigue or shortness of breath, which might be expected, but finding someone to watch the baby while the mother takes a well-deserved break. Postpartum recovery times vary greatly. If the delivery has been normal, walking is encouraged in the hospital the day after delivery. This can be continued when the woman returns home. Rest, good nutrition, and a progressive walking program will make recovery faster than will complete inactivity or resuming prepregnancy activity levels too soon. You should not rush into impact activities such as jogging or pursue flexibility increases until you have given loosened joints (due to the hormone relaxin) a chance to recover—6 to 16 weeks. Abdominal curls are important for toning overstretched abdominal muscles and preventing back problems. Also, do Kegel exercises to strengthen pelvic floor muscles.

A nursing mother needs to avoid fatigue and dehydration, which may reduce milk production. Drink fluids liberally, and nap when the baby does to ensure adequate rest. Wear a good supportive bra, with pads to absorb leaks, and nurse before exercise for greater comfort. There is no conflict between nursing a baby and doing moderate exercise. Both help a mother regain her prepregnancy figure.

BREAST SUPPORT

Does bouncing cause breasts to sag? Some believe that breast movement stretches the skin and ligaments that support the breasts. There is no evidence to support this claim; the main culprits are genetics and pregnancy. Still, a good bra makes exercise more comfortable by reducing breast movement during activity. The best designs flatten breasts to redistribute their mass across the chest wall. This results in less mass for gravity to affect. Racerback and crossback straps prevent slippage off the shoulder. Certain designs are more suited to small-breasted women, while others are more comfortable for large-breasted exercisers. A woman should try different styles to decide what is best for her. A good exercise bra should (1) limit breast movement, (2) have wide straps that do not slip off the shoulders, (3) have a wide band at the bottom to prevent the bra from riding up, (4) have no rough seams or uncovered fasteners to prevent chafing, and (5) be made of nonabrasive materials and be seamless or at least have seams that do not cross the nipple area.

◆ MALES AND EXERCISE

Participation in sports and physical activities no longer ends with graduation from high school or college. Large numbers of men are continuing or beginning lifetime exercise programs.

Exercise appears to lower the hormonal levels of males as it does that of females. In one study, testosterone levels of men who ran 40 miles a week averaged 30 percent less than the levels of nonexercisers. The runners' levels were still in a normal range, and the effect was reversible. Sperm count and libido were not affected. While it may lower hormonal levels, overtraining is not associated with decreased fertility in male athletes unless it is accompanied by anorexic behavior and a high-stress lifestyle.

A more common male fertility problem results from constantly wearing tight undershorts. For the testicles to maintain normal sperm production, they must be a few degrees cooler than normal body temperature. Their position outside and slightly away from the body accomplishes this. When the testicles are overheated by consistently being held close to the body, sperm production temporarily decreases. A switch to boxer shorts solves the problem.

Male bicyclists have additional concerns. Males who ride for extended periods (i.e., 2 to 3 hours or more) have an increased risk of reduced perineal (crotch) area circulation. It is caused by compression of the bike saddle. This can lead to pain; numbness; and, in severe cases, male impotence. Females are not exempt from this problem. Reduced perineal circulation in females may result in sexual and urinary tract dysfunction. Male bicyclists traveling over rough terrain may also experience pain and injury to the testicles. The following tips will help avoid these problems:

- ✓ Level the seat or point the nose downward to reduce pressure on the perineum.
- ✓ Lower the seat so that the legs support more weight. (Knees should bend slightly at the bottom of the pedal stroke.)
- ✓ Avoid handlebar extensions because they place more body weight on the nose of the seat.
- ✓ Stand up and pedal every 10 minutes to encourage blood flow in the perineum.
- ✓ Rise out of the seat when going over bumps.
- ✓ Avoid crush injuries involving the top tube by riding a bike of proper size. The top tube of a mountain bike should be 3 to 4 inches below the crotch when one is standing over it; for road bikes, clearance should be 1 to 2 inches.
- ✓ Consider replacing a narrow racing-style saddle with a wider seat or a seat designed to reduce compression on the perineum. Special "male" seats are available.
- ✓ Switch to a recumbent bike.

◆ EXERCISE ADDICTION

Exercising is unconditionally great for the body, the soul, and the mind, right? Almost, but not quite. Even the most benign or beneficial elements can cause harm when taken to an extreme. Although exercise is highly recommended for health and vigor, it is not protected from this universal truth. When a commitment to exercise crosses the line to dependency and compulsion, it can create physical, social, and psychological havoc for those involved.

A "positive addiction" can be a healthy adaptation to the barriers to exercise in life because commitments to work, family, and other healthy pursuits must compete with time to work out. Sometimes the line between commitment and compulsion is crossed. There can be a negative side to exercise that gradually, insidiously takes over from the positive. Other addictions, such as compulsive gambling and compulsive shopping and substance abuse, are discussed in Chapter 14.

Exercise addiction is not just another term for overtraining syndrome. Healthy athletes training for peak performance and competition can experience overtraining symptoms, the short-term result of too little rest and recovery. **Exercise addiction,** in contrast, is a chronic loss of perspective of the role of exercise in a full life. A healthy athlete and an exercise addict may share similar levels of training volume. The difference is in the attitude and the consequences. An addicted individual isn't able to see value in unrelated activities and pursues the activity even when it is against his or her best interest.

The exercise addict has lost balance, allowing exercise to become overvalued compared to elements widely recognized as giving meaning to a full life (e.g., school, work, friends, family, community involvement). When emotional connections are passed up in favor of additional hours of training; when injury, illness, and fatigue don't stop a workout; when all free time is consumed by training—*exercise addiction* is the diagnosis. Withdrawal symptoms such as anxiety, irritability, and depression, which appear when circumstances prevent exercise, are the warning signs of addiction.

To the addict, there is no exception to the rule "the more, the better." Anything that interferes with the quest for more exercise is resented.

The paradox inherent in exercise addiction is the blurred boundary between what is healthy, admirable, and desirable and behavior that is over the edge and dependent. The addict answers poor performance with more exercise and less rest. A healthy athlete looks at the big picture and adjusts training programs, allowing for rest and recovery among the training variables.

Remember that working out should always have an element of play. If exercising loses all aspects of fun, something has gone wrong. The most competitive athletes still love their sport. They love it because it gives pleasure, not because it has become a compulsive need. Take the self-assessment in Table 7-3 to see if you are losing your perspective on exercise.

TABLE 7-3	Are You Addicted to Exercise?

Directions: Rate yourself as honestly as you can on the following checklist.

Yes	No	
____	____	1. I have missed important social obligations and family events in order to exercise.
____	____	2. I have given up other interests, including time with friends, to make more time to exercise.
____	____	3. Missing a workout makes me irritable and depressed.
____	____	4. I feel content only when I am exercising or within the hour after exercising.
____	____	5. I like exercise better than sex, good food, or a movie—there's almost nothing I'd rather do.
____	____	6. I work out even if I'm sick, injured, or exhausted. I feel better when I get moving.
____	____	7. In addition to my regular exercise schedule, I exercise more if I find extra time.
____	____	8. Family and friends have told me I'm too involved in exercise.
____	____	9. I have a history (or family history) of anxiety or depression.

Scoring: If you checked yes on three or more of the statements, you may be losing your perspective on exercise.

◆ EXERCISE AND DISEASE RESISTANCE

During exercise, 75 to 85 percent of the energy produced is released in the form of heat, producing an increase in body temperature. Much of this heat is dissipated at the skin, but body temperature still is elevated during exercise. This regular increase in body temperature, it is speculated, is inhospitable to some viruses and might decrease the incidence of viral infections in exercisers. Moderate exercise has also been found to boost the immune system. However, overtraining leading to exhaustion might weaken the system and increase susceptibility to colds and minor infections. Studies on the relationship between the immune system and physical exercise have produced contradictory results. Non-exercisers who start a new program of intense exercise, exceeding their individual exercise limits, or who exercise sporadically may experience weakened immunity for a brief period. Highly trained athletes may weaken their immune systems with acute, exhaustive exercise. Of course, psychological and emotional stress may play important roles here too—whether it be the anxiety felt by the new, out-of-shape exerciser or by the athlete competing for a championship. Few people exercise so strenuously that they need to worry about any possible adverse effects on immunity. The problem for most Americans is too little exercise rather than too much. For anyone in doubt, a consistent and regular program of moderate exercise is a key component of overall health and well-being, including the immune system. However, the optimal level of exercise for each individual's immune system is unknown. See the "Immune System Function" section in Chapter 4.

Should you exercise when you have a cold or feel ill? Many professionals recommend that you decrease the intensity and frequency of workouts or take some days off when you have a cold or feel one coming on. Illness affects lung and heart function as well as skeletal muscles. As a result, performance may be reduced. Some people find that exercising when they have a mild cold makes them feel better. Illnesses vary in severity and people react differently to them, so listen to your body. If you have only a minor head cold and otherwise feel fine, it is probably acceptable to work out. Avoid exercise to the point of exhaustion. Avoid exercise if you have the flu, have a fever, feel achy, feel extremely tired, are heavily congested, or have swollen glands. Exercise does not cure illness. The old adage that "you can sweat out a cold" with exercise is untrue. When you recover from illness, do not start exercising at the same level as before. Give yourself a few days to build back to normal levels.

◆ ENVIRONMENTAL CONSIDERATIONS

Exercising in the Cold

Your friends think you're crazy for sharing a narrow roadway with cars that spray you with slush as you exercise on a chilly winter day. Walking, running, and cycling are more complicated in the winter. Still, there is something liberating about a good workout on an icy winter day. Cold-weather workouts can be invigorating, comfortable, and safe if you follow these tips:

1. *Layer clothing:* Dress in several thin layers so that you can remove or add a layer as needed. Wool and polypropylene clothing wick moisture away from the skin to keep you dry. The outer layer of clothing should be breathable and windproof.

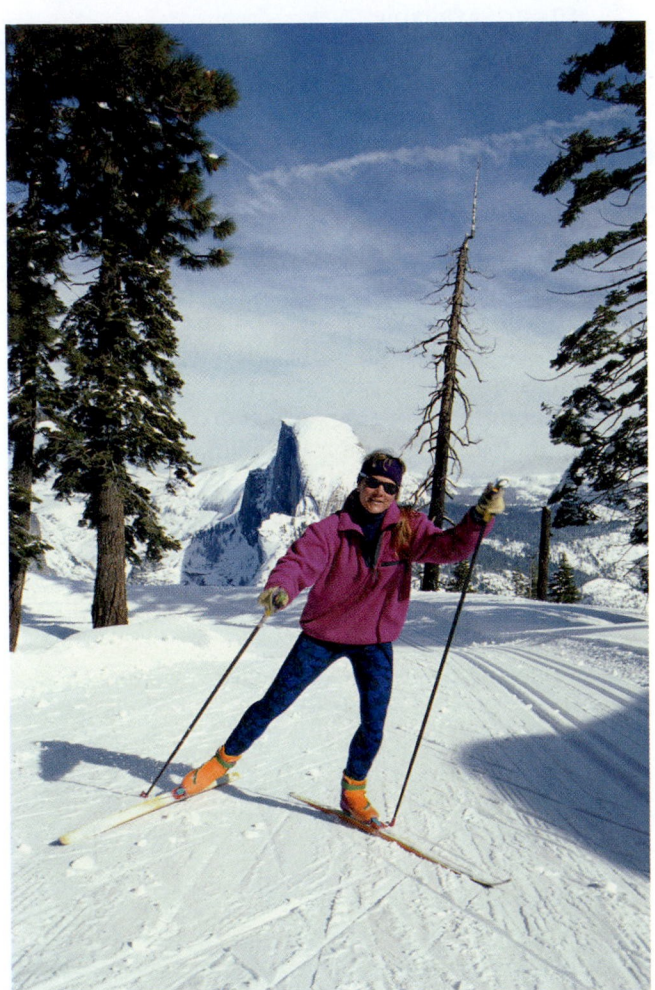

There is no possibility that you will freeze your lungs or throat. The air is warmed as it passes through your mouth and throat. Wear a mask or scarf over your nose and mouth if the cold air bothers you.

2. *Avoid overheating:* Don't overdress or you'll overheat. You should feel a little cool until you warm up. Check weather conditions on the Internet or on the TV weather channel. Do take the windchill factor into account when preparing for a workout (Figure 7-1).

3. *Avoid overexposure:* There is a possibility of frostbite if you don't dress properly. Frostbite can occur on outer body areas such as the fingers and toes when your skin temperature drops below 32°F. Frostbite can easily be avoided by covering exposed areas and by getting inside and warming up if any body parts feel numb or tingly. **Hypothermia** is a life-threatening condition in which body temperature drops to a dangerously low level. Medical attention should be sought immediately.

4. *Protect exposed parts:* Fingers and toes receive the smallest blood supply and experience winter's chill fastest. Mittens are more effective than gloves, which allow cold air to circulate around the fingers. On extremely cold days you may need to wear two pairs of socks or a thermal insole to keep your feet from getting too cold. Exposed ears or face can lead to windburn or chapping. To avoid discomfort, wear a hat and spread a thin layer of petroleum jelly on exposed skin areas.

5. *Work with the wind:* Plan out-and-back workouts, heading into the wind on the way

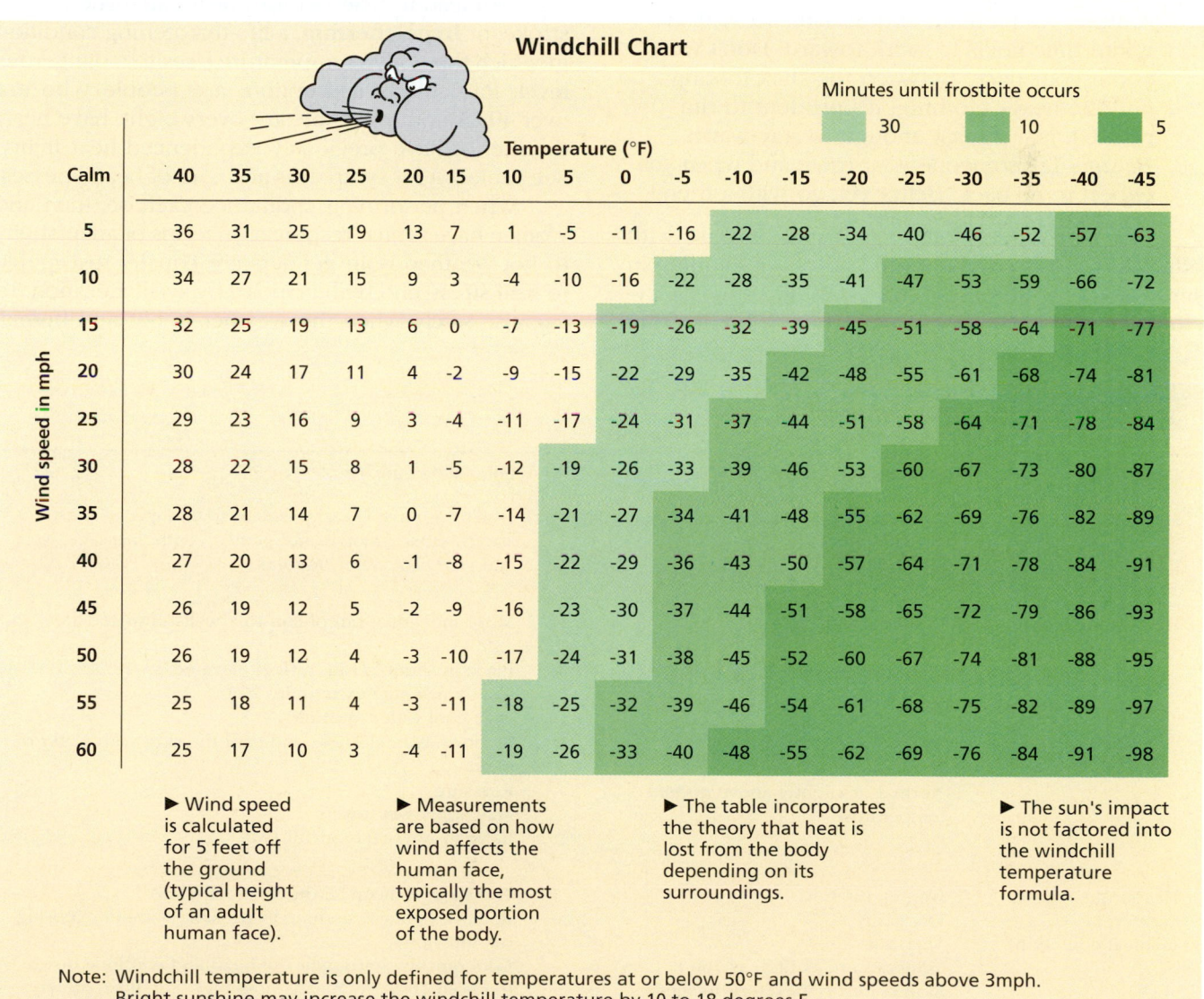

FIGURE 7-1   Windchill chart.

SOURCE: National Weather Service.

out so that you can return with the wind to your back. Not only will you appreciate the push when you're tired, you'll be less likely to be chilled by your sweat during the return.

6. *Exercise with caution:* Winter weather changes the safety rules for outdoor exercise: Fewer daylight hours, icy roads, and snowy nights lower visibility for drivers. Exercise at midday as often as possible. Avoid high-volume traffic areas, wear bright clothing, and be prepared for potential hazards by remaining alert. Wear waffled or ridged shoe soles to provide extra traction on icy roads.

7. *Stay motivated:* Winter exercising demands greater personal motivation than exercising at any other time of the year. Winter holidays, less daylight, and poor weather can disrupt a routine. To maintain enthusiasm, set realistic wintertime goals to work toward. Don't worry about your pace. Between the slick footing and the heavy clothing, it's prudent to run relaxed. Just go fast enough to stay warm.

8. *Be safe:* Tell someone your route and when you expect to be back. Better yet, go with a friend.

Don't hesitate to mix your usual exercise with other activities—cross-country skiing or sledding in snow country, aerobics, stair climbing, indoor cycling, or water exercise if you crave a break from the cold. Your heart will benefit as long as you stay in your training zone, and the cross training will work new muscle groups.

Exercising in the Heat

Given a couple of weeks and plenty of water, the human body can adapt well to exercising in the heat. Hot weather workouts make the body work harder than it does in cool weather. The heart must pump enough blood to not only fuel working muscles but also carry heat to the skin to be dissipated, reducing work capacity. Drinking plenty of cold fluids is critical to maintain sweating, your body's air-conditioning system. The body can acclimatize to heat but not to dehydration. Overexertion in hot weather, particularly when coupled with dehydration, can lead to heat cramps; heat exhaustion; heatstroke; or **hyperthermia,** a life-threatening condition in which the body's temperature rises to a dangerous level. Particularly susceptible are people who are over 40, are out of shape, are overweight, have heart disease, or have previously experienced heat injury. See Table 7-4 for symptoms and care of heat illnesses.

When performing endurance exercise, men and women have similar responses in terms of adaptability to hot weather. Both genders are equally susceptible to heat stress, and both respond by acclimatization. To exercise safely when the weather is hot and humid,

TABLE 7-4	*Heat Illnesses*	
Condition	**Symptoms**	**Immediate Care**
Heat cramps	Painful muscle spasms (calf is common) Sweaty skin Normal body temperature	Isolate cramps: Direct pressure to cramp and release, stretch muscle slowly and gently, gentle massage, ice, and give cool water or colas
Heat exhaustion	Profuse sweating Cold, clammy skin Flulike symptoms Dizziness Weak, rapid pulse Shallow breathing Headache Normal or slightly above normal temperature	Move individual out of sun to a well-ventilated area Place in shock position (feet elevated 12–18°) Gently massage extremities Give cool water to drink Remove extra clothing and cool the skin with water or a fan Reassure May apply wet towels Refer to physician or call EMS
Heatstroke (this is an extreme medical condition)	No perspiration Dry skin Very hot Temperature as high as 106°F Skin color bright red or flushed (African American—ashen) Rapid strong pulse Unresponsiveness (may be confused, stagger, or be agitated)	Transport to hospital quickly (call EMS) Remove as much clothing as possible without exposing the individual Cool quickly, starting at the head and continue down the body (use any means possible—fan, hose down, pack in ice) Wrap in cold, wet sheets for transport Treat for shock (place in a semireclining positon)

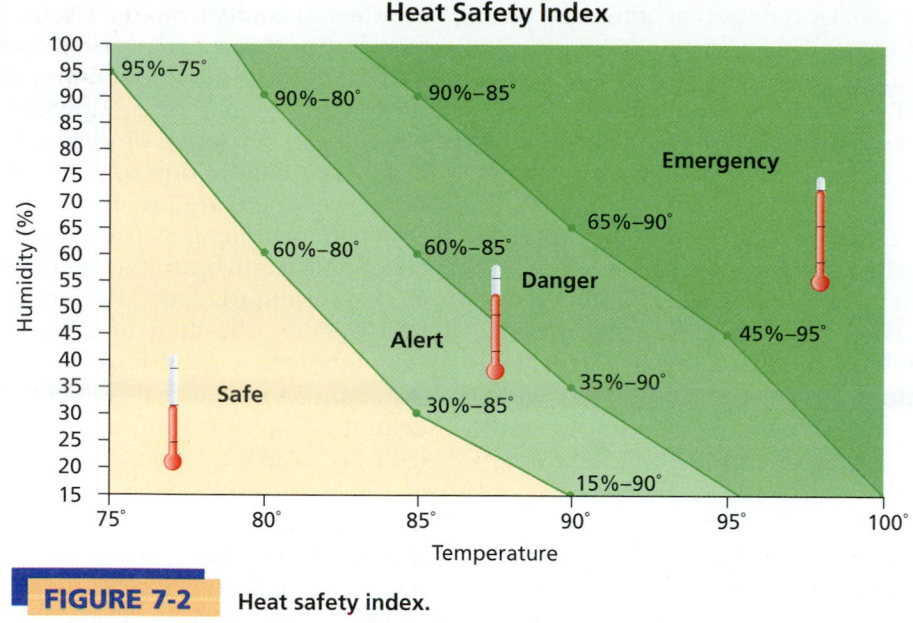

FIGURE 7-2   Heat safety index.

SOURCE: Ball State University Weather Station, Department of Geography.

follow the Top 10 "Guidelines for Hot Weather Exercise" and postpone the workout when the heat safety index is in the danger zone or above (Figure 7-2).

TOP 10 LIST

Guidelines for Hot Weather Exercise

1. Respect the heat. Hot, humid, sunny weather can be deadly.
2. Monitor weather conditions before exercising and adjust your workout accordingly. Postpone exercise when the heat safety index is in the danger zone or above.
3. Drink plenty of fluids to avoid dehydration (see Figure 7-3).
4. Weigh yourself before and after a workout. A sudden loss of weight may signal dehydration.
5. Wear loose-fitting clothing that allows air to circulate and expose as much skin to the air as possible to promote sweat evaporation.
6. Wear light colors because they reflect rather than absorb sunlight.
7. When acclimating to warmer weather in the spring, decrease exercise intensity and duration. Allow 2 weeks to acclimate to normal exercise levels.
8. Check with your doctor about the effects of any medications you take because some can reduce heat tolerance.
9. Do not wear vinyl or rubber sweat suits to lose body weight. They can lead to dehydration and death.
10. Stop exercising at the first sign of heat illness. See Table 7-4.

HEAVY SWEATING DURING EXERCISE

One of the hazards of exercising in hot, humid weather is dehydration caused by excessive loss of body water in the form of sweat. Overheating while exercising indoors at any time of the year can be as dangerous as outdoor exercise due to low levels of air movement. Sweat cannot evaporate effectively, and this may result in a heat illness. Dehydration disturbs cellular fluid and electrolyte balance, thus interfering with muscular contraction. Water losses of as little as 2 to 3 percent of body weight have been shown to impair exercise performance, reduce the amount of time a person can exercise, reduce cardiac stroke volume (volume of blood pumped out with each heartbeat), and reduce cardiac output (the amount of blood pumped by the heart over time). Water loss can also interfere with the body's ability to regulate internal temperature, resulting in overheating, which can be deadly.

Sweat is primarily water, but a number of major **electrolytes** (essential minerals in the form of salts) and other nutrients may be found in varying amounts. Sodium, chloride, and potassium are the predominant electrolytes found in sweat. They help maintain normal body fluid volume and are involved in nerve impulse transmission and muscle contraction (this includes the heart muscle).

ELECTROLYTE REPLACEMENT

Is profuse sweating likely to create an electrolyte deficiency? No. That is not likely to occur even during prolonged exercise, such as marathon running. This is not to say that electrolyte replacement is not important and that electrolyte deficiency is impossible. After prolonged exercise with heavy sweating, the body's stores of electrolytes are diminished and could eventually become deficient. However, with a normal diet, it is difficult to create an electrolyte deficiency.

Salt tablets are not recommended to replace lost sodium and chloride because these electrolytes are abundant in a normal diet. Tablets may be prescribed for those who cannot replace them through normal dietary means. Keep in mind that diets high in sodium have been associated with high blood pressure. Citrus fruits, fruit juices, and bananas are foods recommended for electrolyte replacement.

FLUID REPLACEMENT: WATER OR SPORTS DRINKS?

Rehydration (replacing body fluid volume) is critical to safe, effective exercise involving heavy sweating indoors or outdoors. For years we were told that water is the best drink to replace fluids, because that is mainly what you lose when you sweat during a hard workout. But science is dynamic, and conventional wisdom sometimes becomes history in the light of new discoveries. Water is still considered one of the most effective ways to rehydrate and works fine for the fitness exerciser and those exercising for *less than 1 hour.* Also, water is convenient and free. New information concerning exercise of *1 hour or more* now gives the slight edge in fluid replacement to electrolyte-containing beverages such as the popular sports drinks. This is the case because fluids containing electrolytes are more readily retained in the body's tissues. Why? Because plain water tends to increase urination slightly so that fewer fluids remain in the body's tissues. Also, when fluids taste good (as sports drinks do), they are more readily consumed. Thus the intake is increased. Due to these new findings, many commercial beverages have been produced to help in the process of rehydrating the body. These drinks are commonly known as carbohydrate-electrolyte replacement solutions (CES) or sports drinks. Other than water, the major ingredients in these solutions are carbohydrates in the form of glucose and/or sucrose and some of the major electrolytes. The glucose/sucrose content varies with the different brands, ranging from 1 percent to more than 10 percent. Studies show that sports drinks containing carbohydrates boost endurance and energy, as well as help delay fatigue during exercise. Select a sports drink carefully. Drinks with high carbohydrate concentrations are slow to empty from the stomach, interfering with rehydration, and can cause bloating and nausea. Avoid sports drinks containing carbohydrate concentrations higher than 8 percent (4 to 8 percent works best). Experiment during training to find out if you can handle one of these drinks. You should drink early and frequently during your workouts. Don't do anything new for competitive events. If you are a competitive athlete or marathoner or if you are exercising for several hours at a time in hot humid weather, the fluid of choice for most effective rehydration or prevention of dehydration is a sports drink (not to exceed 8 percent carbohydrate concentration). Water is the next best fluid, followed by fruit juices diluted with 50 percent water. All three are preferable to caffeinated sodas. Caffeine promotes urination, and the carbonation gives you a feeling of being fuller than you are. This information, which gives sports drinks a slight edge in terms of rehydration, does not mean that drinking water is not a good way to replace lost fluids.

Whatever you drink, drink it cold. Cold drinks are better than warm ones because they help cool down the core temperature of the body and empty from the stomach faster. Athletes/exercisers drink substantially more when fluids are cold. See the Fluid Pyramid in Figure 7-3 for fluid replacement guidelines.

Water: Are Americans Dehydrated?

Probably not. New research has reexamined the old question of how much water we should consume daily. Until recently it was believed that most Americans were dehydrated and in danger of all kinds of health problems because of that. Is there anyone on the planet who has not heard of the longtime standard health rule "drink at least eight 8-ounce glasses of water every day"? That's 64 ounces! Where did that advice originate? Is this the recommendation today?

The "8 × 8 rule" originated from a 1945 Food and Nutrition Board report recommending 1 milliliter of water for every calorie consumed, averaging eight cups for a 2,000-calorie diet. The medical community at the time bought into that report, and the notion that the body needs at least eight 8-ounce glasses of water a day became a firmly established rule.

Later research found no evidence to support the notion that it is mandatory to consume eight 8-ounce glasses of water. Water is essential, and 64 ounces is fine. However, most people can stay perfectly healthy with six or perhaps even three glasses of fluids a day, depending on how active they are, how hot it is, what the altitude is, and

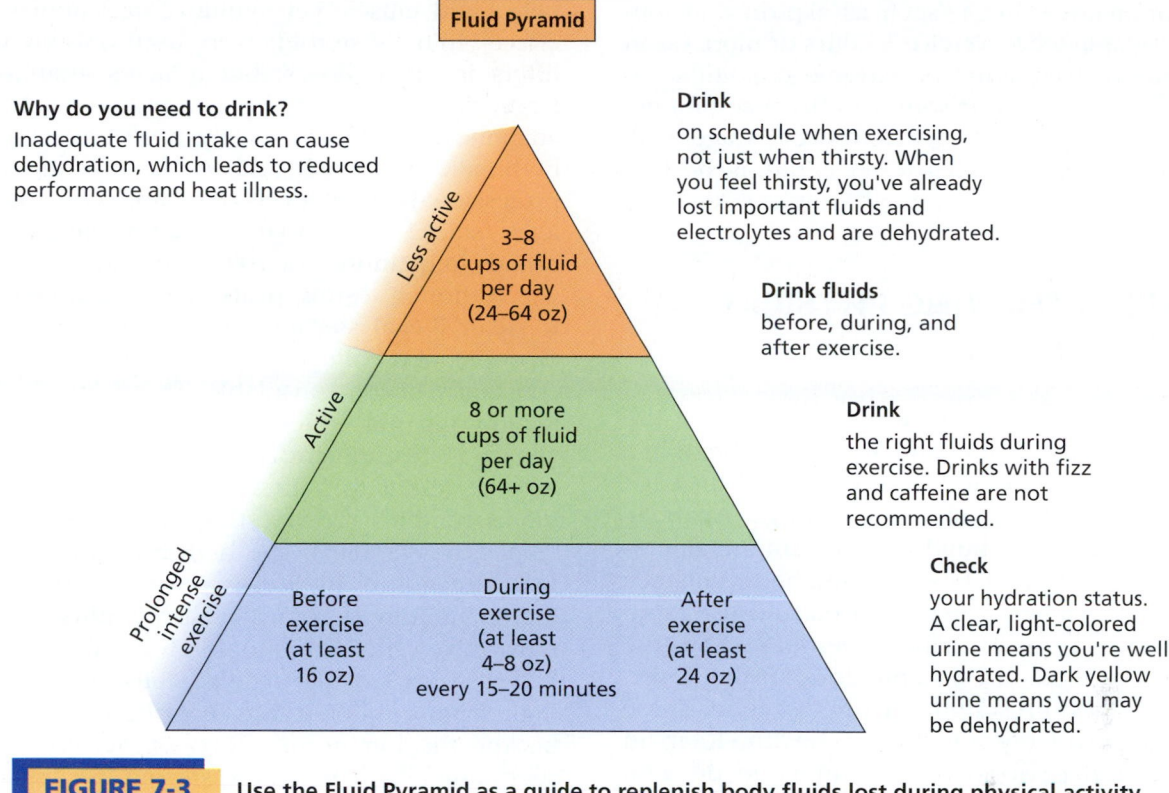

Fluid Pyramid

Why do you need to drink?
Inadequate fluid intake can cause dehydration, which leads to reduced performance and heat illness.

Less active

Active

Prolonged intense exercise

3–8 cups of fluid per day (24–64 oz)

8 or more cups of fluid per day (64+ oz)

Before exercise (at least 16 oz)

During exercise (at least 4–8 oz) every 15–20 minutes

After exercise (at least 24 oz)

Drink
on schedule when exercising, not just when thirsty. When you feel thirsty, you've already lost important fluids and electrolytes and are dehydrated.

Drink fluids
before, during, and after exercise.

Drink
the right fluids during exercise. Drinks with fizz and caffeine are not recommended.

Check
your hydration status. A clear, light-colored urine means you're well hydrated. Dark yellow urine means you may be dehydrated.

FIGURE 7-3   Use the Fluid Pyramid as a guide to replenish body fluids lost during physical activity.

what else they are consuming (see Figure 7-3). Body size also enters into the picture. Larger people need more fluids than do smaller ones.

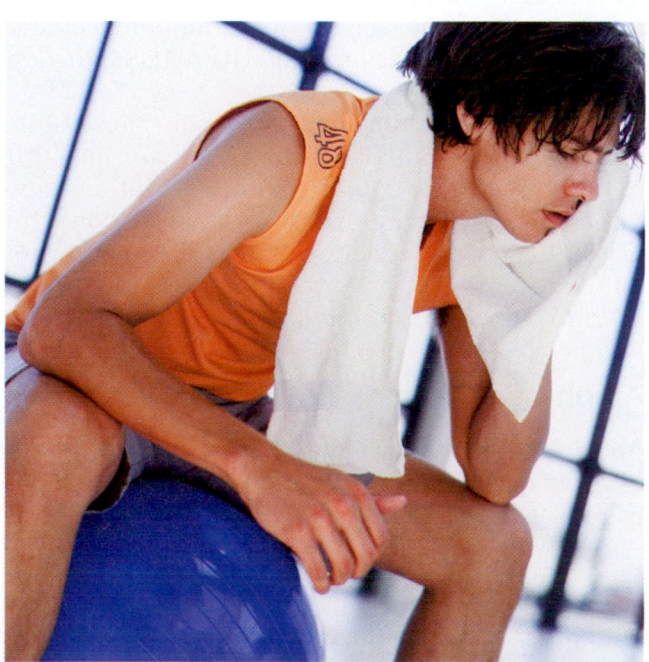

Weigh before and after exercise and finish within 2 percent of your starting weight.

The body is very good at regulating fluid balance, and thirst is generally a reliable indicator of water needs. Under normal circumstances there is no reason to tote a water bottle around all day. When you are exercising strenuously or doing hard physical work, especially of long duration and in hot weather or in high altitudes, you should make an effort to drink even if you don't feel thirsty.

Does the water in other beverages and foods (such as fruits and soup) count toward meeting the body's total fluid requirement? Yes. Milk, soup, fruits, and vegetables consist almost entirely of water, so they count. Even meat has some water. Caffeinated beverages such as coffee, tea, and cola tend to promote urination, but they also count, in part, as fluid intake.

Do not lose sight of the fact that while water is a vital component of good health (every organ and body function depends on it), it is not magic. Plain old tap water is fine, and it's convenient and free.

Note: Though uncommon, it is possible to drink too much water. When your kidneys are unable to excrete the excess water, the electrolyte content of the blood is diluted, resulting in a condition called **hyponatremia** (low sodium levels in the blood) or water intoxication. Hyponatremia risk is higher among females, exercisers using non-steroid anti-inflammatory drugs (such as aspirin and ibuprofen), people who exercise 3 hours or more (as in marathons or triathlons) in extreme conditions or high altitudes, and exercisers who because of a genetic condition produce very salty sweat. In general, though, drinking too much water is rare in healthy adults who consume an average American diet.

◆ DRUGS AFFECTING PHYSICAL PERFORMANCE

In the world of competitive athletics, where the margin between winning and losing may be only a fraction of a second, athletes looking for an edge are tempted by legal and illegal drugs. Anabolic steroids are taken to build muscle. Amphetamines may be taken to mask fatigue, caffeine to enhance performance. Diuretics may be used to cause rapid weight loss or to mask anabolic steroid use. See the material in Chapter 14 on ephedrine in the "Over-the-Counter and Prescription Drugs" section. These drugs can adversely affect your health. Keep in mind physical performance has more to do with skill and hard work than with popping a pill, injecting a drug, or drinking a superdrink.

Anabolic Steroids

Anabolic steroids are an artificial form of the male hormone testosterone. These drugs function like testosterone to produce increases in weight, strength, endurance, and aggressiveness. Steroids were first developed in the 1930s to build body tissues and prevent the breakdown of tissue that occurs in some diseases. In the 1950s, a few foreign countries experimented with giving testosterone to their male and female athletes. Because those athletes dominated many international competitions, a U.S. doctor developed a form of anabolic steroid that could

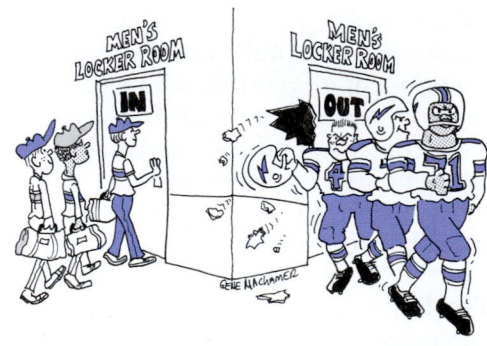

Overly aggressive behavior or 'roid rage is a symptom of steroid use in males.

help build muscle yet minimize masculinizing side effects. Initially steroids were used only by weightlifters in small doses, but athletes assumed that larger doses would build even more muscle. Today anabolic steroids are widely used and abused by both male and female athletes, from young teens to professionals, at all levels of competition. Many athletes "stack" them—that is, take a combination of brands in quantities of 100 mg or more daily.

Although testing procedures are now in place to deter illegal steroid abuse among professional, Olympic, and college athletes, new designer drugs constantly become available. These can escape detection and put athletes willing to cheat one step ahead of testing efforts. The dynamic, however, may be about to shift if the saving of urine and blood samples for retesting at a future date becomes the standard. The high probability of eventual detection of the newer designer steroids, once the technology becomes available, plus the fear of retroactive sanctions, should give athletes pause.

Steroids can be deadly. Unfortunately, to the high school junior trying to make first-string linebacker, the long-term effects of steroids may not seem important. However, steroid use can lead to early heart attack, strokes, liver tumors, kidney failure, sterility, bleeding ulcers, cancer, high blood pressure, lowered high-density lipoprotein, and death. One surprising risk to the user who injects anabolic steroids is the exposure to HIV/AIDS and hepatitis B and C. See Table 7-5. The primary medical uses of anabolic steroids are to treat delayed puberty and some types of impotence, and wasting of the body caused by HIV/AIDS infection or other diseases.

Although steroids may be easily accessible through health clubs and spas, they are illegal if purchased without a physician's prescription. New research suggests the drugs can cause a powerful psychological dependency and stopping them requires careful medical oversight. Withdrawal can lead to severe depression lasting for months.

Amphetamines

Amphetamines (*speed, uppers, L.A. turnaround, bennies,* or *black beauties*) are powerful central nervous system stimulants. Biphetamine and dexedrine are commercial names for these drugs. They are controlled drugs, meaning legislation has severely restricted even medical use. Their use without a prescription is illegal. Amphetamines include closely related compounds: methamphetamine and dextroamphetamine. The sharp increase in the use of methamphetamine is a serious concern today. Currently, amphetamines are legitimately used for

TABLE 7-5	*The Bad News*
About Steroids	

Men may develop
   Breast development
   Baldness
   Shrunken testicles
   A higher voice
   Infertility
Women may develop
   A deep voice
   An enlarged clitoris
   Increased body hair
   Baldness
   Increased appetite
Both men and women might experience
   Severe acne
   Liver abnormalities and tumors
   High blood pressure
   Increased low-density lipoprotein (LDL) cholesterol
      (the "bad" cholesterol)
   Decreased high-density lipoprotein (HDL) cholesterol
      (the "good" cholesterol)
   'Roid rage or uncontrollable aggressive behaviors,
      rage, or violence
   Psychiatric disorders, such as depression
   Drug dependence
   Increased chance of injury to muscles, tendons, and
      ligaments
   Death

short-term diet control in persons with obesity, **narcolepsy** (uncontrollable attacks of deep sleep), and attention deficit/hyperactivity disorder (ADHD). They increase blood pressure, heart rate, respiratory rate, and metabolic rate; suppress the appetite; and place the body in a state of stress. The ability of amphetamines to relieve sleepiness and fatigue; decrease appetite; and increase alertness, confidence, aggressiveness, and short-term performance has led to extensive nonmedical use, particularly by people involved in activities that demand stamina and long periods of wakefulness: long-distance truck drivers, pilots, flight attendants, and entertainers. They have also been used by students cramming for exams and athletes trying to enhance their performance. These drugs do not increase maximal oxygen uptake. Although these stimulants can boost physical performance and promote aggressiveness, they have side effects that can impair athletic performance. Nervousness and irritability make it hard to concentrate on the game, and insomnia can prevent an athlete from getting needed sleep. Also, a person using amphetamines in competition may be seriously injured and not be aware of it.

Common side effects include headaches, mood swings, rapid heartbeat, restlessness, insomnia, and anxiety. Use of amphetamines over a prolonged period increases tolerance of the drug and results in a need for larger doses. Large doses can lead to high blood pressure, anorexia, convulsions, and psychosis. Use of amphetamines during exercise in a hot environment may result in an elevated body temperature and death. Amphetamine injections, when needles are shared, may expose the user to diseases such as hepatitis and AIDS.

Diuretics

Diuretics cause the body to pass water by increasing urine output. They are useful in treating edema and mild hypertension. Diuretics are useless in producing true weight loss because they result in loss of water, not fat. Any water lost is quickly regained over the next 24 hours. When used by wrestlers to decrease weight temporarily in order to compete, the resulting dehydration produces weakness and fatigue, along with increased susceptibility to heat illness. Diuretics have also been used, ineffectively, by some athletes to mask anabolic steroid use. Urine tests for steroids are sufficiently sensitive to detect amounts as minute as a drop in a swimming pool of water.

   Using diuretics may cause

✓ Muscle cramps
✓ Exhaustion
✓ Decreased ability to regulate body temperature
✓ Potassium deficiency
✓ Heart arrhythmias

Caffeine

Caffeine is probably the most common drug used by adults and children in our society. It occurs naturally in coffee, tea, colas, cocoa, and chocolate and is added to some prescription and nonprescription drugs. Table 7-6 lists average amounts of caffeine found in commonly used drinks, food, and drugs. Caffeine is a powerful central nervous system stimulant. In healthy, rested people, a dose of 100 milligrams (about 1 cup of coffee) increases alertness, banishes drowsiness, quickens reaction time, enhances intellectual and muscular effort, increases heart and respiratory rates, and stimulates urinary output. One well-conducted study linked regular coffee drinking (two to five cups a day) with a longer life.

   Ingestion of one to two cups of coffee an hour before prolonged exhaustive exercise produces a glycogen-sparing effect by promoting fat use, which may enhance performance in endurance activities. It also tends to mask fatigue. This effect decreases as fitness increases, however, resulting in little or no benefit for highly trained athletes. If a competitive edge is desired, an athlete is wiser to drink a sports drink or plain water. Caffeine produces dehydration and, in some individuals, abnormalities in heart electrical function, both of which hinder performance.

While moderate use of caffeine is generally harmless, overconsumption can produce a toxic reaction known as *caffeinism*. Too much caffeine produces insomnia, nervousness, irritability, restlessness, muscle twitches, headaches, heart palpitations, and gastric disturbances. Large amounts of caffeine increase the excretion of calcium, which might weaken bones. It also may lead to low birth weight in babies and can interfere with several medications including certain antidepressants and antipsychotics, increasing the risk of side effects. Unfiltered coffee, such as that made in French press coffeemakers, contains a fat-like substance called *cafestol*, which can raise levels of LDL (bad) cholesterol.

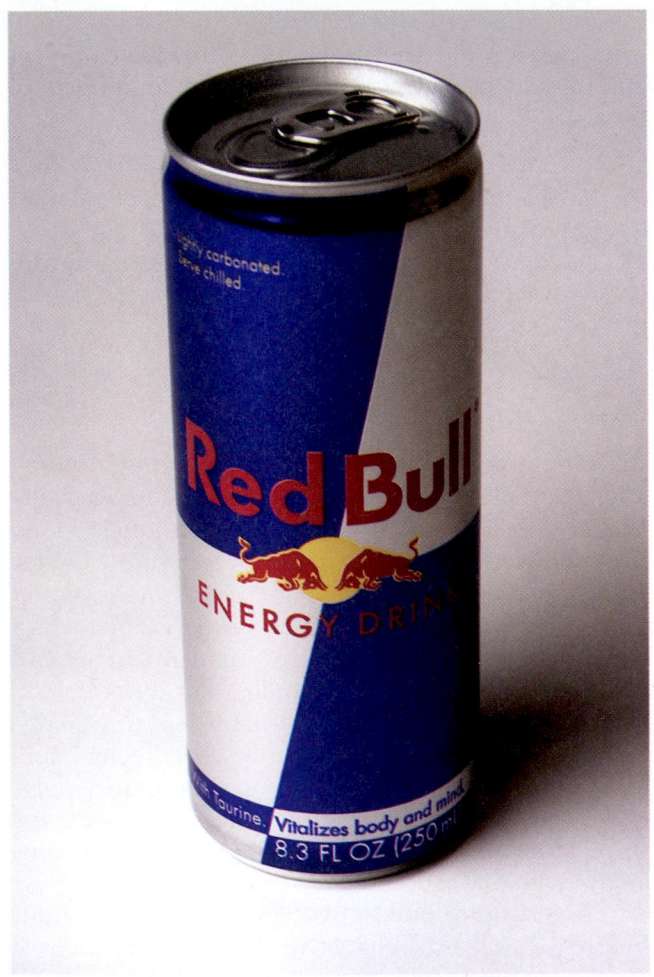

How many milligrams of caffeine does Red Bull or Monster have? How many does a 12 oz. and 16 oz. Starbucks have?

Tips for Behavior Change for Caffeine Consumption

Refer to the Stage of Change flowchart on page 226. What is your stage of change after answering the questions and tracing the flowchart?

Refer to Figure 2.2 (page 36) to see which processes of change are most effective for facilitating your transition from your current stage to the next stage (or *maintaining* your behavior if you are already in the maintenance stage). Here are some behavioral examples for selected processes of change:

- Consciousness-raising: Investigate the pros and cons of caffeine consumption.
- Emotional arousal: Identify the amount of caffeine in the foods, beverages, and medications you commonly consume.
- Self-liberation: Sign a behavior change contract to reduce your caffeine consumption by 25 percent by a specific date.
- Reward: Plan specific rewards when the goal is achieved (a new water bottle, new exercise outfit, etc.).
- Environment control: Switch to half-and-half coffee, drink decaffeinated beverages, and remove medications and over-the-counter drugs containing caffeine from your living area. Instead of relying on caffeine to keep you awake while studying, take a break and go for a walk/jog.

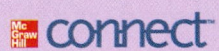 **Go online to Connect to complete this activity.** http://connect.mcgraw-hill.com

How much caffeine is too much? Although tolerance varies from one person to another, intake of less than 200 milligrams per day is a wise limit. People with certain heart problems are sometimes advised to avoid it.

Caffeine use is habit-forming, and those who try to abruptly stop a long-term pattern of heavy consumption often experience withdrawal symptoms. Headaches, lethargy, irritability, and difficulty concentrating are common symptoms that will gradually diminish over a few days to 2 weeks.

Recent studies have linked caffeine to a reduced risk of several diseases: type 2 diabetes, Parkinson's, gallstones, liver damage, and colon cancer. It has also been found to help preserve the

TABLE 7-6 — *Common Sources of Caffeine*

	Milligrams			Milligrams
Coffee (6-oz. cup)		Mountain Dew		55
Starbucks 12 oz. "tall"	279–300	Mellow Yellow		52
Starbucks 16 oz. "grande"	400–500	Coca-Cola		35
McDonald's 12 oz.	109	Diet Coke		47
Brewed, drip method	80–150	Pepsi-Cola		35
Decaffeinated, brewed	3	Diet Pepsi		36
Instant	60–100	Pepsi One		55
Decaffeinated, instant	2	Water, caffeine enhanced (12 oz.)		60–125
Espresso (2 oz.)	90–120	Tea (8-oz. cup)		
Hot chocolate (8 oz.)	5–20	Brewed		20–100
Chocolate milk (8 oz.)	5	Oolong		36
Chocolate		Green		32
Dark chocolate (1 oz.)	5–35	Ice		5–9
Chocolate cake (1 slice)	20–30	Analgesics (Excedrin, Anacin, Midol)		30–70
Milk chocolate (1 oz.)	1–10	Cold/allergy remedies		16–30
Chocolate-flavored syrup (1 oz.)	4	Maximum Strength No-Doz		200
Energy drinks		Weight control drugs		50–200
Red Bull (16 oz.)	160	Diuretics		100–200
Monster (16 oz.)	160	Stay Alert gum		100
5-Hour Energy (2 oz.)	250	Jolt gum		13
Rockstar Energy shot (2.5 oz.)	200	Gels		20–25
Fixx Extreme (0.17 oz.)	400	Caffeine tablets		200
Soft drinks (12 oz.)				
Jolt Cola	110			

cognitive skills of older men and women (i.e. lessens risk of Alzheimer's). So, the drug has both benefits and negative consequences.

AGING AND PHYSICAL ACTIVITY

Is your body older than you are? Scientist and well-known physical educator T. K. Cureton estimated that middle age begins for the average person at age 26, because at that age he or she has the physical capacity our ancestors did when they were 40. When we retire, we are expected to slow down and take it easy. This often produces disastrous results as atrophy and disuse take their toll. Exercise is probably the single most important thing we can do to age successfully. Even in moderate amounts, exercise has been found to help us enjoy life and avoid diseases that many people mistakenly believe come automatically with age. Regular physical activity cuts risk of

✓ Heart attack
✓ Stroke
✓ High blood pressure and high cholesterol
✓ Diabetes
✓ Osteoporosis

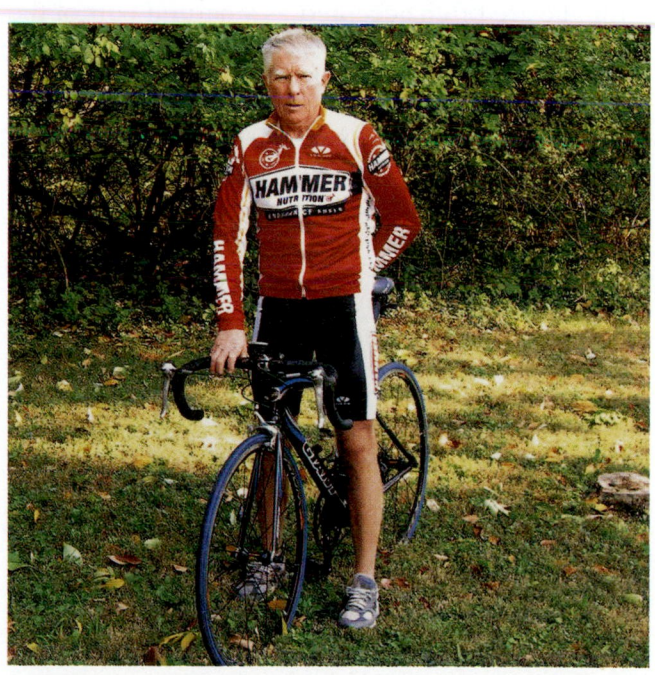

Studies show that aerobic exercise reverses the shrinkage of memory regions of the brain.

✓ Depression and anxiety
✓ Falls and broken bones
✓ Some kinds of cancer
✓ Alzheimer's disease/dementia

We now think that these health problems are more related to physical inactivity. The body adapts to whatever load is placed on it, and the ability to do work is reduced if the load lessens. Attitudes are changing. Older adults, encouraged by their doctors and by research revealing the benefits of exercise, are biking, swimming, jogging, lifting weights, and walking in ever-increasing numbers. We know that older adults (even up to age 100) are remarkably responsive to exercise, reaping health benefits. As the health-conscious baby-boom generation matures, its members are likely to redefine the concept of aging.

Aging and Performance

Some say, "Growing old isn't so bad if you consider the alternative." James Dean's "Live fast, die young, and leave a good-looking corpse" does have its proponents, but they are quickly weeded out of the genetic pool. At birth, we each have an 80-plus-year warranty, but the maintenance is up to us. Just like any machine, the human body grows less efficient as it ages. The decline in aerobic fitness among the sedentary is about 1 percent every year after age 25. Decreases in strength, flexibility, and endurance and increases in body fat proportion with age are often accepted as a natural part of the aging process. These changes may be common, but they are not inevitable. The most significant factor contributing to declines in physiological capacity at any age is *lack of regular exercise.* The "use it or lose it" rule applies. As much as 50 percent of the functional decline seen in aging is related to disuse and can be prevented with regular aerobic exercise. Unused muscles atrophy, lose elasticity, and grow weak. Ligaments and tendons shorten and tighten, decreasing range of motion and causing aches and pains as they pull across joints. As muscle tissue atrophies, basal metabolism drops, resulting in an increase in body fat even when a person is not eating enough to maintain adequate nutritional levels.

Other adverse changes that occur with aging can also be favorably affected by exercise. For example, exercise can enhance insulin sensitivity, reduce blood pressure, and improve psychological well-being.

Osteoporosis has become a national health priority—one in two women and one in four men over the age of 50 will have an osteoporotic fracture in their lifetime. See "The Numbers." As the population ages, osteoporosis here and around the world will result in an epidemic of life-diminishing, life-threatening fractures. To develop optimal bone strength and mass and to ward off osteoporosis,

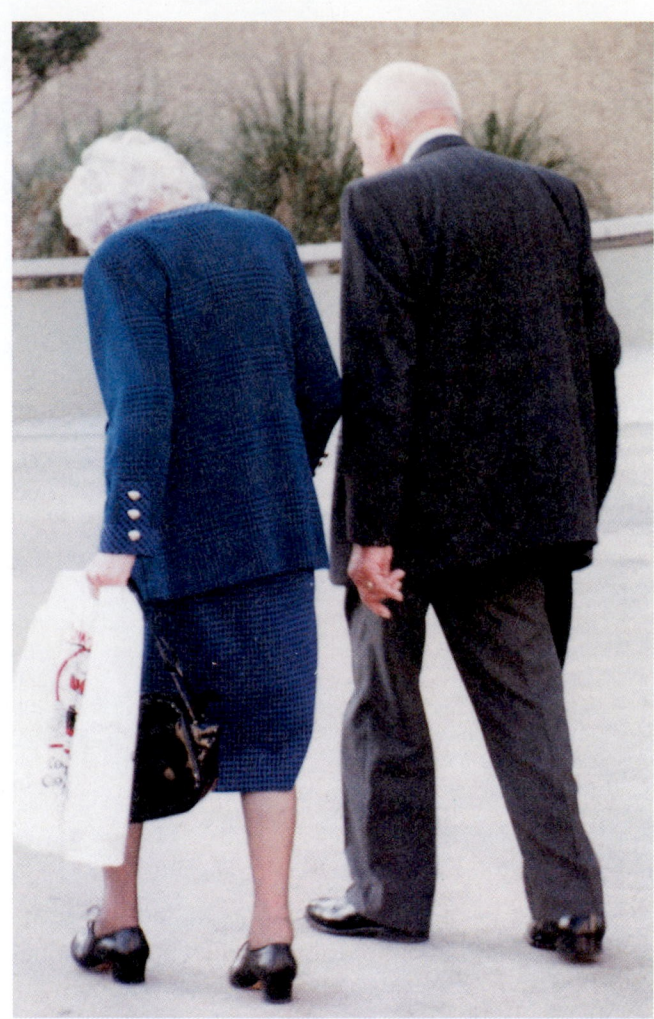

Postmenopausal women (and men) can maintain and may increase their bone density by regularly doing weight-bearing and resistance exercise.

women need adequate amounts of calcium in the diet, estrogen in the bloodstream, and weight-bearing exercise in their lifestyle. Exercise acts synergistically with estrogen to develop bone strength. Inactivity accelerates bone mineral loss and increases the risk of osteoporosis. Bone mass usually peaks between the ages of 25 and 30 and then gradually declines. The decline is hastened by menopause. While exercise alone cannot prevent osteoporosis, it may help premenopausal women build their bone densities so that they enter menopause ahead of the game. Ideally, women and men should exercise early in life to build bone and later in life to keep it strong. Weight-bearing exercise and strength training that stresses the bone help increase bone content and is better increased by a combination of the two than it is by strength training alone. Once osteoporosis has developed, women and men should

THE NUMBERS

43%	Amount of lean muscle tissue on the male body.
23%	Amount of lean muscle tissue on the female body.
2%	College-age women who already have osteoporosis. Another 15% have significant losses in bone density. (Data from a University of Arkansas study.)
24 million	Number of Americans (8%) who are living with diabetes. Of these, 14.6 million do not know they have it. Another 57 million have prediabetes.
1 in 3	American adults who have hypertension.
40%	Decreased risk of death attributed to seniors who participated in a brisk activity once a week compared to that of their inactive peers.

still be encouraged to exercise except while a fracture is healing. Men are also affected by osteoporosis, but at later ages than women. Studies show that men and women 60 and older who train with weights, exercise bands, and resistance machines several times a week can quickly double their total body strength. See the exercise band photo in the osteoporosis section later in the chapter. This helps fight osteoporosis by keeping skeletons sturdy. Also, such strength gains have major implications for maintaining independence in later years. Muscle weakness can advance to the stage where an elderly individual cannot do common activities of daily living. Household tasks such as getting out of a chair, sweeping the floor, and taking out the trash may become impossible. Reduced functional ability may then increase the chance of nursing home placement. Lifelong exercise may also help protect the elderly against falls and the devastating effects of hip fractures. It's never too late to start exercising. Starting late in life is far preferable to not starting at all.

While aging is unavoidable, declines in functional capacity with age are not inevitable. How you age is largely up to you. Cardiologist George Sheehan has said that growing older isn't so bad; it is inactive people who give aging a bad name.

As one physician observed, "So many things we think are linked to aging . . . actually have to do with lifestyle. Exercise produces a 40-year age offset. A fit person of 70 is the equal of an unfit person of 30 in regard to bones, muscles, heart, brain, sex, and everything else. I see an immense energy in old people who continue [exercise]." Exercise intensity appears to be the key to getting the greatest benefit. A group of master athletes (ages 40 to 75) studied over an 18-year period showed no significant decline in aerobic capacity if they maintained training intensity.

The effect of true nonpreventable aging involves a gradual loss of the speed and vigor with which we do activities, but it should not prevent us from doing them. As one older runner observed, "I can do everything I used to. It just takes longer to do it and longer to recover."

Exercise is adult play. At what point was our childhood eagerness to get out and romp replaced by hours of sitting in front of the TV watching others play? Whether aging is an extension of a full and active life or a gradual wasting away is determined by how you choose to live your life.

Department of Health and Human Services (DHHS) Physical Activity Guidelines for the Older Adult

The DHHS recently published exercise guidelines for all Americans. It is the first time physical activity recommendations for all ages and special needs groups have been published in one document. The overriding recommendation is . . . for *all* Americans to avoid inactivity! Older adults (age 65 and older) are advised to follow the same guidelines as those

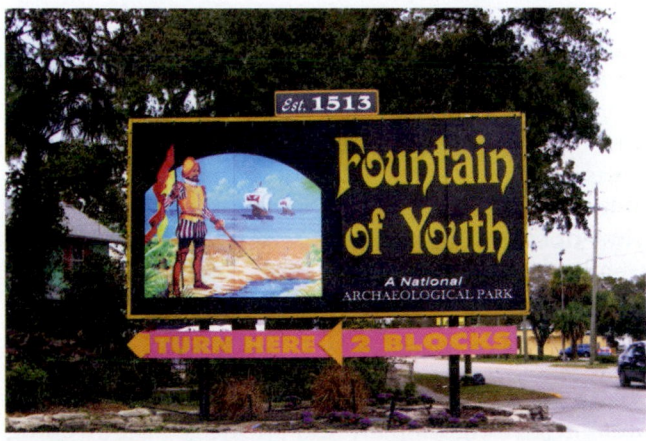

Instead of looking for the "fountain of youth," Ponce de Leon would have been better off docking his ship, remaining on land, and starting a fitness program. Research confirms that exercise truly is the "fountain of youth."

recommended for healthy younger adults (age 16 to 64), as described in the Exercise Guideline box in Chapter 4, unless chronic conditions prohibit activity. Older adults should be as physically active as their abilities and conditions allow.

The main difference in the guidelines for the two groups involves balance activities. Older adults, who are at risk for falling, should include balance improving exercises in their weekly workouts. This is good advice for younger people too.

Does Exercise Increase Life Span?

While the length of your life may have a strong genetic component, study after study has shown that exercise helps lower the risk of major chronic diseases and premature death. Research conducted at the Cooper Institute for Aerobics Research in Dallas found that exercise of *moderate* intensity improved the overall *quality* of life (e.g., enhanced the ability to perform daily tasks, helped with weight control, enhanced psychological well-being) and perhaps increased the *quantity* of life by postponing a heart attack or stroke. A second study, part of the famous ongoing research of male Harvard alumni, reported that exercise of moderate intensity improved the quality of life but that it took exercise at a *vigorous* intensity level to add years to one's life. The Harvard men who had expended at least 1,500 calories a week in vigorous physical activity had a 25 percent lower death rate than did sedentary men. Vigorous activity was defined as fast walking, jogging, playing singles tennis, swimming, and performing heavy, sustained household chores. Studies such as these illustrate that any exercise has health benefits, but more exercise, enough to give your heart and lungs a real workout, is better. While a healthful lifestyle is no guarantee of a longer life, it does stack the odds in your favor.

Are you ever "too old" to begin exercise? No! While the overall impact you can make on the quality of your life is greater if you start exercising young and continue throughout life, there is no age at which the benefits of exercise stop. The older you are, the more you need exercise. See the Top 10 "Benefits of Exercise for Older Adults."

◆ EXERCISE AND CHRONIC HEALTH CONDITIONS

The general FITT principles of exercise prescription apply to individuals with and without chronic disease. Also, it is essential to include flexibility and strength-training exercises in all well-designed exercise programs. However, certain conditions may require differences or modifications in exercise programming to maximize effectiveness, avoid complications, and increase enjoyment of the activity. Each of the following conditions is highlighted with a brief overview and special exercise considerations to ensure safety and enjoyment: arthritis, asthma, diabetes, hypertension, and osteoporosis. If you have any of these conditions, it is important to check with your physician before participating in an exercise program. Have your doctor fill out the Exercise Clearance Form in Chapter 3.

Arthritis

Arthritis and rheumatoid disease cause muscle weakness, fatigue, pain and stiffness, and swelling in joints and other supporting structures of the body such as muscles, tendons, ligaments, and bones. The two most common forms are osteoarthritis and rheumatoid arthritis. Fourteen percent of

---

TOP 10 LIST

Benefits of Exercise for Older Adults

1. Helps maintain the ability to live independently and reduces the risk of falling and fracturing bones.
2. Increases energy and helps the individual perform daily routines with greater ease.
3. Decreases risk of dementia, frailty, and Alzheimer's disease that spell the end of independence.
4. Helps maintain healthy bones, muscles, and joints; helps control joint swelling and pain associated with arthritis.
5. Enhances cardiorespiratory function and improves peripheral circulation; decreases the risk of arteriosclerosis and other circulatory problems.
6. Reduces constipation.
7. Reduces symptoms of anxiety and depression and fosters improvements in mood and feelings of well-being.
8. Helps people with chronic, disabling conditions improve stamina and muscle strength.
9. Reduces the risk of dying from coronary heart disease and of developing high blood pressure, colon cancer, and diabetes.
10. Improves a person's posture, decreases backache, enhances appearance, and helps control weight.

Americans have arthritis and rheumatoid disease. Osteoarthritis is a degenerative joint disease that typically affects the knees, hips, feet, spine, and hands. Rheumatoid arthritis is a chronic, systemic inflammatory disease that affects the synovial membranes of joints. The complications of arthritis may lead to a less active lifestyle.

Scientists stress that physical activity of the type and amount recommended for health has not been shown to cause or worsen arthritis. While rest is important during flare-ups, lack of physical activity is associated with increased muscle weakness, joint stiffness, reduced range of motion, and fatigue. Whether you should exercise during general or local flare-ups is up to you and your doctor. Consider working through the flare-up by doing mostly range of motion exercises, just to keep the body moving. It is true that arthritic joints cannot be cured, but staying active will help alleviate much of the pain of osteoarthritis.

The goals of an exercise program for people with arthritis are to preserve or restore range of motion and flexibility around affected joints; increase muscle strength and endurance; and increase cardiorespiratory endurance conditioning to improve mood and decrease health risks associated with a sedentary lifestyle.

Recommendations/modifications for exercise for those with arthritis include the following:

✓ Begin slowly and progress gradually.
✓ Avoid rapid or repetitive movements of affected joints.
✓ Perform flexibility exercise one to two times daily, using pain-free range of motion exercises. These can be done on land or in water such as a pool, hot tub, or warm bath. Physicians should provide specific stretches to be done instead of saying, "just stretch." Yoga and Tai Chi are good activities for increasing flexibility.
✓ Perform cardiorespiratory endurance exercise initially in short bouts (i.e., 10 minutes each time). Work up to 30 minutes. Performing three 10-minute sessions per day is also acceptable. Aquatic, walking, and cycling activities are advised.
✓ Perform resistance training two to three times per week. Do not exercise with pain.
✓ Include functional lifestyle activities (e.g., climbing stairs, standing up from a sitting position, buttoning clothes) daily.
✓ Stop exercise if you have continuing joint pain that lasts more than an hour after exercise, unusual fatigue, increased weakness, decreased range of motion, or increased joint swelling.

✓ Morning exercise may not be advised for those with significant morning stiffness.
✓ Consider applying heat to joints before exercise and ice after exercising.

Asthma

Years ago, it was thought that strenuous physical activity was dangerous if you had asthma, but now we know better. Exercise is not only safe if done properly, it is an integral part of treatment. Studies show that physically fit people have fewer attacks, need less medication, and lose less time from work or school. Seventeen million Americans are living with asthma.

Activities that involve short, intermittent periods of exertion such as volleyball, baseball, half-court basketball, and tennis are generally well tolerated by individuals with asthma. Activities that involve continuous exertion such as jogging, field hockey, and cycling as well as cold weather sports (e.g., cross-country skiing, ice skating, jogging in winter) may be less well tolerated. However, with proper precaution, most people with asthma are able to participate fully in these activities. Swimming is well tolerated because of the warm, moist air environment. Other beneficial activities include both indoor and outdoor cycling, aerobics, walking, or running on a treadmill.

To make sure asthma doesn't interfere with your ability to exercise, keep it under control. If your doctor has prescribed medications for daily use, use them faithfully. Take necessary steps to control allergies. Visit the doctor on a regular schedule, follow instructions about monitoring your condition at home, and be sure to report any problems promptly.

People with well-controlled asthma can exercise following the FITT prescription for exercise outlined in Chapter 4. For balanced fitness, also include strength training and flexibility components. Follow the guidelines described in Chapters 5 and 6. However, if your asthma is exercise-induced, pay special attention to avoiding environment "triggers" such as cold, dry, dusty air and/or inhaled pollutants and chemicals. Even if your asthma is well controlled, you may develop coughing, shortness of breath, chest pain, or nausea if you exercise without taking precautions. Do not exercise during an acute asthma attack; wait until the symptoms have subsided. For safe exercise participation follow these guidelines:

✓ Exercise regularly. Acute attacks are more likely if you exercise only occasionally.
✓ Drink plenty of water before, during, and after a workout, even in cool weather, to moisten the airways.

✓ Warm up and cool down thoroughly.
✓ Avoid exercising in cold, dry air. In the winter, work out indoors or if you are active outside, cover your mouth and nose with a scarf or breathing mask to warm the air you breathe.
✓ Don't exercise on days when your symptoms are bothersome, such as when you are wheezing or coughing.
✓ Avoid areas where air pollution is high (e.g., near highways or during high-traffic times of the day). On days when pollution is worse than normal or the pollen count is particularly high, exercise indoors or not at all.
✓ If your doctor recommends it, use medications as prescribed before exercising.
✓ If you develop symptoms during exercise, don't try to push your way through them. Stop what you are doing and follow the directions on your inhaler. If this doesn't bring relief within 15 to 20 minutes, seek medical help.

Diabetes Mellitus

Diabetes mellitus (both type 1 and type 2) is a chronic disease characterized by the body's inability to produce insulin or use the hormone properly. See Chapter 9 for expanded information about diabetes, especially Table 9-5. The treatment goal for diabetes is blood glucose control, which includes exercise, diet, and medications. One of the best things diabetic individuals can do is to stay active. Moderate to intense exercise may cause blood glucose levels to diminish for the 24 hours following exercise. Before beginning an exercise program, they should undergo an extensive medical evaluation, particularly for the cardiovascular, nervous, renal (kidney), and visual systems because these are at high risk for diabetic complications.

Exercise increases vulnerability to two major diabetes-related problems: hypoglycemia (a rapid drop in blood glucose level) and foot sores (caused by peripheral vascular disease). Hypoglycemia is initially characterized by sweating, hunger, dizziness, anxiety, a rapid heart rate, and tremor. Without proper attention, the sufferer may lose consciousness and go into shock. Foot sores that are not properly treated can rapidly worsen, sometimes within a matter of hours, and lead to infection. Severe cases may require amputation. Individuals with advanced diabetic neuropathy should choose low-impact activities like swimming, rowing, water exercise, and cycling rather than high-impact ones like jogging. Everyone with diabetes should inspect the feet for signs of irritation before and

TOP 10 LIST

Exercising with Diabetes

1. Get proper medical advice before starting an exercise program.
2. Monitor blood glucose levels before, during, and after exercise, especially in the early stages of exercise training. Check twice prior to exercise, 30 minutes before and immediately before; and every 20 to 30 minutes during prolonged exercise. **If your blood glucose level is 300 mg/dl or higher, do not exercise.**
3. Don't exercise when you are sick. Exercising when you are sick can make your blood glucose levels fluctuate dramatically, and it may take longer to get well.
4. Keep fluid levels well up before, during, and after exercise, especially during hot weather. Dehydration can affect blood glucose levels and heart function.
5. Be aware of signs of hypoglycemia (low blood glucose) even several hours after exercise. Have a carbohydrate-based snack or drink handy.
6. Exercise 1 to 2 hours after a meal.
7. Avoid injecting insulin in a muscle that is about to be used for exercise.
8. Wear correct footwear. Peripheral vascular disease is relatively common in diabetics and it often affects the feet.
9. Exercise at the same time each day. Exercise at a similar time, intensity, and duration each day helps you get to know your own blood glucose response to exercise training.
10. In case of emergency, wear an identification bracelet or shoe tag while exercising.

after exercise. Activities like scuba diving and rock climbing can be dangerous if there is any possibility of hypoglycemia.

Diabetics with retinopathy and nephropathy should avoid activities that sharply raise blood pressure. This means that when these individuals strength train they should lift lighter weights and a higher number of repetitions instead of heavier weights and a lower number of reps. Avoid exercise that causes jerky motions (e.g., bouncing on a trampoline); increases eye pressure (e.g., scuba diving or mountain climbing); or places your eyes below the level of your heart (e.g., toe touching).

With proper training, most diabetics can exercise as much as they wish. Follow the FITT prescription for cardiorespiratory endurance fitness and include flexibility and strength-training components for balanced fitness. See the Top 10 "Exercising with Diabetes."

Hypertension

Hypertension (or high blood pressure) is defined as a blood pressure (BP) equal to or exceeding a systolic BP of 140 mm Hg and/or a diastolic BP of 90 mm Hg. Hypertension is one of the most prevalent forms of cardiovascular disease. It is the major contributor to strokes, heart attacks, congestive heart failure, peripheral vascular disease, and kidney failure. The risk of many of these diseases increases at levels of blood pressure well below the diagnostic threshold of 140/90 mm Hg. Therefore, lowering blood pressure may benefit individuals with any elevation above optimal levels. See Chapter 9 for important blood pressure information.

The American College of Sports Medicine advises that exercise should be the cornerstone of therapy for the prevention, treatment, and control of high blood pressure. Most aerobic, resistance, and flexibility types of exercise are recommended, but the primary form of exercise should be the aerobic type. The FITT prescription for cardiorespiratory endurance exercise should be adhered to but with the following adaptations:

✓ The preferred intensity of the aerobic exercise should be at the moderate-intensity level (below 70 percent HRR) because it appears to reduce BP as much as, if not more than, exercise at higher intensities. Walking, cycling, and swimming are good choices. The intensity level of running may be too high.

✓ The preferred frequency of the aerobic exercise is 7 days per week because BP is lowered for several hours after a single bout of exercise. Lowering BP just a few days per week with aerobic exercise is not sufficient.

Here are additional special exercise guidelines for those with high blood pressure:

✓ Do not exercise if resting systolic BP is greater than 200 mm Hg or diastolic BP is greater than 110 mm Hg.

✓ Vigorous activities done with high force, such as sprinting, rowing, or heavy lifting or straining, are not advised for hypertensive individuals.

✓ Downhill skiing may exaggerate an elevated BP response from the cold and elevation.

✓ Be aware of heat. Some BP medications impair the ability to regulate body temperature or can cause dehydration.

✓ Cool down. Extend the cool-down period because some BP medications may cause BP levels to drop after abruptly stopping exercise.

✓ Weight loss, even a few pounds, helps to lower BP.

Resistance training should not be the only or main mode of exercise for individuals with hypertension, but it should be combined with an aerobic exercise program. Use lower resistance (i.e., 30 to 60 percent of maximal effort) with higher repetitions (i.e., 12 to 15). Follow these guidelines when performing resistance exercise:

✓ Avoid isometric types of exercise.

✓ Do not hold your muscle at the point of full muscle contraction.

✓ Avoid "holding" your breath while exercising (valsalva maneuver), especially during resistance types of exercise.

✓ Avoid tight gripping.

Osteoporosis

Osteoporosis literally means "porous bone." It is a skeletal disease characterized by low bone mass, increased bone fragility, and increased risk for bone fracture. Osteoporotic fractures commonly occur in the hip, spine, and wrist but can occur at other sites. Osteoporosis is a silent disease in that a fracture is frequently the first indication of bone loss. This disease has a debilitating effect on independence and quality of life, especially for older adults. Risk factors for osteoporosis are family history, female gender, estrogen deficiency, low weight, dietary factors, prolonged use of corticosteriods, and physical inactivity. Bone mass attained early in life is perhaps the most important determinant of lifelong skeletal health. Young women who suffer from female athlete triad are at risk of bone loss and osteoporosis. Exercise can positively affect peak bone mass in children and adolescents, maintain or even modestly increase bone mass in adulthood, and assist in minimizing age-related bone loss in older adults. See Aging and Physical Activity in this chapter.

How does exercise help prevent osteoporosis? If bones are not used, they weaken. Studies on astronauts and injured athletes have shown that even well-conditioned individuals suffer from a reduction in bone mass and density during prolonged periods of inactivity. The detrimental results of little or no activity may be heightened as we get older. When force or stress is applied to a bone, the bone bends. This sets up a cascade of events that stimulates cells to strengthen the bone. The bone can adapt to stress or the lack of it by forming or losing mass. For the bone to become bigger and more dense, the stress must be above and beyond normal levels. The bone will continue to grow and adapt until it is restructured to handle the new imposed stress.

Each bone in the body must be stressed to grow strong. If the leg bones are stressed by running and

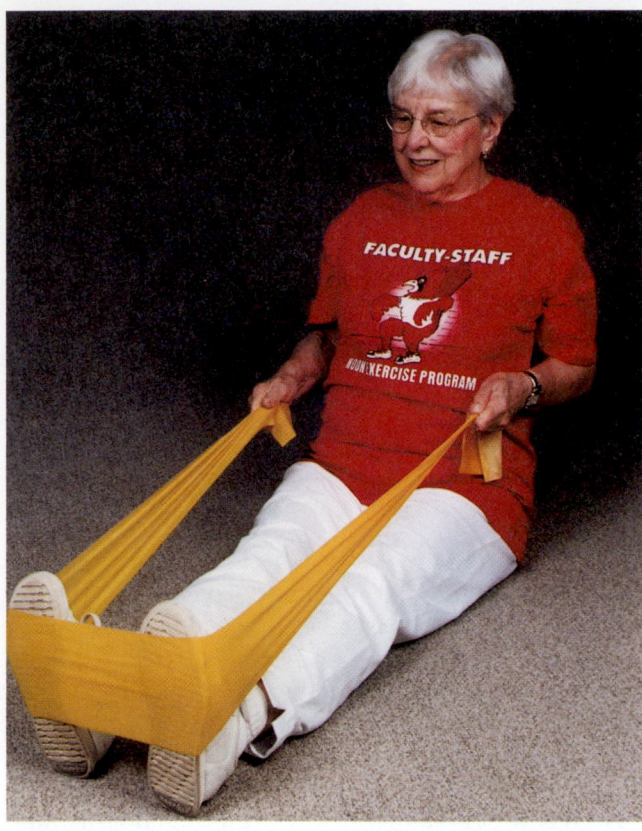

Use the exercise band workout found on the back cover of this book. Proper strength training offers numerous benefits to people of all ages and fitness levels.

jumping, the arm bones will not benefit unless they too are stressed with specific exercises (e.g., weight lifting). Thus a good exercise program to prevent and treat osteoporosis involves all of the major muscle and bone groups in the entire body.

Young bone is more responsive to exercise stress than old bone. Given that approximately 60 percent of the final skeleton is built during adolescence, vigorous physical exercise during childhood and adolescence is more important than at any other time in life.

If you already have osteoporosis or low bone density, consult your doctor before starting an exercise program. Depending on the status of your condition, your doctor may or may not recommend certain exercises and will inform you of precautions that are necessary when you exercise or perform regular activities. Avoid exercise when a fracture is healing. Use extreme caution when performing exercise that involves the following movements, as they may be dangerous:

✓ *Forward bending.* Avoid activities and exercise that involve bending forward excessively at the waist because they increase the risk of compression fractures of the vertebrae.

✓ *Heavy lifting.* Avoid heavy lifting, especially when bending forward at the waist. This may include lifting loads of laundry, bags of groceries, or exercise weights.

✓ *Twisting.* Twisting movement can place unusual force on your spine. Golfing and bowling are two common sports that involve twisting and may be harmful. Check with your doctor about whether you can safely participate in these sports.

✓ *High-impact activities.* Activities that involve higher-impact movements, sudden stops and starts, and abrupt weight shifts put too much stress on your spine and can lead to falls and knee injuries. Such activities include sprinting, soccer, racket sports, volleyball, and basketball.

Sometimes you cannot avoid certain movements such as bending forward or reaching overhead. But you can use caution and practice good posture and body mechanics to decrease risk of injury.

If you don't have osteoporosis and are otherwise healthy, exercising to prevent osteoporosis is generally safe. Once osteoporosis has developed, exercise is still encouraged except while a fracture is healing. The following types of exercises are recommended for osteoporosis prevention:

1. *Weight-bearing and impact exercise.* Weight-bearing exercise means your bones and muscles are working against gravity as you exercise. These involve activities you do on your feet with your bones supporting your weight. Examples include brisk walking, jogging, skipping, jumping rope, stair-climbing or step-type exercises, racket sports, aerobic dance, dancing, hiking, and team sports. *Swimming and bicycling are not weight-bearing* because your body is supported by the water or the bike rather than your legs. Recent research reveals that for many, walking may not adequately stress the bones to improve their strength. Activities with more impact and higher intensity may be necessary. This, however, would not be the case for the frail elderly. For osteoporosis prevention, weight-bearing/high-impact activities are best and weight-bearing/low-impact activities are good, but less so. This latter category includes low-impact aerobics and most cardiovascular machines (stair climbers, rowers, elliptical trainers, treadmill walking). Yoga and Pilates are nonimpact and are least beneficial for osteoporosis prevention.

2. *Strength training.* Strength training uses resistance, such as free weights, weight machines, resistance bands, and water activities to strengthen muscles. Strength-training activities for the legs, abdomen, and back should be emphasized to improve lower-body strength and posture to help prevent falls and broken bones. Because of the increase in gravitational force on bone in a weight-bearing position, strength-training exercises performed on the feet are considered to be more effective at stimulating bone than are machine-based exercises performed in a seated position. In the on-the-feet weight-bearing position, there is an increased load at the hip and greater demand for postural control and balance, which in turn optimizes bone health. Also, push-ups and exercises performed on the feet (with or without hand weights), such as forward, backward, and sideways lunge; squat; chair raise; heel and toe raise; stepping; and jumping are also recommended.

3. *Back strengthening.* Back-strengthening exercises should be included in exercise programs for the treatment and prevention of osteoporosis. Strengthening the muscles of the back may help improve the health of people with osteoporosis and low bone mass by improving posture and decreasing risk of compression fractures caused by the stooped posture commonly seen in people with the disease. Exercises that gently arch the back, the opposite direction of a stooped posture, can strengthen back muscles while minimizing back stress. See the Exercises for the Lower Back pullout at the back of the book.

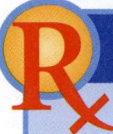

PRESCRIPTION FOR ACTION

You've read the chapter. Now go do one or more of these:

✓ Make a list of reasons why you didn't exercise outside last winter and ways you can counter this during the cold months this year.

✓ Get up during TV commercial breaks and do 30 seconds (about the length of one commercial) of each of the following exercises:
  - jumping jacks (or jog in place)
  - push-ups
  - abdominal curls or planks
  - squats

✓ Show your grandparents or another older person how to use an exercise band.

✓ Weigh yourself before and after your workout today and see how much water you lost.

✓ Write down three reasons why you will want to exercise across your life span.

✓ Keep a log of how much water you drink today.

✓ Keep a log of how much calcium you get today.

✓ Do you consume caffeine? Keep a log to measure how much caffeine you are getting a day. Which of the products you consume contain the most caffeine?

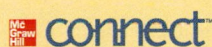 **Go online to Connect to complete this activity.**
http://connect.mcgraw-hill.com

Frequently Asked Questions

Q. True or False? Most of your body heat is lost through the head.

A. False. You lose heat from whatever is uncovered. There is nothing special about the head. This myth originated from a 50-year-old military study. Subjects in extreme cold lost the most heat from their heads—but the head was the only exposed body part.

Q. Is THG a vitamin or an anabolic steroid? As a college athlete, should I be taking it?

A. No! Do not take it. Tetrahydrogestrinone, or THG, is one anabolic steroid that is receiving a lot of attention. Until recently, THG was marketed as a dietary supplement for enhancing athletic performance. However, researchers have found that THG is actually a chemically altered version of an anabolic steroid that is banned by most sports organizations. THG is referred to as a "designer" steroid because it is undetectable by traditional steroid testing techniques. THG is not approved by the Food and Drug Administration and carries their health warning.

Q. Can healthy people do anything to boost their immunity?

A. There is nothing more powerful than *regular, moderate exercise.* When unfit, sedentary people work out for 45 minutes at a moderate intensity most days of the week, the number of days they are sick falls by about half. The natural killer cells and neutrophils of the immune system that provide the first defense against bacteria, viruses, and other invaders start circulating at a higher level. These remain elevated for about 3 hours after the workout and then return to normal until the next time you exercise.

Q. Can I work out when I have a cold or upper respiratory infection?

A. It depends. Studies suggest that *moderate* exercise training (at 70 percent HRR) during an upper respiratory infection (URI) does not appear to extend the length or increase the severity of the illness. However, exercising during a URI should be considered carefully. Use the following guidelines to decide if it is OK for you to exercise during a cold or URI.

- If you are not experiencing extreme tiredness, malaise, fever, or swollen lymph glands, you may safely exercise at an intensity level lower than that of your regular workouts.
- Also, perform a "neck check." Assess cold symptoms and classify them as either above or below the neck. If symptoms are "above the neck" (i.e., runny nose, sneezing, or scratchy throat), you may exercise at a lower intensity. Exercise is not advised when you have "below the neck" symptoms (i.e., fever, aching muscles, productive cough, vomiting, or diarrhea).
- If you begin feeling better during the workout, increase the intensity of the workout accordingly.

Q. True or false? All alcoholic beverages are dehydrating.

A. False. Although nonalcoholic beverages are recommended for rehydration, especially when you are exercising or working in hot weather, beer, many mixed drinks, and wine are fairly diluted and thus add to the total fluid intake. Concentrated alcoholic beverages such as vodka and brandy, if drunk undiluted, are very dehydrating.

Q. True or false? "Oxygenated" water, which is infused with 5 to 10 times as much oxygen as regular water, will help your muscles and improve your performance. So will vitamin-enriched water.

A. False and false. Studies show that oxygenated water does not improve aerobic performance or increase oxygen levels in the blood. The only way to get oxygen into the blood and muscles is through the lungs. Vitamin-enriched waters and those containing herbs will not improve performance or benefit your health in any way. However, "sports drinks" containing low levels of sugar and sodium can help conserve carbohydrate stores and delay fatigue during a prolonged workout.

Q. Does exercise affect the cognitive ability of older adults?

A. Yes. Older adults who stay fit may be better equipped to deal with situations that require quick or multitask thinking. Research reveals that active seniors have increased "executive control function" (ECF). ECF is a type of complex thinking needed to handle a sudden unexpected change (such as a car darting into your lane) and in multitasking situations (such as talking on the telephone and checking e-mail simultaneously). Fit seniors have sharper thinking, a reduced risk of cognitive decline, and improved motor preparation. So do fit *young* people.

Q. What is sarcopenia?

A. Pronounced sark-ko-PEEN-ya, this is a word you are likely to begin hearing more often. It means not only loss of muscle and strength but also decreased quality of muscle tissue. Most people lose 20 to 40 percent of their muscle tissue as they get older. Strength training can restore muscle mass and strength or at least slow this loss.

Q. Is it ever too late to start strength training?

A. No. In several recent studies, even elderly nursing home residents saw marked improvement after undertaking an 8-week program that significantly improved their balance, strength, and walking speed. It also helped lower cholesterol.

Summary

Exercise is meant to be enjoyed throughout life. Regardless of gender or age, the body improves with use and degenerates with disuse. People don't wear out; they rust out. For the greatest benefit from an exercise program, it is helpful to be aware of special concerns, such as how to exercise safely in hot and cold weather and how to avoid high-risk exercises. You have learned in this chapter that women respond to exercise the way men do but perhaps a little slower and to a lesser extent, and, with a physician's approval, pregnant women can safely exercise. This means training principles are approximately the same, regardless of gender. You have also learned that water is a fine rehydrater after exercise but that sports drinks are recommended for rehydration after prolonged exercise (60 to 90 minutes) and profuse sweating. Sports drinks contain electrolytes, which enhance fluid retention, contain carbohydrates, delay the onset of fatigue, and boost energy, and they taste good, which increases the likelihood that we will drink more when working out. You now understand that moderate exercise intensity strengthens the immune system and that, unfortunately for some, exercise can become addictive. As you adjust to a physically active lifestyle, you will find that the benefits far outweigh the effort involved. Exercise will become a habit, and you will begin to look forward to your workout as an important part of your day. You have also become aware of the health consequences of using performance-enhancing drugs.

Let the words of Don Ardell inspire you to maximize your potential to be the best you can be: "Excellence ain't easy. If it were, everyone would be doing it and it would be ordinary. Know that, in lots of ways, the deck is stacked against anyone who wants to excel. Do it anyway."

Terms

- amenorrhea
- amphetamines
- anabolic steroids
- caffeine
- diuretics
- dysmenorrhea
- electrolytes
- estrogen
- exercise addiction
- female athlete triad
- hemoglobin
- hyperthermia
- hyponatremia
- hypothermia
- Kegel exercises
- menarche
- narcolepsy
- oligomenorrhea
- 'roid rage
- sarcopenia
- stress incontinence

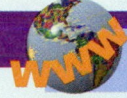 ## Internet Resources

AARP Health
www.aarp.org/health

Information on drugs, insurance, and staying healthy at 50 plus.

Administration of Aging
www.aoa.dhhs.gov

Department of Health and Human Services site that contains links on aging-related topics.

Alzheimer's Association
www.alz.org

Learn about what you can do to maintain a healthy brain.

American Diabetes Association
www.diabetes.org

Has an exercise section with FAQs, and information about cycling and walking events. It also provides news on the latest research, nutritional information, and even recipes.

Arthritis Foundation
www.arthritis.org

Has information on health and exercise tips concerning arthritis. Also provides tips about living with arthritis, and the latest research.

Cooper Institute for Aerobics Research
www.cooperinst.org

Provides information about exercise research.

Department of Health and Human Services Physical Activity Guidelines for Americans
www.health.gov/paguidelines

Summarizes the latest physical activity guidelines for Americans; for all age groups and virtually all populations.

Health A to Z
www.healthatoz.com

Includes health and medical search engines.

Healthfinder
www.healthfinder.gov

Consolidates official government health resources and offers links to over 500 health sites.

Mayo Clinic/Mayo Health Oasis
www.mayoclinic.com or www.mayohealth.org

A complete health and wellness library. Search by major subject area.

Medline Plus

www.medlineplus.gov

The National Library of Medicine's health information portal.

National High Blood Pressure Education Program

www.nh/bi.nih.gov

Learn how to lower high blood pressure.

National Institute on Aging

www.nih.gov/nia

Provides information on healthy aging and aging concerns.

National Osteoporosis Foundation

www.nof.org

Gives information and exercises.

National Osteoporosis Society

www.nos.org.uk

Provides information, exercises, and can answer questions.

National Women's Health Information Center

www.4women.gov

Contains women's health information.

Shape Up America

www.shapeup.org

Run by former surgeon general C. Everett Koop. Dedicated to educating and empowering consumers to improve their health.

Steroid Abuse

www.steroidabuse.gov

Provides information on steroid abuse.

U.S. Anti-Doping Organization

www.usantidoping.org

Information on the full list of banned drugs.

Name _____ **Class/Activity Section** _____ **Date** _____

Exploring Special Exercise Considerations Challenge

1. Your sister's gynecologist just told her she is pregnant. Knowing you are taking a college fitness/wellness course, she asks you for advice concerning the fitness walking program she began 2 months ago to help her get back into shape and lose a few pounds. Give her three or four tips.

2. At dinner, two of your friends were debating whether to use a popular sports drink to replace the sweat they expected to lose in the July 4 12-mile run, which they estimated would take *more* than 1 hour to complete. The July 4 festivities are tomorrow, with the race beginning at noon in Old Town and ending at the top of Heartbreak Hill. What advice would you give them?

3. Your grandparents (age 65) were advised by their neighbor to stop that "foolish" exercising, slow down, and start acting their age. They ask you your opinion about this advice. What can you tell them about the benefits of staying physically active?

4. In Speech 101, your topic for the final exam speech is "The Difference Between Men's and Women's Exercise Performance Levels: Are They More Alike Than Different?" List three similarities and three differences you want to highlight in your speech.

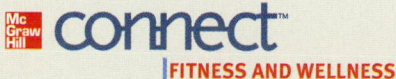

http://connect.mcgraw-hill.com

5. Take the "Are You Addicted to Exercise?" self-assessment in this chapter. How many "yes" statements did you check? _____ Discuss your assessment score. Have a friend you think may be becoming addicted to exercise also take the self-assessment in this chapter. How can you help a friend who may be becoming addicted to exercise?

6. Is there anything healthy people can do to boost their immunity?

7. Many of my friends are afraid to exercise outside during cold weather because they think they might freeze their lungs. How do you respond to that?

8. You suspect that your roommate, who is on the football team, is using steroids. He is really "bulking up" and bursts into a rage at the slightest irritations. What are other signs of anabolic steroid use? What are the health consequences?

9. Your grandmother has been diagnosed with osteoporosis and your grandfather has been taking medication for hypertension for several years. They want to begin an exercise program. List three or more dos and don'ts for each condition for them to follow.

CHAPTER 8

Preventing Common Injuries and Caring for the Lower Back

STUDY QUESTIONS

You will have successfully mastered this chapter if you can answer the following:

1. Can you identify four main reasons injuries occur?
2. Can you give three tips for avoiding an overuse injury?
3. How do muscle weakness and inflexibility contribute to injuries?
4. What are four common muscle imbalances?
5. Can you list and explain the general recommended treatment for common injuries (P.R.I.C.E.)?
6. What are the basic causes and treatment of ankle sprain, blisters, bursitis, chafing, heel spur syndrome, iliotibial band syndrome, muscle cramp, muscle soreness, muscle strain, patellofemoral syndrome, plantar fasciitis, shin splints, side stitch, stress fracture, and tendinitis?
7. What are the symptoms of injury that indicate the need for medical attention?
8. What are two vital components of rehabilitation needed to resume activity safely without injury?
9. What are the two most important keys to preventing lower back pain?
10. Can you describe exercises recommended to reduce the risk of lower back pain?

You will find the answers as you read this chapter.

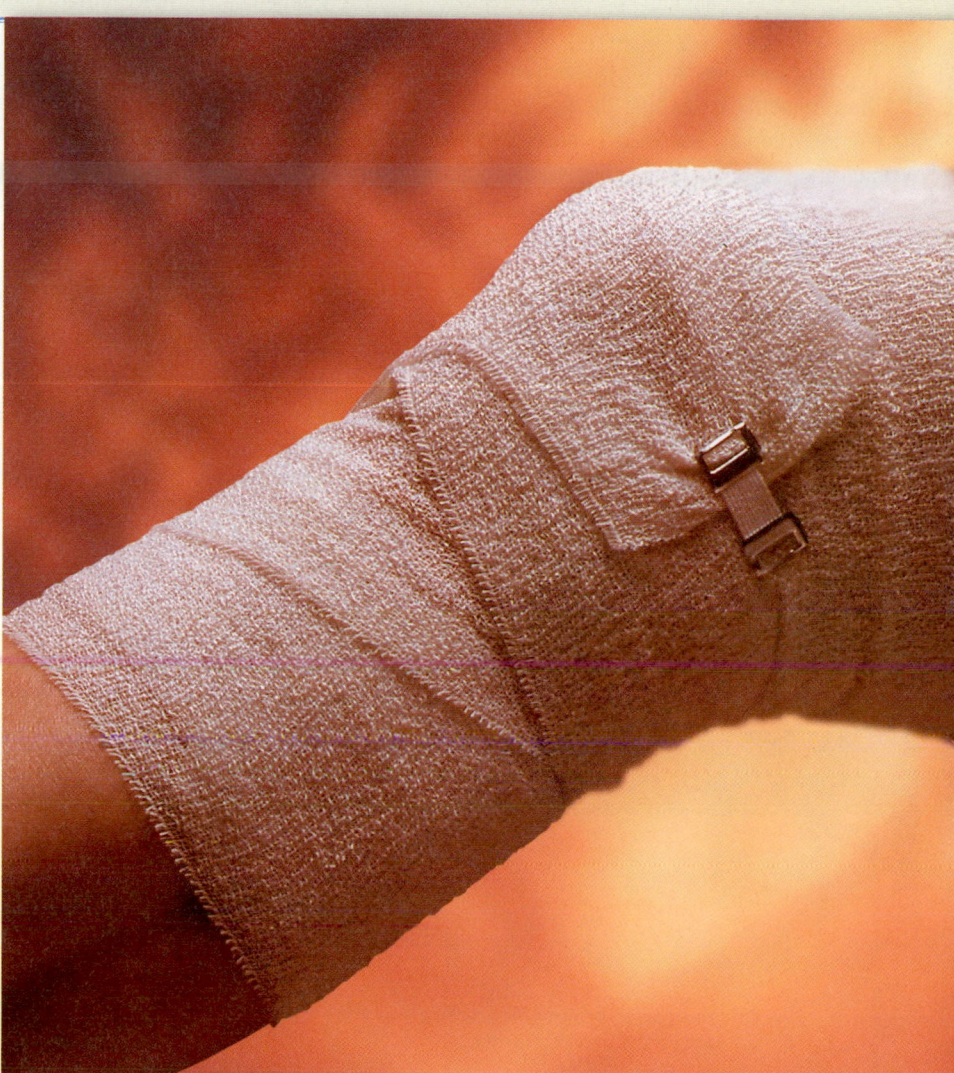

“ *An ounce of prevention is worth a ton of cure.* ”
—Anonymous

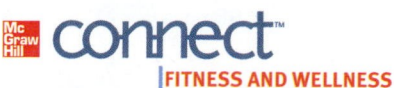

FITNESS AND WELLNESS

http://connect.mcgraw-hill.com

You walk into your first jogging class, eager to improve your fitness. You have not exercised regularly, and you hope this class will help you get in shape. Your instructor begins with a warm-up and an easy jog around campus. After your run, you feel great and invigorated. The next morning, you wake up and your whole body aches. You don't remember having been run over by a truck. "What should I do now? Withdraw from class? Stay in bed? Buy stock in Ben-Gay? When will I be able to move again?"

Participation in fitness activities offers many benefits. These benefits far exceed the risk of injury. When you exercise, you intentionally use certain muscles to increase their strength and endurance. As your body adapts to these efforts, you may experience minor aches and soreness. Physical activity also carries some risk of overuse or injury. Fortunately, many of these discomforts are minor, and you will be able to continue or quickly resume your workouts. Everybody is built differently and varies in physical potential, so "listen to your body" to improve your personal fitness level safely—and avoid the pain of injury. This chapter discusses how to prevent injuries, how to recognize their signs and symptoms, and what treatments are recommended. It also examines how to maintain a healthy back, because chronic back pain is a common problem. Finally, factors that affect the musculature of the spine and ways to avoid lower back injury are covered.

◆ INJURY PREVENTION

Prevention is the key to reducing the frequency of injuries. Ninety percent of injuries include slow wear and tear, strains, sprains, and inflammations. Understanding the causes of injuries allows you to stop minor problems before they turn you into the "walking wounded." Prevention is far more conducive to wellness than is any patch and repair job. There are four main reasons injuries occur:

1. *Overuse:* doing too much too soon or too often, causing a breakdown at the weakest point—ankle, Achilles tendon, shin, knee, or back.
2. *Footwear:* wearing improper or worn-out shoes.

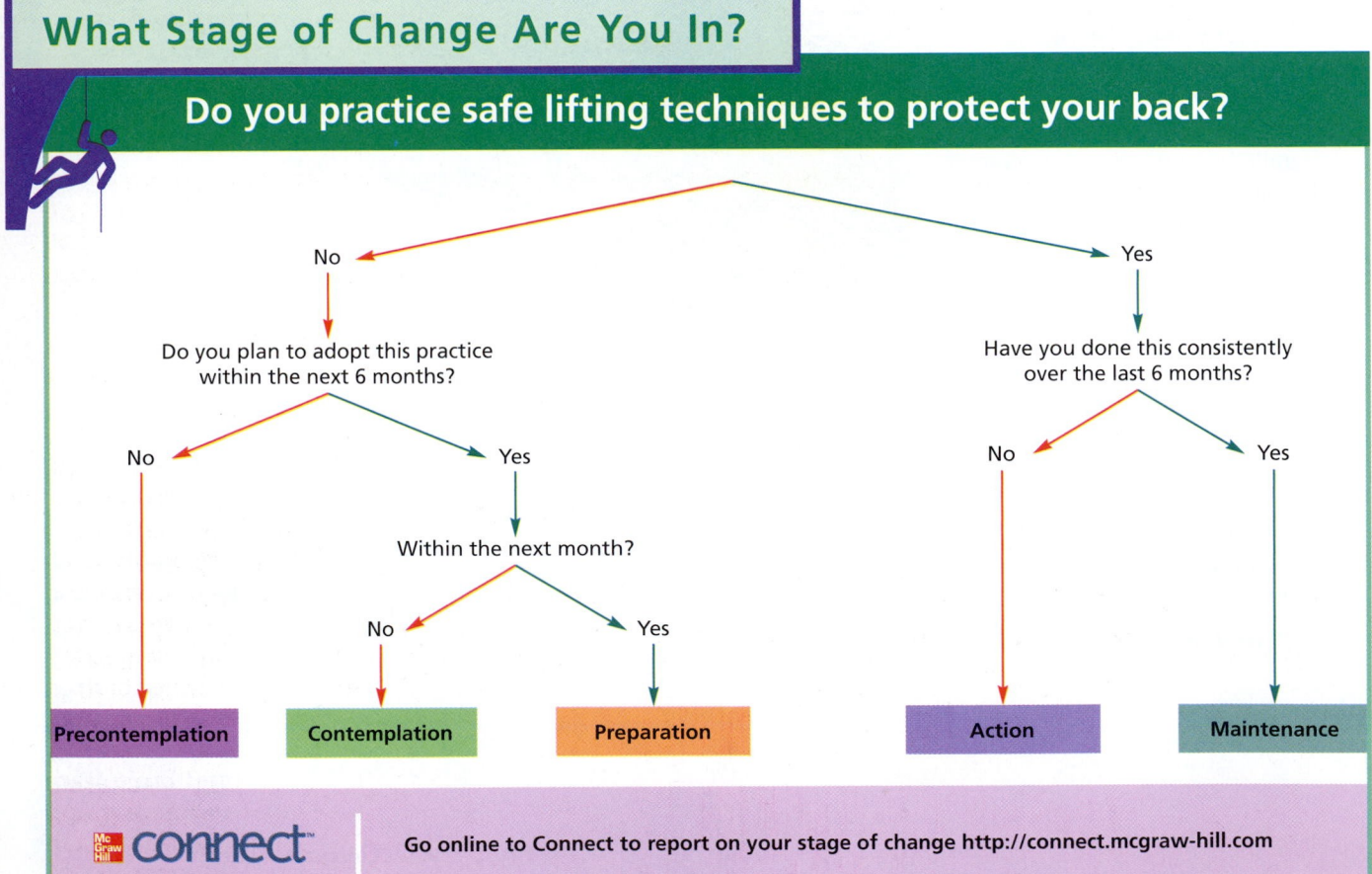

What Stage of Change Are You In?

Do you practice safe lifting techniques to protect your back?

- No
  - Do you plan to adopt this practice within the next 6 months?
    - No → **Precontemplation**
    - Yes
      - Within the next month?
        - No → **Contemplation**
        - Yes → **Preparation**
- Yes
  - Have you done this consistently over the last 6 months?
    - No → **Action**
    - Yes → **Maintenance**

Go online to Connect to report on your stage of change http://connect.mcgraw-hill.com

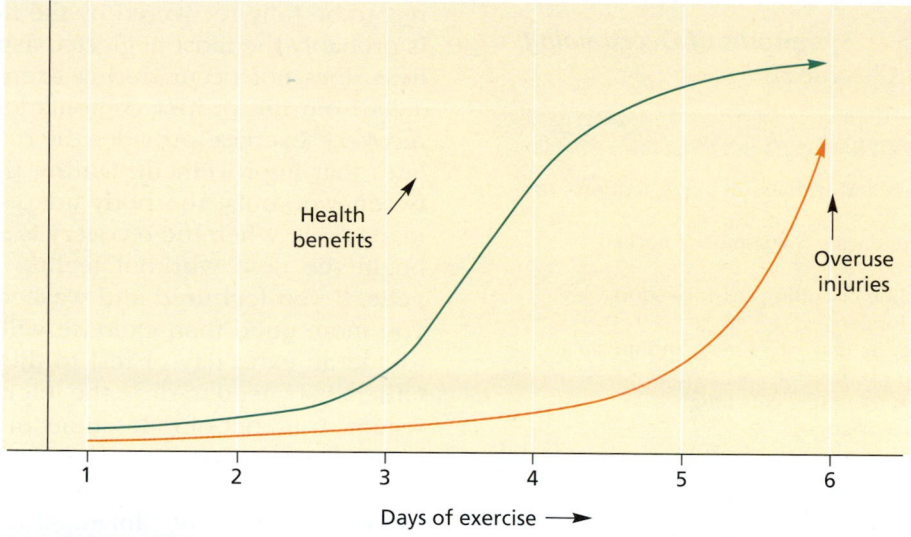

Health benefits

Overuse injuries

Days of exercise →

1 2 3 4 5 6

FIGURE 8-1   Overload is good up to a point. Overuse may cause injury. Health benefits accrue rapidly with 3 to 5 days per week of exercise. The risk of injuries increases with more than 5 days per week of exercise.

3. *Weakness and inflexibility:* muscles so weak or tight that the slightest unusual twist strains them.
4. *Mechanical problems:* the result of biomechanical/anatomical problems (the way the foot hits the ground, body build, etc.) or using poor form while exercising.

An individually adjusted workload, well-made and well-kept shoes, supplemental toning and stretching exercises, and mechanical improvements will prevent the majority of injuries.

Overuse

To improve or maintain fitness, you must overload, or push beyond normal demands. Progressive overload following the guidelines in Chapter 3 is necessary and good to a point, but you must be able to recover between workouts. The goal is to exercise so that you improve but not so much that you cause **overuse,** excessive overload leading to injury or illness (Figure 8-1). Overuse problems commonly occur at the beginning of a new exercise program and account for 25 to 50 percent of injuries. The first 2 months of a new program are the most critical. The body and muscles must be given time to adapt gradually to the new demands.

Set realistic goals early in a fitness program. Your instructor will help you determine an appropriate entry-level conditioning program and progression. Gradually increase your exercise intensity and duration to attain your personal goals. Try not to compete or compare yourself with friends who may be

able to exercise for a longer duration or at higher intensity. You will be able to catch up in time, but if you attempt to keep up with them before your body is ready, you risk an overuse problem.

A good rule of thumb when building your program is to increase the duration of the workout no more than 10 percent weekly. A beginner should not jump from a 20-minute workout up to 40 minutes. Also, do not increase both intensity and duration during the same week. Total time spent training per week is a pretty good predictor of injury. If

THE NUMBERS

17,000,000	Average annual number of Americans who sustain an exercise-related injury.
500	Miles of use in which your shoes will maintain their ability to absorb shock.
85%	Americans affected by low back pain at some time in their lives.
82%	Injuries that occur in the lower extremities.
78%	Injuries that are attributable to overuse.
10%	Maximum amount of time to safely increase exercise weekly.

TABLE 8-1   Symptoms of Overtraining, Overuse, and Chronic Fatigue

Signs in Your Training

- Persistent soreness and stiffness in joints, tendons, or muscles
- Labored breathing during a workout of normal intensity
- Performance decline or cutting sessions short
- Recovery taking longer
- Persistent lethargy, fatigue, weakness, and unusual lack of interest in exercise
- "Giving up" when the going gets tough
- Impaired muscular strength

Signs in Your Life

- Increased tension, anger, irritability, depression, mood changes
- No interest in activities you usually do, general apathy
- Poor concentration (general clumsiness, tripping, poor auto driving) and easily distracted
- Not sleeping well

Signs in Your Health

- Increased infections and colds
- Increases of six to eight beats per minute in morning resting pulse
- Swelling or aching lymph glands in neck, underarm, or groin area
- Skin eruptions in nonadolescents
- Constipation or diarrhea
- Loss of appetite, frequent nausea
- Chronic thirst
- Cuts and scars taking a long time to heal
- Inexplicable weight changes, either up or down
- Anemia or amenorrhea (in women)

training volume or intensity is too high and the recovery inadequate, tissue repair may be incomplete, resulting in overuse syndrome. Many fitness buffs and athletes have a feeling of invulnerability. They think their bodies can adapt to increased exercise workloads without any problem. Realize that more is not always better. By allowing your body to adjust gradually to new exercise demands, you will greatly reduce the risk of suffering an overuse injury. See Table 8-1 for symptoms of overtraining, overuse, and chronic fatigue.

Consider alternating an impact activity with a low-impact or nonimpact activity. This alternation gives the muscles a period of rest and recovery and switches the demands to a new muscle group. It is repetitive stress on the body that causes problems.

If you are getting the right amount of exercise, you should look good, feel good, and be alert and productive. After a workout, you should get enough rest to be fully recovered by the next workout. Rest is probably the most neglected aspect of fitness. Fitness does not occur during exercise alone but results from the proper combination of training and recovery. Exercise provides the overload that stimulates that improvement. During the rest period between workouts, the body adapts to the demands made on it. When the recovery is adequate, you will begin the next workout feeling strong and energetic. If you feel tired and washed out, rest will do you more good than exercise will. Some may need to add an extra day of rest to the weekly program. Others may need to drop the intensity of exercise or volume (number of miles, time, or number of sets or reps). Dehydration can be a major contributor to fatigue. Drink plenty of water daily—especially if you exercise in a hot climate. Also keep in mind that exercise isn't the only source of overstress. Other aspects of daily life, such as poor nutrition; emotional tension; job, social, or family problems; and lack of sleep, can contribute to chronic fatigue.

There is a difference between the pain of injury and the pain of hard effort. The concepts of "no pain, no gain" and "going for the burn" are useful in athletics but inappropriate for fitness exercisers whose goal is health, not athletic performance. Pain is the body's natural way of informing you that something is wrong. Do not try to exercise through pain or injury. Previous injury is a strong risk factor for future injuries. Allow time for healing, and correct mechanical problems before resuming activity.

Footwear

While many injuries are due to overuse, that is only part of the problem. Wearing improper or worn-out shoes places added stress on your hips, knees, ankles, and feet—the sites of up to 90 percent of sports injuries. The feet are the most abused and neglected part of the body. Good footwear can prevent many injuries and is the best investment you can make in an exercise program. Each time your foot hits the ground when you are jogging, the force of impact is three to five times your body weight. Your feet, ankles, shins, knees, hips, and lower back must absorb a tremendous amount of stress. If the stress is too great, breakdown occurs at the weakest link in the chain. A well-fitted pair of shoes is the first line of defense against impact injuries.

Shoes should provide good shock absorption, support, and stability yet maintain a reasonable degree of flexibility. In a normal footstrike, the initial contact and main wear area is the outer heel of the shoe. Your foot will naturally roll inward from outer heel contact to big toe pushoff when you jog;

therefore, the heel counter (the rigid plastic insert in the shoe's heel) must be firm to prevent excessive heel movement. The bottom of the shoe must have good traction to prevent slipping. Shoes are manufactured to be used for a certain number of miles, and they can lose their cushioning ability even if the uppers still look good. Each step compresses the sole, causing it to flatten and gradually lose shock absorbability. Exercise shoes typically lose about one-third of their ability to absorb shock after 400 to 500 miles of use. The upper part of the shoe stretches and weakens, decreasing lateral support. This happens so gradually that you may not notice it until you try on a new pair of shoes. With less cushioning and support, there is a greater chance of injury. If you wear the shoes 5 to 10 hours a week during exercise (walking, jogging, aerobics, etc.), you should probably replace them every 6 months to retain adequate cushioning. Runners would be well advised to keep a log of their mileage as a reminder of when to buy new shoes.

Weakness and Inflexibility

Sit down with your feet extended in front. Slowly reach toward your toes. Can you touch them without bending your knees? Many exercisers who neglect flexibility exercises cannot pass this test for minimal flexibility. Their legs are too tight, and this increases susceptibility to muscle and tendon injuries. Aerobic activities are great for the cardiorespiratory system, but they alone do not develop balanced fitness. They tend to shorten and tighten muscles that are used repetitively, leaving opposing, relatively unused muscles weak. This can lead to muscle imbalance. If some muscles are too tight, joint movement is restricted. Table 8-2 lists some common muscle imbalances. The solution to this problem is to stretch the tight muscles and strengthen the weak ones. A balance of strength and flexibility is important in injury prevention.

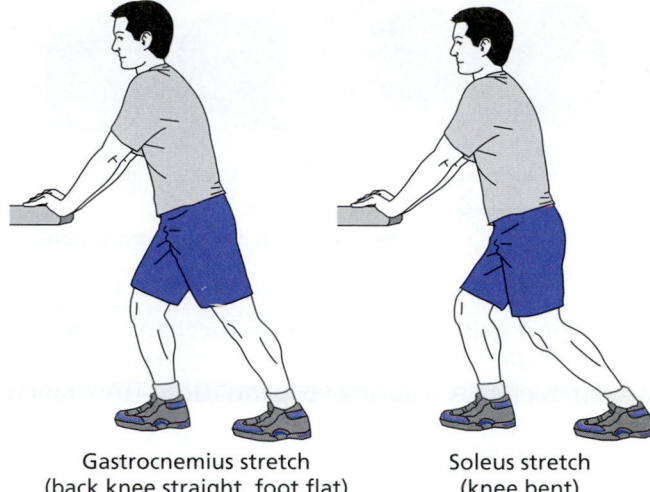

Gastrocnemius stretch
(back knee straight, foot flat)

Soleus stretch
(knee bent)

Good calf flexibility reduces the risk of Achilles tendinitis, plantar fasciitis, and shin splints.

Incorporate a basic stretching routine into each workout, preferably during the cool-down. (See Chapter 5 for recommended flexibility exercises.) Concentrate on event-specific exercises. For example, if you are a swimmer, you will want to spend additional time stretching the shoulders and arms. If jogging or aerobics is your activity, concentrate on stretching the hamstrings, quadriceps, lower back, and calves. Muscle strength may be more important in injury prevention than flexibility. Studies of tennis players show that those who do not do resistance training have more frequent injuries such as "tennis elbow." In swimmers, poor rotator cuff strength is a predictor of shoulder injury, and strengthening it reduces the frequency of shoulder problems. Abdominal curls are an important supplement to any fitness workout. Strong abdominals and a flexible lower back are critical in preventing lower back problems. See Chapter 6 for specific resistance training programs.

Mechanics

Structural weaknesses, affecting mainly the legs, knees, ankles, and feet, are often revealed when a beginner starts a new exercise program or when overuse occurs. Biomechanical difficulties often arise in the feet. The foot is a marvelous structure of 26 bones, with almost double that number of ligaments and muscles. It strikes the ground about 80 to 90 times a minute during exercise. When a weak foot pounds the ground several thousand times a day, the potential for injury is great. Slight **pronation** of the foot is natural—that is, your foot will roll inward slightly after the outer edge of the heel strikes the ground. All bodies are not created equal, so different

TABLE 8-2 Imbalances	Common Muscle
The rule of thumb in avoiding injuries is to *stretch* the muscles that are tight and *strengthen* the opposing muscles that are weak.	
Tight	**Weak**
Gastrocnemius (calf)	Tibialis anterior (shin)
Quadriceps (front of thigh)	Hamstrings (back of thigh)
Erector spinae (lower back)	Abdominals (stomach)
Pectorals (chest)	Rhomboids (Upper back)

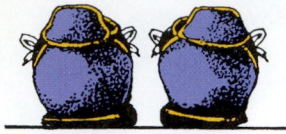 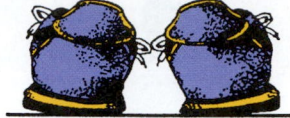

Underpronation   Overpronation

FIGURE 8-2   Underpronation and overpronation.

foot types, gait styles, and body mechanics vary in susceptibility to injury. For example, knock knees or flat feet may cause **overpronation**—too much inward roll when the foot should be pushing off (Figure 8-2). This twists the foot, shin, and knee and can cause tendinitis, plantar fasciitis, or knee strain. Observing the wear pattern on your shoes can help you select a shoe designed for your specific mechanics. Set your shoes on a flat surface. If they tilt inward and if there is excessive shoe wear on the inside of the forefoot, your feet may overpronate. If, in contrast, the outside of the shoe is overstretched and tilts outward and there is excessive wear on the outside of the shoe, your feet may pronate too little. **Underpronation** is insufficient inward roll of the foot upon contact. People with high arches and tight Achilles tendons tend to underpronate. When the foot hits the ground, it does not roll inward enough to absorb the shock of impact, increasing the risk of shin splints, stress fractures, iliotibial band syndrome, tendinitis, and plantar fasciitis. Underpronation causes excessive wear on the outside of the shoe sole.

Moderate pronation problems can be corrected through wise shoe selection. Most exercise shoes are designed to limit overpronation, not eliminate all inward rotation. A person who overpronates needs motion-control shoes with a straight or semicurved last and features that limit pronation. The best shoe for an underpronator has a curved last to allow normal pronation. Employees in many sports shoe stores are trained to help you select a proper shoe. If discomfort persists, you may want to consult a physician or podiatrist who will check your foot mechanics. He or she may prescribe **orthotics,** shoe inserts molded to your foot, to correct abnormalities. They allow the foot to operate with mechanical efficiency. They are highly effective for alleviating excessive foot under- or overpronation.

Regardless of your body type, pay attention to form when participating in any aerobic activity. In this way, many injuries and discomforts can be avoided. You will find technique and safety tips for a variety of aerobic activities in Chapter 4. You may also want to refer to the contraindicated exercises listed in Chapter 5.

The body is a marvelous mechanism. Considering its complexity, it is a wonder it doesn't break down more often. Exercise is vital to maintain wellness. Illness and injury are less common in those who maintain peak performance through regular exercise than it is in those who exercise sporadically. Even when injuries do occur, few are debilitating. Many simply cause some inconvenience. For a summary of tips on preventing injuries, see the accompanying Top 10 list. If we can't prevent all injuries, it is important to be able to recognize the signs and symptoms of those most commonly encountered by exercisers. This gives you an opportunity to take corrective action in the early stages and limit downtime.

◆ P.R.I.C.E.

Acute injuries to muscles, joints, and tendons are often accompanied by swelling. Swelling causes pain and decreased range of motion. Rapid recovery

TABLE 8-3	*Recommended Treatment for Common Injuries*
P =	Protect from further injury
R =	Rest to allow healing and avoid tissue irritation
I =	Ice to reduce pain and swelling
C =	Compress with a wrap to control swelling
E =	Elevate to reduce swelling

requires keeping the swelling to a minimum. The aim of treatment is to assist the healing process. The recommended treatment for many injuries, whether mild or severe, is protect, rest, ice, compress, and elevate, or **P.R.I.C.E.** (see Table 8-3).

P = Protect

The classic advice of old-time coaches was to "run it off." On the contrary, it is important to protect the injured area from further tissue damage. Don't let the problem get worse. Look for the cause of the injury and remedy the situation. A medical professional might recommend that a more severely injured limb be protected with crutches, a splint, or sling. The aim is to minimize irritation, tissue bleeding, inflammation, and pain and provide optimal healing conditions.

R = Rest

The injured area should be rested for 24 to 72 hours or more, depending on the severity of the injury. A few days of rest from the activity in which the problem occurred might be sufficient to protect irritated tissue from reinjury while healing from a minor strain. Switching to a different activity, such as

swimming, cycling, or deep-water running, can rest a sore area and maintain your conditioning. A minor complaint can become a major problem if you keep aggravating the situation. Healing progresses more rapidly when stress to the area is reduced. Frequently, people will start back into their usual activity before they are ready, and will reinjure themselves. Wait until most of the pain and swelling have subsided and you have regained 80 percent of your normal range of motion compared with the uninjured side. If you are unable to exercise for a week, when you return to your usual workout routine, reduce your duration, frequency, and/or intensity by at least 25 percent. Do not resume your normal workout level until you are free of pain during and after exercise.

I = Ice

Apply ice to the injured part immediately. A convenient way to apply ice is to put ice cubes or crushed ice in a plastic freezer bag and place it on the injured area. A pound bag of frozen peas or corn also works well. You may apply the ice directly to the skin without risking freezing the skin. The ice may make the injured part ache for the first 5 to 10 minutes. Keep it on! When the area feels numb, discontinue the ice. This will give immediate pain relief and reduce inflammation and tissue damage.

How long will you need to leave the ice on? It varies with the amount of fat and muscle in the area being treated. Apply ice for about 10 minutes to areas with little fat and muscle, like fingers and toes. Apply the ice for 15 to 30 minutes to larger areas like an ankle or knee. Areas with a lot of fat and muscle, like a thigh, may need to be treated for up to 30–45 minutes for greatest effectiveness. Allow the area to rewarm for 45 minutes to an hour

For a serious injury, a medical professional may recommend a splint to protect and rest the area while healing.

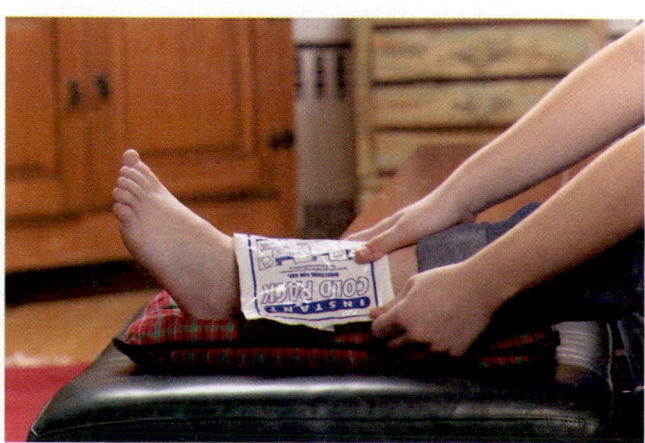

Apply ice to the injury immediately. This will give pain relief and reduce inflammation and tissue damage.

before icing again. What about frozen gel packs? Gel packs should be left on for only about 10 minutes because they are much colder than ice packs and have potential to cause tissue damage (frostbite). Ice is preferred because as it cools, it melts, and it is not likely to cause tissue damage. Ice the injured area every 3–4 hours for 48–72 hours or longer if pain and swelling persist. Ice should not be used by anyone who has diabetes, sensitivity to cold, or a medical condition with reduced blood flow to the arms or legs. These individuals need to seek medical advice for care of minor injuries.

If you feel mild discomfort when exercising and suspect an overuse injury such as tendinitis, you should apply ice to the tender areas right after you work out and reapply it several times a day for the next 48 hours or longer if pain lingers. Remember: You can never go wrong with ice. Sports medicine physician Francis G. O'Connor states, "Ice is indicated as long as inflammation persists—from the onset of the injury, through rehabilitation, and into sports return."

C = Compress

When not icing the injury, wrap the part with an elastic wrap to prevent fluid buildup in the injured area. Wrap it snugly but not tightly enough to interfere with circulation. If the part starts throbbing, the wrap may be on too tight. Remove the wrap and reapply it more loosely. Do not sleep with the wrap on.

E = Elevate

Raise the injured area above the level of the heart whenever possible. This will reduce the swelling by combating the effect of gravity pulling blood and fluids down to the injured area. Most people with an injured ankle or knee will place it on a pillow for elevation when going to sleep. However, you may move during the night and lose the elevation. Instead, place three or four books under the mattress to raise it approximately 6 to 8 inches.

◆ HEAT AND PAIN RELIEVERS

Many people mistakenly apply heat to an acute injury. Heat applied too early stimulates blood flow and increases swelling and inflammation. Stick with ice for at least the first 48–72 hours or more after an injury, and only then, *after swelling has completely subsided,* should heat be applied. At that point heat

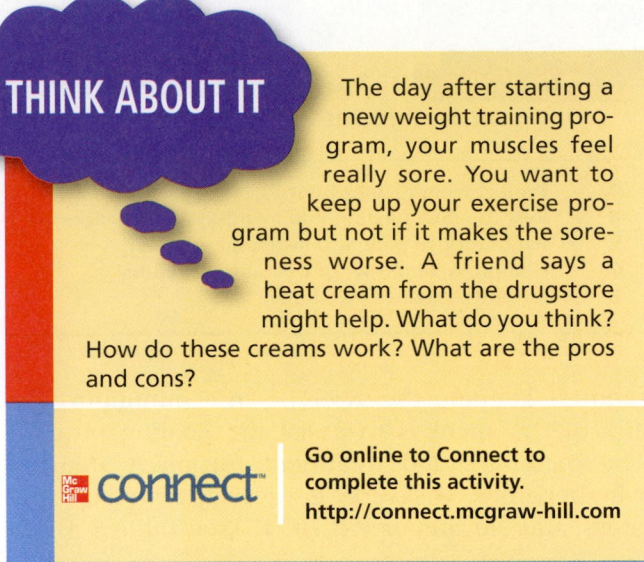

THINK ABOUT IT

The day after starting a new weight training program, your muscles feel really sore. You want to keep up your exercise program but not if it makes the soreness worse. A friend says a heat cream from the drugstore might help. What do you think? How do these creams work? What are the pros and cons?

connect™   Go online to Connect to complete this activity. http://connect.mcgraw-hill.com

may speed healing, relax muscles, and reduce stiffness. Either dry heat (heating pad or lamp) or moist heat (a hot bath, whirlpool, hot-water bottle, damp heat pack) will do. Apply the heat for 10–20 minutes, two or three times a day. You can also use it for 5–10 minutes before exercising to reduce stiffness.

Over-the-counter liniments and balms are popular methods for producing a warm feeling in muscles. The effect of these products is only superficial—the active ingredients stimulate sensory nerve endings in the skin to produce a sensation of heat. This has no healing effect and may mask the pain.

Aspirin or ibuprofen (such as Motrin or Advil) can reduce the pain and inflammation of minor sprains, strains, and tendinitis. Acetaminophen (such as Tylenol) is less helpful because it has no anti-inflammatory effect. Do not use anti-inflammatories to mask pain so that you can continue to work out—this will worsen an injury. Do not use the maximum recommended dose of these pain relievers more than 2 or 3 consecutive days because they increase risk of stomach bleeding. Consult your doctor before using any drugs.

◆ COMMON INJURIES

In pursuit of wellness, you may occasionally push yourself beyond the current capabilities of your structure. Finding your peak and keeping it is a challenge and part of a process of learning about your body's unique strengths and weaknesses. While some acute injuries are obvious, others can creep up slowly and gradually worsen. If, in your zeal to experience peak performance, you develop an athletic ailment, it will usually be minor and you will be able to resume

TABLE 8-4	Common Injuries, Symptoms, and Treatments	
Injury	**Symptoms**	**Treatment**
Ankle sprain	Pain, swelling, tenderness on the side of the ankle	P.R.I.C.E., anti-inflammatories Move in pain-free range, strengthen when pain and swelling subside
Blisters	Small fluid-filled skin swelling at a site of friction	Remove source of irritation, protect area, do not pop unless painful, use antiseptic and bandage, leave skin in place
Bursitis	Pain, swelling, loss of movement near a joint	Rest area, ice, anti-inflammatories
Chafing	Skin irritation from friction	Remove source of irritation Protect with petroleum jelly, clothing, or bandage
Heel spur	Pain underneath heel	Rest, anti-inflammatories, heel pad in shoe, calf stretch
Iliotibial band syndrome	Snapping, pain on side of hip or knee	Rest from causative activity, ice, iliotibial band stretch
Muscle cramp	Muscle spasm, tightness, and pain	Gently stretch and massage muscle Drink fluids, rest or decrease intensity of activity, increase dietary calcium and potassium
Muscle soreness	Muscle aching with movement 1 to 4 days after increased exercise	Hot shower to area, gentle stretching, heat, anti-inflammatories help somewhat
Muscle strain	Tightness, sharp pain, swelling Weakness, loss of use Usually began during activity	Rest from activity that caused strain, ice, stretch and strengthen after pain decreases
Patellofemoral syndrome	Knee pain, stiffness walking up and down stairs or after sitting	Ice, strengthen quadriceps
Plantar fasciitis	Heel or arch pain Usually worse in morning	Ice, stretch arch, heel lift, arch support, stretch calf
Shin splints	Pain in lower third of front of lower leg	Rest from activity that caused injury, ice, stretch calves, strengthen anterior tibialis
Side stitch	Pain in side during activity	Stop activity, stretch side, press on sore area
Stress fracture	Pinpoint pain, swelling along bone	See physician Discontinue causative activity until healed
Tendinitis	Swelling, tightness, pain with movement near a joint where muscle attaches to bone	Rest from causative activity, ice, gentle stretching when pain abates

activity within a few days. Here we discuss the potential causes of, symptoms of, and treatments for the most common injuries listed alphabetically. Table 8-4 gives a summary of these common injuries, their symptoms, and their treatments.

Ankle Sprain

A **sprain** is a partial or complete tear of a **ligament**, the fibrous connective tissue that binds bones together to form a joint. A sprain is most often a result of a sudden force, typically a twisting motion that surrounding muscles are not strong enough to control. Both ankles and knees are vulnerable to sprains. An ankle sprain will produce swelling and tenderness on the outside of the ankle. The amount of swelling depends on the severity of the injury. In severe cases, discoloration or bruising will develop. Range of motion in the ankle may be decreased by swelling and pain. P.R.I.C.E. for the first 72 hours is the best treatment for sprains. It is extremely important to control the amount of swelling in the joint in order to return to activity quickly. Strong, flexible muscles help protect against sprains. For example, to prevent ankle sprain, strengthen ankles with flexion, inversion, and eversion exercises. High-top shoes or a commercial ankle wrap will not reduce the risk of reinjury and can provide a false sense of confidence. When you start back into activity, progress gradually. A sprained ankle can take 1 to 2 months to heal.

Ankle sprains injure ligaments and the proprioceptors within them. **Proprioceptors** are sensory receptors found in muscles, tendons, and joints that enable you to sense the position and movements of your limbs. This position sense is important in balance. Studies have indicated that 4 weeks of balance training can reduce the risk of ankle sprains by one-third. A good start would be to stand on one foot while you are brushing your teeth. If that is too easy, stand on the ball of the foot, or close your eyes and try to balance for 60 seconds. Using tools like a balance board, bosu, or disc also can be helpful.

Blisters

Blisters are a common problem, especially for beginning exercisers. They are an accumulation of fluid under the skin due to excess friction. They are usually a problem only if they become infected or cause you to limp. The most common areas for blisters are the bottom of the foot, the sides of the big and little toes, and the back of the heel. Blisters can be prevented by eliminating the friction that causes them. Keep the feet as dry as possible and wear 100 percent acrylic (Orlon) socks. Acrylic is best at dissipating moisture and preventing blisters from forming. Cotton socks produce twice as many blisters, and even worse is a cotton-acrylic blend. One trick for preventing a blister is to apply a piece of duct tape over "a hot spot" *before* a blister forms. Also, cover or remove the irritation from inside the shoe. Never wear new shoes for a workout without first breaking them in by walking around in them at home for a few days. Should a blister be opened? Some say no; let the fluid reabsorb into the system because an open blister invites infection. Others say to pop the blister if it is painful and causes you to limp. The best treatment is to apply a donut pad and lubricant to the blister to reduce friction and pressure. To prevent blisters, some runners wear their socks inside out to avoid the abrasion of the rough interior seam. It may also help to wear two socks on the affected foot—a thin nylon sock inside an acrylic sock. If the blister is lanced, leave as much of the skin as possible covering the wound, and keep the area clean to prevent infection. Consult your physician if you think it may be infected.

Bursitis

Bursitis is inflammation of a bursa, a fluid-filled sac that lies between tissues and allows tendons, ligaments, muscles, and skin to glide smoothly over one another during activity. There are over 150 bursae, but the most commonly affected lie in the knee, elbow, shoulder, and hip. When a bursa becomes irritated because of overuse or training, it begins producing extra fluid. The sac swells, often within 24 hours, causing pain and limiting motion in the affected area. The recommended treatment is to protect the area, rest from activity, ice, compress with an elastic bandage to reduce swelling, and take anti-inflammatory medication. Do not wrap the knee tightly, however, as this could lead to blood clots by compressing the large vein behind the joint.

Chafing

When skin rubs against skin or against clothing, it becomes irritated and can crack and bleed. The most common problem areas are between the thighs, under the armpits, and on the nipples (runner's nipples). While chafing can happen to anyone, its frequency increases with greater body fat percentage. Treat chafing by applying petroleum jelly to the affected area. To prevent chafing, select clothing of smooth, nonabrasive material with few or well-covered seams. Synthetics are best. Avoid cotton because it stays wet, causing friction.

Avoid clothing that is tight or that bunches under the arms or between the legs. Wearing tights or knee-length exercise shorts can protect chafed thighs. Nipple chafing can be decreased by going shirtless in warm weather or by applying petroleum jelly and adhesive bandages to the nipples. Women should select a good exercise bra that has flat or covered seams.

Heel Spur

A **heel spur** is a bony growth on the underside of the calcaneus (heel bone) at the insertion of the plantar fascia. The pull of fascia on the heel can remodel the bone into a spur pointing toward the toes. Heel spurs are common and are not necessarily the sign of a problem. They do not always cause pain unless there is significant fat pad atrophy or unless they are caused by chronic irritation of the plantar fascia at its insertion. The heel pain of plantar fasciitis is sometimes associated with a heel spur. Treatment involves rest; anti-inflammatory medications; and insertion of a heel pad in the shoe to protect the heel, alleviate inflammation, and distribute impact during activity.

Iliotibial Band Syndrome

Tightness, burning, snapping, and pain on the side of the knee or hip may be related to inflammation of the **iliotibial band,** a long tendon that begins in the buttocks, runs down the side of the thigh, and attaches to the side of the lower leg just below the knee. Common in runners, an overtight iliotibial band may become inflamed from the friction of rubbing against the outer knee or hip bone as the knee repetitively flexes and extends. Pain may increase with running hills and is most intense at heel strike. Cyclists may experience ITBS due to a bike seat that is too high or bike cleats rotated inward. This is primarily an overuse injury and can be treated with decreasing or changing activity, ice, anti-inflammatories, strengthening hip abductors, and stretching the iliotibial band, hamstrings, and quadriceps (see stretches in Figure 5-1).

Muscle Cramp

A **cramp** is a sharp, involuntary muscle contraction. It may occur during exercise or at rest. The calf is the most common area for a muscle cramp to occur, but cramps may occur anywhere in the body. Muscle cramps may be caused by fatigue, which causes the nervous system to overstimulate muscles. Cramps may also be related to a strength imbalance, an electrolyte imbalance, or dehydration. Occasionally, low levels of circulating calcium or potassium in the blood can contribute to cramps. Cramps can be treated with fluid intake and with gradual stretching of the muscle. A calf cramp may be treated by extending the foot to a 90-degree angle. Occasionally, gentle massage may help.

Muscle cramps may be prevented by taking precautions when exercising in the heat. Wear light, loose clothing; drink water freely; gradually acclimatize yourself to the heat; and exercise during the cooler hours of the day. Improve fitness gradually and get plenty of potassium and calcium in your diet. Extra salt is not needed. A regular program of stretching may also help prevent muscle cramps.

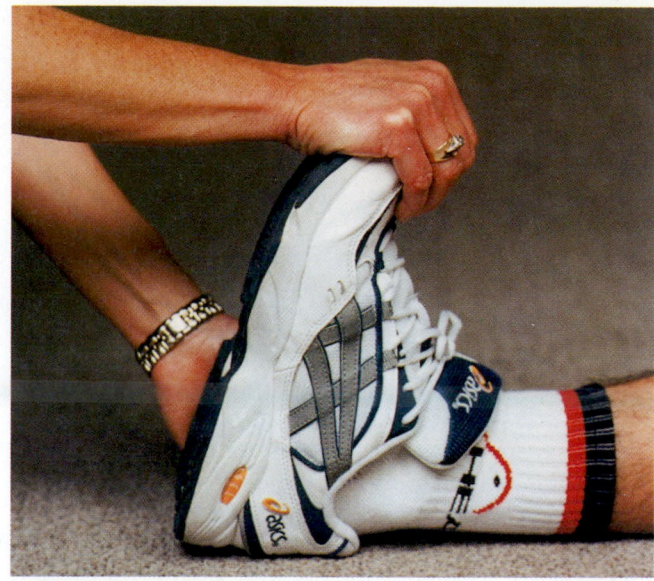

A calf cramp may be relieved by extending the foot and stretching the calf.

Muscle Soreness

Muscle soreness is discomfort or tenderness after an increase in workout level. It may be fairly mild and usually is just a reminder that you had a good workout. For example, a person who has not recently lifted weights will develop muscle soreness following the first workout. There is no real pain but rather a mild achiness when you move the major muscle groups used in the activity. After several sessions of the same activity, soreness will diminish or disappear. Intensity of muscle soreness is related to intensity of exercise, duration, and eccentric (lengthening) contractions. For example, running downhill repeatedly will produce more quadricep soreness than will an equal amount of flat or uphill running. Muscle soreness is thought to be caused by microscopic tears or spasms of the connective tissue. There is no long-term damage from this. Muscle soreness may develop immediately or over a 24- to 36-hour period following unaccustomed exercise and will usually disappear within 2 to 4 days. Other than following a sensible progression in activities and intensity, there is no real prevention for muscle soreness. This is a normal response to an increase in exertion and part of an adaptation process that causes muscles to recover and build, leading to greater strength and endurance. There is little that can be done for mild muscle soreness. While stretching is beneficial for flexibility, it has little effect on reducing soreness. If there is sharp pain rather than soreness during activity, the problem may be a muscle strain.

Muscle Strain

A muscle **strain** is a tear of muscle fibers or a tendon and is sometimes referred to as a *pull*. Symptoms include sharp pain, weakness with possible loss of function, spasm or extreme tightness, and tenderness to the touch. There are many different causes, but it most often results from a violent contraction of the muscle. A strain may be caused by fatigue, overexertion, muscle imbalance or weakness, or electrolyte or water imbalance.

A strain may range from mild (more painful than just soreness) to a complete rupture of the muscle. The muscles most likely to be affected are the hamstrings, gastrocnemius, Achilles tendon, erector spinae, groin, and the rotator cuff muscles of the shoulder. Rest, ice, and anti-inflammatories are used to treat muscle strain. Reduce or eliminate activity until the injury starts to heal. The severity of the injury and which muscle is injured will affect the recovery time. The hamstrings usually take the longest to heal and rehabilitate. If the strain is severe, it will heal with a significant amount of scar tissue, leaving it more susceptible to reinjury. Scar tissue is not elastic like muscle, so stretching and strengthening exercises are important to return to normal function. To prevent strains, complete a full warm-up before working out, take care not to overdo it, and work toward balancing the strength and flexibility in opposing muscles.

Patellofemoral Syndrome

Pain around and under the kneecap, along with knee stiffness, is characteristic of **patellofemoral syndrome.** Symptoms include a dull pain when walking up and down stairs, squatting, or after sitting with the knees bent for a period of time ("theater sign"), and occasionally mild swelling or a feeling that the knee is "giving way." Patellofemoral syndrome is associated with overuse, worn-out shoes, always running in the same direction on the track, excessive downhill running, and rapid ballistic movements such as those done in aerobics. One common cause is structural. Wide hips tend to make the quadriceps pull the kneecap out against the femur, producing inflammation. Loose kneecaps or a quadriceps muscle not strong enough to keep the patella in its groove may also lead to patellofemoral syndrome. The knee will not get better if you continue your activity during the injury.

Rest, ice, and anti-inflammatories are the conventional treatments for this injury. If the knee swells significantly, see a physician. Swelling can indicate a major problem and take much longer to heal.

To prevent recurrence, the knee must be rehabilitated. Low-impact activities are recommended to strengthen muscles, for example, swimming and bicycling. To stabilize the knee and assist in correcting the tracking mechanism of the patella, strengthen the quadriceps. Stretching should increase hamstring and iliotibial band flexibility. In severe cases, surgery may be indicated.

Plantar Fasciitis

Plantar fasciitis causes heel or arch pain. It is most painful when a person takes the first few steps in the morning, but in severe cases, pain may continue throughout the day. It results from micro tears of collagen fibers of the plantar fascia, a long thick band of connective tissue on the underside of the foot that attaches the base of the calcaneus to the base of the toes. Micro tears may result from excessive impact, worn shoes, or poor foot mechanics. Anatomical problems frequently cause plantar fasciitis—tight Achilles tendon, high arches, flat feet, or excessive pronation. Also, with age and repeated weight-bearing stress, the fat pad under the heel becomes flattened and less shock-absorbent. Rest, night splints,

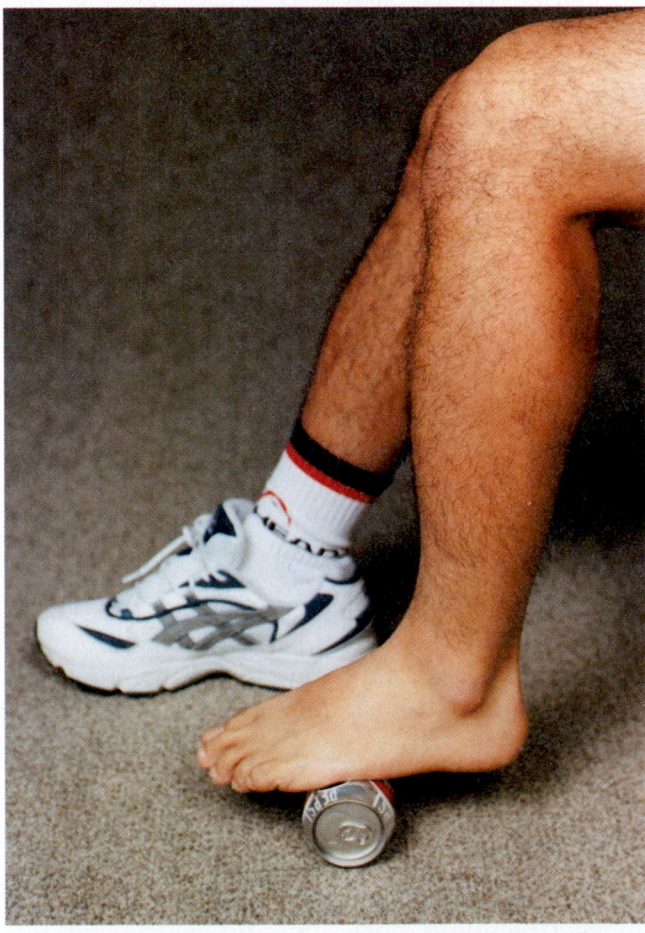

To treat plantar fasciitis, roll a cold can of soda under your arch to ice and stretch the fascia.

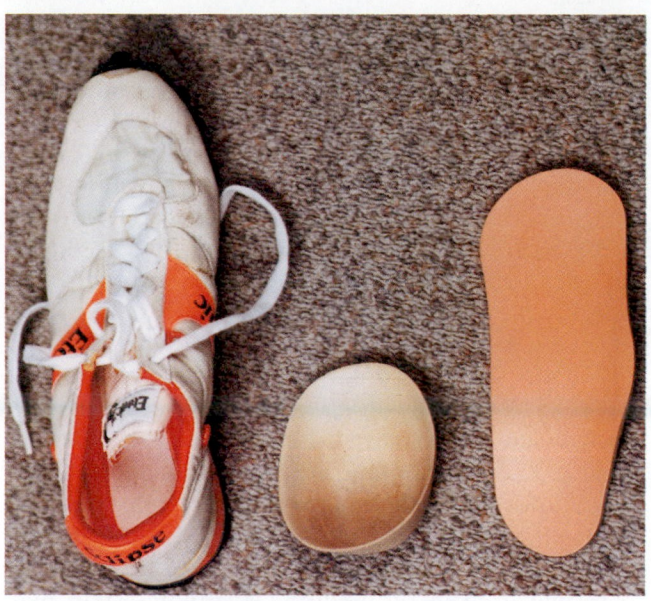

Orthotics or heel cups may reduce symptoms in persistent cases of plantar fasciitis.

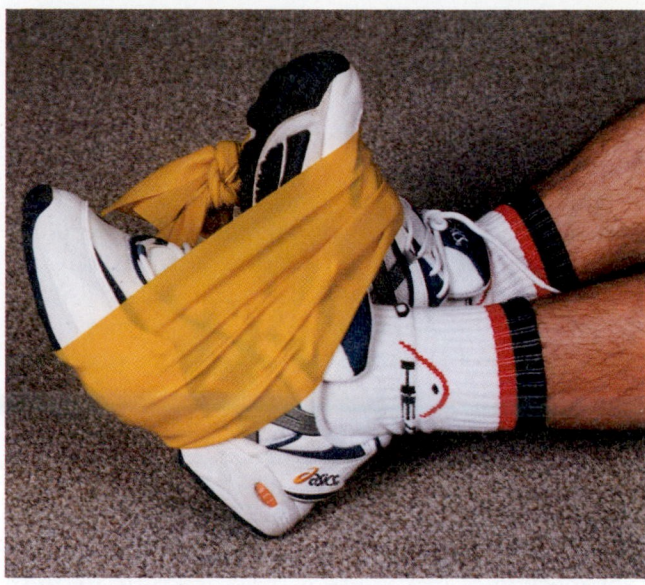

To decrease risk of shin splints, strengthen shins with a set of 15 to 20 toe pulls twice a week using an elastic band.

stretching the toes toward the face, calf stretching, ice, and arch supports or heel cups are the recommended treatments. Rolling a can of chilled soda or a frozen plastic bottle of water back and forth under the arch is a good way to apply cold to the area. Orthotics are often recommended to reduce symptoms in persistent/recurrent cases of plantar fasciitis.

Shin Splints

A **shin splint** refers to pain in the front of the lower leg (shin). Early signs are acute burning pain or irritation in the lower third of the anterior tibialis. This may progress to slight swelling, redness, warmth, and inflammation. A variety of factors contribute to shin splints. They often come early in an exercise program and are particularly common in those who are out of shape, overweight, wide-hipped, knock-kneed, or duck-footed. Working out on very hard or very soft surfaces can bring on shin splints even if a person is well conditioned. Switching from a hard to a soft surface or vice versa, excessive mileage, improper footwear, poor foot mechanics, running on a road slope, and running in the same direction all the time on an indoor track may cause them. Women, particularly those who wear high heels, are affected nearly three times more often than are men.

Shin splints may be a sign of a long arch problem in the foot. As the long arch begins to sag, it stretches lower leg muscles and causes pain. Another cause is a muscle imbalance between the strong calf muscle and the weak anterior tibialis, which may lead to inflammation of the membrane between the tibia and the fibula. This imbalance can be corrected with toe pulls to strengthen the anterior tibialis and by stretching the calf (see the photos in this chapter). These should be done each workout. If mechanical problems are not corrected, shin splints tend to recur.

To treat shin splints switch to a low- or nonimpact activity and rub ice on the affected area for 15 to 20 minutes three to four times a day. Aspirin therapy may be indicated for a few days to reduce inflammation. If the pain is persistent, consult a physician to rule out a stress fracture.

Side Stitch

A **side stitch** is a sharp pain just under the ribs, typically on the right side. It may result from participating in vigorous activity before the body has had a sufficient warm-up. It may be related to a lack of conditioning, weak abdominals, shallow breathing, consuming a meal too near the time of exercise, dehydration, excessive exercise intensity, or **ischemia** (inadequate oxygen) to the diaphragm. Side stitches tend to occur in unfit or new exercisers. Better conditioning brings more efficient blood flow and oxygen delivery to the respiratory muscles. To prevent side stitches, warm up well, increase exercise intensity gradually, and avoid eating 1 to 2 hours before a vigorous workout. Side stitches can be treated by stopping activity and stretching, massaging, or pressing on the painful area. After cessation of the activity for a few minutes, the pain and spasm should subside. Taking a deep breath may also break the spasm. Once the pain has dissipated, activity may resume.

Stress Fracture

A **stress fracture** is a microscopic break in a bone caused by overuse. While it can occur anywhere in the lower legs and feet, it is most common at the end of the tibia near the ankle and in the metatarsals of the feet. Unlike a broken bone that occurs with a distinct traumatic event, a stress fracture is the result of cumulative overload that occurs over many days or weeks. Overtraining and overly rapid increases in training are the major causes. Bone is living tissue that adjusts to the exercise force demands placed on it. As force is applied, bone will remodel itself to handle the force better. If too much force is applied, the bone may fracture before it can successfully remodel. Running excessive mileage, overdoing impact aerobics, wearing worn-out shoes, exercising on hard surfaces such as asphalt or concrete, and having poor foot mechanics may cause a stress fracture. Because they have smaller, lighter bones, women are more susceptible to stress fractures than are men. Especially when combined with hard training, an inadequate intake of calcium and vitamin D can predispose one to the onset—and recurrence—of stress fractures.

A stress fracture may be confused with a case of severe shin splints, but stress fractures are more likely to cause pinpoint pain on the sore bone. Stress fractures are difficult to detect clinically. Frequently, they will not show up on an X ray until 3 to 4 weeks after the onset of symptoms. A bone scan can detect a stress fracture much earlier in the injury because it reveals the active bone formation that occurs while the fracture is healing. The pain of a stress fracture will not go away with conventional treatments (ice, ultrasound) or medication. Only rest will decrease the pain.

The best treatment for a stress fracture is rest from the activity that caused it. This does not mean elimination of exercise altogether. Nonimpact activities such as riding a bicycle and swimming are good alternatives during the healing phase. Depending on the severity of the stress fracture, activity may be resumed within 2 to 6 weeks of diagnosis. "Running through the injury" is not recommended. This may lead to a nonunion fracture of the bone and a 6- to 8-week recovery period in a cast.

Tendinitis

Anytime you see "-itis," think inflammation. **Tendinitis** is the inflammation of a tendon from repetitive stress. Common signs of inflammation include pain, redness, heat, and swelling. **Tendons** are the fibrous cords that connect muscles to bones. They are vulnerable to inflammation because the force of muscle contractions is transmitted through them. The most commonly affected in runners, walkers, and aerobic

dancers is the Achilles tendon, which connects two calf muscles, the gastrocnemius and soleus, to the back of the heel bone. Other areas commonly affected are the knee, shoulder, and elbow ("tennis elbow"). When a tendon is inflamed, normal daily activities, such as opening a door and walking up the stairs, can be painful. Tendinitis is often brought on by muscle tightness or increasing the workload too quickly. Achilles tendon problems are often due to tight calf muscles. When the foot flexes to push off, the powerful Achilles pulls the heel up. If the calf is too tight, it yanks the heel up prematurely, stressing the Achilles tendon. Rest from the activity that caused the injury and stretching the calves to alleviate excessive tightness are recommended. Over-the-counter anti-inflammatory medications (ibuprofen, aspirin) may also help. It may take 2 to 3 weeks to heal and rehabilitate completely. Continuing activity will only delay healing. Meanwhile, you may include alternative activities to maintain fitness. A regular program incorporating stretching and strengthening can help prevent tendinitis.

 ## WHEN TO SEEK MEDICAL HELP

Not all injuries can be self-treated. If symptoms are severe or if self-treatment is not working, you need professional medical treatment. You should seek medical assistance for an injury if you experience any of the symptoms in Table 8-5.

Once injured, whom should you see? Your family doctor will be able to treat common sprains and strains. However, there are other sports injury

TABLE 8-5	*Medical Help*

Seek medical help when:

1. The injury is extremely painful or the pain has not decreased in intensity within a day or two. You are unable to bear complete weight on that part or are unable to walk more than three or four steps without significant pain.
2. There is joint pain lasting more than 2 days or significant tenderness when you press on a specific spot in a joint, muscle, or bone, such as a bony part of the foot.
3. There is a loss of strength or range of motion (compared with the uninjured side) and loss of the ability to do normal tasks.
4. The limb gives way when you try to use it.
5. You heard a distinct "pop" or "snap" when the injury occurred.
6. The injured area, compared with the uninjured side, looks misshapen or has unusual lumps (other than swelling).
7. There is numbness or tingling in the injured area, which may indicate nerve compression.

TABLE 8-6	*Injury Specialists*

Physical Therapists: These therapists are licensed by the state to administer rehabilitative techniques—from ultrasound to strength and flexibility exercises. Some states require a doctor's referral before visiting a registered physical therapist.

Athletic Trainers: Many colleges, universities, and sports medicine clinics have athletic trainers who have extensive knowledge of and experience in dealing with injuries. They are highly trained and must pass rigorous written and practical examinations to become certified.

Sports Medicine Clinics: Many clinics have "walk-in" hours and are likely to include some of the specialists already mentioned as part of their staffs.

Orthopedists: These MDs with specialized surgical training treat injuries to any part of the musculoskeletal system. Many specialize in athletic injuries.

Podiatrists: These DPMs (doctors of podiatric medicine) treat foot-related problems common to fitness-related injuries. Though not MDs, they receive special training and are state-licensed. They can prescribe medications, design orthotics, and perform some surgeries.

Chiropractors: These DCs (doctors of chiropractic), believing that the alignment of the spine and proper nerve function are essential to body functioning, use manual manipulation and other techniques to relieve pain and structural disorders.

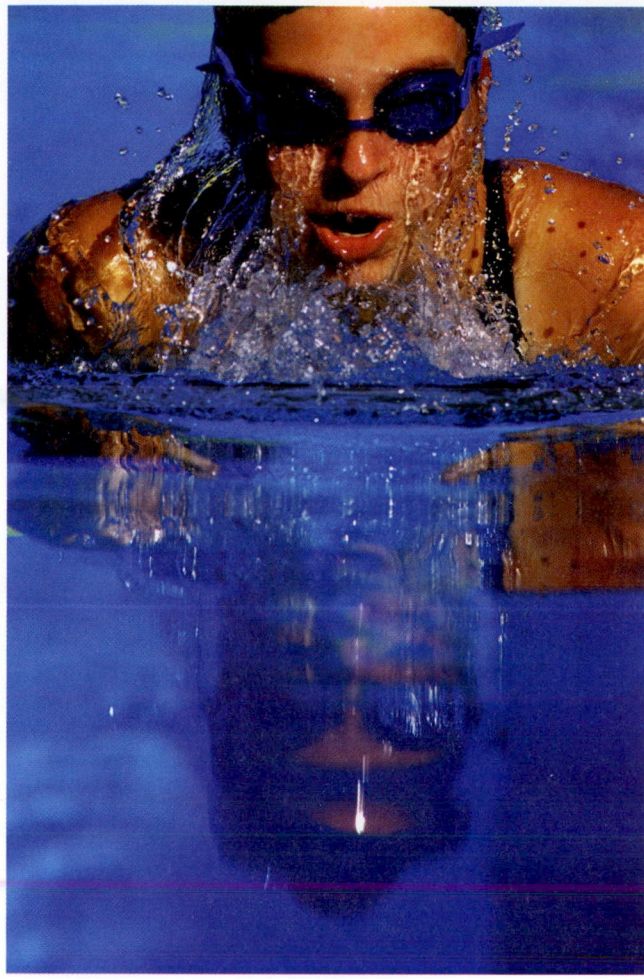

While recovering from an injury, switching to a nonimpact activity such as swimming can maintain your aerobic fitness.

specialists who can help. Table 8-6 describes some of these specialists.

Communicating with a doctor is an important step in assuming an active role in your health care. Be sure to tell the physician how the injury occurred: what you felt, signs and symptoms, and any additional information to aid in diagnosing the injury. Do not feel rushed or intimidated by confusing terminology and tests. You are the consumer and are paying for the doctor's time and services. Do not rely on the nurse, the receptionist, or a friend to explain your injury and treatment. Make sure you completely understand everything you must do to speed your recovery.

◆ GETTING BACK INTO ACTION

There are three steps to getting back into action after an injury. First, move the injured part as early as possible, within a pain-free range, to regain flexibility. This motion will increase circulation and reduce stiffness and swelling. As you are able, work all the

motions of a joint. For example, in an ankle injury, move the ankle up and down, in and out, 10 to 20 times, three to four times a day. Gradually increase the range of motion. If you feel pain after moving the part, it should subside within 1 hour. Apply ice and reduce the amount of repetitions in the next session. You may be doing too much too soon.

Second, after obtaining at least 80 percent pain-free range of motion, begin to build strength. Gradually increase the strength of a part to equal that of the uninjured side. You can use partner resistance, free weights, rubber tubing, or weight machines. If possible, work under the supervision of a qualified physical therapist or another rehabilitation professional, especially in the early stages of rehabilitation, because this is when you are most susceptible to reinjury.

Third, gradually work your way back to your former activity level. Do not expect to start where you stopped. Frequently, exercisers will try to begin working out at their previous level after merely reducing swelling and pain. Healing may not yet be complete. The result is often reinjury because the weakened area is unable to withstand the stress. Overload should be gradual, with the realization that *more* is not always *better*. If in doubt, start at the lowest level for your activity in Chapter 4 and increase that time by no more than 10 percent per week. While recovering from an injury, participating in a nonimpact activity such as deepwater running, swimming, and stationary cycling can maintain endurance.

◆ CARE OF THE LOWER BACK

Without question, back pain is one of the most common conditions affecting Americans—second only to the common cold as a reason for seeing a physician. Eighty percent of Americans will experience back pain some time in their lives. Back pain affects a largely youthful population, with the first back pain episodes afflicting people in their twenties and thirties. One of the main contributors to this epidemic of poor back health is a sedentary lifestyle (and spending hours hunched over a computer or working at a desk). Fortunately, most back pain is preventable with exercise, good posture, and good lifting mechanics.

Ways to Avoid Lower Back Pain

Why does back pain occur? How can risk of back injury be reduced? We often take a healthy back for

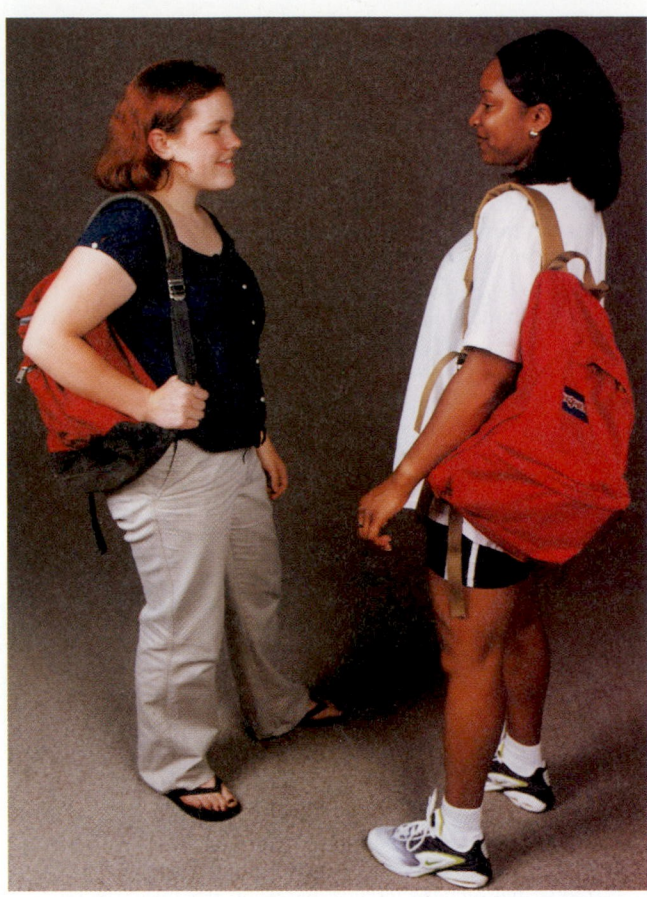

Habitually carrying a heavy backpack on one shoulder may cause back pain.

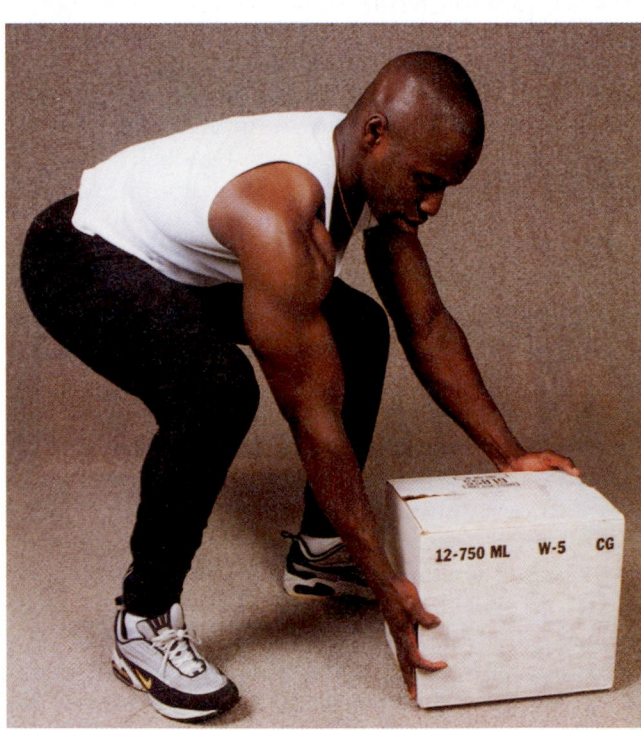

Correct lifting technique.

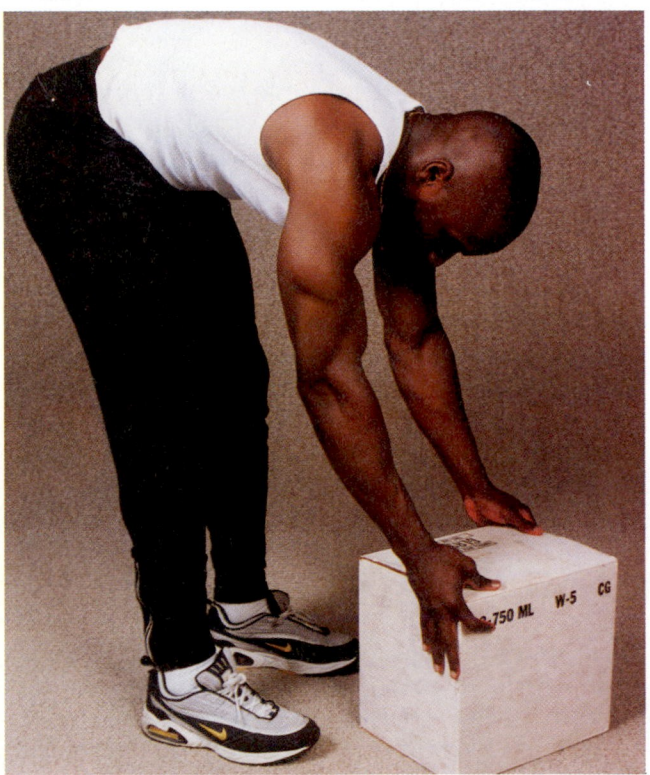

Incorrect lifting technique.

granted until something goes wrong. Back problems are rarely caused by a single, isolated factor. The 32-year-old computer programmer who hurts his back while pulling the lawn mower chain prefers to blame the lawn mower. His condition may actually be a result of several years of abuse and neglect. The pull on the lawn mower chain merely "triggered" the condition. During high school and college years, our bodies are relatively flexible. As we age, muscles begin to shorten and tighten, decreasing flexibility, especially in the back. Combine this with possible weight gain and declining overall fitness and it becomes evident why back pain afflicts millions. With few exceptions, back problems can be prevented with improved fitness, living and work habits, and posture.

The most important key to preventing lower back pain is maintaining strong abdominal muscles and back flexibility. Studies show that people who are physically fit have almost 10 times less back pain. Many of those who suffer back pain are overweight and have weak, sagging abdominals and short, tight back muscles. This puts additional stress on the spinal column. Maintaining normal weight and keeping abdominal muscles strong and tight reduces strain on the spine. Strong abdominals keep the pelvis and spinal column stabilized in a normal position. At the same time, it is important to keep the opposing back muscles and hamstrings flexible. People with chronic back problems need to stretch and strengthen regularly, using the exercises in Figure 8-3. Exercise, not rest, is recommended for most people with back problems.

Sleeping position plays a role in back health. The one-third of your life you spend sleeping should help, not harm, your back. This makes it important to select a firm but not extremely hard mattress. Sleeping on a mattress that is too hard will leave the back unsupported. Sleeping on a sagging mattress places the back in an unbalanced position. Water beds, properly adjusted, may provide satisfactory back support as an alternative to a traditional mattress.

The fetal position is the best sleeping position for maintaining a healthy back. Lie on your side, pull your knees up to your chest, and put a pillow between your knees. This will round the lower back and alleviate back stress. If you must sleep on your back, place a pillow or similar object under your knees to relax the lower back. Sleeping on your stomach increases the arch of the back, shortening the back muscles. Placing a small pillow, or even your arm, under your pelvic bone (abdomen) may help reduce strain on your back.

To decrease back stress when getting out of bed, roll to one side and sit up sideways, using your arms to help. This will eliminate using all your back and abdominal muscles to get out of bed. This tip is especially helpful if you currently have a back problem.

Good lifting mechanics can reduce the risk of lower back injury. When lifting a heavy weight, bend your knees as if sitting down; keep your head up and looking straight ahead. Your trunk should be held as erect as possible to maintain a neutral spine, and you should use the large muscles of the buttocks and legs to lift. It is also important not to let the knees pass the toes as you squat in order to avoid excessive knee stress. Combining lifting with a twisting force is one of the most common causes of back injury. Instead, lift the object and pivot with your feet rather than your waist.

Keep your body close to the object. Standing far away from the object will place undue stress on the lower back. Lift with your back straight rather than bent at the waist. When carrying heavy objects such as books, backpacks, and groceries, try to distribute the load equally and close to the body. Do not carry a backpack on one shoulder, as this puts uneven stress on back muscles and is a common cause of back pain. Finally, obtain help when lifting heavy objects. See the Top 10 "Ways to Improve Back Health."

Back Tips for Sitting, Standing, and Driving

Many Americans spend the majority of their time behind desks or in cars. Sedentary jobs and lifestyle make us vulnerable to back pain. How can you maintain a healthy back if you spend a lot of time sitting at a desk? Sit close to your work and keep your hips and knees at a 90-degree angle. Your head should be positioned in line with your shoulder, and your chin should be parallel to the floor. This will straighten the lower back and prevent slouching. When you sit in a chair, place both feet on the floor. If the chair is too low, it will increase your back curvature excessively. Use a chair that

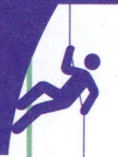

Tips for Behavior Change

- Read the section in this chapter on safe lifting and observe the photos.
- Bend your knees when you lift.
- Lift with your head up and shoulders erect.
- When lifting, pivot with your feet. Do not twist your back.
- Keep your feet hip width apart for stability.

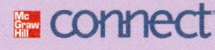 Go online to Connect to complete this activity. http://connect.mcgraw-hill.com

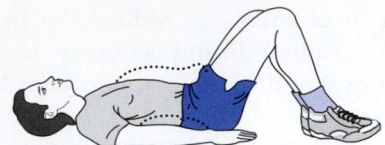

1. Pelvic tilt. Lie on back, knees bent. Press small of back firmly down to floor by tightening the abdominal muscles. Hold for a count of 5.

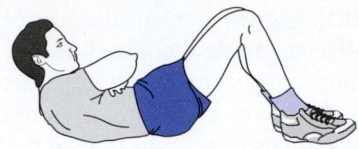

2. Abdominal curl. Do a pelvic tilt and, while holding this position, curl head and shoulders up until shoulder blades have been lifted from the floor. Hold briefly. Lower slowly.

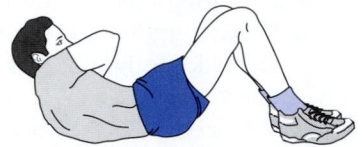

3. Oblique abdominal curl. Do a pelvic tilt and, while holding this position, curl head and shoulders up, twisting right shoulder toward left knee. Hold briefly. Lower slowly. Repeat on other side.

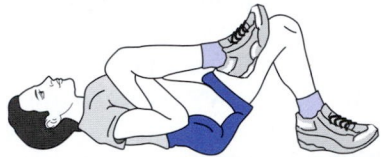

4. Low back stretch. (a) Lie on back. Pull one knee toward chest. Hold for a count of 5. Repeat with other leg. (b) Double knee pull. Pull both knees to chest; hold for a count of 5.

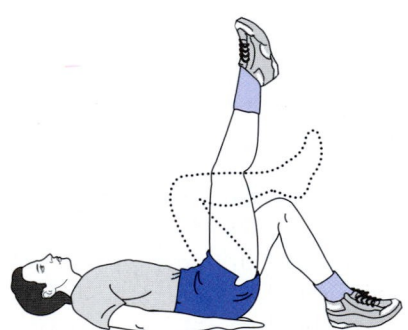

5. Lying hamstring stretch. Lie on back. Bring knee toward chest and extend leg toward ceiling. Flex foot. (You may grasp the back of your thigh with your hands.) Hold 20 seconds. Repeat with other leg.

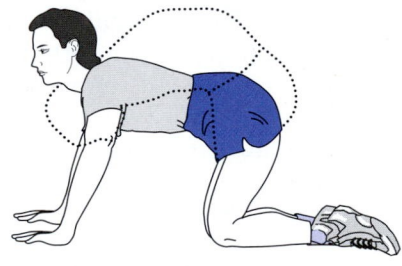

6. Cat stretch. Start on all fours. Round the back upward like a cat. Tighten abdominals. Hold for 5 seconds. Relax and return to starting position. Do not let back sag.

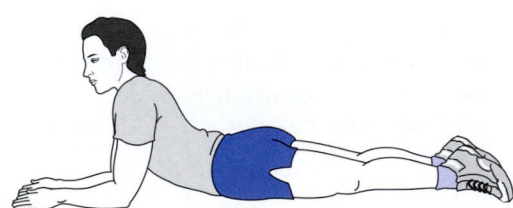

7. Upper back lift. Lie on your stomach with forearms flat on the ground. Tighten abdominals. Lift upper body by using back muscles. Do not press with arms. Hold for a count of 5.

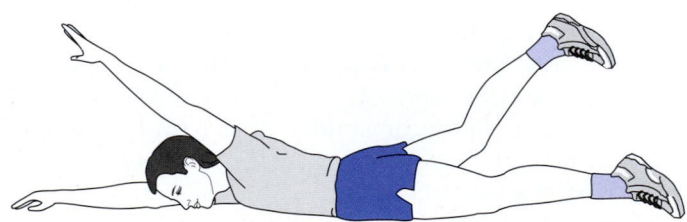

8. Alternate arm/leg lift. Lie on your stomach with arms extended in front. Raise one arm overhead toward ceiling while simultaneously lifting the opposite leg. Hold for a count of 5. Repeat with the other arm and leg.

FIGURE 8-3   **Exercises for the lower back.**

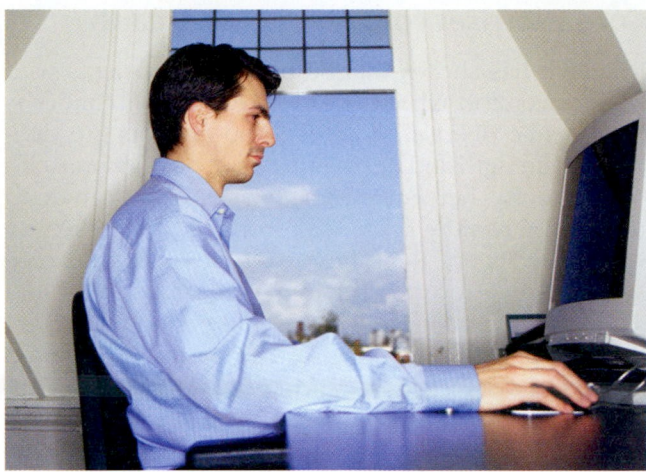

If you spend a lot of time behind a desk, sitting with good alignment can reduce the risk of back, neck, and shoulder pain.

supports your back in its normal slightly arched position, or you can place a small pillow or towel against your lower back. Remove this low back support for a few minutes every half hour to allow your back to change position.

Maintain good posture while driving, especially when driving long distances. Sitting for extended periods in an automobile is a common cause of back pain. To maintain normal spinal curvature, place a small pillow between your lower back and the seat. Sit close enough to reach the accelerator and steering wheel without slumping.

If your job requires long periods of standing, you can minimize stress on the back by putting one foot on a low stool. Frequently shift your weight from one leg to the other. Some occupations put unusual physical stress on the back. Dentists, nurses, and musicians may sit, lift, or move in twisted, awkward positions.

Wearing high-heeled shoes is unhealthy for the lower back. This shortens the Achilles tendon and hamstrings, throws the back into an overarched position, and overstretches the abdominals. Wear low-heeled shoes to maintain back health.

A common cause of pain farther up the spine is holding the phone between your ear and shoulder, which is usually done to free the hands. When your neck is scrunched to one side frequently throughout the day, it can cause headaches and neck and upper back or shoulder pain. If you use the phone a lot, to prevent neck and shoulder problems, try this:

✓ Use a hands-free receiver or buy an inexpensive phone rest that holds the receiver on your shoulder so that you don't have to twist your neck.

TOP 10 LIST

Ways to Improve Back Health

1. **Stretch and strengthen.** Weak, tight muscles invite injury. Strengthen the abdominals with abdominal curls and do back stretching/strengthening exercises to maintain a strong, flexible spine (see Figure 8-3).

2. **Use good sitting posture.** Sitting for hours hunched in front of a computer screen can overstress back muscles. Sit erect, knees level with hips, feet flat on the floor. Add a towel roll behind your back to maintain the natural spinal curve.

3. **Use good standing posture.** To decrease back stress, stand with one foot elevated a few inches on a box to relax the back.

4. **Change positions frequently.** When sitting, take frequent breaks—1 to 2 minutes every 30 to 60 minutes. Stand up, stretch, move around. When standing, vary your body position and shift weight frequently.

5. **Use good sleeping posture.** Sleep on your side with knees bent and a pillow between your knees to relax your back. If you prefer sleeping on your back, put a pillow under your knees to reduce back stress. Avoid sleeping on your stomach.

6. **Use good lifting techniques.** Stand close to the object and bend your knees as if sitting down, keeping the back straight and head up. Tighten your abdominals and lift with your legs, keeping the object close to your body. Avoid bending from the waist and twisting as you lift.

7. **Don't overdo it.** Know your limits. Weekend bouts of yard work, such as 2 to 3 hours of gardening and raking the lawn on Saturday, and playing 2 hours of basketball when you've been sitting behind a desk all week overstress the back. Spread out the work and play in shorter bouts over a few days to give your muscles a chance to adjust.

8. **Keep active.** Maintaining a base of fitness throughout the week enables you to go canoeing, play ball, or do that yard work on the weekend with less risk of a stiff, sore back compared with a couch potato.

9. **Manage your weight.** Carrying extra pounds in front increases the load your back must support. Losing weight decreases back stress 24 hours a day.

10. **Distribute the load.** Habitually carrying a heavy bag, books, or backpack on one side creates uneven spinal stresses. Evenly distribute the load or switch sides to even out the stresses.

✓ Use a clipboard to secure your papers so that your hands are free.
✓ Try a speaker phone or headset.
✓ Hold the phone in the hand opposite the one you usually write with and make a conscious effort to avoid twisting your neck.

If you must sit, stand, or work in one position for an extended time, get up, stretch, and walk for several minutes. You will feel better, and your back will benefit from the change.

Not to be overlooked is the effect of emotional stress on back health. Stress produces tension, which increases sensitivity to pain, which creates more stress. The stress → tension → pain cycle can exacerbate the symptoms of any injury. Stress reduction and relaxation techniques can play an important role in the treatment of low back problems and other injuries.

Lower Back Injuries

The lower back is made up of many tiny ligaments that hold the vertebrae together from the skull to the tailbone. A sudden twisting force can injure these ligaments. Several groups of muscles, called the *erector spinae muscle group,* also parallel the spinal column. These muscles may be injured by lifting a heavy weight, excessively bending and twisting, or sleeping on a sagging mattress.

If your back aches, press the sore area with your fingers. If this does not cause pain, the injury is probably deeper. For sore, achy back muscles, lie on a bag of crushed ice or a cold pack for 20 minutes, or alternate 20 minutes of ice with 20 minutes of heat. If you have back pain, what symptoms indicate that you should see a physician? If the pain is severe, doesn't decrease with a few days of home treatment, radiates from the back into the buttocks or legs, or is accompanied by numbness or tingling, it may indicate an **intervertebral disc** injury. The intervertebral disc is a cushion that separates the bony vertebrae. Discs are filled with fluid and are flexible through early adulthood but thin and lose their resiliency as we age. A ruptured intervertebral disc may compress nerves, causing pain down the buttocks and legs. Consult a physician who specializes in back pain for these injuries.

Core Exercises for Lower Back Health

Research has shown that 80 percent of patients with back discomfort who visit physicians have no underlying organic disease. Most of these patients are deficient in strength and flexibility of core postural muscles of the trunk. There are several exercises you can do to maintain a healthy back. We recommend the exercise routine in Figure 8-3. These exercises focus on core strengthening for the abdominals *and* stretching and strengthening the back. Practice this series daily to get the best results. The exercises can easily be included as part of your exercise warm-up or cool-down routine. These exercises should not cause any pain, numbness, or tingling in the back and legs. If they do, discontinue them and consult your specialist.

Other exercise programs that can develop muscular fitness in core stabilizers include Pilates and stability ball exercises. Yoga and Tai Chi may also reduce back pain by increasing flexibility and reducing stress. For information on these exercise programs and additional core stability exercises, see Chapters 5 and 6.

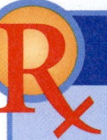

PRESCRIPTION FOR ACTION

You've read the chapter. Now go do one or more of these:

✓ Check the inner side of the midsole of your shoes for wrinkles, which indicate they have been compressed by daily impact and need to be replaced.

✓ While waiting in line, clasp hands behind your back and pull elbows back to strengthen postural muscles.

✓ While watching TV, do 20 to 30 abdominal crunches or 5 to 10 back extensions.

✓ Put on your favorite music and do the back exercise program in this chapter.

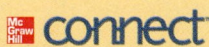 Go online to Connect to complete this activity.
http://connect.mcgraw-hill.com

Frequently Asked Questions

Q. My joints pop and crack a lot when I move. Is there something wrong with them?

A. Joints can be noisy for a lot of reasons, mostly benign. If there is pain or swelling along with the popping, see your physician. If your joints feel fine, a little noise is common and harmless.

Q.   I've been working out for 4 months and am not doing anything different. Why are my knees starting to bother me?

A.   Are you wearing the same shoes you started with? If so, it is time to replace them because the soles compress over time, leaving you with less cushioning. Check your workout—are you running on hard surfaces, constantly going the same direction on a track or crowned roads, or repeatedly stepping up on curbs with the same leg? Finally, outside of workouts, have you added any new activity such as weekend yard work or carrying unaccustomed loads? Switch to a nonimpact activity for a few days to give your knees a chance to recover, then modify your workouts to reduce excessive impact or repetitive stresses on your knees.

Q.   Every time I start a running program, I get shin splints. What can I do to keep this from happening next time?

A.   First, check your shoes. Are they less than 6 months (500 miles) old, and are they good running shoes? Well-cushioned shoes designed for the stresses of running are your first line of defense against impact injuries. If your shoes are OK, the problem may be overuse—doing too much too soon. Many beginners, in their zeal to get in shape, try to run a mile in the first workout and increase from there. Start with several weeks of walking. Once you can walk 2 to 3 miles without discomfort, alternate jogging and walking. Review the progression in Chapter 4, and do not try to progress faster. Try the shin-strengthening exercise in Chapter 6, and stretch the calves. Consider alternating days of running with cycling or another nonimpact activity, and do not try to run through the shin splints. If your shins start to ache, switch to a nonimpact activity until they heal. When you start back after a layoff, decrease your workout by 25 to 50 percent, do more walking, and build back slowly.

Q.   Which is better for an injury—heat or ice?

A.   Ice is the treatment of choice for any acute injury. It decreases pain, limits swelling, and penetrates deep tissues better than heat does. Heat applied too early can increase swelling. Once swelling has subsided, heat can be relaxing and can decrease stiffness.

Q.   I was told that I shouldn't pedal backward on an indoor cycling machine. Why not?

A.   Pedaling backward can increase risk of knee injuries. When you pedal, the greatest pressure is exerted in the middle of the downstroke. Pedaling forward, this occurs in front of your body with your foot in the 3 o'clock position, a mechanically stable and safe position for the knee. Pedaling backward, the greatest force occurs in the 9 o'clock position, where the knee is less mechanically stable, putting you at increased risk of injury.

Q.   Does exercise cause arthritis?

A.   No. Exercise increases joint lubrication, helps joint range of motion, and strengthens muscles that support joints. Gentle range-of-motion and low-impact aerobic exercises are recommended as a way to decrease the stiffness and pain of arthritis, either rheumatoid or osteoarthritis. Osteoarthritis from joint wear and tear is common in those over 40, may have a hereditary component, and can be brought on by joint injury, jogging, or doing other high-impact activities that stress aging joints. So if arthritis runs in your family or if you have had joint injuries, it is even more important to keep your joints strong and flexible with regular exercise such as walking, swimming, and stretching.

Q.   I've read that wearing magnets can relieve back pain. Do they work?

A.   Every year a new fad comes along, promising results that don't pan out. The body has natural healing ability, so if you buy a product and get relief, it is easy to attribute it to that product, when you would have gotten better without it. A randomized, double-blind crossover study of chronic back pain patients found no difference in pain relief between those using real and sham magnets. Don't waste your money.

Summary

Much soreness and injury can be prevented. Stretching, strengthening, proper warm-up, sensible progressions, and avoiding overuse are the keys. It is better to block injuries at the source than to pay doctors' fees to treat breakdowns. The pursuit of excellence involves learning to balance your strengths and weaknesses and cooperating with your body instead of assaulting it.

You can prevent lower back problems with proper care and treatment. Maintain leg and back flexibility, strengthen abdominals, use correct lifting mechanics, and reduce sources of lower back stress. This is all within your control.

Terms

- blisters
- bursitis
- cramp
- heel spur
- iliotibial band
- intervertebral disc
- ischemia
- ligament

- orthotics
- overpronation
- overuse
- patellofemoral syndrome
- plantar fasciitis
- P.R.I.C.E.
- pronation
- proprioceptors

- shin splint
- side stitch
- sprain
- strain
- stress fracture
- tendinitis
- tendons
- underpronation

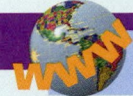

Internet Resources

About.com Sports Medicine

http://sportsmedicine.about.com

Includes articles about sports, sports medicine, injury prevention, diagnosis, and treatment.

American Academy of Family Physicians

www.familydoctor.org

Check out the patient site with information on all types of conditions, including common sports injuries and their diagnosis, treatment, and prevention.

American Academy of Orthopaedic Surgeons

www.aaos.org

Contains information about orthopedic conditions, including sports injuries and their diagnosis, treatment, and prevention.

American College of Sports Medicine

www.acsm.org/sportsmed

Has information on sports research and on health and fitness, aerobic exercise guidelines, and a quarterly fitness newsletter. "Current Comments" gives information on a variety of exercise topics of recent interest.

eMedicine from WebMD

www.emedicine.com

An open-access comprehensive textbook for all clinical fields. Features a keyword search for injuries, prevention, and treatment.

Free MD.com

www.freemd.com

Virtual MD interviews can be accessed for many medical conditions. For example, if you have injured your ankle, you can access an interactive evaluation of your symptoms.

Mayo Clinic

www.mayoclinic.com/health

Includes information on first aid for injuries, blisters, bursitis, ankle sprains, muscle cramps, muscle strain, knee pain, plantar fasciitis, heel spurs, shin splints, tendonitis, and stress fractures.

Medline Plus: Sports Injuries

www.nlm.nih.gov/medlineplus/sportsinjuries.html

Covers sports injuries, screening, prevention, frequently asked questions, and treatment options.

The Physician and Sports Medicine

www.physsportsmed.com

Contains articles on exercise, nutrition, injury prevention, personal fitness, and rehabilitation.

Sports Injury Bulletin

www.sportsinjurybulletin.com

Information, prevention, and rehabilitation of sports injuries.

Virtual Sports Injury Clinic

www.sportsinjuryclinic.net

Includes self-help advice and a virtual diagnosis for common sports injuries. Also covers rehabilitation, stretching, and strengthening for injury prevention.

Back and Neck Pain Videos

Causes of Back Pain http://mayoclinic.com/health/back-pain/DS00536

Neck pain information http://mayoclinic.com/health/neck-pain/DS00542

Neck Stretches for the Office http://mayoclinic.com/health/neck-stretches/MM00708

Overview on back pain causes, treatments, and prevention http://mayoclinic.com/health/back-pain/DS00171

Sleeping Positions That Reduce Back Pain http://mayoclinic.com/health/sleeping-postions/LB00003_D

Name _____ **Class/Activity Section** _____ **Date** _____

Phil A. Case Study

Phil is a 20-year-old student at State College. He has kept himself in good shape and has been running road races for the last 4 years. This morning, while running on White River Road, he stepped into a chuck hole and sprained his ankle. He was able to limp home. You are one of his best friends, and he has come to you for advice. He says "My ankle is sore. Do you think I should see a doctor?"

1. According to your text, what are five symptoms that indicate a person needs to seek medical help for an injury?

   a.

   b.

   c.

   d.

   e.

2. Phil says none of these symptoms apply to him, and there is only mild swelling. He asks, "What do you think I should do to minimize swelling?" List and describe five treatments recommended for common injuries.

   a.

   b.

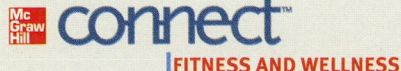

McGraw Hill **connect** | **FITNESS AND WELLNESS**

http://connect.mcgraw-hill.com

c.

d.

e.

3. Phil wants to keep in shape and plans to start running again as soon as possible. He asks, "I wonder if I should try to run tomorrow?" List three steps in the progression of getting back into action. Also, what is a good nonimpact activity to use while the ankle recovers?

a.

b.

c.

d.

LAB Activity 8-2

Name _____ Class/Activity Section _____ Date _____

Action Plan for the Back

BACK EXERCISES

Complete the series of back exercises that are described in Figure 8-3.

1. Describe how your lower back area felt at the completion of the exercise session.

2. Explain how you will fit this exercise regimen into your daily schedule.

BACK CARE

Explain how you will perform the following tasks using proper body mechanics/alignment:

1. Lifting a garage door to open it:

2. Lifting a heavy box to put in the back of a station wagon:

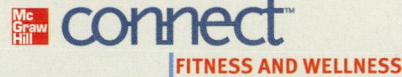

http://connect.mcgraw-hill.com

3. Sitting several hours at a desk studying:

4. Driving a car for 5 hours:

5. Standing/working at a checkout counter for 5 hours:

6. Sleeping:

CHAPTER 9

Maximizing Heart Health

STUDY QUESTIONS

You will have successfully mastered this chapter if you can answer the following:

1. What are the 10 primary cardiovascular disease (CVD) risk factors? How does each affect heart health?
2. What are the 6 secondary CVD risk factors? How does each affect heart health?
3. What are the 12 controllable and 4 uncontrollable risk factors for CVD?
4. To cut CVD risk, what four lifestyle factors should be addressed?
5. How are *arteriosclerosis, atherosclerosis, angina pectoris, myocardial infarction,* and *stroke* defined?
6. What are the differences between cardiovascular disease (CVD) and coronary heart disease (CHD)?
7. What are the symptoms of a heart attack and a stroke, and what is the S.T.R. approach to stroke awareness?
8. What are the roles of HDL and LDL in heart health?
9. How does smoking cigarettes increase heart disease risk?
10. What are prehypertension, normal blood pressure range, and the blood pressure reading that indicates hypertension?
11. What cholesterol reading indicates high blood cholesterol?
12. Which CVD risk factors are positively affected by exercise?
13. What are the positive and negative effects of alcohol on CVD?
14. What is the importance of lifestyle for cardiovascular disease and how does the mind–body connection affect it?

You will find the answers as you read this chapter.

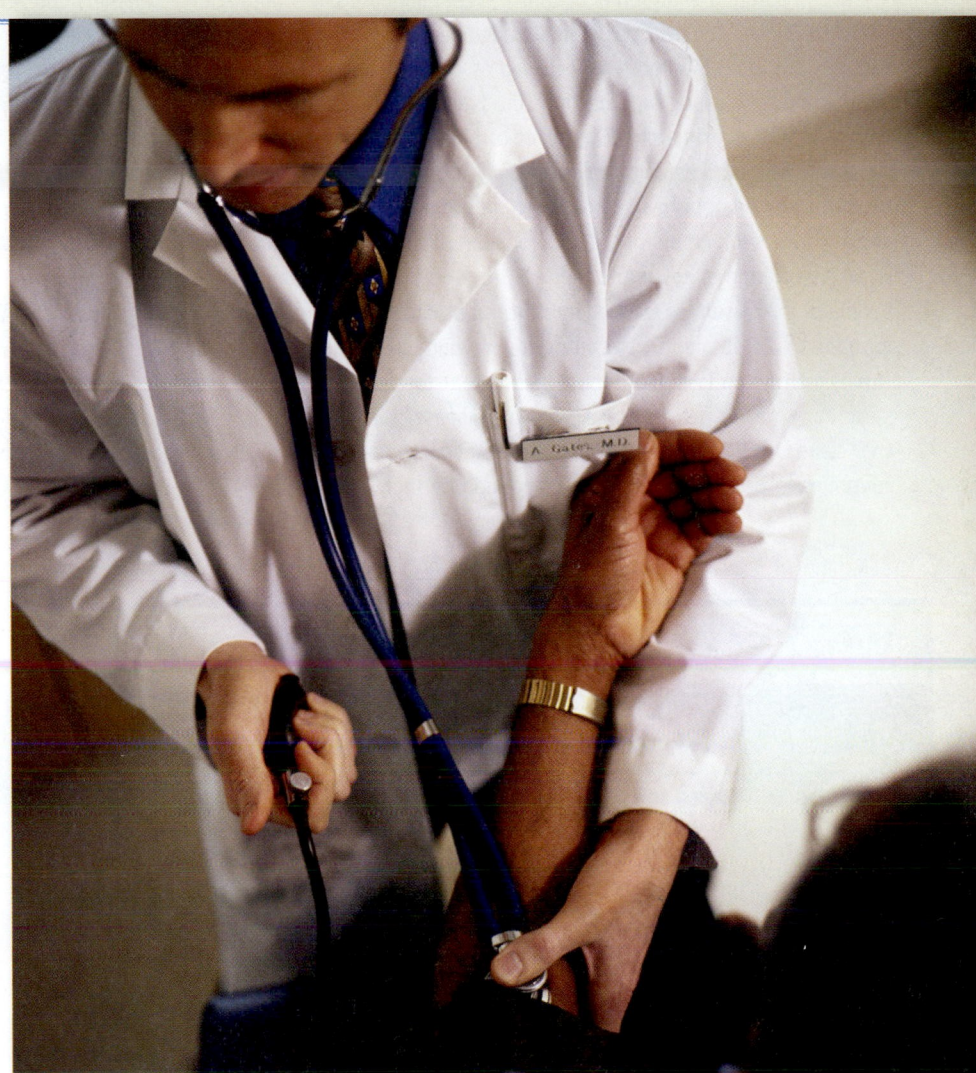

" *This is not a dress rehearsal. This is it.*"
—Tom Cunningham

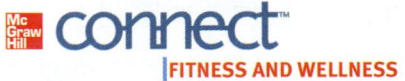
FITNESS AND WELLNESS

http://connect.mcgraw-hill.com

The number one killer in America is not cancer, accidents, or AIDS. It is cardiovascular disease (CVD) (Figure 9-1). Make no mistake: cancer and other diseases are real threats, but cardiovascular diseases claim more lives each year than cancer, chronic respiratory diseases, accidents, and diabetes *combined!* If all major forms of CVD were eliminated, U.S. life expectancy would rise by 7 years. In contrast, if all forms of cancer were eliminated, the gain would be 3 years. The tragedy is compounded because cardiovascular diseases are often inaccurately perceived as diseases of the elderly. On the contrary, based on data from the Framingham Heart Study (Chapter 1), approximately 45 percent of heart attack victims are under age 65 and 5 percent are under age 40. Young adults are not exempt from the grim heart disease picture either—most teenagers already have two or more risk factors for heart disease. The American Heart Association states that one in six teenagers and one in three people in their twenties showed evidence of atherosclerosis. This information was obtained from autopsies of young accident victims. This is alarming information and confirms that the disease process starts early in life. "Heart disease is a man's disease" is another myth. CVD claims the lives of as many, or more, women as men, and the gap continues to widen. These diseases demand attention because they are killing too many Americans in the prime of life. Don't become complacent! The way you live your life now determines your future heart health. Many cardiovascular disease deaths are preventable. You can reduce your chances of developing CVD by assessing your current level of risk and learning ways to reduce those identified risk factors. Education and behavior change are the keys.

The importance of lifestyle and knowledge for the heart health picture is emphasized by the remarks of the world-renowned CVD expert Dr. Jeremiah Stamler when he was asked, "Are diet and exercise enough to cut CVD risk?" He responded, "Yes, along with not smoking and a healthy weight. Only 3 percent of the population have all four healthy lifestyle characteristics. Americans are pushed to solve problems with pills—for cholesterol, for diabetes, for blood pressure. But pills often fail to lower risk to optimum levels. They are costly and have side effects. They ameliorate but don't cure the underlying problem. *Heart disease is caused by adverse lifestyles. If you want to get rid of the disease, get rid of these lifestyles."*

Are you at risk for heart disease? Would you know what to do if you were? Read the Top 10 "Ways to Protect Your Heart." This chapter provides you with valuable information about each of those items and guides you toward maximizing your heart health.

What Stage of Change Are You In?

Do you check your blood pressure on a regular basis? (i.e., about once per month)

- No
  - Do you plan to adopt this practice within the next 6 months?
    - No → **Precontemplation**
    - Yes
      - Within the next month?
        - No → **Contemplation**
        - Yes → **Preparation**
- Yes
  - Have you done this consistently over the last 6 months?
    - No → **Action**
    - Yes → **Maintenance**

◆ IMPACT OF CARDIOVASCULAR DISEASE (CVD)

Cardiovascular disease (including stroke) accounts for nearly 37 percent of deaths in the United States, according to American Heart Association (AHA) statistics. In other words, about 1 in 3 Americans who die each year does so from CVD. How do the death rates from cancer and other causes compare to that from CVD? See Figure 9-1. **Cardiovascular disease** (from *cardio* meaning "heart" and *vascular* meaning "blood vessels") refers to diseases of the heart and blood vessels. Common forms of CVD include coronary heart disease (i.e., heart attack, angina pectoris, atherosclerosis in the heart's blood vessels), congestive heart failure, rheumatic heart disease, congenital heart disease, stroke, high blood pressure, pulmonary (lung) disease, diseases of the arteries and veins, and renal disease. More than one in three Americans suffer from some form of CVD. See Figure 9-2 to see the toll taken by these various forms of CVD. Which type of CVD claims the most American lives? Studies show that lower educational levels are directly associated with increased incidence of death from CVD.

Coronary heart disease, the most prevalent form of CVD, is still the single largest killer of American men and women (about one of every five deaths). The cost of all CVD in 2010 was estimated by the AHA at $475.3 billion. This figure includes the costs of physician and nursing services, hospital and nursing home services, medications, and lost productivity resulting from disability. While costs for treatment

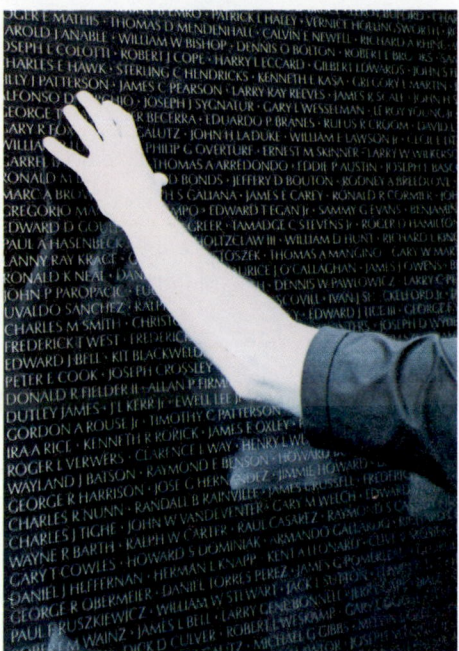

More Americans die each year from cardiovascular disease than would have been killed in 10 Vietnam wars.

of CVD are spiraling upward, the death rate for these diseases appears to be declining. Advances in medical treatment and education and healthy lifestyle changes can be credited for the declining death rate. However, don't become too complacent about these facts. We still have a long way to go. Cardiovascular disease is the *number one* health concern in the United States. It is a killer. Someone still dies every 37 seconds; more than 2,400 Americans die each day of CVD.

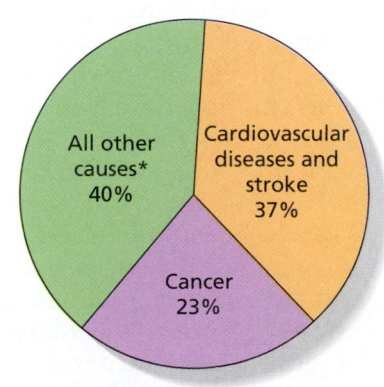

*Includes accidents, diabetes, chronic respiratory diseases, and other diseases and conditions.

FIGURE 9-1   Cardiovascular disease is still the number one cause of death in the United States.

Source: American Heart Association 2010 Heart Disease and Stroke Update.

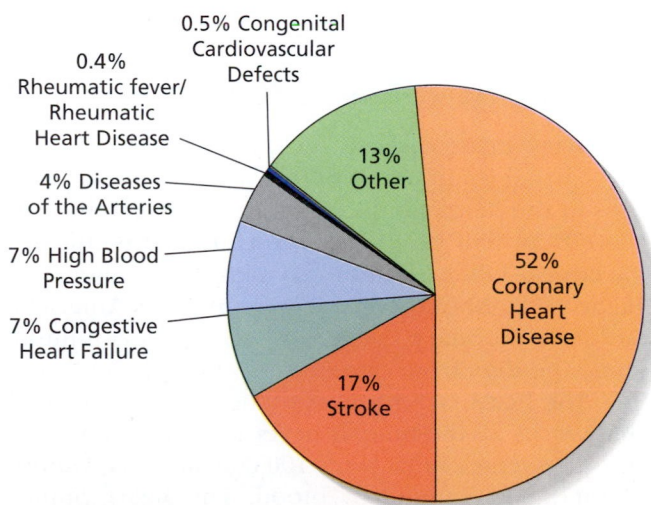

FIGURE 9-2   Percentage breakdown of deaths from cardiovascular diseases; one in three Americans has some form of CVD. United States, 2010.

Source: American Heart Association.

TOP **10** LIST

Ways to Protect Your Heart

1. Exercise regularly. Aim for at least 30 minutes, at least 5 days of the week. Performing aerobic exercise regularly helps protect coronary arteries by reducing heart rate, blood pressure, cholesterol level, and body fat.
2. Maintain blood pressure level within normal limits.
3. Maintain blood cholesterol levels within acceptable limits.
4. Don't smoke.
5. Keep your weight within reasonable limits. Weighing too much (especially if you carry the extra pounds in your waistline) raises the risk of a heart attack.
6. Keep blood sugar (glucose) level close to normal.
7. Don't let your triglyceride level exceed 150 mg/dl (or 100 mg/dl if you have other coronary risk factors).
8. Control stress and hostility. Learn and practice stress management strategies and know how to diffuse anger/hostile behaviors.
9. Know the early warning symptoms of angina pectoris and the symptoms of a heart attack and a stroke.
10. Be aware of your genes. If one or more close blood relatives have had a heart attack before age 60, your risk rises substantially. Accordingly, the need to control the primary risk factors for cardiovascular disease is heightened.

Note: In addition to the Top 10 "Ways to Protect Your Heart," eat healthy. This will provide added protection against CVD. Recommendations include reducing homocysteine levels by eating five servings of fruits and vegetables and six servings of grains per day. Also, consuming foods high in antioxidants (vitamins C, E, and beta carotene) helps prevent heart attacks by preventing LDL oxidation (which increases clotting and plaque rupture).

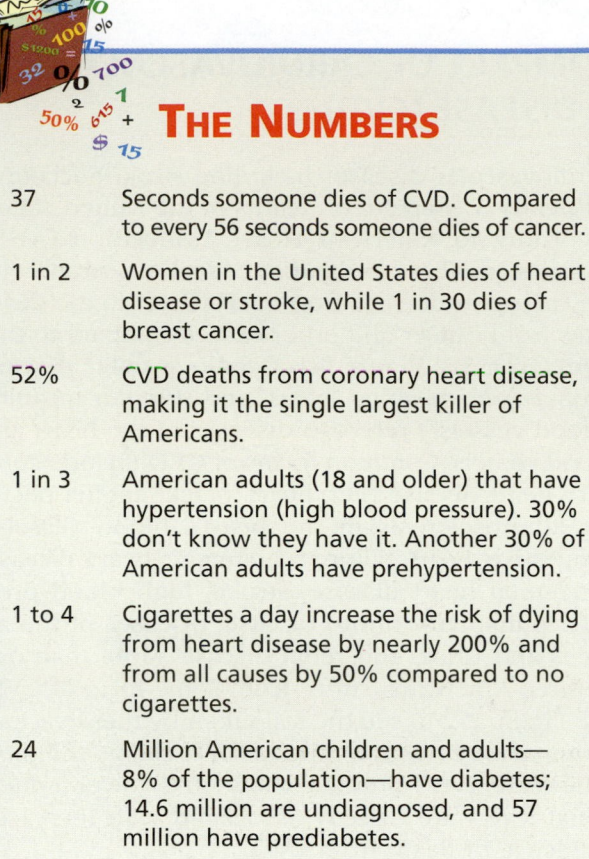

THE NUMBERS

37	Seconds someone dies of CVD. Compared to every 56 seconds someone dies of cancer.
1 in 2	Women in the United States dies of heart disease or stroke, while 1 in 30 dies of breast cancer.
52%	CVD deaths from coronary heart disease, making it the single largest killer of Americans.
1 in 3	American adults (18 and older) that have hypertension (high blood pressure). 30% don't know they have it. Another 30% of American adults have prehypertension.
1 to 4	Cigarettes a day increase the risk of dying from heart disease by nearly 200% and from all causes by 50% compared to no cigarettes.
24	Million American children and adults—8% of the population—have diabetes; 14.6 million are undiagnosed, and 57 million have prediabetes.

Coronary Heart Disease (CHD)

Coronary heart disease includes angina pectoris, myocardial infarction, and the atherosclerotic process in the heart's blood vessels. CHD accounts for more than half of all cases of CVD and is the *single* largest killer of American men and women. See Figure 9-2. About every 25 seconds an American suffers a coronary event, and about every minute someone dies from one.

The heart is a muscle (a little larger than a fist) that works all the time. It never stops beating. Each day, the average heart beats 100,000 times and pumps about 2,000 gallons of blood. The heart pumps blood continuously through the circulatory system, which includes the lungs and blood vessels (i.e., arteries and veins). The arteries, arterioles (small arteries), and capillaries (very tiny blood vessels) carry oxygen- and nutrient-rich blood to all parts of the body. Veins and venules (small veins) carry oxygen- and nutrient-depleted blood back to the heart and lungs. If all the vessels were laid end-to-end, they would extend for about 60,000 miles. That's enough to encircle the earth more than twice.

Besides providing oxygen and other nutrients to all tissues of the body, the heart must supply itself with oxygen. This is accomplished by a separate circulatory system, which nourishes only the heart muscle. The two coronary arteries (the right coronary artery and the left coronary artery) branch off the aorta and then divide into many smaller arteries that lie in the heart muscle and feed the heart (see Figure 9-3). The most important factor in your heart's health is the efficiency of your coronary arteries to transport blood to your heart. The heart requires a steady supply of oxygen-rich blood to function properly. The most common barrier to that supply is coronary artery disease, in which the arteries become blocked or narrowed. Coronary heart disease is most commonly the result of atherosclerosis.

You supply the ingredients for what damages or protects the blood vessels of the heart through what you eat, how you exercise, and how you react to stress. You have the power to make your heart stronger.

ATHEROSCLEROSIS

What is commonly known as "hardening of the arteries" is **arteriosclerosis,** a general term for the

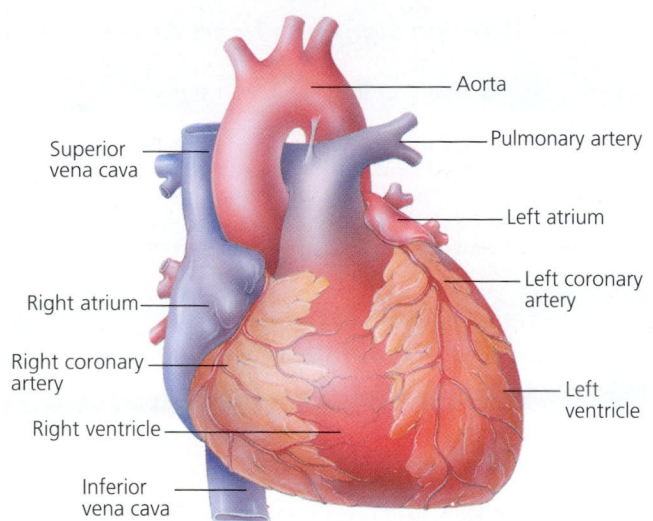

tion in which fatty patches (deposits of cholesterol and other lipids) accumulate under the lining of coronary arteries or arteries in other places in the body. This buildup is called **plaque.** Scientists now know that the atherosclerotic process is initiated by injury to the innermost layer of the artery wall—the endothelial cell layer, or endothelium. The fatty patches (or streaks) of plaque impede blood flow by causing arteries to become thick and rigid. An atherosclerotic patch is actually like a "blister": soft on the inside, with a thin skin that can easily rupture when it becomes inflamed and unstable. When a blister ruptures, debris (like a blood clot) is sent into the bloodstream where it can enter an artery in the heart or the brain causing a heart attack or a stroke.

How does the inflammatory response to an injured artery wall work? When these delicate endothelial cells are injured, they pull away from each other and form a gap. This "nick" or injury has to be closed quickly to protect and keep the blood vessel lining smooth. The body tries to repair the "nicks" by covering them with cholesterol (especially the "bad" type) and other substances. To counter, the body's immune system sends in white cell protectors to attack the plaque buildup. In trying to heal the damaged area, inflammation develops at the site. The inflamed plaque gets irritated, becomes unstable, then cracks, and a clot is released into the bloodstream. A heart attack or stroke may result (see Figure 9-4) if the clot flows to the heart or brain. We now know this is what generally happens in a heart attack or stroke rather than plaque growing so large that it blocks an artery.

FIGURE 9-3   **Blood supply to the heart.** Blood is supplied to the heart from the right and left coronary arteries, which branch off the aorta. If a coronary artery is blocked by a blood clot caused by a ruptured fatty patch, a heart attack occurs; part of the heart muscle may die due to lack of oxygen.

SOURCE: Paul M. Insel and Walton T. Roth. *Core Concepts in Health,* 10th Edition Update. New York: McGraw-Hill, 2008, p. 448. Reproduced with permission of The McGraw-Hill Companies.

thickening and hardening of arteries. Some hardening of arteries normally occurs as we age. **Atherosclerosis** (*athero* from the Greek work for "paste" and *sclerosis* for "hardness") is a type of arteriosclerosis. It is an inflammatory and a progressive condi-

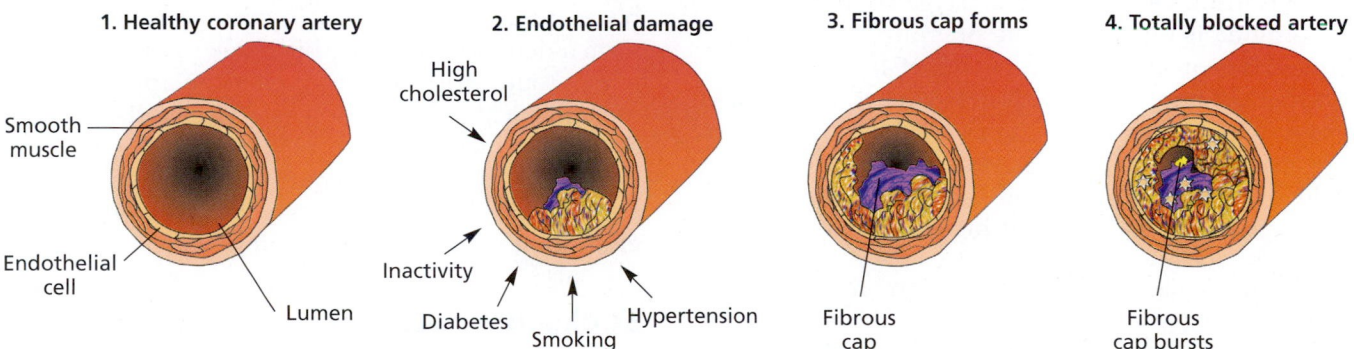

FIGURE 9-4   **Progression of atherosclerosis.**
1. Healthy coronary artery. The lumen is not narrowed by atherosclerotic plaque patches, so blood can flow easily through the artery.
2. Beginning stage of atherosclerosis. Plaque builds up when the endothelial cells, which line the arteries, are damaged by an unhealthy lifestyle. Circulating cholesterol and other debris in the blood begin to collect, forming fatty patches at the injured area.
3. Advanced atherosclerosis leads to diminished blood flow. Due to the damage and fatty patch buildup, plaque continues to accumulate, and then a fibrous cap or blister forms over the site.
4. Totally blocked artery. The body interprets plaque as an injury to the blood vessel wall. The immune system sends white blood cells to attack the plaque. The plaque can become inflamed, unstable, and may result in the fibrous cap rupturing, creating a blood clot that can block the lumen and lead to a heart attack or stroke.

What injures the endothelium lining of the arteries, especially the coronary arteries, and leads to atherosclerosis (and inflammation)? While there is a strong genetic component to atherosclerosis, you can largely control many contributing factors: high blood pressure, smoking, high blood cholesterol (the "bad" type and triglycerides), diabetes, high blood levels of some compounds like homocysteine, and chronic imflammation. Chronic inflammation can also develop from things as diverse as sexually transmitted diseases, your reaction to perceived emotional stress, anger, and gum (periodontal) disease. All of these factors are influenced by lifestyle. To reduce the risk of atherosclerosis and inflammation, become physically fit, consume a diet high in omega-3 fats (fish), don't smoke (and avoid secondhand smoke), control blood pressure, and reduce weight (if overweight). Inflammation of the gums can be prevented by practicing good oral health (i.e., flossing every day and brushing your teeth for two minutes twice a day).

Atherosclerosis, a major cause of CVD, coronary heart disease, and stroke, does not suddenly develop at age 65. It is a long, progressive process beginning in childhood.

ANGINA PECTORIS

Atherosclerosis may lead to **angina pectoris,** or chest pain/discomfort due to CHD. This pain/discomfort occurs when a coronary artery becomes partially blocked, causing an oxygen debt in the heart muscle. Often, angina pectoris is brought on by sudden exertion or vigorous exercise, emotional stress, or even extreme temperatures when the blood flow to the heart is insufficient to meet its oxygen demands. Typical angina is uncomfortable pressure, fullness, and squeezing or pain in the center of the chest. The discomfort may also be felt in the neck, jaw, shoulder, back, or arm. Many types of chest discomfort are not related to angina, such as that caused by acid reflux (heartburn) and lung infection. Angina is a sign that someone is at higher risk of heart attack. The AHA estimates that over 6 million people suffer from angina pectoris, with 350,000 new cases occurring each year.

MYOCARDIAL INFARCTION (MI)

Myocardial infarction (MI), or heart attack, results when one or more of the coronary arteries is partially blocked by atherosclerotic deposits called plaque. Plaque blisters can rupture, causing a blood clot (thrombus) to form, which chokes off the supply of blood to the heart muscle.

The portion of heart muscle beyond the blockage is deprived of oxygen, resulting in injury or death

Warning Signs of a Heart Attack

"Classic" or more common signs

- Uncomfortable pressure, fullness, squeezing, or pain in the center of the chest that lasts more than a few minutes or that goes away and comes back.
- Pain or discomfort in other areas of the body: shoulder, neck, jaw, back, or stomach, one or both arms.

Less common signs

- Atypical chest pain, stomach or abdominal pain.
- Nausea or dizziness.
- Shortness of breath and difficulty breathing.
- Unexplained anxiety, weakness, or fatigue.
- Palpitations, cold sweat, or paleness.

Not all of these signs occur in every heart attack. If some of these symptoms do occur, don't wait. Get help immediately! Call 911.

NOTE: Women don't always have the crushing chest pain type of heart attack seen on TV. They may experience less dramatic, lighter symptoms such as fatigue or a burning feeling in the back.

of that portion. If a damaged area is large enough or in a vital area of the heart, the individual will die. However, many people do survive a heart attack and are capable of living productive lives. See the box "Warning Signs of a Heart Attack."

A number of studies have shown that in some damaged hearts, new blood vessels develop to nourish the area that is being starved of oxygen and other nutrients. This is called **collateral circulation.** Everyone has collateral blood vessels, which are microscopic and are closed under normal conditions. However, in some people with coronary heart disease, these vessels seem to enlarge and form a detour around the blockage to provide alternative routes for the blood. *Exercise* appears to be one practical way to increase myocardial oxygen demand, which in turn may stimulate the development of collateral vessels. In some cases, coronary angiography (X ray) has revealed increased collateralization after exercise training.

Stroke (Brain Attack)

A **stroke** occurs when blood flow to the brain is interrupted either by a blockage (ischemic stroke) or by a burst blood vessel (cerebral hemorrhage). More than 80 percent of strokes are ischemic. The brain needs a continuous supply of oxygen-rich blood to function. When a blood clot interrupts the flow of oxygen, the brain does not receive the nourishment it needs, and brain cells die. When considered separately from other CVDs, stroke, primarily caused by atherosclerosis, is the *third* leading killer

Most Common Warning Signs of Stroke

- Sudden numbness or weakness of face, arm, or leg, especially on one side of the body.
- Sudden confusion, trouble speaking or understanding.
- Sudden trouble seeing in one or both eyes.
- Sudden trouble walking, dizziness, loss of balance or coordination.
- Sudden severe headaches with no known cause.

Not all warning signs occur in every stroke. If any or some start to occur, get help immediately. Call 911.

of Americans (behind CHD and cancer). About 700,000 Americans will have a stroke this year—that's someone every 40 seconds. See the box listing "Most Common Warning Signs of Stroke."

Many Americans, however, cannot name a single warning sign or do not know that a stroke is treatable if caught early. So, a group of researchers developed the S.T.R. approach to stroke awareness by determining the top three symptoms; then identified them by the first three letters in stroke (STR); and combined them with the most important action step. See the box "S.T.R. Approach to Stroke Awareness." The S.T.R. Approach is a first step in the assessment process or sign of a stroke. If the person has trouble with any of these simple commands, emergency services (911) should be called immediately. The first 60 minutes after symptoms appear is referred to as the *Golden Hour.* If a person gets advanced medical care in the Golden Hour, the chances of surviving with less permanent damage is greater.

Stroke is the chief cause of serious disability and a major contributor to dementia later in life. A stroke can result in paralysis of one side of the body, loss of ability to speak or understand the speech of others, loss of memory, and behavioral change. Because brain cells can't heal, modification of risk factors is important in the prevention of this disease that kills about 150,000 Americans every year. It is not solely a disease of the elderly; more than

S.T.R. Approach to Stroke Awareness

SMILE: Ask the person to SMILE. Does the smile sag or droop on one side?

TALK: Ask the person to TALK or repeat a simple sentence: "The sky is blue." Is the speech slurred or jumbled?

RAISE: Ask the person to RAISE BOTH ARMS. Is one arm weaker? Can both be raised easily and evenly?

Action Step: Call 911 immediately if the person has trouble with ANY ONE of these tasks, even if there is improvement in condition.

NOTE: Another sign of stroke: Ask the person to stick out their TONGUE. If the tongue is crooked, if it goes to one side or the other, that is an indication of a stroke.

28 percent of stroke victims are under age 65. Your risk of stroke increases with these factors:

✓ *Hypertension:* If you have high blood pressure, you are two to four times more likely to have a stroke than is someone with normal blood pressure. It is the most important risk factor for stroke.

✓ *Heart disease:* Risk escalates if you have carotid artery disease, had a pervious stroke, disease of the leg arteries, or sickle cell anemia. Sometimes blood clots forming in the heart can move up to the brain and block blood flow.

✓ *Gender:* Stroke is more common in men than in women, but because women live longer than men, more women die of stroke each year. Women account for 6 out of 10 stroke deaths. Use of birth control pills, pregnancy, and child birth pose special risks for women.

✓ *Diabetes:* Those with diabetes have almost double the risk of stroke.

✓ *Age:* The incidence more than doubles in each decade after age 55 (for women) and 45 (for men).

✓ *Smoking:* Smoking (or living or working with people who smoke) doubles the risk of stroke by making blood vessels stiff.

✓ *Race:* African Americans have nearly *twice* as many fatal strokes as whites and more than *twice* as many as other minorities. Hypertension, obesity, and diabetes are the suspected causes. American Indians, Alaska natives, and Mexican Americans have a higher than average risk.

✓ *Lifestyle:* These factors can be controlled: high-fat, high-cholesterol diet; smoking; sedentary lifestyle; and alcohol or drug abuse. More than two drinks a day for men and more than one for women can lead to multiple medical problems. Cocaine, methamphetamine (and all other amphetamines), and heroin have all been linked to stroke.

✓ *Family history:* Risk increases if your mother, father, sister, brother, or grandparents have had a stroke.

To reduce your risk of stroke:

✓ Exercise regularly.
✓ Keep blood pressure at optimal or normal level.
✓ Do not smoke.
✓ Keep diabetes under control if you have diabetes.
✓ Be evaluated by a sleep specialist if you have sleep apnea.
✓ Keep homocysteine levels at optimal levels by consuming plenty of produce and grains.

THINK ABOUT IT

You may have noticed the increase in advertisements encouraging healthy people to undergo "full body scans" to look for early signs of disease, such as heart disease and cancer. Many types of imaging technology can be used to perform these scans, including X ray, CT, (computed tomography), MRI, and ultrasound. What do we know about the potential risks of diagnostic imaging scans? In a healthy individual with no symptoms of disease, what are the pros and cons of preventive full body scans?

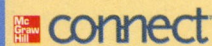

Go online to Connect to complete this activity.
http://connect.mcgraw-hill.com

✓ Keep infection and inflammation down. Be tested for C-reactive protein, a marker for inflammation in the blood.
✓ Reduce chronic stress, anger, and hostility. Exercise and meditation (or other stress management techniques) are good ways.
✓ Don't drink alcohol excessively.

◆ RISK FACTORS

Risk factors are the conditions, situations, and behaviors that increase the likelihood that an undesirable outcome (injury, illness, or death) will occur. The risk is established by multiple scientific studies. A risk factor does not cause the undesirable outcome 100 percent of the time, but among those people who engage in the behavior (or experience the condition), a certain number will experience the undesired outcome. The stronger the risk factor's link with a negative outcome, the more likely it is that an individual will experience the undesired result.

Researchers have identified several risk factors that may lead to the development of CVD. The more risk factors you possess, the greater your chances are of developing CVD. While no one can accurately predict whether you will have a heart attack, you can estimate your odds by evaluating your risk factors. Take the *Are You at Risk for Heart Disease?* test in Lab Activity 9-1 to determine your risk and how to reduce it. Complete Lab Activity 9-2 also.

Primary risk factors are linked directly to the development of CVD; they increase the possibility of having a heart attack and stroke. Notice: *Most primary risk factors are controllable.* Even type 1 diabetes, which is generally considered uncontrollable due to its genetic link, can be managed and usually controlled. Type 2 diabetes can be prevented for many years by a healthy lifestyle (i.e., regular exercise, diet, and weight management). Notice: Only 4 of the 10 risk factors are *uncontrollable!*

Primary	
Controllable Factors	**Uncontrollable Factors**
1. Inactivity	1. Positive family history
2. High blood pressure	2. Male gender
3. High blood lipid level	(+ postmenopausal
4. Cigarette smoking	women)
5. Obesity	3. Race
6. Diabetes mellitus	4. Age
(type 1 and type 2)	
and prediabetes	

The **secondary risk factors** contribute to the development of CVD, but not as directly as the primary risk factors do.

Secondary
Controllable Factors
1. Individual response to stress
2. Emotional behavior (anger and hostility)
3. Excessive alcohol (+ some illegal drugs)
4. Metabolic syndrome
5. C-reactive protein
6. Homocysteine

Notice: All of the secondary risk factors are *controllable!* The choices you make and the way you live have a profound impact in reducing your total number of risk factors. If you possess several uncontrollable risk factors, it is imperative that you adopt a healthy lifestyle as soon as possible.

Primary Risk Factors (Controllable)

1. INACTIVITY

Inactivity is a real killer. It affects just about everything: brain, heart, blood vessels, bones, liver, gut, sleep, anxiety, mood, self-esteem, and your body's ability to process sugar.

Countless studies link inactivity to CVD. The surgeon general's report confirmed that physical inactivity is a major health problem in the United States. The report warns couch potatoes: "Beware, sitting around is hazardous to your health." Additionally, the Centers for Disease Control and Prevention (CDC) in Atlanta has named physical inactivity as our nation's most common cardiac threat. Why? Because only 30.8 percent of Americans engage in physical activity at intensity levels recommended for fitness and health benefits. This leaves close to two-thirds of our population either entirely sedentary or not active enough to reap health benefits. Consequently, it is not surprising to learn that approximately 250,000 deaths (12 percent of deaths) every year in the United States can be attributed to lack of exercise. Remember, the heart is a muscle, and muscles have to be used or they will atrophy. Many experts believe that today's best buy in the prevention of CVD is *exercise* (Figure 9-5). Equally important, however, is overall lifestyle and how long you have been exercising. News from the U.S. surgeon general's report provides strong support for physical activity in the prevention of heart disease, high blood pressure, high cholesterol, diabetes, obesity, and cancer.

In yet another ongoing inquiry into the relationship between physical activity and mortality, the Harvard Alumni Study continues to produce results that have led its director, Dr. Ralph S. Paffenbarger, to conclude, "There's no doubt whatever that insufficient activity will shorten your life." Even exercise of moderate intensity (brisk walking or gardening) is beneficial in improving health and well-being. It is vigorous exercise (using the FITT prescription), however, that produces the greatest health benefits and is linked to increased longevity.

The most convincing support for exercise and improved health and increased longevity was recently published in the American Heart Association journal *Circulation*. This "blockbuster study" found that long-term exercise may have anti-aging properties due to its effect at the chromosomal level, specifically on the telomeres. Telomeres are the protective caps found on the ends of each chromosome that help cut DNA decay. They have been compared with the protective caps on the ends of shoelaces. Each time a cell divides, its telomeres shrink or deteriorate. The shrinkage is thought to be the basic cause of aging. When telomeres become too short after repeated cell divisions, cells die. As people get older, telomeres get shorter, and some research has linked shortened telomeres to higher rates of chronic health issues such as heart disease, infections, cognitive problems, and even cancer. This study and other recently published key findings show that vigorous, lifelong exercise is associated with a significant reduction in telomere shortening. The conclusion is that a sedentary lifestyle may accelerate the aging process. Do you want to stave off CHD and other age-related health problems? The Rx . . . get moving! See Chapter 10 for how stress affects telomeres.

The American lifestyle is sedentary. We no longer have to hunt and grow our food, build our homes, or walk to school and work. Our ancestors did not have to build physical activity into their daily lives; it was a part of their lifestyle. Modern conveniences and technology have eliminated physical activity from our lives. The culprits are the automobile, television (with remote control), elevators, escalators, riding lawn mowers, cell phones, and computers and computer games. You can probably add to this list.

University of Tennessee researchers examined the lifestyle of an Old Order Amish community in Canada who still live like most Americans did years ago (i.e., no modern conveniences like electricity, telephone, automobile, etc.). They found that the men accumulated approximately 18,000 steps per day, and the women about 14,000 steps per day. This is far and above the 2,000–4,000 average steps typical of most Americans today. The recommended step goal is around 10,000 steps in a day, which is approximately 5 miles. The lifestyle of the Amish definitely reaches this goal and more. Refer to Chapter 4 for more information on the 10,000-step lifestyle goal. Do you know how many steps you take in a day?

How much exercise do you need? The answer is, it depends on you: how fit you are, whether you are overweight, and what your goals are. To figure out what is right for you review the FITT. Prescription and the DHHS. Activity Guidelines sections in Chapter 4.

The old saying "Use it or lose it!" is true. You don't have to run marathons to be physically active.

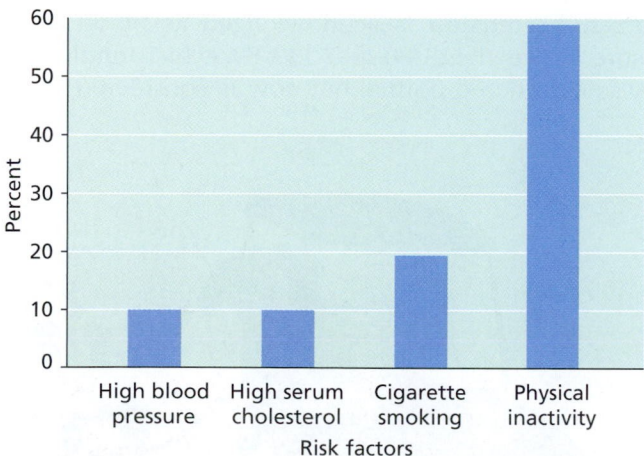

FIGURE 9-5 Estimated percentage of U.S. population having selected risk factors for CVD. More Americans are at risk for heart disease because of physical inactivity than because of any other manageable risk factor.

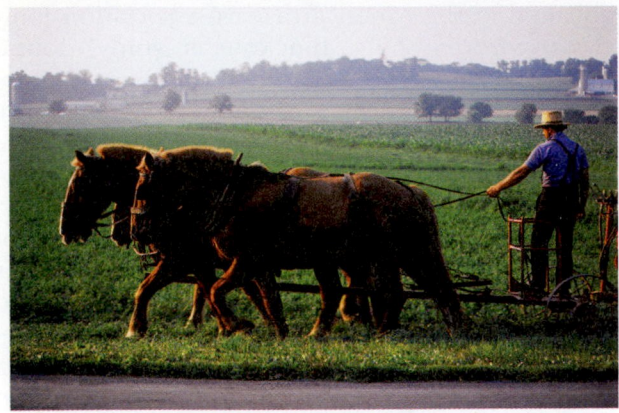

The Amish have no trouble accumulating 10,000 steps a day. This explains why the Amish have an obesity rate of less than 10 percent.

Small increases in daily activity can significantly burn up excess calories, make the heart muscle a stronger and more efficient pump, lower blood pressure, alleviate stress, increase HDL levels, and build self-confidence. Exercise does more than build strong muscles and help prevent heart disease. New science shows that it also boosts brain power and may offer hope in the battle against Alzheimer's.

The American Heart Association reports that regular vigorous exercise protects against coronary heart disease and even improves the survival rate after a heart attack. That is life insurance that money cannot buy. The most important thing you can do to improve your health and well-being is to *exercise*.

Exercise is so important for several reasons. It

✓ lowers both systolic and diastolic blood pressure
✓ lowers LDL (the "bad") cholesterol
✓ raises HDL (the "good") cholesterol
✓ decreases inflammation
✓ helps in weight management
✓ reduces stress
✓ reduces risk of type 2 diabetes
✓ evens out emotional behaviors
✓ calms feelings of hostility and anger
✓ reduces risk of metabolic syndrome
✓ prevents telomere shortening

The message is this: 30 minutes of moderately intense exercise nearly every day is essential for significant health benefits. Exercising for 20 to 60 minutes a day at a higher intensity level provides a higher level of fitness and health benefits and achieves the government guidelines too. The point is that to get to 60 minutes, you have to get to 30 minutes first. Get moving!

Ride your bike, walk to school, and play tennis instead of watching others doing these activities.

Park at the back of the parking lot instead of right next to the building. Get a step pedometer and try to accumulate 10,000 steps in a day. There are many ways to add activity to your daily life. Remember, it doesn't have to be exhausting!

2. HIGH BLOOD PRESSURE (HYPERTENSION)

Blood pressure is the term used to define the pressure exerted by blood on the inner walls of the arteries. It is also the force exerted by the heart while pumping blood through the body.

What was once considered normal blood pressure (120/80) is now labeled prehypertension, and treatment is recommended. Hypertension nearly triples CVD risk for men and doubles it for women. Also, CVD risk doubles with each 20/10 mmHg measure over 119/79.

There are two blood pressure levels, recorded as two separate numbers in fraction form (for example, 120/80). When the heart contracts and pumps blood into the arteries, the pressure increases. This is the **systolic,** or pumping, **pressure,** recorded as the upper number. The **diastolic,** or resting, **pressure** is the force of the blood against the arteries when the heart relaxes and fills with blood between beats. It is recorded as the lower number. Both the systolic and diastolic numbers are important. High levels of either or both mean greater risk for heart attack and stroke.

Normal blood pressure is 119/79 or below. However, *many experts contend that the new gold standard or "optimal" blood pressure should be 115/76 because damage to the arteries from the pressure of blood pounding through them begins to increase at this point.* This means your risk of CVD increases! **Prehypertension** is acknowledged as blood pressure between 120/80 and 139/89, which until 2003 was considered normal but now is considered to be

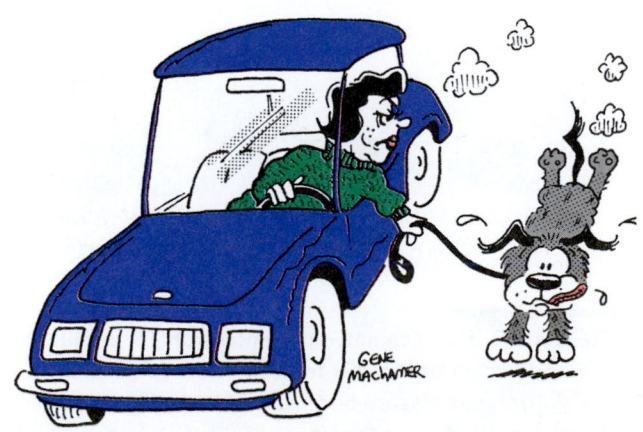

Americans are ingenious at avoiding activity.

TABLE 9-1	Blood Pressure Stages (Adults 18 Years Old or More)		
Blood Pressure Classification	Systolic Blood Pressure (mmHg)	Diastolic Blood Pressure (mmHg)	Recommendation
Normal	less than 120	less than 80	Encourage or maintain lifestyle modifications (healthy diet, maintain healthy weight).
Prehypertension	120–139	80–89	Begin lifestyle modifications and monitoring and possibly treatment. (Begin weight reduction, healthy diet such as DASH, increase activity, limit alcohol.)
Stage 1 Hypertension	140–159	90–99	Lifestyle modifications, medical evaluation, and possibly drug treatment.
Stage 2 Hypertension	>160	>100	Lifestyle modifications, medical evaluation, and drug treatment.

What was once considered normal blood pressure (120/80) is now labeled prehypertension, and treatment is recommended. Hypertension nearly triples CVD risk for men and doubles it for women. Also, CVD risk doubles with each 20/10 mmHg measure over 119/79.

in the "danger zone" before full-blown hypertension develops. This unsafe condition calls for lifestyle changes and monitoring. **Hypertension,** or high blood pressure, measures 140/90 or more and requires medical treatment. Look at the stages of hypertension listed in Table 9-1.

High blood pressure causes the heart to overwork. Over time, the overworked heart weakens, enlarges, and has difficulty keeping up with the demands of the body. High blood pressure also causes blood vessels to become inelastic, severely reducing the amount of blood flow to the body's vital organs. Decreased levels of oxygen and other nutrients can produce heart, brain, and kidney damage. Remember, high blood pressure also leads to heart attacks and strokes.

One in three American adults has high blood pressure, and about 38 percent have prehypertension. In 90 percent of the cases there is no known cause. However, factors that can increase your chances of developing high blood pressure are heredity, cigarette smoking, male gender, age, being an African American, obesity, sensitivity to sodium, heavy alcohol consumption, use of oral contraceptives, stress, and a sedentary lifestyle. In a small number of cases, hypertension is caused by a specific condition, such as kidney disease, a tumor of the adrenal gland, or a defect in the aorta. This is called **secondary hypertension.** The cause of secondary hypertension can be identified and treated successfully.

How do you know if your blood pressure is too high? The only way to know is to have it checked. (See What Stage of Change Are You In? flowchart.) You cannot feel high blood pressure—and usually there are no symptoms until complications develop. That is why hypertension is called the "silent killer." You can be hypertensive for years and be unaware of the damage occurring. Even warning signs associated with advanced hypertension may go unnoticed but may include headaches, sweating, rapid pulse,

Tips for Behavior Change for Reducing Blood Pressure

Refer to the Stage of Change flowchart on page 284. What is your stage of change after answering the questions and tracing the flowchart?

Refer to Figure 2.2 (page 36) to see which processes of change are most effective for facilitating your transition from your current stage to the next stage (or *maintaining* your behavior if you are already in the maintenance stage). Here are some behavioral examples for selected processes of change:

- Consciousness-raising: Check your blood pressure once a month for the next 6 months. Investigate what foods/beverages you currently consume that have an impact on blood pressure.
- Social liberation: Identify places on campus that have free blood pressure checks. Attend lectures/workshops on subjects that affect blood pressure (nutrition, alcohol consumption, smoking, etc.).
- Emotional arousal: Imagine yourself in the future after you have developed high blood pressure and it resulted in a heart attack or stroke.
- Countering: Follow the DASH eating plan for one month (Chapter 11).
- Helping relationships: Ask a friend or group of friends to exercise with you everyday. Have them make a commitment to it.

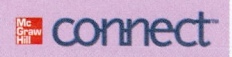 Go online to Connect to complete this activity. http://connect.mcgraw-hill.com

TOP 10 LIST

Nondrug Approaches for Reducing Blood Pressure

1. *Maintain a healthy weight.* Losing even 5 or 10 pounds, if you are overweight, can reduce blood pressure.

2. *Exercise regularly.* Exercise helps you lose weight and keep it off. See specific recommendations described earlier in the chapter.

3. *Do not smoke.* Smoking does not cause hypertension but does promote CVD. A hypertensive who smokes is at serious risk.

4. *Keep your sodium intake low (below 2,300 milligrams daily—about 1 teaspoon).* Many people are salt-sensitive, meaning that salt (sodium chloride) elevates their blood pressure.

5. *Avoid alcohol; if you drink alcohol, do so in moderation.* Have no more than one drink daily if you are a woman or two if you are a man.

6. *Eat a well-balanced diet rich in fruits, grains, and vegetables.* This will help you cut back on the consumption of fats and high-calorie foods and lose some excess weight. Reduce caffeine and cola intake. See the DASH eating plan described in Chapter 11.

7. *Increase your calcium intake.* Calcium has been linked to reduction in blood pressure. A daily consumption of 800–1,500 milligrams is recommended. (One glass of milk has approximately 300 mg.)

8. *Increase your intake of potassium.* Studies document that an increased potassium intake in people with mild hypertension can lower blood pressure. Do not exceed 6,000 mg. per day. (Bananas are high in potassium.)

9. *Increase fiber intake.* Plant fiber has been observed to lower blood pressure in hypertensive individuals by an average of four to eight points.

10. *Practice a stress management technique such as meditation* or one of those discussed in Chapter 10. Harvard Medical School studies confirm the value of stress management in the reduction of high blood pressure.

shortness of breath, dizziness, nosebleeds, and visual disturbances. It is imperative that you know your blood pressure, because high blood pressure, while it cannot be cured, can be controlled or prevented through specific lifestyle changes. See the Top 10 "Nondrug Approaches for Reducing Blood Pressure."

3. HIGH BLOOD LIPID PROFILE (CHOLESTEROL AND TRIGLYCERIDES)

Research has firmly linked high levels of cholesterol and other blood fats to the development of arterial plaque, a major cause of atherosclerosis and CVD. About half of all Americans have elevated cholesterol levels. Only 35 percent of those with high levels are aware of it, and only 12 percent are being treated for it.

Cholesterol is not a true fat but a waxy substance found in the bloodstream. Because it is soluble in fats rather than in water, it is classified as a lipid, as fats are. About 75 percent of total body cholesterol is manufactured in the liver, while 25 percent comes from dietary sources—mainly from foods of animal origin.

From all the bad press cholesterol gets, you would think cholesterol is our body's enemy. Not true. It is vital for our existence. Cholesterol is necessary for healthy cell membranes, brain cells, digestion, and adrenal glands. The problem with cholesterol is that your body makes most of what it needs, and the normal American diet adds much more. Health experts recommend that we keep dietary cholesterol consumption to less than 300 milligrams per day (less than 200 if you have high blood cholesterol). **Hypercholesterolemia** is the term for high cholesterol levels in the blood. See the Diversity Issues box "Who Has High Cholesterol?"

When evaluating your blood lipid profile for risk of CVD, consider two factors: (1) the total amount of cholesterol/triglycerides found in the blood and (2) the way cholesterol/triglycerides are transported in the bloodstream.

Total Amount of Lipids Knowing your total cholesterol level provides you with a *rough* estimate of your heart disease risk. Blood cholesterol is measured by analyzing a small blood sample in a laboratory. Total cholesterol level includes the amount of cholesterol carried by high-density lipoprotein, low-density lipoprotein, and very low-density lipoprotein. The National Heart, Lung, and Blood Institute relates blood cholesterol level to CVD risk, as illustrated in Table 9-2.

Transportation of Lipids Like oil and water, cholesterol and blood (because it is mainly water) do not mix. Cholesterol must attach to a protein molecule to be carried through the bloodstream. This combination is called a *lipoprotein*. This amazing system is also in place to assure that cholesterol is circulated wherever it is needed. However, some cholesterol-carrying lipoproteins play central roles in the development of atherosclerotic plaque and CVD. The action begins in the liver where cholesterol is packaged for delivery. The two main types of lipoproteins basically work in opposite directions. The first is **low-density lipoprotein (LDL)** cholesterol, and the second is **high-density lipoprotein**

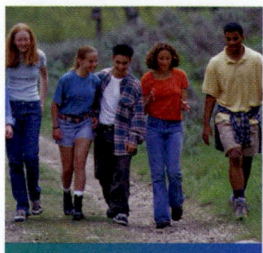

DIVERSITY ISSUES

Risk Factors for Cardiovascular Disease

Who Uses Tobacco?

	Males (%)	Females (%)
White	23.1	18.8
African American	25.0	17.1
American Indian/ Alaska Native	35.6	29.0
Hispanic/Latino	20.1	10.1
Asian	15.9	4.6

Studies show that smoking prevalence is several times higher among those with less than 12 years of education than it is among those with more than 16 years of education.

Who Has High Blood Pressure (HBP)?

- Men have a greater risk of HBP than do women until age 45. From ages 45–54, the percentage of men and women is similar. Beyond that age, the percentage of women is much higher.
- African Americans, Puerto Ricans, and Cuban and Mexican Americans are more likely to suffer from HBP than are whites.
- The prevalence of hypertension in African Americans in the United States is among the highest in the world and is increasing.
- 43% of African American males and 45% of African American females have HBP.
- 34.3% of white males and 31.3% of white females have HBP.
- 25.9% of Mexican American males and 31.6% of Mexican American females have HBP.
- 19.5% of Asians and 28.5% of Native Americans/Pacific Islanders have HBP.
- 33% of the U.S. population have HBP; other published sources give a higher estimate—37%.
- Ages 20–34: 12.2% of males and 6.6% of females have HBP.

Who Is Physically Inactive?

- People with lower incomes and less than a 12th-grade education are more likely to be sedentary.
- Adults with a graduate degree are about twice as likely (80.6%) as adults with less than a high school diploma (41%) to engage in at least some leisure-time activity.

Who Is Physically Active in Leisure Time?

	(%)
Total	30.8
Males	33.9
Females	28.9
Whites	33.9
Blacks	22.9
Hispanics	23.8

Who Is Overweight or Obese?

	Prevalence of Overweight and Obesity (%)	Prevalence of Obesity (%)
Total	66.7	33.9
Males (M)	73.3	32.7
Females (F)	60.5	35.0
Whites		
Male	72.4	32.3
Female	57.5	32.7
Blacks		
Male	73.7	36.8
Female	77.7	52.9
Mexican Americans		
Male	74.8	26.8
Female	73.0	41.9
Hispanic/Latino	67.8	27.5
Asians	38.1	8.9
American Indian/ Alaska Native	67.1	32.4

Overweight in adults is BMI = 25.0 to 29.9. Obesity in adults is BMI = 30.0 or higher.

Who Has Metabolic Syndrome?

	Males (%)	Females (%)
Total	35.1	32.6
White	37.2	31.5
Black	25.3	38.8
Mexican Americans	33.2	40.6
Ages 20–39	20.3	15.6

SOURCE: American Heart Association, *2010 Heart and Stroke Facts Statistical Update* (National Center, 7272 Greenville Ave., Dallas, TX 75231–4596).

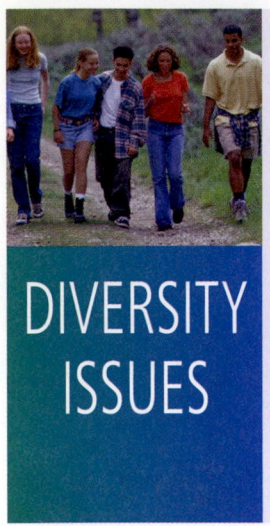

DIVERSITY ISSUES

Who Has High Cholesterol?

	Total Cholesterol 200 mg/dl or Higher	Total Cholesterol 240 mg/dl or Higher	LDL Cholesterol 130 mg/dl or Higher	HDL Cholesterol Less Than 40 mg/dl
Total	45.1%	15.7%	32.8%	15.5%
White males	42.6%	13.8%	33.8%	24.9%
White females	47.7%	18.1%	33.7%	6.5%
Black males	35.6%	7.9%	36.2%	13.5%
Black females	41.4%	13.4%	27.4%	6.1%
Mexican American males	52.1%	17.5%	45.0%	30.6%
Mexican American females	48.0%	14.5%	30.3%	10.5%

SOURCE: *2010 Heart Disease and Stroke Statistics*, American Heart Association.

(HDL) cholesterol. Additional information about LDLs and HDLs follows:

1. **Low-density lipoprotein (LDL).** LDLs are considered "bad" because they carry a large amount of cholesterol. They carry cholesterol from the liver out to the rest of the body. The lower density of the lipoprotein allows it to attach easily to the inner wall of the blood vessel, thus accelerating the atherosclerotic process. A *high* LDL cholesterol level increases your risk for atherosclerosis, CVD, and stroke (Table 9-2). It is recommended that LDL levels be kept below 100 mg/dl. How can you lower LDLs?
   - ✓ Don't smoke.
   - ✓ Manage stress.
   - ✓ Reduce consumption of saturated and trans fats.
   - ✓ Lose weight, if necessary.
   - ✓ Consume more fiber and omega-3 fats.

   Very low-density lipoproteins (VLDL) are even more dangerous. They carry triglycerides.

2. **High-density lipoprotein (HDL).** HDL carries cholesterol from the blood back to the liver where it is broken down for elimination from the body or sent out again as needed. It is considered the "good" cholesterol because of the dense structure of the lipoprotein. It is thought that HDL acts as a garbage collector in clearing away plaque and other debris as it flows through the bloodstream to the liver to be excreted from the body. The higher your HDL cholesterol level, the better and the more protection from CVD it provides. HDL also acts as an anti-inflammatory agent. See Table 9-2. HDL levels above 40 mg/dl are recommended. How can you increase your level of HDL?

- ✓ Exercise regularly.
- ✓ Don't smoke.
- ✓ Reduce weight and/or maintain a normal weight.
- ✓ High-fiber and low-fat diets may also increase the HDL cholesterol level.
- ✓ Use monounsaturated fats (e.g., olive oil, canola oil, sunflower oil) as primary fat, while keeping total fat intake low.

TABLE 9-2 *Interpreting the Numbers: Cholesterol Guidelines*

Total Cholesterol	Risk Category
Below 200 mg/dl	Desirable
200–239 mg/dl	Borderline high
240 mg/dl and above	High
LDL Cholesterol	
Below 100 mg/dl*	Optimal
100–129 mg/dl	Near optimal
130–159 mg/dl	Borderline high
160–189 mg/dl	High
190 mg/dL and above	Very high
HDL Cholesterol	
Below 40 mg/dl	Bad
40–59 mg/dl	Better
60 mg/dL and above	Best
Triglycerides	
Below 150 mg/dl	Desirable
150–199 mg/dl	Borderline high
200–499 mg/dl	High
500 mg/dl or above	Very high

*Achieving a goal of less than 170 is recommended if there is a high risk for CVD.

SOURCE: National Heart, Lung, and Blood Institute. Cholesterol levels are measured in milligrams (mg) of cholesterol per deciliter (dl) of blood.

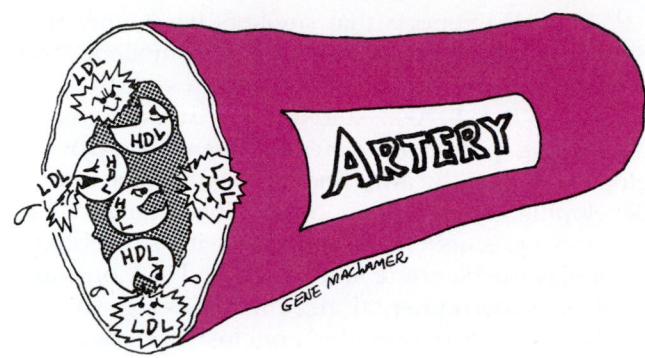

HDL cholesterol clearing away plaque in arteries.

TABLE 9-3	Ratio of Total Cholesterol to HDL Cholesterol	
Optimal ratio (very low risk)		3.5:1
Near optimal ratio (low risk)		4:1

A lipoprotein analysis gives a more accurate picture of your CVD risk than does total cholesterol alone. A lipoprotein analysis breaks down the total cholesterol into its components, or lipoproteins. Problems occur when there is too much LDL cholesterol for the HDLs to pick up promptly, or if there are not enough HDLs to do the job.

What causes LDL and HDL to get out of balance in some people? There is genetic variability in how efficiently (or inefficiently) a person metabolizes dietary saturated fat and cholesterol. Some people can eat almost anything and their blood cholesterol levels remain stable. Others find that even a small amount of dietary fat makes their blood cholesterol levels increase. Most of us are somewhere in between on this spectrum. An unhealthy combination of "good" and "bad" cholesterol quadruples the risk of heart attack.

Drs. Michael Brown and Joseph Goldstein won the 1985 Nobel Prize in Medicine for their discovery of **LDL cholesterol receptors.** Located primarily in liver cells, these receptors bind and remove cholesterol from the blood. The more cholesterol receptors you have, the more efficiently you can remove cholesterol from the blood. The number of cholesterol receptors is in part genetically determined. Lifestyle factors also influence the number. A diet high in saturated fat and cholesterol produces what Brown and Goldstein termed "double trouble." It not only saturates the receptors, it also decreases their number—a bad combination. So, to lower your level of LDLs, reduce your consumption of saturated and trans fats. Only about 5 percent of the population has genetically high cholesterol levels that remain elevated regardless of lifestyle.

Total Cholesterol/HDL Ratio Scientists believe that the ratio of total cholesterol to HDL cholesterol is a better indicator of risk for cardiovascular disease than is the total value alone. To determine your ratio, take a laboratory blood test that will reveal your total cholesterol and HDL cholesterol levels.

Next, divide the total cholesterol level by the HDL cholesterol level to find the ratio. For example, if the total cholesterol measures 160 and the HDL cholesterol 40, your ratio would be four to one (4:1) (160 ÷ 40 = 4). This would place you in the near optimal category, as you can see in Table 9-3. Everyone should strive for a ratio that is 4:1 or lower. The lower this ratio, the lower the risk for CVD. A ratio above 4:1 increases your CVD risk.

Average HDL levels in adult Americans are about 45 to 65 mg/dl, with women averaging higher values than men. The female sex hormone estrogen tends to raise HDL levels, which may explain why premenopausal women are usually protected from heart disease. Studies suggest that HDL levels above 70 may protect against heart disease, while those below 35 signal coronary risk.

Triglycerides **Triglycerides** are manufactured in the body to store excess fats. They are also known as *free fatty acids,* and in combination with cholesterol, they accelerate the formation of plaque. Triglycerides are carried in the bloodstream by very low-density lipoprotein (VLDL). These fatty acids are found in poultry skin, lunch meats, and shellfish. However, they are mainly manufactured in the liver from alcohol, starches, and refined sugars (honey included). Alcohol, starches, and sugars are not fats, but the body can convert them into fats and then dump those fats into the bloodstream. To lower triglycerides,

✓ Decrease consumption of alcohol, sugar, and refined carbohydrates.
✓ Reduce weight if overweight.
✓ Reduce consumption of animal fats in the diet (poultry skin, lunch meats, shellfish).
✓ Get regular aerobic exercise.
✓ If necessary, take prescribed medications.

As a general rule, you should keep your triglyceride level below 150 mg/dl of blood. However, some reports indicate that triglyceride levels over 100 should be cause for concern, especially if you have other CVD risk factors. See Table 9-2.

You should know your cholesterol level and have it checked annually, especially if you have a positive family history of CVD. The best way to do this is to have a 12-hour fasting blood test that is analyzed by a reputable laboratory. Over-the-counter tests that don't require fasting are not as reliable. Since cholesterol levels are greatly influenced by diet and lifestyle, follow these guidelines to reduce high levels:

✓ A diet rich in cholesterol—or, worse, one rich in saturated fat (saturated fat is highest in vegetable oils such as tropical and palm, in meat, and in high-fat dairy products) and trans fats (hydrogenated oils in many crackers, cookies, cakes, pies, and pastries)—can increase your blood cholesterol level. Keep total fat less than 30 percent of total calories per day and dietary cholesterol below 300 mg per day. This small modification in dietary fat can reduce cholesterol levels by 10 to 15 percent. (See Chapter 11 for other dietary strategies that affect heart health.)

✓ Reduce body weight if overweight. Weight reduction alone can lower cholesterol and triglyceride levels.

✓ Lowering your stress level also helps offset high cholesterol. See Chapter 10.

✓ Increase daily aerobic exercise. Try to walk more, use escalators and cars less, and be a participant rather than a spectator.

✓ Reduce alcohol, sugar, and caffeine consumption.

✓ Increase consumption of fiber-rich foods such as oatmeal, dried beans and peas, whole-grain breads and cereals, raw fruits and vegetables.

✓ Take your medication, if prescribed.

4. CIGARETTE SMOKING

Cigarette smoking is a primary risk factor. Nicotine increases heart rate and blood pressure and constricts blood vessels. Carbon monoxide also creates cardio-vascular stress by impairing the transport of oxygen in the blood. Smoking kills more than 400,000 Americans a year, and 35 percent of those deaths are CVD-related. About one in five deaths from CVD is attributable to smoking. Some health professionals are calling tobacco use a "weapon of mass destruction." Every cigarette package is required by law to carry a consumer warning. One such warning is "Cigarette Smoking Can Kill You."

Even Ann Landers, the nationally syndicated columnist, gave a warning: "Beware, cigarettes are killers that travel in packs." Numerous studies have proved that cigarette smoking causes oral cancer, lung cancer, and emphysema, and in women it is linked to cervical cancer, early menopause, and damage to the fetus during pregnancy. It also leads to the development of wrinkles in men and women. The number of Americans killed each year from smoking is greater than the number killed during World War II and the Vietnam War combined. No level of smoking is safe!

The AHA reports that smokers have more than twice the risk of heart attack of nonsmokers. Even limited smoking (four to five cigarettes per day) increases CVD risk. Also, smoking increases the risk of developing peripheral vascular disease (narrowing blood vessels in the arms and legs), which may lead to developing gangrene and, eventually, to amputation.

Passive smoke, synonymous with secondhand smoke, is the cigarette smoke inhaled by nonsmokers from environmental air. The U.S. surgeon general's new report provides conclusive evidence of the alarming public health threat posed by secondhand smoke. It declares smoking bans are the only way to protect nonsmokers. The research reveals that secondhand smoke is remarkably effective in damaging the cardiovascular system:

1. Nonsmokers may be *more* susceptible to heart and vascular damage from secondhand smoke than smokers are even though they absorb much smaller doses of the smoke's toxins. That is because smokers develop compensatory responses to some of the adverse cardiovascular effects of cigarette smoke—but nonsmokers do not get the "benefit" of these adaptive responses.

2. Carbon monoxide, a substance in secondhand smoke (and in inhaled cigarette smoke), damages (causes injuries or "nicks") the smooth inner lining of blood vessel walls. This accelerates the atherosclerotic buildup. Carbon monoxide, higher in the blood of smokers but also found in nonsmokers, decreases the amount of oxygen carried in the blood. It also reduces the heart's ability to use the oxygen it does receive.

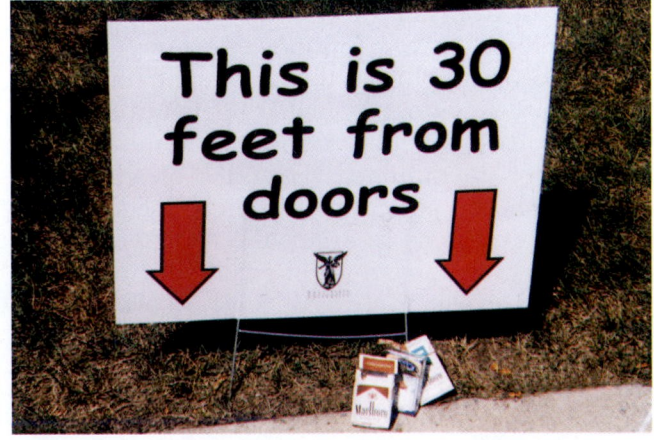

The science is clear: secondhand smoke is not mere annoyance—it's lethal. Some states ban smoking outdoors— from within 15 to 30 feet of all public buildings. They even post signs to indicate the specific distances. Others ban smoking on beaches and in parks.

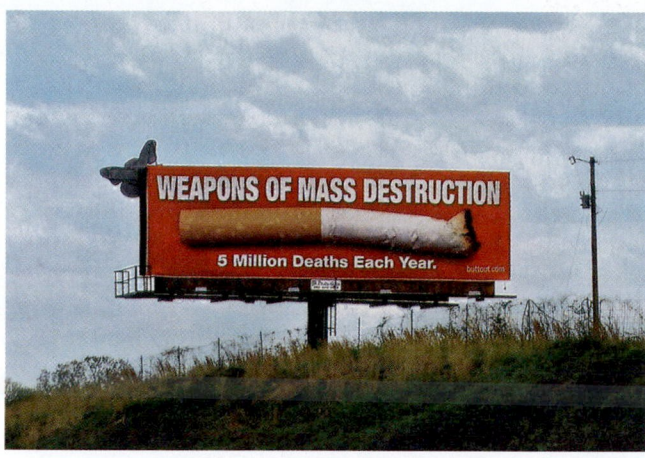

Smoking is the only legal form of suicide.

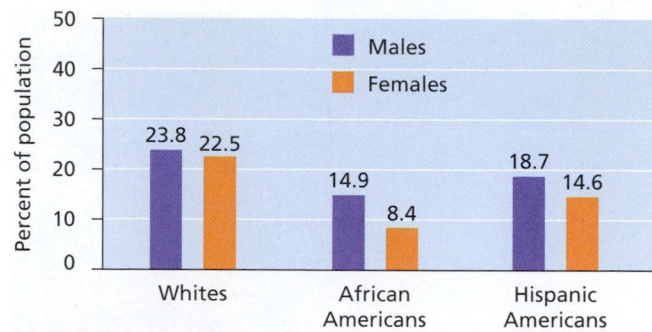

FIGURE 9-6   Prevalence of high school students smoking cigarettes by race/ethnicity and sex: United States, 2010.

SOURCE: AHA.

3. Even short exposure to secondhand smoke can cause blood platelets to become stickier in nonsmokers, making it more likely that a clot will form in the narrowed arteries, which can ultimately lead to a heart attack or stroke.
4. Secondhand smoke increases atherosclerosis by lowering HDL cholesterol and increasing LDL cholesterol buildup.
5. It increases chronic inflammation.
6. Nonsmokers exposed to secondhand smoke at home or work have a 30 percent higher risk of dying from CVD than do other nonsmokers.
7. It increases insulin resistance.
8. Secondhand smoke is a human carcinogen, killing about 3,000 nonsmokers a year through lung cancer.
9. The population burden associated with passive smoking and CVD is estimated to be 50,000 deaths annually in the United States. The simplest and most cost-effective control measure to reduce cost is to *mandate* smoke-free workplaces, schools, and public places.

While studies show that smoking has declined by more than 49 percent since 1965, this downward trend appears to be leveling off. There are still 4,000 new smokers every day. About 80 percent of people who use tobacco begin before age 18 (see Figure 9-6). A nonsmoker should not begin to smoke. Smokers should stop *now*. Don't hesitate, do it! Ninety percent of smokers who quit do so on their own! See Chapter 14 for tips on how to quit smoking.

5. OBESITY

Obesity has escalated to epidemic proportions in the United States and is continuing to increase at an alarming rate. Weight wise, Americans are evenly divided. Slightly more than one-third are obese, one-third are overweight, and one-third are normal or under weight. The goal of *Healthy People 2010* was for the percentage of obese people to drop to 15 percent. That goal was set at a time when nearly 25 percent of all adults were obese. According to the latest federal statistics, about 34 percent of adults are now obese. See the Diversity Issues box on page 295. Obesity is uncomfortable; increases the burden on the vital organs, especially the heart; and is directly linked to CVD. Obesity is expensive too. Annual medical costs for an obese person are 37.7 percent more than those for someone of normal weight.

It is especially risky to have excess body fat in the waist and abdominal area even if you are not overweight! Abdominal obesity more than doubles the risk of dying of heart attack (and even of cancer). Abdominal fat, called visceral fat, is located deep within the abdomen, around the internal abdominal organs. Visceral fat appears to be metabolically more active than fat elsewhere, and it pumps fatty acids, appetite-stimulating hormones and inflammation-fueling chemicals into the bloodstream. It interferes with liver function, hampers processing of cholesterol and insulin, and may compromise the functions of other systems and tissues. Visceral fat is linked to insulin resistance (a precursor to diabetes).

Waist measurement, the ratio of your waist to hip measurement and body mass index (BMI) are ways to estimate one's body fat and to assess CVD risk. A high-risk waistline is 35 inches or more for women, 40 inches or more for men—even if you are at normal weight. See Chapters 3 and 12 for instructions on how to measure your waist and hip and determine your waist-to-hip ratio. What is your ratio? What is optimal for men and women? Skinfold calipers (discussed in Chapter 3) more accurately measure percent of bodyfat. The CDC considers anyone above 30 pounds over target weight to be obese.

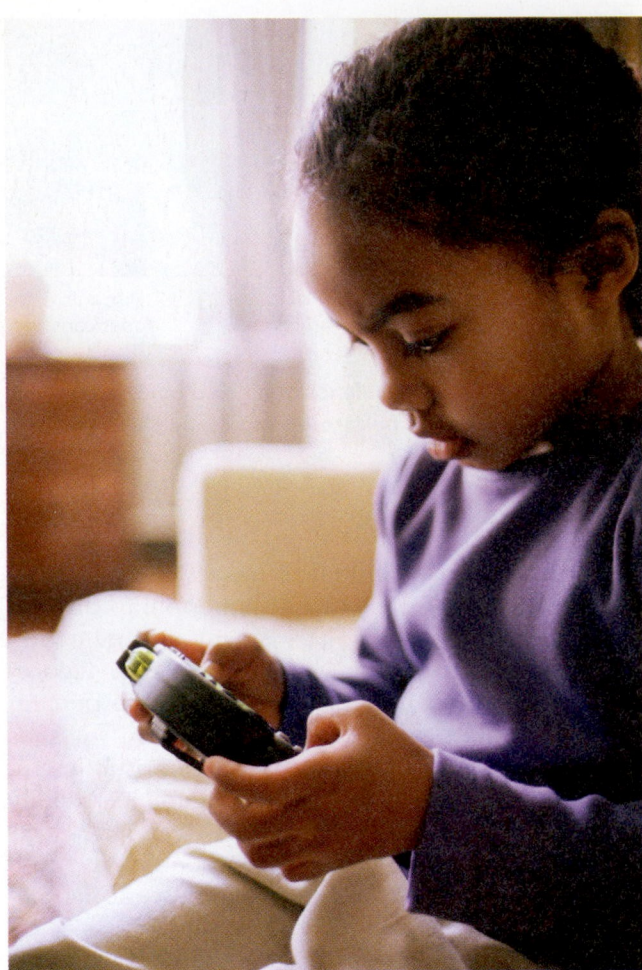

Health experts recommend that school-age children get at least 60 minutes of exercise daily. Today, too many children spend their time in nonphysical activities such as playing video games and watching TV. Former President Bill Clinton states, "Our children may grow up to be the first generation with shorter life spans than we had."

Besides all the other negative aspects of obesity, too much fat unleashes a flood of molecules called cytokines that trigger systemwide inflammation. Obesity is a pro-inflammatory state. Chronic inflammation causes widespread tissue damage. The plumper and more abundant a person's fat cells, the greater the number of cytokine-releasing macrophage cells in the fat tissue. Macrophages play an important role in the development of fatty plaques that lead to atherosclerosis. Visceral fat is thought to be a high producer of cytokines—another reason to lose the belly fat.

More than 66 percent of the U.S. population is now obese or overweight. In 1980 the number was only 46 percent, up steadily from the 1970s. Childhood obesity rates have more than tripled since the late 1970s. Ninety percent of people with type 2 diabetes are overweight. Obesity, considered a chronic

disease, causes more than 300,000 premature, preventable deaths per year.

In addition, obesity puts women in particular at increased risk of CVD. A study conducted by the Harvard Medical School of 115,000 women ages 30 to 55 found that of all the women in the 8-year study who developed CVD, 40 percent had no other risk factors except being 20 percent or more over their ideal weight. Women who had been slim at age 18 and gained weight in adulthood seemed to be at increased risk. The first step in medical treatment for these conditions is usually weight reduction. Obesity is controllable and can be reversed. You can eliminate the obesity risk factor by maintaining a reasonable weight (see Chapter 12). Even modest weight reduction (5 to 10 percent of body weight) can help reduce your risk of CVD and stroke.

Physical inactivity is a major factor in the development of obesity in men, women, and children. Watching too much television is one of the main culprits. The number of television hours watched per person in this country averages about 4 per day. Some call this "death by TV." Americans should limit TV viewing to about 1 hour or less a day to prevent physical and mental inactivity. Of course, consuming more calories than are used in daily activity also contributes to obesity. NOTE: Accumulating 10,000 steps expends approximately 500 calories!

6. DIABETES MELLITUS (TYPE 1 AND TYPE 2) AND PREDIABETES

What do blindness, hearing loss, gangrene, kidney failure, heart attack, and stroke have in common? They can all result from diabetes, which eventually strikes one in three people in the United States. See the Numbers box.

Diabetes mellitus (which includes both type 1 and type 2) is a disease that affects how the body

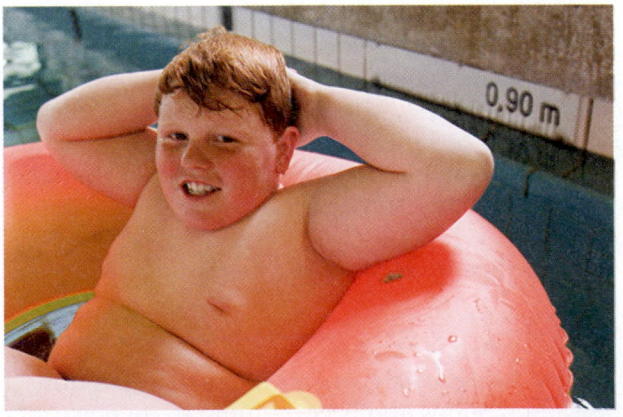

Diabetes has increased at an alarming rate in the United States in the last decade due to escalating obesity rates. Health experts are blaming a wired-up, couch potato culture for this escalation.

uses *glucose,* a sugar that is the body's main source of fuel. This chronic disease is characterized by the body's inability to produce enough of the hormone *insulin* or use it properly. In the normal digestive process, the food you eat is changed to glucose. Insulin (which is produced in the pancreas) carries the glucose in the blood to the body's cells so that the body the gets the energy it needs. In diabetes, this normal process is interrupted. When glucose doesn't reach the cells, it accumulates in the blood and the underfueled cells are starved for energy. This surplus glucose is eliminated by the kidneys, which pass it off in the urine. Too much sugar in the urine and in the blood is a classic sign of diabetes.

Diabetes is found in two forms, type 1 and type 2. Genes have a hand in both types, but more so in type 1. Yet, research on identical twins reveals that just because one twin develops type 1 diabetes the other twin doesn't always develop it. The other twin has only a 30–50 percent chance of coming down with it. If genes were the only factor involved as a type 1 diabetes cause, both identical twins should get it. Something else, in addition to genes, has to be at work. Individuals with a genentic tendency to develop type 1 diabetes appear to be fine until something "triggers" the onset of the disease. It may be a virus that attacks the pancreas that triggers the onset, or it may be something in the environment. Type 2 results from a combination of environmental and genetic factors and is heavily influenced by obesity. Scientists believe that a genetic predisposition for type 2 can be warded off, even prevented, by lifestyle interventions of weight management and exercise.

Insulin-dependent diabetes, also known as type 1 or juvenile onset, occurs when the immune system attacks and permanently disables the insulin-making cells in the pancreas. In this form, the pancreas makes little or no insulin. The diabetic must receive insulin injections every day to stay alive and must carefully watch his or her diet and exercise regularly. It occurs most often in children or young adults. Symptoms develop rapidly, usually within a period of months or even weeks. Approximately one million Americans have type 1 diabetes. Medically supervised medication and lifestyle strategies are key to controlling (or managing) type 1.

More common (90 to 95 percent of diabetics) is non-insulin-dependent diabetes, once known as adult-onset or type 2, in which the pancreas makes insulin but either the amount is insufficiently released or the body cannot properly use what is available. This type of diabetes can often be controlled without insulin injections through other medications, diet, and weight management. This form of the disease usually occurs in people over 40 years old and is associated with aging and obesity. New data,

however, show a dramatic rise of type 2 in children and young adults, making the term "adult-onset diabetes" obsolete. Because the onset of type 2 is gradual, the disease may go undetected for years. Diabetes seriously increases the risk of developing cardiovascular disease. About 75 percent of people with diabetes die of some form of heart, stroke, or blood vessel disease. Part of the reason for this is that diabetes affects cholesterol and triglyceride levels by producing a different kind of LDL that is even worse for the arteries than is ordinary LDL. This accelerates atherosclerosis. Even so, type 2 diabetes can be delayed or averted by weight management and physical activity. One condition shared almost universally by type 2 diabetics is obesity. Not all obese people become diabetic, but *90 percent of people with type 2 diabetes are overweight or obese.*

The surge in youth obesity in this country has paralleled a rise in childhood type 2 diabetes. At one time type 2 diabetes was almost unheard of in children. They almost always had type 1. A new advisory from the American Academy of Pediatrics and the American Diabetes Association (ADA) calls for diabetes testing of overweight children with any two other risk factors starting at age 10 or at puberty, if it comes earlier. See the projected diabetes rates for those born in 2003 in Figure 9-7.

Many people know their blood pressure and cholesterol levels, but few know their glucose level. A substantially elevated glucose level is the chief diagnostic sign of diabetes. Unfortunately, far too few people are properly tested. As a result, researchers

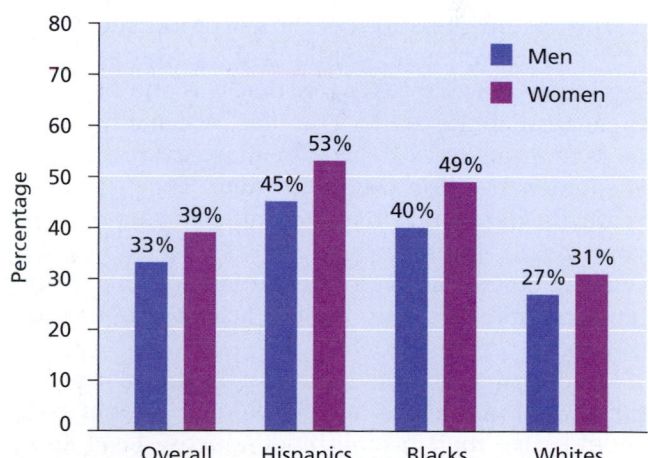

FIGURE 9-7   *Children born in 2003: Who will have type 2 diabetes?* A third of the people born in the United States in 2003 will develop diabetes. The chances of developing diabetes are highest among women and minorities. Minorities have a combination of genetic predisposition and higher obesity rates that puts them at risk.

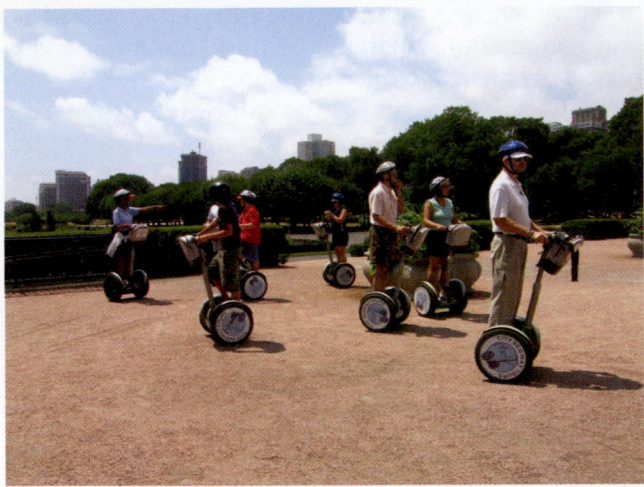

Our culture has minimized physical activity and maximized convenience and inactivity.

say that millions of people who have type 2 diabetes don't know it.

Now we have identified a condition called **prediabetes** (or insulin resistance), which is a precursor to diabetes. It is defined as a fasting blood glucose between 100 and 125 mg/dl. Millions of Americans have this metabolic condition where the blood-glucose level is only slightly elevated. Prediabetes should not be taken lightly. It means you are on course to develop type 2 diabetes, heart disease, and stroke, and even if you don't, you face a higher risk of cognitive decline and certain cancers. The millions of people with prediabetes can be protected from developing full-blown diabetes—and its life-threatening complications—by losing weight and, if necessary, taking medications to lower their blood sugar.

The main reason public health experts are urging wider glucose testing is that it is the only way to catch diabetes early. The disease usually causes no symptoms for a decade or more even though it is silently festering the entire time. That's 10 to 12 years during which diabetes quietly eats away at your vision, injures your kidneys and nerves, and sets the stage for CVD. This is damage that would be preventable if only people learned sooner that they have type 2 diabetes.

According to the American Diabetes Association's new guidelines, all people age 45 and older should have their fasting blood-glucose level tested at least every 3 years. Several groups of people are at greater risk and should be checked for diabetes at least once a year. Get tested, starting at age 35, if you

✓ Are overweight, especially with extra belly fat.
✓ Have a brother, sister, or parent with diabetes.
✓ Are not white (i.e., African American, Hispanic, and Native American, especially the Pima tribe of Arizona).

TABLE 9-4	*Blood-Glucose Levels*
Normal	65 to less than 100 mg/dl
Prediabetes:	100–125 mg/dl
Impaired fasting glucose or insulin resistance	
Diabetes	126 mg/dl or more

✓ Had a baby weighing more than 9 pounds or had gestational diabetes (diabetes during pregnancy).
✓ Have an HDL cholesterol of 35 or less or a triglyceride level of 250 or more.
✓ Have hypertension or take antihypertension drugs.
✓ Had a minimally elevated glucose level on a previous test.

Two readings of *126 mg/dl or more* on a fasting blood-glucose test taken on different days means you have diabetes. Less elevated reading, from *100 to 125,* indicate impaired fasting glucose, which means you have prediabetes or are insulin resistant and face a sharply increased risk of diabetes (see Table 9-4). Regardless of your glucose level, you are probably prediabetic if you have low HDL, high triglycerides, high blood pressure, or excessive abdominal fat (i.e., a waist measurement of more than 35 inches for a woman and 40 inches for a man). Numerous studies have concluded that a large waist is a better predictor of CVD and type 2 diabetes risk than body weight, body mass index, or other measures.

Certain lifestyle changes such as

✓ regular moderate exercise,
✓ losing weight (5 percent to 7 percent of body weight),
✓ stopping smoking,
✓ eating a high-fiber diet, and
✓ eating a diet low in simple carbohydrates (sugar and other sweets) and alcohol or following the DASH diet

can improve insulin resistance; they may also help improve the associated HDL, triglyceride, and blood pressure problems. Those steps can also help people who have type 2 diabetes (and sometimes even those with type 1) control their glucose level.

Two symptoms that occur in many people with diabetes are increased *thirst* and *frequent urination.* That's because excess glucose circulating in your body draws water from your tissues, making you feel dehydrated. To quench your thirst, you drink a lot of water and other beverages, and that leads to more frequent urination. Other signs and symptoms of type 2 diabetes are

✓ Flu-like symptoms. Since glucose is not reaching your cells, you may feel tired and weak.
✓ Weight loss or weight gain
✓ Blurred vision
✓ Frequent hunger
✓ Dry skin
✓ Slowly healing wounds
✓ Itching, tingling, or numbness in the extremities
✓ Frequent vaginal or skin infections
✓ Combinations of these symptoms

Unless detected and controlled, diabetes can ultimately lead to stroke, heart disease, kidney failure, blindness, amputation of limbs from gangrene, and death. See Table 9-5. According to the ADA, the disease is a leading cause of death in this country and diabetics are two to four times as prone to heart attack and stroke as are nondiabetics. Three out of every five people with type 2 diabetes suffer at least one significant complication of the disease. Assess your risk of developing diabetes by completing "Are You at Risk for Diabetes?" Lab Activity 9-4.

Primary Risk Factors (Uncontrollable)

1. POSITIVE FAMILY HISTORY

A family history of heart disease in brothers, sisters, parents, or grandparents increases your risk of developing CVD. Tendencies toward high blood pressure, stroke, peripheral blood vessel disease, rheumatic fever, high blood lipid levels, obesity, and early heart attack appear to be somewhat hereditary. This is why your physician is so interested in your family history. A family's lifestyle also may contribute to heart disease and stroke. For example, family members may be overweight, smoke, eat large amounts of cholesterol and saturated fat, or be physically inactive. You should find out as much as possible about your family's medical history. You can be alerted early to a possible risk and take preventive measures.

2. MALE GENDER (+ POSTMENOPAUSAL WOMEN)

Although CVD is the leading cause of death for both men and women, males have a higher risk of heart attack, especially earlier in life. The gender factor exists because men have heart attacks 10 years earlier than women. Until age 55, men also have greater

TABLE 9-5	Complications of Diabetes

Over time, untreated or poorly controlled diabetes can cause debilitating and even life-threatening complications. Diabetes quadruples the risk of heart attack for women and doubles it for men.

	What happens	Complications
Eyes	Retinopathy. The small blood vessels of the retina become damaged. Also, cataracts and glaucoma are more likely to develop.	Decreased vision and ultimately blindness. Diabetes is the leading cause of blindness in people 20 to 74.
Blood vessels	Plaque builds up and blocks arteries in major organs, such as the heart and brain. The walls of blood vessels are damaged so that they cannot transfer oxygen normally.	Poor circulation causes wounds to heal poorly and can lead to heart disease, stroke, gangrene of the feet and hands, and infections. Diabetics have two to four times the usual rate of CVD.
Kidneys	Nephropathy. Blood vessels thicken; protein leaks into urine; blood isn't filtered normally.	Poor kidney function; kidney failure. Nearly one-half of new cases of end-stage kidney disease stem from diabetes.
Genitals	Poor circulation in blood vessels in genitals can lead to impotence.	Eighty percent of diabetic men experience impotence.
Nerves	Neuropathy. Nerves are damaged because excess glucose injures the walls of the tiny blood vessels that nourish the nerves and interferes with the blood supply to them.	Leg weakness; reduced sensation, tingling, and pain in the hands and feet; chronic damage to nerves. Nerve damage and poor blood vessel circulation may lead to leg amputations.

risk for hypertension than women do. The incidence of stroke is higher for males than females under age 65. The increased male risk is not clearly understood. Some credit the increased risk to the male sex hormone testosterone, which triggers the production of low-density lipoproteins, thereby clogging blood vessels. Others say a male's lifestyle may be the culprit.

We do know that a female's hormonal makeup is protective until menopause. Female hormones signal the liver to produce more "good" cholesterol (HDL) and make blood vessels more elastic than a male's blood vessels, especially during childbearing years. Once women reach menopause (usually in their early to middle fifties), their rate of heart-related problems equal or surpass those of men. Part of the explanation for this is that women tend to go up in waist size after menopause due to increased visceral fat (the kind that promotes inflammation). This is due to a hormonal shift: decreased levels of estrogen which are no longer needed to sustain pregnancy, and increases in testosterone and the male tendency to bulk up around the middle as opposed to the pre-menopausal tendency for females to store excess fat in the buttocks and thighs. Lower estrogen may increase appetite and trigger cravings for sweets and fatty foods. Other factors that come into play for postmenomausal women at this time include a sharp rise in LDL cholesterol, which remains higher during this transition, a more sedentary lifestyle, and weight gain, especially in the belly area. It is crucial that women in their early to mid-forties begin to gradually increase physical activity. How much? At least an hour of moderate-intensity exercise is needed according to the most recent studies. Second, they must become more aware of dietary habits to help offset metabolic changes that can lead to weight gain with menopause.

It is imperative that males and postmenopausal women modify other risk factors to protect their cardiovascular systems (i.e., increase physical activity, maintain a healthy weight, don't smoke, keep blood

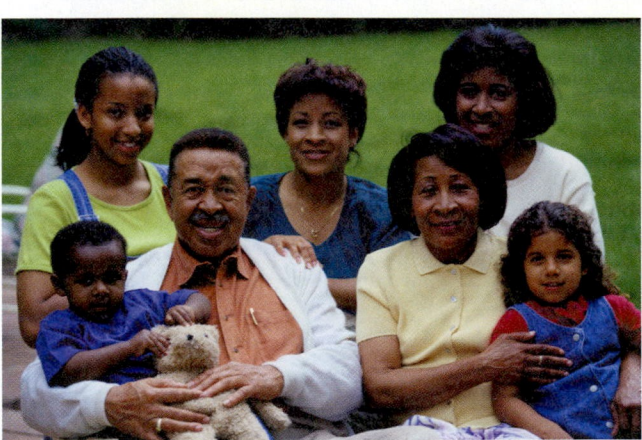

African Americans have increased risk for heart attack, stroke, and diabetes

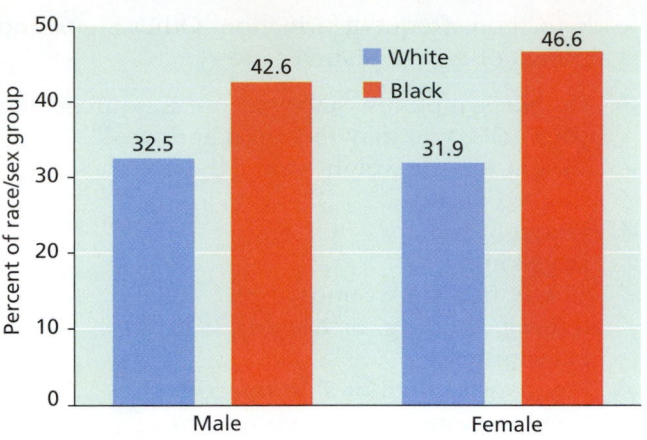

FIGURE 9-8 Estimated percentage of population with hypertension by race and sex among U.S. adults. Hypertensives are defined as persons with a systolic level ≥140 and/or a diastolic level ≥90 or those who reported using antihypertensive medication.

pressure and cholesterol levels at recommended levels, manage stress, modify emotional behaviors, and don't drink excessive amounts of alcohol).

3. RACE

According to the AHA, African Americans have the greatest risk of all races for heart attack and stroke. High blood pressure develops earlier in life in blacks than in whites and is generally more severe (see Figure 9-8). One explanation for this higher incidence is that many African Americans share a mutation in a gene that helps control blood pressure. A hereditary intolerance to sodium may also account for the danger. African Americans' and Mexican Americans' risk of diabetes and obesity is twice that of any other ethnic group in the United States (see Figure 9-7). Social and economic stresses may also contribute to increased cardiovascular disease risk. It is paramount that early heart health intervention and education programs be supported for African American populations. Also, being aware of these risks, African Americans should adopt a healthy lifestyle early. See the Diversity Issues box on page 295 for additional population information.

Heart disease and stroke risks are also high among Mexican Americans, American Indians, and Native Hawaiians. Again, this increased risk is due to higher rates of obesity and diabetes.

4. AGE

Being older has some advantages (wisdom and experience), but protection from CVD is not one of them. As you age, your risk for developing heart disease increases. This does not mean that coronary heart disease is *only* a disease of the old. You don't suddenly drop dead one day at age 45 from a "heart attack." At any age and certainly at age 18, you have atherosclerotic plaque in your arteries. It accumulates over time, and by the time you've gained "age," you've also increased the private stash of cholesterol in your arteries. There is little that can be done to stop the calendar. Adopting a healthy lifestyle early in life may add years to your life and life to your years.

Secondary Risk Factors (All Controllable)

These factors are associated with increased risk of CVD, though not as directly as the primary risk factors.

1. INDIVIDUAL RESPONSE TO STRESS

We all feel stress, but we each feel it in different amounts and react in different ways. Too much stress over a long time and unhealthy responses to it can damage our health. Stress is unavoidable. It includes happy, wonderful, and positive events as well as sad, destructive, and negative ones. For example, the death of a family member and the birth of a child, while perceived differently, are stressors that produce the same physiological response in the body. Job stress may be particularly unhealthy. High blood pressure is three times more common among people who have jobs with high demands but little control (assembly line worker, waitress), or people who are unrecognized for their efforts. Stress has been found to cause a rise in heart rate, blood pressure, depression, and blood cholesterol, and it can lead to excessive smoking or eating—all linked to CVD. Stress (and depression) almost triples the risk of heart attack. Note these examples: Indianapolis 500 race car drivers have higher cholesterol levels after they race than before; tax accountants have increased cholesterol around April 15; and students have higher cholesterol levels during exams. Research shows that social isolation increases

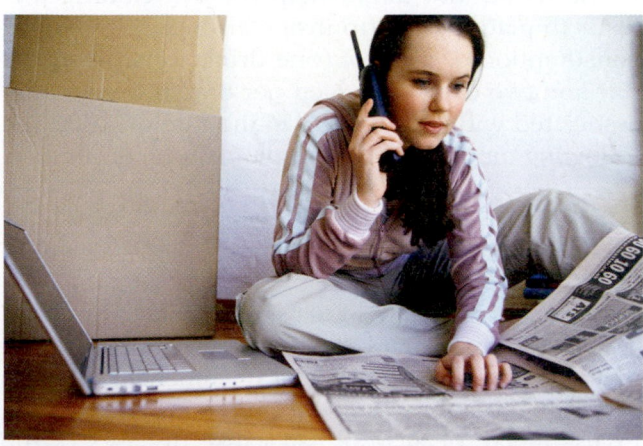

Doing several things at the same time (multitasking) is an excellent example of how hectic life in the twenty-first century has become.

feelings of stress and its negative health consequences. One of the most important antidotes for dealing with social isolation is a good social support system (i.e., family and friends, church membership, etc.). Low educational and socioeconomic levels may also increase stress for many, due to causes such as dangerous living environment, poor access to health care, unhealthy lifestyle, and poor nutrition.

Stress causes chemical wear and tear on the body by releasing stress hormones into the bloodstream. Large amounts of stress hormones are found in the bloodstreams of people who react to stressful situations with hostile and angry behavior. However, low levels of stress hormones are found in the bloodstreams of people who react normally to stressful events. How you respond to stress seems to be the critical factor. You should recognize stress in your life (the positive and the negative) and learn to handle the stressful situations in a healthful manner. Coping with stress successfully is vital in today's hectic, in-the-fast-lane lifestyle. Exercise, relaxation techniques, and behavioral modification are excellent methods for reducing stress.

We need to change the way we look at or perceive stressful situations. Problems are to be solved, not worried about. Read more about ways to reduce stress in Chapter 10.

2. EMOTIONAL BEHAVIOR (ANGER AND HOSTILITY)

Several studies have linked emotional behavior to increased risk of heart disease. Until recently there were just three emotional behavior patterns or **personality types—Types A, B, and C.** Now a newly coined personality type, **Type D** (which stands for "distressed"), has been identified and may be the type with a dangerous risk for CVD. The Type A individual exhibits aggressiveness, competitiveness, and impatience and is a workaholic. Type As demonstrate a high degree of time urgency—a tendency to do two or three things at the same time. The Type B individual is more relaxed, noncompetitive, patient, and slow to anger. Type Cs are actually classified as Type As but learn to cope with emotional stress by using the five Cs: control, commitment, challenge, choices in lifestyle, and connectedness. Such people welcome change, considering it a challenge. They are committed to goals, gaining confidence as a result (see Chapter 10). Type Cs are called *"hardy" stress resisters*.

Early studies identified Type A people as the ones at greater risk of having heart attacks. However, more recent research indicates that it is only when a Type A person exhibits the behaviors of *hostility* and *anger* that a serious risk is apparent. These behaviors arouse the fight-or-flight response, significantly elevate blood pressure, overstimulate the production of stress hormones, and have been documented to increase coronary artery atherosclerosis. Some studies found that hostility levels are a more accurate predictor of heart disease than high cholesterol, hypertension, smoking, or obesity. The other Type A behaviors do not seem to be as significant but may eventually lead to hostile, angry reactions to stress. That's why Type A behavior should be recognized. Types B, C, and D will also suffer adverse health consequences when angry, hostile behaviors are exhibited.

Type D people possess negative emotions and tend to be depressed, anxious, irritable, insecure, and distant. They have a joint tendency toward "negative effectivity" (worry, irritability, gloom) and "social inhibition" (discomfort in social interactions, reticence, and a lack of social poise). Some scientists believe that the social and emotional problems associated with Type D personality can increase the chances of developing cardiovascular disease. Hypertension and CHD have been linked to those identified as Type Ds. They seem to have more inflammation throughout the body and exaggerated blood pressure and other negative reactions to stress. Among people who already have heart conditions, those with Type D personalities are less responsive to treatment, have poorer quality of life, and also are more likely to die prematurely.

Twenty percent of apparently healthy people experience extreme surges in blood pressure when confronted with the challenges of everyday life. They are called **hot reactors** because their systolic blood pressure can rise from 120 to a deadly 300 when they are stressed. They often go untreated until felled by a stress-induced heart attack or stroke. Hot reactors can be found in all emotional behavior types.

We are not born with hot reacting, angry, and hostile behaviors. These behaviors are learned, and for the sake of our health, we can unlearn them. Learning to modify negative emotional behaviors with the antistress methods found in Chapter 10 (such as exercise, yoga, etc.) is not difficult and may add years to your life. How does a "hostile heart" become less angry and cynical—and become a "trusting heart"? Try these suggestions:

1. *Stop angry, cynical thoughts.* Every time you have a cynical thought, think to yourself, "STOP!" This is called *thought stopping* and is an effective behavior modification technique when practiced regularly.
2. *Practice laughing at yourself.* Once you realize how silly your anger is in many situations, laughing at yourself will quickly replace fuming.
3. *Be empathetic.* Put yourself in the other person's shoes. Often the other individual is a victim of circumstances too.
4. *Reason and understand your anger.* There will be times when anyone would be angry in the same situation, but you must say, "I have this trait, and it is bad for my health." Cognitively decide whether the situation warrants your attention and whether you have an effective response. If not, take a "time out" from the situation.
5. *Learn to relax.* Practice the excellent "stress busters" (such as exercise, meditation, etc.) in Chapter 10.
6. *Practice patience and trust.* Instead of getting irritated while standing in a line, concentrate on a relaxing word (such as "quiet") until your anger subsides. Trust that others are not out to cheat you.
7. *Become a good listener.* Pay attention to what others are saying and do not interrupt. This may help you understand the situation better *before* you jump to an angry response.
8. *Live as if you had a serious disease.* You will soon see that the little problems that once riled you up aren't really so important.
9. *Learn to forgive.* Compassion is the strongest medicine for anger. Blame leads to anger; forgiveness heals.

3. EXCESSIVE ALCOHOL (+ SOME ILLEGAL DRUGS)

Drinking too much alcohol raises blood pressure and triglyceride levels, damages the heart muscle, and increases risk of stroke and heart failure. The American Heart Association reported recently that binge drinking in college raises C-reactive protein levels and may lead to heart disease later in life.

Alcohol consumption, especially of red wine, has received attention as a protective factor against CVD because it is thought to raise HDL cholesterol in the blood and might help prevent clotting that leads to plaque buildup inside arteries. *"Moderate"* consumption of alcohol (one drink for women per day and two drinks for men per day) is the amount associated with a reduction in the rate of CVD. The following amounts are examples of one drink:

✓ 1½ oz. of bourbon, scotch, vodka, gin
✓ 4 oz. wine
✓ 12 oz. beer

If you don't drink, don't start. A protective effect of alcohol consumption has not been proven, but many adverse effects are well documented. Besides causing automobile accidents and social disruption, excess intake of alcohol can cause diseases of the liver, pancreas, and nervous system, and increase breast and colon cancer risk. To put the benefit of moderate drinking in perspective, the reduction in heart disease risk is comparable to what you might achieve by exercising regularly or by cutting blood cholesterol levels through a low-fat diet.

Stimulant illegal drugs such as cocaine, methamphetamine ("meth"), and MDMA ("Ecstasy") can also cause serious CVD problems, including heart attack, stroke, and sudden cardiac death. Fatalities have been recorded even in first-time users of cocaine. Intravenous drug use carries a high risk of infections of the heart (endocarditis) and stroke.

4. METABOLIC SYNDROME (SYNDROME X)

Also known as syndrome X, insulin-resistance syndrome, and prediabetes syndrome, **metabolic syndrome** is a dangerous cluster of symptoms that raise the risk of heart disease, stroke, diabetes, and some cancers. It is defined as having three or more of the following five risk factors:

✓ Elevated blood pressure: blood pressure higher than 130/85
✓ Elevated glucose: fasting blood sugar of at least 100 mg/dl (a sign of insulin resistance)
✓ High triglycerides: triglycerides of 150 or higher
✓ Low HDL ("good") cholesterol: HDL cholesterol less than 40 for men and 50 for women
✓ Obesity: a waist measurement of more than 35 inches for women and 40 inches for men

Do you have metabolic syndrome? It is a silent disease that affects approximately 25 percent of white Americans and even more African Americans, Mexican Americans, and Native Americans. Scientists know a lot about the components that make up metabolic syndrome, but they know less about the overall syndrome. The key element seems to be insulin resistance, but that is largely a result of obesity (especially abdominal or visceral fat) and lack of exercise. Thus, the root cause is hard to determine.

The best treatment for metabolic syndrome is a healthy diet, regular exercise, and weight loss, even if you don't lose much. See the Diversity Issues box on page 295.

5. C-REACTIVE PROTEIN (CRP)

Scientists have known for some time that inflammation in the blood vessels can trigger heart attacks and strokes by causing the plaque buildup in the arteries to become inflamed and unstable. This can result in the plaque rupturing and and a clot developing that induces a heart attack or stroke. Inflammation can be measured with a blood test that checks for a substance called **C-reactive protein,** a marker for this inflammation. CRP is produced by the liver in response to inflammation somewhere in the body and is now recognized as an important factor in heart disease, Alzheimer's, cancer, and diabetes. Elevated levels of CRP are linked to an increased risk for heart attack and stroke. A person can have no outward signs of inflammation but still have subtle inflammation and hence elevated CRP.

Twenty-five percent of Americans who have heart attacks have no identifiable risk factors. That is why scientists have been searching persistently for another piece of the puzzle; CRP looks to be one of the missing pieces.

Doctors are not recommending universal blood testing for CRP because even something as simple as the common cold (or minor injuries) can boost it. What causes the inflammation?

✓ Unhealthy diet, especially high in saturated and trans fats
✓ Obesity (fat cells release proteins that cause low-level inflammation) and excessive eating (the bigger the meal, the higher CRP levels climb)
✓ High LDL and low HDL
✓ High blood pressure and smoking (both damage the lining of blood vessel walls)
✓ Lingering infections (such as chronic gum disease, sinus infections, urinary-tract infections, and sexually transmitted diseases).

What can be done?

✓ Regular exercise. Physically fit people have lower CRP levels.
✓ Cholesterol-lowering drugs called statins also reduce CRP, as do aspirin and some other medications. Low doses of aspirin (e.g., a "baby" aspirin) are recommended for patients with coronary disease who are not taking other anticoagulants and do not have contraindications to aspirin. Also, antibiotics work.
✓ Not smoking. Smoking harms the entire cardiovascular system.
✓ Diet. People who eat a diet with a high-glycemic load have higher CRP. See Chapter 11 for information on a high-glycemic diet. Also, eat foods rich in omega-3 fatty acids (salmon, tuna, sardines, flax seeds, lots of fruits and vegetables, and whole grains).
✓ Brush and floss your teeth thoroughly, and get dental checkups.
✓ Tame stress and depression.
✓ Protect against irritants (minimize unprotected exposure to the sun, drink alcohol in moderation).
✓ Rein in infections. Get vaccinated against flu, pneumonia, hepatitis B, and HPV (for women), and treat sexually transmitted disease and gum and sinus infections.

6. HOMOCYSTEINE

Homocysteine is an amino acid in the blood and a natural by-product of protein metabolism. The consumption of protein from meat or vegetable sources (such as soy) starts a series of biochemical reactions that ultimately lead to the production of homocysteine. Normally homocysteine is converted into nondamaging amino acids by folacin (often called folate or folic acid) and vitamins B_6 and B_{12}. However, in some individuals these processes are impaired, and homocysteine accumulates in greater quantities than it would normally. Studies have shown that too much homocysteine in the blood is related to a higher risk of CHD, stroke, peripheral vascular disease, and cognitive decline (or dementia). Further, it is known that homocysteine causes injuries (or "nicks") and inflammation in cells lining the arteries, makes the blood more prone to clotting, and promotes the oxidation of low-density lipoprotein which makes it more likely that cholesterol will be deposited as plaque in the blood vessels. A high homocysteine level is considered to be a risk factor for CVD and to be in the same league as cholesterol.

Homocysteine levels in the blood are strongly influenced by diet as well as genetic factors. The dietary components with the greatest positive effects are folic acid and vitamins B_6 and B_{12}. Folic acid and the B vitamins help break down homocysteine and thus lower concentrations in the blood. Also, studies reveal that low blood levels of folic acid are linked with a higher risk of fatal CHD and stroke.

Along with diets high in protein and low in B vitamins, heavy smoking has been linked to high homocysteine levels. Heavy smokers have up to 50 percent higher homocysteine levels than nonsmokers.

Although evidence for the benefit of lowering homocysteine levels is lacking, people with high risk should be strongly advised to get enough folic acid and vitamins B_6 and B_{12} in their diets. Foods high in these nutrients include

✓ Folacin: leafy greens, broccoli, wheat germ, beans, whole grains, fortified oatmeal
✓ Vitamin B_6: whole grains, bananas, potatoes, beans, fish, meat, poultry
✓ Vitamin B_{12}: meat, poultry, liver, eggs, dairy, fish, fortified cereals, soy products

It has been suggested that laboratory testing for homocysteine levels can improve the assessment of CHD risk. It may be particularly useful in people who have a personal or family history of CVD, but in whom the well-established risk factors (inactivity, smoking, high blood pressure, obesity) do not exist.

◆ TREATMENT FOR BLOCKED CORONARY ARTERIES

As you have discovered, most of the risk factors linked to coronary heart disease can be controlled. The way you live, the choices you make, can have a profound impact on the health of your cardiorespiratory system. When coronary arteries become blocked, usually the first treatments prescribed are diet modification (low fat) and exercise therapy. These are two major areas of one's life that, if maximized, can have positive results. When these methods are unsuccessful, the following procedures may be required.

Drug Therapy

This involves drug treatment affecting the supply of oxygen to the heart muscle or the heart's demand for oxygen. Some drugs (coronary vasodilators) cause the blood vessels to relax, enlarging the opening inside them. Blood flow then improves, and more oxygen reaches the heart. Nitroglycerine is the most commonly used drug in this category. Another category of drugs (beta blockers) slows down the heart rate or reduces blood pressure, thus decreasing the heart's need for oxygen, reducing its workload. There are many other classifications of drugs used to treat CVD as well (e.g., the statins).

Angioplasty (or Balloon Angioplasty)

The AHA describes this treatment as a nonsurgical procedure that improves the blood supply to the heart by dilating a narrowed coronary artery. The blocked part of the coronary artery must be identified

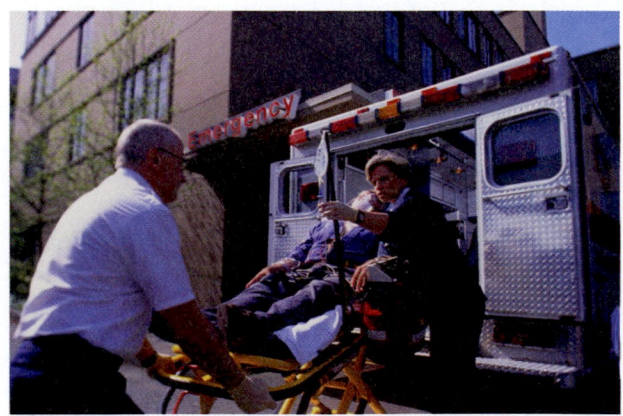

Many U.S. companies are adopting "Shape-Up or Pay-Up" programs where employers penalize their unfit employees by requiring them to pay higher health insurance premiums (than their more fit coworkers) if they smoke, are overweight, or don't control blood pressure, diabetes, or cholesterol. Do you support this idea? Why or why not?

before this technique is performed. During this process (cardiac catheterization), a doctor guides a thin plastic tube (catheter) through an artery in the arm or leg into the coronary arteries. A liquid dye, visible in X rays, is injected into the catheter, and X-ray movies are taken as the dye flows through the arteries. Doctors can identify obstructions in the arteries by tracing the flow of the dye. Once obstructions are identified, a catheter having a balloon tip is inserted inside the first; the balloon tip is inflated at the obstruction site. This compresses the plaque and enlarges the opening of the blood vessel. The balloon is deflated, and both catheters are removed. The process injures the vessel wall, causing the area to grow new cells. Some people grow too many cells, reclogging the artery. About 20 percent of people who have this treatment have renarrowed arteries within 6 months. The introduction of stints (cylinders that prop the arteries open) has substantially reduced the risk of arteries closing again. However, the reclosure risk is still 10 to 20 percent within the first year.

Coronary Bypass Surgery

This is a surgical technique in which doctors take a blood vessel from another part of the body (usually the leg) and use it to detour around a blockage in the coronary artery. Blood flow to the heart is restored.

THE FUTURE . . . FOCUS ON LIFESTYLE

The cost of treating cardiovascular diseases in this country is staggering. Many scientists believe we will be more successful if we focus on prevention rather than rely on expensive, high-tech treatments. "An ounce of prevention is worth a pound of cure" will in all likelihood be the slogan of the twenty-first century. Heart disease prevention in our future will focus primarily on lifestyle changes and approaches that involve "mind and body" concepts. Many scientists are already substantiating these trends in their research and medical practices.

One example is Dr. Dean Ornish, cardiologist, clinical professor of medicine at the University of California at San Francisco, and pioneer in the treatment of CVD. He found that after treating his patients with the current, recommended medical procedures—medication, angioplasty (balloon technique), and coronary bypass surgery, all expensive and dangerous—most did not stay well. Despite the procedures, some died and many returned for further treatment. He began to question the wisdom of such dramatic medical care for heart disease. He

found it interesting that lifestyle factors could trigger all mechanisms known to cause CVD. The lifestyle choices we make each day, such as what we eat, how we respond to stress, how much we exercise, and whether we use tobacco, have a profound impact on the heart's health. With this concept in mind, he developed a plan that focuses on lifestyle. His program, "Reversing Heart Disease," is having significant success in reducing atherosclerosis without medication or surgical procedures. The program involves the following lifestyle changes:

1. A special diet is recommended. The Reversal Diet is 10 percent fat, 70 to 75 percent carbohydrate, 15 to 20 percent protein, and 5 milligrams of cholesterol per day. In comparison, the typical American diet is 40 to 45 percent fat, 25 to 35 percent carbohydrate, 25 percent protein, and 400 to 500 milligrams of cholesterol per day. The Reversal Diet allows, but does not encourage, moderate alcohol consumption (less than 2 oz. per day). It excludes caffeine, allows moderate use of salt and sugar, and is not restricted in calories.
2. Smoking is prohibited.
3. Thirty minutes a day or 1 hour every other day of moderate exercise is prescribed.
4. Stress management methods are prescribed every day. These include yoga stretches, progressive relaxation, abdominal breathing, meditation, and imagery.
5. Psychological support should be enhanced. This involves increased time spent talking about feelings with friends and family and participating in spiritual and religious activities.

Mind and Body Connection

The traditional risk factors explain only a portion of the known causes of heart disease. Why do some people develop heart disease while others do not? Clearly, all the risk factors are important, but could there be something more? Are there common psychological—and perhaps even spiritual—factors that lead to or prevent coronary heart disease? Is there an unconscious connection between mind, body, and spirit that would explain the unknown causes of heart disease?

Scientists are examining these questions: Is laughter good for you? Can prayer bring down blood pressure? Does a bad marriage or a divorce suppress your immune system? Does listening to others lower blood pressure? Is a cynic more likely to have heart trouble? To each of these questions there is a scientist able to answer "YES!" and provide data to back it up. There is a whole field of mind–body research tapping into the interaction between our immune systems and our bodies, minds, moods, and spirit. Just as we learned the importance of exercise and nutrition to our health, we are discovering ways to go deeper into inner wellness. Ponder these studies that support the mind–body concept:

✓ Norman Cousins, author, philosopher, and former professor at the Department of Psychiatry and Bio-behavioral Sciences at UCLA Medical School (now deceased), found that laughter heals because it replaces fear and stress with serenity and homeostasis.

✓ Scientific studies citing the benefits of a good laugh have piled up:
  • A Japanese study found it can reduce glucose levels in diabetics and increase immune system activity.
  • A Stanford University study found it has good effects on the CV system (i.e., blood pressure and arteries).

✓ Larry Scherwitz, professor of psychology at the University of California, found that people who overuse the self-centered pronouns "I," "me," and "mine" are twice as likely to have heart attacks. These people are hostile, have a low level of trust in others, and put their self-centered interests and pleasures ahead of others.

✓ Redford Williams of Duke University found that cynics, being full of contempt for other people, and angry hostile people have more than their share of heart trouble.

✓ Many scientists have developed psychological tests to measure levels of anger that bring on heart attacks. Studies linking social support (i.e., loving family, happy marriage, one or two close friends, support groups) to vitality, longevity, lowered blood pressure, and healthier immune systems confirm that emotions may regulate health. These head and heart factors are powerful medicine.

✓ Dean Ornish, MD, is convinced that one cause of blocked coronary arteries stems from three kinds of loneliness (or isolation): (1) we feel isolated from ourselves, (2) we lack "connectedness" and intimate relationships with others, and (3) we have a cosmic loneliness of the spirit (or higher part of ourselves). He feels that isolation leads to chronic stress and to illnesses such as heart disease and that real intimacy and feelings of connectedness with others can be healing. He argues that the ability to be intimate with ourselves, with others, and with a higher spirit—within ourselves—is the key to emotional health and essential to the health of our hearts as well.

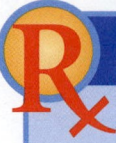

PRESCRIPTION FOR ACTION

You've read the chapter. Now go do one or more of these:

✓ Write down the top two reasons your last fitness program didn't work. Then, write down what you'll do this time to avoid those same pitfalls.
Reasons failed: Strategies to counter:
  •   •
  •   •

✓ Get your blood pressure checked.

✓ Do two of the following to maintain a healthy blood pressure or reduce hypertension:
  • Have a high-fiber snack (something with at least 5 or more grams of fiber).
  • If you smoke, cut in half the number of cigarettes smoked today.
  • Avoid alcohol.
  • Reduce caffeine.

✓ Measure your waist.

✓ Calculate your BMI.

✓ Read food labels and avoid all trans fats (anything hydrogenated or partially hydrogenated).

✓ Get 30 minutes of exercise today.

✓ Floss and brush your teeth for 2 minutes today.

✓ Reflect on the meaningful people in your life. Connect with two of them today via e-mail or telephone, or write a letter.

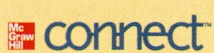

Go online to Connect to complete this activity.
http://connect.mcgraw-hill.com

✓ Mind–body connection authority Jon Kabat-Zinn advocates meditation as a technique to bridge the gap between the mind and the heart to improve health, ease pain, and reduce stress.

✓ Another authority on the mind–body connection, Bill Moyers, author of *Healing and the Mind,* explored the latest research in the field of medicine known as psychoneuroimmunology. He found evidence supporting the ways in which thoughts, feelings, and emotions influence our health. Moyers documents the importance of mind–body interactions in the prevention and treatment of illness.

Frequently Asked Questions

Q. How can do take control of my heart health?

A. CVDs affect hundreds of millions, but staggering numbers of people are completely unaware that they are even afflicted. You cannot fight a problem if you don't know you have it. Take control! No matter how old you are or how well you feel, see a health care professional about some basic screening tests. Not knowing your numbers won't make them go away, but getting tested puts your fate in your own hands.

Q. How many people in the United States adhere to a lifestyle that reduces the risk of coronary heart disease?

A. It is somewhat difficult to pinpoint the exact number, but findings from the Nurse's Health Study (involving more than 80,000 women) may give us some insight. The study revealed that women in this low-risk category make up only *3 percent of the population,* a pitifully low number. That means 97 percent of the U.S. population does not! The study confirmed that the risk of heart disease can almost be eliminated if we follow a few rules. The heart-healthy lifestyle defined in this study involves four factors:

- Engaging in moderate to vigorous physical activity for at least half an hour per day
- Not smoking
- Eating healthy and consuming a diet
  - Low in saturated fat (found in animal products) and trans fat (found in cookies, crackers, pies, cakes, donuts, candy, margarine)
  - High in fiber
  - High in folate (found in green leafy vegetables, orange juice, fortified cereals, legumes, and whole grains)
  - High in omega-3 fatty acids (found in fish)
  - Low in glycemic foods (found in sweets, etc., which raise glucose levels)
  - Averaging at least half a drink of an alcoholic beverage a day
- Avoid being overweight

Q. True or false? Your good lifestyle choices counteract your bad ones.

A. False. Sorry, but eating lots of fruits and vegetables or being at your target weight, for example, cannot compensate for smoking or not exercising. You have to look at all your risk factors and address each one individually.

Q. The United States is such a diverse nation with many different ethnic populations. Are the leading causes of death the same for each?

A. Look at Figure 9-1. You can see at a glance that CVD disease is by far the number one killer of all people in the United States, regardless of ethnicity. Far down the list is cancer, followed by accidents. Every 37 seconds someone in this country dies of CVD, whereas every 56 seconds someone dies of cancer.

Q. I recently had my cholesterol tested. Why didn't the figures for LDL and HDL cholesterol add up to the total cholesterol number?

A. Because the total includes several other substances. About 10 to 15 percent of the total consists of other particles, notably very low-density (VLDL) and intermediate-density lipoprotein (IDL). While these also contribute to clogged arteries, there hasn't been enough research to correlate specific VLDL and IDL numbers with heart risk, so doctors generally don't consider them. As you know, more important than total cholesterol, since it is a combination of different substances, are the HDL and LDL numbers. The isolated LDL and HDL numbers, with diametrically different effects on the heart, are the best indicators of coronary risk. Ask your doctor for those scores, available on a blood test called total lipid profile.

Q. My friend, who just had a full body scan, suggested that I should get one too. Is a full body scan recommended? What are the pros and cons?

A. Full body scans are CT (computed tomography) examinations of the entire body that are being offered to healthy people to look for early signs of disease. Diagnostic CT scanning to examine specific parts of the body when there is a problem has been used for decades. But scanning almost the entire body for screening is a new concept.

Full body CT screening is controversial. The potential benefit is the early detection of significant disease, such as tumors or plaque in the coronary arteries. The risk is that of radiation exposure. X rays can cause damage to cells in your body. Even at low doses there is a risk of causing cancer. That's too high a risk for a test that is not medically necessary, especially if you have one every few years.

Another downside is the likelihood that the scan will reveal some abnormality in the body that is benign or inconsequential. But because the abnormality has been "seen" on the scan, you may have to have additional anxiety-provoking tests. The exam also has its limitations—it can't detect every abnormality, so it does not absolutely rule out the possibility of cancer or other disease.

Cost is a factor too. These scans are not cheap, and they are not covered by health insurance. The American College of Radiology does not sanction full body scans for screening healthy people.

Q.   Is it really OK to eat eggs two or three times a week even though I'm on medication to keep my cholesterol down?

A.   Yes, it is. Research shows that two or three eggs weekly are not apt to raise blood cholesterol. The real villain is saturated animal fat, found in whole milk, fatty meat, cheese, and butter as well as trans fats. A Harvard study of 120,000 men and women found that a daily egg did not boost the risk of heart disease or stroke. Eggs are rich in choline, needed for proper brain functioning, and the antioxidant lutein, believed to help protect eyes from macular degeneration.

Q.   Why does exercise prevent heart disease?

A.   Here's at least part of the answer. In addition to lowering blood pressure, cholesterol, and body fat, certain components in the bloodstream called cytokines act to either promote atherosclerosis (atherogenic) or prevent it (atheroprotective). Research published in the *Journal of the American Medical Association* studied the effect of long-term exercise on those blood factors. The participants worked out for an average of 2½ hours per week for 6 months. After the exercise program, production of the atherogenic blood factors fell by 58.3 percent and the level of atheroprotective factors rose by 35 percent. In any individual, the amount of change was proportional to the level of activity. In other words, the participants who exercised more enjoyed more of the beneficial effects in their blood levels. Those who exercised less had a smaller response. It appears that with every extra minute you exercise, your body is producing more protection and causing less destruction of your arteries. Although there is likely an upper limit (or point of diminishing returns), this study gives you one more reason to exercise.

Q.   Don't more women die from breast cancer than heart disease?

A.   No. Across nearly all racial and ethnic groups, heart disease is the number one killer of women just as it is the number one killer of men.

Q.   How long do most people have type 2 diabetes before it is diagnosed?

A.   On average, people have diabetes for 8 years before it is diagnosed. Regular visits to your doctor and regular fasting blood sugar tests can help detect the disease early (see Tables 9-4 and 9-5).

Q.   I can find all kinds of information on high blood pressure but not much on low blood pressure. How low is too low?

A.   Within limits, the lower your blood pressure, the better. For most people, blood pressure is not too low unless it causes signs and symptoms such as lightheadedness or fainting. Normal blood pressure is less than 120/80 millimeters of mercury (mmHg). Unusually low blood pressure should be evaluated by a physician. Unlike high blood pressure, there are no clear-cut standards for the diagnosis of low blood pressure. Low blood pressure is not a specific disease. It is usually a sign of an underlying problem.

Summary

Heart disease is the number one killer in the United States. Extensive studies have identified 16 factors that increase the risk of developing CVD. These factors lead to the development of atherosclerosis. The most significant factors are inactivity, high blood pressure, a high blood lipid profile, cigarette smoking, obesity, diabetes, and prediabetes. These 7 are labeled *primary* and all can be controlled. Four additional primary risk factors for CVD are positive family history, male gender (+ postmenopausal women), race, and age. These primary risk factors are all uncontrollable. There are 6 more CVD factors labeled *secondary*. These are all controllable. They are stress, emotional behavior (especially negative emotional behaviors such as hostility and anger), excessive alcohol consumption (+ some illegal drugs), metabolic syndrome, C-reactive protein, and homocysteine. The more risk factors you have and the longer they are present, the greater the chance you have of developing heart disease. By age 20, you already have fatty deposits in your coronary arteries. If your risk of CVD is low, keep up the good work by maintaining a healthy lifestyle. (See Frequently Asked Questions.) However, if your coronary risk is high, now is the time to act. You can't do anything about your race, heredity, sex (gender), or age. However, you can choose to act on the 13 risk factors under your control.

Several treatments are available for coronary arteries that become blocked due to advanced atherosclerosis. These include exercise and diet modification, drug therapy, angioplasty, and coronary bypass surgery. The cost of treating CVD continues to spiral upward every year. To counter this trend, many scientists are convinced that preventing CVD through lifestyle change is the key to maximizing heart health.

Adopting a healthy lifestyle early in life can add years to your life and life to your years. In addition, great discoveries await us as the field of mind and body research gains wider acceptance in the quest for increased well-being.

Let the words of Don Ardell inspire you to maximize your potential to be the best you can be:

"Excellence ain't easy. If it were, everyone would be doing it and it would be ordinary. Know that in lots of ways, the deck is stacked against anyone who wants to excel. Do it anyway."

Terms

- angina pectoris
- arteriosclerosis
- atherosclerosis
- cardiovascular disease
- cholesterol
- collateral circulation
- C-reactive protein
- diabetes mellitus
- diastolic pressure
- high-density lipoprotein (HDL)

- homocysteine
- hot reactors
- hypercholesterolemia
- hypertension
- LDL cholesterol receptors
- low-density lipoprotein (LDL)
- metabolic syndrome
- myocardial infarction (MI)
- plaque
- prediabetes

- prehypertension
- primary risk factors
- risk factors
- secondary hypertension
- secondary risk factors
- stroke
- systolic pressure
- triglycerides
- Types A, B, C, and D personalities

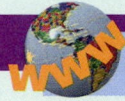

Internet Resources

America On the Move

www.americaonthemove.org

Help to add 2,000 steps a day and reduce calories by 100 calories a day.

American Diabetes Association

www.diabetes.org

National nonprofit organization providing diabetes research, information, and advocacy.

American Heart Association

www.americanheart.org

Includes statistics and information on heart disease and stroke risk information.

American Stroke Association

www.strokeassociation.org

Provides information on strokes.

Centers for Disease Control and Prevention

www.cdc.gov

Provides links to health and disease information. Lead federal agency for enhancing and promoting disease prevention and health education.

Cooper Institute for Aerobics Research

www.cooperinst.org

Has exercise and health research information.

DASH: Dietary Approaches to Stop Hypertension

www.nhlbi.nitt.gov/health/public/heart/hbp/dash

Provides dietary information to lower high blood pressure.

Harvard Medical School Health Publications

www.health.harvard.edu

Consumer-friendly site features a Heart Letter, Mental Health Letter, Women's Health Letter, Men's Health Letter, and special health reports.

My Optimum Health

www.myoptumhealth.com

You can search for information on general health topics.

Healthfinder, U.S. Government

www.healthfinder.gov

Lists government health resources and offers links to over 500 consumer health sites.

Healthy People 2020

www.health.gov/healthypeople

Has information and guidelines for a healthy America. You will soon be able to find the *Healthy People 2020* publication at this site.

Journal of the American Medical Association

www.ama-assn.org

Provides abstracts and news update summaries of latest *JAMA* reports.

Mayo Clinic

www.mayoclinic.com

You can search by major health/disease subject area.

MedlinePlus

www.nlm.nih.gov/medlineplus

National library of medicine.

National Coalition for Women with Heart Disease

www.womenheart.org

Provides CVD information for women.

National Heart, Lung, and Blood Institute

www.nhlbi.nih.gov

Gives information and statistics about heart and lung disease.

National Institutes of Health

www.nih.gov

Has links to a vast number of health sites and provides up-to-date research about disease prevention and treatment. Part of the U.S. Department of Health and Human Services.

National Library of Medicine

www.nlm.nih.gov

You can search for published scientific medical literature.

National President's Challenge

www.presidentschallenge.gov

Provides a personal activity log with exercise programs to pick from, encouragement to exercise for 30 minutes, and more advanced programs for those who want a more strenuous workout.

U.S. Surgeon General

www.surgeongeneral.gov/topics/obesity

Provides information on weight management.

Web MD

www.webmd.com

Has news items, advice, and articles on health.

Your Disease Risk

www.yourdiseaserisk.wustl.edu

An interactive site to assess your disease risk factors.

LAB Activity 9-1

Name _____ **Class/Activity Section** _____ **Date** _____

Are You at Risk for Heart Disease?

Your chances for developing CVD depend on a variety of habits and risk factors. Smoking, physical activity, diet, stress management, blood pressure, waist measurement, and cholesterol are some of the important prognosticators for heart disease. Read each question and circle the most appropriate response as it relates to your lifestyle. Finally, add the points associated with your response to obtain your total score and risk of developing heart disease. Evaluate your risk by completing Lab Activity 9-2.

1.	Do you smoke cigarettes?	Yes	10
		No	0
2.	Do you use other tobacco products (pipe, cigars, chewing, snuff)?	Yes	3
		No	0
3.	Do you usually exercise vigorously at least three times a week for 20 to 60 minutes?	Yes	0
		No	10
4.	How would you describe your lifestyle?	Sedentary (inactive)	6
		Somewhat active	2
		Very active	0
5.	What is your blood pressure?	High 140/90+	8
		Normal	0
		Don't know	2
6.	What is your total cholesterol?	High 240 mg/dl+	8
		Desirable	0
		Don't know	2
7.	Has anyone in your family ever been told he or she had any form of heart disease (parents or siblings <55 years)?	Yes	5
		No	0
8.	Have you ever had any of the following?		
	a. Pain or discomfort in chest and surrounding areas?	Yes	2
		No	0
	b. Unaccustomed shortness of breath with mild exertion?	Yes	2
		No	0
9.	What is your gender?	Female	0
		Male	4
10.	If you are male, what is your age?	Under 40	1

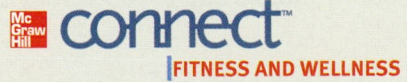

http://connect.mcgraw-hill.com

|FITNESS AND WELLNESS

	If you are female, what is your age?	40+	3
		Under 50	0
		50+	3
11.	Have you ever been told you have diabetes or prediabetes?	Yes	6
		No	0
12.	Is your waist measurement (measured with a tape measure) greater than 40 inches or more for males; 35 inches or more for females?	Yes	3
		No	0
13.	Have you suffered a personal loss or misfortune in the past year that had a serious impact on your life? (e.g., job loss, disability, romantic break up, divorce, jail term, or the death of someone close to you)?	No	0
		Yes, 1 serious loss or misfortune	1
		Yes, 2 or more	2
14.	Do you feel you handle everyday stress well?	Yes	0
		No	2
15.	Would you describe yourself as a Type D or an angry/hostile person?	Yes	2
		No	0
16.	What is your race?	White	0
		African American	3
		Hispanic	1
		Other	1
17.	How would you describe your weight?	Normal/below	0
		Normal to +30 lb.	1
		+30 lb. or more	3
18.	Do you consume alcohol excessively (i.e., more than 14 alcoholic beverages per week for males; more than 7 per week for females), or do you use any illegal drugs?	Yes	2
		No	0
19.	Do you consume meat, eggs, cheese, butter, whole milk, and fried foods?	0 to 5 times/week	0
		5–10 times/week	2
		2 to 3 servings/day	3
		Over 3 servings/day	6
		Your Total Score	___

SCORING

Scores of 0 to 16
Your risk is **low** for developing heart disease at this time. Evaluate your risk every year since risk factors such as blood pressure, cholesterol levels, and age change from year to year. If you have any uncontrollable risk factors, you would be wise to modify other risk factors to protect your cardiorespiratory system.

Scores of 17 to 29
Your risk is **average** or moderate. Your score indicates there is room for improvement on some risk factors. If you have any uncontrollable risk factors, it is imperative to modify other risk factors to protect your cardiorespiratory system.

Scores of 30+
You have a **high** risk of developing heart disease. You should take action **immediately** to modify all controllable risk factors.

LAB Activity 9-2

Evaluation of "Are You at Risk for Heart Disease?"

After completing the *Are You at Risk for Heart Disease?* assessment, answer the following questions:

1. List the factors you identified that contribute to your risk of coronary heart disease.

2. List at least five personal lifestyle changes you can make to lower your risk for heart disease. Be specific; don't say, "Eat better," for example.

3. Take the *Are You at Risk for Heart Disease?* assessment for a parent or friend. What is his or her score? What advice would you give to help to lower his or her score?

4. List **your** personal controllable risk factors. How can you make changes in each one to become more heart healthy?

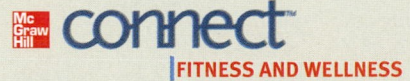

http://connect.mcgraw-hill.com

5. List **your** personal *uncontrollable* risk factors.

6. What if some physicians refused to treat people when they discover that they smoke or don't exercise or have diets high in fat. Discuss how you feel about this decision.

7. "You've got to die of something, so why worry about a healthy lifestyle?" Argue against.

8. "My grandmother lived to be 90 years old and never thought about a healthy lifestyle. So I won't either." Why is this *not* such a good idea?

9. "I don't smoke cigarettes, so cigarettes don't affect me." Respond and explain your response.

10. Do you have more than one alcoholic drink per day (if you are female) or more than two per day (if you are male)? Do you have more than 14 drinks per week for men or more than 7 per week for women? Do you ever binge drink (more than four for women and more than five for men in one sitting)? Discuss how alcohol affects your personal risk for CVD.

LAB Activity 9-3

Lifestyle Scenario: Critical Thinking

Read the opening scenario concerning Rob in Chapter 1 of your text. You were the physician on call when he was brought in. Complete a medical history on this patient and answer his wife's questions.

1. List Rob's five primary risk factors for heart disease given in the scenario.

2. List Rob's two secondary risk factors for heart disease.

3. What three or four lifestyle changes will you tell Rob to make to reduce his heart disease risk?

Rob's wife has read the chart. She is distraught and has several questions for you. Please respond.

4. "Doctor, I really don't understand some of the words used on the chart. What is angina? Myocardial infarction? What is atherosclerosis, and will it ever go away?"

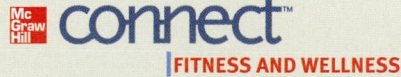
http://connect.mcgraw-hill.com

FITNESS AND WELLNESS

5. "I saw that his cholesterol was 280, his HDL level was 28, and his LDL level was 174. His cholesterol and HDL ratio was 10, and his triglycerides were 325. What do each of these mean? What is normal or desirable for each?"

a

b

c

d

e

6. "Rob doesn't want to quit smoking—he's smoked for 20 years. Why is smoking bad for his heart?"

7. "A nurse said Rob needs a special exercise program to aid in recovery. Won't exercise strain his heart? What good will it do?" (Give three benefits.)

8. "Rob enjoys having an occasional glass of wine. Will he have to give this up?" How much alcohol will he be allowed, if he wishes to consume it? What about his wife, what is the recommendation for women and alcohol consumption?

LAB Activity 9-4

Are You at Risk for Diabetes?

Directions: Answer the questions in Part I to evaluate your risk for developing diabetes. Complete Part II to learn more about diabetes and the connection it has to heart disease.

PART I

Yes	No		
____	____	1.	I am overweight (body mass index greater than 27; to calculate your BMI, multiply your weight in pounds by 705, divide the result by your height in inches, then divide that result by your height in inches again). What is your BMI? _____. And/or do you have a high-risk waistline (35 inches or more for women; 40 inches or more for men)? What is yours? _____
____	____	2.	I get little or no exercise.
____	____	3.	I have a parent with diabetes.
____	____	4.	I am African American, Hispanic American, or Native American.
____	____	5.	I am over 40 years of age (counts as one "yes" answer; if over 65 years of age, counts as two "yes" answers).
____	____	6.	I am a woman who had diabetes during pregnancy or delivered a baby weighing more than 9 pounds.
____	____	7.	I have a brother, sister, or parent with diabetes.
____	____	8.	I have high blood pressure and/or high cholesterol.
____	____	9.	I had a minimally elevated glucose level on a previous test (100–125 mg/dl)

Scoring: Each "yes" answer increases your risk of developing diabetes.

PART II

1. How many "yes" answers did you have?

2. Discuss your potential risk for developing diabetes.

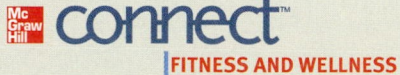

http://connect.mcgraw-hill.com

3. List the warning symptoms of type 1 and type 2 diabetes.

4. Discuss the difference between type 1 and type 2 diabetes.

5. What can you do to prevent or reduce your risk of developing diabetes?

6. Why is diabetes such a serious disease?

7. Why does diabetes increase the risk for heart disease?

8. What segments of the U.S. population are at increased risk of diabetes?

9. How does diabetes affect the eyes, blood vessels, kidneys, genitals, and nerves?

CHAPTER 10

Coping with Stress

STUDY QUESTIONS

You will have successfully mastered this chapter if you can answer the following:

1. What is the definition of *stress, stressor,* and *stress response?*
2. What are the three stages of the stress response?
3. What is the definition of eustress, distress, optimal stress, acute stress, and chronic stress?
4. How are perception and control involved in stress?
5. What is your score on the Life Event Stress Test? What is your potential for a stress-related illness?
6. What is the difference between daily hassles and daily uplifts? How does each affect overall health?
7. Why is too much stress harmful?
8. What are the characteristics of Type A, Type B, Type C, and Type D personalities? Which is the most effective at handling stress?
9. Why is a hot reactor's behavior harmful?
10. What four questions can you ask yourself to manage and modify angry/hostile behavior?
11. What are the six strategies for managing stress?
12. How is the relaxation response described? What are five of its benefits?

You will find the answers as you read this chapter.

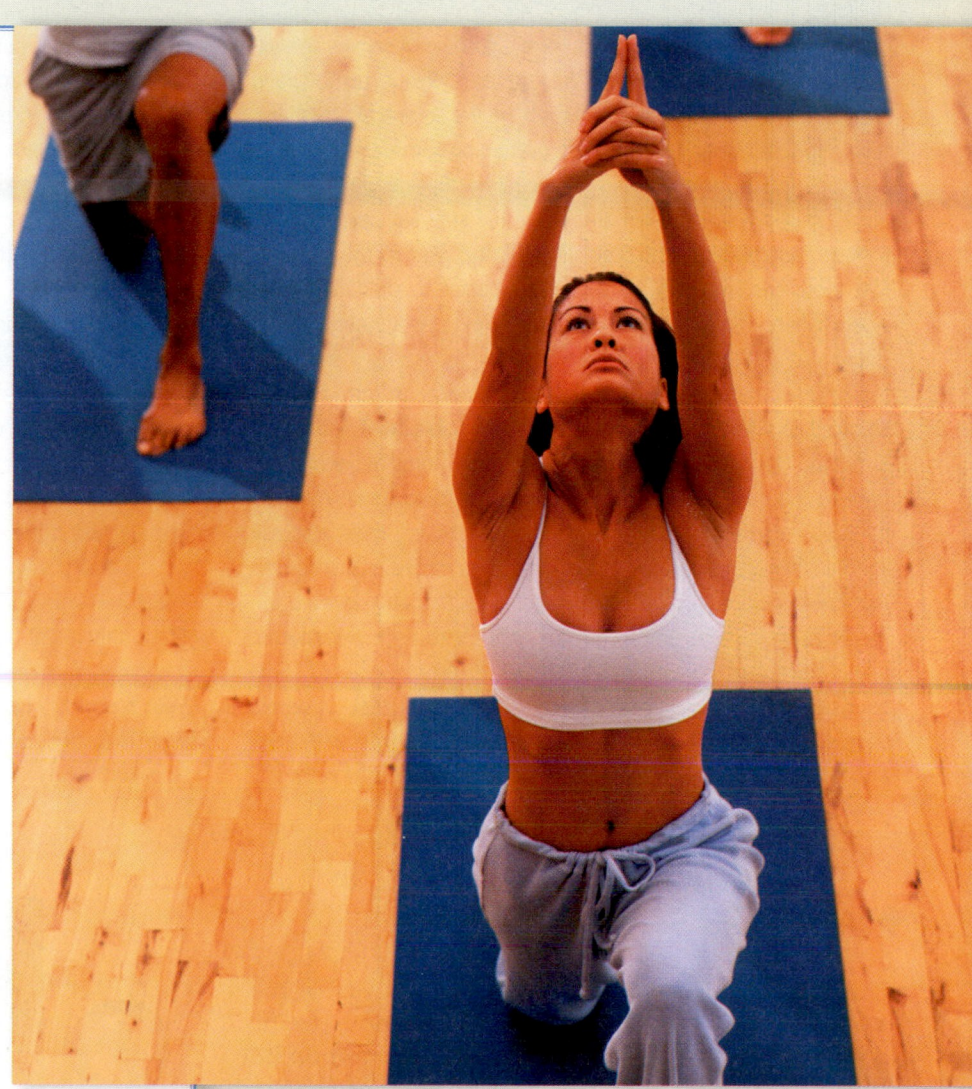

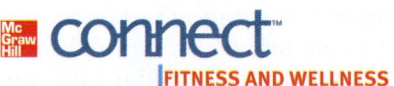

66 *Happiness is an inside job.* 99
—H. Jackson Brown Jr., ed.
A Father's Book of Wisdom

connect
FITNESS AND WELLNESS

http://connect.mcgraw-hill.com

Lisa was the oldest child of three and the first in her family to go to college. Living on campus was wonderful—it meant new friends, open visitation in the residence hall, and no curfew. But by the end of the school year, her life had changed for the worse.

Her GPA was barely above a C average, which was far below her high school performance. There never seemed to be enough hours in the day to keep up with all the reading. Also, she felt exhausted most of the time and had trouble waking up for early classes. It was no wonder: The "action" never settled down on her hall before 12:30 or 1:00 A.M. The parties on the weekends were awesome. There were so many, she couldn't decide which one to go to, so she went to them all. She would stay out partying until 6:00 A.M., grab a bite, and then sleep all day. With all the partying, fast food, and beer, her waistline also began to slip, 15 pounds worth! Then, just before final exams, her parents announced that they were getting a divorce. Had her college expenses created a financial burden on the family budget and contributed to the divorce? She felt guilty and partially responsible for her parents' problems. Now she would have to move back home and work full-time at the local big box store to help pay for college. Would it be possible to finish the nursing degree by taking night classes? Antonio, her boyfriend, was pressuring her to drop out of school so that they could get married. He complained that she devoted too much time to schoolwork and not enough to him. Her mother would now have to go back to work and would expect Lisa to help take care of her younger brothers and assist with the household chores. Feeling fatigued and stressed out, she wondered, with work and family obligations, when she would study. Would she have any time for herself? Was she the only one in college with such problems? How complicated her life had become.

This scenario is not uncommon on the typical college campus. The many challenges faced by college students are stressful and can cause feelings of anxiety. Stiff competition for grades, career choices, selection of classes, test anxiety, sense of loss of family and home, balancing work and school, peer pressure, inadequate sleep, poor nutritional habits, low physical fitness levels, and increased social involvement contribute to high levels of stress. Clearly, college is a stressful environment that makes demands on you physically, socially, intellectually, and emotionally. It's no wonder that you sometimes feel anxious, irritable, and stressed out.

Contrary to what many college students believe, stress does not "evaporate" after graduation. The amount of time the average person spends at work has increased rather than decreased in the last two decades. Many people have second jobs or work extended hours in demanding professional jobs. Also, nearly three times as many married women with children work full-time now as did in 1960. Experts call today's young adults the "overworked Americans." A great majority of adults have enough time for work, chores, and sleep but not enough time for friends, self, spouse, and children.

Stress is a normal part of life, so why do so few people understand it or know how to manage it? Improvement in the quality of life is dependent on *balancing* the demands made on you and developing effective ways to *manage* stress. Look back at "Assessing Your Wellness," Lab Activity 1-2. How balanced was your wellness wheel? Balance in the seven dimensions of wellness has implications for how well you cope with the demands of life.

◆ WHAT IS STRESS?

Dr. Hans Selye, the foremost stress authority of the twentieth century, defined **stress** as the "nonspecific response of the body to any demand made upon it." It is the response of the body to any type of change or challenge and to any new, threatening, or exciting situation. *Nonspecific* means that the body reacts the same way regardless of the cause. Stress comes in two forms: *acute* and *chronic*.

✓ **Acute stress** is the most common type of stress. It is the short-term response to imminent danger (like dodging a car in traffic) or to an event in the immediate past or future (like preparing for an exam). (See fight-or-flight response.) Acute stress can be healthy when it helps the immune system fight off infections and disease. Acute stress normally passes quickly, but if it happens a lot, over time it can cause health problems.

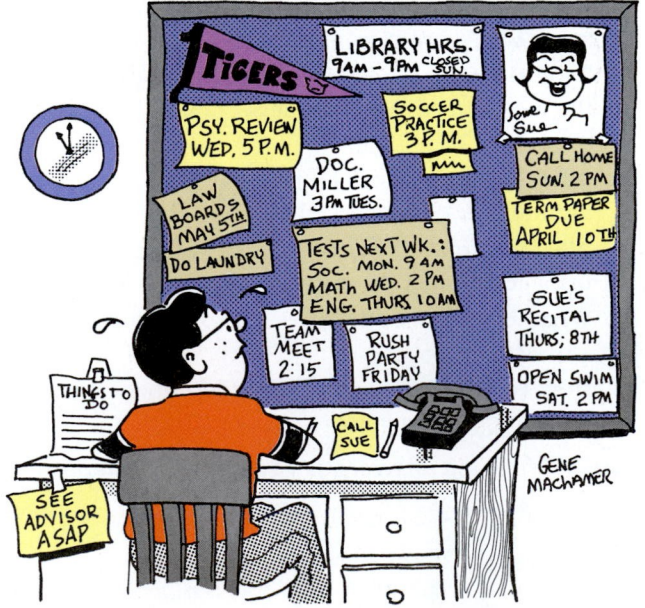

College students have many demands on their time and must plan wisely.

What Stage of Change Are You In?

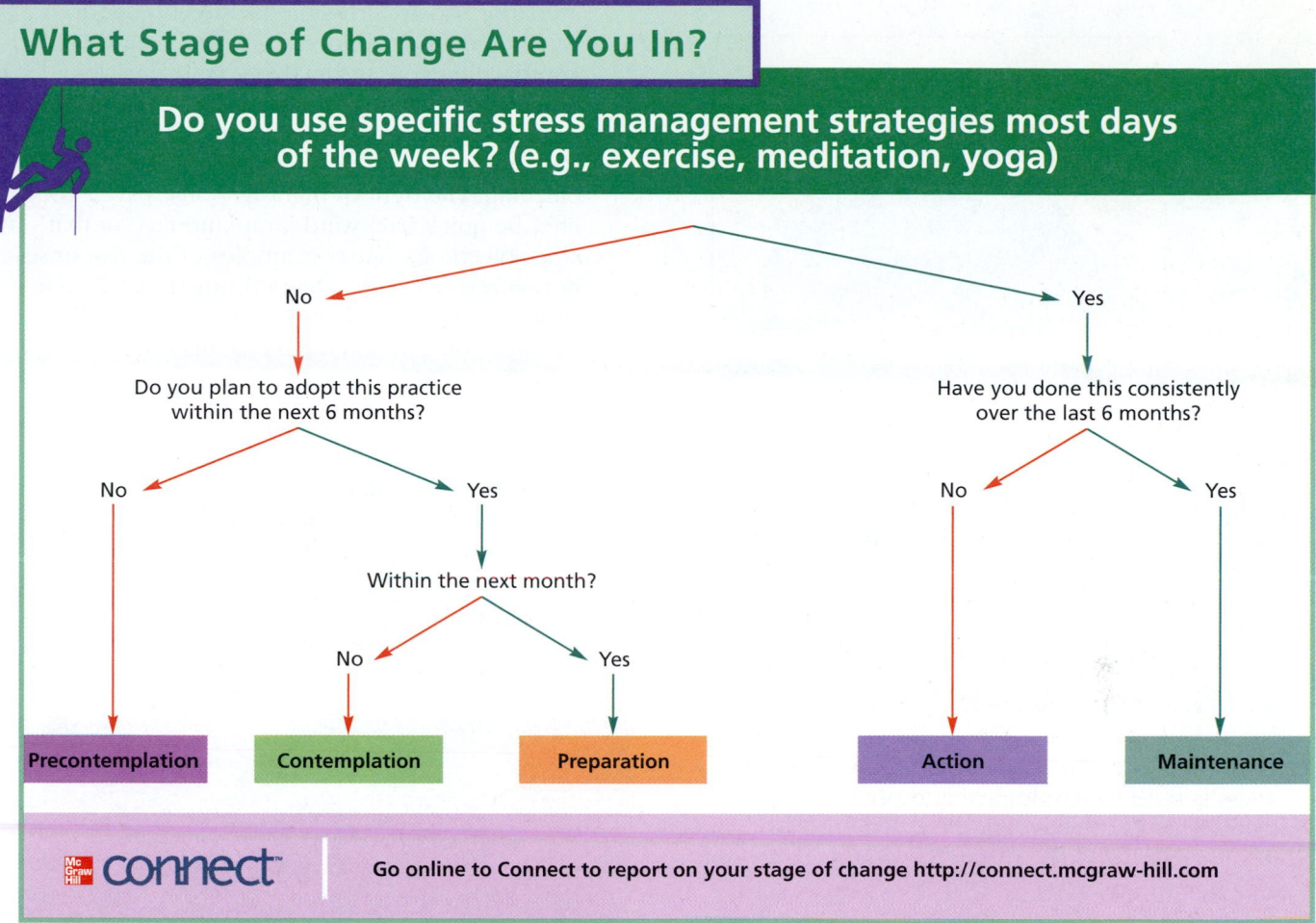

Do you use specific stress management strategies most days of the week? (e.g., exercise, meditation, yoga)

No → Do you plan to adopt this practice within the next 6 months?
- No → **Precontemplation**
- Yes → Within the next month?
  - No → **Contemplation**
  - Yes → **Preparation**

Yes → Have you done this consistently over the last 6 months?
- No → **Action**
- Yes → **Maintenance**

Go online to Connect to report on your stage of change http://connect.mcgraw-hill.com

✓ **Chronic stress** is continuous. It is prolonged stress, more than an individual can cope with or control. Examples are the stress caused by living in poverty, long-term school or work overload, or being in a bad marriage. It is the most serious type of stress and the type most prevalent today. People affected by it may see no way to escape its oppressive, never-ending hold on them. Chronic stress sends the body into a constant state of inflammation. (See "Harmful Effects of Stress" on page 330.)

Stressors, factors causing stress, can be pleasant or unpleasant, real or imagined, and can be of different types. All cause the body to adapt. For example, *physical* stressors include illness, accidents, injury, lack of sleep, heat, cold, and noise. *Psychological* or *emotional* stressors involve pressures and deadlines with work or school, problems with loved ones, the need to pay bills, getting ready for the holidays (or vacation), parenting, final exams, rejection, depression, divorce, and marriage.

Dr. Selye described the ways in which we react to stress as either *eustress* (good) or *distress* (bad). In both cases the physiological response is the same. In the case of **eustress,** which refers to happy, pleasant events (holidays, getting married, etc.), health and performance improve even as stress increases. In contrast, **distress** refers to unpleasant or harmful stress (flunking an exam, breakup of a relationship, etc.) under which health and performance begin to decline.

Optimal stress is a point at which eustress and distress are intense enough to motivate and physically prepare us to perform optimally yet not intense enough to cause the body to overreact or sustain harmful effects. Figure 10-1 illustrates this concept. Optimal stress gives athletes the competitive edge and public speakers the enthusiasm to project with charisma. Overstress results in poor performance and produces overreaction, poor concentration, test anxiety, and health problems. When experiencing positive stress, individuals feel in control. Negative stress causes out-of-control feelings. *Note:* One basic fact is that stress is cumulative. The total amount of stress ("bad" plus "good") is the critical factor.

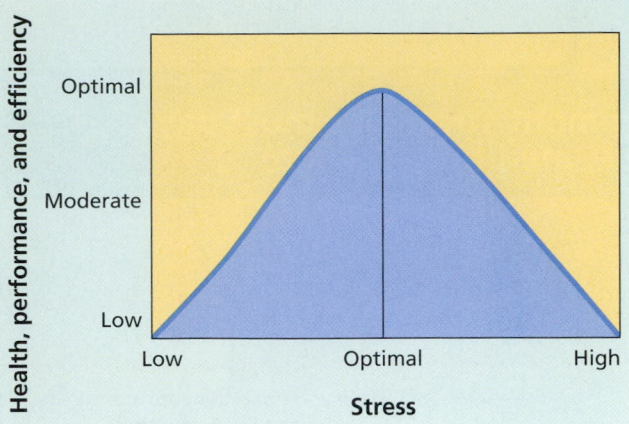

FIGURE 10-1 Optimal stress and the relationship to health and performance. Everyone has a point at which the "right" amount of stress improves health, performance, and efficiency.

THE STRESS RESPONSE: A THREE-STAGE PROCESS

Regardless of the cause, the adaptation (or reaction) to stress is both psychological and physiological and leads to what Dr. Selye called the **General Adaptation Syndrome (GAS).** Today, the GAS is called the **Stress Response.**

1. **Fight-or-Flight Response (Alarm Reaction Stage)**
   The first stage is the **fight-or-flight response (alarm reaction stage).** Here the body prepares to cope with a stressor (real or perceived). The response is a warning signal that a stressor is present. Physiological and psychological responses appear.

   This wonderful system gives us the capacity to do extraordinary things under extraordinarily stressful circumstances (see Figure 10-2). It is rapid, intense, and short-lived, and it comes in real handy when, for example, there is a true emergency, like those bulleted below. In reality, our stress responses were programmed for life in our primitive state, thousands of years before we became "civilized." It gave early humans the energy to fight aggressors or run from predators (i.e., the caveman or woman could escape the jaws of a hungry lion [stressor] by running swiftly [fight-or-flight]). Now, unfortunately, that same system is activated, to a lesser degree, when we face the day-to-day dramas of life. This is when the system can be very damaging.

   Many examples of the fight-or-flight response can be found even in today's world. Imagine this

scenario: You are crossing the street on your way home when suddenly you see a car quickly approaching you. Instinctively, your muscles tense, and you jump back onto the curb with such force that you fall back into a newspaper stand and cut your head, which quickly stops bleeding. The fight-or-flight response saved your life (the quick backward jump and the cut that stops bleeding). Other examples of the response, normally described as "superhuman" acts, are in reality the fight-or-flight response in action. Perhaps you can add others to this list:

✓ A person lifts an automobile off an injured individual at an accident scene.
✓ A young hiker amputates his arm to save his life after getting it caught between two boulders in a climbing accident.
✓ A mother knocks down a locked bedroom door to rescue her children from a burning house.
✓ A student outruns a mugger on a dark corner of the campus.

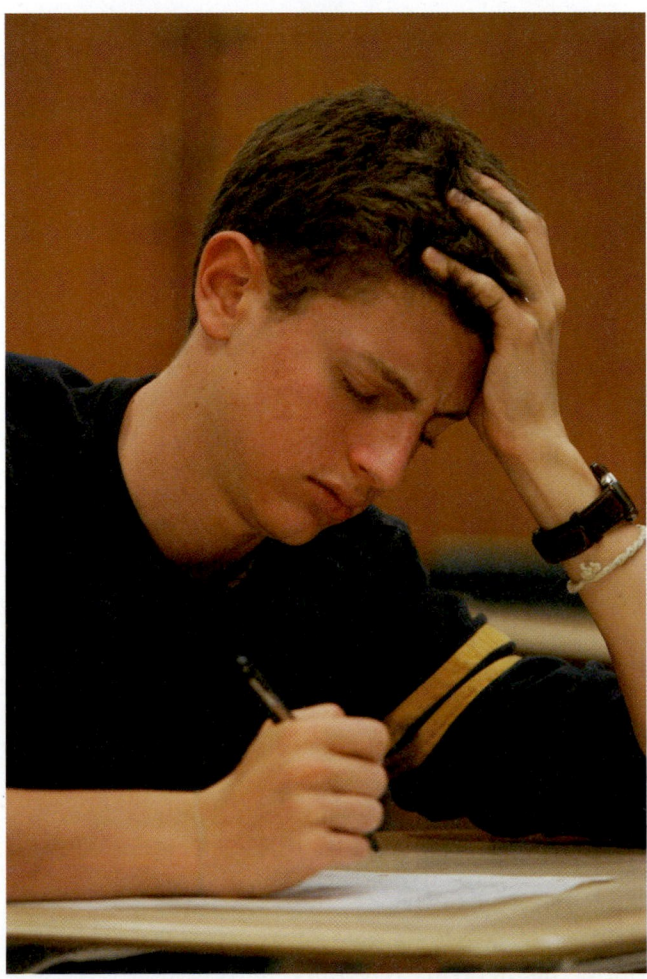

Chronic arousal of the fight-or-flight response causes chemical wear and tear on the body.

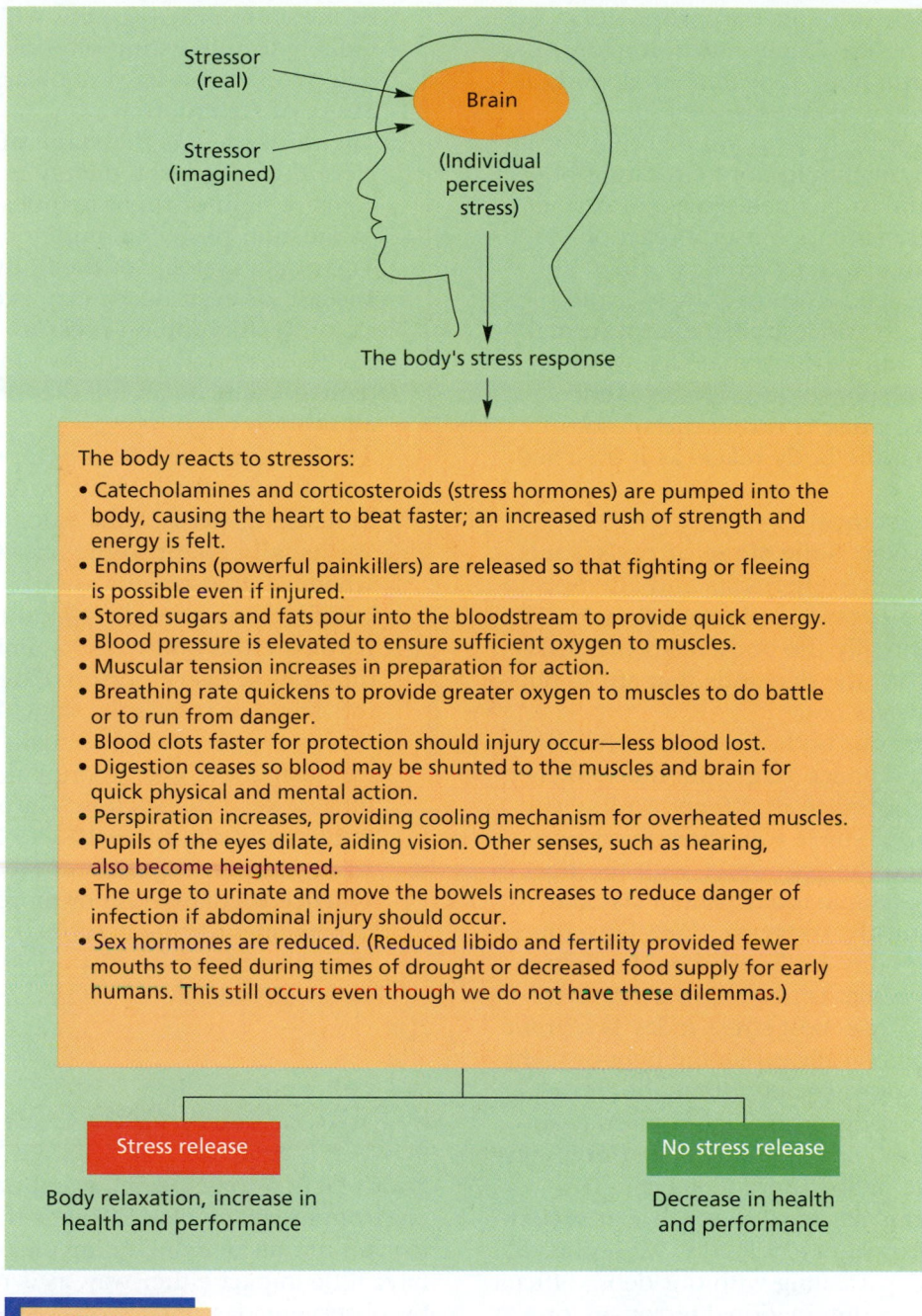

The body's stress response

The body reacts to stressors:
- Catecholamines and corticosteroids (stress hormones) are pumped into the body, causing the heart to beat faster; an increased rush of strength and energy is felt.
- Endorphins (powerful painkillers) are released so that fighting or fleeing is possible even if injured.
- Stored sugars and fats pour into the bloodstream to provide quick energy.
- Blood pressure is elevated to ensure sufficient oxygen to muscles.
- Muscular tension increases in preparation for action.
- Breathing rate quickens to provide greater oxygen to muscles to do battle or to run from danger.
- Blood clots faster for protection should injury occur—less blood lost.
- Digestion ceases so blood may be shunted to the muscles and brain for quick physical and mental action.
- Perspiration increases, providing cooling mechanism for overheated muscles.
- Pupils of the eyes dilate, aiding vision. Other senses, such as hearing, also become heightened.
- The urge to urinate and move the bowels increases to reduce danger of infection if abdominal injury should occur.
- Sex hormones are reduced. (Reduced libido and fertility provided fewer mouths to feed during times of drought or decreased food supply for early humans. This still occurs even though we do not have these dilemmas.)

Stress release

Body relaxation, increase in health and performance

No stress release

Decrease in health and performance

FIGURE 10-2   Physical reactions to stressors. (The fight-or-flight response.)

These are only a few examples that have required action to prevent or minimize physical harm. A few minutes after the frightening event (acute stressor), the individuals return to their normal physiological state.

Other stressors, the kind you encounter every day, such as noise, arguments, keys locked inside the car, missed deadlines, traffic jams, planning a wedding, final exams, holidays, or any new situation that causes us to adapt, have the same potential for eliciting the fight-or-flight response. Ironically, the

strains and hassles of life in a civilized world have transformed this lifesaving mechanism into a potentially life-threatening one.

We are designed to cope with acute stress much better than with chronic stress. Unfortunately, physical and emotional stress in modern times tends to be chronic rather than acute. We often do not have time to recover from one stressful situation before we face another one. The buildup of unused stress products produces excessive wear and tear on the body and even increases the rate of aging. When stressors inappropriately provoke the fight-or-flight reaction many times a day, the body repeatedly responds as if experiencing real emergencies.

The fight-or-flight response is often appropriate and should not be thought of as always harmful. It is a necessary part of our physiological makeup, a useful reaction to many situations in our current world. However, we need to learn how to avoid triggering the stress response except in real emergencies and develop effective ways to play out the response once it is evoked.

Our stress today is rarely the life-or-death type but the body reacts as if it is. See Figure 10-2.

2. **Stage of Resistance**

The second stage is the **stage of resistance.** Here the body actively resists and attempts to cope with the stressor and to regain normal balance. Eventually the body loses the ability to keep up with the demands that stress puts on it and it wears out.

The longer our bodies stay in a chronic "on guard" resistance stage, the more likely we are to experience ill effects. Unlike the caveman whose stress was short-lived—he either survived the encounter with the tiger or he didn't—people today cannot slay the stressor so quickly. Today we don't have much opportunity to physically play out the fight-or-flight response that is needed in *acute stress* situations, because most stress today is *chronic.* Though we chronically evoke the fight-or-flight response, modern society does not accept the natural response associated with it. For example, you do not run away from or hit your boss when he or she reprimands you. Our innate reactions have not changed, but society has. Stress reappears repeatedly. We report to work every day. Dealing with our debt, difficult family members, international terrorism, or a busy school schedule is continuous and ongoing. Unfortunately, our bodies have not developed an automatic off switch for the flood of hormones responding to the modern, extended version of the alarm response. As a result, the body remains in the resistance stage for longer periods. Our sedentary lifestyles decrease the outlets for the fight-or-flight hormones that are pumped into the body. Stress becomes harmful when it is prolonged and/or perceived as negative to the recipient.

Learning stress management skills is important in coping with the stresses of life. People who have learned these skills may still overreact to a stressor but will relax more quickly to the resting physiological state than will people who have not learned these skills.

3. **Stage of Exhaustion**

The third stage is the **stage of exhaustion.** Here the adaptation energy is exhausted, and signs of fight-or-flight reappear. During the exhaustion phase, immunity breaks down. The organ systems of the body malfunction. Disease or even death may occur. For example, high blood pressure (caused by excessive stress) promotes kidney and heart damage, which can kill the individual if allowed to continue.

Thankfully, the final point of this stage is not often reached. If our bodies are successful in resisting stress, exhaustion does not follow. We usually adapt to the stress and make whatever adjustments are necessary to cope whether the stress is physical or psychological. However, the body has its limits and they are different in every person. Extended time in the alarm or resistance stage means the body cannot repair itself; eventually it becomes exhausted and even more vulnerable to illness. Read the section "Harmful Effects of Stress," and see Table 10-1 to learn how many stress warning signs you have. Learn and practice regularly one or more of the stress management skills described in this chapter to reduce the unhealthy consequences of stress in your life.

PERCEPTION AND CONTROL

Your reaction to a specific event (stressor) is different from everyone else's. Things that are distressful for you can be an exhilarating pleasure for others or have little impact either way, as is readily illustrated by observing passengers on a steep roller coaster ride. Whether a particular stressor causes a negative reaction depends on whether the person *perceives* that stressor as being negative. How do *you* perceive snakes, public speaking, the announcement of an exam, competition, being cut off in traffic, being called in to see the boss, a doctor's appointment, being called on to contribute to class discussion, and a professor requesting to speak with you after class? These situations do not bother some individuals but are agonizing to others.

Faulty perception occurs when an individual assesses a situation (or stressor) as threatening regardless of its actual threat. It is unnecessarily seeing a situation as hopeless, harmful, or negative.

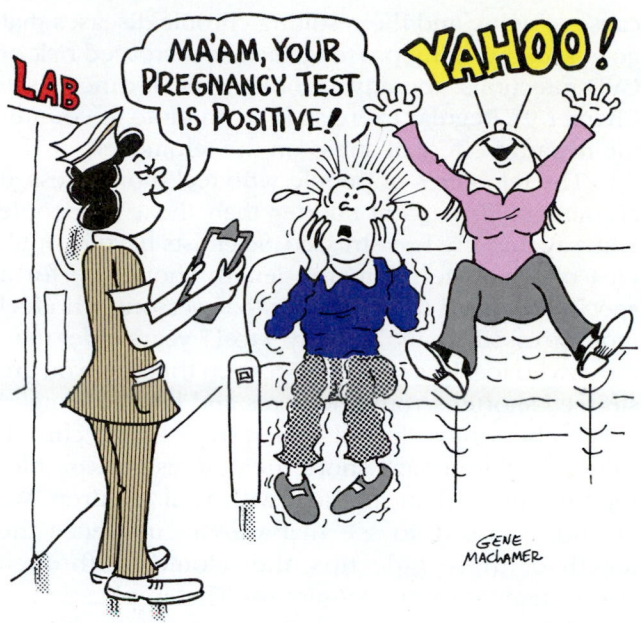

We perceive stressors differently.

Faulty perception of stress often is the real culprit and is the cause of most people's problems. The faulty perception of stress most times results in negative health consequences. Be aware we are, after all, thinking, cognitive creatures. We are able to assess the positive and negative consequences of any situation or threat and apply a coping strategy (such as problem solving) that may provide us with a sense of control (actual or perceived) that may affect our perception of stress.

Before gearing up to fret, fight, or flee when facing a stressor, ask yourself, "Does a threat really exist? Is the issue important to me? Can I make a difference?" If the answer to any of these questions is no, do not waste your energy. It is not worth it. Some situations are truly threatening and require high-energy stress responses. When the threat you perceive in a situation is real, go ahead and gear up. You can then benefit from the energy generated by your natural stress response by applying it to the situation at hand.

Control is also a major factor in the total stress picture. The core cause of much stress is the sense that one is "not in the driver's seat." The *perception (real or unreal) of not having control* is very stressful. (The "control freak" who is obsessed with being in control over everything in his or her life is *not* healthy and is *not* what is meant in this discussion.) The way to turn a stressful incident into something that is not stressful is to gain a sense of control over it. Managing stress means empowering yourself to take control rather than relinquishing the control to events, to other people, to your environment, or to

the calendar. People who handle stress best tend to control their lives and look for active solutions to the problems and circumstances of their lives.

You are responsible for allowing stressful situations to raise your blood pressure and heart rate. We can all recall events that made us angry one time but did not even faze us the next. Why is this? It is because we *allowed* ourselves to become upset. Perhaps the situation was complicated by nasty weather, lack of sleep, or a buildup of particular events. The bottom line is that this particular time we *allowed* the event to provoke an angry response.

Here are some important ways to gain control over your life:

✓ *Recognize and understand what causes your stress.* Find ways to avoid the stressful situation. If you can't, learn how to develop your own coping mechanisms and problem-solving skills (see "Building Skills for Stress Management").
✓ *Make healthy lifestyle decisions*—get regular exercise and adequate sleep. Not smoking, eating nutritionally, and not overindulging in alcohol allow you to exert control.
✓ *Learn and implement time management skills.* Getting organized helps spread stress out instead of having it pile up. See Strategy 3b and Lab Activity 10-5 Online.

THE NUMBERS

1st	Rank of stress among the top health concerns of Americans today.
75% to 90%	All visits to health care providers that result from stress-related disorders.
2nd	Rank of suicide as a leading cause of death in the college population. It is often linked to untreated depression and triggered by major life change events.
75%	College students who feel "really stressed" at least one day of the week.
30%	Reduction of cardiovascular disease risk that has been linked to the regular practice of meditation. Cortisol is decreased by 20% in those who meditate.
1 of 3	People who get enough sleep.

✓ *Learn when to say no.* Only you know when to take on added duties and assignments and when your "plate is full" and you must say, "No, sorry, not at this time. I have too many irons in the fire." This puts you in charge of your precious time.

✓ *Regularly practice relaxation techniques* and employ often the other stress-coping strategies found later in this chapter. Commit to restoring a sense of control, and reduce symptoms of stress in your life. See Lab Activity 10-1.

The key to surviving and even thriving on stress is improving cognitive problem-solving skills to better cope with faulty perception. Take charge of *you—for you.*

◆ HARMFUL EFFECTS OF STRESS

Stressors (i.e., all events, emotions, or situations, good or bad) cause you to react and force you to adapt. This adaptation to the stresses of life isn't harmful unless you are overloaded with too much in a short time—too many life change events and hassles, especially the ones perceived as undesirable or uncontrollable. In today's society, stress has increased dramatically. In essence, your fight-or-flight responses stay aroused 24 hours a day, 7 days a week. This is *chronic stress* and it travels with us daily, everywhere we go. The high price we pay for not dealing with chronic stress (or long stretches of acute stress) can lead to a psychosomatic disease.

A **psychosomatic disease** (*psych* refers to the mind; *somatic* refers to the body) is a physical ailment that is mentally induced. The mind and the body are an interrelated whole—what affects one ultimately affects the other. **Psychoneuroimmunology** is a specialized branch of medicine that studies the mind–body connection. Harvard's Dr. Herbert Benson has determined that 75 to 90 percent of visits to health care professionals are "in the stress-related, mind–body realm."

The long-term activation of the stress response system can disrupt almost all your body's processes, increasing your risk of aging, obesity, insomnia, digestive complaints, heart disease, diabetes, and depression. The following paragraphs summarize the impact stress has on the body.

Chronic stress can speed up the aging process. It has a huge influence not only on how cells divide but also on the length of telomeres on chromosomes inside the cells. As you read in Chapter 9, a telomere is protective cap at the end of each chromosome of the body and slows DNA decay. These caps are like the little plastic tips covering the ends of shoelaces. The deterioration of DNA is the basic cause of aging and the resulting chronic diseases that goes with the aging process, such as increased risk of CVD infections, cognitive problems, even cancer (see Chapter 9). Regular exercise is an antidote to counter the negative effect of stress on the telomeres.

The telomeres of people who feel more stressed are almost 50 percent shorter than those in people who say they are less stressed. Scientists have a rough idea of what the telomere's length should be for a specific age, and they estimate that persons who feel more stressed are biologically 9 to 17 years older than those who feel less stressed. So, even thinking you are stressed shortens your telomeres and is a major ager! Researchers have found that mothers with chronically ill children have shorter telomeres and are biologically older than mothers with well children. We are now starting to see that we can influence the length of those little tips, the telomeres, through stress management techniques. The implication is that if you can reduce the effects that stress has on you through such techniques as meditation or exercise (see "Building Skills for Stress Management"), you can even increase your chance of rebuilding telomeres and decrease the rate of aging and other negative health problems. *Note:* Lifelong vigorous exercise also increases the length of telemeres and slows aging.

Long-term stress suppresses your *immune system,* making you more susceptible to colds and other infections. In fighting infection, substances that cause inflammation are released. Prolonged stress doesn't allow the body to turn off the inflammatory responses once the infection is cleared. This can lead to high C-reactive protein levels, and increase plaque buildup and the risk of cardiovascular disease. In some cases, stress can have the opposite effect, making the immune system overreactive. The result is an increased risk of autoimmune diseases, in which the immune system attacks different cells and organs of the body. Examples include, but are not limited to, type 1 diabetes, crohn's disease, psoriasis, rheumatoid arthritis, fibromyalgia, and colites. Stress also worsens the symptoms of autoimmune diseases.

If your fight-or-flight response never shuts off as in chronic stress, the *nervous system* is negatively affected. A wide variety of adverse psychological symptoms may be produced, ranging from severe depression, persistent feelings of anxiety and helplessness, to impending doom. Behavioral problems such as sleep disturbances, loss of sex drive, disordered eating, and excessive drinking, along with nervous habits (e.g., nail biting), phobias, and addictions may occur.

The negative effects of chronic stress on the *cardiovascular system* include increased blood pressure, cholesterol, and triglyceride levels. These are all linked to heart attacks and strokes, and increased accumulation of abdominal fat—a marker for higher risk of heart disease and diabetes. Chronic stress is linked to the development of insulin resistance—a risk factor for diabetes.

Chronic stress damages other body systems as well. It often affects the *digestive system,* causing countless gastrointestinal problems (e.g., stomachache, diarrhea, and irritable bowel syndrome). Research has shown that among overweight persons, stress leads to overeating, whereas among thin people it tends to lead to loss of appetite.

Managing stress in our lives means adapting and changing as circumstances demand and learning to *listen.* Listen to our bodies, our feelings, and our relationships and be *aware* of the common signs of stress. See Table 10-1.

TABLE 10-1	*Stress Warning Signals*

Check the signs of stress that you have experienced in the last month. Stress affects many dimensions of your life.

Physical

_____ Headaches	_____ Allergy flare-up, asthma attack, rashes, hives
_____ Gastrointestinal (constipation and/or diarrhea, indigestion, stomach cramping or bloating, nausea or vomiting)	_____ Muscle twitches or eye twitches
	_____ Heart pounding, racing, or beating erratically
	_____ Restlessness
_____ Acne or fever blister flare-up	_____ Fatigue
_____ Frequent colds, flu, low-grade infections/herpes flare-ups	_____ Tight or stiff neck/shoulders
_____ Chest pain	_____ Difficulty sleeping (insomnia, sleeping too much, sleeping too little)
_____ Increased perspiration (excess sweating, cold or sweaty hands)	_____ Weight gain or loss

Emotional/Behavioral

_____ Depression	_____ Eating more or lack of appetite
_____ Unhappiness for no reason	_____ Mood swings
_____ Easily upset	_____ Feeling powerless to change things
_____ Feeling burned out or overwhelmed	_____ Paying less attention to appearance
_____ Edginess, ready to explode	_____ Being accident-prone
_____ Questioning your personal worth	_____ Impulsive actions
_____ Feeling sensitive to criticism	_____ Bouts of anger/hostility
_____ Bossiness	_____ Social withdrawal or need to be with people most or all of the time
_____ Crying	
_____ Irritability, nervousness, anxiousness	_____ Trouble getting along with others
_____ Increased smoking	_____ Increased drinking (or drug use)

Cognitive

_____ Disorganization (losing things, making dumb mistakes)	_____ Negative attitude and/or negative self-talk
_____ Trouble thinking clearly	_____ Lethargy
_____ Difficulty making decisions	_____ Inability to get things done
_____ Lack of creativity	_____ Loss of sense of humor
_____ Constant worry	_____ Thoughts of running away
_____ Forgetfulness (memory problems)	

Spiritual

_____ Emptiness	_____ Looking for magic
_____ Lack of purpose	_____ Loss of direction
_____ Doubt	_____ Cynicism
_____ Being unforgiving	_____ Apathy
_____ Martyrdom	

Relational

_____ Lack of intimacy	_____ Clamming up
_____ Isolation	_____ Lowered sex drive
_____ Resentment	_____ Nagging
_____ Loneliness	_____ Distrust
_____ Lashing out	_____ Fewer contacts with friends

Sure, a few weeks in a crisis mode won't kill us, but the earlier we learn coping skills and change unhealthy habits, the healthier and more productive we will be throughout our lives. See the stress-coping strategies later in this chapter if you are experiencing many of the symptoms in Table 10-1 (or feel particularly "stressed out") so that you can avoid a serious psychosomatic disease. The sage advice of Eubie Blake, the famous jazz musician who lived to be 100 years old, is applicable here: "If I knew I was going to live this long, I'd have taken better care of myself."

◆ MEASURING YOUR STRESS

In 1967, two psychiatrists at the University of Washington School of Medicine, Thomas H. Holmes, MD, and Richard H. Rahe, MD, observed that certain life events coincided with illness. According to these doctors, change, whether for "good" or "bad," causes stress, leaving humans more susceptible to illness. Even simple changes, such as in eating habits, job routine, and extra schoolwork, can increase one's susceptibility to stress-related diseases. Remember, it is the sum of both "good" and "bad" stress that is important. After studying the medical histories and personal biographies of patients, the doctors found a curious link between life-changing events and illnesses such as heart disease, gastrointestinal problems, and even psychological problems (depression, anxiety, etc.); they developed a list of life changes that range from minor to severe and assigned points to each one based on the amount of stress evoked. The list includes both the positive (eustress), such as a vacation trip or marriage, and the negative (distress), or, the most stressful, the death of a child, spouse, or other loved one. The original test was revised recently to keep pace with the new millennium and to more effectively reflect the stress of college/school. Take a few moments to complete the *Life Event Stress Test,* identifying the events that have occurred in your life during the last year. See Table 10-2. The total score on this self-test offers some insight into one's risk for illness as a result of recent life events. Stressful change in itself won't necessarily harm you; that depends, at least in part, on how you perceive the event, and whether you feel in control of the situation; the support you can rely on from family and friends; and your stress coping skills. Lab Activity 10-1 provides an excellent evaluation of your score on this self-test. Be sure to complete it after taking the test.

The test can be an effective tool when used to anticipate major life events so that you can take *control* of the stress they produce. No one would

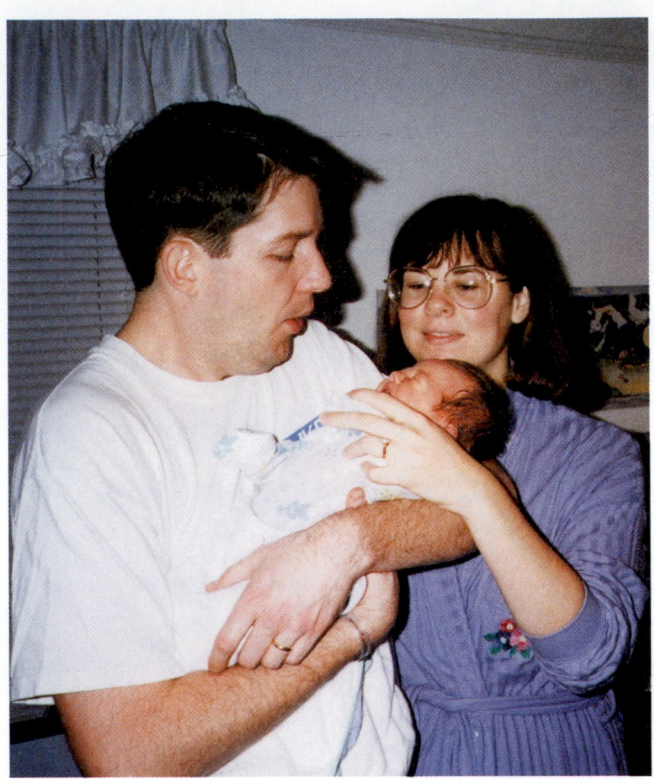

Even happy life events add to our total stress picture.

suggest that we get rid of holidays, vacations, and weddings. But we should take all life changes, including these positive ones, into account when planning our lives. Realizing there are certain life events you cannot control is equally important in stress reduction. Remember, change is inevitable; that's what living is about. But keep in mind that you can plan ahead for change and regulate the timing of many events (stressors) to prevent them from stressing you out. Spread change over time. Change in life situations alone may not be enough to cause illness. When these changes are perceived as distressing and result in prolonged emotional and physiological wear and tear, your risk of illness increases. Some people are more vulnerable to certain types of stress than others are. If you would like to find out what type of stress you are most susceptible to and how well you cope with stress, take the *Measuring Your Stress and Coping Skills* test (Lab Activity 10-4). This test also measures coping skills for dealing with stress.

Establishing coping strategies such as the ones discussed later in this chapter is a positive way to block the development of a stress illness. Well-timed social support is one of the best coping mechanisms we have. When you are experiencing many life changes but have family and friends with whom you can discuss your problems, you probably will avoid a stress illness. An individual experiencing fewer

TABLE 10-2   *Life Event Stress Test*

Directions: To get a feel for the possible health impact of the recent changes in your life, think back over the last year and circle the "stress points" listed for each of the events you experienced during that time. Then total your points. Your score is termed your life change units (LCU). This is a measure of the amount of significant change in your life to which you have had to adjust. In other words, your LCU is a measure of the stressors you have encountered this year. If an event has occurred more than once, multiply the score for that event by the number of times it has occurred.

Life Change Event

Home and Family

Death of spouse	119
Death of other family member:	
child	123
brother or sister	102
parent	100
other family member	60
Divorce	96
Separation from spouse:	
due to marital problems	76
due to work	53
Gain of a new family member:	
birth of a child	66
adoption or remarriage	65
a relative moving in with you	46
Change in the marriage status of your parents:	
divorce	59
remarriage	50
Major change in health or behavior of family member	55
Marriage	50
Change in arguments with spouse	50
Change in residence:	
move within the same town or city	25
move to different town, city, or state	47
Change in living conditions (visitors in the home,	
remodeling house, change in roommates)	42
Spouse beginning or ending work	46
Child leaving home:	
to attend college	41
due to marriage	41
for other reasons	45
In-law problems	38
Vacation (or presently in winter holiday season)	38

Health

An injury/illness which:	
kept you in bed a week or more or sent you to	
the hospital	74
was less serious than above	44
Pregnancy (or causing pregnancy)	67
Miscarriage or abortion	65
Major change in your usual type and/or amount	
of recreation	28
Major change in eating habits	27
Major change in sleeping habits	26
Major dental work	26
Any drug/alcohol use	26
Sleep less than 7–8 hours per night	25

School/College

Beginning or ending school/college	38
Expelled from school	35
Change of school/college	35

Working while attending school	35
Failing an important course	22
Increase in class workload	20
Lack of enough money	18
Change of major	11
Lower grade(s) than expected	10

Work

Loss of job:	
fired from work	79
laid off from work	68
Retirement	52
Change to a new type of work	51
Change in your responsibilities at work:	
demotion	42
transfer	32
promotion	31
more responsibilities	29
Change in your work hours or conditions	35
Troubles at work:	
with coworkers	35
with persons under your supervision	35
with your boss	29
other work troubles	28
Taking course(s) to help you in your work	18

Financial

Major change in finances:	
decreased income	60
investment and/or credit difficulties (or credit card debt)	54
increased income	38
Foreclosure on a mortgage or loan	58
Loss or damage of personal property	43
Going into debt (you or your family)	30

Personal and Social

Being held in jail	75
Death of a close friend	70
Major decision regarding your immediate future	51
An accident	48
"Fall out" of a close personal relationship	
(or broken engagement)	47
Engagement to marry	45
Sexual difficulties	44
Girlfriend/boyfriend problems	39
New, close personal relationship	37
Major personal achievement	36
Change in religious beliefs	29
Change in social activities	27
Change in personal habits	26
Change in political beliefs	24
Vacation	24
Minor violation of the law	20

Total Score _____

Score	Rating	Implication for Illness
≤249	Low Stress	37% chance of getting a stress-related illness in the next year or two. Consider yourself fortunate.
250–500	Moderate Stress	51% chance of getting a stress-related illness in the next year
≥501	High Stress	80% chance of getting a stress-related illness in the next year

Note: These predictions are not absolute. Your final score is influenced by individual perception of these events, your coping/stress management skills, and the social support of family and friends. Adapted from T. E. Holmes, & R. H. Rahe, "The Social Readjustment Scale." *Journal of Psychosomatic Research* 11 (1967): 213–219.

life changes but with less support may become ill. You understand that change is inevitable and have managed stress successfully before and you can do it again. And remember, during times of extreme stress or crisis, or when self-care measures aren't working, consider getting professional help.

◆ DAILY HASSLES AND UPLIFTS

Stress research suggests that it is not only the major "life events" that have a negative impact on health but also other factors called *daily hassles,* and these may be even more harmful. **Daily hassles** are the events or interactions in your daily life that you find bothersome, annoying, or negative in some way. These irritating demands include common problems such as losing things, chronic car problems (or running out of gas on the way to work/school), time demands/deadlines, exams (i.e., preparing for, taking), traffic jams, arguments, and family concerns. Various studies show that hassles are strongly related to episodes of illness, even when there are no major life events to consider. Having too many things to do, roommate problems, not enough sleep, parking problems on campus, and money difficulties were the most frequently reported hassles of students at Ball State University. Examine the Top 10 "Hassles of College Students" to see how the hassles in your life compare.

Everyday hassles can be the "straw that broke the camel's back" when they are added to your life at a time when it is already overloaded with stressful events. The average person is as likely to be "nibbled to death" by everyday hassles as to be overwhelmed by tragedies. The way you handle daily hassles depends to a large degree on your score on the *Life Event Stress Test.* When scores are high (i.e., you are

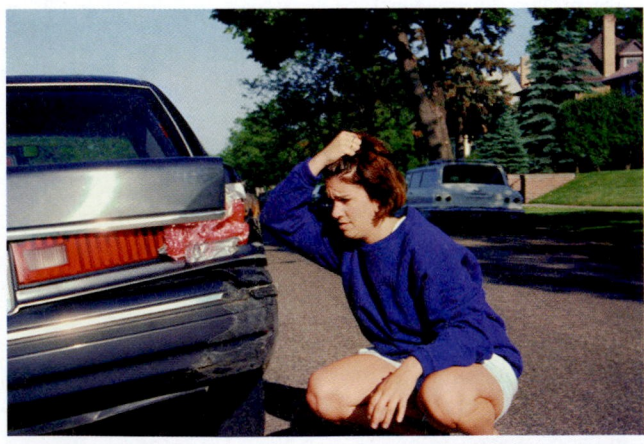

Everyday hassles can "nibble" us to death. Sometimes it's not the mountain in front of you but the grain of sand in your shoe that brings you to your knees.

TOP (10) LIST

Hassles/Uplifts of College Students

Hassles

1. Misplacing or losing things
2. Troubling thoughts about your future
3. Not getting enough sleep
4. Money problems
5. Social obligations
6. Concerns about weight and physical appearance
7. Too many things to do (registration for classes, exams, extracurricular groups, everyday chores, chronic car problems)
8. Concerns about meeting high standards (not living up to expectations, getting low grades)
9. Being lonely (relationship issues)
10. Child care problems

Uplifts

1. Being visited, e-mailed, phoned, or sent a letter
2. Visiting, phoning, or writing someone
3. Having fun (socializing, partying, being with friends)
4. Completing a task
5. Recreation (sports, games, etc.)
6. Hugging and/or kissing (relating well with spouse or lover)
7. Getting enough sleep
8. Being complimented
9. Having someone to listen to you
10. Eating out

---

overstressed), you are more likely to react to daily hassles with less tolerance and a shorter fuse. As with any stressor, the way you perceive it is critical. What constitutes a hassle or an uplift varies greatly from person to person. Concern about weight may not be a hassle to you but may be a real problem to a person for whom physical appearance is a top priority.

The counterpart to daily hassles are **daily uplifts.** These are positive events that make us feel good. Fridays, payday, going shopping, and having a date were the uplifts most often listed by students at Ball State. Research has shown that these little daily uplifts can reverse the negative effects of daily hassles. An appropriate balance between hassles and uplifts may be the important ingredient in your overall health and well-being. These daily uplifts may protect you from stress-related illnesses.

List the events in your everyday life that you find bothersome. How many of them can you eliminate? How many will you have to deal with in some manner? List the daily uplifts you find enjoyable. Can you find ways to add to this list? How does your list compare to the Top 10 "Hassles/ Uplifts" list?

◆ TYPES A, B, AND D PERSONALITIES AND STRESS

We all know people who have the "hurry-up-itis" syndrome. They are always rushed, never have enough time, usually need more than 8 hours a day to complete a day's work, could not survive without a cell phone or laptop computer, and appear to be doing four or five things at one time. Are these behaviors unhealthy?

The **Type A personality's** hallmark characteristic is *time urgency* and *impatience.* They are often described as competitive and ambitious too. Type A's put big demands on themselves to accomplish more in less time. They have little time for or interest in hobbies or leisure pursuits and have few intimate friends. The key problem with Type A behavior is stress. Type A's put themselves under constant pressure, and their bodies react by producing extra amounts of stress hormones.

The **Type B personality** is the opposite—relaxed, casual, and patient. Most Type Bs build time into the day for absorbing activities such as exercise, hobbies, and friendship. They speak more softly, are less obsessed with success, and tend to deal more effectively with stressful situations.

Research led many to believe that the individual who exhibits Type A behavior is prone to developing coronary heart disease, with increased risk of suffering a heart attack. However, today it is known that the personality behaviors of *hostility, cynicism, and anger are the major culprits that increase the risk of heart disease and not the Type A personality itself.* People exhibiting hostility, cynicism, and anger in response to stress produce greater amounts of hormones that damage the cardiorespiratory system. Hostile people often alienate others or spend too much time on work and focus too little on relationships, putting them at risk of social isolation and the increased stress that comes with it. Some studies have found that hostility levels are a more accurate predictor of heart disease than high cholesterol, hypertension, smoking, or obesity. The problem is that the components of Type A behavior can be harmful if they lead to the development of hostile, angry behavior. This is especially true in the case of chronic hurrying, a hallmark characteristic of Type A behavior. *Chronic hurrying,* synonymous with Type A behavior and

life in the twenty-first century, is especially stressful when we want to hurry but are stuck in situations where all we can do is wait, such as heavy traffic and long lines. The frustration boils over into stress and *anger.* It is now clearly understood that Type B's exhibiting angry, cynical, and hostile behaviors suffer the same negative effects as do Type A's.

- ✓ Do you become angry when a car in front of you cuts you off?
- ✓ Do you find it frustrating to wait in lines?
- ✓ Do you lash out with gestures and raised voice when someone does something that seems incompetent, messy, selfish, or inconsiderate to you?
- ✓ Do you often instigate arguments with others?
- ✓ Do you get upset over small things?
- ✓ Do you frequently feel other people aren't doing their part to solve a problem?

People with a hostile personality trait that leads to a heightened risk of heart disease typically can answer "yes" to the questions above.

Are we born a Type A? Most researchers believe that Type A personality characteristics are a reaction to environmental factors, or tendencies toward certain behaviors, and are influenced by our culture rather than genetics. So while some have a natural tendency toward being more intense, this tendency can be exacerbated by environmental stress, or mitigated by conscious effort and lifestyle changes. Our increasingly complex world fosters the development of the Type A personality. We reward the student who excels in the classroom, the winning athlete, the "superwoman" (with career and family), the youngest-ever CEO, the secretary who never takes a break, the executives who talk business over lunch, and the college student who works, carries a full load of classes, is an A student, and volunteers at church.

Continuing studies strengthen the dangers of truly harmful emotions and has led to the identification of a new personality called **Type D.** The Type D is at increased risk of cardiovascular disease and is potentially lethal to those who have already suffered a heart attack or stroke. Type D (for "distressed" personality) people possess negative emotions and tend to be depressed, anxious, insecure, and distant. A newly developed 14-question personality test defines overall distress in terms of two emotional states: "negative affectivity (worry, irritability, gloom)" and "social inhibition (discomfort in social interactions, reticence, and a lack of social poise)." "Yes" or "no" responses to questions like those following (a brief version of the 14-question test) might reveal if you are a Type D personality with negative affectivity and social inhibition:

✓ I make contact easily when I meet people.
✓ I often talk to strangers.
✓ I am often unhappy.
✓ I am often irritated.
✓ I take a gloomy view of things.
✓ I find it hard to start a conversation.
✓ I would rather keep people at a distance.
✓ I often find myself worrying about something.
✓ When socializing, I don't find the right things to talk about.

Don't panic if you think you might be a Type D. Type D personality is not a mental illness. It is a collection of normal human traits. There are many Type D individuals who are living healthy lives and functioning quite well. Even the most distress-prone person can learn to cope with stress and beat back anxious thoughts. If you think you may be distress-prone, you can take practical steps to make it less toxic. Exercise, a wholesome diet, and relaxation techniques such as meditation will reduce almost everyone's risk of cardiovascular disease. These lifestyle changes that protect your heart can improve your emotional state as well.

The Hot Reactor

A further example of how the combination of angry behavior and stress can be lethal has been discovered. Many apparently healthy individuals are prime candidates for stress-related heart attacks or strokes because of the extreme reactions they demonstrate in response to daily stress. These people are labeled **hot reactors** because when stressed, they produce astronomical amounts of powerful hormones called catecholamines (adrenaline and norepinephrine) that damage the cardiovascular system and disrupt the electrical rhythm of the heart. Abnormally high blood pressure and dangerous heart muscle lesions are the results of the massive doses of these stress hormones being released into the bloodstream. (Systolic readings can rise from 120 to a deadly 300.) Venting anger by "blowing off steam," losing your cool, and lashing out can be dangerous to your health. Many people ask, "Isn't it better to express anger—to let it out rather than bottle it up inside?" Now you know that the answer is NO! It is healthier to diffuse these harmful feelings by using the techniques described in Chapter 9.

Hot reactors are guilty of faulty perception. They perceive nearly every stressor as a life-and-death issue and constantly perceive a loss of control in their daily lives. Daily challenges at work or school (deadlines, friendly competition, dealing with the kids, disagreement with a neighbor) trigger an overblown fight-or-flight reaction. The fight-or-flight reaction is a human response meant to be used only in real life-or-death situations. Squandering doses of these powerful hormones on mundane situations (e.g., missing a green light, standing in a checkout line, and running out of dental floss) is a characteristic of a hot reactor. Hot reactors may be either hard-driving Type A's, more placid Type B's, or the distressed Type D.

◆ ANGRY/HOSTILE BEHAVIOR MODIFICATION

Assess your reaction to stress by taking the behavior quiz in Table 10-3. OK, what if you have angry/hostile tendencies? What can you do about it? Life-threatening overreaction to stress is neither innate nor inevitable. People are not born with this trait. We know many angry/hostile behaviors are learned and become habits. We also know that they can be unlearned.

Anger/hostile behavior management training programs that reduce anger/hostility and its adverse effects have found great success by teaching participants to be more aware of situations that make them angry. This includes such things as having the participants ask themselves four questions when feelings of life-threatening anger start to mount:

1. Is this situation really important?
2. Is this anger appropriate for this situation?
3. Is this action modifiable?
4. Is this situation worth dying for?

Reframing is an excellent way to calm hot, angry reactions to stress too. Read more about reframing

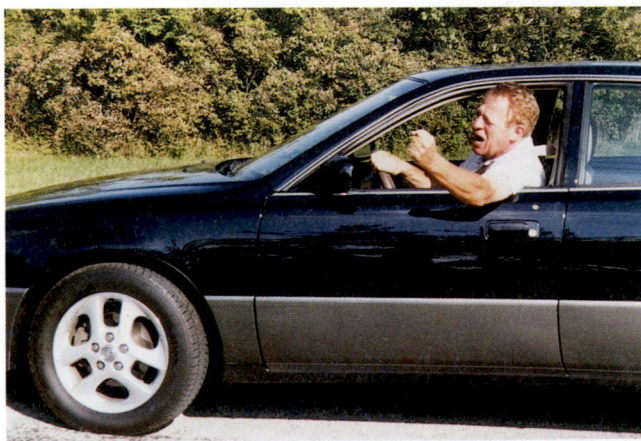

Being a "hot reactor," as in road rage, can be deadly.

TABLE 10-3	*Quiz to Identify Your Type A, Angry/Hostile, Hot Reactor Behavior*

Answer **yes** or **no** to the following statements:

Part I: Are You A Type A?

Yes **No**

___ ___ 1. I hate to wait for anyone or anything.
___ ___ 2. I often interrupt others when they are speaking.
___ ___ 3. I am usually rushed. There's never enough time in the day.
___ ___ 4. I feel guilty when I have nothing to do or when I play.
___ ___ 5. I get impatient when others perform tasks incompetently.
___ ___ 6. I eat faster than most of my friends do.
___ ___ 7. I feel stretched to my limits at the end of the day.
___ ___ 8. I think about other things during conversations.

Scoring

Part I: Statements in this section demonstrate Type A behavior. If you said yes to *three* or more of these statements, you probably fall into the Type A category.

Part II: Are You Too Angry?

Yes **No**

___ ___ 1. I am quick-tempered.
___ ___ 2. When driving, I get irritated at drivers who cut me off or drive too slowly. I frequently blow my horn, tailgate, and try to pass them.
___ ___ 3. I have been so mad that I have thrown things or slammed a door.
___ ___ 4. I remember irritating incidents and get mad again.
___ ___ 5. I am annoyed when others are incompetent at their job.
___ ___ 6. I get angry when I am affected by others' mistakes.
___ ___ 7. I get annoyed by the slowness of waiters and the rudeness of sales clerks.
___ ___ 8. I feel my anger is justified. I feel an urge to punish people—to get back at them.
___ ___ 9. I frequently feel irritated when I stand in line or drive in heavy traffic.
___ ___ 10. I like to have the last word in an argument.
___ ___ 11. In a checkout express line, if the person in front of me has more items than the limit, I get annoyed.
___ ___ 12. I feel upset when I am not given recognition for doing good work.
___ ___ 13. When I am angry, I keep things inside, pout, and sulk.
___ ___ 14. When I get angry, I say nasty things.

Scoring

Part II: Statements in this section demonstrate angry/hostile/cynical/hot reactor behavior. Even one yes response to any of these statements is too many and may be raising your risk of heart disease. Have a friend or loved one who knows you also check the statements for you. Was there a change in any of the answers to the statements?

---

later in this chapter. Take a few minutes now to read the Top 10 "Stress Reduction Tips." You can take charge and be in control of your life—and your health!

THE STRESS-RESISTANT HARDY PERSON

Have you ever imagined what George Washington or any of our other founding fathers would think about our modern, high-tech, fast-paced world? They might be surprised by our 24-hour information society driven by the Internet and round-the-clock global news channels, computers, fax machines, cell phones, heart transplants, overcrowded calendars, never-ending deadlines, and chronic shortages of time.

Certainly they would agree that we have just cause to feel overwhelmed by our daily schedules and would be glad not to be participating in the twenty-first century with us. Yet we all know some people who, in spite of it all, seem relatively insulated from the potential negative effects of their hectic pace. Their lives are as full as ours, but they seem to carry on, taking "everything in stride"—often with a sense of enjoyment and fun. Who are these effective copers? Are they born this way, or are they bred—learning strategies for coping with stress that protect them from being overwhelmed and feeling stressed out?

While researching these questions, it was discovered that even when highly stressed, many individuals have a lower incidence of physical illness, lower amounts of anxiety and depression, and increased longevity. These stress-resistant individuals

TOP 10 LIST

Stress Reduction Tips

(After Implementing the Five Stress Management Strategies Outlined in This Chapter)

1. Simplify. Organize your time so that you do things that are most important first. Let less important things go. Remind yourself that you are not the general manager of the universe. Someone else has that job and doesn't need any help.

2. Identify things that cause you the most stress. Plan ways to get around them.

3. Concentrate on doing one task at a time. Once you have finished, take a moment to let yourself feel good about getting it done. Take a rest if you need it, and then move on.

4. If you are constantly running late, make some changes. Plan to be early to classes, appointments, etc. Allow extra time to do things and get places.

5. Learn to say "No."

6. Live within your budget and don't use credit cards for ordinary purchases.

7. Worry constructively and only about things you can control. Don't sweat the small stuff. It's all small stuff.

8. Weed out trivia. Write down important things and forget unimportant details. Don't overburden your memory. Unclutter your life. Start with cleaning out your wallet (or purse). Then your desk, or study area, then a drawer or closet.

9. Live in the present. Clear your mind of unpleasant experiences and emotions. Let it go!

10. Every night, think of one thing for which you are grateful and record it in your journal.

SLOW DOWN!

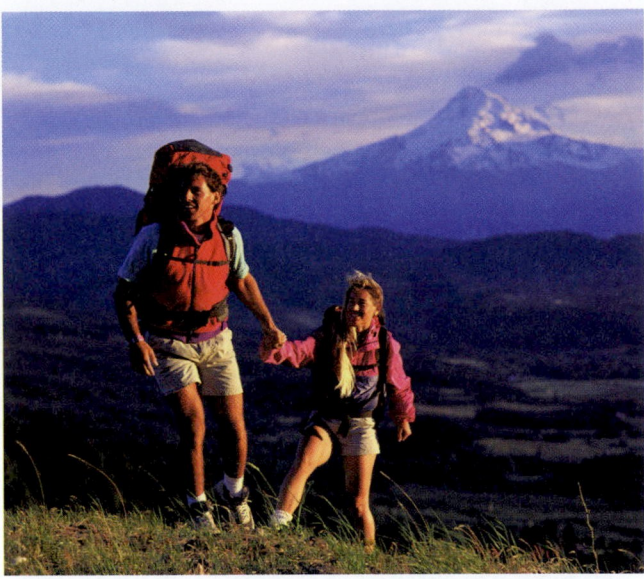

The stress-resistant hardy person makes healthy lifestyle choices and has a sense of connectedness to others.

were labeled "hardy." **Hardiness** is an ability to resist the ill effects of stress. The hardy have strong immune systems and are optimists. The same study found that people lacking "hardiness" were more prone to illness in the face of stress. They are pessimists with weak immune systems. A hardy soul is in reality a Type A who has been relabeled a **Type C personality** because of the five unique personality traits he or she possesses for adapting to life stress. We call the Type C traits the *Five C's:*

✓ *Control:* Control is the opposite of helplessness. The hardy person has a sense of internal control (influence) over life events and their outcomes. These people take daily hassles in stride. They think ahead, plan, and make lists of what needs to be done. They seek active solutions to problems. Do you feel "in control" of your life? If not, what plan can you implement that will help you gain more control?

✓ *Commitment:* Commitment is the opposite of alienation and is typified by meaningful involvement in life (i.e., with one's family, job, and community). The hardy person has a sense of purpose in life and sets short- and long-term goals. Rearing one's children, having friends, participating in community projects, having religious values (or spirituality in some form), reaching career goals, and working to complete your degree are examples of personal commitments that help us unstress. List one or two goals to which you have made a commitment.

✓ *Challenge:* The hardy person perceives life change as a potential opportunity and a challenge rather than a threat. These people continue to learn from positive and negative experiences. Hardy people are highly confident in their ability to do their work. They accept setbacks as a part of life and as an opportunity for growth. They are positive thinkers and view bad situations as temporary and changeable.

✓ *Choices in lifestyle:* Hardy individuals make lifestyle choices that enhance health and reduce stress. They reduce their use of caffeine, nicotine, alcohol, and sugar and incorporate aerobic exercise and relaxation activities into their lives. How much caffeine do you consume every day? Do you practice any of the relaxation techniques in this chapter? Sydney J. Harris said it best: "The time to relax is when you don't have time for it."

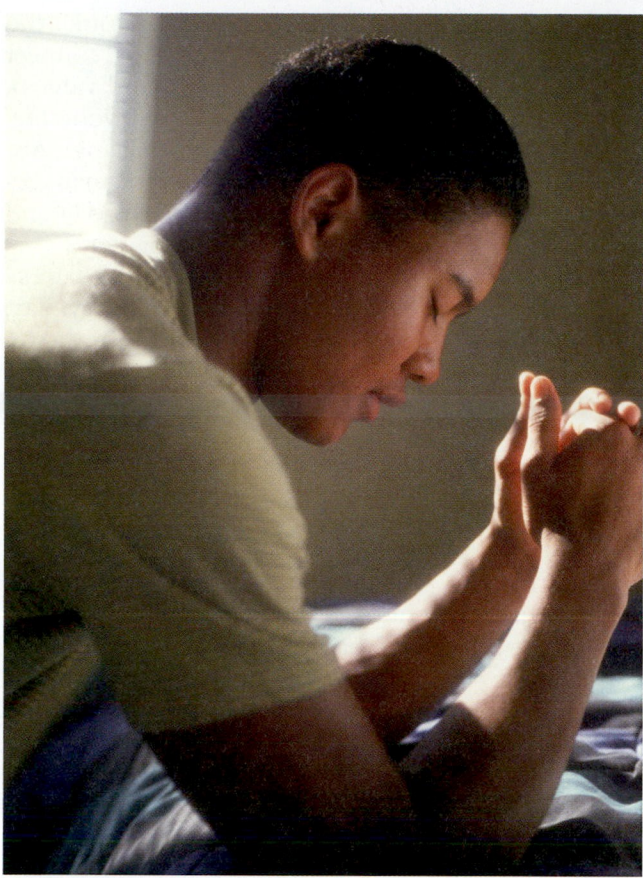

A growing body of evidence links spirituality with enhanced health—including cardiovascular and immune function. Spirituality has been found to reduce the risk of disease, increase the rate of recovery from surgery, and lower the overall death rate.

✓ *Connectedness:* Hardy people develop a network of social support that includes helping and being helped by others. They have developed a sense of "connectedness" to others. They are actively involved with others. Studies show that social interaction is important. It may lower the pulse rate and blood pressure, enhance the immune system, and boost the production of endorphins. When you're in a caring relationship with another person, these health benefits accrue. Do you have a church group or one or more close friends to whom you feel "connected" (i.e., sharing troubles, ambitions, and desires) or whom you can count on for emotional support?

Research on the hardy, stress-resistant Type C personality has made it clear that the five interrelated traits are important factors that buffer us from the ravages of our modern lifestyles and help us adapt and even flourish in the face of them. How many of these hardiness traits do you possess? Lab

Activity 10-3, *Becoming Stress-Resistant and Hardy,* will help you strengthen these traits in your life. Can you think of two ways you can apply the knowledge of these five traits to your life, bolstering your "hardiness" rating?

◆ BUILDING SKILLS FOR STRESS MANAGEMENT

In stress management the goal is to get the body to send out fewer stress hormones so that the body functions efficiently and comfortably, and we can feel at peace. We need this restful state so that we can rejuvenate our body and mind.

The Relaxation Response

Relaxation training is recommended, in combination with nutrition and exercise, not only to reduce stress but to treat chronic pain and illness, such as heart disease, high blood pressure, diabetes, infertility, and cancer. Relaxation is also used in easing depression, painful AIDS symptoms, headaches, and back pain. The concept of relaxation as "good medicine," once dismissed by scientists, is now accepted, thanks to the work of several pioneers in the mind–body field.

As you have learned, when an individual is stressed, the body responds with an outpouring of hormones to prepare him or her to either fight or take flight (the Stress Response). Performance and work decline when you feel stressed out. When you are relaxed and feel in control, mind and body function efficiently and effectively. Dr. Herbert Benson of the Harvard Medical School, the founder of the Mind/Body Medical Institute at New England Deaconness Hospital in Boston, discovered that with effort and training in the use of meditation, we can learn to quiet down and summon at will the healing changes in body chemistry called the **relaxation response.** Benson found that the relaxation response is the body's built-in defense mechanism against the harmful effects of the inappropriate elicitation of the fight-or-flight response caused by everyday living.

The innate physiological changes produced by the relaxation response, which we can elicit to counteract stress, include the following:

✓ Decreased oxygen consumption and metabolic rate, lessening strain on the body's energy resources
✓ Increased intensity and frequency of alpha brain waves associated with deep relaxation
✓ Reduced blood lactates (substances in the blood associated with anxiety)

✓ Decreased anxiety, fears, and phobias and increased positive mental health (i.e., less anxiety and greater feeling of control)

✓ Slowed rate of aging (less shortening of telomeres)

✓ Significant decreases in blood pressure in hypertensive individuals (which remained lowered throughout the day)

✓ Reduced heart rate and slowed respiration

✓ Decreased muscle tension

✓ Increased blood flow to the arms and legs

✓ Improved quality of sleep

Dr. Jon Kabat-Zinn, another stress pioneer, is known for using stress-reduction programs, especially mind–body interactions and mindfulness meditation, to help patients suffering from chronic pain and stress-related disorders at the University of Massachusetts Medical Center. While traditional meditation involves training the mind on a single point of focus, such as a word or phrase, **mindfulness meditation** (i.e., non-mantra meditation) is the practice of paying attention to what is happening to you from moment to moment. To be mindful, you must slow down, do one activity at a time, and bring your full awareness to both the activity at hand and to your inner experience of it. Multitasking is not advised or should be kept at a minimal level. This type of meditation can be done while you are walking to your car, having an unpleasant encounter with someone, typing on a computer, or any other type of activity.

We often start and finish everyday activities almost automatically, not even remembering the in-between of what we just did. Being mindful and present is about being there for the in-between. Also, mindfulness helps you pay more attention to emotions, thought, and sensations without reacting strongly to them. It helps you acknowledge them and their negative emotions in order to let them go. Mindfulness provides a potentially powerful antidote to the common causes of daily stress, whether pleasant or unpleasant.

Those who practice meditation of any type can produce the relaxation response and benefit from all of its antistress effects. Recent research involving brain scans reveals that meditation calms the brain's emotion center. This is powerful evidence supporting the practice as a true stress-buster.

The Six Strategies

OK, what if you have a high "Life Change" score, have angry, hostile tendencies, are a hot reactor, or maybe a type D personality? Do you feel anxious and overwhelmed?

You can't change the complexities of life, but you can develop strategies that enable you to cope more effectively. You can learn to relax, to quiet the mind and body (so you can "get in touch" or "connect to" your inner thoughts, feelings, goals, and values), and to successfully manage the stress in your life. Complete the flowchart "What Stage of Change Are You In?" (page 325) to assess your stress management skills. Then read the Tips box (page 341) and review the behavior change model in Chapter 2.

By following one or more of the six stress management strategies in this chapter every day, you will be well on your way to becoming a relaxed, stress-hardy person. Enjoy!

The six stress management strategies described here are

1. Exercise
2. Relaxation techniques
3. Lifestyle change
4. Reframing
5. Laughter and humor
6. Create a memory bank

STRATEGY #1 EXERCISE

Get physical. An avalanche of research reveals that aerobic exercise promotes health and energy and is a powerful antidote for stress, anxiety, and even moderate depression. It has even been found to lead to lowered levels of perceived stress. Another benefit of exercise is that it counters the aging effects of stress by maintaining longer telomeres. Many physicians recommend exercise to their "stressed" patients instead of medications such as tranquilizers. Exercise allows us to play out the inappropriate (or over used) fight-or-flight response, use the muscles that are tensed for action, and reduce the adrenaline being pumped into the bloodstream. A number of studies suggest that exercise reduces the intensity of the stress response, shortens the time it takes to recover from stress, and helps ward off illness in people experiencing stress. While stress increases blood pressure and platelet stickiness (the factor that increases clotting), exercise reduces them. Regular exercise also helps reduce abdominal obesity, improves insulin sensitivity, decreases inflammation, and slows the progression of artery disease.

Exercise is a natural way to relax and renew energy. When hassles and problems begin to pile up in the office or at school, change into your workout clothes and take a vigorous run, a swim, or a brisk walk. The effect is amazing. Headaches, tension, anxiety, aggressiveness, and irritability are diminished. Vigorous exercise increases the release of *endorphins*, brain chemicals that may alleviate the harmful effects of stressors by producing a more relaxed state.

Tips for Behavior Change For Stress Management

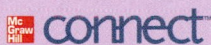

Refer to the Stage of Change flowchart on page 325. What is your stage of change after answering the questions and tracing the flowchart?

Refer to Figure 2.2 (page 36) to see which processes of change are most effective for facilitating your transition from your current stage to the next stage (or *maintaining* your behavior if you are already in the maintenance stage). Here are some behavioral examples for selected processes of change:

- Consciousness-raising: Assess your level of stress (take the Life Event Stress Test [Table 10-2] in this chapter).
- Social liberation: Identify stress management self-help groups/workshops on campus.
- Emotion arousal: Read about the long-term ill effects of stress on the body.
- Countering: Do a deep breathing exercise when you feel anxious, angry, or stressed out.
- Helping relationships: Join the stress management support group in your residence hall or on campus. (Or ask a friend who also has stress issues to "work together" to healthfully manage your stress.)

Mc Graw Hill connect | Go online to Connect to complete this activity. http://connect.mcgraw-hill.com

Besides better stress management, the psychological benefits of exercise, documented by research, are increased self-esteem, increased alertness, and decreased depression and anxiety.

Although aerobic vigorous exercise is best, even a 30-minute walk can do wonders to relieve tension. What is the "number one reason" people give for not exercising? "I don't have the time to exercise." Anyone can squeeze in 20 minutes, the minimum amount of time recommended for an aerobic workout! (The FITT prescription is 20–60 minutes of moderate to vigorous aerobic exercise. See Chapter 4 and Lab Activity 4-4, *"I Have No Time" . . . Overcoming Obstacles.*) For basic health benefits 30 minutes of moderate-intensity exercise is recommended. Play tennis or racquetball, golf, dance, bowl, swim, rake leaves, garden, bike, or do whatever. Wear a pedometer. Just wearing one reminds people to walk more. Enjoy physical activity. It is the healthiest thing you can do for yourself, and it's inexpensive.

STRATEGY #2 RELAXATION TECHNIQUES

Practice the following relaxation techniques to find the ones that you feel most comfortable using and that work for you. For best results, set aside some time every day for relaxation. The seven relaxation techniques described here are meditation, autogenic training and imagery, Jacobson's progressive relaxation, abdominal breathing, Hatha yoga, massage, and biofeedback training.

2a. Meditation

Meditation is a mental exercise that affects body processes, producing physical benefits. The purpose of meditation is to gain control over your attention—to internally quiet down, allowing *you* to choose what to focus on and block out distracting thoughts.

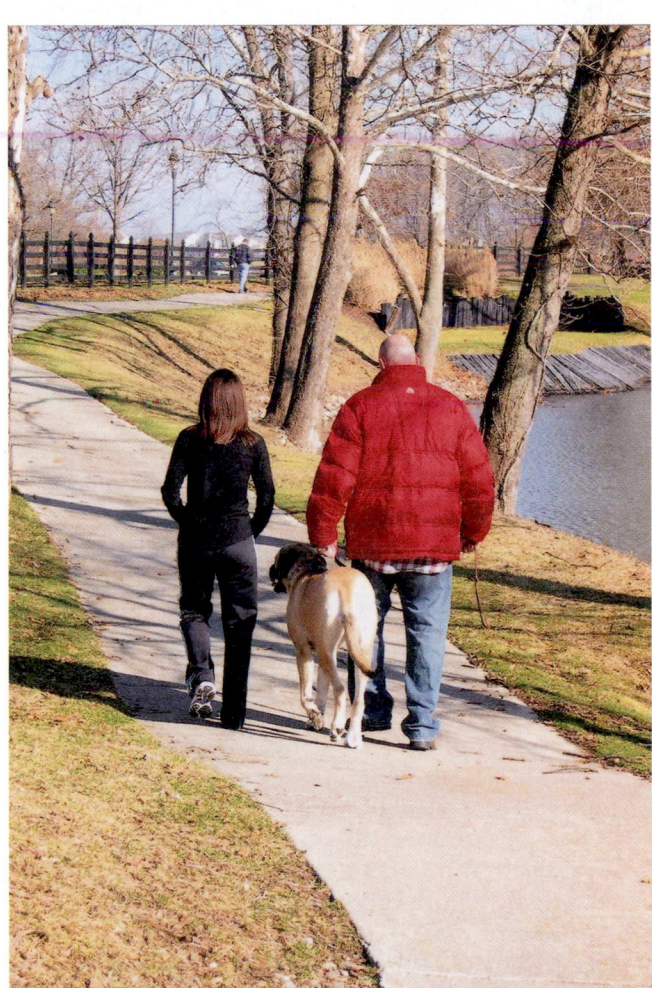

Better than any pill, physical activity de-stresses the mind.

Meditation actually dates back to biblical times, but the type practiced in the Eastern cultures of India and Tibet was exported to the Western world by the Maharishi Mahesh Yogi. The Maharishi popularized the **transcendental meditation (TM)** method. In recent years, TM and meditation in general have been subjected to a battery of scientific studies. Especially revealing and conclusive were the experiments conducted at the Harvard School of Medicine by Dr. Herbert Benson and at the School of Medicine, University of California, San Francisco, by Dr. Dean Ornish. They found that meditation in general was a simple yet powerful, easy-to-learn, nonchemical stress reducer that produced the relaxation response. They call meditation the "universal stress antidote" and assert that it is compatible with modern medicine. Other experts agree that meditation is now mainstream. They believe that a proficient meditator develops a sense of wholeness and is able to face stress, pain, and illness with equanimity and triumph over his or her problems. Meditation is merely a discipline for training the mind to focus, for developing greater calm, relief, and understanding. This, in turn, leads to a greater sense of control and happiness.

To bring the relaxation response benefits into your everyday life, learn to meditate. Meditation ideally should be practiced for 10 to 20 minutes, twice a day. Soon you will be enjoying the relaxing periods of stillness and quietness of the mind that meditation produces. (Use Online Lab Activity 10-4 to learn how to meditate in nine steps.) Meditation involves the following four essential elements:

1. *A quiet, comfortable spot.* A place where you will not be disturbed is essential. However, once you become experienced, you will be able to meditate almost anywhere.
2. *A comfortable position.* A position that will allow you to remain in the same posture for approximately 20 minutes is necessary to avoid any undue muscular tension. Lying down or sitting in a recliner may cause you to lose your focus and fall asleep.
3. *Focusing your attention on something repetitive or unchanging such as a mantra, a mental device, or the breath.* For starters, you can keep it simple by focusing on your breathing, feeling the air as it moves in and out. Use your breath as an anchor to bring you back when your attention is disrupted. A mantra can also be used. A mantra is a silently repeated word, phrase, sound, or thought such as *one, love, peace,* or *omh.* The mantra should be easy to pronounce and short enough to repeat silently as you exhale. Or use a mental device, an unchanging object such as one in the room

where you meditate. Select any one of the three methods to help you maintain your focus, shut out outside stimuli, and keep you calm. The method may vary but the relaxation benefits do not.

4. *A calm, relaxed attitude.* Relax. Let it happen. The harder you try, the more tense you get. Disregard outside noise and thoughts. When distracting thoughts and noise intrude—it is normal that they will occasionally—calmly return your focus to the slow, steady repetition of the breath or mantra or the mental device.

2b. Autogenic Training and Imagery

Autogenic means "self-generating" or "self-induced." The **autogenic training and imagery** technique uses mental concentration exercises to bring about sensations of warmth and heaviness in the limbs and torso and then uses relaxing images to expand the relaxed state. Both meditation and autogenic training lead to the relaxation response. Many who find meditation too easy and boring enjoy autogenic training because of the switches of focus from one part of the body to another and the use of imagery. Otherwise, the physiological and psychological benefits are similar to those of meditation.

Autogenic training should be done with the eyes closed while you are lying down or in a seated position. Whatever position you choose, be sure that you are relaxed and comfortable. Eliminate muscle tension in any part of the body by changing position slightly. Practice for 10 to 30 minutes, one or two times a day, to become skillful at this technique.

The six steps to autogenic training follow:

1. Concentrate on heaviness of arms and legs, beginning with dominant side.
2. Concentrate on warmth of arms and legs, beginning with dominant side.
3. Concentrate on warmth and heaviness of heart and chest.
4. Concentrate on breathing rhythm.
5. Concentrate on warmth of abdominal area.
6. Concentrate on coolness of forehead.

After the six stages of autogenic training have been mastered, transfer body relaxation to mind relaxation by using images of relaxing scenes, such as the following:

✓ Sinking into a mattress
✓ A sack of sugar melting away in the rain
✓ Floating out to sea
✓ A feather floating in the sky
✓ A soaring bird
✓ Clouds drifting by

✓ Ocean surf splashing on the sand
✓ A warm, relaxing fire burning in the fireplace
✓ A sailboat drifting on a calm lake

Use images you find relaxing. They may be different from those used by your friends.

2c. Progressive Relaxation

Edmund Jacobson, a physician, designed for his tense patients a series of exercises called **progressive relaxation** that emphasize the relaxation of voluntary skeletal muscles—that is, the muscles over which you have control. He taught his patients to contract a muscle group and then relax it, progressing from one muscle group to another until the entire body was relaxed. The idea was to learn to recognize tenseness and be able to relax consciously whenever needed. This method, named after its developer, generally does not produce the relaxation response. However, if practiced regularly, it is beneficial in helping people relax.

There are many routines of contract-relax exercises for progressive relaxation. Try the progressive relaxation routine in this chapter (Table 10-4) that begins at the head and ends at the feet, or develop your own routine. Progressive relaxation is a popular "in-class" activity because it is so easy to do. Enjoy!

2d. Abdominal Breathing

Most of us breathe in short shallow breaths, expanding only the chest, especially when we're under stress. This is called *thoracic breathing* and is not the proper way to breathe. It does not allow the lungs to fill and empty completely, and it can increase muscle tension.

During stressful situations, it is even more important to breathe from the abdomen. This method allows more oxygen to enter the body and relaxes the muscles. You can practice the steps described in this chapter at almost any time or in any place, even on the telephone, in class, or at a meeting. Practice at least once a day so that it becomes natural when you use it in stressful or fatiguing situations. This procedure has produced excellent results for many (Table 10-5). Try it now:

2e. Hatha Yoga

Yoga is a 5,000-year-old practice that continues to evolve into many different styles. The most familiar form of yoga is **Hatha yoga,** or physical yoga. This discipline involves the use of various exercises or postures (called *asanas*) in combination with proper breathing rhythm to remove tension and inflexibility in the body. It also improves muscular strength,

TABLE 10-4   Progressive Relaxation Routine

Note: Instructor (or a friend) may read, slowly, the following 14 steps to help you experience this stress antidote.

1. Lie on your back on the floor in a quiet place with the lights dimmed. Remove shoes. Let feet relax and rotate outward. Arms should be beside body, palms turned upward.
2. Proceed slowly over the body, tensing a muscle group and then relaxing it. Stop if cramping or pain develops.
3. Face: Squint eyes, wrinkle nose, make a face, and then relax. Open mouth wide and stick out tongue. Close mouth and clench teeth. Now relax.
4. Neck: Nod head downward to touch chin to chest. Relax.
5. Head: Try to touch right ear to right shoulder and left ear to left shoulder. Relax and center head over torso.
6. Shoulders: Shrug shoulders up toward ears; pull shoulders down from ears; press hard against floor. One at a time. Relax.
7. Hands and arms: Squeeze fingers together, making a fist. Relax. Raise right arm, bending at elbow, and "make a muscle" with biceps. Relax. Repeat with left arm. Relax. With arms on floor, stiffen both arms, making a fist. Relax.
8. Back: Try to squeeze shoulder blades together. Relax. Press lower back area into floor. Relax.
9. Abdomen: Suck in abdominal muscles. Relax.
10. Buttocks: Contract buttock muscles. Relax.
11. Thighs: Contract thigh muscles, one at a time and then both at the same time. Relax.
12. Calves: Flex toes back toward head and then extend or point toes away from head, using right leg and then left leg. Relax.
13. Toes: Curl toes under, first right foot and then left foot. Relax.
14. Be aware of relaxed state of body.

TABLE 10-5   Abdominal Breathing

1. Inhale and exhale fully through the mouth.
2. Inhale slowly and push out your abdomen (stomach) as though it were a balloon inflating. Move your chest as little as possible.
3. Exhale *slowly* and allow stomach to flatten.
4. Repeat the pattern. On each "in" breath, let belly balloon, and on each "out" breath, let it flatten.
5. Each "out" breath is an opportunity to rid the body of tension.

muscular endurance, and body alignment. Hatha yoga should not be associated with religious or spiritual groups. The physiological and psychological benefits of Hatha yoga received thorough research, confirming

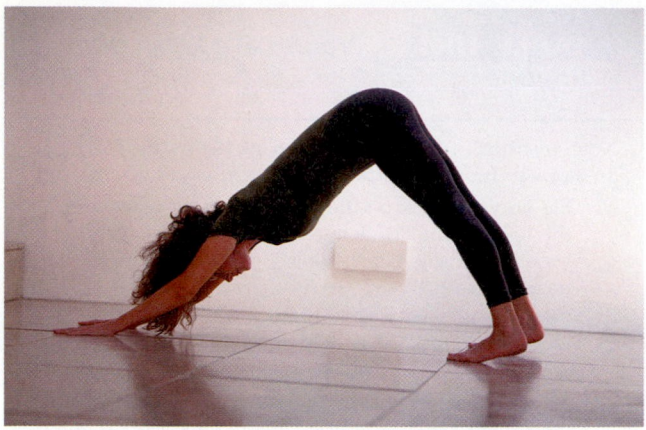

Yoga is a relaxing form of exercise. See Lab Activity 5-2 in Chapter 5 for a sample yoga routine. The Sun Salutation is one of the most practiced yoga routines.

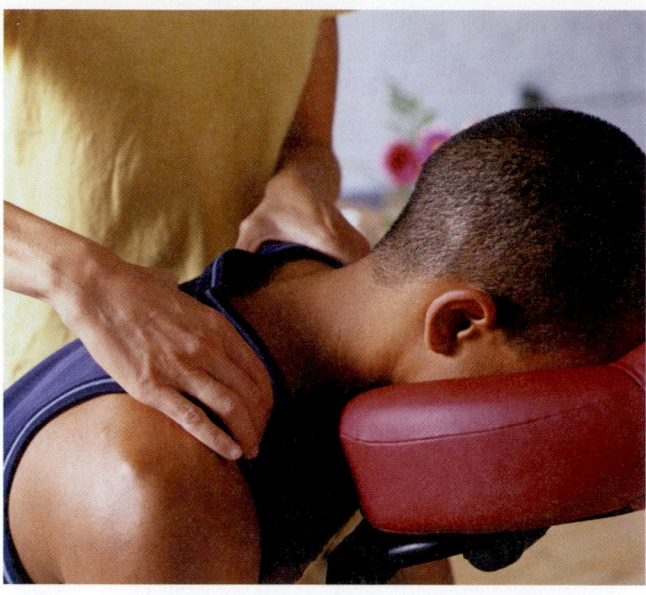

Massage is one of the most enjoyable stress relievers.

it to be an excellent form of exercise and an aid to improving the health and well-being of those who practice it.

2f. Massage

When you are bombarded with too much stress, the muscles in the neck, shoulders, and back can become tight and stiff to the point of pain. Without relaxation, these muscles can become chronically tight and can cause much distress. One of the most enjoyable ways to relieve this condition is to have a massage.

There are several popular forms of massage:

1. *Swedish massage,* the most familiar form, involves kneading and stroking the muscles to decrease tension and increase circulation.
2. *Shiatsu,* originating in Japan and China, is a technique that is a form of acupressure. Pressure is applied with the thumbs or fingers along acupuncture meridians. The idea is to restore balance so that "chi" (an energy believed to be linked to the life force) flows freely and in a balanced manner.
3. *Sports massage* combines Swedish strokes and stretching to help prevent injuries and facilitate flexibility.
4. *Deep tissue massage* uses slow strokes and deep finger pressure to reach deeper layers of muscle to relieve painful areas.
5. *Hot stone massage* involves placing heated stones on different areas of the body to relax the muscles and prepare them for massage.

Massage given by a spouse or friend can be just as pleasant. You can even massage yourself when tight neck and shoulder muscles are tense. Put on your favorite music and enjoy.

2g. Biofeedback Training

Biofeedback training is a technique in which machines measure certain physiological processes of the body. The machines then convert this information to an understandable form and feed it back to the individual. Biofeedback teaches you to identify the early signs that stress is starting to get to you and to bring down your stress reaction before it causes physical symptoms. The point is to calm your body's autonomic nervous septem. Proponents of biofeedback believe that by mentally recognizing involuntary biological responses, such as heart rate and blood pressure, you can control them. With feedback training, stressors are not removed but the response to them is controlled. Control of physiological arousal is an important step in stress management. A major drawback of biofeedback is the cost and availability of the machines and the lack of trained professionals to operate them.

◆ STRATEGY #3 LIFESTYLE CHANGE

Seven important elements are involved in helping us successfully cope with the daily stresses of our hectic, fast-paced lives: the impact of diet; improve time management skills; reduce or eliminate alcohol, drugs, cigarette use; get plenty of restful sleep; develop satisfying relationships; learn when to seek the help and support of others; and schedule "me time" and listen to music. This is an area that you control . . . take charge!

3a. The Impact of Diet

Proper diet is an important part of your stress management program and an area in which you can definitely exert *control*. A nutritious diet will help you look and feel good, plus it will strengthen your immune system. Many believe that poor diet can increase susceptibility to stress by causing fatigue and irritability. This is especially true for individuals who eat too many meals away from home, miss meals, or eat on the run. Unfortunately, there are no miracle foods to boost energy and reduce stress. The best advice for surviving the stress of modern life is to eat three nutritious meals a day and follow these guidelines to help keep you from feeling irritable and uptight:

1. Reduce (below 250 milligrams per day) or eliminate the caffeine in your diet. Caffeine is a stimulant and magnifies the effects of stress. Also, avoid or minimize the use of stimulating drugs (diet pills and oral decongestants) that may cause added agitation.
2. Limit foods containing sugar, especially if you have been skipping meals. Sugar robs the body of B-complex vitamins and may induce anxiety and failure to cope with stressful situations.
3. Limit your intake of salt because excessive fluid buildup leads to discomfort and increased stress. Too much salt can also increase blood pressure due to the fluid buildup. Keep salt consumption below 2,400 milligrams a day—about 1 teaspoon.
4. Limit alcoholic beverage consumption. Alcohol makes people feel relaxed and less stressed while drinking it but leaves them feeling more tired the next day.

3b. Improve Time Management Skills

Insufficient time appears to be the plague of the twenty-first century. College students frequently complain about the lack of this precious commodity. How well you manage your time plays a large role in how much pressure you feel. You should manage your time as if your life depended on it, because it does. The goal of time management should not be the elimination of leisure time (relaxation, etc.); rather, it should be the elimination of life's real time wasters. Use Online Lab Activity 10-5, to practice this important stress management lifestyle strategy. Also, review Top 10 "Tips on How to Reduce College Stress by Improving Studying and Test-Taking Skills." Time management experts suggest these time-saving tips:

1. Analyze how you spend time and then evaluate that use of time. Keep a diary. You may find you are wasting too much time.

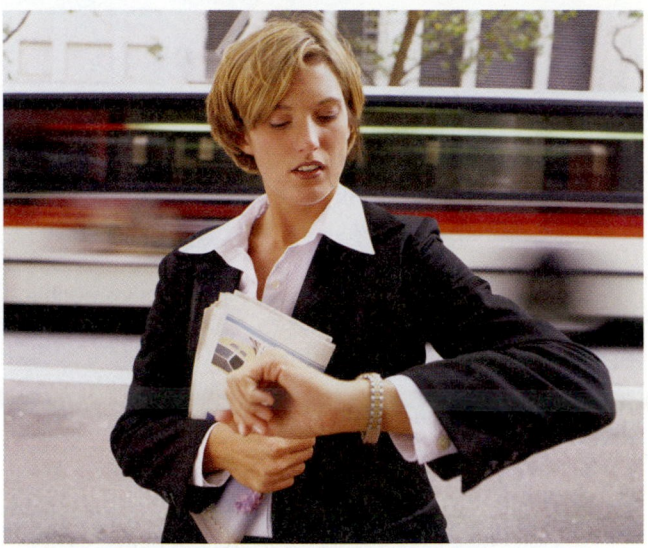

How well do you manage your time? Those who always feel rushed are less likely to be happy than those who almost never feel rushed.

2. Learn to set short- and long-range goals. Write them down. This helps you plan for today and for the future.
3. Learn how to set priorities. Not everything you do is number one on your list of important things. With goals in mind, you will know how to prioritize your activities. Items on the "Do" list must get done; items on the "Maybe" list are those you would like to take care of today, if possible; and those on the "If Possible" list are those you would like to do once the activities of the first and second lists are completed.

THINK ABOUT IT

Many drug commercials on TV make it appear as if their drugs are a cure-all for depression, stress, anxiety, and sleep problems. How does the use of prescription and over-the-counter medication compare to practicing stress management (i.e., taking a walk/jog or doing yoga)? Why do you think the idea of "fixing" a problem with medication might be so appealing to someone suffering from stress or anxiety? What could stress management practices do for this individual that drugs would not?

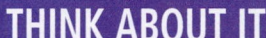

Go online to Connect to complete this activity.
http://connect.mcgraw-hill.com

TOP 10 LIST

Tips on How to Reduce College Stress by Improving Studying and Test-Taking Skills

1. Choose a quiet place—no friends, stereo, telephone, TV, and so on.
2. Learn to manage your time. Follow a daily schedule that includes time for classes, completing reading and writing assignments, exam preparation, meals, exercise, a job, "me time," and so on.
3. Plan on doing 2 hours of studying for each hour you spend in class.
4. Take short breaks after each hour of studying.
5. Don't skip classes.
6. Don't give in to peer pressure to join midweek get-togethers.
7. Don't rely on cramming.
8. Master test-taking skills:
   - Read all directions carefully.
   - Survey the test. Will certain sections take more time, count more?
   - Outline answers for essays.
   - Work on one question at a time.
   - Mark difficult items and return to them later.
9. Don't hesitate to seek help if you are having difficulty with a course.
10. Encourage yourself with positive thinking ("I can do well in this course").

4. Use a planner calendar to schedule your priorities into your day, week, and year. This will help you organize and simplify your life by keeping track of important dates, appointments, and meetings. By systematically planning your day, you can see more clearly what needs to be done. Minor tasks need no longer overshadow major ones. A few minutes of planning can control hours of chaos. A planned day allows you to schedule stress-reducing breaks and rest periods and to have time for family, friends, personal development, and hobbies.

5. Take 5 to 10 minutes at the end of the day to evaluate how well you managed your time. How many of your goals did you check off today? Good time managers use this technique daily to assess time wasted, reprioritize goals (even dumping some), and maintain progress in achieving their short- and long-range goals.

6. Adopt the following time-saving strategies:
   - Learn how to stop being inefficient. This is an art that anyone can learn. Go through mail one time only. Start a task with the intention of completing it now. Don't look it

over and put it aside for later. You will have wasted time looking it over the first time.
- Learn to say "no" to nonessential tasks! Know your limits. Don't allow too many demands to be made "on your time." Learn to delegate certain activities to others when possible.
- Practice quick relaxation tricks frequently throughout the day. Get up and go for a drink of water. Massage your neck, shoulders, and forehead. This energizes you to complete tasks more efficiently.

3c. Reduce or Eliminate Alcohol, Drug, and Cigarette Use

Alcohol is a powerful depressant drug that temporarily masks but doesn't solve your problems. It can increase stress by creating new problems—hangovers, arrests, traffic violations, fights, and accidents. Taking illegal drugs can only increase stress. Why risk ruining your physical and mental health and experiencing the stress of being arrested? Do not smoke cigarettes or use other tobacco products (snuff, chewing tobacco). Nicotine is a stimulant that increases stress.

3d. Get Plenty of Restful Sleep

Take care of yourself. Most people need 7 to 9 hours of restful sleep each night. Getting enough sleep can make you more alert, less irritable, and better able to cope with stressful situations. Cumulative sleep loss has debilitating and even fatal effects. For starters, it elevates levels of the stress hormone cortisol, which strains the heart. According to an Institute of Medicine report, people who sleep less than 7 hours a night tend to be more obese than those who get more than 7 hours of sleep. Insufficient sleep appears to affect hormones that regulate appetite and body weight. Leptin, which suppresses

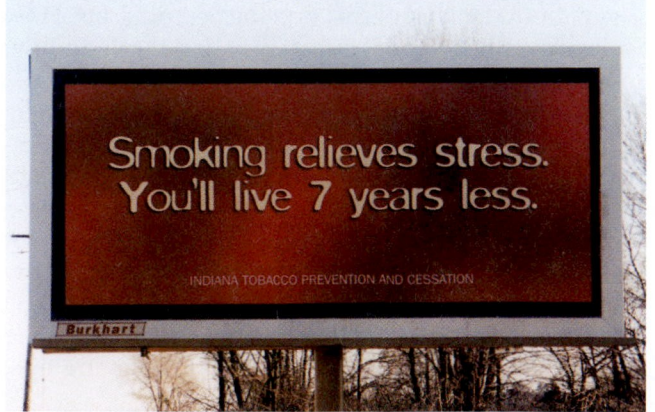

Some individuals use smoking as a way to cope with everyday stress.

appetite, is lowered; ghrelin, which stimulates appetite, gets a boost. These hormone changes combined with more awake time to eat and feeling too tired to exercise all contribute to weight gain. Poor judgment and other declines in cognitive performance lead to increased risks of accident and injury when sleep is shortchanged. Driving while sleep-deprived (getting 6 hours of sleep or less the night before), according to researchers, is nearly as risky as driving while intoxicated! Quality of life decreases dramatically if fatigue dominates the day. Tired people are less productive at work and in the classroom, less patient with others, and less interactive in relationships. Good sleep is as important as regular exercise and good nutrition to cope with life's stresses and keep the body functioning in top form physically, mentally, and spiritually. You can have too much of a good thing, however. Regularly getting more than 9 hours sleep a night disrupts blood sugar levels, which makes type 2 diabetes a concern.

You know if you are getting enough sleep if you wake up in the morning before the alarm goes off, feel refreshed and rested, and are alert throughout the day. If you have any of the following signs and symptoms, you may not be getting enough sleep:

✓ You routinely ignore the alarm clock or snatch a few extra minutes to snooze before getting up.
✓ You look forward to catching up on your sleep on the weekend.
✓ You have to fight to stay awake during class, during long meetings, in overheated rooms, or after a heavy meal.
✓ You're irritable with friends, family members, or coworkers.

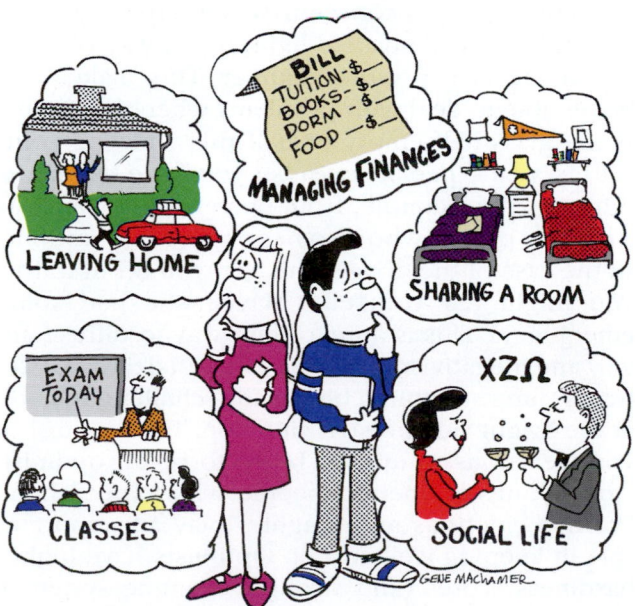

College students face many stresses.

✓ You have difficulty concentrating or remembering.
✓ It takes you more than 30 minutes to fall asleep at night.
✓ You wake repeatedly throughout the night.
✓ You wake up groggy and not well rested.
✓ Your roommate, spouse, or partner complains about your snoring or fitful sleeping.

Review the guidelines in Table 10-6 if you have concerns about the quality of your sleep.

3e. Develop Satisfying Relationships

Having close friends with whom to share the joys and sorrows of living is a huge asset in protecting your health. Recent research confirms that loneliness is bad for your heart. It is linked to blood vessel problems that may lead to high blood pressure in younger adults and greatly increases blood pressure in men and women over 50 years of age. Club

TABLE 10-6   *Improve Your Quality of Sleep*
To improve your quality of sleep, implement the following helpful guidelines:
• Stick to a regular schedule for sleeping and waking. Go to sleep and wake up at the same time. Try to stick to that schedule even on weekends. Consistency helps your body to know when it's time to go to sleep and wake up.
• Don't eat or drink a lot before bedtime.
• Sleep primarily at night. Avoid frequent daytime naps—they may disrupt sleep at night.
• Develop a soothing bedtime routine. A warm bath or shower before bedtime relaxes tense muscles.
• Create a dark, quiet, and comfortable place to sleep. A slightly cool room is ideal.
• Get adequate exposure to bright light each day. Get outside as much as possible, especially at midday during short winter days.
• Exercise regularly—but not within a few hours of bedtime. Don't overtrain, though; this has the opposite effect on sleep.
• Check your medications. Many contain ingredients (such as caffeine) that can cause insomnia (e.g., pain relievers, decongestants, asthma/cold/antihistamine medications, exercise and diet aids).
• Acknowledge the sources of stress in your life and devise a plan to eliminate the ones you can.
• Practice relaxation techniques—especially in the evening—such as meditation.
• Modify your lifestyle. Reduce or eliminate caffeine, tobacco, and alcohol, especially before bedtime. While alcohol may help people fall asleep, it usually produces a light restless sleep, often causing the individual to awaken suddenly during the night, unable to sleep again.

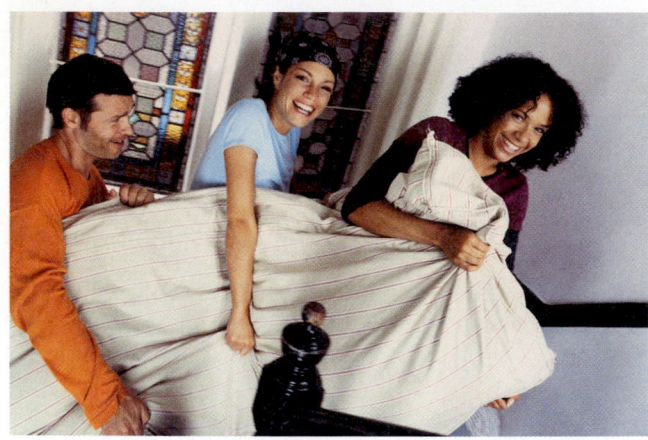

Having friends you can rely on (like helping on moving day) can enhance the immune system. Social support is a key factor in reducing the distress in our hectic lives.

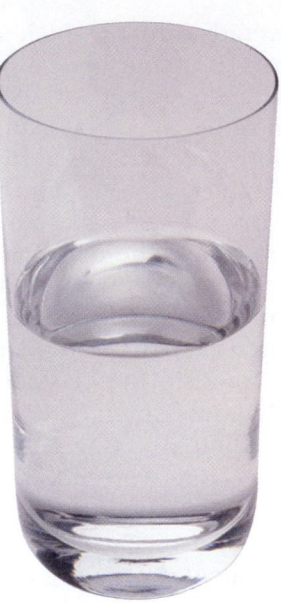

Reframing: Is the glass half empty or half full?

membership, religious or civic activities, and volunteer work have been shown to protect against the physical effects of stress. Unhappiness, depression, and feelings of isolation can be caused by lack of close emotional bonds with friends, a spouse, or family members. Intimate relationships and social support can become a powerful life-support system when internal resources have fallen short. Social support can provide direct reinforcement for healthy behaviors and indirectly buffer disappointments that would otherwise lead to excessive stress. Friends are not just nice, they are a necessity. You have to *be a friend to have a friend.* Make the effort. It's good health and happiness insurance.

3f. Learn When to Seek the Help and Support of Others

There will be stressful situations you will not be able to deal with alone. Don't be embarrassed about seeking professional help. Developing a variety of support groups such as family, friends, coaches, counselors, or physicians can be helpful. Talking to someone gives you a different perspective on worries and concerns.

3g. Schedule "Me Time" and Listen to Music

Do something that soothes you every day, whether for 10 minutes or an hour or two. Schedule it on your calendar if necessary. Make this time inviolate. Let nothing else interfere. This is an excellent way to balance the stresses of work or school. "Me time" can include learning to do nothing (loafing) at times and feeling OK about it. Many people enjoy listening to their favorite music during their "me time."

Music can be therapeutic, relaxing, and an excellent way to calm the mind. Music triggers the brain to release endorphins, the chemicals that ease stress and improve blood flow. According to a study at the Cornell Center for Complementary and Integrative Medicine, music can lower stress hormones by as much as 25 percent when you listen for 15 minutes or more a day.

 ### STRATEGY #4 REFRAMING

Reframing means consciously reinterpreting a situation in a more positive light. It is a way of looking at life in a positive manner. This makes you better able to deal with problems when they come. Is the glass half empty or half full? Viewing yourself as a sick person because you have asthma is different, for example, from perceiving yourself as a healthy person who also happens to have asthma. In the case of the driver who cuts you off in traffic, you might tell yourself, "Maybe she had some emergency." This is an excellent way to diffuse anger and negativism. See if you can learn to "reframe" life's stumbling blocks into challenges. Look at the bright side of each situation. Take control of your reactions to events. Learn to be an optimist. Good things happen to people who expect them. Positive emotions and laughter play an important role in keeping well and fit. Optimists have higher hardiness scores (and stronger immune systems), whereas pessimists are more likely to resort to anger and hostility.

STRATEGY #5 LAUGHTER AND HUMOR

Laughter and its subtle companion humor can provide psychological relief from tension, anxiety, anger, hostility, and emotional and physical pain. Laughing is like "internal jogging"—it causes endorphins (pain-relieving chemicals) to be released in the brain. A hearty belly laugh decreases stress hormones in the blood. Laughter is a natural tranquilizer with no negative side effects. It helps relax the blood vessels and boosts blood circulation. In one study, laughter increased blood flow 22 percent; under stress, it decreased 35 percent. Laughter and humor reduce anger and anxiety, increase joy, reduce food cravings, provide a greater sense of control, lower production of stress hormones, and improve immune function. Note: There is an emerging therapeutic field known as humor therapy to help people manage health-debilitating stress. It is called "Laughercise" because the benefits are as much like those of physical activity. Laughercise has been shown to increase the levels of good HDL cholesterol and decrease levels of C-reactive proteins (a measure of inflammation).

Make an effort (and practice it too) to see the humor in everyday situations. Don't be afraid to laugh at yourself whenever you make a silly mistake. After all, we are only human. Smile and laugh more, even if it is fake. Studies show the positive effects of smiling, whether the smile is fake or real; fake laughter also provides positive benefits. Scientific evidence is beginning to support the biblical axiom that "a merry heart doeth good like a medicine." Bob Hope, a Hollywood comedian who lived to be 100 years old, is a good example of this axiom. When asked about his life's work he answered: "I have seen what a laugh can do. It can transform almost unbearable tears into something bearable, even hopeful."

STRATEGY #6 CREATE A MEMORY BANK

Happiness comes from noticing and enjoying the little things in life. Take 5 minutes of your day, every day, to savor the special experiences of your life. Store them in your memory bank. Journaling will help you remember them. When you look back over your day (and your life), what special memories do you fondly recall: roasting marshmallows over a campfire, watching the sunset, smelling a rose, the glow after a satisfying workout, birds singing

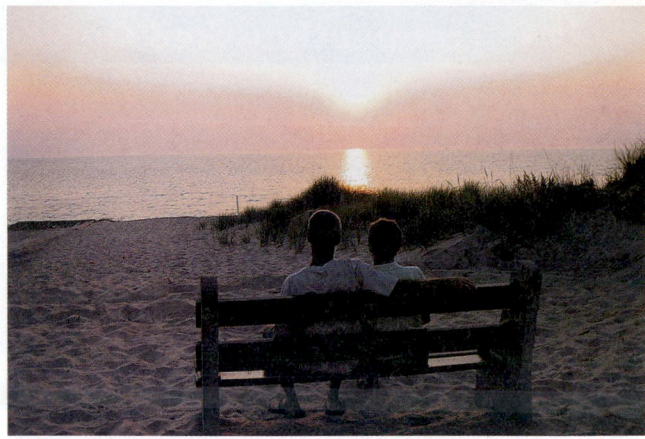

Create a memory bank. Create memories of special moments you'll savor later.

early in the morning, a beautiful morning sunrise, newborn animals, a hug that said "I care"? What can you do today to increase your store of pleasant memories?

PRESCRIPTION FOR ACTION

You've read the chapter. Now go do one or more of these:

- ✓ Think of an act of kindness and then do it for a stranger.
- ✓ Get 8 hours of sleep tonight.
- ✓ Go to a humorous or uplifting movie (or get a video/DVD of one).
- ✓ Reflect on the meaningful people in your life. Connect with two of them today via e-mail, telephone, or letter.
- ✓ Watch a sunset tonight and/or a sunrise tomorrow.
- ✓ Get your study area organized.
- ✓ Write in a journal. Record the best things that have happened to you this week.
- ✓ Volunteer your services to a worthy project/group that interests you.
- ✓ Arrive early to every class/job and all appointments tomorrow.
- ✓ Take a break from e-mailing/texting today.

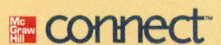

Go online to Connect to complete this activity.
http://connect.mcgraw-hill.com

Frequently Asked Questions

Q. Can stress really cause premature aging?

A. Yes! Just look at any U.S. president after a few years in office. A groundbreaking study found that chronic stress appears to accelerate the aging process by shortening the life span of the immune system cells and telomeres on our chromosomes. The cells of people under lots of stress aged the equivalent of 9 to 17 years more than the cells of people under little stress. What's more, it wasn't just the stress itself but the perception of stress (or how the person perceives the stress) that can lead to faster aging. The researchers suspect that stress hormones such as cortisol are to blame. They also believe it may be more or equally important how you view your life and cope with demands, and what kind of support you have. The meaning is clear: people at risk for high stress can slow down cell aging through exercise, meditation, prayer, or other stress reducing strategies. Health can indeed be an example of "mind over matter."

Q. Is mindful meditation or "living in the moment" hard to do?

A. Of course it can be, but it's a behavior that you can learn with practice. It takes some time and effort, but in the end, the act of living in the moment rewards not only you but the people around you.

Q. Can spirituality uplift one's health?

A. Modern medicine, with its high-tech wizardry, can do wonders for the body but little for the soul. And until recently medical research avoided spirituality.

In the last decade a growing number of researchers have put spirituality and religion under the microscope. The research so far suggests that having a spiritual dimension in your life may help you get healthy when you are sick and stay healthy when you are well.

There are several plausible explanations for a faith–health link: Religion and spirituality may encourage healthy habits and help reduce stress, perhaps by promoting social support, an optimistic outlook, and deep relaxation during prayer, meditation, or another relaxation technique.

Q. I think my boyfriend might be depressed. How large a problem is depression (more than just "the blues") among college students? What are the symptoms of depression?

A. Combine the academic pressures of college life with the fact that the age of onset for mental disorders is often 18–25, and it is not a surprise that students are especially vulnerable. The following can be symptoms of depression:
- A persistent feeling of sadness, anxiety, or "emptiness"
- Feelings of hopelessness and worthlessness

- Loss of interest in activities
- Fatigue or lack of energy
- Trouble concentrating
- Insomnia, early morning awakening, or oversleeping
- Thoughts of suicide (or actually *saying* they are thinking about it)

Seek professional help immediately if you, loved one, or a friend exhibit signs of depression.

Q. I sleep 5 to 6 hours a night and don't feel tired during the day. Am I getting enough sleep?

A. Probably not. Roughly 5 percent of people claim that's all the sleep they need to function well during the day. But getting so little slumber may harm your health even if it doesn't impair your performance. Without enough sleep,
- Your ability to learn; your problem-solving, speaking, and writing skills; your reaction time; and your stamina can decline.
- You are more likely to become tense and moody and to have trouble getting along with others.
- The body's immune system may weaken. People who report daytime sleepiness have worse overall health and higher mortality rates than do well-rested people.
- The risk of developing insulin resistance and obesity increases. This may predispose people to diabetes, high blood pressure, coronary heart disease, stroke, and possibly cancer.
- Weight gain and reductions in muscle mass may occur due to inhibited nocturnal surges of growth hormone.

Q. Last year I thought it was a good idea to attend a college in another state. Now that I am four states away from home I'm not so sure. I don't know anyone in my residence hall much less on campus. All my friends went to in-state schools. Last week I felt like I was getting sick. Can loneliness affect my health?

A. It sure can. Research at Carnegie Mellon University studied college freshmen coping with their first semester away from home. They found that freshmen who felt the loneliest and most socially isolated had the weakest immune response to the flu virus. Their studies show that loneliness and social isolation can have an impact and that the first semester of college can be "really stressful." College students aren't the only ones whose health may suffer with those feelings. Loneliness and social isolation have previously been associated with immune detriments in other age groups.

Q. I heard on TV that stress can make you fat. Is this true?

A. Yes! The fight-or-flight reaction, which is triggered on an almost continuous basis in some people, causes a release of stress hormones. One of them is cortisol. High cortisol levels are associated with overeating, craving high caloric fatty and sugary foods, and relocating fat from the circulation and storage depots to the deep internal abdominal area. Research has demonstrated that moderate to vigorous exercise and stress management activities can offset the negative effects of cortisol and reduce the health risks associated with stress-induced obesity.

Q. What is Tai Chi? Is it a beneficial form of exercise?

A. Tai Chi is an ancient Chinese exercise form that combines relaxed, slow movement with a calm, alert mental state. The practitioner keeps his or her body relaxed and upright, focusing throughout the exercise sequence on natural diaphragmatic breathing. The Chinese have long touted Tai Chi's medical benefits, practicing it for health, vitality, relaxation, and self-defense. Medical research has begun to confirm that Tai Chi practice has a positive effect on health by
- Reducing diastolic and systolic blood pressure
- Improving strength and balance
- Improving emotional health (i.e., reduced tension, depression, anger, improved general mood)
- Possibly positively affecting the immune system

Q. The nation seems to be in the middle of an anger epidemic. Why is this?

A. Bad tempers are everywhere. The media report incidents of road rage, airplane rage, cell phone rage, grocery store rage, parking lot rage, and youth sports activities rage. Leading social scientists confirm that the nation is in the middle of an unsettling and deadly anger trend. This all-too-frequent display of rage is described as a fuming, unrelenting sense of anger, hostility, and alienation that simmers for months, even years, without relief. Eventually, all it takes is a triggering incident, usually minor, for a hostile person to go ballistic. Why?
- Stress is a hallmark of the anger epidemic, and the major contributing factors are lack of time and intrusive technology. Cell phones, pagers, and so on allow us to be interrupted anywhere, at any time. This constant accessibility and compulsive use of technology fragments what little time we have, adding to our sense of urgency and overload.
- Multitasking. People feel the need to do several things at the same time (drive and talk on the phone).
- High expectations and entitlement. Pressure to achieve more and live the "good life." People feel they are entitled to fulfillment at any cost because of materialism and consumerism.
- Lack of manners. Rude and selfish behavior has increased, and so has anger at the bad behavior of others.
- Lack of connection. Families are not doing things together the way they used to. Social support also has diminished.
- Media. Television programs (talk shows such as *The Jerry Springer Show*; crime shows; shows such as *Dateline* and *20/20,* and the evening news) continually show examples of rage outbursts, almost convincing the viewing public that it's OK or at least normal.
- We feel it's normal. We are exposed to more violence, which makes it mainstream.

Summary

No one is exempt from stress. Stress is unavoidable. Optimal levels of stress improve health and performance, but excess levels, especially when chronic and perceived as negative, can be hazardous to your health. Major life events—death of a spouse, marriage, and divorce, for example—are significant stressors. Other, more common stressors are daily hassles (missed sleep, rush-hour traffic, losing things). We learn to cope with major life events and daily hassles in a variety of ways. Some are healthy; some are not. Healthy stress management strategies include exercise, relaxation techniques, lifestyle changes, reframing, laughter and humor, and creating a memory bank. Hassles can be countered with the giving and receiving of daily uplifts (compliments, hugs, and getting enough sleep). These strategies are worth the effort because stress is cumulative; the more stress you have, the worse the attack on your immune system.

Four stress-coping behavior types—Types A, B, C, and D—have been identified. Type A's are described as rushed, competitive, and impatient. These behaviors often lead to angry, hostile, and cynical reactions when the individual is stressed, which are, in turn, the lethal risk factors for coronary heart disease. Type B's are more relaxed than Type A's, but if they demonstrate anger and hostility, they also will develop negative health consequences. Hot reactors perceive every stressor as a life-or-death situation and may be either Type A or Type B. Type D's are "distressed" and exhibit two emotional states: negative affectivity (worry, irritability, gloom) and social inhibition (discomfort in social interactions, reticence, and a lack of social poise). Type D's are especially at risk for cardiovascular disease. Type C's are often referred to as "hardy." Type C's possess the Five C's: They accept challenges, feel they are in control of their lives, have a strong commitment or purpose in life, make healthy lifestyle choices, and have a strong sense of connectedness to others.

Your wellness is dependent on how well you balance the stress in your life, how well you can modify your angry and hostile behavior, and how successfully you take charge of your life. As one wise person said, "If you can't fight and you can't flee, flow."

Terms

- acute stress
- autogenic training and imagery
- biofeedback training
- chronic stress
- daily hassles
- daily uplifts
- distress
- eustress
- faulty perception
- fight-or-flight response (Alarm Reaction Stage)
- General Adaptation Syndrome (GAS)
- hardiness
- Hatha yoga
- hot reactors
- meditation
- mindfulness meditation
- optimal stress
- progressive relaxation
- psychoneuroimmunology
- psychosomatic disease
- reframing
- relaxation response
- stage of exhaustion
- stage of resistance
- stress
- stressors
- Stress Response
- transcendental meditation (TM)
- Type A personality
- Type B personality
- Type C personality
- Type D personality

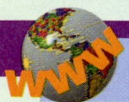 Internet Resources

ABC of Yoga

www.abc-of-yoga.com

For all the basics, from terminology to postures.

American Foundation for Suicide Prevention

www.afsp.org

Provides information about depression and suicide.

American Institute of Stress

www.stress.org

Dedicated to advancing our understanding of the role of stress in health and illness, nature and importance of mind–body relationships, and the inherent and immense potential for self-healing.

American Massage Therapy Association

www.amtamassage.org

Provides a list of certified massage therapists in your area and advances the art, science, and practice of massage therapy.

American Psychological Association

www.apa.org

A scientific organization's site provides studies of the mind and behavior.

American Yoga Association

www.americanyogaassociation.org

Gives information on how to start practicing yoga and how to choose a yoga teacher. Has an online store for books, DVDs, videos, etc.

Association for Applied Psychophysiology and Biofeedback

www.aapb.org

Provides information about biofeedback and mind–body interactions.

Anxiety and Panic Recovery Resources

www.stressrelease.com

Provides resources to help manage and regain control of your life.

Health Behavior News Services

http://www.cfah.org/hbns/

Resource for most recent research about how people can change their behaviors to improve their health. Topics include stress, diet, exercise, cardiovascular health, diabetes, HIV/AIDS, and addictions.

Healthfinder

www.healthfinder.gov

Consolidates official government health resources and offers links to over 500 consumer health sites.

The Humor Project

www.humorproject.com

Provides articles, speakers' bureau, discussion boards, and publications on utilizing humor for the release of stress.

Mayo Clinic

www.mayoclinic.com

Provides reliable health and wellness information, including information on stress.

Meditation Center

www.meditationcenter.com

Provides simple instruction and information about a variety of meditation techniques.

Benson-Henry Institute for Mind Body Medicine (BHI)

www.massgeneral.org/bhi

Harvard's Dr. Herbert Benson provides the latest information about mind–body stress reduction.

Mindfulness Meditation

www.mindfulnesstapes.com

Provides information about mindfulness, Jon-Kabat-Zin, and mindfulness CDs that are available.

National Institute of Mental Health (NIMH)

www.nimh.nih.gov

Part of the National Institutes of Health (U.S. Department of Health and Human Services). Provides up-to-date research and information pertaining to a wide variety of wellness topics.

Stress, Depression, Anxiety, Sleep Problems, and Drug Use

www.teachhealth.com

Provides information on recognizing stress, a stress test, biological bases of stress, and stress management techniques.

Stress Less

www.stressless.com

Provides sources for over 1,000 stress-reducing products.

Transcendental Meditation

www.tm.org

Provides information on TM.

Yoga Basics

www.yogabasics.com

Provides information on newsletters and articles, has a yoga products section.

Yoga Journal

www.yogajournal.com

Provides video demonstrations of the Sun Salutation and other postures. Gives information on yoga conferences, yoga products, videos, etc.

LAB Activity 10-1

Evaluation of the Life Event Stress Test and Relaxation

After completing the *Life Event Stress Test* (Table 10-2) in this chapter, answer the following questions:

1. What was your score? _____
2. What was your rating? _____
3. Discuss the results of this test in terms of its implication for your having a stress illness this year. List at least *four* or *five* factors that influence this implication.

4. List and discuss *three* stress management strategies you could incorporate into your current lifestyle. How will you do so? Be specific.

5. What role does diet play in the total stress picture in your life? List *three* ways you can improve the diet–stress connection in your daily life.

6. List the top *two* daily hassles and the top *two* daily uplifts in your life.

Relaxation

Relaxation is an important stress management strategy. You cannot simply wish to become a more relaxed person. Becoming relaxed is a skill that takes commitment and practice. Make the commitment now.

1. How often do you practice a relaxation technique now? (See Strategy #2 in the chapter for a list of the six relaxation techniques.)
   Circle one: **Never**   **Once in a while**   **Every day**
   Discuss your response:

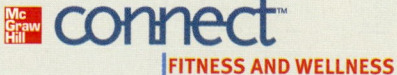
http://connect.mcgraw-hill.com

2. Do you think you could benefit by improving your ability to relax? Explain.

3. (A) List the six relaxation techniques discussed in this chapter. (B) Name one of the relaxation techniques (in Strategy #2) that you would enjoy practicing on a regular basis:

   (A) The six are:

   (B) Describe it:

   Why did you select this one?

4. **Practice the relaxation technique you identified (in #3 above) for 20 minutes a day for 3 days.**

5. Describe your experience with this technique (i.e., how you felt before and after; what time of day you practiced it; where, etc.).

6. Is this a skill you can use to manage the stress in your daily life? Explain.

7. Would you like to try any of the other techniques?

   If so, which one(s) and why?

8. Do you think relaxation is important in the management of your stress?

   Why or why not?

LAB Activity 10-2

Becoming Stress-Resistant and Hardy

List two ways your "hardiness" can be strengthened in each of the following categories:

1. *Control:* Do you feel you are in control of your life? List at least two ways you can gain more control. (Example: Plot out the courses you need to complete your degree, semester by semester; or plan to be early to every appointment and class for a month.)

2. *Commitment (task involvement):* How can you build commitment in your life (e.g., family, friends, studies, work, community)? List at least two ways to improve commitment. (Example: I will complete my nursing degree by age 20.)

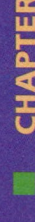

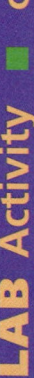

http://connect.mcgraw-hill.com

357

3. *Challenge:* Do you see changes and/or setbacks as challenges instead of stumbling blocks? Give at least two recent examples or list two strategies you can use in the future. (Example: So I didn't do well on this anatomy pop quiz. . . . Now I know that I need to study daily, go for tutoring, and/or go to study sessions for this course.)

4. *Choices in lifestyle:* How healthy is your current lifestyle? List at least two improvements you can make in your lifestyle. (Example: I will get at least 8 hours of sleep every night for 2 weeks.)

5. *Connectedness:* Do you have anyone you can count on for emotional support? Do you feel *connected* with at least one other person or group? Do you have close friends and family members? List at least two ways to improve connectedness. (Example: Twice a week I will either e-mail, telephone, or write a note to a friend to keep in touch with friends I rarely get to see.)

LAB Activity 10-3

Measuring Your Stress and Coping Skills

This is a four-part test. The first three parts are designed to give you an indication of how vulnerable you might be to certain types of stress and make you aware of how they might affect you. The last part of the test will provide you with information on how to cope with stressful situations.

Part I

Choose the most appropriate answer for each of the 10 questions.

	a. Almost always true	b. Usually true	c. Usually false	d. Almost always false
1. When I can't do something "my way," I simply adjust and do it the easiest way.	—	—	—	—
2. I get upset when someone in front of me drives slowly.	—	—	—	—
3. It bothers me when my plans are dependent on others.	—	—	—	—
4. Whenever possible, I tend to avoid large crowds.	—	—	—	—
5. I am uncomfortable when I have to stand in long lines.	—	—	—	—
6. Arguments upset me.	—	—	—	—
7. When my plans don't flow smoothly, I become anxious.	—	—	—	—
8. I require a lot of space in which to live and work.	—	—	—	—
9. When I am busy at a task, I hate to be disturbed.	—	—	—	—
10. I believe that it is worth waiting for all good things.	—	—	—	—
Total score				—

SCORING

For 1 and 10, a = 1, b = 2, c = 3, d = 4; for 2 through 9, a = 4, b = 3, c = 2, d = 1. This test measures your vulnerability to stress from being frustrated or inhibited. Scores in excess of 25 seem to suggest some vulnerability to this source of stress.

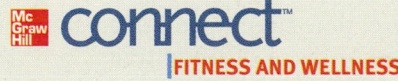

http://connect.mcgraw-hill.com

Part II

Check or mark the letter of the response that best answers the following 10 questions. How often do you

	a. Almost always	b. Very often	c. Seldom	d. Never
1. Find yourself with insufficient time to complete your work?	—	—	—	—
2. Find yourself becoming confused and unable to think clearly because too many things are happening at once?	—	—	—	—
3. Wish you had help to get everything done?	—	—	—	—
4. Feel your boss/professor expects too much from you?	—	—	—	—
5. Feel your family and friends expect too much from you?	—	—	—	—
6. Find your work/school infringing on your leisure hours?	—	—	—	—
7. Find yourself doing extra work to set an example to those around you?	—	—	—	—
8. Find yourself doing extra work to impress your superiors?	—	—	—	—
9. Have to skip a meal so that you can get work completed?	—	—	—	—
10. Feel that you have too much responsibility?	—	—	—	—
Total score				—

SCORING

a = 4, b = 3, c = 2, d = 1. This test measures your vulnerability to overload, that is, to having too much to do. Scores in excess of 25 seem to indicate vulnerability to this source of stress.

Part III

Answer each question as it is generally true for you.

	a. Almost always true	b. Usually true	c. Usually false	d. Almost always false
1. I hate to wait in lines.	—	—	—	—
2. I often find myself racing against the clock to save time.	—	—	—	—
3. I become upset if I think something is taking too long.	—	—	—	—
4. When under pressure I tend to lose my temper.	—	—	—	—
5. My friends tell me that I tend to get irritated easily.	—	—	—	—
6. I seldom like to do anything unless I can make it competitive.	—	—	—	—
7. When something must be done, I'm the first to begin even though the details may still need to be worked out.	—	—	—	—
8. When I make a mistake, it is usually because I've rushed into something without giving it enough thought and planning.	—	—	—	—
9. Whenever possible, I try to do two things at once, such as eating while working or planning while driving or bathing.	—	—	—	—
10. When I go on a vacation, I usually take along some work to do just in case I get a chance.	—	—	—	—
Total score				—

SCORING

a = 4, b = 3, c = 2, d = 1. This test measures the presence of compulsive, time-urgent, and excessively aggressive behavioral traits. Scores in excess of 25 suggest the presence of one or more of these traits.

Part IV

This scale was created largely on the basis of results compiled by clinicians and researchers who sought to identify how individuals cope with stress. This scale is an educational tool, not a clinical instrument. Its purpose therefore is to inform you of ways in which you can effectively and healthfully cope with the stress in your life. At the same time, through a point system, it will give you some indication of the relative desirability of the coping strategies you are using. Simply follow the instructions given for each of the 14 items listed. Total your points when you have completed all the items.

1. Give yourself 10 points if you feel that you have a supportive family.   _____

2. Give yourself 10 points if you actively pursue a hobby.   _____

3. Give yourself 10 points if you belong to a social or activity group (other than your family)   _____
    that meets at least once a month.

4. Give yourself 15 points if you are within 5 pounds of your ideal body weight, considering   _____
    your height and bone structure.

5. Give yourself 15 points if you practice some form of deep relaxation at least three times a   _____
    week. Deep relaxation exercises include meditation, imagery, and yoga.

6. Give yourself 5 points for each time you exercise 30 minutes or longer during an average week.   _____

7. Give yourself 5 points for each day you consume at least five servings of fruits and vegetables   _____
    during an average week.

8. Give yourself 5 points if you do something just for yourself that you really enjoy during an   _____
    average week.

9. Give yourself 10 points if you have a place in your home/department/residence hall you   _____
    can go to in order to relax and/or be alone.

10. Give yourself 10 points if you practice time management techniques in your daily life.   _____

11. Subtract 10 points for each pack of cigarettes you smoke during an average day.   _____

12. Subtract 5 points for each evening during an average week that you take any form of   _____
    medication or chemical (including alcohol) to help you sleep.

13. Subtract 10 points for each day during an average week that you consume any form of   _____
    medication or chemical substance (including alcohol) to reduce your anxiety or calm you down.

14. Subtract 5 points for each evening during an average week that you bring work home—work   _____
    that was meant to be done at your place of employment. (This does not include schoolwork.)

Total score _____

SCORING

Now calculate your total score. A perfect score would be 115 points or more. If you scored in the range of 50 to 60, you probably have an adequate collection of coping strategies for most common sources of stress. You should keep in mind, however, that the higher your score, the greater your ability to cope with stress in an effective and healthful manner.

SOURCE: Daniel Girdano/George S. Everly, *Controlling Stress and Tension: A Holistic Approach,* © 1979, pp. 62, 67, 108–109. Adapted by permission of Prentice-Hall, Englewood Cliffs, New Jersey.

CHAPTER 11

Eating for Wellness

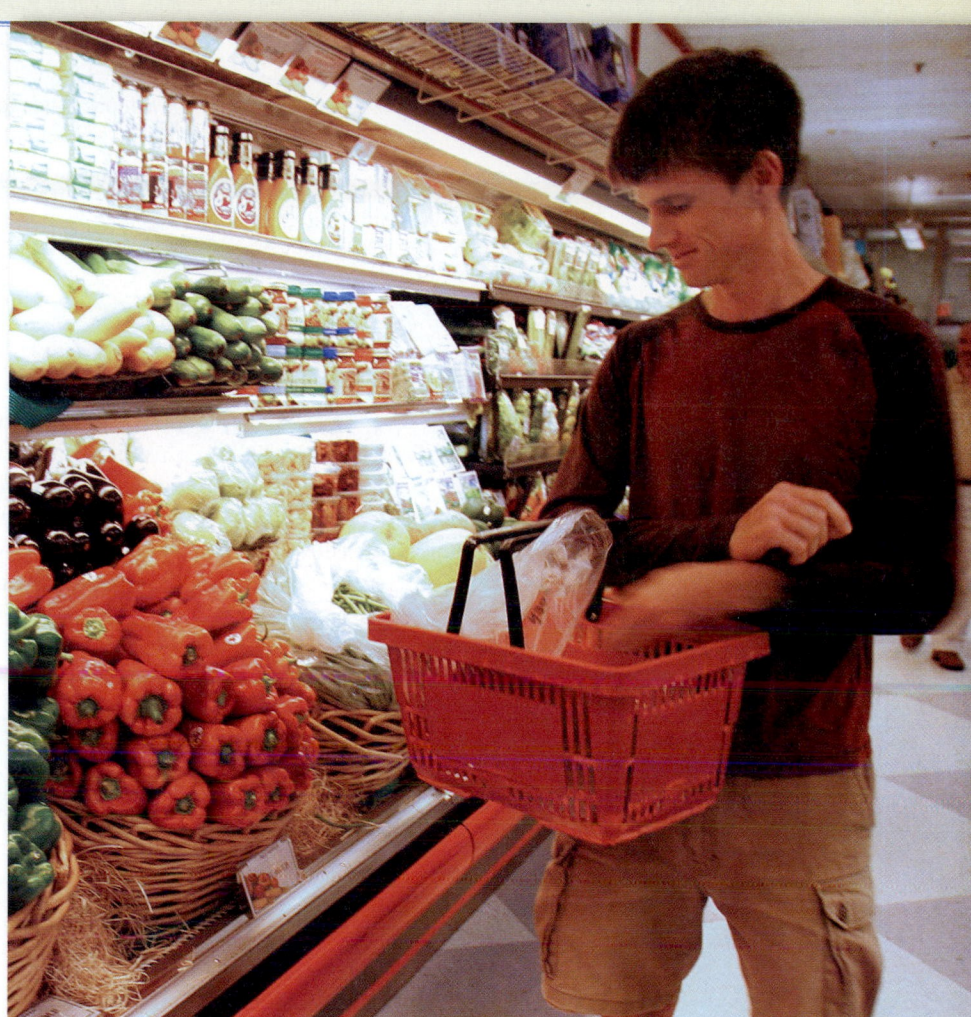

STUDY QUESTIONS

You will have successfully mastered this chapter if you can answer the following questions:

1. What is the purpose of the federal government's *Dietary Guidelines?*
2. Can you list the six major nutrients and describe their main function in the body?
3. What are the percentages of calories recommended in the diet for carbohydrates, proteins, and fats?
4. Can you identify the health benefits of fiber and list good food sources of fiber?
5. What are the differences between complex and simple carbohydrates?
6. Can you identify the correct descriptions of cholesterol, saturated fats, monounsaturated fats, polyunsaturated fats, and trans fats?
7. Are you able to calculate fat gram allowances for specific daily calorie intakes?
8. Can you describe the role phytochemicals and antioxidants play in nutritional health, and identify foods high in these compounds?
9. What are four preventive factors relating to osteoporosis?
10. Can you describe the USDA's MyPyramid food guidance system?
11. Can you give 10 specific examples of small changes that you can incorporate into daily food selections and preparations that could make a significant change in your nutritional wellness?
12. Are you able to look at a food label and identify the largest ingredient; calculate the percentage of calories that come from fat, carbohydrate, and protein; and identify the sources of fat?
13. Can you identify three ways to eat nutritiously in a fast-food restaurant?

You will find the answers as you read this chapter.

“ *Let your food be your medicine, and your medicine be your food.* ”
—Hippocrates

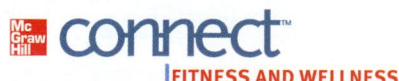

connect™
|FITNESS AND WELLNESS

http://connect.mcgraw-hill.com

n a world where so many things seem out of our hands, taking control of what you eat is an important personal way to affect how you feel. Fundamental knowledge about nutrition can make a tremendous contribution to your level of wellness. It can help you make food choices that will enhance your health and vitality. This knowledge can also help you decipher social influences and messages related to eating. This is another step toward assuming self-responsibility for your well-being and health. Learning about nutrition can be exciting. Eating is a daily activity, so you have many opportunities to affect your wellness in a positive way. Food not only sustains life but also has a clear link to *disease prevention*. Scientists are finding that certain foods (especially fruits, vegetables, and whole grains) are directly associated with the prevention of cardiovascular disease and certain cancers—the leading causes of death in our country. We are fortunate to live in a country where food is plentiful; we have wide and varied choices. We must learn, however, to make healthy choices because we live in an environment where unhealthy choices are also plentiful.

We tend to see diet as affecting only the physical dimension of wellness. Food, however, can be associated with all the dimensions. Much of our social life revolves around food. Providing food is an important sign of caring. Eating and being fed are intimately connected with our deepest feelings. Table 11-1 gives examples of how food relates to all seven dimensions of wellness. Perhaps you can think of other connections.

After reading this chapter, you should be able to make responsible food choices in your pursuit of high-level wellness. You have heard it before, but it is remarkably true: You are what you eat.

◆ CHANGING TIMES

In the agricultural lifestyle of the past, most people grew and prepared their food. Foods were fresh and simple. Early Americans consumed much greater amounts of fresh fruits, vegetables, and grains and lesser amounts of salt, fats, refined sugars, and processed foods than Americans do today. Today's fast-paced technological society has contributed to drastic changes in the way we eat. While juggling careers, child care, social and professional obligations, education, and recreation, we often skip meals, eat on the run, or throw meals together quickly. More than ever, meals are consumed behind the wheel

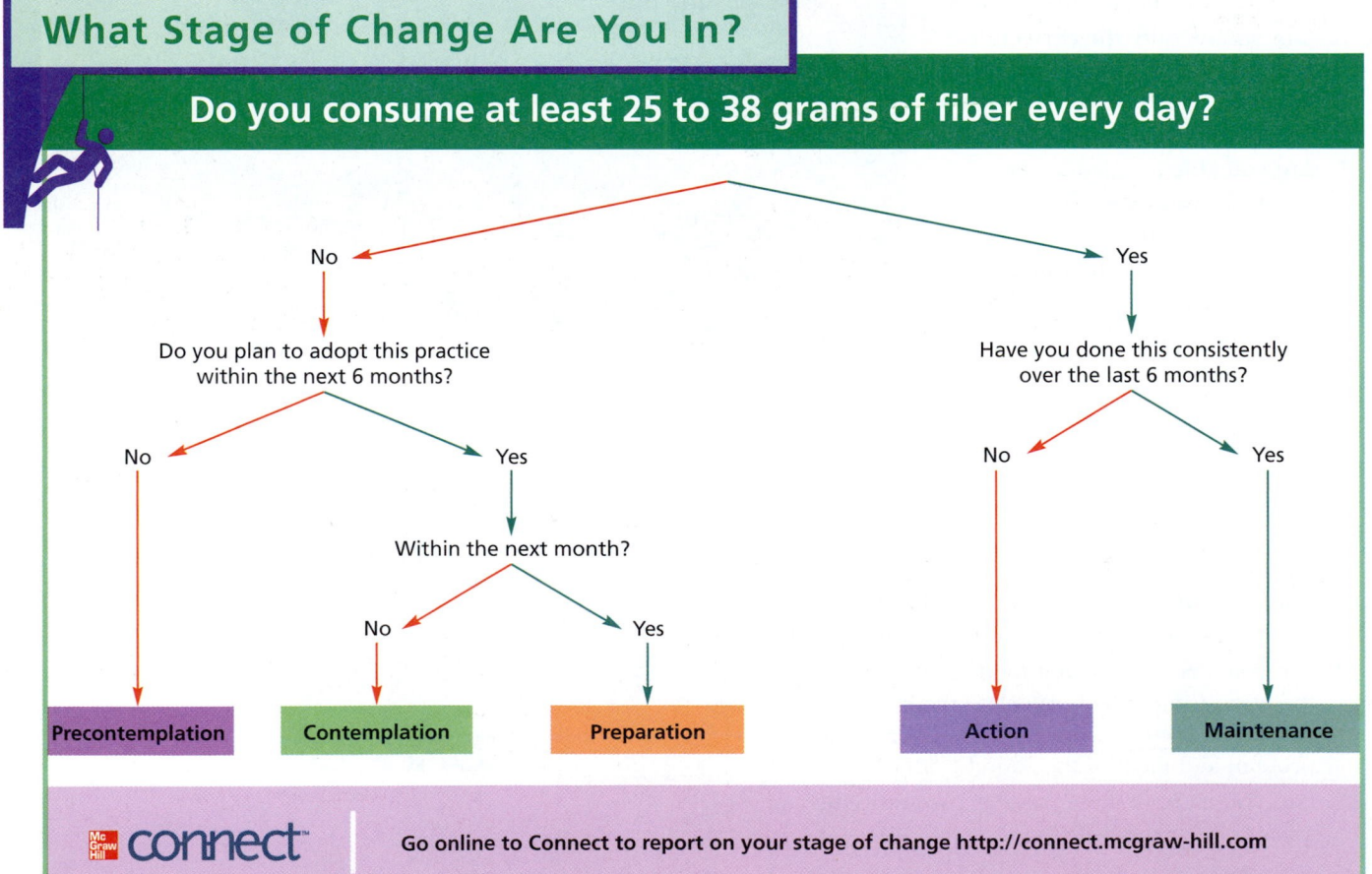

What Stage of Change Are You In?

Do you consume at least 25 to 38 grams of fiber every day?

No → Do you plan to adopt this practice within the next 6 months?

Yes → Have you done this consistently over the last 6 months?

No → Precontemplation

Yes → Within the next month?
- No → Contemplation
- Yes → Preparation

No → Action

Yes → Maintenance

Go online to Connect to report on your stage of change http://connect.mcgraw-hill.com

TABLE 11-1   *Food Is Associated with Every Dimension of Wellness*

Dimension	How Food Is Associated
Physical	Food is required for physiological nourishment, genetic growth, and survival.
Emotional	Food is often used as a reward, to please, to soothe feelings, and to ease depression or stress.
Social	Food is often at the heart of social events, celebrations, and family interactions.
Intellectual	Having a healthy relationship with food requires informed consumerism, knowledge about the science of nutrition and sound dietary principles, and the ability to read food labels.
Spiritual	Food is used in rituals and is part of spiritual cleansing. Abstention from eating or from eating particular foods often accompanies spiritual growth experiences. Food is used in many death rituals throughout the world.
Environmental	The human need for food demands food and crop quality and protection from contamination, protection of the food chain, and strategies for combating world hunger.
Occupational	Food is often a part of business meetings and social gatherings and breaks at work. Also, the income generated by our occupations determines our food choices. Institutional food preparation is big business. The business of "food" provides a lot of jobs.

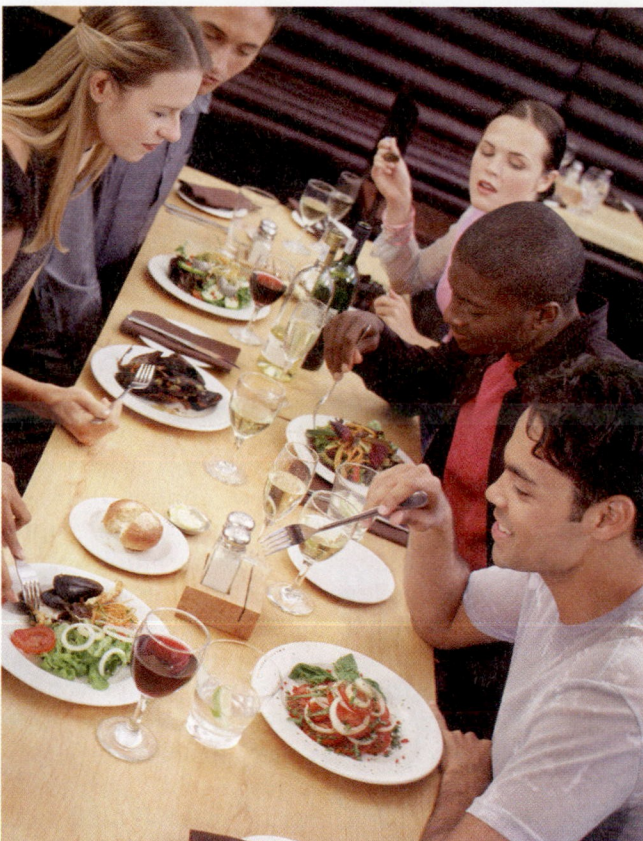

Eating is one of life's pleasures, and the choices we make can have a dramatic impact on our present and future well-being.

of a car, in what food industry experts call "dashboard dining." Most gas stations have become mini-foodmarts. As a result, the food preparers are often fast-food restaurants or manufacturers of frozen, processed, or snack foods. In the last 30 years our daily intake of food has dramatically shifted from at-home sit-down meals to snacking, with chips, sodas, hamburgers, french fries, and pizza leading the charge. Food preparation and advertising are big business, and the purpose of mass advertising is to sell products, not necessarily to enhance our nutrition. Supermarket shelves are lined with packaged food products bearing little resemblance to the original farm product. Most are highly processed, often stripped of key nutrients. The result is a new form of malnutrition—not caused by a lack of food, but by our eating too much of the wrong foods. As we have progressed from eating wheat and berries to consuming tacos and french fries, the incidence of heart disease, obesity, type 2 diabetes, and cancer has increased. This progression has also cost us our vitality and seriously compromised our immune systems.

Poor diet is said to contribute to 4 of the top 10 leading causes of death in our country. Studies repeatedly identify five shortfalls in our eating habits:

1. Too few fruits and vegetables
2. Too little fiber
3. Too much saturated fat
4. Too many refined sugars
5. Too much food overall (i.e., calories)

Take a serious look at these habits. How many of them relate to you?

Public awareness of the importance of nutrition continues to grow with the help of all types of media and educational materials. Many people admit that their diet is poor but believe that healthful eating is too complicated or that they'll have to give up their favorite foods. According to government statistics, only 10 percent of the population can be classified as having a "good" diet. Television contributes to the problem by presenting mixed messages about diet and nutrition. We are exposed to hundreds of commercials for sugary, high-fat snacks, often featuring enchanting music, jingles, and appealing characters. In prime-time programming, nutrition is anything but balanced—grabbing a snack is the norm.

In college, you are faced with the perhaps new responsibility of buying and preparing your meals or making daily cafeteria or food court selections. Unfortunately, many college students are unaware of or apathetic about the implications of poor dietary habits on the future development of chronic diseases. Many young adults have been raised in the "happy meal" world of snacks and fast foods. Studies show that a majority of college students do not consume the recommended five to nine servings of fruits and vegetables a day, do not eat enough fiber, and eat too much saturated fat. In one study, 59 percent of students said they know their diet is worse since they started college. Unfortunately, many of these habits often continue into later adulthood. Since maintaining healthy dietary habits is essential to lifelong wellness, the college years can be a crucial time to develop healthy practices.

Healthful eating *can* be enjoyable and is easier to sustain than most people think. The underlying approach for dietary choices should be to combine basic nutrition *knowledge* with positive and practical *action*. Small, gradual changes can collectively produce substantial and sustainable dietary improvements. The purpose of this chapter is to help you begin adopting these improvements.

Dietary Guidelines

As a service to the American people, the U.S. Department of Health and Human Services publishes the *Dietary Guidelines*. Revised every 5 years, these guidelines help answer the question, "What should we eat to stay healthy and prevent chronic diseases?" The guidelines reflect the newest research on diet and health relationships, with the purpose of giving *practical* suggestions on how to make healthy diet adjustments. It is impossible to specify the perfect diet for every individual. However, these guidelines point out positive directions for everyday food selections that can help you maintain optimal health. The guidelines also recognize the value of physical activity and the importance of weight management. The *2010 Dietary Guidelines* can be found at www.dietaryguidelines.gov. The Institute of Medicine (the scientific advisory group to

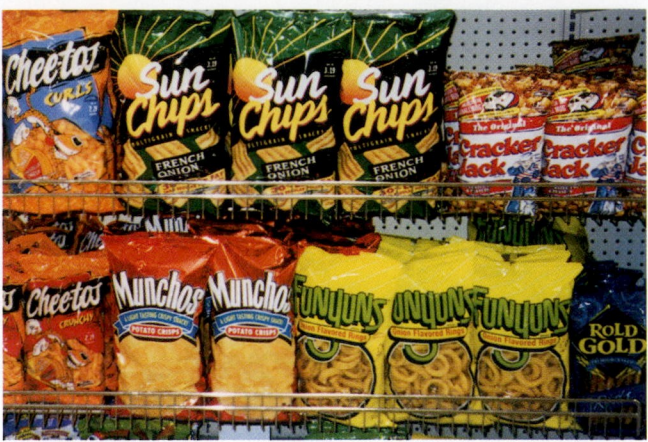

We have become a "snack food nation," consuming over $50 billion in snacks each year.

the National Academy of Sciences) has identified specific recommendations for us to follow as well (see Table 11-2).

Nutritionists concur that simply issuing guidelines and disseminating recommendations is obviously insufficient to produce change in most people's eating behavior. As in making most lifestyle changes, you need

✓ *Knowledge* (to identify problem diet behaviors and how to improve them)
✓ *Motivation* (to make healthy changes)
✓ *A supportive environment* (to maintain changes in restaurants, supermarkets, worksite and school food services, nutrition labeling, and nutrition education in the schools)

For many, the dietary guidelines seem difficult to attain in this fast-food, grab-it-and-go world. Rather than viewing them as impossible and unrealistic, let them inspire you, not intimidate you! Remember that these are *goals*. Look for ways to shift from wherever you are now, up a few notches. For example, add an extra serving of fruit to your day;

TABLE 11-2	Daily Diet Recommendations
Cholesterol	Less than 300 mg
Carbohydrate	45–65% of calories
Protein	10–35% of calories
Total fat	20–35% of calories
Saturated fats/trans fats	Less than 10% of calories
Fiber	25 grams for women, 38 grams for men

SOURCE: National Academy of Sciences, Institute of Medicine. "Dietary Reference Intakes for Energy, Carbohydrates, Fiber, Fat, Fatty Acids, Cholesterol, Protein and Amino Acids." 2005.

try a new vegetable at dinner; substitute low-fat yogurt for cake as a dessert; walk an extra 15 minutes after classes.

So, where are the trans fats? What constitutes a "serving" of vegetables? What qualifies as a "whole" grain? Where are the "good" fats? How do you eat out healthfully? These questions are addressed in the following sections, and we give practical suggestions for making daily food choices that will enhance your nutritional wellness and get you closer to reaching the *Dietary Guidelines*.

◆ NUTRITION BASICS

Your body is a priceless machine that needs fuel. This fuel should be comprised of six major nutrients: carbohydrates, proteins, fats, vitamins, minerals, and water. These nutrients fulfill three main functions in the body:

1. Provide energy
2. Build and repair body tissues
3. Regulate body processes

Only the carbohydrates, fats, and proteins contribute energy or calories (kcal) to your diet. To function at optimal efficiency, you need a balance of all six of the essential nutrient groups.

Carbohydrates

Carbohydrates are the major source of energy for the body. They are the body's preferred form of energy. In fact, some cells, like brain cells, use only carbohydrates for fuel. Carbohydrates are stored in the liver and in muscles in the form of **glycogen.** It is recommended that our daily caloric intake be 45 to 65 percent carbohydrate. Carbohydrates have mistakenly earned the reputation of being fattening even though they provide only 4 calories per gram. Of course, any calories consumed in excess of body energy needs are stored as body fat. If we analyze the two types of carbohydrates, this unearned reputation can be understood. Carbohydrates, with the exception of milk sugar, come from plants. The two types are **simple carbohydrates** (sugars) and **complex carbohydrates** (starches).

SIMPLE CARBOHYDRATES (SUGARS)

When you see the suffix *-ose* as an ingredient on a package label (as in sucrose, fructose, dextrose, and maltose) or see *corn sweetener, corn syrup, molasses, sorbitol, brown rice syrup, evaporated cane syrup, juice concentrate, agave nectar,* or *honey,* think *sugar.* The presence of these refined and processed sugars in our diet accounts for carbohydrates' "fattening" reputation. Instead of consuming the natural simple sugars found in fruits and milk, we consume too much of these hidden processed sugars.

The major sources of added sugars in Americans' diets are

1. Soft drinks
2. Cakes, cookies, pies
3. Fruit drinks, such as fruit punch, sports drinks, and lemonade
4. Dairy desserts, such as ice cream
5. Candy

These refined sugars have been extracted from their natural sources and have little nutritional value other than the calories they contain—hence the name "empty calories." Excess sugar throws the entire body chemistry off balance, causes fatigue, and dramatically weakens the immune system for up to 6 hours after ingestion. Simple carbohydrate foods can cause extreme surges in blood sugar levels, which also increase insulin release. This can increase appetite and the risk of excess fat storage. Some new studies even link excess sugar to heart disease. Even if you profess not to eat sweets, you probably consume more sugar than you realize because it is hidden in so many processed foods, such as pasta sauces, ketchup, barbecue sauce, cereals, energy bars, and juice drinks. Proclaimed "low-fat" foods are often loaded with added sugars. A 12-ounce cola drink contains 10 teaspoons of sugar. A fast-food chocolate shake has 13 teaspoons of sugar. Jell-O is 83 percent sugar. Check your breakfast cereal. Some are nothing more than "candy" fortified with vitamins. Look for cereals with no more than 3 or 4 grams of added sugar per serving.

It is recommended that a woman get no more than 100 calories (about 25 grams or 6 teaspoons) a day from added sugars, and a man no more than 150 calories (about 38 grams or 9 teaspoons). For reference, consuming a 20-ounce Gatorade and a package of cheese crackers would be about 40 grams of added sugars. A 16-ounce Snapple Lemon Tea with 2 Hostess Twinkies is 78 grams of added sugars. Seeing these numbers, it is evident that many people are on a daily sugar high! How many grams of sugar do you consume each day? Keep a log of your sugar grams for a few days to see your numbers.

COMPLEX CARBOHYDRATES (STARCHES)

The starches are potatoes, rice, whole grains, beans, and vegetables. These foods are low in calories. They are nutritionally dense, a rich source of vitamins and minerals that provides a steady amount of energy for many hours. What *is* fattening are the

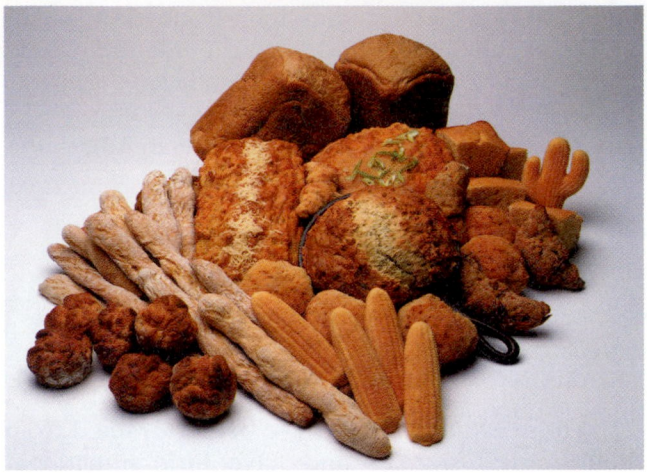

Whole-grain products are better for your health than those made with refined flours.

calorie-rich additives we often add to these foods (butter, sour cream, jams, gravies, sauces). Complex carbohydrates should constitute 35 to 55 percent of our total caloric intake, while simple sugars should be limited to only 10 percent. Carbohydrates supply many vital nutrients, such as vitamins, minerals, and water. In addition, they supply an important nonnutrient: dietary fiber. **Fiber** is the part of plant food that is not digested in the small intestine, where most other foods are digested and absorbed into the bloodstream. Fiber is not a single substance but a large group of widely different compounds with varied effects on the body. Formerly called *roughage* or *bulk,* fiber was once thought of primarily as a filler—it takes up room, leaving less space for high-fat, high-calorie items. That is still one of fiber's potential benefits. Even though fiber does not provide vitamins or minerals, foods that are high in fiber are often rich in vitamins and minerals. Researchers recognize that fiber plays a role in reducing the risk of heart disease, diabetes, obesity, and some types of cancer. Look at the Top 10 "Reasons to Eat More Fiber." As you can see, a high-fiber diet contributes to health in a multitude of ways. There are two types of fiber: insoluble and soluble. Both play important roles in your nutritional health.

Insoluble fiber comes from the cell walls of plants and is not digested by the body. Insoluble fiber absorbs water as it passes through the digestive tract, increasing fecal bulk. It quickens the passage of food through the system, helping to prevent constipation. This type of fiber may act as a deterrent to digestive disorders, including possibly cancers of the colon and rectum. Whole-wheat bran is the richest source of insoluble fiber. This valuable bran is lost when whole-wheat flour is refined to produce white flour and wheat flour (used in most

breads, crackers, and cereals). Lentils, skins of fruits and root vegetables, and leafy greens are other good sources of insoluble fiber.

Soluble fiber travels through the digestive tract in a gel-like form, pacing the absorption of carbohydrates. This prevents dramatic shifts in blood sugar levels and can help control diabetes. A diet rich in soluble fiber has also been shown to reduce blood cholesterol levels, especially LDL, thus reducing the risk of cardiovascular diseases. However, this effect occurs primarily when fiber is coupled with a diet low in saturated fats. Oat bran, beans, vegetables, and fruits are rich sources of soluble fiber, though most plant foods contain both types of fiber. Animal foods never contain fiber.

According to the American Cancer Society, approximately one-third of cancer deaths are related to what we eat. Eating between 25 and 38 grams of fiber daily is recommended (about double the amount in the current American diet). Not enough is known

TABLE 11-3   *Fiber in Selected Foods*

Food	Fiber (grams)
Bran cereal (1/2 c.)	10
Beans, lentils, peas (1/2 c.)	6–9
Spaghetti, whole wheat (1 c.)	6
Mini-wheat cereal (1 c.)	5
Chex cereal (1 c.)	5
Cauliflower (1/2 c. cooked)	5
Pear (1 med.)	5
Sweet potato (1 med.)	5
Peas, frozen (1/2 c.)	4.5
Quick oatmeal (1/2 c. dry)	4
Popcorn (6 c.)	4
Potato, baked (1 med.)	4
Brown rice (1/2 c. cooked)	4
Berries (1/2 c.)	4
Pork and beans (1/2 c.)	4
Almonds (1/4 c.)	3.9
Apple (1 med.)	3.5
Whole-wheat bread (1 slice)	3
Broccoli (1/2 c. cooked)	3
Orange (1 med.)	3
Triscuit crackers (7 crackers)	3
Spinach, canned (1/2 c.)	3
Banana (1 med.)	3
Cheerios (1 c.)	2
Corn, canned (1/2 c.)	2
White bread (1 slice)	.6
Iceberg lettuce (1 c.)	.5
Cornflakes (1 c.)	.5

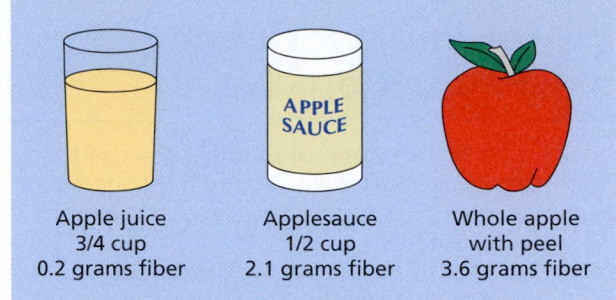

Apple juice
3/4 cup
0.2 grams fiber

Applesauce
1/2 cup
2.1 grams fiber

Whole apple
with peel
3.6 grams fiber

A fiber profile.

houses, whereas refined flours have little nutritional value. Many experts believe that Americans' overconsumption of refined flours is contributing to the explosion of obesity and type 2 diabetes, since these refined products play havoc with our insulin levels. Unfortunately, fiber has been eliminated from most snack and fast foods. Americans average less than one serving a day of whole grains.

The *Dietary Guidelines* encourage the consumption of whole grains. Look for whole-grain breads, bagels, pasta, cereal, crackers, and rice. Even though the outer package of a product may say "multi-grain," "seven-grain," "made with whole grain," or even "wheat," carefully check the ingredient list. Look for the words "whole grain," "whole wheat," "whole oats," "wheat bran," "oat bran," "bulgur," or "oatmeal" as the first ingredient. These are whole grains! Wheat flour, enriched wheat flour,

about how each kind of fiber (soluble and insoluble) works, so there is no set recommended dietary ratio for either type. How much is 30 grams of fiber? If you were to eat 1 cup of bran cereal, ½ cup of carrots, ½ cup of beans, a medium-size apple, and a medium-size pear in 1 day, you would have consumed 30 grams of fiber. Table 11-3 shows the fiber content of some common foods.

For busy students and adults, breakfast is one of the best meals to get a jump start on fiber consumption for the day. Check the labels of various breakfast cereals. Many have 5 or more grams of fiber per serving. Add some fresh fruit and you have a great start toward those 25 to 38 grams.

WHOLE GRAINS VERSUS REFINED FLOURS

Whole grain consists of three parts: bran (outer layer), endosperm (middle layer), and the germ (core). When grains are refined through processing, the bran and germ are removed. This takes away most of the nutrients and fiber. These refined flours are then used to make white bread, rolls, pasta, rice, bread sticks, pizza crusts, crackers, cereals, cookies, pretzels, etc. As a result, not all grains are created equal. Whole-grain products are nutritional power-

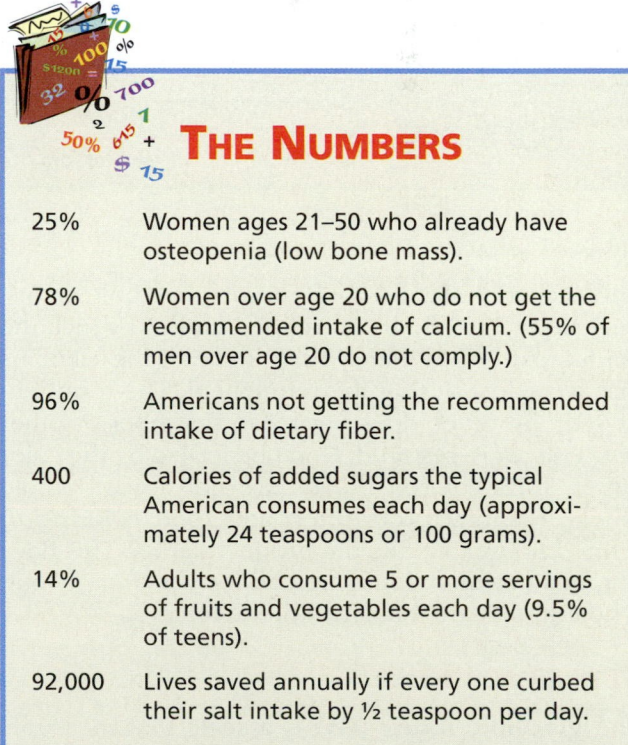

THE NUMBERS

25%	Women ages 21–50 who already have osteopenia (low bone mass).
78%	Women over age 20 who do not get the recommended intake of calcium. (55% of men over age 20 do not comply.)
96%	Americans not getting the recommended intake of dietary fiber.
400	Calories of added sugars the typical American consumes each day (approximately 24 teaspoons or 100 grams).
14%	Adults who consume 5 or more servings of fruits and vegetables each day (9.5% of teens).
92,000	Lives saved annually if every one curbed their salt intake by ½ teaspoon per day.

Tips for Behavior Change for Better Nutrition

Refer to the Stage of Change flowchart on page 364. What is your stage of change after answering the questions and tracing the flowchart?

Refer to Figure 2.2 (p. 36) to see which processes of change are most effective for facilitating your transition from your current stage to the next stage (or *maintaining* your behavior if you are already in the maintenance stage). Here are some behavioral examples for selected processes of change:

- Consciousness-raising: Investigate and make a list of foods that are high in fiber that you would find appetizing.
- Social liberation: Identify the meal services on campus that offer the most high-fiber foods on their menus (e.g., whole grains, fresh fruits, and vegetables).
- Self-liberation: Map out a plan for increasing your fiber consumption (e.g., add berries to bran cereal at breakfast; carry an apple and almonds in backpack for snacking; eat two green vegetables at every dinner).
- Reward: For each week of averaging 25–38 grams of daily fiber, treat yourself to a fruit pastry.
- Environment control: Keep high fiber snack foods available in your room—granola bars, trail mix, popcorn, and so forth.

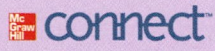 Go online to Connect to complete this activity.
http://connect.mcgraw-hill.com

unbleached flour, and oat flour *are not* whole grains. Enriched wheat flour is a refined grain to which the manufacturer has added back some of the vitamins that were lost during the refinement. The term "enriched," however, does not mean that fiber or other nutrients were restored. Don't be fooled by the color either. Dark-colored breads are not always whole wheat. Manufacturers often add food coloring to refined flours to make the product darker. This does not mean refined flours are bad for you. Simply put, whole grains are a far healthier choice.

GLYCEMIC INDEX

The **glycemic index (GI)** is a scale that measures the extent to which a food affects blood-glucose (sugar) levels. A food that quickly raises blood-glucose levels is said to have a *high*-GI (e.g., white bread and buns). In the long run, a diet with a lot of high-GI foods may cause type 2 diabetes, an increased chance of some cancers, and heart disease. *Low*-GI foods (e.g., brown rice) result in a small rise in blood sugar and can help reduce the chance of type 2 diabetes as well as raise the levels of good HDL cholesterol in some people. Low-GI foods create more of a feeling of fullness. High-GI foods include cornflakes, rice cakes, white potatoes, white-flour bagels, instant white rice, pretzels, Pop-Tarts, doughnuts, and the like. Low-GI foods include sweet potatoes, wholewheat breads, beans, peanuts, bran cereals, apples, yogurt, and the like. For a more comprehensive list of the glycemic index of foods, log on to www.glycemicindex.com or www.nutritiondata.com (look under "topics").

If you have ever felt hungry or felt a sudden drop in blood sugar 1½ hours after eating pancakes, you've experienced the impact of eating a high-GI food. Not all nutrition experts have embraced the glycemic index as a calculator of "good" and "bad" foods. To people who suffer from fluctuations in their blood-sugar levels, however, the glycemic index may be helpful in selecting foods.

Proteins

Hundreds of different kinds of proteins make up the cells of the body. **Protein** is the major substance used to build and repair tissue, maintain chemical balance, and regulate the formation of hormones, antibodies, and enzymes. Protein can also be used as a source of energy, but only if there are not enough carbohydrates or fats available. It is not an efficient source of energy, however. When protein is broken down, the nitrogen part of the protein molecule is left. The kidneys are overworked trying to excrete this excess nitrogen. Also, if your body must rely on protein for energy, the protein is not available for building and repairing tissue—its real function.

Each gram of protein provides 4 calories of energy. We need protein daily, and most of us consume more than enough. The Institute of Medicine recommends that the amount of protein adults eat for good health can be 10–35 percent of total daily calories. Protein needs vary throughout the life cycle due to different growth stages. Growing children need more protein per body weight than adults do. Pregnant or lactating women, competitive athletes, and people over age 55 may need a little extra protein. Persons age 19 and older can approximate their daily protein need in grams by multiplying their weight (in pounds) by 0.36.

Example: 130-lb. person $\times$ 0.36 = 46.8 or 47 grams of protein daily

> To give you an idea of how little food this is, 47 grams of protein would be:
> 4 oz. of meat (a piece roughly the size of your palm)
> 2 cups skim milk

Example: 180-lb. person $\times$ 0.36 = 64.8 or 65 grams of protein daily

> Sixty-five grams of protein could be fulfilled with:
>
> 1 cup oatmeal
> 1½ cups macaroni and cheese
> 1½ cups skim milk
> 1 large bowl of chili with beans

Most Americans meet or exceed the amount of protein needed. (Average consumption is about 100 grams per day.) Excessive protein (especially excessive red meat consumption) has been linked to kidney disease and several cancers (colorectal, breast, prostate, stomach).

Good sources of protein are found in animal and plant foods. Meat, poultry, fish, eggs, and milk products are good sources of animal protein. Many of these sources also contain high amounts of fat and cholesterol, so you are wise to select some plant sources of protein: legumes (beans and peas), whole grains, pastas, rice, and seeds. These plant proteins are also a great source of fiber.

Fats

Fat is the most concentrated form of food energy, providing 9 calories per gram, more than twice the energy provided by carbohydrates and proteins. Fat adds texture and flavor to food. It helps satisfy the appetite because it is digested more slowly. Also known as *lipids,* fats are necessary for growth and healthy skin and for transporting fat-soluble vitamins in the body. Fats are also linked to hormone regulation. Because of their concentrated form, fats are an efficient way to store energy. Like protein, however, fats are not a good *single* source of energy. Fats burned for energy in the absence of carbohydrates produce a toxic waste product called *ketone bodies. Ketosis,* a buildup of poisonous **ketone bodies,** causes fatigue and nausea and overtaxes the kidneys. Extreme cases can cause brain damage. Fat is burned more completely in the presence of carbohydrates, another reason to have a diet high in complex carbohydrates (and to avoid weight-loss diets that promote very low carbohydrate and calorie intake).

An important distinction should be made among the three types of fatty acids. Dietary fats comprise a combination of three forms—saturated,

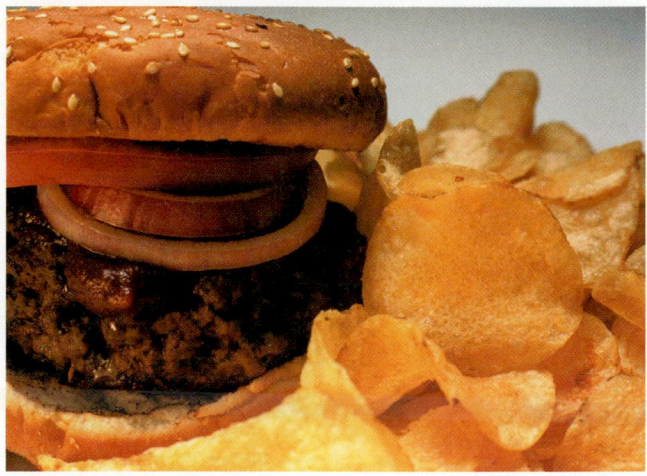

Our love for fats contributes to heart attacks, strokes, and several cancers.

monounsaturated, and polyunsaturated. Even though they are complex mixtures, they are classified simplistically by their overall saturation and chemical structure. Canola oil, for example, is classified primarily as a monounsaturated fat, even though it is also made up partially of polyunsaturated fatty acids. Table 11-4 identifies and compares types of fats according to their primary fatty acid structure.

An easy observation shows that with a few exceptions, **saturated fats** are primarily in foods of animal origin (e.g., red meats, cheese, whole milk, hot dogs, luncheon meats), whereas most vegetable fats are unsaturated. Additionally, all animal fats contain cholesterol. (Vegetable foods have no natural presence of cholesterol.) Diets high in saturated fat have a strong link to heart disease and stroke. They elevate blood cholesterol levels, which in turn can lead to clogged arteries (atherosclerosis). **Polyunsaturated fats** come mostly from plant foods and are a healthier fat to consume. **Monounsaturated fats** also come from plant foods and are healthier choices. When "mono" fats replace saturated fats in the diet, they not only decrease total and LDL cholesterol but also appear to raise HDLs—an added benefit.

Regardless of the types of fats, we need to be more discriminating in our selections. We have a tendency to eat too much total fat, saturated fat, and trans fats. Most nutritionists recommend that our daily calories consist of only 20–35 percent fat, keeping saturated and trans fats under 10 percent of our calories. The excessive fat in our diet is the main reason Americans have so many heart disease deaths. Thirty to 40 percent of cancers in men and 60 percent of cancers in women have been attributed to diet, with excessive saturated and trans fats being prime culprits. The amount and type of dietary fat

TABLE 11-4   Comparison of Fats

		Characteristics	Examples
Limit in the Diet	**Saturated**	Raises total cholesterol. Raises "bad" LDL cholesterol. Increases risk of heart disease. Increases risk of some cancers.	Red meats; poultry skin; coconut and palm oils; butter; cheese; luncheon meats; whole milk; hot dogs; chocolate; bacon; lard
	Trans	Raises total cholesterol. Raises "bad" LDL cholesterol. Lowers "good" HDL cholesterol. Increases risk of heart disease. Increases risk of some cancers.	French fries and other deep-fried foods; many fast foods; stick margarine; shortenings; cookies; crackers; doughnuts; candy; pies and cakes; dips; some boxed foods like ramen noodles
Use Only Small Amounts	**Polyunsaturated**	Lowers total cholesterol. Lowers "bad" LDL cholesterol. May reduce risk of heart disease.	Corn, soybean, safflower, and sunflower oils; tub margarines; mayonnaise; salad dressings
Preferred Choices, But Use in Moderation	**Monounsaturated**	Lowers total cholesterol. Lowers "bad" LDL cholesterol. May raise "good" HDL cholesterol. May reduce risk for heart disease. May reduce risk for some cancers.	Olive, peanut, and canola oils; avocado; olives; most nuts; peanut butter (without added hydrogenated oils)
Preferred Choices	**Omega-3 (considered a special type of polyunsaturated fat)**	Lowers total cholesterol. Lowers risk for heart disease and stroke. Inhibits atherosclerosis and inflammation in blood vessels. May lower blood pressure. Reduces blood clots. Can reduce occurrence of cancerous tumors.	Cold-water fish (salmon, tuna, halibut, mackerel, sardines, herring). Lesser amounts: walnuts; flaxseed and flaxseed oil; green leafy vegetables; canola oil; wheat germ; soybeans

eaten—not the amount of cholesterol consumed—have the greatest impact on the blood cholesterol level. Dietary cholesterol also affects the level of blood cholesterol but to a lesser and more variable extent than does the fat content of the diet.

Monounsaturated fat and polyunsaturated oils are often turned into solid unhealthy saturated fats by a manufacturing process called **hydrogenation.** This technique adds hydrogen atoms to these fats as a way to prolong the shelf life of a product and improve the texture of some foods (e.g., pastries, pie crusts, cookies). Avoid completely and partially hydrogenated oils! Like saturated fats, they elevate the blood cholesterol level. During the process of hydrogenation, some fatty acid molecules become rearranged and convert to a **trans-fatty acid** (sometimes called **trans fats**). Trans fats are linked to coronary artery disease and some cancers. Scientists now believe that trans fats may be more harmful than saturated fats to artery health because they

raise "bad" LDL cholesterol and lower "good" HDL cholesterol in the blood—the worst possible combination! In studies at the Harvard School of Public Health, researchers discovered that persons who consumed the most trans-fatty acids had a 50 percent greater risk for heart attacks than those who consumed the least. Trans fats were also linked to increased waist size—another risk factor for heart disease. Regardless of the number of calories consumed, trans fats appear to affect the body in a specific way to increase this harmful abdominal fat. Foods typically high in trans fats include margarine, crackers, cookies, doughnuts, pies, french fries, chips, cakes, taco shells, frostings, peanut butter, some cereals, and candy. And because foods can still be called "cholesterol-free," implying a certain healthfulness, this is misleading if they contain hydrogenated oils and trans-fatty acids. Because trans-fatty acids are present in so many manufactured foods, the U.S. Food and Drug Administration mandated

that a food's level of trans fats be listed on its label beginning in 2006. The Institute of Medicine has not established a safe or recommended level of trans fat intake. However, people are urged to eat as little as possible. Many manufacturers have already begun eliminating heart-hazardous trans fats from their products as evidenced by the margarines, snacks, and baked goods that advertise on their labels "zero trans fats."

Be a wise consumer and watch out for "hidden" fats in commercially prepared foods. Whereas it is obvious that butter, oils, and the visible fat on meats have a high fat content, the fat in crackers, peanut butter, pastries, dips, sauces, and deep-fried fast foods is less obvious. It is important to be able to decipher food labels and understand where the fats are in our heavily processed food supply. Remember, "completely" or "partially hydrogenated oils" equals trans-fatty acids.

Fat substitutes (such as Olestra and Simplesse) are being used in many commercially prepared foods. These substitutes are made from soybeans or various milk and egg proteins with the purpose of duplicating the taste and texture of fat—without the caloric fat content. Read the food labels for any side effects or contraindications from these substitutes. Some can cause abdominal distress.

Regardless of the source, it is important to moderate your overall fat intake because all fats are high in calories. If a little oil is needed in food preparation, choose small amounts of olive oil or canola oil. Choose fish over red meat. And remember that a small handful of nuts can supply health benefits. Table 11-5 shows you how to figure your daily fat allowance to adhere to recommended fat-calorie guidelines.

With so much emphasis on low-fat eating, some people may try to cut their fat grams to almost zero. Remember that a little dietary fat is necessary for basic metabolic functions, especially for the absorption of fat-soluble vitamins. A minimum of 10 to 20 grams per day should satisfy these requirements.

FISH OILS

Studies of the diets of Eskimos and Asian fishers have revealed interesting information about fats. Their diets provide 40 percent of daily calories from fats. Yet Eskimos are listed among the people with the lowest rates of heart disease in the world. Why? They eat lots of fish, and fish are rich in **omega-3** fatty acids. A diet rich in omega-3 fatty acids inhibits atherosclerosis in coronary arteries and can reduce the blood cholesterol level. Populations in countries that consume high amounts of omega-3 fatty acids from fish have lower incidences of breast, prostate, and colon cancer than people in

TABLE 11-5 — Determining Your Fat Gram Allowance

It is recommended that we consume no more than 35 percent of our daily calories from fat. For better artery health and weight loss, 20 to 30 percent consumption is preferred. If you know your approximate daily caloric intake, it is easy to calculate your desired fat grams.

Example: Terry consumes 2,000 calories per day. He wishes to stay at a 30 percent fat-calorie guideline.

$30\% \times 2,000$ calories = 600 fat calories
600 calories $\div$ 9 (calories per gram of fat) = 66.6 or 67 grams of fat

An easy way to estimate your fat gram limit per day is to divide your ideal weight in half. Keep your number of fat grams per day under this number. (If your ideal weight is 140 lb., your fat gram limit should be 70 g per day.) For people with higher weight this estimate is not quite as accurate (e.g., someone whose ideal weight is 220 lb. should probably *not* be eating 110 grams of fat each day).

Fat Grams per Day for Specific Calorie Intakes and Percentages

Daily Calories	20%	25%	30%	35%
1,200	27g	33g	40g	47g
1,400	31g	39g	47g	54g
1,600	36g	44g	53g	62g
1,800	40g	50g	60g	70g
2,000	44g	56g	67g	78g
2,200	49g	61g	73g	86g
2,500	56g	69g	83g	97g
2,800	62g	78g	93g	109g

countries that consume less omega-3s. More and more research is emerging that suggests a diet high in omega-3 fatty acids assists in preventing memory decline, arthritis, macular degeneration, and autoimmune diseases. The American Heart Association recommends eating fish twice a week to get heart-healthy

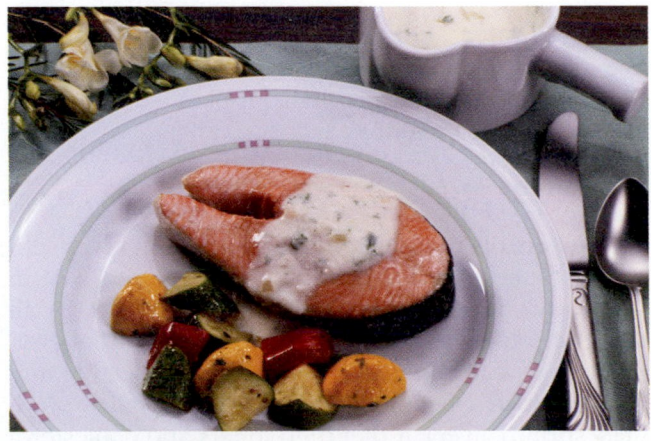

Cold-water fish like salmon are rich in omega-3 fatty acids.

TABLE 11-6 Vitamins and Minerals

Vitamins	Functions	Sources	Daily Value (DV)*	Upper Level (UL)†
Fat Soluble				
A (Retinol)	Promotes growth and repair of body tissues; keeps skin cells moist; builds resistance to infection; promotes bone and tooth development; aids in vision	Green leafy vegetables, yellow fruits and vegetables, eggs, butter, margarine, cheese, milk, liver	5,000 IU‡ or 1,500 mcg	10,000 IU
D	Regulates absorption of calcium and phosphorus; promotes normal growth of bone and teeth	Vitamin D-fortified milk products, fish, eggs, fortified margarines, sunlight (absorbed through the skin)	400 IU	2,000 IU
E (Alpha-tocopherol)	Essential in preventing oxidation of other vitamins and fatty acids; maintains cell structure	Vegetable oil, green and leafy vegetables, whole grains, egg yolks, nuts, wheat germ	30 IU	1,100 IU (synthetic) 1,500 IU (natural)
K (Phylloquinone)	Aids in blood clotting	Cabbage, cauliflower, spinach, green vegetables, liver, cereals	80 mcg	30,000 mcg
Water Soluble				
C (Ascorbic acid)	Builds resistance to infection; aids in tissue repair and healing; involved in tooth and bone formation	Citrus fruits, strawberries, tomatoes, potatoes, melons, broccoli, peppers, cabbage	60 mg	2,000 mg
B_1 (Thiamin)	Needed to convert carbohydrates into energy; promotes normal function of nervous system	Whole grains, fortified grain products, milk, pork, legumes, nuts, meats	1.5 mg	50 mg
B_2 (Riboflavin)	Combines with proteins to make enzymes that affect function of eyes, skin, nervous system, and stomach	Meat, dairy products, whole grains, green leafy vegetables	1.7 mg	200 mg
B_3 (Niacin)	Aids in energy production from fats and carbohydrates	Meat, poultry, fish, liver, nuts, whole grains, legumes	20 mg	35 mg
B_6 (Pyridoxine)	Aids in protein metabolism and red blood cell formation	Whole grains, meat, fish, poultry, legumes, milk, green leafy vegetables	2.0 mg	100 mg
Folic acid (Folacin)	Aids in red blood cell formation; aids in synthesizing genetic material	Meat, poultry, fish, eggs, broccoli, asparagus, legumes	400 mcg	1,000 mcg
B_{12} (Cobalamin)	Aids in function of body cells and nervous system	Animal foods only; meat, poultry, fish, eggs, dairy products	6 mg	3,000 mcg

omega-3 fatty acids. The best omega-3 sources are salmon, mackerel, herring, tuna, and sardines. Omega-3s are also available from plant sources such as flaxseed and walnuts.

CHOLESTEROL

Cholesterol is not a true fat. It is a fatlike waxy substance found in animal tissue. It plays a vital role in the body's functioning. Your liver manufactures all the cholesterol that you physically need. However, most of us consume more cholesterol by eating animal products (meat, egg yolks, cheese, dairy products, shrimp, liver). A diet high in fats and cholesterol

has been linked to atherosclerosis; therefore, you are prudent to limit animal products in your diet. It is recommended that you restrict cholesterol consumption to 300 milligrams per day. (One egg yolk equals approximately 213 mg cholesterol; a hamburger patty or chicken breast has approximately 80 mg.) Remember, vegetable foods contain no cholesterol unless it is added in processing or food preparation.

Vitamins

Vitamins are the organic catalysts necessary to initiate the body's complex metabolic functions. Although these chemical substances are vital to life,

TABLE 11-6   Vitamins and Minerals (continued)

Vitamins	Functions	Sources	Daily Value (DV)*	Upper Level (UL)†
Macrominerals				
Calcium	Aids in bone and tooth formation, aids in use of phosphorus, helps muscle contraction and heart function	Dairy products, green leafy vegetables, broccoli, fish	1,000 mg	2,500 mg
Phosphorus	Aids in metabolism and energy production	Dairy products, eggs, meat, fish, poultry, legumes, whole grains	1,000 mg	4,000 mg
Magnesium	Activates important enzyme reactions	Whole grains, nuts, legumes, green vegetables	400 mg	350 mg from supplements only
Potassium	Regulates body fluids and the transfer of nutrients across cell walls	Citrus fruits, juices, bananas, potatoes, spinach	4,700 mg	None
Sodium	Regulates fluid balance in cells; aids in muscle contraction	Table salt, milk, seafood (abundant in most foods except fruits)	1,500 mg	2,300 mg
Trace				
Iron	Essential for oxygen transport in the blood	Liver, meat, poultry, fish, dried fruit, whole grains, legumes, green vegetables	18 mg	45 mg
Zinc	Aids in metabolism and growth of tissue	Seafood, poultry, eggs, whole grains, vegetables	15 mg	40 mg
Copper	Involved with iron in the formation of red blood cells, affecting overall metabolism	Liver, nuts, shellfish, meat, poultry, vegetables	2 mg	10 mg
Iodine	Forms thyroid hormone	Iodized salt, seafood	150 mcg	1,100 mcg
Selenium	Necessary for normal growth and development, and for use of iodine in thyroid function; has antioxidant properties	Seafood, meat, liver, grains	70 mcg	400 mcg
Chromium	Works with insulin to help the body use blood sugar	Whole grains, bran cereals, meat, poultry, seafood	120 mcg	1,000 mcg

*Daily Value (DV): These levels, also called U.S. Recommended Daily Allowances (USRDAs), appear on food and supplement labels. There is only one DV for everyone over age 4.
†Upper level (UL): These levels are the highest levels that pose no risk. As intake increases above the UL, so does the risk of adverse effects.
‡IU = International Units.

SOURCE: National Academy of Sciences, 2004.

they are required in only minute amounts. Because of our adequate food supply, symptoms of vitamin deficiencies are rare. However, some factors may alter one's requirements (aging, illness, stress, pregnancy, smoking, dieting). Vitamins fall into two categories: fat soluble and water soluble. Vitamins A, D, E, and K are **fat-soluble vitamins,** which means they are transported and stored by the body's fat cells and liver. They are stored in the body for relatively long periods (many months). Vitamin C and the B complexes are **water-soluble vitamins.** They remain in various body tissues for a short time (usually only a few weeks). Excesses are excreted.

Minerals

Minerals are inorganic substances that are critical to many enzyme functions in the body. Two groups

of minerals are necessary to the diet: macrominerals and trace minerals. **Macrominerals** are needed in large doses (more than 100 mg daily). Examples are calcium, phosphorus, magnesium, potassium, and sodium. **Trace minerals** are needed in much smaller amounts. Examples are iron, zinc, copper, iodine, fluoride, and selenium. Table 11-6 lists vitamins and minerals, their functions, good food sources of each, and adult recommendations.

Three minerals deserve special attention: calcium, iron, and sodium.

CALCIUM

Calcium is the body's most abundant mineral and is critical to many body functions. If the calcium supply in the blood is too low, the body withdraws calcium from the bones. This inadequate supply of

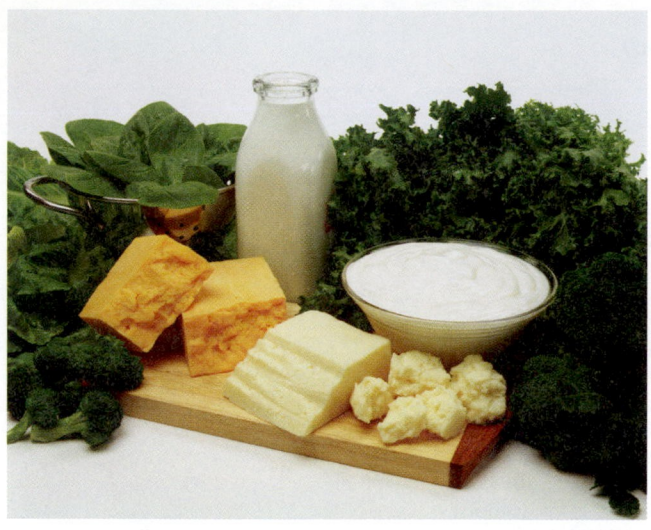

Dairy products are not the only sources of calcium in the diet.

calcium is a major factor contributing to **osteoporosis,** an age-related condition of insufficient bone mass. Healthy bone is living tissue that is continuously being replenished. Most of the adult skeleton is replaced about every 10 years. In osteoporosis, the formation of bone fails to keep pace with lost bone tissue. The result is porous, brittle bones susceptible to fracture. Women are more susceptible to osteoporosis because they have smaller, less dense bones. However, men are also at risk. In fact, one in four men over age 50 will break a bone as a result of osteoporosis.

According to a report from the Surgeon General, roughly 10 million Americans over age 50 have osteoporosis (brittle bones). Another 34 million have **osteopenia**—a bone density that is lower than normal. "The bone health status of Americans appears to be in jeopardy, and left unchecked it is only going to get worse as the population ages," says the surgeon general. By 2020, it is predicted that half of all Americans over age 50 will be at risk for fractures from weakened bones. Osteoporosis is a "silent" condition because many are unaware that their bones are thinning until one breaks. Some bone loss is normal with aging in both males and females. However, osteoporosis is *not* part of normal aging. Therefore, it is vitally important that you build strong bones during young adulthood. Strong bones begin in childhood. With good nutrition and physical activity, bones can remain strong throughout a lifetime. Consumption of adequate dietary calcium from preadolescence through young adulthood is one critical factor in building bone mass. Current calcium consumption is dangerously low. It's estimated that most Americans consume only 500 to 800 milligrams of calcium daily.

Your current habits determine your bone density later in life. Up to about age 25, as calcium is added to the diet, the rate at which bone is replaced is greater than the rate at which it breaks down. By age 25 to 30, you've reached your peak bone mass—the point at which your bones are as dense and strong as they'll ever be. Forty to 60 percent of this peak bone mass is built during the teenage years. By age 40, bone mass begins to decline slowly in both men and women. After menopause, women lose bone mass rapidly due to a drop in the estrogen level. Osteoporosis cannot be cured—it can only be prevented, or its progression delayed. That is why it is critical that teens and young adults take action to build as much bone mass as possible while they are young to slow the rate of bone loss later in life. The number of cases of osteoporosis will continue to skyrocket if today's young adults don't adjust their diets and exercise habits. See Table 11-7 for the recommended calcium intake for various age groups. A negative balance of only 50–100 mg of calcium per day over a long period of time is sufficient to produce osteoporosis.

TABLE 11-7   *Optimal Calcium Requirements (Recommendations of the National Institutes of Health)*

Age	Calcium (mg/day)
1–3	500
4–8	800
9–18	1,300
19–50	1,000
51 and older (men)	1,200
51 and older (women)	1,500

For your information:

1 cup yogurt = 300 mg	1 cup cottage cheese = 150 mg
1 cup milk = 300 mg	1½ oz hard cheese = 350 mg
1 cup cooked broccoli = 90 mg	3 oz sardines = 370 mg
1/2 cup ice cream / frozen yogurt = 100 mg	4 oz tofu = 145 mg
1/2 cup spinach = 100 mg	1 slice whole-wheat bread = 25 mg
8 oz orange juice with calcium = 350 mg	1 packet instant oatmeal = 150 mg
1/3 cup nonfat dry milk = 300 mg	1 cup kale = 180 mg
3/4 cup Total cereal = 1,000 mg	1 Viactiv soft chew = 500 mg

Note: Your body absorbs only 500 mg of calcium at a time, so spread your intake throughout the day.

Food labels list calcium content as "% Daily Value." To convert to milligrams (mg) of calcium add a zero. For example, if one serving has 15% DV for calcium, it has 150 mg.

TOP 10 LIST

Ways to Keep Your Bone "Banks" Filled

1. Eat calcium-rich foods every day—low-fat dairy products, spinach, hard cheeses, broccoli, fish with edible bones (salmon, sardines). Sprinkle nonfat dry milk into casseroles, soups, meat loaf, and sauces.
2. Get regular vigorous exercise. Exercises that create muscular contraction and gravitational pull on the long bones, or create weight-bearing impact are the best (jogging, aerobics, weight training, tennis, jumping rope).
3. Ingesting an adequate amount of vitamin D is essential for bones to absorb calcium. Recent research has found that 1,000–1,500 mg of calcium combined with 1,000 IU of vitamin D not only helps bones but plays an important role in reducing cancer risk.
4. Do not smoke. Smoking reduces the production of estrogen and negatively affects calcium absorption.
5. Avoid excesses of alcohol and sodium. Both increase urinary loss of calcium.
6. Watch your protein intake. Eating excessive protein can cause urinary calcium excretion if calcium and vitamin D intake is low. Because of this, the popular high-protein, low-carbohydrate diets can contribute to dissolution of bone if inadequate amounts of calcium and vitamin D are consumed.
7. Limit consumption of soft drinks. Today's young adults have tripled their consumption of soft drinks and cut their consumption of milk by more than 40 percent, robbing them of bone-building calcium during this critical stage of bone formation. The risk? More bone fractures and a future of osteoporosis.
8. If you have lactose intolerance (trouble digesting dairy products), lactose-free products are available at some stores. Or experiment with dairy foods lowest in lactose: ricotta, mozzarella, Parmesan, American, and cheddar cheeses; tofu; some yogurts; sherbet; 1 percent low-fat cottage cheese.
9. Look for calcium-fortified foods such as orange juice and cereals.
10. Consider a calcium supplement—ideally in the form of calcium citrate, the most readily absorbed form.

Recent studies show that calcium isn't the only factor in creating strong bones. Other dietary and lifestyle habits contribute to bone health. Check out the Top 10 list for "Ways to Keep Your Bone 'Banks' Filled."

IRON

Iron deficiency is a nutritional problem for some people, particularly women, teenagers, and endurance athletes. Due to menstruation, women need to ingest more iron than men do. Iron deficiency may cause chronic fatigue and listlessness. To increase your iron intake, take the following steps:

1. Eat foods rich in iron (lean meats, poultry, fish, fortified cereals and grains, green vegetables, beans, peas, and nuts).
2. Consume iron-rich foods with foods high in vitamin C to triple iron absorption (a hamburger and tomato; cereal and orange juice).
3. Keep consumption of tea and coffee under 3 cups per day (caffeine reduces the absorption of iron).
4. Use cast-iron cookware (iron is absorbed into the food in a form readily assimilated into the body).

Iron supplementation should not be done indiscriminately. Prolonged consumption of large amounts can cause a disturbance in iron metabolism for some people, contributing to atherosclerosis and heart attacks. This excessive iron buildup is more prevalent in men than in women, because women lose blood through menstruation each month. Individuals concerned about their iron level should consult a physician.

SODIUM

Many people can reduce their chances of developing high blood pressure by consuming less salt. The American Heart Association and the National Academy of Sciences recommend no more than 1,500 milligrams of sodium per day for healthy adults. (One teaspoon of table salt contains 2,400 milligrams of sodium.) Most Americans consume much more than that daily, some up to 10,000 milligrams! We consume sodium most commonly in the form of table salt and in the processed foods we eat. Even if you never salt your food, 90 percent of processed foods contain sodium—even milk does. In this way, sodium becomes "hidden" in our diet. Boxed rice dishes, pizza, soups, frozen dinners, luncheon meats, and many snacks are loaded with salt. Sodium is also present in other popular condiments, such as monosodium glutamate (MSG), meat tenderizer, ketchup, salsa, soy sauce, mustard, barbecue sauce, and salad dressings. It is even present in many medications— antacids, for instance. Fast-food restaurants are "salt mines." Eating a breakfast biscuit with egg and sausage adds up to 1,200 mg of sodium. Excess sodium consumption has been one factor linked to hypertension in some sodium-sensitive individuals. Excesses of sodium also increase calcium loss in urine, which is detrimental to bone density. Excess salt in the diet has also been linked to stomach cancer. Therefore, be conscious of your sodium intake and try to keep it within the recommended range.

Water

Water is often called the forgotten nutrient. However, it is *the most important* nutrient because it serves as the medium in which the other nutrients are transported. Almost all the body's metabolic reactions occur in this medium. Water also helps rid the body of wastes, aids in metabolizing stored fat, and helps control body temperature. Water composes approximately two-thirds of your body weight. Your exact percentage of water weight varies depending on your body composition. Lean tissue contains more water than does fat tissue. Lean muscle tissue is about 73 percent water; fat tissue is only 20 percent water. Being dehydrated can result in feelings of fatigue, stress, headaches, constipation, and hunger. You should drink before you feel thirsty, because thirst is a sign that you're already dehydrated. One's water needs vary, dependent on body size, activity level, and climate.

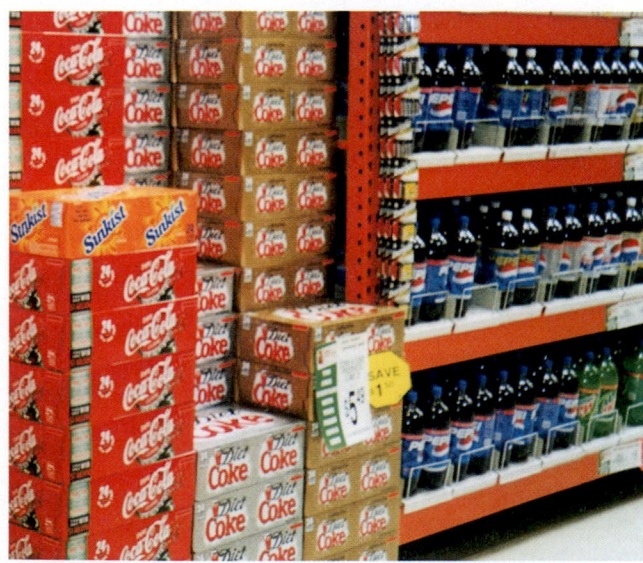

The average teenager consumes three cans of carbonated soft drinks every day. Twice as much soda as milk is consumed today; 20 years ago the reverse was true. The result? Fat teens and brittle bones.

Drinking water is important, but also remember that water is a component of many foods (apples, lettuce, melons, potatoes, soups, tomatoes, fruit juices, etc.). Caffeinated beverages such as coffee, tea, and colas have a slight diuretic effect but also count. Alcohol, however, dehydrates you because your body uses up water to metabolize it. Are you getting enough water? If so, your urine is clear, almost colorless. (See Chapter 7 for more information on water consumption.)

◆ PHYTOCHEMICALS AND ANTIOXIDANTS: DISEASE FIGHTERS

Research is exploding in a new area of dietary study: examining the power of specific food components to ward off chronic diseases. These food components, known as **phytochemicals** (meaning "plant chemicals"), are present in foods such as fruits, vegetables, grains, legumes, and seeds. Phytochemicals are also in garlic, licorice, soy, and green tea. Phytochemicals have been associated with the prevention and treatment of at least four of the leading causes of death in the United States: cancer, cardiovascular diseases, diabetes, and hypertension.

There are hundreds of helpful phytochemicals. These plant pigments and enzymes interact with hormone receptors, suppress malignant changes in cells, enhance immune function, and reduce cholesterol levels. Excitement is building in this new area of nutrition research as scientists continue to uncover the relationship between these plant chemicals and disease prevention. Phytochemicals, with peculiar names such as carotenoids, pectins, lignins, flavonoids, indoles, lycopene, quercetin, and lutein, translate into a cornucopia of fruits and vegetables. Eating a wide variety of colorful fruits and vegetables gives you a full range of these powerful internal bodyguards that help fight off everything from cataracts to cancer to arthritis.

One particular group of phytochemicals, called **phytoestrogens** (plant estrogens), have a structure similar to that of the body's own hormones. Found particularly in soy products (soy milk, soy nuts, tofu, etc.), they may reduce the long-term harmful effects of the body's own hormones, commonly associated with breast, colon, and prostate cancers. Soy products may also be linked to the reduction of blood cholesterol.

Phytochemicals, along with certain vitamins (A, C, E, and selenium), are known as antioxidants. **Antioxidants** are compounds that come to the aid of every cell in the body that faces an ongoing barrage of damage because of the normal aging and oxygenation process (living and breathing), environmental pollution, chemicals and pesticides, additives in processed foods, stress, and sun radiation. As aging and exposure occur, our body creates **free radicals,** singlet oxygen molecules that damage our cells and tissues. This free radical assault on the body contributes to a number of chronic diseases, such as atherosclerosis, arthritis, cancer, cataracts, heart disease, stroke, and an array of other degenerative diseases. Antioxidants (phytochemicals, carotenoids, vitamins C and E, etc.) that are plentiful in fruits and vegetables neutralize these free radical chemical reactions, thereby suppressing cell deterioration and slowing the aging process.

Realizing the power of these substances, Americans need to take action by eating a wide variety of fruits and vegetables—at least five servings per day. Check out these antioxidant "all-stars":

✓ apples	✓ grapes
✓ broccoli	✓ strawberries
✓ green and red peppers	✓ kale
✓ cantaloupe	✓ brussels sprouts
✓ spinach	✓ blueberries
✓ carrots	✓ sweet potatoes
✓ tomatoes	✓ cabbage
✓ raspberries	✓ raisins
✓ onions	✓ oranges

How many of these have you eaten in the last 3 days? Remember, an apple a day may indeed keep the doctor away! Use the Top 10 list to learn ways to add more fruit and vegetables to your day.

TOP 10 LIST

Answers to "How Am I Supposed to Eat All Those Fruits and Vegetables?"

To further promote healthy eating, the National Cancer Institute initiated a national campaign encouraging all Americans to eat five to nine servings of fruits and vegetables every day. Contrary to what most people say, with some planning it is surprisingly easy to do. Here are some suggestions for adding produce to your life:

1. Start your day with a glass of 100 percent fruit juice (not fruit "drink"). Six ounces is a serving.
2. Top your cereal or pancakes with sliced bananas, berries, apples, or raisins.
3. Create a veggie omelette, pizza, pita sandwich, or burrito.
4. Iceberg lettuce is the least nutritious of vegetable greens. Try romaine, spinach, red leaf, chicory—add other veggies.
5. Add chopped fruits to yogurt or pudding and as an ice cream topping; make a fruit smoothie using skim milk and fruit.
6. Add tomatoes, carrots, zucchini, peppers, spinach, or broccoli to pasta and rice salads and pasta sauces. Frozen or canned veggies work fine.
7. Top baked potatoes with assorted cooked veggies or salsa.
8. Fortify stews, soups, and casseroles with extra veggies (e.g., add broccoli, peppers, or peas to your standard macaroni and cheese).
9. Replace chips with raw veggies for dipping.
10. Keep dried fruits, raw veggies, and fresh fruits available for quick snacks.

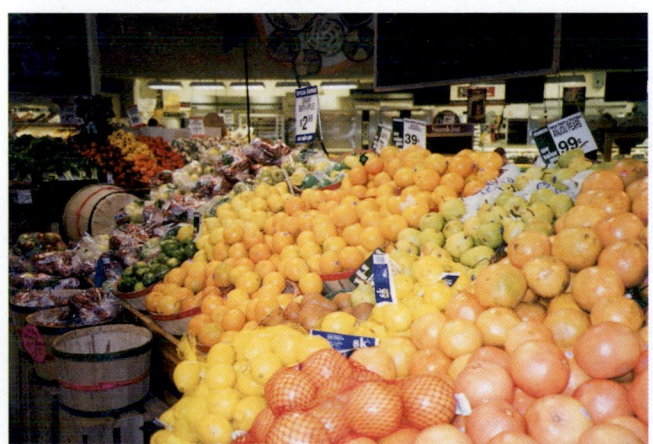
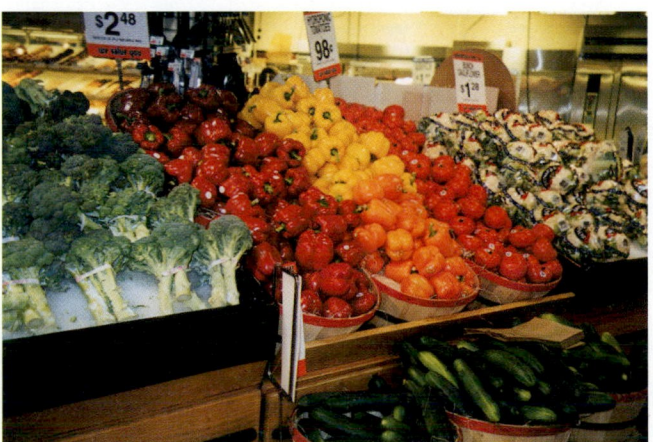

Fruits and vegetables are true "disease fighters." Yet a majority of adults admit to eating only one or two servings per day.

Nutritional Supplements

Are vitamin supplements necessary? Vitamins do not contain energy or calories. Therefore, extra vitamins will not provide more energy or power. Eating a variety of foods is a preferred way to maintain an adequate intake of vitamins, minerals, fiber, and other nutrients. However, with today's lifestyle, most people are not consuming a varied and balanced diet. Manufacturers' processing and preserving, food irradiation and chemical pollution, nutrient-depleted soil, and shipping and storage practices have significantly reduced the nutritional value of foods. Other lifestyle factors, such as smoking, consuming alcohol, stress, and using drugs such as aspirin and oral contraceptives, may increase the need for vitamin or mineral supplementation. Most medical authorities have been reluctant to recommend supplements on a broad scale for healthy people who eat healthy diets. After all, the benefits from food are more complex than merely delivering so many milligrams of this or that nutrient. However, the accumulation of research in recent years has shown that extra amounts of certain vitamins (especially the antioxidants) may play a significant role in preventing chronic diseases such as heart disease and cancer. Also, because most Americans aren't eating enough fruits, vegetables, and whole grains, supplements of vitamin B_{12}, vitamin D, folic acid, vitamin E, and calcium are most common. And frankly, some of these nutrients are hard to get in sufficent quantities from food alone. Anyone with irregular diet patterns, those on a weight-reduction regimen, pregnant or lactating women, strict vegetarians, and elderly people should consider a nutritional supplement or multivitamin. This could offer some nutritional insurance.

In fact, the *Journal of the American Medical Association* issued a report based on more than 30 years of scientific review that recommends a daily multivitamin for most adults. This statement is a startling reversal of the medical community's past denial of the need for dietary supplements. However, it is also important to realize that not all supplements are created equal. Not only are people taking vitamin and mineral supplements, but herbs, enzymes, amino acids, human growth hormones, energy and sexual enhancers, and diet pills are flying off drugstore shelves. In the United States supplements are not considered "drugs," thereby escaping the scrutiny of the U.S. Food and Drug Administration (FDA). However, a 2003 ruling by the FDA forces manufacturers to label their products accurately to ensure that what's written on the label is what's actually contained in the product. In the past, approximately 15 percent of supplements contained either too much or too little of the stated ingredients or contained contaminants. Companies are also now prohibited from making disease claims in their advertising or on their labels, such as "cures cancer" and "lowers cholesterol." More regulations are pending in Congress because illnesses and deaths have occurred as a result of people misusing supplements. Remember that dietary supplements are not a substitute for a healthy diet. Nutrient and nutrient–food interactions are so complex that merely relying on pills to fill in all the gaps would be a mistake. Therefore, consider the following suggestions if you choose to take a supplement:

1. Look for the seal from the United States Pharmacopoeia (USP) that sets safety and purity standards.
2. Buy from an established company rather than from a late-night infomercial provider.
3. Check the label for a company Web site or telephone number. Does the company have a Current Good Manufacturing Practices (CGMP) certification and/or a National Nutrition Foods Association (NNFA) rating?
4. Educate yourself about the supplements you take (see Internet Resources at the end of this chapter).
5. Talk to your physician, because some supplements may interact with the prescription medicines you are taking.

◆ THE WELL-BALANCED DIET

Eating healthy is exciting. Nutritious eating does not doom you to "nutrition martyrdom"—eating flavorless foods, counting grams, or passing up favorite desserts. Eating right means having a wide variety of foods, some in moderation, throughout

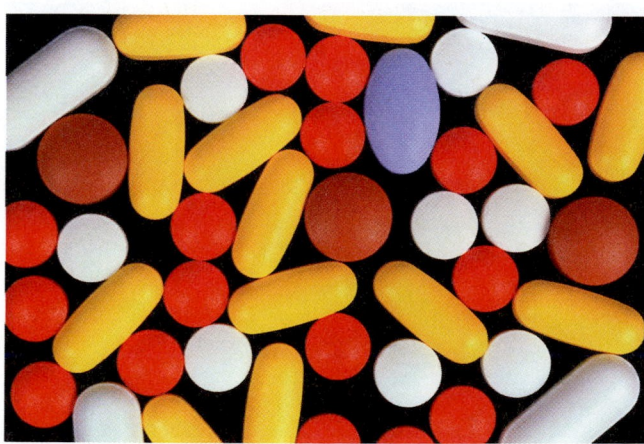

Taking supplements cannot replace a balanced diet but can fill some specific nutritional gaps for some people.

the week. There are no "forbidden" or "bad" foods—only bad eating habits. If you have a high-fat snack one day, make sure to balance it with low-fat foods at other meals. Eating should remain one of life's pleasures. Americans are fortunate to have food choices that are varied, plentiful, and safe to eat. Nutritionists often refer to three words when attempting to simplify the principles of good nutrition: *variety, moderation,* and *balance.* Do you eat the same thing for breakfast every day? For lunch? For snacks? Despite our access to diverse foods, we have a tendency to consume relatively few types of foods and often become locked into standard meals that often are culturally influenced. Why not have rice, chili, or yogurt for breakfast rather than eggs, bacon, and doughnuts?

USDA's MyPyramid

In 2005, the U.S. Department of Agriculture (USDA) introduced a new food guidance system. Called My-Pyramid, the graphic replaces the old food guide pyramid. The multicolored stripes that run from the bottom of the pyramid up to its apex represent the spectrum of food choices, with the width of each stripe approximating the quantity of food each of us should consume from each group (e.g., the green "vegetables" stripe is much wider than the purple "meat & beans" stripe). By showing a person climbing the steps at the side of the new pyramid, physical activity is emphasized as an essential link with healthy eating as key components of healthy living. MyPyramid is actually 12 different pyramids. It was designed to be personalized, based on varying ages, genders, and activity levels.

The Web site, www.MyPyramid.gov, allows you to enter your personal data and then view your customized pyramid. Figure 11-1 shows the USDA MyPyramid with a few example guidelines—based on 2,000-, 2,400-, and 2,800-calorie diets. In viewing the pyramid, pay attention to the recommended serving sizes. For an example, a single restaurant serving of pasta may actually be 5 ounces of grains (2½ cups)! And, if it is made of refined flour, it does not count as a "whole" grain. MyPyramid.gov has many interactive tools to help you plan your diet—lists of foods in each striped category, tracking worksheets, specific serving size guidelines, and more. Visit MyPyramid.gov to learn more about your personalized eating plan. Lab Activity 11-1 allows you to explore your pyramid in depth.

MyPyramid is not meant to be a rigid prescription but a general guide for eating a variety of foods. Fats and sugars are sometimes added to grains, fruits, and vegetables (with sauces, toppings, and preparation methods), making them less healthy choices. For example, having a buttery alfredo sauce on pasta is not as healthy as having a tomato-rich marinara sauce. In the dairy group, a glass of skim milk would be healthier than a milk shake. For a fruit, apple pie has more fat and calories than an apple. Also remember that there are "good" fats such as omega-3s and that whole-wheat grains are healthier than white flour grains. Thus, it is up to you to make wise choices within each food group.

As you evaluate your diet, realize that most people underestimate the size of their food portions. Since excess in portions lead to weight gain, learn to train your eye to estimate what a cup, an ounce, or a tablespoon is. You will find helpful tips on how to quickly estimate your portions in Chapter 12.

DASH Eating Plan

Because high blood pressure affects nearly one in three American adults, the National Heart, Lung, and Blood Institute has developed an eating plan that is a slight modification of MyPyramid. Called DASH (Dietary Approaches to Stop Hypertension), this eating plan has received accolades from the medical community for its effectiveness in lowering blood pressure. Since individuals with *normal* blood pressure at age 55 have a 90 percent lifetime risk of developing hypertension, the DASH plan should be considered seriously by everyone. DASH is based on the following principles:

- ✓ Reduction of overall fat, saturated fat, and cholesterol
- ✓ Reduction of sweets and added sugars
- ✓ Increased fruits, vegetables, and low-fat dairy foods
- ✓ Increased fiber by including whole grains
- ✓ Restriction of sodium
- ✓ Increased magnesium, potassium, and calcium (which help the body excrete excess salt)

Check out Table 11-8, which describes the DASH eating plan. Everyone could benefit by adopting many of the DASH guidelines.

Mediterranean Diet

There has been increasing interest in the health benefits of eating a Mediterranean-style diet, but there is no one, typical "Mediterranean diet." At least 16 countries border the Mediterranean Sea, and diets vary among these countries based on culture, ethnic background, and agricultural production. Nevertheless, the Mediterranean-style diet is typically high in fruits, vegetables, whole grains, beans, nuts, and seeds. Olive oil is an important source of fat. Fish and poultry are eaten rather than red meat, processed meats, dairy, or eggs. Red wine is consumed in moderation.

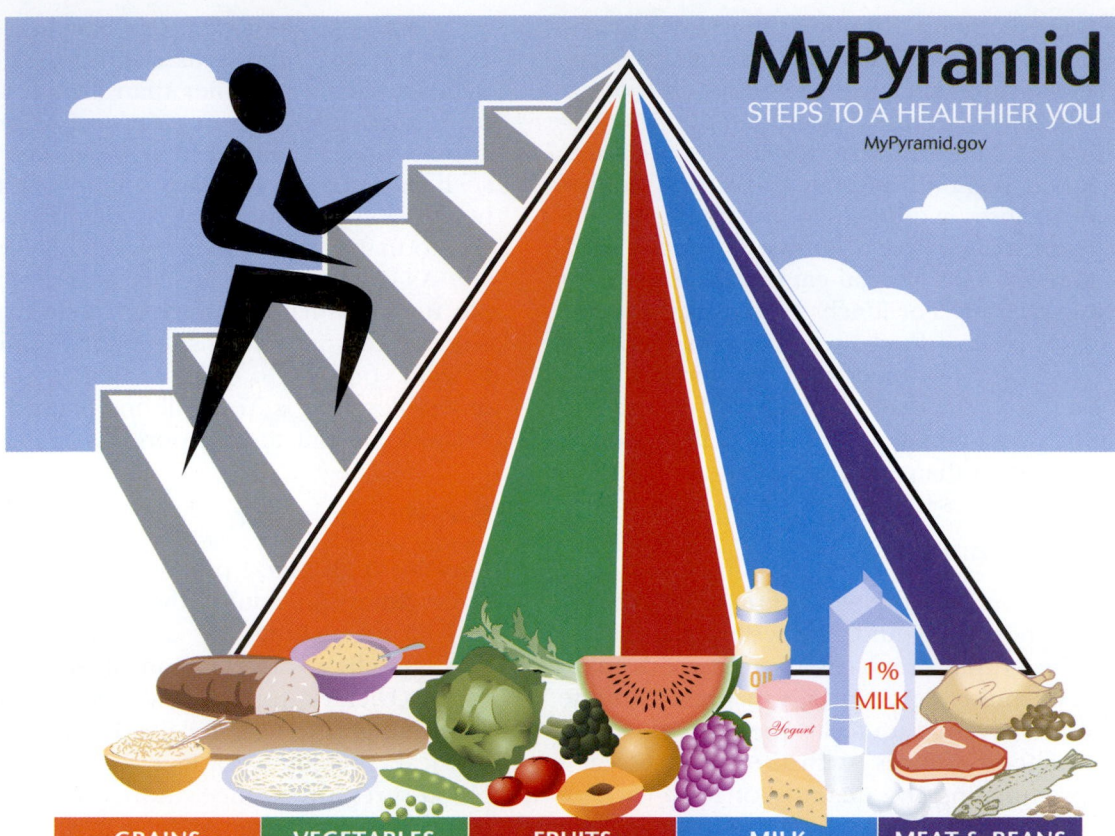

GRAINS	VEGETABLES	FRUITS	MILK	MEAT & BEANS
Make at least *half* your grains "whole."	Eat a variety of vegetables: dark green; orange; beans, peas, and lentils.	Choose fresh, frozen, canned, or dried fruits rather than fruit juices.	Choose fat-free or low-fat milk, yogurt, and cottage cheese. Choose lower-fat cheeses.	Choose lean meat, poultry, or fish—baked, broiled, or grilled.
1 oz. is equivalent to: 1 slice bread; 1 c. dry cereal; ½ c. cooked rice, cereal, or pasta; ½ bagel, English muffin, or bun; 1 4½" pankcake; 3 c. popcorn; 1 6" tortilla; 1 small muffin	A ½ c. equivalent is: ½ c. raw or cooked vegetables; 1 c. raw leafy vegetables; ½ c. vegetable juice	A ½ c. equivalent is: 1 small whole fruit; ½ c. canned, frozen or fresh fruit; ½ c. 100% fruit juice; ¼ c. dried fruit	1 c. is equivalent to: 1 c. milk or yogurt; 1½ oz. hard cheese; 1½ c. ice cream; 2 c. cottage cheese; ⅓ c. shredded cheese	1 oz. is equivalent to: 1 oz. cooked meat; 1T. peanut butter; ¼ cup dry peas, beans or lentils; 1 egg; ½ oz. nuts
2,000 calorie diet = 6 oz. daily	2½ c. daily	2 c. daily	3 c. daily	5½ oz. daily
2,400 calorie diet = 8 oz. daily	3 c. daily	2 c. daily	3 c. daily	6½ oz. daily
2,800 calorie diet = 10 oz. daily	3½ c. daily	2½ c. daily	3 c. daily	7 oz. daily

Oils:

The USDA recommendation that corresponds to the thin, yellow stripe is that "most of your fat sources come from fish, nuts, and vegetable oils" and that you "limit solid fats like butter, stick margarine, shortening and lard."

Physical activity:

Find your balance between food and physical activity

- Be sure to stay within your daily calorie needs.
- Be physically active for at least 30 minutes most days of the week.
- About 60 minutes a day of physical activity may be needed to prevent weight gain.
- For sustaining weight loss, at least 60 to 90 minutes a day of physical activity may be required.
- Children and teenagers should be physically active for 60 minutes every day, or most days.

FIGURE 11-1 The USDA MyPyramid. Specific pyramids for 12 different caloric levels are available at www.MyPyramid.gov.

SOURCE: U.S. Department of Agriculture, Center for Nutrition Policy and Promotion, 2009. www.mypyramid.gov

TABLE 11-8   *The DASH Eating Plan*

The DASH eating plan is based on 2,000 calories a day. The number of daily servings in a food group may vary from those listed, depending on your caloric needs. Use this chart to help you plan your menus, or take it with you when you go to the store.

Food Group	Daily Servings (except as noted)	Serving Sizes	Examples and Notes	Significance of Each Food Group to the DASH Eating Plan
Grains and grain products	7–8	1 slice bread 1 oz dry cereal* 1/2 cup cooked rice, pasta, or cereal	Whole-wheat bread, English muffin, pita bread, bagel, cereals, grits, oatmeal, crackers, unsalted pretzels and popcorn	Major sources of energy and fiber
Vegetables	4–5	1 cup raw leafy vegetable 1/2 cup cooked vegetable 6 oz vegetable juice	Tomatoes, potatoes, carrots, green peas, squash, broccoli, turnip greens, collards, kale, spinach, artichokes, green beans, lima beans, sweet potatoes	Rich sources of potassium, magnesium, and fiber
Fruits	4–5	6 oz fruit juice 1 medium fruit 1/4 cup dried fruit 1/2 cup fresh, frozen, or canned fruit	Apricots, bananas, dates, grapes, oranges, orange juice, grapefruit, grapefruit juice, mangoes, melons, peaches, pineapples, prunes, raisins, strawberries, tangerines	Important sources of potassium, magnesium, and fiber
Low-fat or fat-free dairy foods	2–3	8 oz milk 1 cup yogurt 1½ oz cheese	Fat-free (skim) or low-fat (1%) milk, fat-free or low-fat buttermilk, fat-free or low-fat regular or frozen yogurt, low-fat and fat-free cheese	Major sources of calcium and protein
Meats, poultry, and fish	2 or less	3 oz cooked meats, poultry, or fish	Select only lean; trim away visible fats; broil, roast, or boil instead of frying; remove skin from poultry	Rich sources of protein and magnesium
Nuts, seeds, and dry beans	4–5 per week	1/3 cup or 1½ oz nuts 2 Tbsp or 1/2 oz seeds 1/2 cup cooked dry beans, or peas	Almonds, filberts, mixed nuts, peanuts, walnuts, sunflower seeds, kidney beans, lentils	Rich sources of energy, magnesium, potassium, protein, and fiber
Fats and oils†	2–3	1 tsp soft margarine 1 Tbsp low-fat mayonnaise 2 Tbsp light salad dressing 1 tsp vegetable oil	Soft margarine, low-fat mayonnaise, light salad dressing, vegetable oil (such as olive, corn, canola, or safflower)	DASH has 27 percent of calories as fat, including fat in or added to foods
Sweets	5 per week	1 Tbsp sugar 1 Tbsp jelly or jam 1/2 oz jelly beans 8 oz lemonade	Maple syrup, sugar, jelly, jam, fruit-flavored gelatin, jelly, beans hard candy, fruit punch, sorbet, ices	Sweets should be low in fat

*Equals 1/2 to 1¼ cups, depending on cereal type. Check the product's Nutrition Facts label.
†Fat content changes serving counts for fats and oils. For example, 1 Tbsp of regular salad dressing equals 1 serving; 1 Tbsp of a low-fat dressing equals 1/2 serving; 1 Tbsp of a fat-free dressing equals 0 servings.

SOURCE: U.S. Department of Health and Human Services. National Heart, Lung, and Blood Institute.

Studies have shown that this diet dramatically reduces the risk of death from both cardiovascular disease and cancer. The Mediterranean-style diet also has been shown to protect against cognitive decline and dementia in older individuals. Since there is convincing evidence that red meat and processed meats like bacon, sausage, ham, salami, and hot dogs contribute to the development of colorectal, pancreatic, stomach, and prostate cancer, following a Mediterranean-style diet gives you a good chance of avoiding the common chronic diseases that afflict many Americans.

Making Positive Changes

All this information about nutrition can seem confusing and sometimes appear contradictory; for example, how do you consume enough meat for iron yet reduce saturated fat? Eggs are a good source of protein, but how do you make sure daily cholesterol milligrams don't exceed 300? You certainly hear enough about what *not* to eat. We believe in a positive approach to a wellness lifestyle, and Table 11-9 gives many general tips to help you eat more nutritiously in today's fast-paced world. These suggestions are ways to incorporate the dietary guidelines into sensible and simple practices. Significant improvements in your nutritional health can be accomplished with *simple* changes. For example, using Prochaska's transtheoretical model for behavior change (see Chapter 2), participants in a research study were successful in lowering and maintaining their dietary fat intake to below 30 percent of their calories by using five specific action-based techniques:

1. Switching to low-fat or nonfat cheeses and dairy products
2. Eating whole-grain breads, rolls, pancakes, and muffins without butter or margarine
3. Eating a variety of fruits and veggies with every meal and as snacks
4. Using low-cal or nonfat salad dressings
5. Taking the skin off chicken

You may want to go back and review Prochaska's behavior change theory to help identify your current stage of change in regard to some of your dietary practices. Look at the specific behavior change strategies that could help you make a healthy dietary change. See Table 11-10 for one example.

TABLE 11-9	***Twenty Tips for Nutritional Wellness***

1. Use fresh, unprocessed foods whenever possible.
2. Remove the skin from poultry (the source of most of the saturated fat).
3. Eat low-fat dairy products.
4. Eat fish twice a week (baked or broiled, *not* fried or breaded).
5. Instead of focusing a meal on a meat, use a small amount of meat (diced, shaved, chopped, sliced) to mix in with vegetables and rice or pasta.
6. Steam, bake, broil, or roast foods, using a cooking rack to allow fat to drain from the food.
7. Select salad oils, cooking oils, and margarines made with unsaturated fats. Soft, tub margarines with liquid oil listed as the first ingredient are good choices.
8. Use a nonstick vegetable oil spray or a small amount of olive oil when sautéing.
9. Use deli luncheon meats such as shaved chicken breast and turkey instead of high-fat bologna, salami, beef, or hot dogs.
10. Use applesauce in place of the oil in brownie, cake, and quick-bread recipes.
11. Use plain low-fat yogurt as a substitute for sour cream in dips and on baked potatoes. Fat-free sour cream and cream cheese are also available. Evaporated skim milk can substitute for cream in recipes.
12. Use lettuce leaves as "wraps" rather than breads.
13. Use ground turkey or soy-based crumbles in casseroles, chili, spaghetti sauce, tacos, and skillet dinners that normally require ground beef.
14. When making scrambled eggs, separate the eggs, eliminating half the yolks. If a recipe calls for one egg, substitute two egg whites to reduce the cholesterol.
15. Decrease at least by half the margarine or butter called for in preparing packaged rice and pasta mixes (with minimal effect on taste).
16. Take advantage of nonfat chips, dips, snacks, cereals, cookies, and crackers that are appearing on grocery shelves almost daily. (Remember, however, that "no fat" doesn't necessarily mean "no calories.")
17. Try canned fruit with natural juices as a tasty topping for pancakes and french toast, rather than butter and syrup.
18. Top pizzas, baked potatoes, and stuffed burritos with broccoli, mushrooms, zucchini, peppers, salsa, or onions rather than meats.
19. Try powdered "nonbutter" sprinkles or "butterlike" sprays as toppings for vegetables.
20. Use breads and cereals that list 100 percent whole wheat or "whole grain" as the first ingredient.

TABLE 11-10 Tips for Behavior Change: Eating Five to Nine Servings of Fruits/Vegetables Every Day

Stages of Change: In What Stage are You?

1. Precontemplation: "I don't like fruits and vegetables, and I'm in good health. So why would I want to eat them?"
2. Contemplation: "I realize fruits and vegetables have a lot of nutritional value and could probably cut my risk of future chronic diseases."
3. Preparation: "I've been spending more time in the produce section of the grocery store, learning more about different fruits. I have even started buying and trying some new kinds."
4. Action: "I have been eating five servings every day for about 2 months."
5. Maintenance: "I eat at least seven servings (sometimes more!) every day and have done so for over 6 months. I can't imagine not eating them every day!"

Processes of Change

After identifying your current stage, try using some of the following selected processes and behavior strategies appropriate for your particular stage to facilitate your transition into the next stage (refer to Figure 2-2).

- Consciousness-raising: Read about health benefits of eating fruits and vegetables.
- Social liberation: Investigate new fruits and vegetables at the grocery and try new recipes.
- Self-reevaluation: Write down pros and cons of making this major dietary change.
- Self-liberation: Map out a plan (e.g., drink a glass of juice and slice a banana onto cereal at breakfast; carry an apple in backpack for a snack; have a green vegetable at dinner every night; snack on grapes, carrot sticks, or other fruits/veggies while studying).
- Reward: Treat yourself to a rich fruit dessert once a week (cobbler, pie, etc.).
- Environment control: Have plenty of fruits/vegetables available in room/apartment.

People eat food, not numbers. So rather than focusing on constant measuring, counting, and weighing, dietary change should involve practical changes that can become lifetime habits. It is not advisable or possible to do a complete overhaul of your diet. It is easier, and usually more lasting, to make small and gradual changes. Realize that no one is perfect or eats perfectly all the time. You do have choices, though. If nothing else, try to select foods high in **nutrient density.** Nutrient-dense foods provide substantial nutrients (vitamins, minerals, phytochemicals, fiber, etc.) with relatively few calories, fat, and sugar. Examples of nutrient-dense foods are fruits, vegetables, legumes, and whole grains. These foods allow you to meet your nutritional needs without overconsuming calories. They fill you up (as opposed to "empty

calorie foods" like pastries, chips, sodas, and alcohol, which are high in calories and lack many nutrients).

A good way to assess your nutritional habits is to record everything you eat for 3 to 7 days in a log. By observing types and quantities of food consumed, you can best judge if your diet is nutritionally sound. Keeping a food log can help you set goals for making positive dietary changes. (There is a sample Food Log form in the Lab Activities section at the end of this chapter.) You may prefer to use one of the many computer programs, Web sites, or the tools that accompany www.MyPyramid.gov for dietary assessment. At the end of this chapter are helpful websites with links to nutritive values of foods, even fast foods. It may be tedious to keep records for several days, but this experience creates an awareness of food choices and quantities as well as of where improvements can be made.

Nutrition Labeling

Now that you understand the basics of nutrition, how do you find out the nutritional content of the foods you are eating? You do this by reading labels. Read about what you are eating. Part of self-responsibility is becoming a nutrition-wise consumer. The federal government regulates food labeling and requires processed and packaged foods to have uniform labels. This uniformity can help consumers make healthy choices. Study the sample label in Figure 11-2 to learn how to read a label.

When reading labels remember these points:

1. Check serving size. If not careful, you may eat two to three servings if the stated serving size is skimpy.
2. Watch for hidden sugars added to a product: syrup, sucrose, molasses, corn sweetener, dextrose, maltose, honey, and so on.

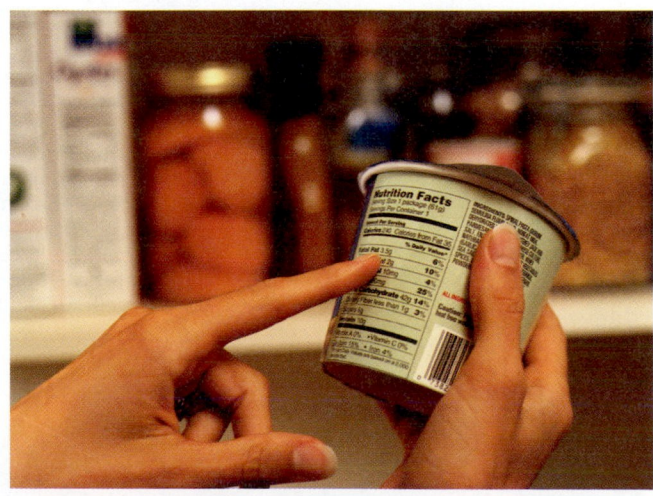

Knowing how to read a food label helps you understand how a particular food fits into your daily allowances.

Serving sizes are standardized to reflect the amounts of foods people actually eat. They are also expressed in common household and metric measures. (You should note whether you are consuming more than one serving.)

With only 5g of saturated fat, and 1.5 g of trans fat, where is the rest of the 13 total grams of fat? It could be unsaturated fats which are not currently required on a label.

This mandatory list of nutrients includes those most important to today's consumers. In the past, the concern was vitamin and mineral deficiencies. Now the worries pertain to fat, cholesterol, sodium, types of carbohydrates, and protein amounts.

This means that in a 2,000 calorie diet 65 grams is equal to 30 percent fat.

This information can help you calculate what percentage of calories of this food comes from fat, carbohydrates, and protein.

CHECK YOURSELF:
What % of calories of this food comes from fat? carbohydrates? protein?
FAT: 13 grams X 9 cal/gram = 117 fat calories. 117/261 = .45 This marcaroni and cheese is 45% fat.
CARBOHYDRATES:
31 grams X 4 cal/gram = 124 carbohydrate calories. 124/261 = .47. This macaroni and cheese is 47% carbohydrate.
PROTEIN: 5 grams x 4 cal/gram = 20 protein calories. 20/261 = .08 This macaroni and cheese is 8% protein.

MACARONI AND CHEESE
Nutrition Facts

Serving Size 1/2 cup (114g)
Servings Per Container 4

Amount Per Serving

Calories 261	Calories from Fat 117

	% Daily Value*
Total Fat 13g	**20%**
Saturated Fat 5g	25%
Trans Fat 1.5g	10%
Cholesterol 30mg	**10%**
Sodium 660mg	**28%**
Total Carbohydrate 31g	**11%**
Sugar 5g	**
Dietary Fiber 1g	4%
Protein 5g	**

Vitamin A 4% • Vitamin C 2% • Calcium 15% • Iron 4%

* Percents (%) of a Daily Value are based on a 2,000 calorie diet. Your Daily Values may vary higher or lower depending on your calorie needs:

	Calories	2,000	2,500
Total Fat	Less than	65g	80g
Sat Fat	Less than	20g	25g
Cholesterol	Less than	300mg	300mg
Sodium	Less than	2,400mg	2,400mg
Total Carbohydrate		300g	375g
Fiber		25g	30g

1g Fat = 9 calories
1g Carbohydrates = 4 calories
1g Protein = 4 calories

** No daily values have been determined for sugars and protein intake.

Ingredients: Enriched wheat flour (contains niacin, reduced iron, vitamin B_1, vitamin B_2, folic acid), cheddar cheese cultures, partially hydrogenated soybean and/or cottonseed oil, non-fat milk, salt, corn syrup, monosodium glutamate, citric acid, natural and artificial flavors, yellow 5 and 6.

% Daily Value shows how a food fits into the overall daily diet. For each item, it shows the percentage or recommended daily consumption for a person eating 2,000 calories a day (e.g., 5 grams of saturated fat is 25 percent of the *recommended* daily value of 20 grams).

No Daily Value for trans fats has been established. If a product lists 0 grams trans fat, it could still contain up to 0.5 grams per serving (but still be advertised as "trans free").

Percentage of daily requirements for selected vitamins and minerals

Recommended daily amounts of each item for two average diets. (If you eat less than 2,000 calories, you will have to adjust the Daily Values.)

Based on 10 percent consumption

Based on 60 percent consumption

Voluntary components that will be allowed on labels are calories from saturated fat, polyunsaturated fat, monounsaturated fat, potassium, soluble and insoluble fiber, sugar, alcohol, other carbohydrates, and other essential vitamins and minerals.

Ingredients are listed in descending order by weight. The ingredient in the largest quantity is always listed first.

FIGURE 11-2   How to read to food label.

THINK ABOUT IT

Food manufacturers invest a lot of money to making their product labels attract consumers to buy their products. They especially like to be able to include health claims such as "Lowers Cholesterol" or "Promotes Heart Health" (such claims are tightly regulated by the FDA and other government agencies). What would it be like if foods high in salt, sugar, fat, or calories were required to have a visible symbol on their label indicating that they were poor nutritional choices—for example, "Promotes Obesity" or "Contributes to Heart Disease"? What are the pros and cons of such a regulation? How realistic is this idea?

McGraw Hill connect™

Go online to Connect to complete this activity.
http://connect.mcgraw-hill.com

3. Check fat content. Avoid hydrogenated fats.
4. Some crackers, pastries, cookies, candies, and instant cocoas are made with coconut and palm oil, which is more saturated than beef fat.
5. Select *whole*-wheat bread ("wheat flour" means refined *white* flour—the bran and wheat germ have been removed). All whole-wheat bread is brown, but not all brown bread is whole wheat.
6. Fortified foods contain added vitamins and minerals not originally in the food or present in lower amounts. Breakfast cereals are commonly fortified. Can you name the vitamin with which milk is commonly fortified?
7. Enriched foods have lost nutrients during processing and then have had them replaced by the manufacturers. For instance, when wheat is turned into white flour, it loses at least 50 to 80 percent of many nutrients. Of these, iron, niacin, thiamin, and riboflavin are replaced, but other nutrients lost in the milling process, such as fiber, zinc, and copper, are not restored.

◆ EATING OUT

Eating out has become routine for many of us. Americans now spend more money in restaurants than in grocery stores. Meal preparation time at home has decreased due to changing lifestyles, and it is evident this trend will not reverse. In this fast-paced world, people want food fast. Many fast-food restaurants pride themselves on the ability to have a meal in your hands 90 seconds after you place your order. The fast-food industry is a multi-billion dollar industry, and there is considerable emphasis by food companies in getting the consumer to form an emotional bond with their products. Even though most people know the connections between diet and health, many still rate price, convenience, and taste of food as the main factors affecting their food choices. For every dollar spent by the World Health Organization on preventing the diseases caused by our industrialized, Western diet, more than $500 is spent by the food industry promoting their unhealthy foods! Most fast-food chains supply nutrient information on their food products on their Web sites, or in brochures. What has this information revealed about the nutrient value of fast food? Are fast foods "junk" foods? Nutritionists have found that fast-food items do have significant amounts of some nutrients (especially protein), but many tend to be low in fiber and high in calories, sodium, and fat. The questions are, How often do you rely on these foods? What other foods are you eating during the day? Occasional visits to fast-food restaurants will have little effect on the nutritive value of your total diet. In response to consumer demand, many chains have become diversified and have added many more items to their menus. Many offer healthier items such as salads and fruits. However, it is still up to you to make a wise selection. For many, it is difficult to get ample amounts of fruits, vegetables, and whole grains by

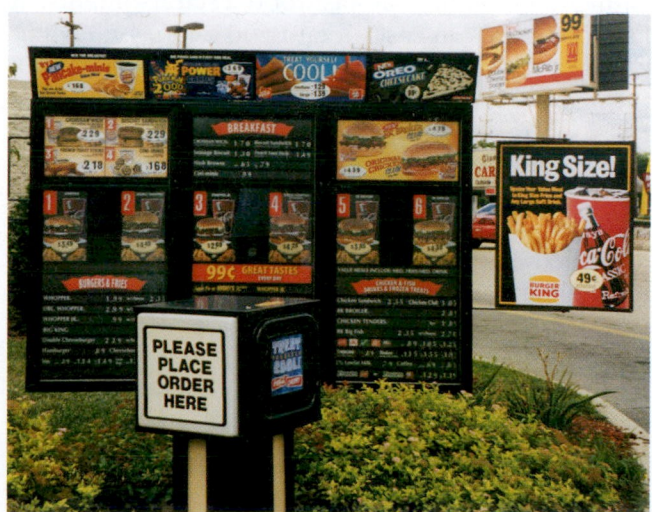

We spend 50 percent of our food dollars taking out, driving through, or sitting down for a restaurant meal. In comparison, in 1980 eating out accounted for only 25 percent of our budgets.

TOP 10 LIST

Fast Tips for Fast Foods

1. At sub shops choose lean meats and avoid tuna salad, bacon, oils, regular mayonnaise, and high-fat cheeses. Try the all-veggie sub.
2. Salad bars are a wise choice for vitamins A and C and fiber; go easy on the dressings, high-fat cheeses, bacon, olives, sour cream, and refried beans. If the bar has pita bread, tacos, or tortillas, why not stuff them with veggies?
3. Potato bars are another good choice if you avoid the heavy cheese and butter-type sauces, bacon, and sour cream.
4. Chicken and fish sound healthy, but many are coated with fat. Select the baked or grilled ones without breading or skin.
5. Pizza is a good choice, especially if the toppings are vegetables; avoid pepperoni, sausage, bacon, and olives.
6. Hamburgers—order the small one instead of the "jumbo" burger. Try the veggie burger.
7. Drink skim milk or juices instead of a shake or soda.
8. When eating Mexican food, emphasize soft corn tortillas, beans, chicken, and vegetables (easy on the cheese).
9. For breakfast, avoid croissants, biscuits, sausage, bacon, butter, and the Danish. Better choices are pancakes, English muffins, bagels, bran muffins, and whole-grain cereals.
10. Ask for salad dressings "on the side" and use sparingly. Select fat-free or low-fat dressings.

eating consistently at fast-food establishments. A fast-food meal can easily total 1,600 calories, 65 grams of fat, and 1,500 milligrams of sodium. Check out the Top 10 list of suggestions for healthy eating at fast-food restaurants.

Restaurant eating in general (not only eating fast foods) has become a way of life for many. Many restaurants offer low-fat, low-calorie dishes, often identified on the menu. Some list fat grams and other nutritional information. Having nutritional knowledge can help you make healthy selections. Ask the server how foods are prepared. Are they baked or fried? Can lower-fat sauces or condiments be substituted? Can the vegetable of the day be substituted for french fries? Salads are not always healthy if loaded with bacon, high-fat cheeses, and full-fat dressings. Check out the à la carte menu. Baked potatoes, salads, vegetables, and soups can often be ordered to make up a meal. Watch portion sizes. Restaurants have a tendency to feed us too much food! Split a meal with a friend or utilize the "doggie

bag." When looking at your overall diet, keep your entire day's and week's intakes in perspective. No foods should be totally forbidden. Everyone enjoys an occasional burger and fries, cheesecake, or pepperoni pizza. Try to live by the "80-20 rule": 80 percent of the time eat nutritionally dense, healthy foods; 20 percent of the time indulge! Remember: *variety, moderation,* and *balance.*

◆ SPECIAL NUTRITIONAL CONSIDERATIONS

High-level wellness means adjusting to life changes and seeking information for special situations. This section discusses dietary considerations for vegetarians, pregnant mothers, the elderly, and those engaging in regular, vigorous exercise.

Vegetarian Diet

For a variety of health and moral reasons, many people prefer a vegetarian diet. A vegetarian diet can be nutritious and healthy. From not eating animal foods, vegetarians normally have lower body fat, blood cholesterol, blood pressure, and rates of coronary heart disease than do meat eaters. They also have a lower than average risk of various cancers and type 2 diabetes because of their high consumption of beans, fruits, and vegetables. There are different vegetarian diets, however. Careful planning and food selection are important to avoid nutritional deficiencies. All vegetarian diets emphasize the use of vegetables, fruits, and grains as main staples. Some diets exclude all animal products, while some include dairy products and eggs.

Here are the types of vegetarians:

1. **Strict vegetarian** (or **vegan**) consumes only plant foods. (Vitamin B_{12} supplementation is recommended because it is not in any plant foods.)
2. **Lactovegetarian** will consume plant foods and dairy products. (No meat or eggs.)
3. **Ovo-lactovegetarian** will consume plant foods, dairy products, and eggs.
4. **Semivegetarian** excludes only red meat.

Meat is not essential to your diet, but protein is. Therefore, following a vegetarian diet requires careful planning and food selection to consume sufficient vitamins and minerals (especially the B vitamins, vitamin D, calcium, zinc, and iron). Search for good-quality protein sources such as legumes (beans), nuts, grains, seeds, and soybean products. A thorough knowledge of nutrition is essential. For

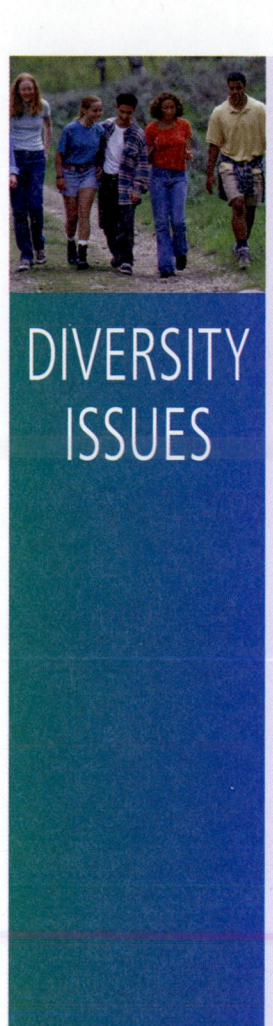

DIVERSITY ISSUES

Ethnic Food Choices

America loves more than burgers and fries. Ethnic foods are popular. Check out these suggestions. (Remember, any foods in huge portions can contribute extra fat, calories, and salt.)

	CHOOSE	AVOID
MEXICAN	rice and beans, salsa, soft tacos, chicken or bean burritos, chicken or vegetable fajitas, corn tortillas, grilled chicken or seafood, fat-free or low-fat refried beans, black bean soup	refried beans made with lard, taco chips and shells, cheese sauces, sour cream, guacamole, fried appetizers, chimichangas, nachos, tostadas, fried ice cream, chili con queso
CHINESE	wonton soup, steamed rice, soft noodles (lo mein), chicken, shrimp, stir-fries, vegetables, Hunan or Szechuan dishes, steamed spring rolls	breaded and deep-fried meats, fried rice, fried noodles, egg rolls, fried wontons, General Tso's chicken, crab Rangoon
ITALIAN	marinara and tomato-based sauces, grilled fish and chicken, minestrone or fagioli (bean) soup, pasta primavera, pasta with red clam sauce, vegetable pizza, steamed clams, marsala or cacciatore	alfredo, carbonara, or other cream sauces, parmigiana dishes, cannelloni, ravioli, manicotti, garlic bread, fried calamari, deep-crust pepperoni pizza, sausage pizza, cannoli
INDIAN	baked breads (chapati), tandoori chicken or fish, yogurt-based curry dishes, dal (lentils), rice pilaf, hummus, kabobs, basmati rice	fried breads (bhatura, poori, paratha), ghee (clarified butter), fried appetizers (pakoras), samosa, korma (meat in cream sauce)
THAI	chicken and seafood dishes (larb, po tak), broiled beef with onions (yum neua), tofu and vegetables, Thai salad	fried fish, chicken or duck, curries, peanut sauces, yum koon chaing (sausage with peppers), crispy noodles, coconut milk curries
GREEK	dolmas (rice wrapped in grape leaves), tzatziki (yogurt and cucumbers), shish kabob, pita bread	moussaka, gyros, baklava, vegetable pies (spanakopita)

example, combining a good source of vitamin C with whole grains and legumes will greatly enhance iron absorption from grain and legumes. Drinking fortified soy milk will help you obtain calcium and vitamin B_{12}. Vegetarians can easily adapt MyPyramid by substituting beans, nuts, tofu, peas, and veggie/soy meats in the meat category. Those who do not consume dairy can obtain calcium from soy milk, broccoli (and other green leafy vegetables), fortified orange juice, tofu, and almond butter. By also consistently selecting whole grains rather than refined flours, vegetarians can consume adequate vitamins and minerals. With care, the vegetarian diet can be nutritionally complete.

Pregnancy

Many women become more nutritionally aware and eat more wisely during pregnancy. This makes

sense. It is an enormous responsibility to be in control of the nutritional well-being of another human. Good nutritional habits before conception give the baby an even healthier start. Good nutrition can improve infant birth weight and reduce infant mortality. It has become recognized that a deficiency in folic acid (a B vitamin) is linked to neural tube birth defects. Therefore, the U.S. Public Health Service has issued a public health recommendation that all women of childbearing age should consume 0.4 milligram (or 400 mcg) of folic acid per day. The evidence is so clear and the concern so great that the FDA has mandated that folic acid be added to "enriched" grain products.

Pregnancy is not a time to diet. Weight gain and some increased fat deposition are necessary and healthy. Be sure to increase calcium, iron, and protein. Your physician may recommend a vitamin supplement because many vitamin needs are increased.

Although some additional vitamins and minerals are needed, only about 300 extra calories per day are necessary for fetal growth and metabolic expenditure. A woman may be "eating for two," but normal energy expenditure is not double. Therefore, it is important to eat nutritionally dense foods. Twinkies, chocolate chip cookies, and potato chips offer few nutrients to a growing baby. Alcohol and caffeine should be limited because they increase nutrient excretion and adversely affect fetal development.

Aging

Many factors may interfere with good nutrition in older adults: economics, isolation, dentures, chronic health disorders, loss of taste, and medications. Nutrient absorption may decrease, especially for calcium and zinc. The widow or widower whose partner had always prepared the meals might start eating fast foods or frozen dinners. The depressed and lonely surviving partner may eat very little. Proper nutrition throughout life and into later life can minimize degenerative changes and help you maintain productivity and wellness. However, your 65-year-old body will not be the same one you fed at age 25. If you decrease activity and your body composition changes (increase in fat, decrease in lean), caloric intake should be decreased. Maintaining an active lifestyle can keep energy requirements from decreasing drastically. Although energy needs may drop as you age, nutrient needs do not diminish significantly. You must make your calories count. Be sure to eat adequate fiber and calcium and fewer fats and refined sugars. In many ways good nutrition (along with proper exercise) can help slow the aging process.

Sports and Fitness

Do you play competitive soccer? Are you training for a half-marathon? Is lap swimming every morning your fitness routine? Nutrition complements physical activity as you pursue a wellness lifestyle. However, the basic nutritional needs of an active person vary little from those of the more sedentary. *Everyone* needs a wide variety of healthy foods. If you are physically active, you burn more calories and have less chance of gaining weight (while eating more). Nevertheless, you do not need a special diet. There are many myths surrounding athletic performance and nutrition. An athlete (even a body builder) does not benefit from consuming massive amounts of protein. The typical American diet contains adequate amounts of protein—even to support an athletic lifestyle. Athletes who train heavily may need a little more. (See Frequently Asked Questions.) These increased protein needs can be satisfied easily through small adjustments in the normal diet—skim milk,

yogurt, skinless chicken breast, and beans can provide excellent high-quality protein.

The main fuel for exercising muscles, glycogen, comes from carbohydrates. The best are the complex ones (breads, pastas, cereals, potatoes, rice, fruit), which provide plenty of vitamins and minerals. Persons engaged in fitness activities should consistently follow a 55 to 65 percent carbohydrate diet-proportion guideline. For those engaging in heavy exercise training, a diet with 65 to 70 percent of its calories from carbohydrates may be necessary to refuel glycogen stores. High-sugar snacks consumed before exercising can decrease performance. Carbohydrate loading (that is, manipulating diet and training to increase glycogen stores in the muscles) has not been shown to be effective for athletes participating in events requiring less than 1½ to 2 hours of continuous, noninterrupted effort.

The benefits of vitamin and mineral supplementation is a current area of study in regard to nutrition for competitive athletes. Large doses of the antioxidant vitamins C, E, and beta-carotene have shown promise in minimizing muscle damage and soreness in hardworking athletes. However, there is no evidence that consuming supplements containing vitamins, minerals, herbs, protein, or amino acids will build muscle or improve sports performance. Muscle overload through training, not supplementation, builds muscle. Research continues to explode in this area.

In regard to nutrition, the key to sports and fitness performance is the same as the key to general wellness and vitality: a balanced diet.

℞ PRESCRIPTION FOR ACTION

You've read the chapter. Now go do one or more of these:

✓ Eat a whole-grain cereal for breakfast and top it with fruit.

✓ Substitute skim milk, water, or 100 percent fruit juice for a sweetened soft drink.

✓ Make sure your dinner plate has two different-colored vegetables on it.

✓ Try an all-veggie pizza, burrito, wrap, or sandwich.

✓ Choose fruit for dessert or for a snack.

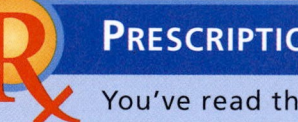

Go online to Connect to complete this activity.
http://connect.mcgraw-hill.com

Frequently Asked Questions

Q. I work out quite a bit: endurance biking and weight training. Don't I need a lot more protein than a casual exerciser does?

A. Many athletes overestimate the amount of protein they need, thinking that more is better. Some studies indicate that more grams of protein than the normal recommendation (i.e., weight in pounds multiplied by 0.36) may help somewhat, while other studies show no improvement in workload capacity or strength. In the studies that recommend more protein, weight in pounds multiplied by 0.54 to 0.64 is the additional amount sufficient for strength and endurance athletes. If you are typical, you probably eat more than enough protein. For example, if you weigh 180 pounds, your recommended protein intake is approximately 65 grams (180 lb. × 0.36). If you increase to 180 lb. × 0.54 or 180 lb. × 0.64, the result is 97 to 115 total grams of protein. To put this in food perspective, 70 grams of protein would be 8 oz of skinless chicken breast and 2 cups of skim milk. An addition of 1 cup oatmeal, 1 cup cottage cheese, and 2 tablespoons peanut butter brings the total to 115 grams of protein. As you can see, the typical American diet contains a sufficient amount of protein to support even the most active lifestyle. Remember, more carbohydrates, *not* protein, are needed for energy fuel, and excessive protein does not build muscle faster. Excessive protein intake puts extra strain on the kidneys.

Q. I hate milk and know I don't get enough calcium. Can't I take a calcium supplement? If so, what kind?

A. It is best to get enough calcium in the diet, but like you, many people struggle with this. There are many types of calcium supplements, some more absorbable than others. The most absorbable form of calcium is calcium citrate, and it can be taken without food. Avoid oyster shell calcium, coral calcium, dolomite, and bone meal products due to possible lead contamination. Calcium carbonate (the type found in antacids) is less absorbable than calcium citrate. Also, you absorb more from divided doses (500 mg or less) than from taking a high dose of calcium all at once. In addition to calcium, it is important to get the recommended levels of magnesium, zinc, and vitamin D to enhance the absorption of calcium. Remember, you can also obtain calcium from nondairy foods: calcium-fortified orange juice, sardines, oatmeal, whole grains, broccoli, and tofu.

Q. I keep seeing more foods labeled "organic" in my grocery store. What does that mean?

A. In the past, "organic" was never officially defined. Growers and manufacturers could slap "organic" on any food they wanted and not be breaking any regulations. This has changed. Under the new USDA federal regulations, "certified organic" means an item has been grown according to strict uniform standards that are verified by independent state or private organizations. These standards include no pesticides, chemical fertilizers, genetic engineering (scientific tinkering with a plant's DNA), or irradiation (a process that uses low levels of radiation to kill bacteria). "Organic" meat denotes that the animals have not been administered antibiotics, have had access to outdoor land, and have been fed organically grown feed. On packaged foods: "100% organic" means all ingredients are organic; "organic" means at least 95 percent of the ingredients are organic; "made with organic ingredients" means at least 70 percent of the ingredients are organic. Sales of organic foods are exploding as consumers become more aware of the health risks associated with pesticides and agricultural chemicals.

Q. Which is better to eat, butter or margarine?

A. It is best to limit consumption of *all* fats, including butter and margarine. Butter is high in saturated fat, which raises "bad" LDL cholesterol. Regular margarine is high in trans-fatty acids (hydrogenated oils), known to increase the "bad" LDL cholesterol *and* decrease the "good" HDL cholesterol. Therefore, if you must use a spread, look for lower-fat or lighter kinds of margarines that say "trans-free" on the label. These are better for you. Both margarine and butter have the same number of calories, approximately 100 calories per tablespoon. You may want to try some of the butter sprinkles, butter-flavored mixes, and butter sprays, which are fat-free.

Q. I don't like many vegetables. Is it okay to get all my phytochemicals strictly from fruit?

A. If you absolutely cannot stand vegetables, eating extra fruit can compensate to some degree, but fruits and vegetables are not nutritionally identical. Both fruits and vegetables contain about the same vitamins and minerals, but vegetables offer a wider array of phytochemicals and carotenoids that help fight cancer, heart disease, and more. How about trying to add some new sauces or spices to vegetables to make them more flavorful? Or add shredded carrots, zucchini, or spinach to pasta sauces or meat loaf. Add steamed broccoli or peas to macaroni and cheese. Throw a handful of veggies into soup. They make great pizza toppings. There are many creative ways to add vegetables to your diet. And you may find you like them!

Q. I love pizza. Is it considered an unhealthy "junk food"?

A. It all depends on the toppings you choose. Ordering a vegetable-topped pizza is generally a pretty healthful choice. Also, a thin crust is better than a thick crust. When you load a pizza with pepperoni, sausage, bacon, or extra cheese, the fat and calories skyrocket. Since an entire large veggie pizza rarely contains even one cup of vegetables, why not add some more on your own? In the 10 minutes you wait for a pizza to be delivered or preheat the oven, you can sauté some mushrooms, onions, peppers, broccoli, or spinach to add to the pizza. Chopped tomatoes or even canned vegetables will do. Use your imagination!

Q. Are fresh fruits and vegetables more nutritious than frozen, canned, or dried?

A. Not really. Most frozen, canned, and dried fruits or vegetables can be as nutritious as fresh produce. The frozen and canned versions are usually processed quickly using fresh-picked produce. To maximize vitamin content, use little water in preparation. Eating fruits and vegetables in a variety of forms will ensure a balance of important nutrients. When choosing frozen, canned, or dried versions, try to choose products without added sauces, sodium, or sugars.

Q. There are so many different artificial sweeteners used in foods. Are they safe?

A. The words "sugar free" can be music to many ears when they want to satisfy their sweet tooth without excess calories or carbohydrates. Saccharin (*Sweet 'N Low*), Aspartame (*Equal, NutraSweet*), Sucralose (*Splenda*), and Stevia (*Truvia, Sweet-Leaf*) are all FDA-approved artificial sweeteners. Despite FDA approval, artificial sweeteners have been suspected to cause everything from mood and behavior disorders to headaches, multiple sclerosis, obesity, heart disease, and cancer. While some individuals may attribute many maladies to artificial sweeteners, there are no published, peer-reviewed, controlled scientific studies to support these accusations. Preliminary studies on animals suggest, however, that high intakes of artificial sweeteners may affect appetite control and cause some to eat more sweet foods—artificially sweetened or not. Because of many unknowns, moderation should be followed in consuming products containing artificial sweeteners. Some dietitians recommend that we consume no more than four daily servings of an artificially sweetened product. Examples of a single serving include:

- 8-ounces diet soda or other beverage
- 1/2 cup sugar-free pudding or gelatin dessert
- 1 cup of fat-free yogurt
- 1 packet artificial sweetener (added to any food or beverage)

Q. Since I have classes during midday, I never have time for lunch. What healthy and filling items can be packed in a backpack to get me through the day?

A. Many of us are busy or on-the-go during lunchtime. The following items can be packed in a backpack, office drawer, or car to fill an empty stomach: fresh or dried fruits, 100% fruit juices, whole-grain bagels, carrots or celery sticks, granola or cereal bars, snack-size boxes of whole-grain cereal or crackers, soy nuts, whole-wheat fig bars, almonds, peanut butter- or cheese-filled whole-wheat crackers.

Summary

Although diet is not singled out as a specific risk factor for coronary heart disease, dietary factors are often interrelated with patterns of physical activity as major contributors to heart disease, stroke, obesity, atherosclerosis, osteoporosis, and some types of cancer. While many dietary components are involved in diet and health relationships, primary factors are our high consumption of fats (especially saturated fats), salt, and sugars. These components are often consumed at the expense of fruits, vegetables, and complex carbohydrates that may be more conducive to health.

Like many, you may admit to having some poor nutritional habits. You may rationalize this with some of the following:

- I'll do better after I get out of school and have more time. (Frankly, you will probably be busier after graduation.)
- But I feel fine! (Like smoking, poor eating habits may not noticeably affect your health for years.)
- I don't have any control over what the cafeteria serves. (However, you do have *choices* in the cafeteria and between meals.)
- I don't have enough money to buy the right foods. (On the contrary, milk is cheaper than soft drinks; a bunch of bananas costs less than a bag of potato chips.)
- I'm going to die anyway, so I might as well eat what I like. (Yes, we are all going to die. However, lifetime dietary habits significantly affect the *quality* of the last 10 to 20 years of your life.)

Wellness involves making informed choices rather than rationalizing. Improved eating habits can positively affect your health—now and later in life. Therefore, learn about the foods you are eating. Read food labels. Good nutrition involves *dietary guidelines*, a *pyramid of choices*, and *three simple words: variety, moderation*, and *balance*.

Terms

- antioxidants
- carbohydrates
- cholesterol
- complex carbohydrates
- fat
- fat-soluble vitamins
- fiber
- free radicals
- glycemic index (GI)
- glycogen
- hydrogenation
- insoluble fiber
- ketone bodies
- lactovegetarian
- macrominerals
- minerals
- monounsaturated fat
- nutrient density
- omega-3
- osteopenia
- osteoporosis
- ovo-lactovegetarian
- phytochemicals
- phytoestrogens
- polyunsaturated fat
- protein
- saturated fat
- semivegetarian
- simple carbohydrates
- soluble fiber
- strict vegetarian (or vegan)
- trace minerals
- trans-fatty acids (trans fats)
- vitamins
- water-soluble vitamins

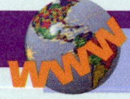

Internet Resources

2010 Dietary Guidelines

www.dietaryguidelines.gov

Published by the U.S. Department of Health and Human Services, these guidelines reflect the latest research on diet and health and provide practical suggestions for making healthy diet adjustments.

American Dietetic Association

www.eatright.org

Provides a vast amount of reliable, objective food and nutrition information, including fact sheets, position papers, and healthy eating tips.

American Heart Association: Delicious Decisions

www.deliciousdecisions.org

Provides basic information about nutrition, tips for shopping and eating out, and healthy recipes.

Ask the Dietitian

www.dietitian.com

Thoroughly covers all areas of nutrition, food, weight issues, and fitness in a question-and-answer format.

Center for Nutrition Policy and Promotion

www.usda.gov/cnpp

Promotes healthy eating and provides dietary guidance that links scientific research to consumer issues: food plans, dietary guidelines, nutrition insights, and up-to-date reports.

Center for Science in the Public Interest

www.cspinet.org

Features the *Nutrition Action Healthletter,* a watchdog of the fast-food and restaurant industry whose mission is to educate the public on healthy eating.

Fast Food Facts

www.foodfacts.info

Has a database of fast-food restaurants with comparisons and the nutritional content of their foods, sorted by calories, fat, cholesterol, and more.

Food-o-Meter

www.webmd.com/diet/healthtool-food-calorie-counter

Provides nutrition facts including calories, fat, carbohydrates, protein, sugar, and fiber in over 37,000 foods and beverages. Includes popular everyday foods and restaurant chains.

Fruits and Veggies Matter

www.fruitsandveggiesmatter.gov

Emphasizes the importance of fruits and vegetable in the diet for prevention of chronic diseases. Gives benefits, recipes, resources, tips, and Q&A.

Glycemic Index

www.glycemicindex.com
www.nutritionaldata.com

A comprehensive list of the glycemic index of foods can be found at these sites.

Harvard School of Public Health

www.hsph.harvard.edu/nutritionsource

Covers current research on all aspects of nutrition, providing tips on healthy eating and dispelling myths. Addresses everything from soft drinks to weight management to exercise.

MyPyramid

www.MyPyramid.gov

A U.S. Department of Agriculture interactive site that helps you choose the foods and amounts that are right for you according to the current *Dietary Guidelines.* Provides tips, tracking sheets, resources, calories for specific foods, and guidelines for healthy eating.

National Dairy Council

www.nationaldairycouncil.org

Provides timely and reliable nutrition information on the health benefits of dairy foods.

National Osteoporosis Foundation

www.nof.org

Covers facts, risk factors, information, and news related to fighting osteoporosis and promoting bone health.

Nutrition.gov

www.nutrition.gov

Everything you need to know about nutrition issues, dietary guidelines, weight management, supplements, and food safety. Provides science-based guidance and reliable information for all ages from a multitude of federal agencies.

Nutrition Data

www.nutritiondata.com

Provides complete nutritional information for any food or recipe and helps you select foods that best match your dietary needs.

Office of Dietary Supplements

http://ods.od.nih.gov

An office of the National Institutes of Health, this site helps consumers, health care providers, and educators find credible scientific information on a variety of dietary supplements.

The Vegetarian Resource Group

www.vrg.org

Covers all issues and topics regarding vegetarianism.

U.S. Food and Drug Administration

www.fda.gov

Provides information about the safety and effectiveness of food, drugs, cosmetics, weight-loss products, and any medical devices intended for human use.

The following restaurants have nutritional information for their foods online:

www.arbys.com	www.longjohnsilvers.com
www.blimpie.com	www.mcdonalds.com
www.bostonmarket.com	www.panerabread.com
www.burgerking.com	www.papajohns.com
www.carlsjr.com	www.pizzahut.com
www.chick-fil-a.com	www.popeyes.com
www.churchs.com	www.quiznos.com
www.dairyqueen.com	www.schlotzskys.com
www.dominos.com	www.sonicdrivein.com
www.dunkindonuts.com	www.steaknshake.com
www.fazolis.com	www.subway.com
www.hardees.com	www.tacobell.com
www.jackinthebox.com	www.whitecastle.com
www.kfc.com	

LAB Activity 11-1

Analyze Your Diet Using MyPyramid

Go to www.MyPyramid.gov and enter your personal data under "MyPyramid Plan." Print your recommended Plan. Then compare your average daily diet to what is recommended in MyPyramid. (See Figure 11-1 for serving size equivalencies.)

MyPyramid daily recommendations

My average daily consumption

GRAINS: _____

_____

Are half your grains "whole grains"? _____

VEGETABLES: _____

_____

FRUITS: _____

_____

MILK: _____

_____

MEAT/BEANS: _____

_____

According to MyPyramid, what are your estimated daily calorie needs? _____

Do you feel you balance your calorie *intake* with your calorie *expenditure* on most days? _____

According to MyPyramid, how many teaspoons of oils are you allowed? _____

According to MyPyramid, how many discretionary calories (i.e., extra fats and sugars) are you allowed? _____

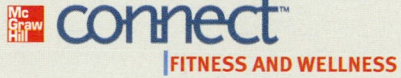

http://connect.mcgraw-hill.com

Identify three positive dietary changes you could implement that would help you come closer to complying with your Pyramid recommendations. Include *what* you could do and a *specific strategy* for how to do it. (The MyPyramid Web site has many healthy eating tips.)

Example: *What?* Eat two more servings of fruit every day.

Strategy? Slice a banana on my cereal every morning; put an apple in my backpack for an afternoon snack each day.

a.

b.

c.

LAB Activity 11-2

Name _____ Class/Activity Section _____ Date _____

How Much Fat?

1. Lisa consumes 2,100 calories per day. To keep her percentage of fat at 30 percent of her calories, figure out how many *grams* of fat she can consume per day. _____ (Show your work.)

   If Lisa wants to eat even *healthier* and limit her fat percentage to 20 percent of her daily calories, how many fat grams per day can she consume? _____ (Show your work.)

2. Robert consumes 2,700 calories per day. To keep his percentage of fat at 30 percent of his calories, how many *grams* of fat can he consume per day? _____ (Show your work.)

   If Robert wants to eat even *healthier* and limit his fat percentage to 25 percent of his daily calories, how many fat grams per day can he consume? _____ (Show your work.)

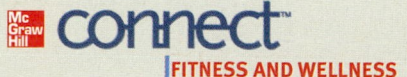

http://connect.mcgraw-hill.com

WHAT ABOUT YOU?

(Multiply your body weight by 15 to approximate your caloric intake for a day.)

_____ lb. × 15 = _____ calories

Number of daily fat grams at 30 percent of calories = _____ (Show your work.)

Number of daily fat grams at 25 percent of calories = _____ (Show your work.)

Number of daily fat grams at 20 percent of calories = _____ (Show your work.)

LAB Activity 11-3

Label Reading Assignment

HONEY WHEAT MUFFIN MIX

Directions
Combine mix with:
1/3 c. whole milk
1 T. oil
1 egg
Stir and pour into prepared muffin tin. Bake 15 minutes at 400°.

Nutrition Facts

Serving Size 1 muffin (from 31g mix)
Servings Per Container 6

Amount Per Serving	Mix	Prepared
Calories	123	162
Calories from Fat	27	54

	% Daily Value**	
Total Fat 3g*	4%	10%
Saturated Fat 0.5g	3%	7%
Trans Fat 0.5g		
Cholesterol 0mg	0%	12%
Sodium 210mg	9%	9%
Potassium 15mg	<1%	1%
Total Carbohydrate 23g	8%	8%
Dietary Fiber <1g	2%	2%
Sugars 12g		
Other Carbohydrate 11g		
Protein 1g		
Calcium	0%	2%
Iron	2%	2%

Not a significant source of vitamin A and vitamin C.

*Amount in mix. As prepared, one serving provides 6g fat (1.5g saturated fat; 1.0g trans fat), 35mg cholesterol, 220mg sodium, 45mg potassium, 24g total carbohydrate (12g sugars) and 3g protein.

**Percent Daily Values are based on a 2,000 calorie diet. Your daily values may be higher or lower depending on your calorie needs:

	Calories:	2,000	2,500
Total Fat	Less than	65g	80g
Sat Fat	Less than	20g	25g
Cholesterol	Less than	300mg	300mg
Sodium	Less than	2,400mg	2,400mg
Potassium		3,500mg	3,500mg
Total Carbohydrate		300g	375g
Dietary Fiber		25g	30g

Calories per gram:
Fat 9 • Carbohydrate 4 • Protein 4

Ingredients: Enriched Wheat Flour, Sugar, Hydrogenated Vegetable Oil (Coconut and/or Palm Kernel), Corn Syrup, Salt, Cellulose Gum, Dextrose, Rice Flour, Artificial Flavor

Look at the muffin mix label and complete the following:

1. What constitutes one serving?

2. Why are there two columns (mix, prepared)?

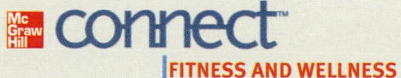

3. How many grams of total fat are there in two prepared muffins? _____

4. In one prepared muffin, figure out the

   a. percent of calories from fat: _____

   b. percent of calories from carbohydrates: _____

   c. percent of calories from protein: _____

5. Give one source of complex carbohydrate in this product:

6. Give one source of simple carbohydrate in this product:

7. Name the source of cholesterol in this prepared product:

8. Name and comment on the sources of fat in this prepared product:

9. What alternatives or substitutes could be made in preparing these muffins to make them healthier?

10. What is your overall assessment of this food (i.e., nutritional density; sodium, fat, cholesterol content; types of carbohydrates; fiber content)?

Name _____ **Class/Activity Section** _____ **Date** _____

Select and Analyze a Food Label

Select a label from a food that you commonly eat. Make sure the ingredients are listed on the label. Attach the label to this form. Analyze the food as follows:

Food: _____

Serving size: _____

Total calories per serving: _____

Total fat grams per serving: _____

Total trans fats per serving: _____

Total carbohydrate grams per serving: _____

Total protein grams per serving: _____

Comment on the amount of cholesterol in this food: _____

_____

_____

Comment on the amount of sodium in this food: _____

_____

_____

Comment on the types of carbohydrates in this food (i.e., complex or simple). Is this food a good source of fiber?

_____

List any source(s) of added sugar: _____

_____

_____

What is your overall assessment of this food (i.e., nutritional value, nutritional density, etc.)? _____

_____

_____

Manufacturer: _____

In your opinion, is this an appropriate portion size?

Why or why not? _____

_____

Percentage of calories from fat: _____

Percentage of calories from carbohydrates: _____

Percentage of calories from protein: _____

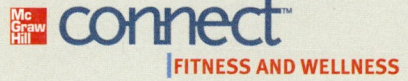

CHAPTER 12

Achieving a Healthy Weight

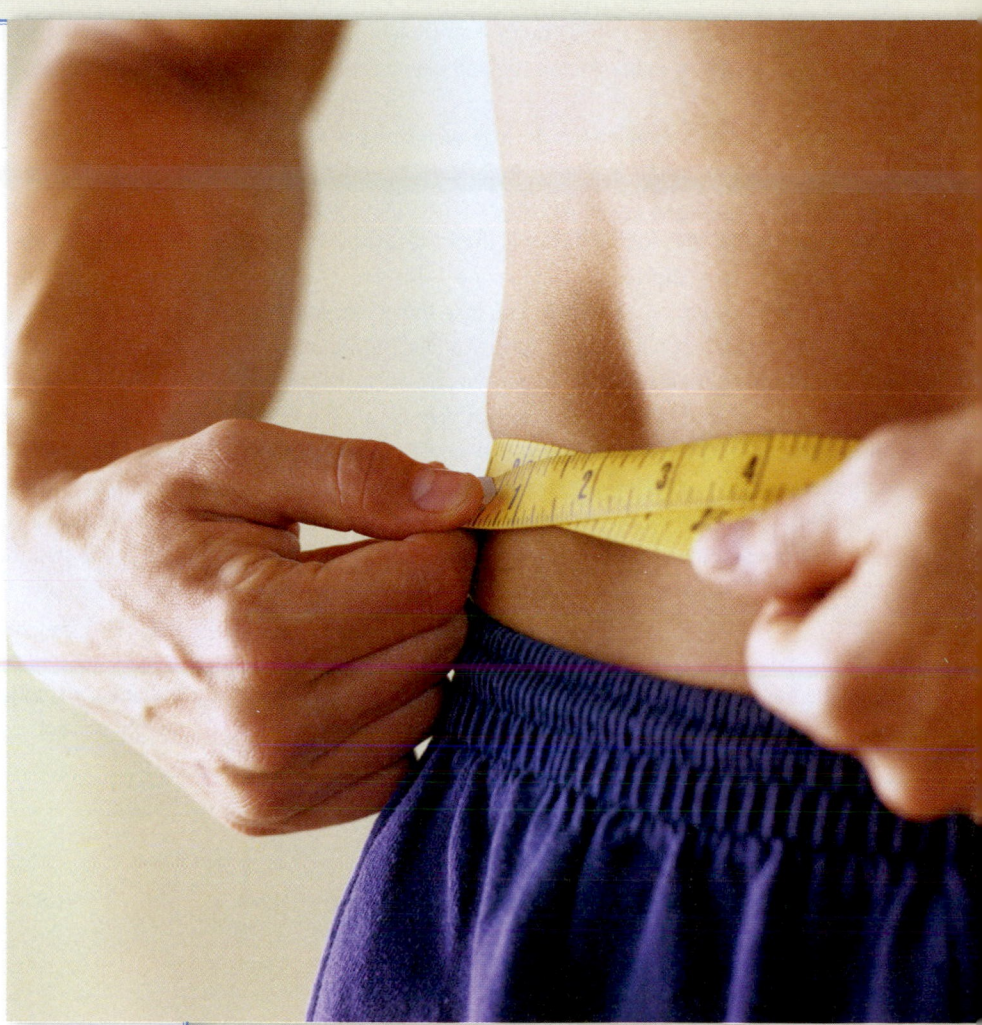

STUDY QUESTIONS

You will have successfully mastered this chapter if you can answer the following:

1. What is the difference between overweight and obesity?

2. Can you identify the percentages of adults over age 20 who are overweight and the percentage who are obese?

3. Can you explain the purpose of the body mass index (BMI) and identify a BMI associated with health problems?

4. What are six health conditions associated with obesity?

5. How is the location of fat on the body linked to health risks?

6. Are you able to calculate waist-to-hip ratios and identify a risky waist-to-hip ratio and a high-risk waist circumference for both men and women?

7. How do each of the following factors contribute to obesity: energy balance, heredity, fat cells, set point, and metabolism?

8. Can you define basal metabolic rate (BMR), and identify five factors that affect it?

9. Are you able to list guidelines that distinguish a healthy weight-loss program from a fad/diet program?

10. What are the three major components of effective lifetime weight management?

11. How does exercise help in weight management?

12. Can you compare and contrast these eating disorders: bulimia nervosa, anorexia nervosa, binge eating disorder, and disordered eating?

You will find the answers as you read this chapter.

> " *More die in the United States of too much food than of too little.* "
> —John Kenneth Galbraith

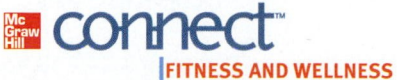

FITNESS AND WELLNESS

http://connect.mcgraw-hill.com

There is an epidemic in the United States, and it is not caused by a virus or a bacteria. It is obesity. This epidemic is associated with increased risk for premature death, reduced quality of life, and increased health care costs. Because the obesity trend is increasing so rapidly, most health professionals believe obesity is the most serious health threat to our nation. During the past 30 years, adult obesity rates have doubled, and childhood obesity rates have more than tripled. These rising rates are one of the major factors behind skyrocketing health care costs.

The paradox is that efforts to lose weight have resulted in a multi-billion-dollar business. Americans spend approximately $59 billion yearly on weight-loss products, programs, and diet aids. The diet-food industry is the fastest-growing food market. Bookstore shelves and magazine racks are crammed with diet plans guaranteed to help you lose those extra inches. Television, radio, and newspapers further advertise a multitude of weight-loss options. In fact, losing weight is so important that 88 percent of dieters say they would give up a job promotion, retirement, or a dream house if they could only reach their target weight!

With all this attention and effort, one would think that the population would be getting leaner. Paradoxically, obesity rates are climbing in all populations in our country. Overweight and obesity account for over 100,000 U.S. deaths per year, second only to tobacco as the most preventable cause of death. Although smoking has had a bigger impact on deaths, obesity has a bigger effect on illness. In addition, the proportion of smokers among U.S. adults declined by 18.5 percent between 1993 and 2008 whereas the proportion of obese adults increased 85 percent. And obesity is increasing in prevalence in both developed and developing countries throughout the world.

The latest national statistics reveal that an alarming 67 percent of American adults age 20 or older are overweight or obese (see Figure 12-1). In fact, more people are obese than overweight! One-fifth of U.S. children are overweight or obese. However, there are disparities in overweight and obesity in some segments of the population (see Diversity Issues).

Although there is tremendous interest in diets and dieting, many dieters fail to achieve their weight goals, and over 90 percent of those who do lose weight are unable to keep the weight off. The paradoxes of these facts reveal the complexity of America's weight issues. The determinants of obesity in the United States are complex, numerous, and operate at social, economic, environmental, and individual levels.

Maintaining a reasonable body weight is a definite wellness issue. Your body is the vehicle by which you function in society. Being overweight can affect you physically, emotionally, socially, and occupationally. The purpose of wellness is to strive toward full potential, so maintaining a reasonable body composition is one step toward achieving wellness. Knowledge gives you the tools to plan your lifetime weight-management scheme. It is important that you understand body composition facts, effective weight-loss principles, weight-management guidelines, and the influence of culture, heredity, environment, and behavior on weight control.

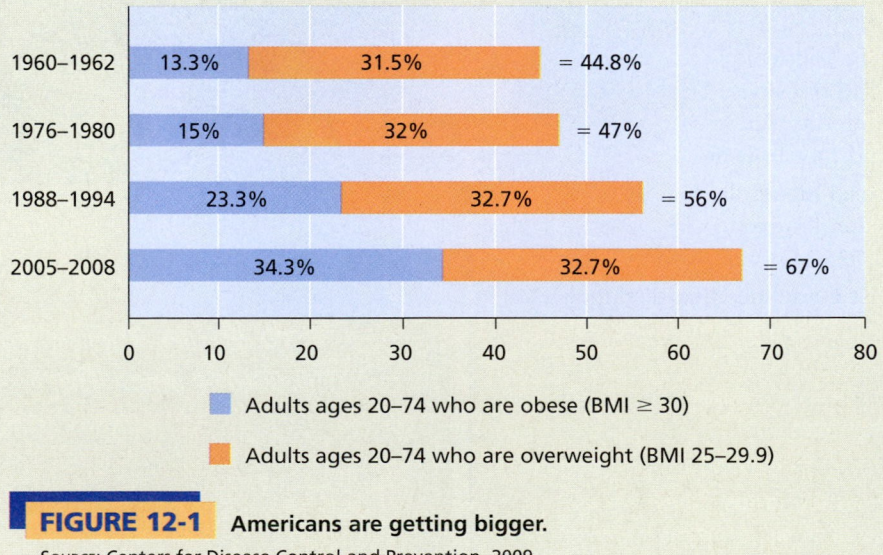

	Adults ages 20–74 who are obese (BMI ≥ 30)	Adults ages 20–74 who are overweight (BMI 25–29.9)	Total
1960–1962	13.3%	31.5%	= 44.8%
1976–1980	15%	32%	= 47%
1988–1994	23.3%	32.7%	= 56%
2005–2008	34.3%	32.7%	= 67%

FIGURE 12-1   **Americans are getting bigger.**
SOURCE: Centers for Disease Control and Prevention, 2009.

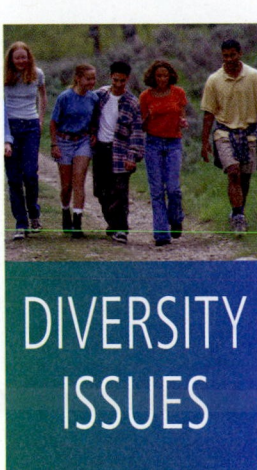

DIVERSITY ISSUES

Weight Issues Among Various Ethnic Groups

- Although overweight and obesity are rising in all age groups, they are substantially more prevalent in women who are members of racial and ethnic minority populations than in white women.
- Among men, Hispanic Americans have a higher prevalence of overweight and obesity than do whites or blacks.
- Smaller surveys indicate a higher prevalence of overweight and obesity in American Indians, Alaska Natives, and Pacific Islander Americans and a lower prevalence in Asian Americans compared with the general population.
- Because of obesity, blacks and Hispanics have a higher incidence of diabetes compared to whites.
- Studies show that racial disparities in diabetes and obesity are linked to behavior, medical care, poverty, and living conditions rather than to genetics.

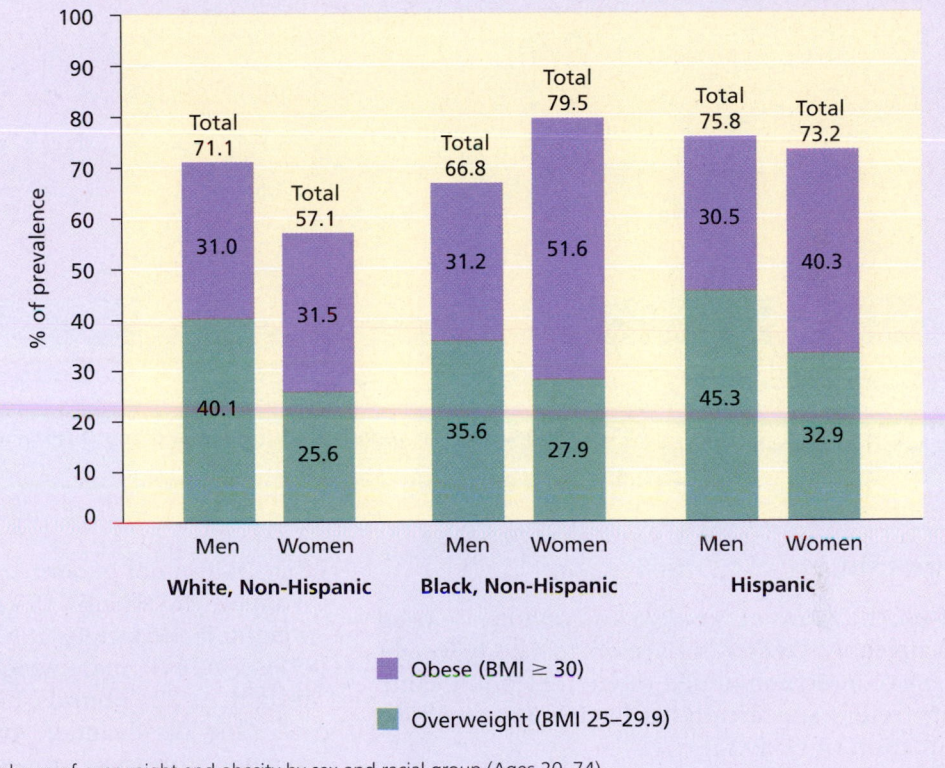

Prevalence of overweight and obesity by sex and racial group (Ages 20–74).
SOURCE: Centers for Disease Control and Prevention, *Health, United States,* 2008.

UNDERSTANDING BODY COMPOSITION

Your body is composed of body fat and fat-free mass. **Fat-free mass** includes muscle, bone, body fluids, and organs. Muscles, part of fat-free mass, are often specifically referred to as **lean-body mass** or **muscle mass. Body fat** is classified as either essential fat or storage fat. **Essential fat,** required for normal body functioning, is stored in major body organs and tissues such as the heart, muscles, intestines, bones, lungs, liver, spleen, and kidneys and throughout the central nervous system. Females have additional essential fat in the breasts and pelvic region for childbearing and other hormone-related functions. **Storage fat** is the extra fat that accumulates in adipose cells (or fat cells) around internal organs and beneath the skin surface to insulate, pad, and protect the body from trauma and extreme cold. As you learned in Chapter 3, there are different ways to assess body composition. Knowing your body composition (especially your percentage of body fat) can help you set realistic weight goals.

What Stage of Change Are You In?

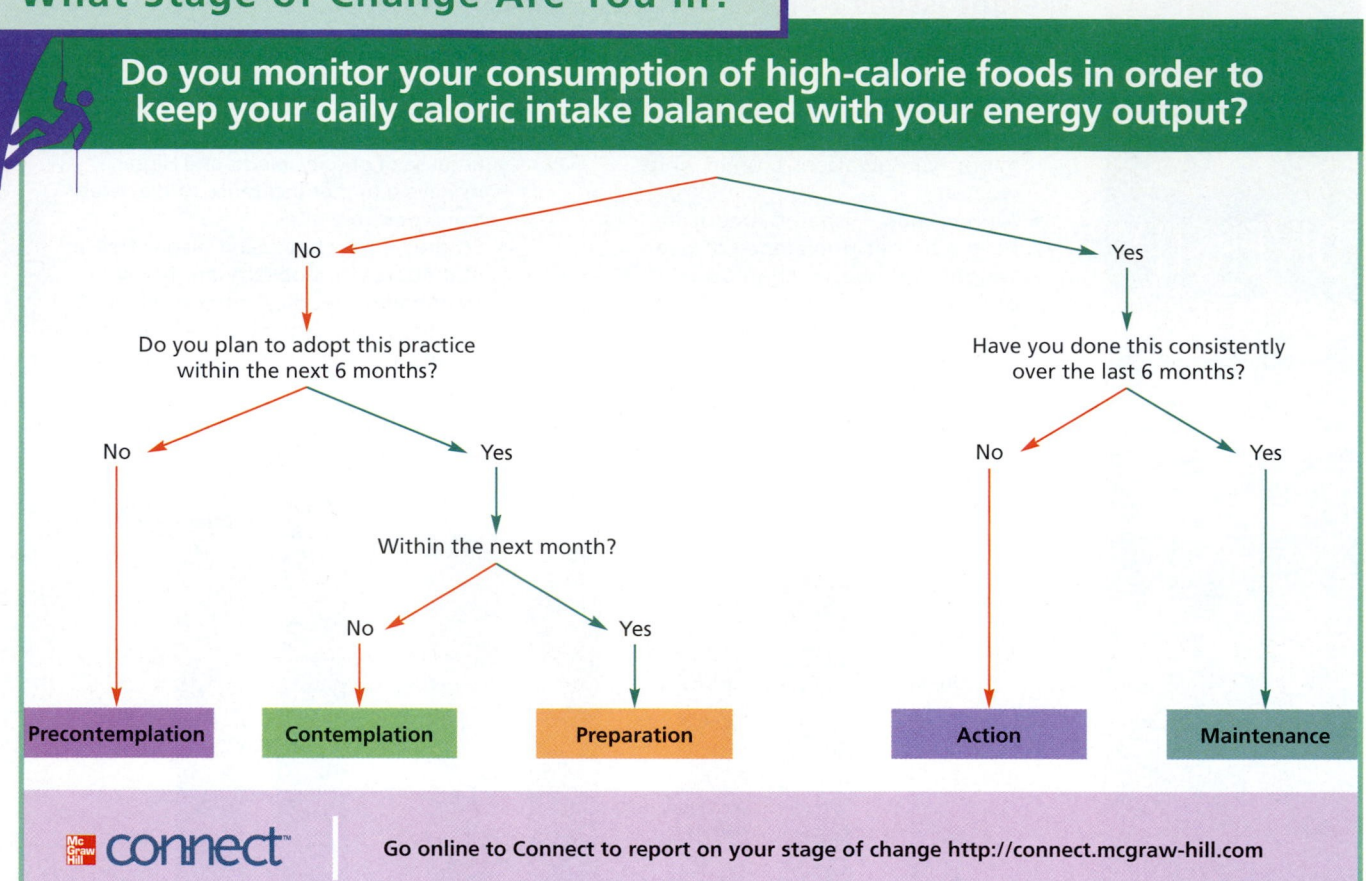

Do you monitor your consumption of high-calorie foods in order to keep your daily caloric intake balanced with your energy output?

No — Do you plan to adopt this practice within the next 6 months?

Yes — Have you done this consistently over the last 6 months?

No / Yes — Within the next month?

No / Yes

No / Yes

Precontemplation | **Contemplation** | **Preparation** | **Action** | **Maintenance**

Go online to Connect to report on your stage of change http://connect.mcgraw-hill.com

Overweight Versus Obesity

Too often, the terms *overweight* and *obesity* are used interchangeably. **Overweight** refers to a body weight in excess of a recommended range for good health. **Obesity** refers specifically to having an excessive accumulation of body fat.

Because these explanations are somewhat vague, the National Institutes of Health has adopted the **body mass index (BMI)** as a method of classifying overweight and obesity. BMI is a direct calculation based on height and weight and has been universally adopted by health professionals to determine healthy weights and risky weights. BMI is computed from the following equations:

$$BMI = \frac{\text{weight in kilograms}}{(\text{height in meters})^2}$$
$$\text{or}$$
$$BMI = \frac{\text{weight in pounds}}{(\text{height in inches})^2} \times 703$$

Table 12-1 allows you to determine your BMI quickly. Note the classifications below the chart. These standards have been adopted worldwide. In this way, overweight and obesity are clearly defined. Notice that BMI is not gender specific. For example, a 5′6″ woman who weighs 155 pounds is considered overweight. If she weighs 186 pounds, she is classified as obese. A 6′0″ man weighing 184 pounds is overweight. At 221 pounds, he is considered obese.

One disadvantage of using the BMI is that it remains a measure of weight and height, not fatness (i.e., it doesn't distinguish between body fat and muscle mass). Nor does it take into account the *location* of fat. Therefore it may not be appropriate for an athlete or body builder with a lot of muscle mass. Also, for the elderly who have lost a lot of muscle mass, their BMI may reflect a "healthy weight," when in actuality they have reduced nutritional reserves. Some research also indicates that there may be race or ethnicity differences in BMI measurements. Regardless of the issues surrounding BMI, it is still considered a useful tool for examining trends and patterns in obesity for the vast majority of people. An analysis of your body fat percentage using skinfold calipers may give a more accurate body composition assessment (i.e., body fat versus lean body mass). For example, a woman over 30 percent body fat and a man over 25 percent are considered obese. (See Chapter 3 for more on skinfold measuring and

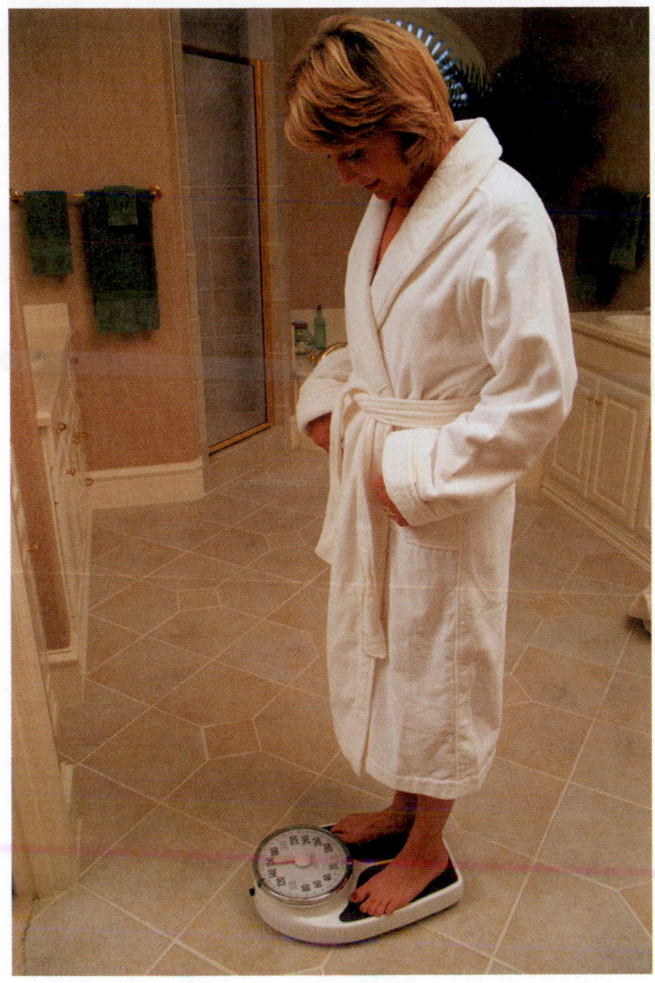

Although people seem concerned about their weight, obesity is on the rise.

body composition.) Other assessment tools such as waist-to-hip ratio and waist size are also useful, indicating that the *location* of fat is an important factor.

Location of Fat

Studies suggest that not only are body fat percentage and BMI related to health, the location of excess fat is a comparable risk factor as well. Fat distributed primarily in the abdominal area (called *apple-shape obesity*) is characteristic of many men (but is also present in some women). This "visceral fat" is deep in the belly and intermingled around the internal organs and is linked to increased risk for coronary heart disease, hypertension, high cholesterol, type 2 diabetes, and several forms of cancer. Fat distributed in the lower extremities, around the hips, buttocks, and thighs (called *pear-shape obesity*), does not present as great a risk. Pear-shape obesity is more common in women. The two types of fat have biochemical differences. Abdominal fat experiences much more enzyme, hormone, and chemical activity, dumping more fatty acids into the bloodstream and

increasing the prevalence of LDL cholesterol. This visceral fat also seems to trigger inflammation throughout the body, which encourages cancer growth. Hip-thigh fat activity is more stagnant. Unfortunately, this hip-thigh fat is more difficult to lose than is abdominal fat. Many obesity experts now think that one's waist-to-hip ratio is more important than the BMI in predicting potential weight-related health problems because abdominal fat is so heavily linked to diseases. A worldwide study revealed that abdominal obesity accounts for 90 percent of the risk for heart attack. A large amount of belly fat is a risk factor for cardiovascular disease even if the rest of the physique is lean. This was true for men, women, all ages, and in all ethnic groups. According to some scientists, if waist-to-hip ratios (rather than BMIs) were currently used to assess the risk of chronic disease, the number of people classified as obese worldwide would increase substantially. Waist-to-hip ratio can be calculated by dividing the number of inches around the waistline by the circumference of the hips. See Table 12-2 for examples of waist-to-hip ratios. For example, someone who has a 30-inch waist and 40-inch hips has a ratio of 0.75. A woman whose ratio is 0.80 or higher is at risk, as is a man whose ratio is 0.95 or above.

Some researchers believe that the waist circumference *alone* can be a predictor of risk. Men with a waist circumference over 40 inches and women with a waist circumference over 35 inches are classified as high risk no matter what their BMIs are. Men with a waist circumference over 40 inches are twelve times more likely to develop type 2 diabetes. An excess of abdominal fat in women has been linked to breast cancer, colon cancer, and heart attack. Whereas the distribution of fat has a genetic link, a comprehensive program of a low-fat, reduced-calorie diet and regular exercise can help reduce body fat stores regardless of where they are located.

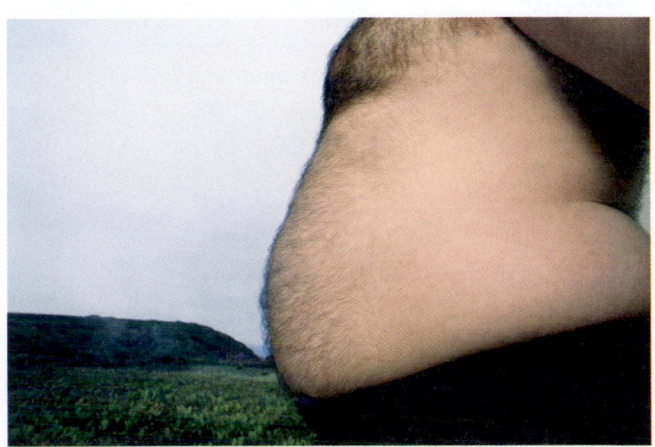

For a man or a woman, having a large amount of abdominal fat substantially increases the risk of heart disease, stroke, type 2 diabetes, and several forms of cancer.

TABLE 12-1   *Find Your Body Mass Index (BMI)*

Find your height, then look across that row. Your BMI is at the top of the column that contains your weight.

Body Mass Index (BMI)

Height	19	20	21	22	23	24	25	26	27	28	29	30	35	40
					Weight (pounds)									
4'10"	91	96	100	105	110	115	119	124	129	134	138	143	167	191
4'11"	94	99	104	109	114	119	124	128	133	138	143	148	173	198
5'0"	97	102	107	112	118	123	128	133	138	143	148	153	179	204
5'1"	100	106	111	116	122	127	132	137	143	148	153	158	185	211
5'2"	104	109	115	120	126	131	136	142	147	153	158	164	191	218
5'3"	107	113	118	124	130	135	141	146	152	158	163	169	197	225
5'4"	110	116	122	128	134	140	145	151	157	163	169	174	204	232
5'5"	114	120	126	132	138	144	150	156	162	168	174	180	210	240
5'6"	118	124	130	136	142	148	155	161	167	173	179	186	216	247
5'7"	121	127	134	140	146	153	159	166	172	178	185	191	223	255
5'8"	125	131	138	144	151	158	164	171	177	184	190	197	230	262
5'9"	128	135	142	149	155	162	169	176	182	189	196	203	236	270
5'10"	132	139	146	153	160	167	174	181	188	195	202	207	243	278
5'11"	136	143	150	157	165	172	179	186	193	200	208	215	250	286
6'0"	140	147	154	162	169	177	184	191	199	206	213	221	258	294
6'1"	144	151	159	166	174	182	189	197	204	212	219	227	265	302
6'2"	148	155	163	171	179	186	194	202	210	218	225	233	272	311
6'3"	152	160	168	176	184	192	200	208	216	224	232	240	279	319
6'4"	156	164	172	180	189	197	205	213	221	230	238	246	287	328
	NORMAL						**OVERWEIGHT**					**OBESE**		

Interpreting Your BMI

- ≤18.9 Underweight
- 19–24.9 Healthy weight (little health risk)
- 25–29.9 Overweight (increased health risk)
- ≥30 Obesity (greatest health risk)

SOURCE: National Institutes of Health; National Heart, Lung and Blood Institute.

TABLE 12-2   *Sample Waist-to-Hip Ratios*

$$\text{Waist-to-Hip Ratio} = \frac{\text{Waist circumference}}{\text{Hip circumference}}$$

(see Chapter 3 for specific measuring instructions)

$$\frac{\text{Waist}}{\text{hip}} = \frac{28''}{38''} = 0.74 \qquad \frac{\text{Waist}}{\text{hip}} = \frac{40''}{42''} = 0.95$$

$$\frac{\text{Waist}}{\text{hip}} = \frac{32''}{40''} = 0.80 \qquad \frac{\text{Waist}}{\text{hip}} = \frac{45''}{39''} = 1.15$$

$$\frac{\text{Waist}}{\text{hip}} = \frac{38''}{42''} = 0.90 \qquad \frac{\text{Waist}}{\text{hip}} = \frac{50''}{40''} = 1.25$$

Higher risk is associated with a ratio >0.8 for women and >0.95 for men.

Risks Associated with Obesity

The health implications of excess weight have become quite clear. Obesity is identified as a risk factor in 4 of the 10 leading causes of death. The major killers associated with obesity are heart disease, several types of cancer, stroke, type 2 diabetes, and atherosclerosis. Obesity contributes to cardiovascular disease by causing changes in the body that increase the risk factors:

✓ Raises levels of LDL ("bad") cholesterol
✓ Raises levels of triglycerides (fats in the blood)
✓ Reduces levels of HDL ("good") cholesterol
✓ Elevates blood pressure

Obesity can aggravate liver disorders and osteoarthritis, and is often found in conjunction with gallbladder disease. Recent statistics show a staggering increase in the number of cases of type 2 diabetes, paralleling the increasing obesity rates in the United States. Although it was once considered an adult disease, the number of overweight children now being diagnosed with type 2 diabetes is staggering. This diabetes and obesity combination can lead to blindness, nerve damage, kidney failure, and cardiovascular disease.

Obesity complicates surgery and pregnancy. Pulmonary problems, sleep apnea, heat intolerance, and reduced fertility are more prevalent in the obese. In fact, after smoking, obesity is the biggest risk factor for cancer. The evidence that overweight and obesity increase the risk of a number of cancers is now even more impressive than in the mid-1990s. Among obese women there is an increased risk of cervical, uterine, colon, breast, and pancreatic cancers. Obese men face an increased chance of colon, stomach, rectal, and prostate cancers. In fact, according to the Institute for Cancer Research, excess weight may account for as much as 20 percent of all cancer deaths in women and 14 percent in men. Obesity restricts mobility, increases fatigue, and decreases overall body efficiency. Figure 12-2 shows the percent increase in the risk of various conditions related to specific BMIs.

The high prevalence of obesity in the United States not only is linked to numerous chronic dis-

eases but is responsible for a substantial portion of total health care costs. Obesity health care costs are $147 billion per year—double what it was nearly a decade ago. This figure does not include the psychosocial costs of obesity—from lowered self-esteem to eating disorders to severe depression. The psychological and social consequences of obesity are often overlooked. Obese people also face a tremendous amount of prejudice and discrimination. Their educational and professional opportunities often suffer.

Until recently, modest weight gains throughout adulthood in initially lean individuals were overlooked and even culturally expected. Results from the ongoing Harvard Nurses' Health Study (a 25-year tracking of more than 100,000 nurses) have revealed that even *modest* (11 to 17 lb.) weight gains after 18 years of age increase one's cardiovascular disease risk. The researchers concluded that a large fraction of the population is falsely reassured that their weight is not a health concern because they are not "overweight." The study found that a person's weight at midlife (30 to 55 years) has the greatest influence on heart disease risk. Those with a BMI of 23 to 27 had a 31 percent increased risk; those with the lowest risk had a BMI below 21. Those with a BMI ≥ 30 have a 50 to 100 percent increased risk of death from *all* causes, compared with those with healthy BMIs (19 to 24.9).

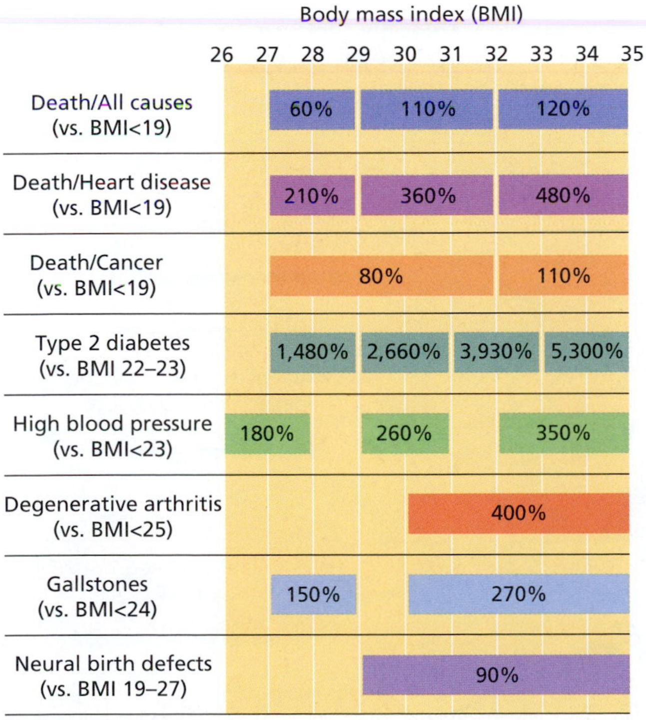

Body mass index (BMI)

	26	27	28	29	30	31	32	33	34	35
Death/All causes (vs. BMI<19)		60%		110%			120%			
Death/Heart disease (vs. BMI<19)		210%		360%			480%			
Death/Cancer (vs. BMI<19)				80%				110%		
Type 2 diabetes (vs. BMI 22–23)		1,480%	2,660%		3,930%		5,300%			
High blood pressure (vs. BMI<23)	180%			260%				350%		
Degenerative arthritis (vs. BMI<25)					400%					
Gallstones (vs. BMI<24)		150%			270%					
Neural birth defects (vs. BMI 19–27)				90%						

FIGURE 12-2   Weighing the risks: Percent increase in risk by level of obesity. At BMIs of 27 and higher, one's risk for various disorders increases significantly.

Sources: New England Journal of Medicine, Annals of Internal Medicine, American Journal of Clinical Nutrition, Journal of the American Medical Association.

◆ WHAT CAUSES OBESITY?

For years the simplistic explanation for obesity was that people became obese because they ate too much. Obesity was viewed as a condition resulting from a lack of self-control around food. In scientific terms, obesity occurs when a person's caloric intake exceeds the amount of energy that person burns. What causes this imbalance between consuming and burning calories is unclear. Evidence suggests that obesity is a complex combination of metabolic, genetic, psychological, behavioral, social, and environmental factors—not solely a result of a lack of individual willpower. It is clear that no single factor results in obesity. In an attempt to explain the causes of obesity, several factors have to be examined. They include energy balance, heredity, fat cells, set point, and metabolism.

The Energy Balance Equation

The energy balance equation states that energy input (calories consumed) must be equal to energy output (calories expended) for body weight to remain constant. Any imbalance in energy input or energy output will result in a change in body weight. If you eat more calories daily than your body expends in activity, you will store the excesses as fat. If you eat fewer calories than you burn, you will lose weight. It is unrealistic to assume that the equation must be exactly equal every day to maintain your weight. Some days you eat more; some days, less. Some days you are more active than you are on other days. Several days of imbalance in one direction will produce a change in body weight.

This explanation assumes that a calorie is a calorie, whether it is from candy or from a vegetable. A **calorie** (actually a **kcal**) is a measure of energy. One pound of body fat equals 3,500 calories of stored energy. Therefore, consuming an extra 3,500 calories will cause you to gain 1 pound of fat. If you burn an extra 3,500 calories with activity, you will lose 1 pound. To cause a reduction in body weight, you (1) reduce calorie intake below the energy requirement, (2) increase the calorie output through additional physical activity above energy requirements, or (3) combine the two methods by reducing calorie intake and increasing calorie output. So how do you lose 10 pounds? By creating a calorie deficit

of 500 calories daily (by increasing exercise or decreasing food intake) for 7 days, you will lose 1 pound (3,500 calories). By maintaining this deficit, you will be 10 pounds lighter in 10 weeks.

However, weight loss is not necessarily this simple. For some people, cutting calories causes feelings of fatigue, resulting in a decrease of energy expenditure. As body weight is reduced, the energy costs of movement go down proportionately, thus reducing caloric output. Also, individual differences in resting metabolic rates, cellular makeup, and lean tissue need to be considered. That is why knowledge about other factors is necessary to fully understand the complexities of weight loss.

Regardless of the problems that come with relying on the energy balance equation as the only way to understand weight loss and weight gain, this equation is the best way of explaining why, in this age of modernization and decreased physical demands, so many Americans are too fat. As Figure 12-3 shows, many factors contribute to our growing girth. Most are not active enough to use the calories consumed.

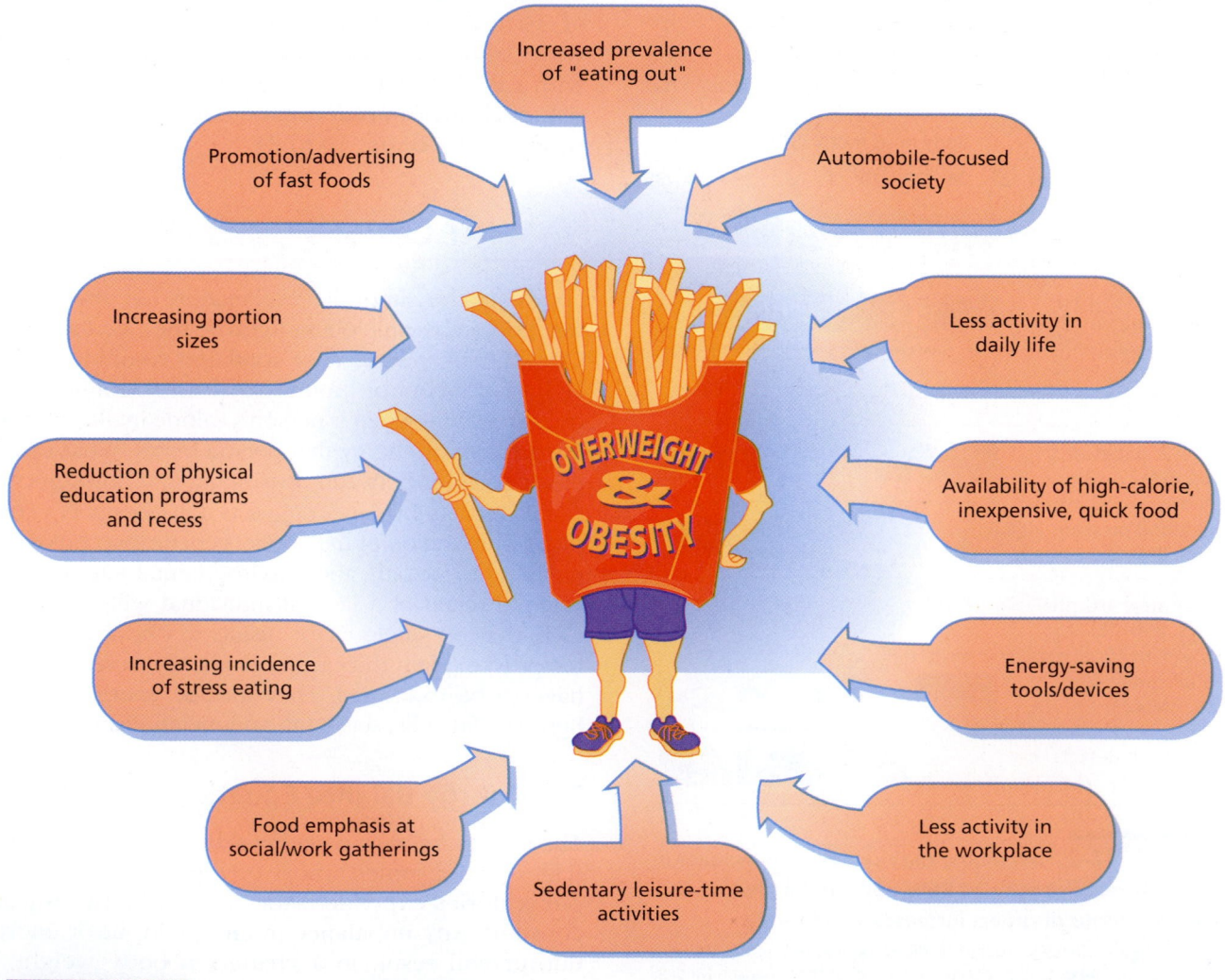

FIGURE 12-3 Many societal factors contribute to overweight/obesity.

TABLE 12-3   "Liquid" Calories and Sugar (per 12-ounce serving)

	Calories	Sugar (grams)
Amp Energy	220	58
Rockstar	280	62
Monster Energy	200	54
Red Bull	220	52
Starbucks Frappuccino	322	43
Starbucks Café Mocha	270	24
Starbucks Caramel Brulee	330	36
Pepsi	150	40
Dr. Pepper	150	39
Mountain Dew	165	46

Note: Alcohol, also a source of "empty calories," is an appetite stimulant and lowers inhibitions and willpower to control food intake.

Food in America is plentiful, available, and relatively inexpensive. It is also high in sugar, calories, and fat. More frequent eating is encouraged by numerous societal changes: The growth of the fast-food industry, 24-hour supermarkets, "pop-in" pantries, the increased incidence of snacking rather than sitting down to eat meals, the number of "all you can eat" buffets, and the growing tendency to socialize with food and drink have all added calories to our day. Although many people are consciously trying to eat lower-fat food items, *low fat* doesn't necessarily mean *low calorie*. The huge soft drink industry and the fast-growing energy drink market contribute to an excess of daily calories for many. Energy drinks are especially popular among young people. These drinks are basically soft drinks with added vitamins, herbs, caffeine, and sugars that are advertised to boost energy and alertness. Coffee drinks are also very popular. Look at Table 12-3 to see the calories and sugar in some of these drinks. Excessive consumption of such drinks can lead to irritability, insomnia, anxiety, heart palpitations, and, of course, weight gain. Surveys indicate that our daily caloric intake is increasing, while our caloric expenditure is decreasing. Countless labor-saving devices at home and at work and our passive leisure-time activities (television, Internet, computer games, videos) have contributed to creeping obesity. Phoning, faxing, e-mailing, online shopping, and express mail don't burn many calories (unless you're the express mail delivery person!). Many neighborhoods lack sidewalks or bike lanes for safe walking and riding, and the automobile is used to travel even the shortest distances. There are fewer opportunities in daily life to burn calories. We live increasingly sedentary lives.

How many calories do you need to maintain a desirable body weight? Table 12-4 helps you estimate your daily caloric need based on your activity level. Remember, this is only an approximation and may vary between individuals. To lose or gain weight, the calorie intake must be adjusted upward or downward. Remember, however, a woman should not eat fewer than 1,200 calories a day, and a man no fewer than 1,600 calories a day. It is difficult to obtain a balanced diet with fewer calories.

Heredity

"I can't lose weight; it's in my genes!" Many would view this exclamation made by many obese persons as an excuse for their physical state. Research about genetic influences on obesity lends some (but not *total*) credibility to this exclamation. Children with obese parents do have a greater tendency to become obese adults. Is this an inherited tendency or a result

TABLE 12-4   *Determining Your Daily Caloric Needs*

The following is a method for estimating the caloric needs for healthy, nonpregnant adults. Older individuals (over age 50) should further reduce calories by 10 to 20 percent. These are only estimates. Individual activity factors and body frames vary from person to person.

Formula: Weight × Activity level = Calories needed daily

Activity Level	Calories Needed per Pound per Day	
	Female	Male
Inactive (little or no regular exercise; desk job; light work)	×12–13	×14–15
Moderately Active (30 minutes of exercise at least 3–4 times per week; or job dictates moderate activity)	×14–15	×16–17
Very Active (45 minutes–1 hour of vigorous, sustained exercise 5–7 times per week; or job dictates considerable activity)	×16	×18

Example: female = 140 lbs × 14.5 (moderately active) = 2,030 calories per day

male = 180 lbs × 14.5 (inactive) = 2,610 calories per day

of inappropriate behaviors learned and reinforced at home? Studies of families (especially twins) have provided insights into this question. A classic study conducted by Claude Bouchard showed that adult identical twins were similar in *total* fat gain and *distribution* of fat gain when consistently overfed for 100 days. There were huge differences between pairs of twins in body weight gains, body composition changes, and waist/hip circumference changes. Between twins, however, there were striking similarities. Similar research shows that adult twins tend to be similar in body weight and body mass index regardless of whether they were raised together in the same home or separated in early childhood and raised in different environments. Heredity seems to influence the number of fat cells in the body, how much fat is stored, where it is stored, and metabolic rates. However, scientists have concluded that genetics is responsible for only 25 percent of these factors.

Some of the body's hormones may also be linked to obesity. One of those hormones is leptin. **Leptin** is a hormone that is secreted by fat cells and informs the brain about how large or small the body's fat stores are. As a result, this leptin-brain connection helps orchestrate complex metabolic actions that regulate appetite. These studies give us more insight into the body's chemistry but do not fully explain the massive increases in weight across all age groups. Cases of obesity based solely on hormone abnormalities are rare. Centers for Disease Control and Prevention (CDC) former director Jeffrey Koplan, MD, concurs: "Genes related to obesity are clearly not responsible for the epidemic of obesity, because the gene pool in the U.S. did not change significantly after 1980."

Although these facts address the role heredity plays in obesity, heredity is only a *tendency* or predisposing factor that can be influenced by environmental components and behaviors. Those people predisposed to be overweight or obese will have more difficulty controlling their weight, but it is certainly not impossible for them to attain and maintain a healthy weight with healthy eating habits and regular exercise.

Fat-Cell Theory

The size and number of fat cells in the body determine degrees of fatness. **Fat cells** (also known as **adipose cells**) are storage sites for energy. The body increases fat storage in two ways: by increasing the *number* of fat cells and by increasing the *size* of fat cells. As might be expected, the body increases its number of fat cells during infancy and puberty growth spurts. Fat cells also expand and

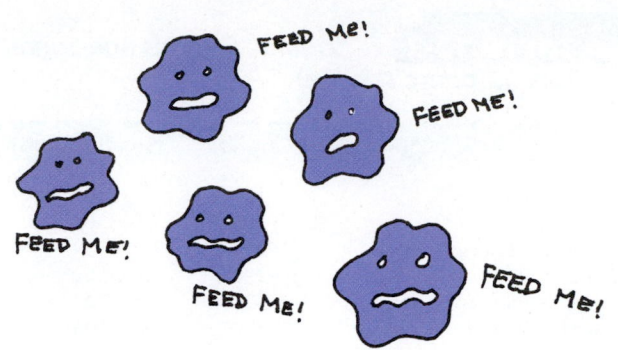

Most fat cells are with you forever.

contract as energy is stored or burned. They can expand to two to three times their normal size, but they cannot enlarge endlessly. At some point, new fat cells can be created in response to the body's need to store more excess energy. This can occur in extremely obese individuals. This capacity to increase cell numbers when a maximum cell size is reached depends on the age and sex of the person and the site of the fat tissue. Unfortunately, fat cells seem to be indestructible. A few studies using rats report that the hormone leptin (which is produced in the fat cells) has triggered the dying of some fat cells, but why this happened is unclear. An individual of normal weight has 30–50 billion fat cells, while an obese person can have as many as 60–100 billion fat cells.

Therefore, the fat-cell theory proposes that weight reduction in adults is a result of decreasing the size of the fat cells, shrinking them by using the energy stored in them or not filling them at all. This theory also explains why people who grow a large number of fat cells during childhood have a predisposition to obesity as adults. They can reduce the

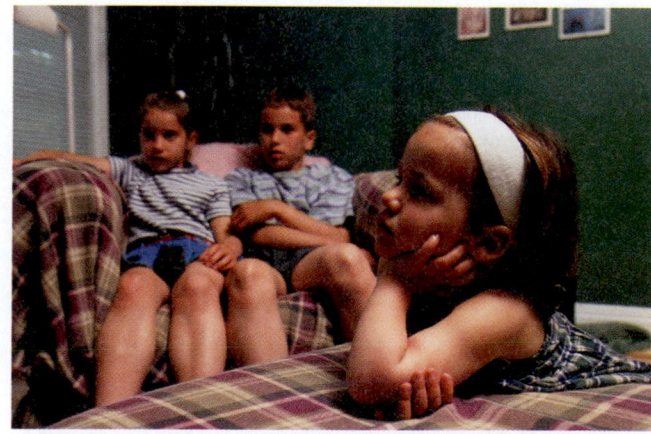

The percentage of obese children in the United States has almost tripled in the last 20 years. The 20-plus hours per week the average child spends watching TV and videos is one of the contributing factors.

amount of fat stored in the cells, but the excess number of fat cells is still there, waiting to be filled again.

It is important to realize that fat tissue is not an inert storage depot. Fat is actually a dynamic organ that produces a multitude of hormones and inflammatory proteins. These chemical messengers travel throughout the body and contribute to a multitude of chronic diseases.

Set-Point Theory

The **set-point theory** maintains that every individual is programmed to be a certain weight and that the body regulates itself to maintain that "set" weight. Studies of people in alternating states of semistarvation and gorging have shown that once intervention ceases, they return to their former weights. What determines your set point? The hypothalamus in the brain may act as a body weight thermostat, lowering body metabolism and increasing hunger if fat levels fall below the set point. Here is where the set-point theory and fat-cell theory merge. The set-point mechanism is thought to respond to signals sent out by the fat cells as to the amount of fat in storage. The weight at which this occurs may depend on the number of fat cells. Consider two 180-pound women. Sara has a normal number of fat cells, which are enlarged. Mary has an excessive number of fat cells of normal size. Sara has a greater chance of weight loss, because she can reduce her cell size and still sustain adequate fat volume. Mary faces a harder battle because her body will work to maintain her cell size. This theory also helps explain why attempts at permanent weight loss by crash dieting are not successful. The body naturally fights against this starvation state.

The set-point theory is based on survival. How else could populations endure famine or our ancestors survive periods of food shortages? Heredity influences the set point too. Some people have naturally higher set points, causing maintenance of higher levels of body fat, whereas other individuals have naturally low set points.

Can you change your set point? Some studies show that sustained consumption of a diet high in fats, refined carbohydrates, and perhaps even artificial sweeteners (the typical American diet?) raises the set point and that regular, vigorous exercise can lower the set point. Exercise stimulates changes in metabolism, causing the body to use fat rather than protect against its losses. Knowing this, it is easy to see how our sedentary lifestyles and dietary habits are connected to America's obesity problem more than are brain thermostat alterations. We've gone from lean to fat because we eat more and exert ourselves less.

Metabolism

Every individual expends a certain amount of energy, even at rest, to sustain vital functions of the body such as brain activities, organ function, and temperature regulation. This energy requirement is called the **basal metabolic rate (BMR)** and accounts for approximately 65 to 75 percent of the calories burned in 1 day. A true measure of basal metabolism is taken when you have been lying quietly but awake and without food for 12 to 15 hours. Most men have a BMR requirement of 1,600 to 2,000 calories daily; most women need 1,200 to 1,500 calories daily. Lab Activity 12-3 provides an opportunity to determine your BMR. BMR is the largest component of your daily energy expenditure, so it can significantly affect body weight over time.

Your BMR is a result of several interrelated factors, including age, gender, body size, nutritional status, musculature, activity level, and genetics. Pay particular attention to Table 12-5, which shows how BMR is affected by each of these factors.

Although some of your BMR is genetically inherited, you can affect it with exercise. An aerobic workout that includes resistance training (free

THE NUMBERS

300	Calories the average American consumes each day above the daily average of two decades ago.
$1,400	The additional annual medical costs for an obese person versus someone of normal weight.
90,000	Yearly deaths from cancer that could be avoided if every U.S. adult could maintain a BMI under 25.0 throughout life.
$147 billion	The direct and indirect costs associated with obesity per year in the United States.
2058	The year when everyone in the United States is predicted to be obese (if current obesity rates continue to rise as they have over the past 25 years).
22%	Reduction in life span for persons in their 20s who are obese.

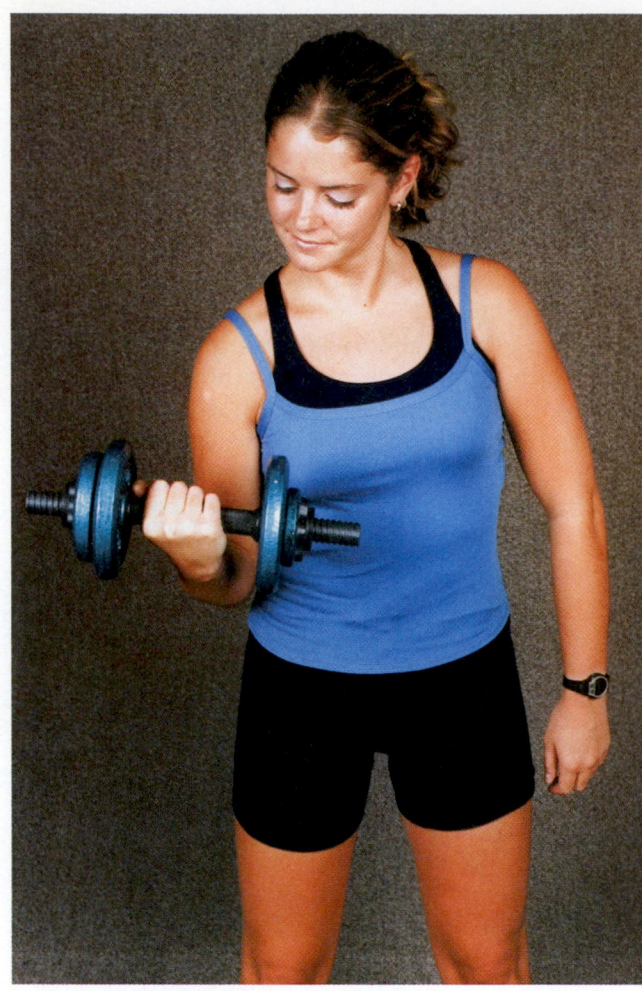

Doing resistance training exercises increases muscle mass, which in turn increases metabolism.

weights, machines, or exercise bands) can increase muscle mass. The more muscle mass you have, the higher your BMR. Fat, being storage tissue, has a low metabolism, whereas muscle tissue is active and has a high metabolism. Women especially can counteract a slow metabolism by participating in exercise programs that include resistance training. In this way, they can increase their muscle mass. Middle-aged women often experience a dramatic slowdown of their metabolisms due to hormonal changes. They too can keep their "energy burners" fired up with regular exercise. The actual workout burns calories too! Your total daily caloric expenditure is influenced by

1. Basal Metabolism = 65 to 75 percent.
2. Digestion = 10 percent (e.g., if you consume 2,000 calories a day, you burn 200 of them by digesting the food).
3. Physical Activity and Exercise = anywhere from 15 to 30 percent (*you* control this!). Remember, *all* physical activity burns calories.

TABLE 12-5	*Factors That Affect Basal Metabolic Rate*
Gender	Women generally have lower BMRs than do men (about 5 to 10 percent lower) due to smaller size, more body fat, and less muscle mass.
Musculature	Increased muscle mass or tone increases BMR. Muscle tissue is more metabolically active than is fat. As muscles atrophy from inactivity, BMR declines.
Age	For both men and women, BMR declines by about 2 to 3 percent per decade after age 25. Loss of lean muscle mass typically occurs with aging as well. Maintaining a regular exercise program (including resistance training) can help prevent a decline of lean muscle mass and BMR as you age.
Body size	Smaller body surface area, smaller build, or short height result in lower BMR.
Nutritional status	Fasting, very low-calorie diets, skipping meals, and long-term undernutrition lower BMR.
Activity level	BMR increases during exercise and may remain elevated somewhat after exercising. The more vigorous the exercise, the longer your metabolism stays elevated.
Genetics	We inherit physiological tendencies, and as a result, BMR is inherently higher in some people and lower in others. Thyroid abnormalities (hypothyroidism or hyperthyroidism) can affect metabolism.

◆ WHAT ABOUT "DIETING"?

Most people who want to lose weight think immediately of going on a diet. This notion is reinforced by the number of new fad diets advertised each year. In this connotation, the word *diet* implies a distinctive way of eating that involves special foods or food combinations; caloric or food restrictions; or special powders, pills, or shakes. In reality, the word *diet* should imply a way of eating for a lifetime. Popular weight-loss diets are viewed by the user as a temporary inconvenience that will be discontinued as soon as the weight goal has been reached. "Going on" a diet implies "going off" it. Dieters assume that weight will be lost quickly and immediately. Chances are, however, that the excess pounds have accumulated gradually over a period of years. These pounds are maintained by ingrained habits. Most fad diets rely on rigid food choices. Food becomes the enemy, and mealtime a battle to be fought. Continual deprivation can result in food cravings, binges, guilt, and self-deprecation. Many popular diets do not emphasize physical exercise. More than half the overweight adults trying to lose weight are doing so by restricting calories. Yet fewer than one-third are increasing physical activity. This is a reflection of our sedentary lifestyle and the emphasis on "going on a diet" as a means to control weight rather than increasing exercise. Diets have special appeal and sound easy. Many of them, however, are nutritionally inadequate, are too low in calories, are potentially dangerous, and, most important, fail to teach lifelong eating habits. Even with programs that result in weight loss, the results are often short-term—and regaining weight is common if habits have not been permanently changed.

If you go on a very low-calorie diet, up to 70 percent of the weight loss during the first 3 days is water. This is predictable because your body needs carbohydrates for energy. Being starved of carbohydrates, it uses **glycogen** (stored carbohydrates) for energy. As you use this glycogen, you lose water, because each gram of carbohydrate is stored with 3 grams of water. Your body also uses protein for energy, resulting in a loss of muscle tissue. Crash dieting can cause headaches, ketosis, and loss of bone mineralization. If you go on a very low-calorie diet (less than 800 calories per day), your body slows its metabolism (BMR) significantly. After all, your body doesn't know that there is a grocery store a block away. It reacts as if you were suffering from starvation. Therefore, your body saves energy by burning fewer calories. This conservation of energy causes the diet to be even less effective. Depression, irritability, fatigue, and feelings of deprivation often follow. The survival urge to eat eventually wins out and weight is regained.

There has been some debate in recent years that the increasing obesity in the United State can be blamed on a shift to a low-fat, high-carbohydrate emphasis in the past few decades. A recent long-range study shows that carbohydrates themselves do not cause weight gain. Excessive *calories* cause weight gain—whether they come from carbohydrates, protein, fats, jelly beans, or soda! Some scientists believe that high-fructose corn syrup added to soft drinks, juice drinks, breads, and some processed foods in the 1980s as an inexpensive sweetener has contributed to the obesity trend. High-fructose corn syrup seems to affect leptin resistance, thus causing weight gain. Similarly, artificial sweeteners used in most diet foods have been found to *increase* one's appetite by affecting leptin levels. Table 12-6 reviews some of the most popular diet plans. It is important to know the facts before trying any specialized plan.

Weight Cycling

Weight cycling is the repeated loss and regaining of body weight. When weight cycling is the result of low-calorie or fad dieting, it is often called the **yo-yo syndrome.** There have been claims that weight cycling may make it more difficult to lose weight or keep it off, increase fat stores, slow metabolism, or even contribute to an increased risk of death from heart disease. Studies have not supported these claims conclusively. Most obesity experts believe that obese individuals should continue efforts to lose weight. Any weight loss is better than facing the potential risks of remaining obese or experiencing weight cycling.

Weight cycling should not affect the success of future weight-loss efforts. As with any attempt at changing behavior, you may experience cycles of success and lapses before finally succeeding. All people, whether they have dieted or not, experience a slowing of metabolism with aging. And a substantial weight loss results in a reduction in caloric needs. Therefore, it is important to monitor caloric intake and exercise habits to prevent weight cycling. This information accentuates even more dramatically the need to learn *skills* for maintaining weight loss and to *prevent* obesity from occurring altogether. Losing weight—and maintaining a healthy weight—is a lifelong commitment.

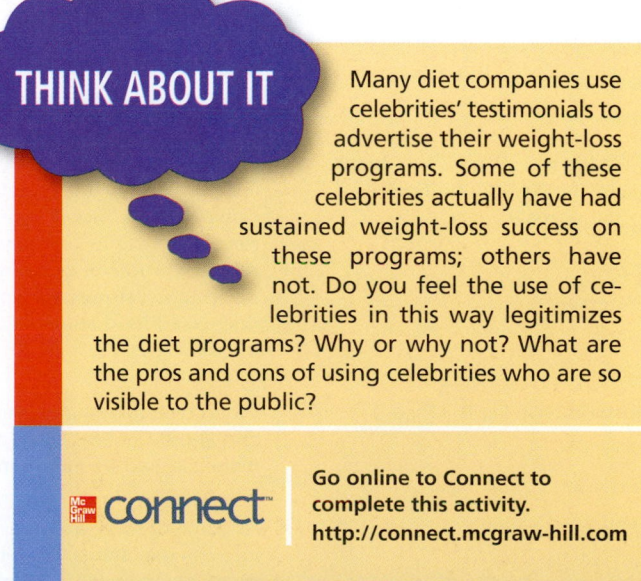

THINK ABOUT IT   Many diet companies use celebrities' testimonials to advertise their weight-loss programs. Some of these celebrities actually have had sustained weight-loss success on these programs; others have not. Do you feel the use of celebrities in this way legitimizes the diet programs? Why or why not? What are the pros and cons of using celebrities who are so visible to the public?

connect   Go online to Connect to complete this activity. http://connect.mcgraw-hill.com

TABLE 12-6 *Diet Plans: Claims and Reality*

Diet Plan	Claims	Reality
Commercial weight-loss companies (Weight Watchers, L.A. Weight Loss, Jenny Craig, NutriSystem, etc.)	Adheres to balanced eating. Provides advice on portions, food choices, calorie intake. Moderate loss of 1–2 lb. per week. Some individual counseling and group support. (Note: Some commercial companies require purchase of their prepackaged foods, which can be expensive and high in sodium.)	Can be safe and effective if healthy lifelong eating habits and portion control are learned. The support system and personalized counseling are helpful. Can be costly.
Meal-replacement drinks/bars (Slim-Fast, Ensure, Boost, Carnation Instant Breakfast)	A liquid shake or bar replaces one or two meals a day. Contain protein and vitamins. Some are low in calories; others are not so low. Most are very high in carbohydrates and sugar.	May still be hungry; less satisfying. Often high in sugar. Lacks fiber. Weight often regained when stopped because proper food selection has not been learned. Some bars are "candy" in disguise. Read the label.
"Fat-burning" diets (cabbage soup diet, grapefruit diet, etc.)	Certain foods can accelerate the body's ability to burn fat. Eating large quantities of these foods results in fast weight loss.	No foods exclusively burn fat. Low in calories (which causes the weight loss). Boring and not nutritionally balanced. Weight is regained easily.
Low-carbohydrate/high-protein diets (Atkins, South Beach, Carbohydrate Addicts, etc.)	Restricts carbohydrates such as bread, cereals, starchy vegetables. Claims that carbs increase insulin, which promotes fat accumulation. Eat a lot of protein and fat. Transitions to phases that add complex carbohydrates and some fruits and vegetables.	Early phase is hard to stick with. Low calories. Loss of water and muscle causes the weight loss. High fat and low calcium can contribute to future diseases. May cause bad breath, fatigue, dizziness, muscle weakness, headaches, and constipation in early phases. Final phases are better balanced.
Low-fat diets (Ornish, Volumetrics, Pritikin)	Fat-free and low-fat foods and a lot of fruits, vegetables, whole grains, beans. Promotes foods high in fiber and water. Weight loss occurs despite eating ample amounts of low-calorie foods.	Healthy for heart and cancer prevention. Effective for weight loss but hard for some to adhere to due to lack of fats and sweets. May be low in calcium and iron if not careful. Exercise is emphasized.
Diet pills	Claim to burn fat, absorb extra fat, increase metabolism, and/or suppress appetite.	Promoted as a "quick fix." May contain amphetamine-like substances (ephedra, yerba mate, caffeine, guarana, bitter orange), which may cause heart irregularities and jitters. Some herbs may help with appetite in some, but safety is an issue. Lifelong eating habits not learned.
Glycemic index ("The Glucose Revolution," "Good Carbs, Bad Carbs")	Carbohydrates that break down quickly (i.e., have a high glycemic index—GI) cause a quick blood sugar and insulin rise, resulting in fat storage. Slow-release carbohydrates (low GI) fill you up, cause a slower release of glucose, decrease blood sugar fluctuations, and burn body fat.	Is a balanced approach of consuming adequate protein, low fat (under 30%), and 60% carbohydrate (of low GI: whole grains, legumes, vegetables, fruits) and reducing refined breads, cereals, rices, potatoes, and snacks). Is sensible and healthy, but requires distinguishing high-GI from low-GI foods.
Blood type (A, B, O, etc.)	Blood type determines what food should and should not be eaten for health, leanness, and overall immune health.	No scientific evidence backs this theory.
Cleansing diets	In place of food; a mixture of lemon juice, maple syrup, ginger, cayenne pepper, and water is drunk, resulting in weight loss and detoxification.	No evidence that detoxification occurs. Lacks protein, fiber, and essential nutrients. Lose lean tissue and water weight.

Reliable Weight-Loss Programs

Are there any reliable weight-loss programs? Yes. There are some good programs available, as long as the dieter understands the purpose and limitations of commercial plans. Enrolling in a weight-control program is an investment of time, energy, and money. Ask yourself if you are ready to lose the weight *and* do what it takes to keep it off. Losing the weight is only half the battle. Keeping it off demands lifestyle changes that are lifelong. It is especially important for the morbidly obese to seek professional help in losing weight. These persons would be wise to consult one of the hospital-based programs available in many communities or meet with a registered dietitian. New fad diets appear almost weekly and disappear almost as quickly, so it is unrealistic to assess every particular diet for strengths and weaknesses. Instead, look at the Top 10 "Guidelines for Evaluating a Weight-Loss Program." Many weight-management specialists view Weight Watchers as a reliable weight-loss program because it incorporates many of the principles that contribute to success: balanced eating, portion control, counseling and support, regular

exercise, and teaching lifelong eating behaviors. It has been around since 1963 and was developed by registered dietitians and specialists in weight management.

The goal of weight loss is fat loss, which takes time and long-term lifestyle change. Remember: It is not necessary for an overweight or obese person to reach an optimal body weight in order to begin experiencing health benefits. Even modest increments of weight loss are associated with improvements in blood pressure and other health parameters. Many diets are variations on the food restriction theme, are unpleasant, and fail to teach modification of eating behavior. Scarcity and deprivation often lead to bingeing and subsequent feelings of guilt and despair. Just about any type of food restriction will result in weight loss. The key is keeping the weight off by learning to live with food—forever!

LIFETIME WEIGHT MANAGEMENT: STAYING LEAN IN FATTENING TIMES

The factors that contribute to obesity are so numerous and complex that it is impossible to pinpoint one cause. Having knowledge of the theories of obesity should help you understand some of these complexities. Fat cells, metabolism, set points, genetics, and energy expenditure all play a role. Behaviors that have developed over time are also intricately involved. One unrefuted truth emerges in nearly all weight-control studies: *Permanent weight control involves a lifelong commitment to good eating habits and regular exercise.*

Dr. James O. Hill, director of the University of Colorado Center for Human Nutrition, states, "You need to use your intellect to *not* gain weight today. Social forces that promote overeating and our modern sedentary lifestyle are so persuasive that you always need to think about what you're buying, what you're eating, and how active you are." Weight management is a *lifestyle*. Maintaining a reasonable body composition is, rather than isolated bouts of crash dieting or sporadic exercise, a result of lifelong integration of three management components:

1. Food management
2. Emotional management
3. Exercise management

(1) Food Management

We must eat to sustain life, and eating is one of life's pleasures. To lose or maintain weight, it is essential to have a good framework for making sensible, well-balanced food choices. Basic weight-management principles are not different from general good nutritional recommendations (low saturated fat, sugar, and salt and high complex carbohydrates, fruits and vegetables, and fiber). Cutting back on the unhealthy fats and sugars in your diet reduces a tremendous number of calories. "I lost weight without eating less!" is often the exclamation of persons who substitute fiber-rich grains, fruits, and vegetables for fats and sugars in their diets. Fiber fills you up and slows the absorption of food, which regulates blood sugar and insulin levels. Eating small amounts of protein with each meal or snack can help with satiety and feelings of fullness. This eating plan not only helps with weight, it helps prevent disease while ensuring adequate intake of all essential nutrients. The *Dietary Guidelines* and MyPyramid (see Chapter 11) describe such an eating plan.

By consistently consuming more calories than are needed, creeping obesity occurs. This is happening in most industrialized countries in the world. Managing food intake in our modern world is a definite challenge. Understanding the following factors that contribute to this caloric imbalance may help you monitor your own food intake.

RECOGNIZING PORTION DISTORTION

A European tourist stared with disbelief at his plate while eating in an American restaurant. "That's not a burrito," he said. "It's a log!"

Many foreign visitors are shocked at the portion sizes in America. Portion and serving sizes have increased tremendously in the past 25 years. As confirmed by a study published in the *Journal of the American Medical Association,* portion sizes since the 1980s have doubled, and in some cases tripled or quadrupled, for most foods served in restaurants and at home. Restaurant plates are larger and are overfilled with pasta, nachos, and chicken wings. Parking lots at all-you-can-eat buffets are packed. And research shows that the more food that is put in front of us, the more we will eat. In 1957, a fast-food hamburger weighed 1 ounce and had 210 calories. Today's average burger is 6 ounces and has 618 calories. A typical serving of a soft drink used to be 8 ounces. Today, a small serving is 12 ounces, and a large serving is 32 ounces. A typical restaurant serving of pasta exceeds the federal recommended serving size by 480 percent! And, with the introduction of fat-free foods, many people erroneously believe that they can eat the entire box of fat-free cookies, neglecting the fact that these foods have calories too. Overall calorie consumption cannot be ignored! It may be helpful to actually weigh and measure your food for several days when eating at home to increase your awareness and help you monitor your intake. It is particularly helpful when dining out to be able to look at your servings and compare them to everyday objects. In this way you can get a quick estimate of your portions and avoid overeating. Check out Table 12-7 for some easy comparisons. Some companies now make prepackaged 100-calorie snacks that are helpful in monitoring calorie intake.

AVOIDING MINDLESS EATING

"I hardly eat anything! Why can't I lose weight?" This question is a common complaint voiced by frustrated dieters. Because we have a culture of snacking and eating on the run, many people underestimate the calories they consume since they seldom sit down

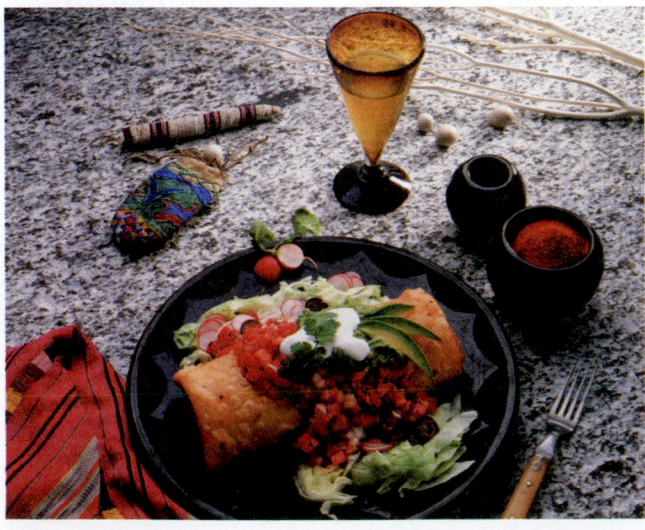

As restaurant portions become larger, Americans are "supersizing" their way to obesity.

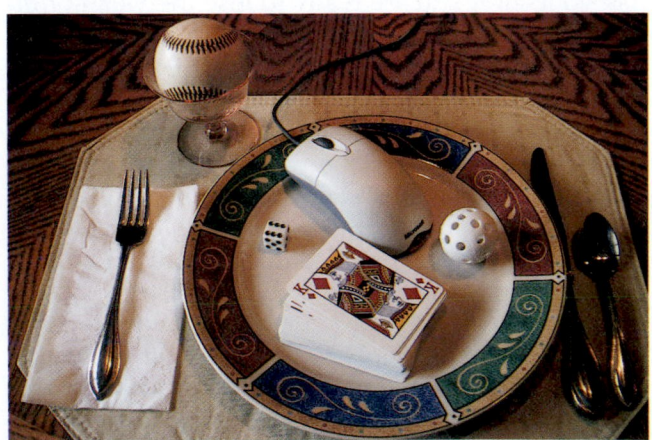

Be aware of serving sizes. Using common everyday references can help you manage your portions.

TABLE 12-7	*Eyeball Your Servings*

1 cup = baseball or closed fist
3 oz. serving of meat = deck of cards or palm of your hand
3 oz. serving of fish = checkbook
1 oz. cheese = 4 dice or size of your thumb
1 baked potato = computer mouse
2 tablespoons peanut butter = golf ball
¼ almonds = 12 almonds
1 pancake = compact disc
1 bagel = hockey puck or 6-oz. can of tuna
½ cup cooked rice or pasta = light bulb
1 oz. lunch meat = compact disc
1 tablespoon butter or spread = poker chip
1 muffin or biscuit = hockey puck
1 tablespoon salad dressing, mayonnaise, or oil = poker chip

for a real meal. The donut in the break room, the mocha coffee from the coffee stand, the chocolate kisses from the candy dish, the taste-testing at the grocery store, and the sack of chips while watching television all count! The 2,000 calories consumed a day from a plate are reasonable, but another 1,000 calories nibbled, grazed on, or grabbed mindlessly throughout the day add up. Even though Americans are consciously consuming less fat as a percentage of total calories, today's average daily calorie intake is up about 300 calories as compared to 1980. Keeping an *honest* food journal for several days (see Lab Activity 12-2 for a sample journal) can help you see what and how much food/calories you are eating and drinking. By becoming conscious of everything you put into your mouth you can begin to eat *mindfully* rather than *mindlessly*!

UNDERSTANDING OUR "TOXIC" ENVIRONMENT

We live in an environment that provides food most everywhere and at any time of the day. It's conveniently packaged, inexpensive, good-tasting, and served in ample portions. Unfortunately much of it is poor quality in terms of nutrition. Dr. Kelly Brownell, director of the Yale Center for Eating and Weight Disorders, has termed our food environment as "toxic." We are surrounded by temptations to eat wherever we go—on street corners, along highways, at gas stations, at the office, at the malls, and in school hallways. We are barraged by over 10,000 food advertisements each year on television—most of which are from fast-food chains or from soft drink and snack food companies. The commercials say, "Eat, eat, eat" but show an actress who is so thin that it appears she never eats! Food messages often drown out health messages. For example, more than $33 billion per year is spent on advertising sugary

soft drinks, candy, and fatty snacks. In contrast, it is rare to see an advertisement for fruits or vegetables. So, what can you do? First of all, tune into your natural hunger signals and vow not to eat just because you are driving past the donut shop, walking past a vending machine, or talking with friends who are snacking. Pay attention to the social and environmental influences that confront you, and do not accept cultural reality as a license to splurge! And finally, become an advocate for environmental change. Education and public information are not enough to change the environment. Support new laws that regulate advertising, prohibit the sale of fast foods and soft drinks in schools, subsidize healthy foods, and require the posting of nutrition information in restaurants.

Whereas many people look to structured weight-loss diets for their "food management," such programs often feature a lot of "can have" and "cannot have"

Tips for Behavior Change for Weight Management

Refer to the Stage of Change flowchart on page 406. What is your stage of change after answering the questions and tracing the flowchart?

Refer to Figure 2.2 (p. 36) to see which processes of change are most effective for facilitating your transition from your current stage to the next stage (or *maintaining* your behavior if you are already in the maintenance stage). Here are some behavioral examples for selected processes of change:

- Emotional arousal: Think about a relative or friend who suffered from multiple health problems and a premature death due to obesity.
- Self-reevaluation: List the pros and cons of reducing the calories in your diet and adding more exercise to your daily life. Make notes on why this change is important to you.
- Self-liberation: Keep a daily journal of calories consumed and calories expended.
- Countering: Substitute the candy and chips in your room that you typically snack on with fruit.
- Helping relationships: Ask your roommate or a friend to join you in this endeavor.

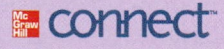 Go online to Connect to complete this activity.
http://connect.mcgraw-hill.com

foods. Sensibility in food choices does not mean that you will never again eat chocolate cake. There should never be guilt or forbidden foods. Instead, lifetime food management means seeing how much or where chocolate cake fits into your total diet. Reduce, don't eliminate, certain foods. Balance your food choices over time. Gradual rather than drastic changes in dietary patterns lead to successful maintenance. Healthful eating does not happen by accident, and it is not always easy. In our "land of plenty" it is essential to learn about the nutritive value of foods, portion sizes, and why we are eating, and devise strategies for making good choices over the course of each day.

(2) Emotional Management

Why do you eat? "Because I am hungry!" you answer. If all people ate only when they were in the physiological state of hunger, few would have a weight problem. Not only are we surrounded with opportunities to eat more than we need to, eating behavior is strongly influenced by psychological, social, and emotional factors. We eat out of emotional needs. We eat when we're happy; we eat when we're sad. Food becomes a substitute for other things. We confuse physical hunger with emotional hunger. Whereas it is true that food affects the brain's production of certain "feel good" chemicals, habitually using food as a "drug" to cope with emotional feelings can be destructive.

Controlling eating habits begins with understanding why you eat and what cues trigger eating. Do you eat when you are bored? Lonely? Angry? Stressed? Do you eat when you turn on the television? Read? Do you eat when something smells good? When others are eating? To avoid studying? Even positive feelings can trigger eating—earning an A on a paper, celebrating the end of final exams, looking forward to the weekend. For emotional eaters, food serves as a comfort. Their "fix" is food, a means of self-nurturing.

For emotional management, spend time observing your eating behavior. Keep a journal, recording the food you are eating and the feelings that accompany that moment. (There is a food journal in Lab Activity 12-2 at the end of this chapter.) Learn to recognize the cues and connections between your thoughts, feelings, and behaviors. Before you eat, ask yourself, "Why am I reaching for food at this time?" Learn to differentiate between hunger and appetite. *Hunger* is an actual physical need for food. *Appetite* is a desire for food that is usually triggered by anxiety, boredom, depression, stress, habit, or the mere availability of food. No diet plan works if it doesn't help you understand

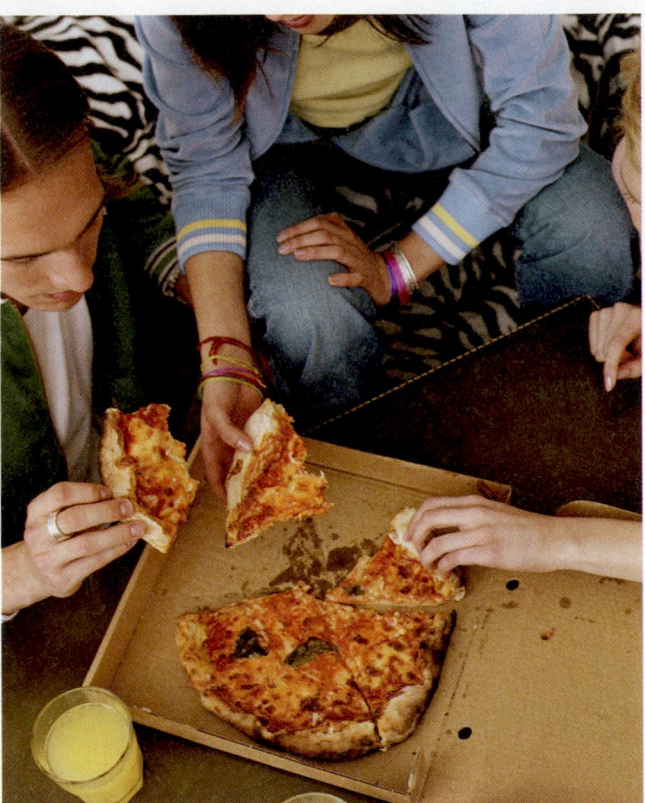

Many times we overeat in social situations even when we're not really hungry.

and resolve the reasons you turn to food when you aren't physically hungry. If you are one of those people who experience occasional food cravings, try using the 3 D'S.

✓ *Delay* at least 10 minutes before you eat so that your action is conscious, not impulsive.
✓ *Distract* yourself by engaging in an activity that requires concentration (e.g., play the guitar, surf the Internet, do a crossword puzzle, read a magazine).
✓ *Distance* yourself from the food.
✓ *Substitute* a small portion or healthier version of the craved food (e.g., a chocolate kiss instead of a whole candy bar, frozen yogurt rather than premium ice cream, veggie pizza instead of pepperoni).

Using behavior modification strategies can help emotional eaters. **Behavior modification** is the use of techniques to enhance awareness or consciousness of a behavior and subsequently alter that behavior. Behavior modification is based on the premise that all behaviors are learned responses to environmental cues or antecedents. In using these techniques, people make eating a more conscious act, and healthier behavior patterns are integrated into the day-to-day routine. These patterns include slowing the act

TABLE 12-8   Behavior Modification Techniques

1. Keep a food journal to maximize awareness of eating.
2. Eat in one room only; sit at a table—don't stand.
3. Prepackage healthy snacks or meals and take them with you.
4. Keep a weight, fat gram, or calorie graph.
5. Never read or watch TV while eating.
6. Use smaller plates.
7. Always leave some food on your plate.
8. Drink a lot of water throughout the day and during meals.
9. Prepare, serve, and eat one portion at a time.
10. Do not place serving dishes on the table.
11. Grocery shop from a list and never on an empty stomach.
12. Leave the table after eating and clear dishes directly into the compost pile or garbage; brush your teeth immediately or chew gum.
13. Keep problem food out of sight or not in the house.
14. Keep healthy food accessible and visible.
15. Make eating a conscious experience (i.e., eat slowly; chew each bite thoroughly; put utensils down between bites; eat with your nondominant hand; cut food into smaller pieces).
16. Rehearse strategies in advance for eating out, special occasions, and high-risk situations.
17. Substitute alternative activities for eating (do a sudoku puzzle; go for a walk; sew; play an instrument; call a friend; etc.).
18. Don't do non-food-related activities in the kitchen; stay out of the kitchen as much as possible; close the kitchen down after a meal.
19. When eating out, plan to share large portions with a companion. Or take extras home for another meal.
20. Eat and snack from a plate, not the package, so you don't absentmindedly eat more than you realize.

TABLE 12-9   Tips for Behavior Change: Losing Weight

Stages of Change: In What Stage Are You?

1. Precontemplation: "As far as I'm concerned I'm not too heavy. I'm just big-boned."
2. Contemplation: "I think I should probably lose some weight; maybe after the holidays I'll try."
3. Preparation: "I am currently planning my weight-loss program."
4. Action: "I have been making the lifestyle changes I need to make to lose weight (dietary change and exercise) for 3 months, and it is working."
5. Maintenance: "I have been successful at losing weight and maintaining that loss for over 6 months."

Processes of Change

After identifying your current stage, try using some of the following selected processes and behavior strategies that are appropriate for your particular stage—to facilitate your transition into the next stage (refer to Figure 2-2):

- Consciousness-raising: Read about people who have lost weight.
- Social liberation: Check out low-fat and low-calorie options at your favorite lunch/dinner spots.
- Self-reevaluation: Assess and write down your feelings and disappointments due to your dependence on food.
- Reward: Treat yourself to a low-fat frozen yogurt or a small piece of chocolate every Saturday after a week of healthy food choices.
- Environment control: Throw out junk-food snacks stored in desk drawer/shelves.
- Helping relationships: Ask roommate to refrain from storing/eating snacks in your room; invite a friend to join you in making dietary/exercise changes.

of eating, altering susceptibility to the cues (separating eating from other activities, such as watching TV), and breaking behavior chains. Set yourself up for success by managing your environment. For example, throw out the cookies stashed in your desk drawer, the chips in your cabinet, and the candy in your glove compartment. It is true that our "food frenzy" culture is a temptation-rich environment, but it is an environment over which *you* have control! Table 12-8 gives examples of some behavior modification techniques.

Changing eating behavior demands commitment and perseverance (unlike the magic potions or easy pitches delivered in many popular magazines). Too often, commercial weight-loss programs reward persons for the total number of pounds lost, creating undesirable behaviors such as going on crash diets,

skipping meals, and using drugs and diuretics. According to some weight-management researchers, the use of rewards for weight loss is inappropriate because weight loss is not a behavior. It is the outcome of a complex interaction of emotions and behaviors over time. As discussed in Chapter 2, behavior change is a complex process that involves stages and coping techniques within each stage. You may want to go back to Chapter 2 and review the transtheoretical model of behavior change to see which techniques can be incorporated into managing emotional eating. Table 12-9 may help you identify your stage of change in terms of weight loss. Some example techniques are listed with selected processes as well. To continue with or maintain weight loss, you must be able to identify your high-risk situations in which difficulties with feelings or social situations can lead to a relapse. Developing and practicing coping strategies for dealing with these situations is an essential part of emotional management. Remove yourself from former patterns of behavior and develop new rituals that will ensure your success. Food stops taking on the role of nurturer when people learn to nurture themselves. Long-lasting change can occur only through kindness to yourself, mindfulness about what you are doing and why, and a willingness to act on your own behalf.

(3) Exercise Management

Dieting alone may help you lose a few pounds, but long-term weight loss requires regular physical activity. Exercise is crucial to losing weight and maintaining weight. Americans have become fatter because calorie output has declined drastically. Most of our work, daily activities, and even some of our leisure pursuits do not burn many calories.

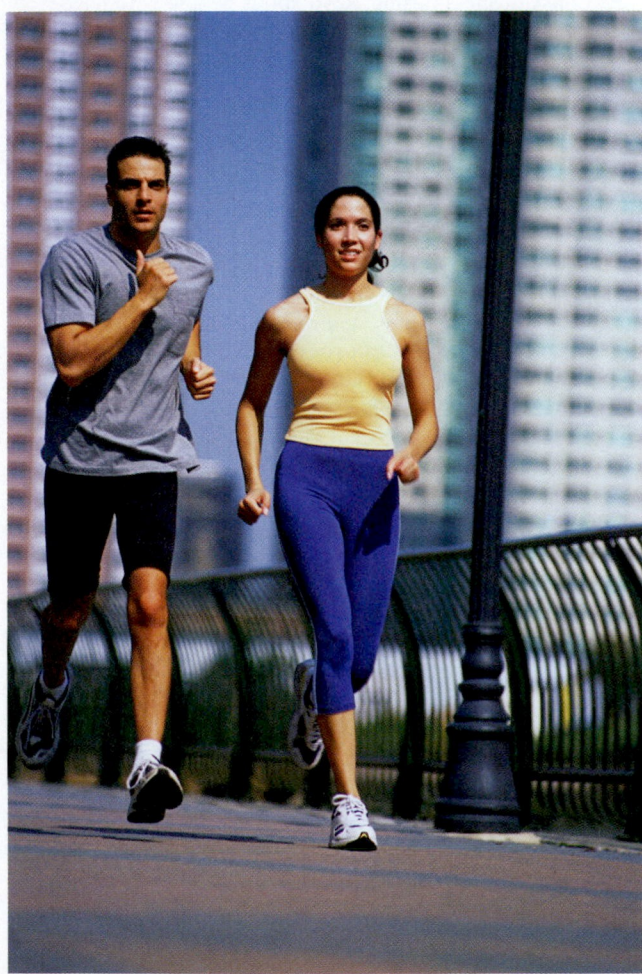

Participating in regular vigorous exercise is essential for lifelong weight management.

Television viewing, which substantially decreases activity levels and may influence diet, is a strong factor in obesity, especially among children and adolescents. In adults there is a direct relationship between the number of hours spent watching television and a person's level of obesity. The Internet, computers, video games, and home movies have decreased overall activity levels. American technology has been ingenious in discovering ways for us to save energy, thus throwing off our energy balance. Electric garage door openers, riding lawn mowers, elevators, and drive-up banks are a few examples of activity-robbing conveniences.

The importance of physical activity in the prevention and treatment of obesity receives less attention than restrictive "dieting." There is certainly no scarcity of diet books and programs. However, for lifetime weight management to occur, exercise (accompanied by dietary management) is imperative. According to the National Weight Control Registry, a group of women and men who have lost at least 30 pounds and maintained that weight loss for at least 1 year, regular exercise is a common trait of successful "losers." This group reports that they average 1 hour or more of moderate- to vigorous-intensity physical activity every day. Although the immediate effects of exercise are sometimes limited, the long-term cumulative effects of small changes in activity level are key components in lifetime weight management. By reengineering some physical activity back into our daily routine (called "lifestyle physical activity") and by fitting in 30–60 minutes of moderate-intensity activity every day, lifetime weight goals can be reached. Plus, living a physically active lifestyle substantially reduces the risk for a variety of other chronic diseases! Look at how regular exercise contributes to fat loss.

✓ **It Burns Calories**   Table 12-10 shows how many calories you burn per minute in various activities. Note that the larger person burns more energy than does the lighter person engaged in the same activity. Also notice how aerobic activities burn considerably more calories per minute than do light, day-to-day tasks. Most people burn approximately 100 calories per mile whether walking or jogging. If this does not seem like a lot, look at it this way: You burn only about 1 calorie per minute while sitting. Remember that weight gain does not occur overnight; nor does weight loss. A pound of fat is lost by burning 3,500 calories. No one ever said it must all be done at once and only by jogging. Liberating large amounts of energy from body reservoirs requires time—typically measured in months, if not years.

TABLE 12-10	*Caloric Expenditure per Minute for Selected Activities*

The figures in this table are only for the *time* you are engaged in the activity (not standing, waiting, resting). Variances may occur if you are running uphill, walking with hand weights, biking into a strong head wind, and so on. There may be small differences between males and females, but not enough to make a significant difference. You can approximate your expenditure if you are between the body weights listed. For information on calories burned in a more expansive list of activities, go to www.caloriesperhour.com or www.caloriccontrol.org.

Body Weight	120	150	180	210
Sitting and writing	1.5	1.9	2.3	2.7
Standing with light work, cleaning, etc	3.3	4.1	4.9	5.7
Aerobic dance	7.3	9.1	10.9	12.7
Basketball (recreational)	6.0	7.5	9.0	10.5
Bicycling (10 mph; 6 min/mile)	5.1	6.4	7.6	8.9
Bicycling (15 mph; 4 min/mile)	8.7	10.9	13.1	15.3
Dancing (active; square; disco)	5.4	6.8	8.2	9.5
Deep water treading/running	12.0	15.0	18.0	21.0
Golf (foursome, carrying clubs)	3.3	4.1	4.9	5.7
Racquetball	7.8	9.8	11.7	13.7
Roller skating (9 mph)	5.1	6.4	7.6	8.9
Running (6 mph; 10 min/mile)	8.7	10.9	13.1	15.4
Running (7 mph; 8:35 min/mile)	10.2	12.8	15.4	17.9
Running (8 mph; 7:30 min/mile)	11.6	14.6	17.6	20.5
Skiing, downhill; cross country (4 mph; 15 min/mile)	7.8	9.9	11.9	13.8
Soccer	7.2	9.0	10.8	12.6
Stair step machine	5.7	7.0	8.7	10.2
Stationary cycling (vigorous)	7.8	9.7	11.7	13.6
Swimming (crawl, 35 yds/min)	5.9	7.3	8.8	10.2
Swimming (crawl, 45 yds/min)	6.9	8.7	10.4	12.2
Tennis (recreational singles)	6.0	7.5	9.0	10.6
Walking (3 mph; 20 min/mile)	3.3	4.1	4.9	5.7
Walking (4 mph; 15 min/mile)	5.1	6.4	7.6	8.9
Walking (5 mph; 12 min/mile)	6.5	8.2	9.8	11.5
Water aerobics	7.2	9.0	10.8	12.6
Weight training	6.2	7.8	9.4	11.2

Whereas 30 minutes of exercise per day is recommended for overall health, recent research reveals that to lose weight and maintain weight loss, much more caloric expenditure from exercise is necessary. Studies indicate that burning approximately 2,800 calories a week with exercise (about 400 calories daily) should be the goal if weight is an issue. This would equate to about 1 hour of moderate-intensity activity per day or walking 4 miles. If more vigorous exercise is preferred (e.g., jogging, aerobic dance, lap swimming), about 40 minutes per day is recommended. As exercise intensity becomes more vigorous, an added benefit is that your metabolism (rate of calorie burning) is increased for several hours after you have completed the exercise bout. However, regardless of intensity level, doing regular, sustained exercise on a consistent basis (on most days of the week) is the best strategy for maintaining weight. And don't forget that doing intermittent activity throughout the day also burns calories.

Find ways to weave increased energy expenditure into day-to-day living: Walk to work or during breaks, take stairs instead of elevators, ride a bike on errands. Wear a pedometer and try to accumulate the recommended 10,000 steps per day.

✓ **It Prevents Loss of Lean Muscle Mass**   As you age, you lose about 2 percent of your muscle mass each year. By the time you are 55, you could be down 15 pounds of muscle and burning about 600 fewer calories per day. Exercise builds and helps maintain muscle tissue. And since muscle cells are metabolically active, they burn more calories in basal metabolism (at rest) than do fat cells. At rest, muscle tissue burns approximately 40 calories per day per pound. At rest, fat tissue burns approximately 2 calories per day per pound. As a result, someone with a lot of muscle mass burns more calories throughout the day *outside* the exercise session. This is a key factor especially for women of all ages (who typically have less

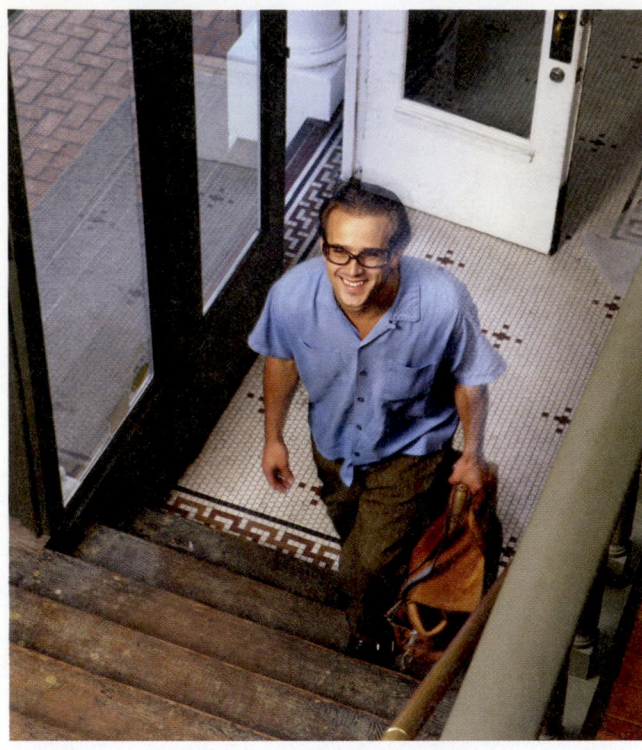

Regularly taking the stairs rather than the elevator is one way to add more activity to your day.

muscle mass and more fat than men) and for *both* men and women during middle age, when metabolism can slow down due to loss of muscle tissue. Doing resistance training exercises 2 to 3 days per week using free weights, machines, or an exercise band, along with daily aerobic exercise can accelerate weight loss.

✓ **It Decreases Abdominal Fat** Excessive fat in the abdominal area (apple-shape obesity) is linked to increased risk of heart disease, many cancers, and type 2 diabetes. Studies show that most of the positive effects of physical activity on heart disease risk factors (especially blood pressure and cholesterol) have to do with reductions in this intra-abdominal fat. This is true for both men and women. Since fat around the abdominal area is easier to mobilize than is fat in the hip/thigh area, regular physical activity attacks abdominal fat very effectively.

✓ **It Is a Natural Appetite Suppressor** Moderate exercise has a tendency to decrease the appetite for a time after the workout because blood is diverted from digestive organs to skeletal muscles. You may feel thirsty but not usually hungry. This is why exercising during a lunch break helps you control weight. After exercising, you feel satisfied with a light lunch. Extremely intense exercise tends to lower blood

sugar, which may stimulate appetite. To burn fat, keep your exercise at a moderate intensity and work to increase the duration. (Be sure not to view exercise as an excuse for eating more!)

✓ **It May Lower Your Set Point** Set-point theorists believe that regular, vigorous exercise is the one sure way to lower your body's fat level. Maintaining an active lifestyle stabilizes the set point at this lower level.

✓ **It Helps Maintain Weight Loss** Most health professionals agree that losing weight is easy; keeping it off is more difficult. To avoid the negative consequences of weight cycling, more attention is being given to *maintenance* of weight loss. Exercise has been shown to be one of the few factors correlated with long-term weight maintenance. A change in lifestyle that includes a consistent exercise regimen across the life span is the fundamental key to successful weight-loss maintenance.

✓ **It Improves Self-Esteem** For overweight, sedentary individuals, exercise may not be a richly reinforcing experience at first. It may be difficult for them to get out and exercise in public. They may feel self-conscious about their bodies. They may have negative feelings about exercise because of past embarrassing experiences. As exercise becomes a satisfying habit, the individual begins to experience a new sense of well-being and power. Anxiety and depression are reduced. As weight comes off, self-image is enhanced. Self-esteem and self-confidence are improved. These psychological benefits received from regular participation in physical activity often supply the additional impetus necessary for adhering to a weight-loss/maintenance program. This positive self-concept helps reinforce all other areas of weight management, including food selection, feelings of anxiety, and feelings of control.

As you incorporate food management, emotional management, and exercise management into your life, you'll forget the "dieting mentality" and incorporate a set of behaviors and attributes that are necessary for permanent weight control. This "non-diet mentality" incorporates looking at your body intelligently (i.e., developing a positive but realistic image of yourself), eating intelligently, and moving your body intelligently (i.e., finding ways to weave daily activity into your life). Check out the Top 10 tips from people who have lost weight and maintained that loss for many years. Like them, when you structure and program your environment and life for success, managing your weight becomes part of your foods at a reasonable cost, and safe places to play and exercise.

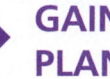

TOP 10 LIST

Tips from Successful Losers and Maintainers

People succeed at weight loss through conscious effort. These tips from successful losers and maintainers address *lifetime* weight management—how to lose weight *and* keep it off forever!

1. Focus on an overall *healthy* eating style, not a specialized "diet."
2. Choose low-fat over higher-fat foods when available (e.g., dairy, salad dressing, sauces, sour cream, cream cheese, cooking spray).
3. Control portions. Everything has calories, even fat-free foods. Take half of that huge restaurant portion home with you or split it with your dining partner.
4. Plan for up to an hour of exercise every day (include both aerobic and resistance training exercises). Look for ways to add additional activity to daily life.
5. Allow favorite foods—in moderation.
6. Fill up on fiber (fruits, vegetables, whole grains) and eat a little protein with each meal.
7. Don't skip meals (especially breakfast). "Grazing" or eating smaller but more frequent meals or snacks improves metabolism and blood sugar levels and reduces cravings and bingeing.
8. Set realistic goals. Working on losing 5 pounds at a time is easier than focusing on losing all 50 pounds.
9. Evaluate your relationship with food. Are you truly physiologically hungry, or are you eating because of stress, boredom, anxiety, or habit? Develop coping and problem-solving strategies.
10. Keep a written or mental record of what is eaten each day and the amount of exercise that is done each day.

Note: If you've eaten one too many chocolate chip cookies or haven't made it to the gym for a few days, don't give up. Take lapses in stride. Try to ascertain why the lapse occurred, learn from it, and move on. Weight management is a lifelong process, not an all-or-nothing contest. Remember, small changes can bring big results.

lifestyle. Through deliberate actions and specific strategies you can learn to quash the saboteurs and temptations that our environment presents.

Undoubtedly the entire nation should assume some responsibility to help make it easier for everyone to adopt these weight-management strategies. A greater emphasis is needed on creating environments and programs that support healthy eating and active living. This is especially important in the lower-income areas of communities. It is much easier to eat healthfully when everyone has access to full-service grocery stores, healthy

◆ GAINING WEIGHT: A HEALTHY PLAN FOR ADDING POUNDS

While many overweight people face the challenge of shedding extra pounds, those who are underweight face the challenge of trying to hold on to each pound and perhaps add more. The key to gaining weight is shifting the body weight equation so that you take in more calories than you burn. Add two to three substantial snacks between three moderate-size meals. Rather than eating high-fat and sugary foods, choose "calorie-dense" foods packed with nutrients. Even skinny people need to be concerned about heart disease and cancer. Here are some dietary suggestions:

- ✓ Mix beans, nuts, cheese, peas, or lean meats into casseroles, side dishes, and pasta.
- ✓ Combine yogurt, fruit, wheat germ, peanut butter, and ice in a blender to make a shake or smoothie.
- ✓ Spread peanut butter on bananas, apples, toast, or bagels.
- ✓ Replace sodas with fruit juices or skim milk.
- ✓ Replace cookies and doughnuts with nuts, raisins, dried fruits, bran muffins, yogurt, puddings, and fruit.
- ✓ Replace hamburgers and fries with thick-crust vegetable-topped pizza.
- ✓ Prepare hot cereals with milk instead of water; add nuts, peanut butter, fruit, and wheat germ.
- ✓ Top cold cereal with bananas or raisins.
- ✓ Eat hearty soups.
- ✓ Add garbanzo beans, seeds, tuna, croutons, cottage cheese, and lean meat to salads.

In addition to dietary alterations, adding strength-training exercises two to three times a week will add muscle mass to your frame. (See Chapter 6 for suggestions.)

◆ CULTURE AND WEIGHT

Why people diet and other weight-related issues are shaped by cultural environments. In earlier times, the female figures painted by Renoir and other artists were soft and fleshy. Rounded bellies and dimpled thighs were the feminine ideal. For both men and women, a surplus of fat was equated with wealth and success. The twentieth century brought about a decline in fatness as a social asset. Insurance companies began observing the increased death rate among the overweight. The socially elite began diminishing the enormousness of banquet menus. Corsets gave way to exercise and raised hemlines. Hollywood stars became the ideals. Thinness became equated with glamour, success, and desirability. As weight reduction became a national pastime, mail-order companies began making large profits with their weight-loss gimmicks. The market eventually gave way to new low-calorie foods and drugs designed to fool the body's hunger sensations. At the same time, labor-saving machines reduced the energy output necessary in daily life. The message that emerged by the 1960s was "Thin is in." The desire for an unrealistic slimness, particularly among women, has caused many to be preoccupied with their bodies and with dieting. Diet books become instant best-sellers.

There She Is . . . Miss Unrealistic America

Open up any fashion magazine or clothing catalog. The models are thin. This thin standard is perpetuated in all channels of social influence: families, peers, and the media. The message is pounded home over and over: "You can never be thin enough." This notion has been documented in studies of *Playboy* centerfolds and Miss America Pageant contestants from 1959 to the present, indicating a shift toward a thinner ideal shape for women in our culture. At the same time there has been a significant increase in diet articles in popular women's magazines. The cultural "ideal" for women's body size keeps getting thinner, though the average woman weighs 144 pounds and wears a size 12 to 14. This cultural index of the "ideal" woman's body is 13 to 19 percent below the expected weight for age and height. A body weight below 15 percent of expected weight is one of the criteria for diagnosing anorexia nervosa, so what does this say about our cultural ideals?

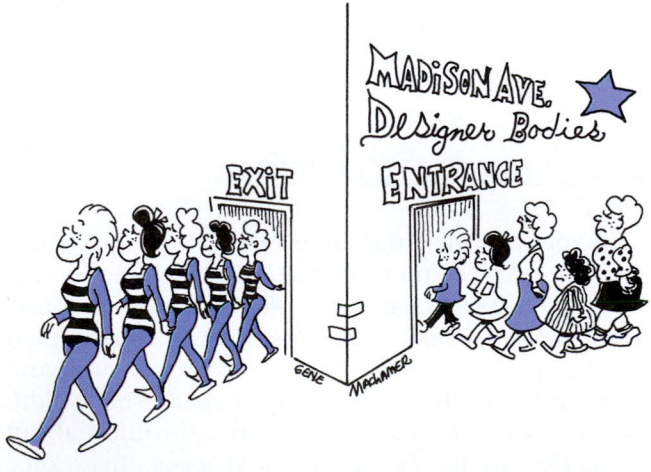

Many feel pressured to pursue a model-like body.

With extreme slimness as a cultural obsession, it becomes clear why fear of fat, fad dieting, surgical fat removal, and eating disorders abound. In a society that puts such a premium on thinness, overweight, obese, and even normal-weight individuals evaluate themselves in that society's mirror, defining themselves as unattractive and as failures. Such harsh evaluations are a result of an acceptance of society's distorted concept of the ideal body. Every day we see pictures of models in magazines that are air brushed and electronically altered—a "manufactured ideal." The readers, however, have "real-life" bodies! One study found that 3 minutes spent looking at models in a fashion magazine caused 70 percent of women to feel depressed, guilty, and shameful. Advertisements suggest that we invest money, time, and hope in trying to reach this ideal. Unfortunately, the results are often feelings of despair and inferiority. The first step toward a healthy weight is acceptance of your body type. Only about 5 percent of the population can look like the models and actresses we are exposed to daily. Twenty-five years ago fashion models weighed 8 percent less than the average woman; today they weigh 23 percent less. Our bodies are genetically programmed to be a certain build—tall, skinny, stout, short, muscular, big-boned, and so on. Everyone needs to accept his or her body type and then maximize it to be the best it can be rather than trying to achieve the impossible.

The media and the fashion industry need to take responsibility for using models who depict fitness and health rather than emaciation. Some already have. With the popularity of fitness and wellness programs in our country, we hope the image is changing. The "one size fits all" standard *must* change.

Men Are Joining In

Body image concerns are no longer confined to women. Millions of teenage boys and men are worried that their muscles aren't big enough or their bodies aren't lean enough. Bombarded with images of muscular half-naked men on the covers of men's magazines and in advertisements, men are facing the cultural pressures that women have felt for decades. Whereas both men and women experience a similar degree of body dissatisfaction, women universally want to lose weight while men tend to be evenly split between those wanting to lose weight and those desiring larger muscle mass. As a result, an increasing number of men are dieting, compulsively weight training, and abusing supplements and steroids as they strive for this ideal. This obsession for some goes beyond working out for health. It can affect schoolwork, jobs, personal relationships, and self-esteem and become a full-blown eating disorder.

◆ EATING DISORDERS

Obsession with weight and the desire to be thin begin early in life. Our culture especially socializes girls to be concerned about their physical appearance. For them, thinness equates with attractiveness and social approval. In contrast, a male's self-concept is linked to physical dominance, power, and sports competence.

Few measure up to the fashion industry's ideal, so dieting is commonplace. At the same time, obesity is dramatically rising. The dilemma of preventing obesity yet avoiding a fostering of "thin mania" presents a tremendous challenge.

The frequency of dieting among young women is alarming. It is estimated that two-thirds of adolescent girls in the United States have dysfunctional or abnormal eating behaviors. One survey of teenage girls revealed that most were more afraid of becoming fat than they were of cancer, nuclear war, or losing their parents! Fear of fat, obsessive dieting, and a distorted body image can lead to a psychological eating disorder. An **eating disorder** is defined as a disturbance in eating behavior that jeopardizes a person's physical or psychosocial health. Bear in mind that preoccupation with weight and dieting are not synonymous with an eating disorder. An eating disorder is an extremely serious psychopathological state. Most professionals agree, however, that dieting precedes the onset of an eating disorder. Eating disorders are viewed as multidimensional in cause and nature. Factors that increase vulnerability can be genetic, biological, psychological, personality, sociocultural, and familial. Thus, the treatment must include all components. Here are some of the general causes for eating disorders:

1. Society's definition of the "perfect body" as unrealistically thin and lean
2. Family characteristics such as overinvolvement and high expectations; overvaluing physical appearance; rigid and cold emotionally
3. Personality traits like "perfectionism"; the desire to achieve; feelings of inadequacy and loneliness
4. A genetic propensity to being overweight
5. Pressure from others to lose weight, including media images
6. Appearance-obsessed friends (dance troupes, school cliques, sororities, cheerleaders)
7. An inherent presence of low self-esteem
8. Family history of eating disorders

It is estimated that 8 to 10 million Americans struggle with eating disorders. One million are men.

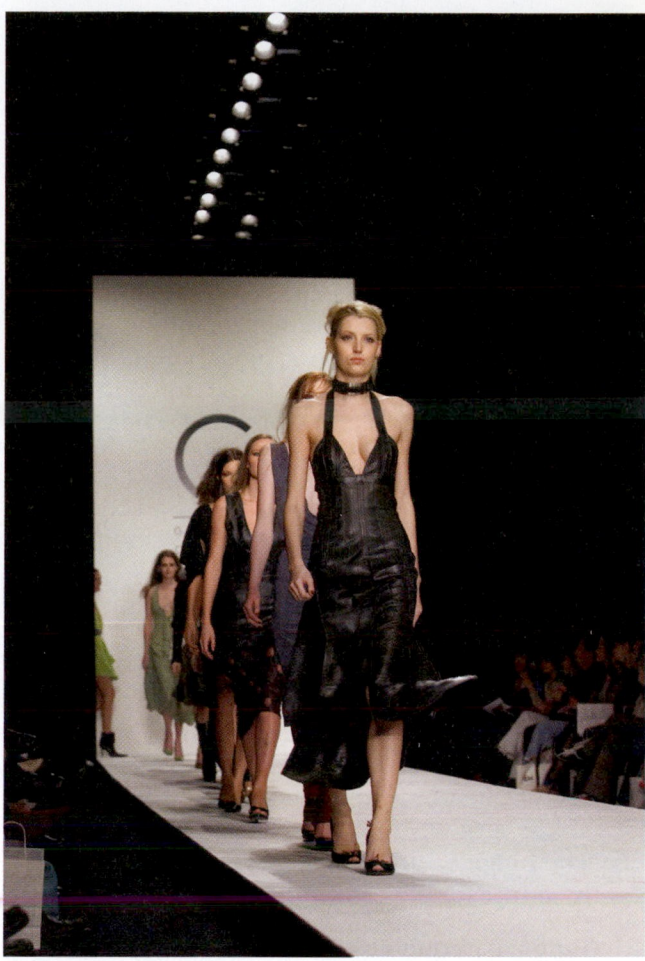

The fashion industry perpetuates the unrealistic ideal of extreme thinness, especially to women.

All segments of society are affected—including minorities—and 86 percent report onset by age 20. However, eating disorders have been reported in children as young as age 6 and individuals as old as 76. Certain populations are especially at risk. They include gymnasts, dancers (especially ballet), cheerleaders, pom-pom performers, distance runners, and models. Although more women than men suffer from eating disorders, there is a higher than normal incidence of eating disorders in certain subgroups of males where slenderness is encouraged: models, dancers, wrestlers, and distance runners. High school and college-age students are also vulnerable due to academic and social stresses and peer pressure to conform. Physical attractiveness is important, and the stresses of growing up and leaving home intensify these pressures. Two of the most common eating disorders are bulimia nervosa and anorexia nervosa, which may occur separately or together. A third eating disorder is called binge eating disorder.

Bulimia Nervosa

Bulimia is a Greek word meaning "ox" and "hunger." The disorder was so named because the sufferer eats like a hungry ox. That is, **bulimia nervosa** is characterized by a compulsive need to eat large quantities of food (bingeing) to the point of gorging, followed by purging through vomiting, use of laxatives, or fasting. Often, the binge is a response to an intense emotional experience, such as stress, loneliness, or depression, rather than the result of a strong appetite. Nevertheless, most bulimics are not aware of what precipitates these uncontrollable binges, and are not able to stop them. The diagnostic criteria for bulimia are

1. Recurrent episodes of binge eating (rapid consumption of a large amount of food in a discrete period).
2. A feeling of lack of control over eating behavior during the eating binges.
3. Self-induced vomiting, misuse of laxatives or diuretics, strict dieting or fasting, or excessive exercise to prevent a weight gain.
4. Two binge episodes a week for at least 3 months.
5. Self-evaluation unduly influenced by body shape and weight.
6. The bingeing and purging are not accompanied by anorexia nervosa.

Bulimia frequently starts as normal, voluntary dieting that later becomes compulsive, uncontrollable, and pathological. The bulimic's eating binge involves a rapid gulping of enormous quantities of food. Preferred foods are high in calories and sweet-tasting and can be eaten rapidly without preparation: ice cream, cookies, candy, bread, cheese, chips, doughnuts. The consumption of this food is not a pleasurable pastime but a compulsion. Up to 10,000 calories can be consumed in one sitting, followed by abdominal pain and discomfort. The binge generates guilt, depression, and anxiety. Purging follows, reducing the anxiety and fear. Then the cycle begins again.

The bulimic is aware of his or her abnormal behavior and has great fear of not being able to stop. He or she has feelings of guilt and shame about the behavior. Bulimia is a secret habit and can continue for many years undetected. The weight of most bulimics is normal or fluctuates within 10 pounds as a result of the binge–purge cycle.

The physical effects of bulimia include electrolyte imbalance (especially potassium), low blood sugar, esophageal lacerations, dehydration, and nerve and liver damage from low potassium. Tooth enamel is eroded by the stomach acid brought up with vomiting. Severe abdominal pain is common. In rare cases, actual rupture of the stomach has occurred. Bone density is lost if the disorder continues for many years.

People with bulimia need professional help. Psychotherapy is necessary to understand the underlying cause of the disorder and to help restore the bulimic's feelings of self-worth and self-confidence. Bulimics tend to be extroverted perfectionists—high achievers—and are often academically or vocationally successful. Yet bulimics have troubled interpersonal relationships, low self-esteem, poor impulse control, and high levels of anxiety and depression and are self-critical and sensitive to rejection. Bulimia is difficult to treat, and some struggle with this disorder for life.

Anorexia Nervosa

Far less common than bulimia, **anorexia nervosa** is a psychological disorder in which self-inflicted starvation leads to a drastic loss of weight. Although anorexia is less prevalent than bulimia, it is associated with more frequent physical problems and greater mortality. The mortality rate from anorexia—estimated at 10 to 20 percent—is the highest of any mental disorder. Whereas the bulimic has a general dissatisfaction with his or her body weight, the anorexic is obsessed with achieving thinness. Individuals with anorexia nervosa have an iron determination to become thin and an intense, irrational fear of becoming fat. They vehemently deny their impulse to eat, their appetite, and their enjoyment of food. The term *anorexia* is a misnomer, because loss of appetite is usually rare until late in the illness. While bulimics feel shameful about their abnormal behavior, anorexics justify their weight-loss efforts.

Found primarily in early and middle adolescent females, anorexia may result in physical deterioration to the point of hospitalization or even death. Anorexia carries a 19:1 female-to-male ratio, with a prevalence estimated at 1 percent among adolescent girls. The diagnostic criteria for anorexia are

1. Refusal to maintain body weight at or above a minimal normal level for age and height (i.e., a body weight that is 15 percent below normal).
2. Intense fear of weight gain or becoming fat despite being significantly underweight.
3. A disturbed perception of body weight, size, or shape (i.e., feeling "fat" although emaciated).
4. In females, amenorrhea (lack of menstrual periods) for at least three consecutive cycles.

Anorexia often starts as innocent dieting that turns into irrational behavior characterized by severe caloric restriction, fasting, relentless exercising, diuretic and laxative use, and, in some cases, self-induced vomiting. The anorexic pursues and maintains thinness despite an emaciated appearance that is apparent to others.

Anorexics display an extraordinary amount of energy for exercise and schoolwork in spite of their starvation state. However, they avoid social relationships, have low self-esteem, and are fearful of change. Despite an aversion for eating, anorexics are preoccupied with food. They may prepare elaborate meals for others, collect recipes, carry or hide snacks, and memorize the caloric content of various foods. Bizarre eating habits are commonplace. Anorexics have been known to cut a raisin in two and chew each half for several minutes. In many situations, they may pretend to be eating while putting food into a napkin or feeding the dog under the table.

Family stress and social pressure contribute to this disorder. Most anorexics come from middle- to upper-class families that place a high premium on achievement, perfection, and physical appearance. Their families are often overcontrolling and overprotective. Anorexics exhibit extreme perfectionism accompanied by a profound sense of ineffectiveness. Only by restricting food intake do they feel a sense of control and feel capable of coping with life's stresses.

Anorexia causes the physiological complications that accompany any malnutritive state: chronic fatigue, dry and scaly skin, hair falling out, lack of menstruation, drops in blood pressure, and cardiac complications. Constipation is commonplace. Bone growth is retarded, increasing the risk of fractures and osteoporosis. Anorexics have an unusual sensitivity to cold due to their low body-fat percentage.

Treatment for anorexia nervosa involves medical, psychological, and nutritional help. The major obstacle to treatment is the patient's denial that any problem exists. The entire family must be involved, because the anorexic's behavior has deep psychological origin: low self-esteem, struggle for control and independence, and fear of physical sexual development.

Binge Eating Disorder

Classified separately from anorexia or bulimia, binge eating disorder (sometimes called compulsive overeating) has become a serious problem. It is now the most common eating disorder. **Binge eating disorder** (BED) is defined as recurrent episodes of eating characterized by eating, in a discrete period, an amount of food much larger than most people would eat in a similar period and accompanied by a sense of lack of control or a feeling that one cannot stop. The criteria for this disorder include

1. Eating much more rapidly than normal.
2. Eating until uncomfortably full.
3. Eating large amounts of food when not hungry.
4. Eating alone because of embarrassment about how much is eaten.

5. Feeling disgusted with oneself, depressed, or guilty about eating.
6. The binge eating occurs, on average, at least 2 days a week for 6 months.

Most people overeat from time to time. Compulsive overeaters, however, experience marked distress regarding their bingeing behavior and engage in binge eating on average at least 2 days a week for 6 months. They tend to overeat when home alone, while normal eaters tend to overeat in restaurants and social situations that are associated with positive feelings.

In some ways, people with binge eating disorder are similar to bulimics. Both engage in frequent binges, are preoccupied with food and body weight, experience intense feelings of body dissatisfaction, and set unrealistically high dieting standards. Both use food to fill an emotional void. However, some important differences distinguish bulimics from people with BED. People with BED do not regularly compensate for their behavior by dieting or purging. Whereas bulimics dwell on the importance of thinness, serious binge eaters would be happy to have an average body weight. Individuals with BED are usually very overweight, and most seek treatment for obesity. Approximately 15 percent of obese people are compulsive overeaters. They eat even if they aren't hungry. Whereas bulimics engage in the extremes of severe dieting and eventual bingeing, people with BED rarely restrict food. Table 12-11 will help you assess whether you have a problem with compulsive overeating.

The goal in treating binge eaters is to normalize eating—to help them say no to overeating. They need help in adopting a plan of healthy eating and overall moderation *without* rigid rules. Binge eaters need help in learning to cope with the underlying emotions that perpetuate this eating problem—anxiety, loneliness, depression, shame, inferiority, and fear of criticism.

Eating Disorders Not Otherwise Specified (EDNOS)

The fact that a person does not meet the exact diagnostic criteria for anorexia, bulimia, or binge eating disorder does not mean that that person does not have an eating problem. As a matter of fact, most people will not meet the full criteria. For example, a person with EDNOS may purge after eating, but with less frequency or intensity than will someone diagnosed with bulimia. Or a person may exhibit occasional anorexic-type behaviors yet be near normal in weight. These varied types of behaviors are called **disordered eating.** The incidence of disordered eating is increasing and far

TABLE 12-11 — Are You a Compulsive Overeater?

1. Do you eat when you're not hungry but don't know why?
2. Do you constantly think about food throughout the day?
3. Do you go on eating binges for no apparent reason and find yourself unable to stop?
4. Do you have feelings of guilt and remorse after overeating?
5. Do you look forward with pleasure and anticipation to the time when you can eat alone?
6. Do you eat sensibly in front of others and then binge when you're alone?
7. Is your weight affecting the way you live your life?
8. Do you eat to escape from worries or trouble?
9. Does your eating behavior make you or others unhappy?
10. Have you tried "dieting," only to fall short of your goal?

If you answered yes to over half these questions, you may want to think seriously about your relationship with food and consult a professional.

exceeds that of the clinically diagnosed eating disorders. Exact statistics are unavailable because most of these behaviors are unreported, secretive, and difficult to define. Since about 80 percent of American women are dissatisfied with their weight, disordered eating behaviors have become a popular way of dealing with food issues. Those who exhibit disordered eating may diet, binge, purge, fast, exercise excessively, eat in secret, or gain and lose weight off and on. A considerable proportion of their lives is consumed by preoccupation with weight, body image, and food. If disordered eating becomes long-lasting and interferes with normal life, help should be sought.

What Can Be Done?

Eating disorders appear to be increasing in incidence, and so implementation of prevention programs is desperately needed. The most obvious and effective site for prevention is the schools. However, all segments of society need to absorb some of the responsibility, including parents, coaches, advertising executives, the media, and the entertainment business. Society needs to send the message of healthy acceptance of self and body. Not everyone is meant to be a size 6. You may want to do Lab Activity 12-4 at the end of the chapter to assess your risk for developing an eating disorder.

If you suspect a friend, roommate, or relative of having an eating disorder, you probably wonder what you can do to help. Eating disorders are not solely about food and eating but are manifestations of emotional distress. Therefore, just begging someone to start eating or put on some weight is futile. Ignoring the situation or waiting to see what happens also will not solve the problem.

The first step to recovery is indisputable: Locate professional help as soon as possible. Congress has mandated that every state establish a system of community mental health centers to assist people with a variety of psychological problems. These centers are a good source for providing treatment or helping you locate professionals who specialize in treating eating disorders. Even though psychotherapy has become more prevalent and accepted in the last 25 years, some still avoid it. For whatever reason, psychotherapy still carries a stigma with some people. Most college campuses have counseling services available as well.

Your anorexic or bulimic acquaintance may deny the condition or balk at your suggestion to seek help; therefore, it may be difficult to persuade her or him to seek help. However, both physical and psychological evaluation are crucial at the onset of treatment. You cannot force someone to get help. It is important, however, to be direct and honest while showing sincere concern and support. You may have to be tough, even make the appointment, and insist on accompanying the anorexic or bulimic to see a specialist.

℞ PRESCRIPTION FOR ACTION

You've read the chapter. Now go do one or more of these:

✓ Keep a food journal to see what, how much, and why you are eating.

✓ Take a favorite recipe and investigate ways to make it less caloric and more nutritious.

✓ Resign from the "clean plate club." Even if it feels somewhat uncomfortable, leave a small amount of food on your plate.

✓ Do some form of exercise that burns a minimum of 300 calories.

✓ Make a rule: No TV or Internet until you've exercised for 30 minutes.

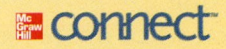 **connect**

Go online to Connect to complete this activity.
http://connect.mcgraw-hill.com

Frequently Asked Questions

Q. Is it true that anything eaten after 8:00 P.M. will be stored as fat?

A. *What* and *how much* you eat affect weight control, not *when* you eat. Your body metabolizes calories eaten after 8:00 P.M. the same way as the calories you ate earlier in the day. If you balance total daily calories consumed with calories burned, it doesn't matter how late you eat. This myth probably stems from the tendency for people to snack "mindlessly" in the evening on high-fat, high-calorie foods such as chips, cookies, and ice cream, which add considerable additional calories to their day. Some people eat sparingly during the day and then consume several thousands of calories at night due to built-up hunger. Going to sleep on a full stomach may make sleeping uncomfortable, because the body is simultaneously shutting down to rest while still exerting energy to digest food.

Q. I have cellulite on my thighs. Is there any special way to remove it?

A. There is no such thing as **cellulite**. It is a slang term used to describe the dimpled fat found primarily on the buttocks and thighs of women. Concentrated areas of fat tend to bulge in some women because, with age, their connective fibers become taut and their skin thin. This fat is like any other fat in that only a comprehensive program of exercise and calorie reduction will remove it. No miracle creams, saunas, diets, or devices specifically break up cellulite. Buying a product that claims to do this reduces only your wallet.

Q. The only place I feel I have too much fat is on my abdomen. Is there any way to just lose fat there? How about trying one of those abdominal muscle stimulators?

A. The concept of *spot reduction* (that is, selectively burning off fat from a particular body area) is a myth. No one can dictate where body fat will accumulate or from where it will be removed. Genetics determine your body build and preferred fat storage sites. Exercising a specific body area does not burn fat in just that area. Fat stores from throughout the body are mobilized during exercise. Thus, your abdomen will lose fat only after a combined program of total-body aerobic exercise and calorie management, not solely by doing 100 crunches a day. It is possible to "spot tone," however. Those 100 crunches create stronger abdominals. As far as those abdominal stimulators go, don't waste your money!

Q. My friend had gastric bypass surgery and lost a considerable amount of weight. What about this and other surgical treatments of obesity?

A. Surgery for obesity should not be taken lightly and should be considered only as a last resort for the morbidly obese (those at least 100 pounds above ideal weight). Even the nonsurgical means of jaw wiring and inserting balloons in the stomach are drastic measures in tackling obesity. Also, their long-term effectiveness is questionable unless a drastic lifestyle change accompanies the procedure. **Liposuction** (suctioning fat from under the skin) has become popular as a method of removing body fat from selected body parts. This surgical procedure is performed by physicians who specialize in cosmetic surgery. Interestingly, liposuction performed on abdominal fat does not eliminate the risks for heart disease, type 2 diabetes, or cancer. Since liposuction removes only the subcutaneous fat, the deeper, more dangerous intra-abdominal fat remains. Therefore, abdominal liposuction does not result in the metabolic benefits that fat loss through diet and exercise accomplishes. As with any major medical procedure, these surgeries have inherent risks and medical complications.

Q. I have been faithfully exercising and monitoring my calorie intake for 6 months. As a result, I have lost 20 pounds. Even though I am sticking with my program, I have stopped losing weight. Since I have 10 more pounds to lose to reach my goal weight, I am frustrated. What now?

A. Weight-loss plateaus are common after several months of consistent progress. First make sure that your weight loss goal is realistic. Maybe your body is telling you that your weight is exactly where you need to be! If that is not the case, try logging your food intake for several days to see if your food portions have begun creeping up. Also realize that your metaboism may have changed and you may not be burning as many calories as you did at your higher weight. To kick-start your metabolism, try some alterations in your workouts: add some strength training; change to a new aerobic activity like swimming, cycling, or using a cardiomachine like an elliptical trainer; incorporate short bursts of high-intensity exercise combined with more moderate intensity throughout your aerobic session to create an "interval" effect. (For example, cycle hard for 45 seconds every 4–5 minutes.) Your body may have gotten used to the same exercise routine, resulting in a stall in excess calorie burning. Making a few changes could make a difference.

Q. I am heavily involved in competitive sports. As a result, I am very muscular. When I stop competing, how do I avoid having all that muscle turn into fat?

A. Your concern is fueled by a common misconception. Muscle can no more turn into fat than a cat can turn into a dog. Neither can fat become muscle. The cellular makeup of each is different. If you stop activity altogether, your muscles will atrophy and lose tone. Calories not needed to fuel your body will be stored as fat. To avoid this, continue doing some regular exercise and modify your calorie consumption, being sure your energy input and output are relatively equal.

Q. **I have heard that I will burn more fat if I work out at the lower end of my target heart rate range rather than at a high intensity. Is this true?**

A. This low-intensity fat-burning idea is a misunderstanding based on an oversimplification. It is true that at higher exercise intensities, the body prefers to use more glycogen rather than fat for fuel. Some have interpreted this to mean that to burn fat, low-intensity exercise is best. However, the type of fuel used during exercise does not make a huge difference. You burn calories *and* fat during both types of exercise. The most important exercise variable is *total* caloric expenditure. Higher-intensity exercise does burn more calories, but you may not be able to sustain that intensity for very long. Because you don't fatigue as quickly when exercising at a lower intensity, you may be able to work out for a longer period and feel more comfortable while doing it. The result is more total calories expended due to the longer workout time. Even though all types of exercise can help in weight management, most people find that a program of regular low- to moderate-intensity activity is easier to maintain over time. The key is doing it every day!

Q. **I am concerned because my sister is very much overweight. She doesn't act like it bothers her, but I think it does. What can I do to motivate her to lose weight?**

A. Often we have relatives or friends who have health-robbing habits (smoking, being overweight, not exercising). Because we care about them, it is natural to want to help. In the case of your sister, do not nag or criticize her. Instead, set a good example and talk about why you do the things you do (select certain foods, behavior

modification tricks, etc.). Try to include her in your practices. Invite her to go on a walk, bike riding, or to an aerobics class. Grocery shop or eat out together. Share recipes and food preparation ideas. Show that you care. Make a pact with her (you will try to stop biting your fingernails, while she tries to lose weight). Be there for her. However, realize that she is ultimately responsible for herself. Nevertheless, be her friend, confidant, and number one cheerleader. A strong support system is essential in any weight-management program.

Q. **I am 26 years old and weigh 40 pounds more than I should. Obesity runs in my family. Is it possible for me to achieve a normal weight or am I always going to fight being overweight because of my heredity?**

A. Yes, you can achieve normal weight, but you will have to work much harder than some people because of your genetics. It may seem unfair, but you will have to exercise for 60 or more minutes a day and be vigilant in your calorie intake. Think positive, though, of the opportunity you have to also lower your risk of heart disease, cancer, and type 2 diabetes. Genetic influences are real, but diet and exercise habits have far more impact on weight than heredity. Embrace your opportunity to take control of what you can—your lifestyle.

Q. **I have heard that it is better for weight loss to eat five or six small meals throughout the day rather than three regular meals. Is that true?**

A. This can be true for some. Because metabolism is increased after eating, you can stoke your metabolism fire with frequent feedings (every 3–4 hours). It is important, however, to keep the caloric intake at about 300 to 400 calories per feeding, and include some protein, carbohydrates, and a little fat for balance and satiety. This means not snacking on chips and junk food. This routine may not work for everyone due to their schedule. No matter what feeding routine you choose, be sure to eat breakfast to jump-start your metabolism to begin the day.

Summary

Obesity is acknowledged as this country's most important nutrition-related disease. It is a national problem that affects the future health and wealth of the nation. It is a complex disorder that no longer is considered only a problem of overeating or lack of willpower. It is caused by multiple factors—some within your control and some beyond it. Environment, culture, and genetics combine to complicate the act of nourishing our bodies. It is important to understand body composition and be able to differentiate between overweight and obesity. Many health problems are associated with obesity, so concern with weight control should begin sufficiently early in life to reduce the risk of developing obesity. Prevention is the treatment of choice. The factors affecting obesity give us insight into the complexities of losing excess body fat.

"Monday I start my diet" is far too often the battle cry for losing weight. This diet mentality has contributed to the obesity problem. Dieting and concerns about appearance have also contributed to the increasing incidence of eating disorders. Because successful weight management has been elusive for many people, the marketplace has provided many legitimate as well as unfounded claims about products and services. Therefore, consumer education is essential. Effective weight management involves food management, emotional management, and exercise management.

Whereas dieting is temporary, restrictive, and negative, lifestyle weight management is a positive, flexible means of dealing with food for life. It is a lifestyle of calorie-controlled, nutritious eating and regular exercise amid established cultural patterns and social and economic forces. No gimmick or gadget can replace this lifestyle approach.

Regular exercise is the key ingredient in maintaining a healthy body composition. Technological advances have increased the quality of our lives in many ways but have eliminated much daily physical exertion. It is a challenge to find ways to fit activity into your life. However, lifelong weight management and total wellness depend on it. Only when we start considering food as fuel, regarding exercise as a daily necessity, and accepting a range of healthy body weights will weight concerns finally disappear.

Terms

- anorexia nervosa
- basal metabolic rate (BMR)
- behavior modification
- binge eating disorder
- body fat
- body mass index (BMI)
- bulimia nervosa
- calorie (kcal)

- cellulite
- disordered eating
- eating disorder
- essential fat
- fat cells (adipose cells)
- fat-free mass
- glycogen
- lean-body mass (muscle mass)

- leptin
- liposuction
- obesity
- overweight
- set-point theory
- storage fat
- weight cycling (yo-yo syndrome)

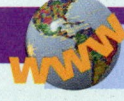 Internet Resources

Calorie Control Council

www.caloriecontrol.org

Loaded with articles on cutting calories and weight management. Has many interactive tools: calories burned during various exercises, BMI, caloric content of foods.

Calories Per Hour

www.caloriesperhour.com

Calculates calories burned for any activity as well as BMI and BMR. Also features a nutrition calculator for food items and a Q & A about diets and dieting.

Food and Nutrition Information Center

www.nal.usda.gov/fnic

A government site that features numerous resources and information on nutrition, including a large section on weight management and obesity.

Medline Plus/Weight Loss

www.nlm.nih.gov/medlineplus/weightcontrol.html

From the U.S. National Library of Medicine, this site is an encyclopedia on a variety of weight-management topics.

National Association of Anorexia Nervosa and Associated Disorders

www.anad.org

Provides comprehensive information and resources (including treatment referrals) on eating disorders.

National Center for Chronic Disease Prevention and Health Promotion—Overweight and Obesity

www.cdc.gov/nccdphp/dnpa/obesity

Covers definitions, BMI, trends, contributing factors, health consequences, and resources for overweight and obesity.

National Eating Disorders Association

www.nationaleatingdisorders.org

A not-for-profit organization working to prevent eating disorders. Offers information on a variety of eating disorders, including body image issues, athletes, prevention, and treatment.

The National Weight Control Registry
www.nwcr.ws/

A registry established in 1994 of individuals who have lost significant amounts of weight and kept it off for long periods of time. Includes research findings and success stories.

Obesity in America
www.ObesityinAmerica.org

A very thorough and up-to-date site covering all aspects of overweight and obesity—facts, trends, causes, surgical options, myths, medications, etc.

Shape Up America
www.shapeup.org

Provides a wide range of information on exercise, healthy eating, lifestyle change, and weight management.

Small Step
www.smallstep.gov

From the U.S. Department of Health and Human Services, gives helpful hints in making lifestyle changes related to weight management.

Something Fishy
www.something-fishy.org

Covers anorexia, bulimia, and compulsive overeating with news, research, dangers, treatment, options, and cultural issues.

Spark People
www.sparkpeople.com

A popular weight loss and fitness site loaded with articles, tips, motivation, success stories, and social networking opportunities to share weight loss and fitness information.

The Calorie King
www.calorieking.com

Has a huge database with nutritional and calorie information for thousands of generic and name-brand foods, including fast foods.

The Diet Channel
www.thedietchannel.com

Loaded with information on a variety of diets, weight-loss programs, and weight-loss strategies.

Trust for America's Health
www.healthyamericans.org

A nonprofit organization that is dedicated to protecting America's health and preventing disease. This site covers a wide variety of health topics and includes obesity statistics for each state.

Web MD Food and Fitness Planner
www.webmd.com/diet/food-fitness-planner-calculator

An interactive site from Web MD that allows you to track your daily foods and exercise in order to reach your goal weight. It also summarizes your fat, carbohydrates, protein, sodium, fiber, and sugar based on what you ate.

Weight-Control Information Network (WIN)
http://win.niddk.nih.gov/

As an information service of the National Institute of Diabetes and Digestive and Kidney Diseases, this site features a wide range of weight-loss and weight-control topics/articles, including dieting tips, suggestions for controlling food portions, and successful weight-loss programs.

Weight Loss Tips
http://video.healthination.com/usnews/better-you-weight-loss.html

A series of short videos with practical tips for weight loss. Includes kitchen strategies, emotional eating, and journaling.

The following restaurants have caloric information for their foods online:

www.arbys.com	www.longjohnsilvers.com
www.blimpie.com	www.mcdonalds.com
www.bostonmarket.com	www.panerabread.com
www.burgerking.com	www.papajohns.com
www.carlsjr.com	www.pizzahut.com
www.chick-fil-a.com	www.popeyes.com
www.churchs.com	www.quiznos.com
www.dairyqueen.com	www.schlotzskys.com
www.dominos.com	www.sonicdrivein.com
www.dunkindonuts.com	www.steaknshake.com
www.fazolis.com	www.subway.com
www.hardees.com	www.tacobell.com
www.jackinthebox.com	www.whitecastle.com
www.kfc.com	

Name _____ **Class/Activity Section** _____ **Date** _____

Weight Management Plan

Date: _____

Current weight: _____

    Goal weight: _____

Current body fat percentage: _____

    Goal body fat percentage: _____

Current body mass index (BMI): _____

    Goal body mass index (BMI): _____

Waist: _____ Hip: _____

Current waist-to-hip ratio: _____ (waist ÷ hip)

Goal waist-to-hip ratio: _____

Goal waist measurement: _____

I. FOOD MANAGEMENT

- Calories per day: _____ (goal)

- Fat grams per day: _____ (goal)

- Snack strategy:

- Food preparation adjustments/alterations:

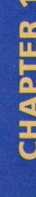

II. EMOTIONAL MANAGEMENT

Behavior modification and coping strategies:

1.

2.

3.

4.

5.

6.

III. EXERCISE MANAGEMENT

Physical activity strategies:

Sunday	Monday	Tuesday	Wednesday	Thursday	Friday	Saturday

LAB Activity 12-2

Analyzing Your Food and Exercise Habits

PART I: FOOD

Use the following food journal to record your food intake for a day. This will allow you to see the number of calories you are eating and analyze the reasons you eat. Knowing the cues and factors that affect eating can help you manage your eating behavior. Don't forget to record "liquid" calories! (Make copies of this log as needed to record multiple days.)

Date: _____

Time of Day	Location	Companion(s) (if any)	Food and liquids	Portion Size/ Quantity	Calories	Hunger Level (0–5) 0 = not hungry 5 = very hungry	Feelings/Mood (before eating)	Feelings/Mood (after eating)

What do you observe about your eating habits? (i.e., portions, hunger levels, feelings/mood, etc.):

List strategies for change:

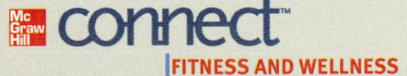

http://connect.mcgraw-hill.com

PART II: EXERCISE

Finding the time to exercise can be a challenge. However, there are several times during a day when you can weave activity into your life (walking rather than driving, riding a stationary bike while watching TV, taking the stairs rather than the elevator, getting up 45 minutes earlier in the morning to jog). Use the following log to keep track of your activity during the day. Use Table 12-10 or go to www.caloriesperhour.com or www.caloriecontrol.org (go to "Exercise Calculator") for the caloric expenditure for various activities. Then answer the questions. (Make copies of this log as needed to record multiple days.)

Date: _____

Activity	Time of Day	Location	Duration	Calories Expended	Positive Outcomes	Negative Outcomes (if any)

1. Assess your activity level today (was it a typical day?):

2. Describe ways you could fit more activity into your day:

3. What obstacles do you face in trying to be active?

4. What are your strategies for combating these obstacles and adhering to a lifetime of activity?

Name _____ Class/Activity Section _____ Date _____

Estimating Your Basal Metabolic Rate (BMR)

Precise measurement of your BMR can be achieved only in a laboratory. However, you can compute an estimate of your BMR by using the following equation from the World Health Organization. Figured into the equation are factors that influence your BMR: age, gender, and weight.

STEP 1

Convert your body weight in pounds to kilograms (kg):

_____ lb ÷ 2.2 = _____ kg

STEP 2

Select the appropriate formula from the table below, using your age and gender:

Age Range	Male Formulas	Female Formulas
10–18	BMR = (17.5 × wt in kg) + 651	BMR = (12.2 × wt in kg) + 746
19–29	BMR = (15.3 × wt in kg) + 679	BMR = (14.7 × wt in kg) + 496
30–59	BMR = (11.6 × wt in kg) + 879	BMR = (8.7 × wt in kg) + 829
60 +	BMR = (13.5 × wt in kg) + 487	BMR = (10.5 × wt in kg) + 596

Example: For a 23-year-old male weighing 195 pounds:

195 lbs ÷ 2.2 = 88.6 kg
BMR ÷ (15.3 × 88.6 kg) + 679 = 2,034.5 calories/day

Now figure your BMR:

BMR = (_____ × _____ kg) + _____ = [_____] Calories/day

Remember, BMR does not include any calorie expenditure from activity or exercise that you do throughout the day. This is just your basal need (i.e., calories needed *at rest* just to sustain vital functions of the body).

If you want to approximate your TOTAL caloric expenditure in a day, use Table 12-10 and accompanying Web sites to calculate the calories you burn in daily activities and exercise. Then:

___ + _____ = [_____]
BMR   activity   total daily
      calories   calories expended

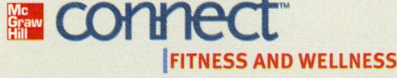

LAB Activity 12-4

Are You at Risk for an Eating Disorder?

Check the following statements that describe you.

____ I feel fat even if people tell me I'm not.

____ If I were thinner, I would like myself better.

____ If I gain weight, I get anxious and depressed.

____ I worry about what I will eat.

____ I feel extremely guilty after eating.

____ I am terrified of being overweight.

____ I often wish I were someone else.

____ I get anxious if I cannot exercise.

____ I find myself preoccupied with food.

____ I am preoccupied with a desire to be thinner.

____ I binge eat sometimes.

____ I have a secret stash of food.

____ I don't like to be bothered or interrupted when I'm eating.

____ I like to read recipes, cookbooks, calorie charts, and books about dieting.

____ I would rather eat by myself than with family or friends.

____ I am hardly ever satisfied with myself.

____ I have dieted to lose weight.

____ I want to be thinner than my friends.

____ I vomit, use laxatives, or take diet pills to control my weight.

____ When I eat, I worry that I may not be able to stop.

____ I have perfectionist tendencies.

____ I have a hard time saying no to others.

____ I avoid eating even if I am hungry.

____ Sometimes I feel worthless.

____ I have a tendency to hide my feelings or have trouble expressing them.

This questionnaire is not meant to be a diagnostic tool, but if you checked many of the statements, that may be indicative of an eating disorder. The more items you checked, the more serious your problem may be. Don't be afraid to seek the advice of a counselor or physician who has experience in treating eating disorders. It takes courage to take this initial step, but it is essential to prevent severe medical and psychological problems.

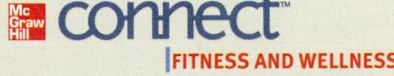

http://connect.mcgraw-hill.com

CHAPTER 13

Preventing Cancer

STUDY QUESTIONS

You will have successfully mastered this chapter if you can answer the following:

1. How do cancer deaths rank in overall death statistics?
2. What are five guidelines for reducing cancer risk?
3. What are four guidelines for preventing sun overexposure?
4. What are four guidelines for selecting foods that reduce cancer risk, and can you apply the guidelines to a menu?
5. What are three early detection factors for cancer?
6. What are cancer's seven warning signals?
7. What are the most common cancers and their risk factors?

You will find the answers as you read this chapter.

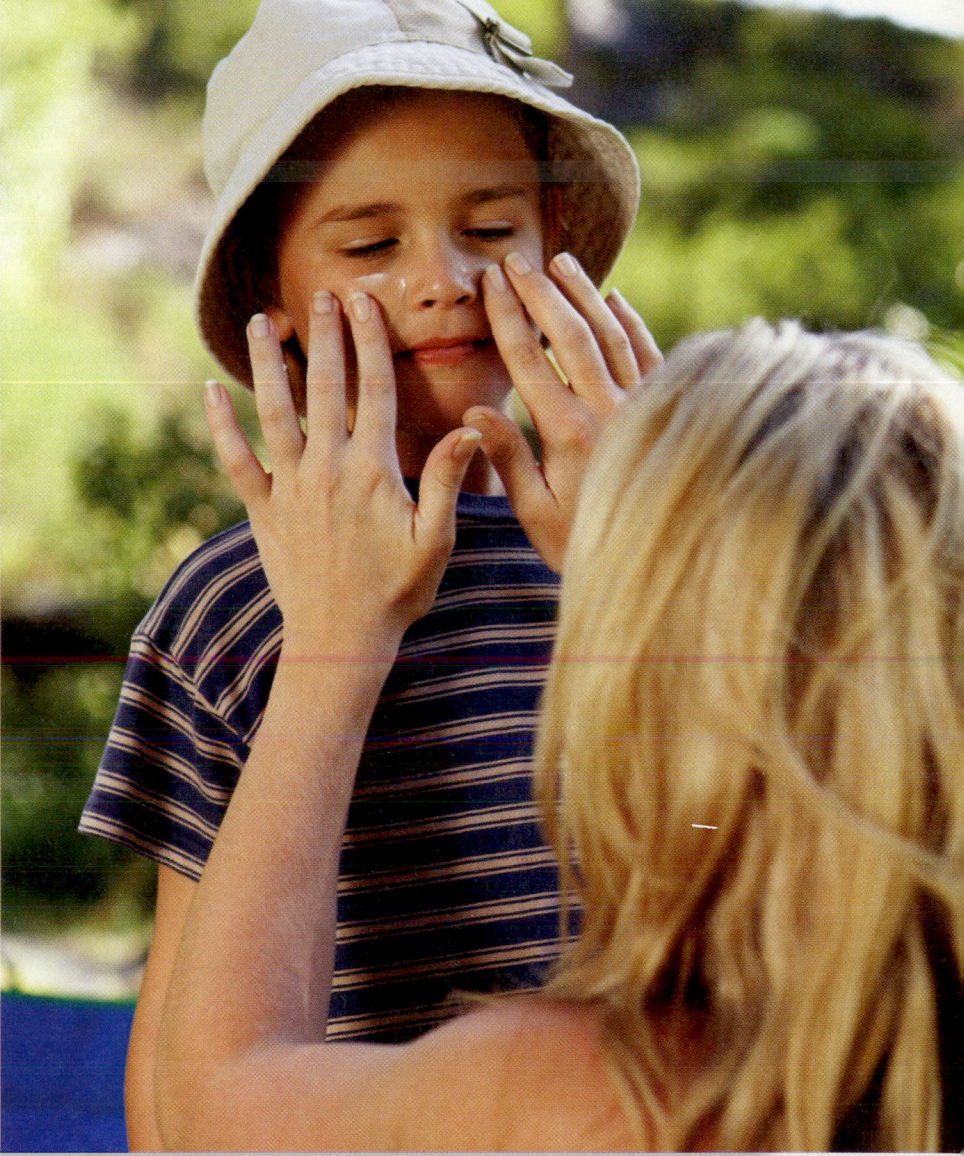

> " *Better to put a strong fence around the top of the cliff than an ambulance down in the valley.* "
>
> —Joseph Malins

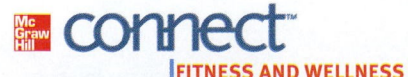

connect™
FITNESS AND WELLNESS

http://connect.mcgraw-hill.com

wellness lifestyle implies taking responsibility for your health and making wise choices. The purpose of this chapter is to discuss how to decrease cancer risk, which is strongly affected by personal lifestyle choices. Adult cancer is largely a preventable disease. While no one would choose to have cancer, a person might choose to use tobacco, tan excessively, or rarely exercise, factors that can initiate and promote

cancer. You will learn which behaviors increase health risks and how to decrease those risks to enhance your state of wellness. This chapter covers what cancer is, its controllable risk factors, early detection, self-exams, common cancers and their symptoms, preventive behaviors, and treatments. Prevention, rather than treatment, is emphasized because it is in prevention that we have the greatest control.

◆ WHAT IS CANCER?

Cancer is not a single disease but a group of over 100 different diseases characterized by abnormal cell growth and replication. Normally, cells grow and are replaced in an orderly manner. Enough new cells grow to replace the ones that are worn out and injured. Cancer cells lack controls to stop the growth process and continue to grow and multiply without restraint. This loss of control of cell growth may be due to a variety of factors. Ultraviolet radiation from sunlight, tobacco smoke, viral infections, diet, and chemicals in food and the environment all have been implicated.

It is possible that all of us at some time experience potentially cancerous changes in our cells.

These **precancerous** cells usually die or are destroyed by the immune system. Few live long enough to cause harm. If one abnormal cell survives, it can replicate into billions of cells, forming a lump or **tumor.** Tumors may be benign or malignant. **Benign** tumors are usually nonthreatening. Although they can grow large enough to interfere with organs and bodily functions, they seldom cause death. They usually resemble surrounding tissue, remain localized, and spread by expansion, like a wart or mole. They do not spread to other parts of the body. They can be removed completely by surgery and are not likely to recur. **Malignant** tumors are cancerous. They differ from surrounding tissue and tend to spread through **metastasis.** In metastasis, cells break away from the primary tumor and migrate to other tissues through

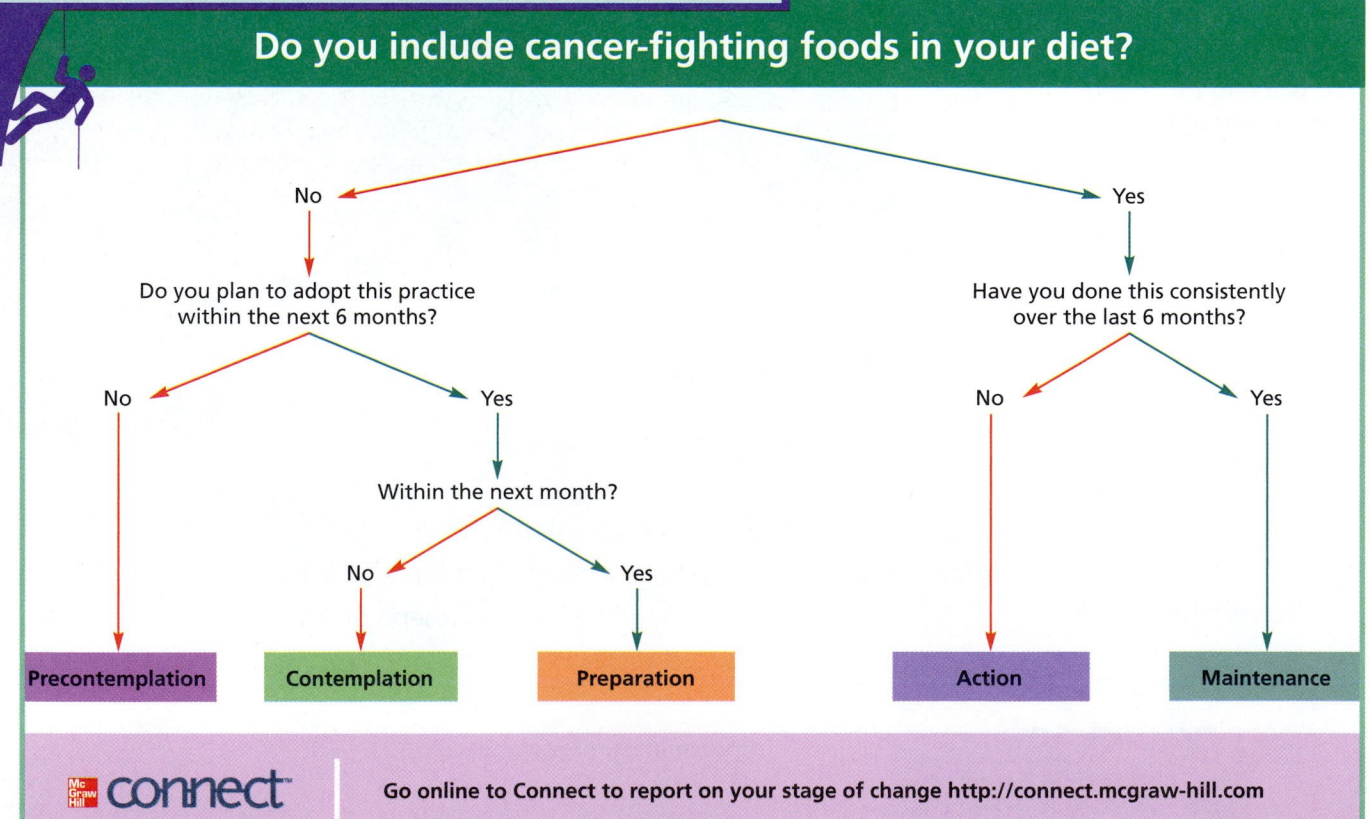

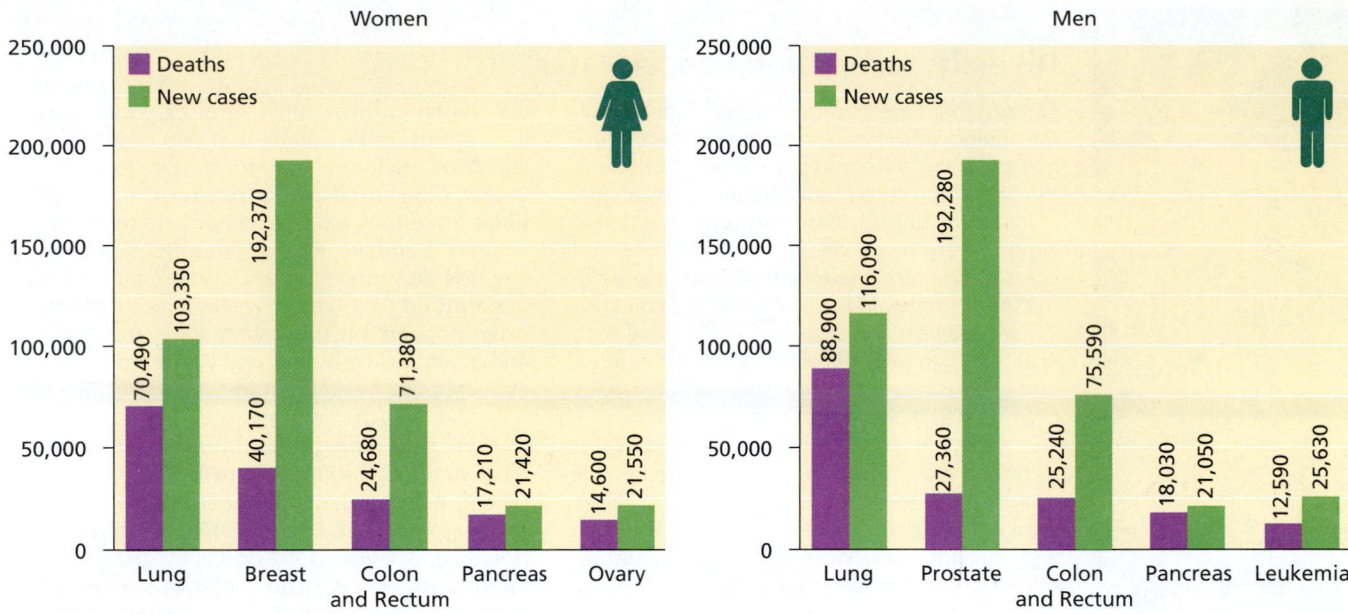

FIGURE 13-1 The most deadly cancers.

SOURCE: U.S. Cancer Statistics Working Group. *United States Cancer Statistics Incidence and Mortality.* Atlanta: U.S. Department of Health and Human Services, Centers for Disease Control and Prevention and National Cancer Institute, 2009.

the lymph or blood system and continue to grow. They have lethal potential because they invade and destroy normal tissues and spread to other parts of the body.

◆ CANCER INCIDENCE

Cancer is the second most common cause of death for Americans, surpassed only by heart disease. Cancer and heart disease rates have been declining steadily, primarily because fewer people are smoking now than in the past. See Figure 13-1 for cancer incidence and death rates by site and gender. According to present rates, about one in three Americans will eventually have cancer. While cancer is most common in people over age 55, it can strike at any age. A diagnosis of cancer is not a death sentence, but early detection is important. The earlier a cancer is detected, the simpler the treatment and the higher the survival rate. The current survival rate 5 years after diagnosis is about 66 percent. Better yet, we know that simple lifestyle changes can cut your risk of cancer. For this reason, it is important to understand cancer risk factors and warning signals and to practice self-exams.

◆ HOW TO REDUCE YOUR RISK OF CANCER

People hear so much about cancer, they often get the feeling that everything causes cancer. If everything causes cancer, there seems to be no use in trying to avoid it. They believe that there is little they can do to make a difference in their cancer risk or that it is not worth the effort. They are wrong. Cancer, like heart disease, is largely preventable. Up to 80 percent of cancers may be related to lifestyle factors over which you have control. Only 5 percent can be blamed on environmental factors. These cancers occur as a result of cumulative exposure to **carcinogens,** substances that cause cancer, and/or a weakened immune system that does not effectively scavenge precancerous

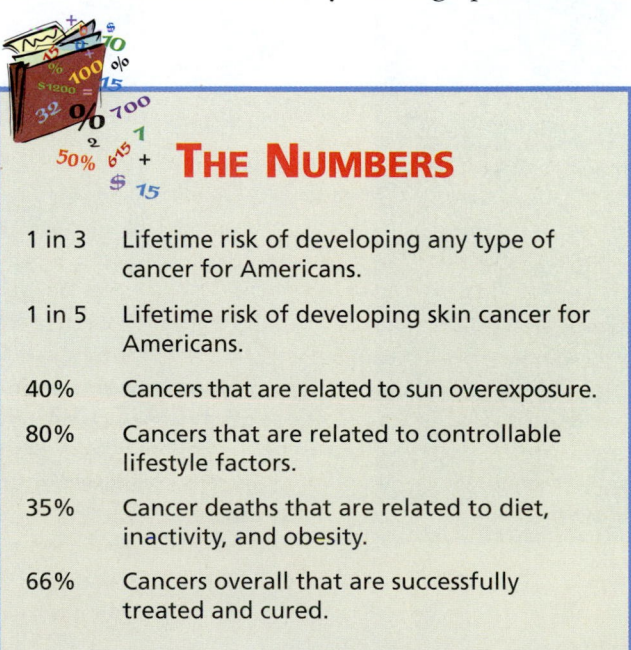

THE NUMBERS

1 in 3	Lifetime risk of developing any type of cancer for Americans.
1 in 5	Lifetime risk of developing skin cancer for Americans.
40%	Cancers that are related to sun overexposure.
80%	Cancers that are related to controllable lifestyle factors.
35%	Cancer deaths that are related to diet, inactivity, and obesity.
66%	Cancers overall that are successfully treated and cured.

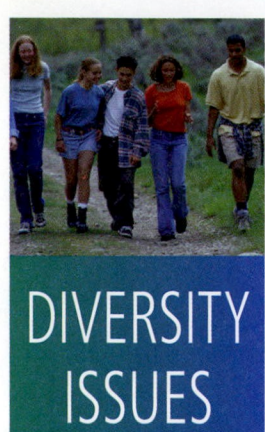

DIVERSITY ISSUES

Diversity Issues and Cancer Rates

Rates of incidence of certain types of cancers differ among countries, races, and socioeconomic groups. Some differences occur because of cultural habits practiced for a lifetime. For example, in Japan and China, where soy foods are eaten at almost every meal, deaths from prostate and breast cancers are one-fourth of what they are in the United States. In the United States, a diet rich in high-fat meat and processed and refined food results in high rates of colorectal cancer, which is rare in countries where the diet consists largely of unrefined grains, fruits, and vegetables.

Likewise, cultural influences affect rates of certain types of cancer among socioeconomic groups. Smoking is an example. At one time, smoking symbolized sophistication, affluence, and maturity and over half the population smoked, but this has changed. Nevertheless, while smoking has declined to less than a quarter of the population, 50 million Americans, mainly the less educated, still smoke. Also, an unacceptably high number of teenagers are using tobacco, which foreshadows grim health problems for that group in the future.

Not only cultural influences but racial background or genetics can affect cancer rates.

People with brown, olive, or black skin have a measure of protection against skin cancer provided by melanin, a natural skin pigment. Darkly pigmented blacks can have up to 30 times more melanin than do people with pale white skin and are less likely to suffer skin damage due to sun exposure. However, blacks are more prone to a type of melanoma that most often appears on the palms, soles, nail beds, and mucous membranes and is often detected at a later, less treatable stage.

Overall, African Americans are more likely to develop and die from cancer than are other racial or ethnic groups (Figure 13-2). The death rate from cancers is about 30 percent greater for African Americans than for white Americans. However, between 1992 and 2005, the cancer death rate for African American men decreased more than it did for other racial and ethnic groups.

While genetics is a factor in cancer risk, behavioral choices are a much more powerful determinant. Following a healthy diet, avoiding tobacco and sun overexposure, and being physically active decrease cancer risk for all populations.

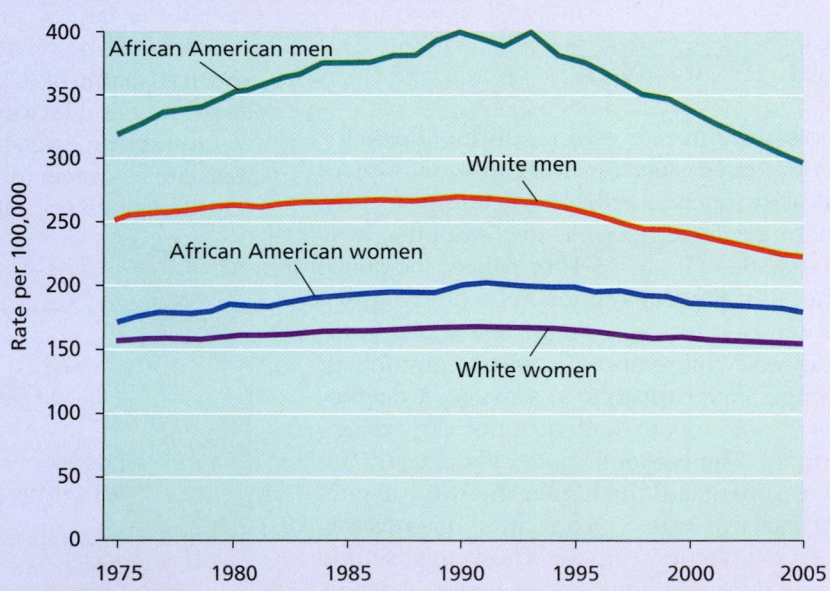

FIGURE 13-2   **Trends in Cancer Death Rates by Race and Sex, 1975–2005.**

Source: National Program of Cancer Registries Centers for Disease Control and Prevention, 2009.

cells. The five primary risk factors for developing cancer are within your control:

1. Tobacco use
2. Sun overexposure
3. Diet
4. Inactivity
5. Obesity

Several other factors contribute to an increased risk of cancer. Secondary risk factors for cancer, some of which are controllable, include

✓ Exposure to some viral infections, for example, hepatitis B or human papilloma virus
✓ Exposure to radiation, workplace hazards, and certain chemicals

Preventable factors that initiate cancer are associated with different death rates. For example, skin cancers, caused mainly by ultraviolet exposure, are the most common form of cancer but are highly curable, and few people die from them. Lung cancer, mainly from cigarette smoking, is far less common but very deadly and kills far more people. The percentage of cancer deaths attributable to preventable causes of cancer is shown in Figure 13-3.

Choices you make daily can greatly cut your cancer risk. It is a matter of education and habit change. What follows is a discussion of what you can do.

1. Don't Smoke or Chew Tobacco

Thirty percent of cancer deaths, and 90 percent of lung cancer deaths, are attributed to tobacco use. This includes cigarettes, pipes, cigars, snuff, and chewing tobacco. Tobacco contains many carcinogens that increase the risk of developing several types of cancers. (See Chapter 14 for additional information

on the effects of tobacco.) Frequent exposure to toxins ingested from tobacco products weakens the immune system and decreases the body's ability to cleanse itself of precancerous cells. In addition, when a smoker is exposed to other carcinogens, there seems to be a synergistic effect that multiplies cancer rates beyond what would be expected from the effect of each carcinogen alone. For example, smoking combined with the use of alcohol increases the risk of cancer 30 fold. The number of smokers is decreasing in the United States. However, the use of smokeless tobacco, especially "dipping snuff," has increased. Whereas tobacco use is most often implicated in lung cancer, tobacco products can produce a variety of oral cancers, including cancer of the lip, tongue, mouth, and throat. Spit tobacco, also known as smokeless tobacco or chew snuff or dip, can cause cancer of the mouth and throat after as little as 3 years of use. Changes in the oral mucosa are found as soon as 7 days after using spit tobacco. Over 2,000 chemical ingredients, including formaldehyde, cadmium, arsenic, and nitrosamines, are in these types of tobacco. Nitrosamines are powerful cancer-causing chemicals that are 50 times higher in spit tobacco than in cigarettes. This makes it even more dangerous than smoking and in less time. Smokeless tobacco use can cause a whitish thickened patch, called leukoplakia, to develop in the mouth where the tobacco is placed between the cheek and the gums. Over half to two-thirds of smokeless tobacco users have these precancerous lesions. Smokeless tobacco users have a 50 percent greater risk of oral cancer compared with nonusers. Other problems include tooth decay, mouth sores, permanent gum recession, tooth loss, bad breath, drooling, and stained teeth. Spit tobacco is *not* a safe alternative to smoking. It is "cancer in a can."

The good news is that cancers caused by tobacco are 100 percent preventable. If you don't use

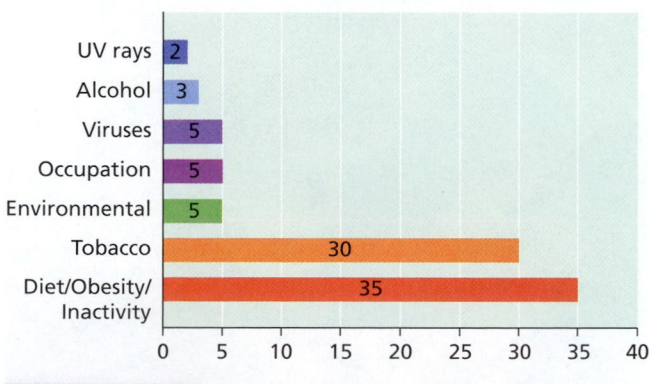

FIGURE 13-3   **Percentage of cancers caused by preventable risk factors.**

SOURCE: Harvard Center for Cancer Prevention.

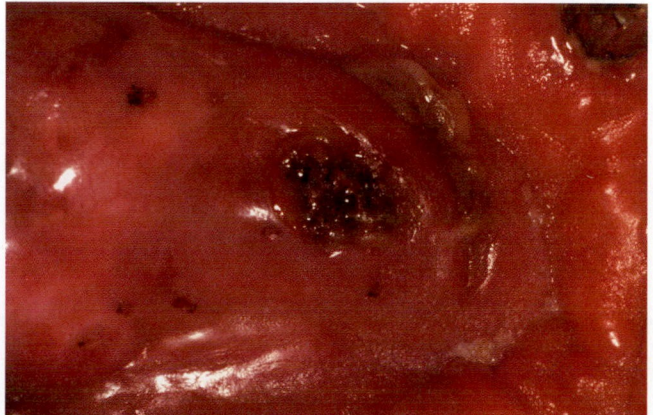

Oral cancers caused by smokeless tobacco are 100 percent preventable.

tobacco, don't start. If you are a tobacco user, quit. People who quit, no matter at what age, live longer, healthier lives than do those who keep using tobacco. For the majority of Americans who don't use tobacco, reducing sun exposure and eating healthfully are the most powerful tools for decreasing cancer risk.

2. Limit Sun Exposure

Overexposure to the sun is the main cause of skin cancer. It is estimated to strike one of every five Americans, making it the most common cancer. We have been a nation of sun worshipers and are seeing the consequences. How ironic that the price of a "healthy" tan can be premature skin aging and wrinkling and skin cancer. It is never good to lie in the sun to tan, but you can still enjoy outdoor activities and minimize the negative effects by following the guidelines in Table 13-1.

While we don't want the sun to roast and prematurely age the skin, we also don't need to totally avoid sun exposure either. Recent studies show that getting plenty of vitamin D cuts risk of several types

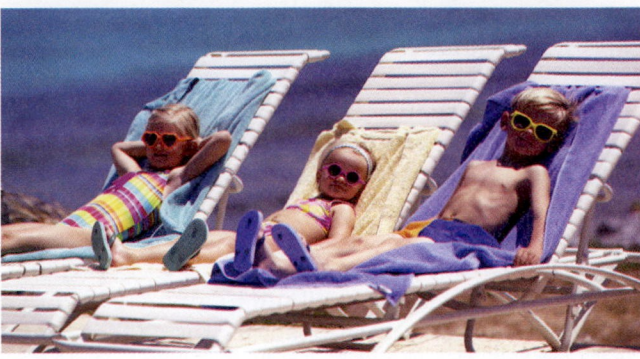

Sun overexposure causes most skin cancers. One blistering sunburn in childhood doubles the lifetime risk of malignant melanoma.

of cancer, including cancers of the colon, prostate, and breast. Many people do not get enough vitamin D, especially people with little sun exposure, those with dark skin, and the elderly. Vitamin D is synthesized by the skin when exposed to UVB radiation. About 15–20 minutes of sun exposure prior to applying sunscreen is sufficient to provide a beneficial dose of vitamin D. It is also provided by food such as fortified dairy products, cereals, fatty fish, and supplements. To reduce health risks, a combination of small amounts of sun exposure and vitamin D–fortified foods or supplementation are recommended, with suggested dosages of 1,000 IU up to 2,000 IU of vitamin D per day.

3. Eat More Plant Foods

About one-third of cancers can be prevented by a healthful diet. Certain foods seem to be related to an increase or decrease in some kinds of cancers; for instance, a diet high in red and processed meats seems to play a role in the development of colon and

TABLE 13-1	*Sun Safety*

1. Avoid prolonged exposure to the sun when ultraviolet (UV) radiation is strongest, between 10:00 A.M. and 3:00 P.M., even on overcast days. Seek shade if your shadow is shorter than you are.

2. Plan activities for early morning or late evening.

3. When you will be working or playing outside for more than 15 to 20 minutes, *apply a sunscreen rated SPF 15 or higher*. This will block 93 percent of the sun's UV radiation, which is primarily responsible for skin cancers. Use at least 1 ounce (about 2 tablespoons). Choose a broad spectrum sunscreen that protects you from both UVB and UVA radiation. Reapply every 2 hours or after swimming or perspiring.

4. Wear protective clothing, i.e. long-sleeved shirt, wide-brimmed hat, sunglasses.

5. Avoid tanning even in tanning parlors or with sunlamps. There is no such thing as a safe tan. Tanned skin is damaged skin. The UVA light emitted by tanning booths can cause sunburn, wrinkles, liver spots, and increased risk of skin cancer. The effects of photoaging (skin aging caused by sun or tanning beds) can be seen as early as age 20.

6. Protect children from too much sun. Skin damage occurs with each unprotected sun exposure and accumulates over a lifetime. Perhaps most of the damage is done in childhood and adolescence. Even one bad burn in childhood can double the risk of skin cancer.

7. Know what skin cancer looks like and examine your skin at least once a month. If you find unusual moles or skin spots, have them examined by your physician. See Online Lab Activity 13-5 to record your skin exam.

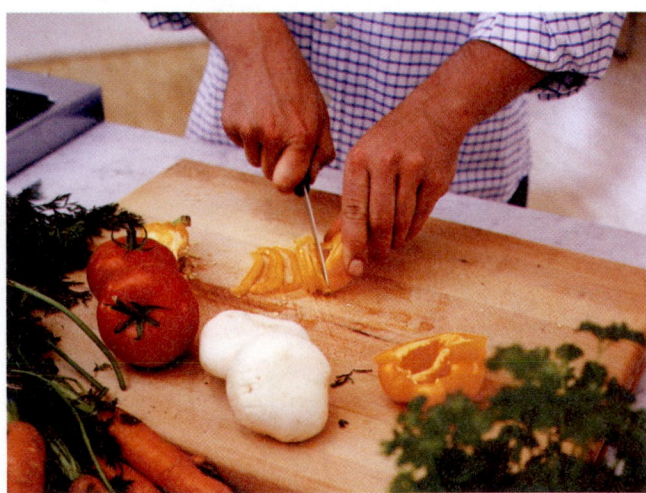

Eating five or more servings of fruits and vegetables a day can reduce cancer risk.

TABLE 13-2   *Cancer Deaths Preventable by a Healthy Diet*

What you eat every day *can* make a difference! Eating more plant foods and less animal fat and meat can greatly cut your risk of cancer. The National Cancer Institute estimates that a healthier diet can reduce your risk of cancer by these amounts:

Colon/rectal	75%
Prostate	75%
Breast, pancreas	70%
Endometrium, gallbladder	50%
Stomach	35%
Lung, mouth, larynx, cervix, bladder, esophagus	20%
Other types	10%
Overall estimate	32%

SOURCE: National Cancer Institute.

prostate cancers. A multitude of studies show that by eating whole-grain foods, fruits, and vegetables and by avoiding high-fat red meat, bacon, and processed meats, we could significantly reduce our overall cancer risk, as shown in Table 13-2. MyPyramid in Chapter 11 and the dietary guidelines are excellent models to follow. However, many Americans are not making these simple dietary adjustments. Only 24 percent of Americans eat the recommended five or more servings of fruits and vegetables a day. Eating a variety of fruits, grains, and vegetables is not only more healthful but less expensive than buying a lot of high-fat meat and highly processed foods such as hot dogs, fries, chips, doughnuts, and junk cereals.

Concerns have been voiced about pesticide and chemical residues in fruits and vegetables, as well as about irradiation of fresh produce and poultry. There is no doubt that the production, processing, and transportation of food in our mass-market world raise concerns that necessitate further research. Nevertheless, we do know that sun exposure, a fatty diet, inactivity, obesity, and tobacco products are highly controllable areas where your behavior has a major impact. Taking positive steps in these areas makes more sense than worrying about food products over which you have little control.

By making positive choices in your daily diet and following the guidelines listed here, you can promote good health now and reduce your cancer risk in the future. Healthy dietary changes you can make can be found in Table 13-3, and a sample

TABLE 13-3   *Healthy Changes*

Improving your nutritional well-being to reduce cancer risk due to diet can be as simple as making healthier substitutions for foods that you eat often. Here are some suggestions.

Eat Less Often	Eat More Often
Meats	
High-fat meat, ribs	Loin, flank steak, roasts, round steak, tempeh
Fried chicken	Chicken with skin removed
Fried fish	Broiled fish
Hamburgers	Soy burgers, ground turkey, tofu in stir-fries
Regular sausage	Vegetarian sausage
Other fried meats	Meats baked, roasted, steamed
Dairy	
Full-fat or 2% milk	1% or fat-free milk
Regular sour cream	Lite or fat-free sour cream or plain yogurt
Full-fat cheese	Fat-free or low-fat cheese
Full-fat cream cheese	Fat-free cream cheese
Fats	
Butter, margarine	Lite or whipped butter or none
Regular salad dressing	Lite or fat-free salad dressing and mayonnaise
Snacks	
Potato chips, corn chips	Low-fat popcorn, pretzels, nuts, baked corn chips
Cookies	Apples, oranges, graham crackers
Ice cream	Frozen yogurt, pudding pops, Popsicles, frozen bananas or grapes
Doughnuts, croissants	Whole-grain bagels with low-fat spread
Candy bar	Fruit, lifesavers, gum, breath mints

TABLE 13-4	*One-Day Sample Menu*
Breakfast	Whole-grain cereal, toast, or low-fat muffin; fat-free or soy milk; and fruit.
Lunch	Tuna or chicken sandwich made with whole-grain bread; low-fat dressing; soup, salad, or vegetables; and fat-free milk.
Dinner	Pasta or rice dish with small amount of meat or tofu; beans; two vegetables; whole-grain bread; and fat-free milk.
Snacks	Low-fat popcorn; fruit; frozen yogurt; and soy nuts or raw vegetables with a low-fat dip.

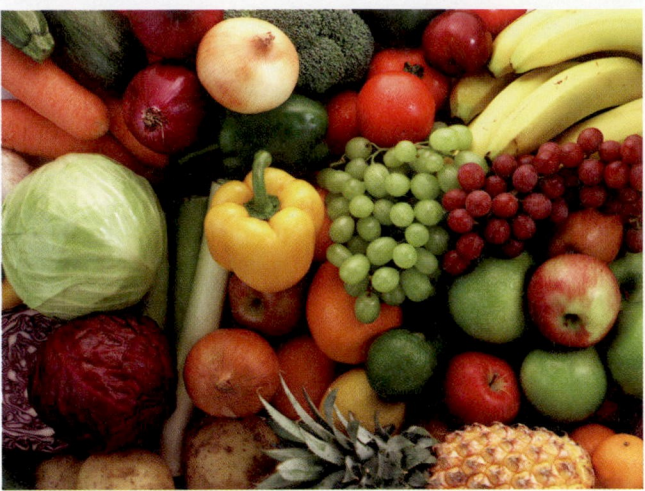

Brightly colored fruits and vegetables are rich in phytochemicals, which bolster the body's cancer defenses.

1-day dietary plan incorporating many of these suggestions is given in Table 13-4.

✓ *Choose most of the foods you eat from plant sources:* Eat 5 to 9 servings of fruits and vegetables a day, as well as 6 or more servings of whole-grain breads, rolls, brown rice, pasta, or beans. A landmark report by the American Institute for Cancer Research (AICR), *Food, Nutrition, Physical Activity, and the Prevention of Cancer: A Global Perspective,* reviewed 7,000 worldwide research studies and found that if people would increase their fruit and vegetable intake to 5 servings a day, it could reduce cancer rates by as much as 20 percent. While a typical American meal might feature an 8-ounce serving of meat, a large serving of potatoes, and perhaps a small serving of peas or corn, the AICR recommends that you fill your plate two-thirds with vegetables, fruits, whole grains, and beans, with a small 3-ounce serving of meat on the side. Diets rich in fruits and vegetables (french fries don't count) protect you against many cancers, particularly those occurring in the gastrointestinal tract. Certainly consuming more plant foods leaves less room for empty-calorie foods, and plant foods are rich in essential vitamins, minerals, and protective **phytochemicals** (plant chemicals), natural plant substances that can ward off cancer. Researchers are still learning how various plant compounds may prevent or stop the development of cancer. Some may neutralize carcinogens before they have a chance to cause cancer, block cell damage, heal damage to normal cells, or stop cancer cells from multiplying or spreading. For greatest benefit, eat a colorful variety of plant foods. See Figure 13-4, Diet and Cancer Risk, for a summary of factors that increase and decrease risk of certain cancers. A more detailed version can be viewed at www.dietandcancerreport.org.

✓ *Eat cruciferous vegetables:* Broccoli, cauliflower, brussels sprouts, cabbage, turnip greens, and other members of the mustard family help prevent certain cancers from developing. Phytochemicals unique to **crucifera** (cabbage, turnip, and mustard family) stimulate liver enzymes responsible for inactivating toxic chemicals.

✓ *Eat a rainbow:* Fill your plate with colorful plant foods. Brightly colored vegetables and fruits are rich in cancer-protective carotenoids and other phytochemicals. Dark-green and deep-yellow fresh vegetables and fruits such as carrots, corn, spinach, winter squash, peaches, and apricots contain up to 500 or more natural carotenoids. While much research has focused on beta-carotene, many other carotenoids are stronger **antioxidants,** and it may be that a combination of these and other phytochemicals makes them cancer-protective. Green and leafy vegetables, whole grains, egg yolks, nuts, and wheat germ contain folic acid, a B vitamin that guards against cell mutations and chromosome abnormalities that may be involved in the initiation of cancer. Folic acid works synergistically with other antioxidant vitamins and phytochemicals to neutralize **free radicals,** potentially dangerous substances that produce precancerous cellular damage. These foods also help strengthen the body's immune system. More information on food sources of these vitamins and minerals is given in Chapter 11.

✓ *Eat whole grains every day:* Consume whole grains daily; substitute whole grain for refined

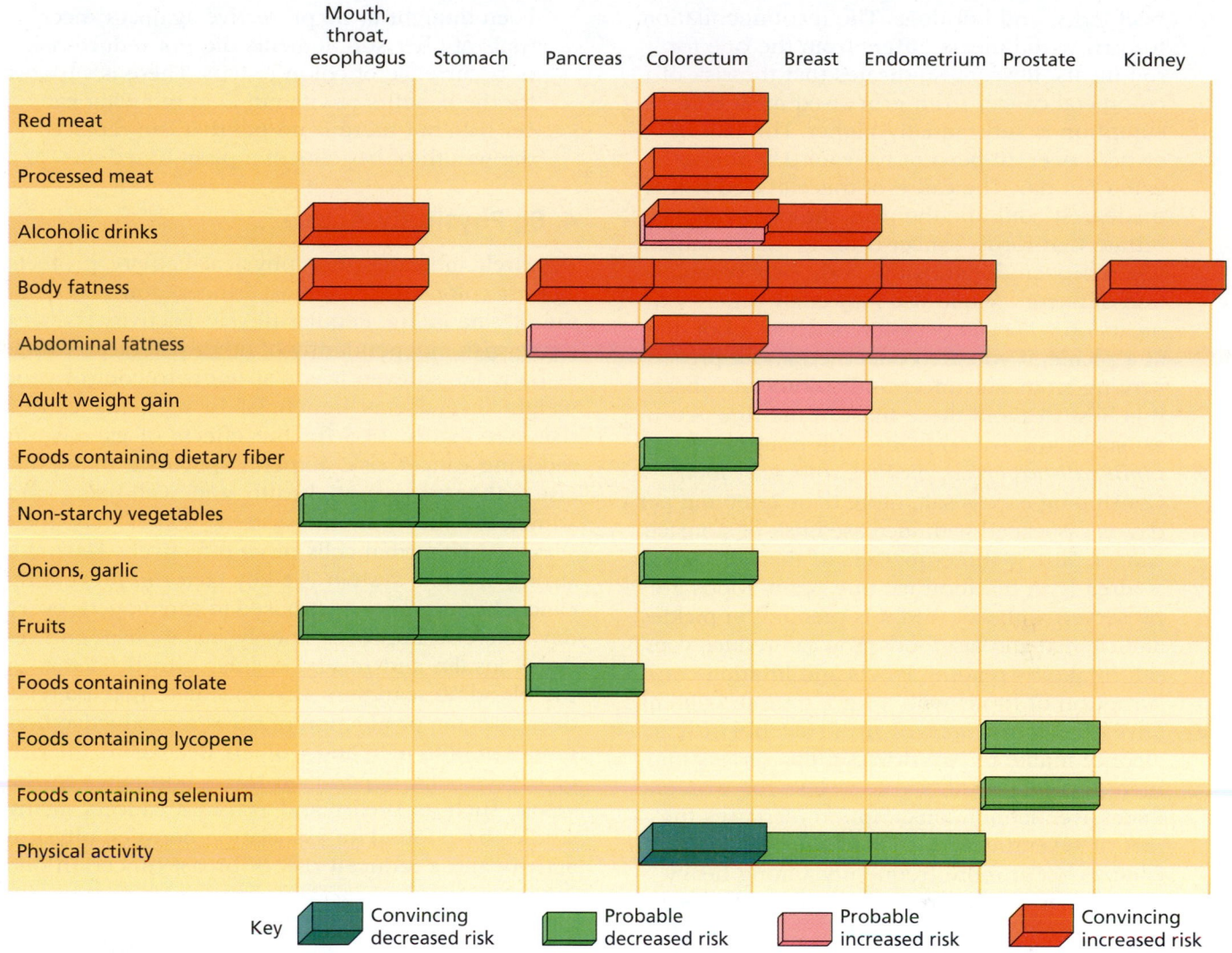

	Mouth, throat, esophagus	Stomach	Pancreas	Colorectum	Breast	Endometrium	Prostate	Kidney
Red meat				Convincing increased risk				
Processed meat				Convincing increased risk				
Alcoholic drinks	Convincing increased risk			Convincing increased risk	Convincing increased risk			
Body fatness	Convincing increased risk		Convincing increased risk	Convincing increased risk	Convincing increased risk	Convincing increased risk		Convincing increased risk
Abdominal fatness			Probable increased risk	Convincing increased risk	Probable increased risk	Probable increased risk		
Adult weight gain					Probable increased risk			
Foods containing dietary fiber				Probable decreased risk				
Non-starchy vegetables	Probable decreased risk	Probable decreased risk						
Onions, garlic		Probable decreased risk		Probable decreased risk				
Fruits	Probable decreased risk	Probable decreased risk						
Foods containing folate			Probable decreased risk					
Foods containing lycopene							Probable decreased risk	
Foods containing selenium							Probable decreased risk	
Physical activity				Convincing / Probable decreased risk	Probable decreased risk	Probable decreased risk		

Key: Convincing decreased risk · Probable decreased risk · Probable increased risk · Convincing increased risk

FIGURE 13-4   **Diet and cancer risk.**

Source: American Institute for Cancer Research.

breads or rolls, and choose whole-grain cereals or oatmeal instead of pastries or sugary cereals. Whole grains are important sources of many nutrients such as folic acid and selenium, which have been associated with a lower risk of colon caner. Refined grains lack the fiber and natural phytochemicals that can fortify the body's defenses against cancer.

✓ *Eat legumes daily:* This includes all types of dried and canned beans, like pinto, red, black, and kidney beans, garbanzos, lentils, and peas. They are rich in fiber, protein, and recently discovered types of phytochemicals with additional health benefits.

✓ *Limit red meats:* When you cut way back on meat, you'll have room for more plant foods in your diet. Research shows that consumption of red meat (pork, beef, lamb) increases risk of colorectal cancer. This may be due to carcinogens that develop when cooking meat at high temperatures, by damage to the lining of the colon by heme iron in meat (it gives meat its red color), or by other processes still under study. Eat low-fat meats and dairy products, as well as vegetarian meals. Cut back on fried foods to one serving or less per day. While you don't have to eliminate animal foods entirely, research suggests a limit of 18 ounces (six 3-ounce servings) of red meat a week for lowest cancer risk. Fish and poultry do not increase cancer risk, so serving them more frequently is recommended for their beneficial nutrients.

✓ *Avoid processed meats:* Processed meats include bacon, sausage, cold cuts, beef sticks, beef jerky, and hot dogs. The recommendation for processed meats differs from the one for red meats. Research indicates that the risk of colorectal cancer from processed meat consumption is substantially higher. The risk increases over 20 percent for each 1½ ounces eaten per day. The cause of this elevated risk is unclear. It could be the iron, the preservative nitrate that forms cancer-causing nitrosamines when broken down by the body, or a combination of factors. While you may enjoy processed meats on a special occasion, such as a hot dog at a picnic, if you are concerned about preventing stomach cancer and colorectal cancer, it is best to avoid these most of the time, even sausages and bacon made with poultry.

✓ *Limit salt-preserved, pickled, and salty foods:* Consuming excess salt, more than 2,400 mg per day, is associated with increased risk of stomach cancer. Nearly three-quarters of the salt we eat is already in the food we buy. Many foods are preserved with salt, and it is plentiful in pickles and canned and fast foods. You can reduce your salt intake by reading labels and limiting consumption of foods with a high sodium content.

✓ *Drink little or no alcohol:* Avoid alcohol or limit alcohol intake to two drinks a day or less for men and one drink a day or less for women. Excessive alcohol consumption increases the risk of several cancers. Esophageal and liver cancers occur more frequently among heavy drinkers of alcohol, especially when the drinking is accompanied by smoking cigarettes or chewing tobacco. Coupled with poor diet, alcohol increases the risk of developing colon cancer because it interferes with folic acid metabolism. Studies have also shown an increased risk of breast cancer in women who regularly consume more than three alcoholic drinks per week. Factors that cause this effect are not yet known, but researchers speculate that the association may be due to the carcinogenic effect of alcohol, its breakdown products in the body, or alcohol-mediated changes in the levels of hormones such as estrogens. Whatever the cause, for those who drink regularly, reducing alcohol consumption is a good way to decrease the risk of cancer.

✓ *Do not rely on supplements to prevent cancer:* Research is ongoing, but we do not yet know exactly what factors in plant foods provide protective benefits. Contrary to expectation, supplements alone have proven ineffective in reducing cancer risk. Trials of beta-carotene supplementation did not reduce lung cancer incidence in smokers, and while fiber has long

been thought to be protective against cancer, trials of fiber supplements did not reduce risk of occurrence of colon polyps. There is support for the benefits of vitamin D in reducing cancer risk, but there is no pill that can replace the wealth of benefits of a plant-based diet.

4. Be Physically Active

Research indicates that physical activity protects against colon cancer, breast cancer, and cancer of the uterine lining. Regular physical activity reduces cancer risk independently of other risk factors such as body fat, so even if you struggle to control your weight, exercise is beneficial in reducing cancer risk. See Figure 13-5 for the effects of exercise in reducing cancer risk. Experts speculate that exercise enhances overall health and well-being and stimulates the immune system, which may then scavenge abnormal cells more effectively. Having a strong immune system is a key factor in preventing cancer because we are exposed to carcinogens every day. Exercise improves energy metabolism and reduces insulin and related cellular growth factors in the blood. Researchers also speculate that exercise decreases the production of some reproductive hormones in both men and women, decreasing the risk of cancers that depend on these hormones to develop, such as breast and prostate cancers. Many studies have found an association between physical activity and a reduced risk of breast cancer. In one

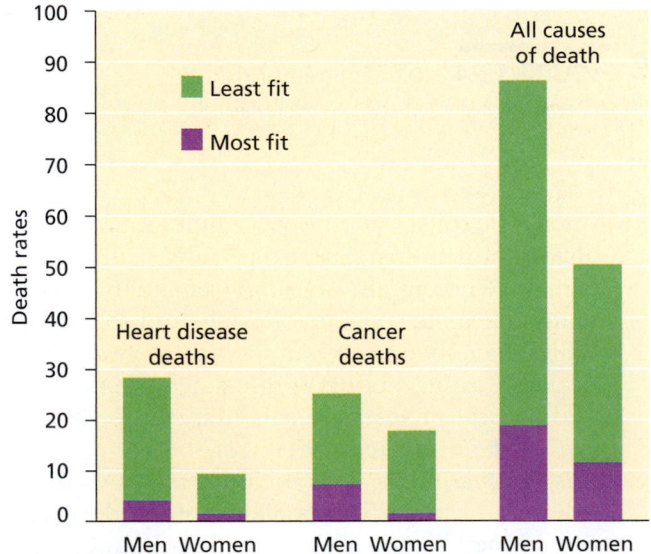

FIGURE 13-5 Exercise and health. An 8-year study of 13,344 people (10,224 men, 3,120 women) shows that physical activity reduces the risk of death from most causes. Charts compare death rates.

Source: Institute for Aerobics Research.

TOP **10** LIST

Cancer-Fighting Foods

Five servings of fruits and vegetables a day is a good start in preventing cancer, but some plant foods are more powerful than others in reducing cancer risk. Here are the best—include them in your weekly shopping list and enjoy them often.

1. Cruciferous vegetables: cabbage, cauliflower, kale, broccoli, collards, brussels sprouts.
2. Dark green leafy vegetables; orange and yellow vegetables.
3. Tomatoes, tomato sauce, watermelon.
4. Red grapes, purple grape juice.
5. Garlic, onions, leeks.
6. Citrus fruits.
7. Prunes, berries (blueberries, strawberries).
8. Legumes: red, black, and pinto beans; garbanzos, lentils, and peas.
9. Whole-grain breads, cereals.
10. Green or black tea.

For more information: www.helpguide.org/life/healthy_diet_cancer_prevention.htm

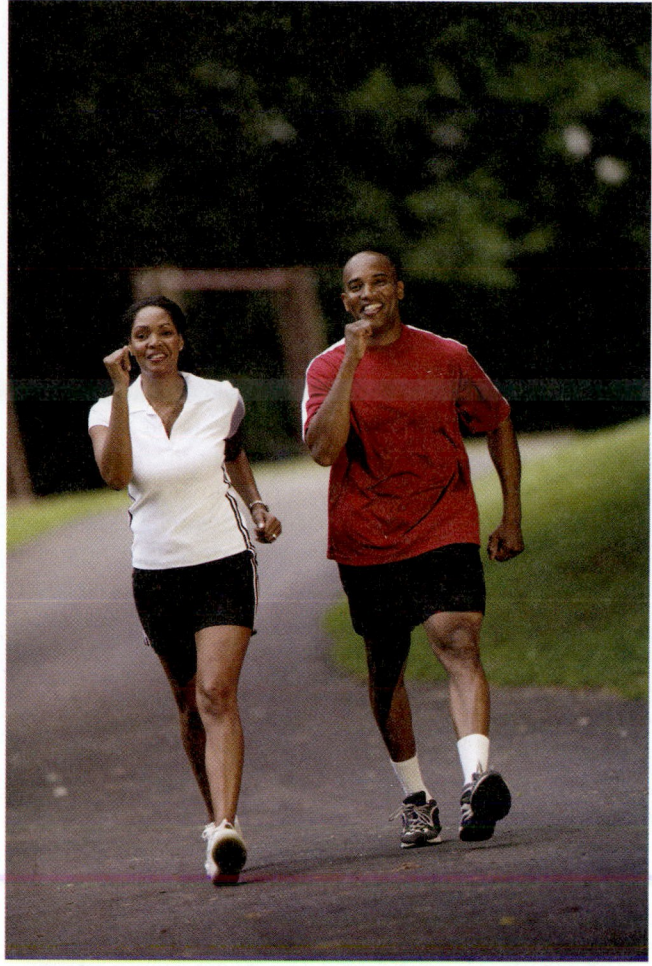

Thirty minutes or more of exercise a day pays big dividends in preventing cancer.

study, women who walked at least 30 minutes a day four times a week had a 37 percent lower risk of breast cancer than did their sedentary peers. A study of Harvard alumni found that men who burned at least 1,000 calories a week in physical activity had half the risk for colon cancer of inactive men. (One thousand calories is the approximate equivalent of walking 2 miles a day, 5 days a week.) This is true for women as well. A Harvard study of women found that for every day a woman walks a half hour, her risk of colon cancer is decreased by 10 percent. The risk of prostate cancer in men appears to be reduced by 10 to 30 percent, and reductions in lung cancer rates of 30 to 40 percent have been reported. Other studies show that the more you exercise, the more protection you get. Exercise appears to prevent colon cancer by helping to speed food through the digestive system, leaving less time for carcinogens to remain in contact with the colon.

Inactivity may be a greater risk than obesity in the cancer equation. Studies done at the Cooper Institute in Dallas show that exercise is beneficial in reducing cancer risk even for those who are overweight. Thousands of people were treadmill tested for cardiorespiratory fitness and then tracked for long-term health. Studies based on that data indicate that physically active individuals who are overweight have a lower risk of cancer than do people who are overweight and sedentary, though they still have a higher risk than do those who are thinner and fit. Whatever your weight, good health habits can pay off. To reduce cancer risk, be moderately physically active for at least 30 to 60 minutes each day, or participate in 20 to 30 minutes of vigorous activity. Also, limit sedentary habits such as computer games or watching television because these contribute to weight gain and obesity.

5. Maintain a Healthy Weight

One of the biggest challenges for many people in reducing cancer risk is reaching and maintaining a healthy weight. Most people become overweight or obese by gaining just a few pounds a year, and at any age, it helps to lose weight if you are overweight. For almost all cancers, the risk increases at the high end of the normal weight scale, before you cross into the overweight category, so the AICR recommends that you be as lean as possible within the normal range. Obese individuals, particularly those who are obese and sedentary, increase their risk of all cancers. The more overweight a person is, the greater the risk. A 16-year study of more than 900,000 U.S. adults indicated that those with the highest body mass index had a death rate from all cancers more than 50 percent higher than that of normal-weight individuals. They estimated that increased body weight was associated with up to one in five cancer deaths in the United States. Increased risk is due to a combination of factors, including sedentary lifestyle, greater caloric intake, greater fat intake, insulin resistance, high insulin levels, and body fat–mediated hormonal factors. A study of nearly 63,000 women by the American Cancer Society indicated that the weight a woman gains after age 18 predicts lifetime risk of breast cancer. Those who gained 20 to 30 pounds had 40 percent increase in breast cancer rates, and those who gained over 70 pounds doubled their risk as compared to women who maintained their weight. The least risk is seen for women who maintain a BMI under 25 throughout adulthood. Fat cells produce estrogen, which makes breast cancer grow. They estimate that weight contributes to one in every two to three breast cancer deaths.

Location of fat, as well as amount, affects cancer risk. People who carry extra weight in the abdomen are at higher risk for breast, colon, and prostate cancer. The good news is that those who are apple-shaped (as opposed to pear-shaped, having bigger thighs and hips) can reduce their risk by losing weight. It appears to be fairly easy for apple-shaped people to lose weight where it counts because fat leaves the abdomen first. Researchers believe that weight loss reduces the amount of sex hormones and insulin-related cellular growth factors available to stimulate possible precancerous cell growth in the reproductive organs. For weight management, avoid sugary drinks and juices; limit calorie-dense foods (more than 65–80 calories per ounce); limit foods high in fats and sugars, especially fast foods; and fill up on unprocessed, high-fiber foods to limit calories. To reach and maintain a healthy body weight, see Chapter 12 for information on how to balance caloric intake with physical activity.

◆ SECONDARY RISK FACTORS FOR CANCER

While the primary factors are the strongest contributors to increased cancer risk, other preventable factors also affect the risk of having cancer:

✓ Exposure to some viral infections
✓ Exposure to radiation, workplace hazards, and certain chemicals

---

TOP 10 LIST

Ways to Cut Your Risk of Cancer

1. Avoid tobacco of any kind.
2. Avoid excessive sun exposure.
3. Eat more fruits, vegetables, beans, and whole grains; decrease red and processed meats.
4. Exercise at least 30 minutes most days of the week.
5. Maintain a healthy weight.
6. Drink little or no alcohol.
7. Use protective measures against STDs.
8. Minimize exposure to radiation, workplace hazards, and chemicals.
9. Know cancer's warning signals.
10. Practice self-exams and see your physician for cancer-related checkups.

Exposure to Some Viral Infections

Some viral infections can initiate inflammation and cellular damage that leads to cancer. For example, human papilloma viruses (HPV) are the major cause of cervical cancer, and may also be a risk factor for penile cancer. These viruses can be passed from one person to another through sexual contact. Most HPV infections are cleared from the body in 2 to 4 years, but those that persist may progress to cancer. The U.S. FDA has approved two vaccines, Gardasil and Cervarix, to prevent HPV infections. Cervarix, recommended for females ages 10 to 25, targets HPV 16 and HPV 18, which cause 70 percent of cervical cancers. Gardasil also prevents infection with genital warts from HPV 6 and HPV 11 and is recommended for males and females ages 9 to 26. Both vaccines help prevent infection, but neither is effective in treating HPV or cervical cancer. Vaccination can help prevent many cervical cancer deaths, but they are effective only if given before infection with HPV.

Chronic viral hepatitis (B or C) is associated with a 34-fold increase in risk of liver cancer, and AIDS-related cancers such as Kaposi's sarcoma are caused by HIV infection. Risk of exposure to these infections can be reduced by behavioral changes. For example, condom use during sex can prevent sexual exposure to hepatitis B, HPV, and HIV. This is particularly important for young adults, because the highest-risk age group for STDs is in the late teens to early 20s. See Chapter 15 for additional information on sexually transmitted infections.

Exposure to Radiation, Workplace Hazards, and Certain Chemicals

Avoid excessive exposure to ionizing radiation. Ionizing radiation includes X rays, radon, and UV radiation. While most medical X rays emit low-dose radiation, it is still wise to use protective shields to cover body areas not being X rayed. There is also a potential problem of radioactive radon gas in the home in certain areas of the country. You can buy an inexpensive radon detector to test for radon, which increases the risk for lung cancer, especially in cigarette smokers. If you detect radon, professionals can advise you regarding steps to take to increase ventilation and seal the home against radon infiltration.

Be aware of hazards in the workplace. Exposure to asbestos and other industrial materials increases the risk, especially when combined with smoking. Minimize exposure to these products by wearing protective clothing and equipment and following standard safety procedures.

Limit your exposure to pesticides and insecticides. Not all chemicals are carcinogenic, but proven carcinogens include benzene, PCBs, DDT, vinyl chloride, arsenic, aflatoxin, chloroform, and formaldehyde. Read and follow label instructions with household and garden chemicals, and use natural products when possible (e.g., soap spray to kill aphids).

◆ EARLY DETECTION

Early detection means taking action to diagnose cancer in its earliest, most treatable stage. This includes three parts:

✓ Knowing cancer's warning signals
✓ Practicing self-exams
✓ Having regular cancer-related checkups by a physician

Once metastases spread from the primary site, cancer becomes much more difficult to cure. Although not all cancers can be detected through self-exams, such exams, along with awareness of cancer's warning signals, can alert a person to the need to consult a physician. The American Cancer Society has developed a list of cancer's seven warning signals:

✓ Change in bowel or bladder habits
✓ A sore that does not heal
✓ Unusual bleeding or discharge
✓ Thinkening or lump in the breasts or elsewhere

TABLE 13-5	Cancer Screening Guidelines
Site	**Recommendation**
Breast	Do a monthly self-exam. Have a clinical breast exam every 3 years from ages 20 to 39. Women age 40 and older should get a mammogram every 1–2 years, scheduled close to the clinical breast exam. Those at higher than average risk of breast cancer should talk to their physicians about whether and how often to have mammograms before age 40.
Colon & Rectum	Beginning at age 50, check with your doctor about the benefits of a screening test: fecal occult blood test, sigmoidoscopy, colonoscopy, double-contrast barium enema, or digital rectal exam. Newer screening tests being studied in clinical trials include a virtual colonoscopy and DNA stool test.
Prostate	See your doctor about a PSA and digital rectal exam beginning at age 50. If at high risk (African American or family history of prostate cancer), begin at age 45.
Skin	Do a monthly self-exam.
Testicles	Do a monthly self-exam.
Uterus & Cervix	Screening should begin about 3 years after a woman becomes sexually active, but no later than age 21. Women should have a Pap test at least once every 3 years. More frequent screening may be needed for women at higher risk due to factors such as HIV infection.

SOURCE: National Cancer Institute, U.S. Preventive Services Task Force, Komen Foundation, ACOG.

✓ Indigestion or difficulty swallowing
✓ Obvious change in a wart or mole
✓ Nagging cough or hoarseness

See your physician for cancer-related checkups. Even if you have no symptoms, it is important for early detection of cancer to have periodic cancer-related checkups (Table 13-5). Until all cancers can be prevented, protect yourself with knowledge about cancer signs, self-exams, early detection, regular checkups, and prompt treatment.

For most people without symptoms, cancer-related checkups are recommended every 3 years from ages 20 to 39 and annually for those over age 40. People who are at high risk for certain cancers may need tests more often.

◆ COMMON CANCERS

Many types of cancers exist, but some are much more common than others. The most common cancers for all age groups combined in frequency of occurrence are

Men	Women
✓ Prostate	✓ Breast
✓ Lung	✓ Lung
✓ Colon/Rectal	✓ Colon/Rectal

For men 15 to 34 years old, testicular cancer is the most common. While lung cancer is second in occurrence for both men and women, it is the leading cause of cancer deaths because of its low survival rate. Although they are the most frequently occurring cancers, affecting nearly one in five Americans, *skin cancers are not usually included in cancer statistics because almost all nonmelanoma skin cancers are easily cured if detected early.* Even so, there are over 11,000 skin cancer deaths yearly. See Figure 13-1 for the most deadly cancers for men and women. Common cancers are discussed here in alphabetical order.

Breast Cancer

Breast cancer is the most common cancer in women, but it is more curable than lung cancer, so it ranks as the second leading cancer killer. It is estimated that the lifetime risk of breast cancer is one in eight. Getting older is the most important risk factor for breast cancer. However, breast cancer can occur at any age. Although rare, about 2 percent of breast cancers are in men. Other risk factors for breast cancer include

✓ Having had breast cancer before.
✓ Having a sister or mother who had breast cancer, especially if she had it before menopause.
✓ Increased breast density.
✓ A long menstrual history (starting menstruation before age 12 and/or experiencing menopause after age 50). This exposes the body to high estrogen levels longer.
✓ Obesity, especially after menopause (fat cells produce estrogen).
✓ Never having a child or having the first child after age 30.
✓ Use of menopausal hormone therapy.
✓ Consumption of one or more alcoholic drinks a day.

Inherited susceptibility accounts for only 5 percent of breast cancers, but if a woman has a strong family history, there is a screening test for the genes that increase the risk. Preventive behaviors include

regular exercise, maintaining a healthy body weight, eating a healthy diet, breastfeeding an infant, and little or no use of alcohol.

The earliest sign of breast cancer is usually an abnormality found on a mammogram. Once the cancer has grown, signs include a breast lump, thickening, swelling, dimpling, tenderness, and nipple pain, discharge, and retraction. Breast pain is generally due to other conditions and is not usually an early sign of cancer.

Mammograms can detect 80–90 percent of early breast cancers, and a woman should have one annually from the age of 40. The breast self-exam (Figure 13-6), which is recommended once a month,

Breast Self-Exam (BSE)

When is the best time to perform the BSE?
- During or right after a warm shower or bath
- Warm, soapy water relaxes and smoothes the skin, making the BSE easier to perform
- Remember to do the BSE once a month just after the menstrual cycle

What are the symptoms?
- A hard, painless lump in the breast tissue (most common sign)
- Pain in the breast
- Discharge from the nipple

Who is most at risk?
- Women age 50 or older
- Women with a complex or abnormal reproductive history
- Women with a family history of breast cancer
- Women of all nationalities, backgrounds and ages are potentially at risk

How do I perform the BSE?

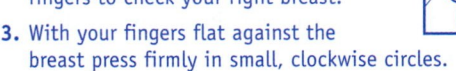

1. Check each breast one at a time.
2. Use your right hand fingers to check your left breast and your left hand fingers to check your right breast.
3. With your fingers flat against the breast press firmly in small, clockwise circles.
4. Start at the outermost top edge of your breast and spiral toward the nipple.
5. Feel for hard lumps or bumps in your breast.
6. Be certain to cover all parts of your breast.
7. Gently squeeze both nipples and look for any discharge.
8. Look carefully for changes in the size, shape, and contour of each breast, e.g., puckering, dimpling, or changes in skin texture.

FIGURE 13-6   Breast self-exam (BSE).

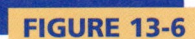

Source: Reproduced with permission from the Oncology Group, New York, New York.

is still useful for those at high risk—a personal history of cancer or a close relative with breast cancer. A self-exam typically detects larger cancers that have been growing for 6 years, whereas a mammogram can detect cancers that have grown for only 2 years and are still too small to be felt. Early detection increases survival rates. Treatment involves some combination of surgery, radiation, and chemotherapy.

Colon and Rectal Cancer

In populations where fruits and vegetables are consumed in abundance and animal foods are scarce, colon cancer is a rare disease. In the United States, however, it is the third leading cancer killer. A genetic tendency to develop noncancerous polyps in the colon, combined with a diet high in red or processed meat and low in fruits and vegetables may cause half, perhaps all, colon cancers. Chronic exposure to carcinogens in red and processed meats can eventually stimulate precancerous changes in cells. This does not mean that you are doomed by poor childhood eating habits, but many studies consistently indicate that eating a Mediterranean-style diet rich in fruits, vegetables, whole grains, beans, and fish can protect you against many forms of cancer. High levels of physical activity are also associated with a lower risk of colon cancer—by increasing intestinal motility and limiting exposure of colon cells to potentially carcinogenic compounds. Other studies have indicated that obesity is associated with doubling the risk of colorectal cancer.

Risk factors for colon cancer include

✓ Age: Over 90 percent of cases occur after age 50.
✓ Having a personal or family history of colon cancer, colon polyps, or inflammatory bowel disease.
✓ Smoking.
✓ Heavy alcohol consumption.
✓ Obesity.
✓ A diet high in red or processed meat but low in fruits and vegetables.
✓ Physical inactivity.

Preventive behaviors include not smoking, maintaining a healthy weight, eating five to nine servings or more of fruits and vegetables daily, consuming little or no alcohol, and exercising 30 minutes or more most days of the week. In addition, research indicates that consumption of milk, calcium, and regular aspirin use may have an anti-inflammatory effect.

Early-stage colon cancer usually has no symptoms. Screening beginning at age 50 is recommended to detect it. Late-stage disease may cause blood in the stool, a change in bowel habits, and lower abdominal cramping. There are several tests that can detect

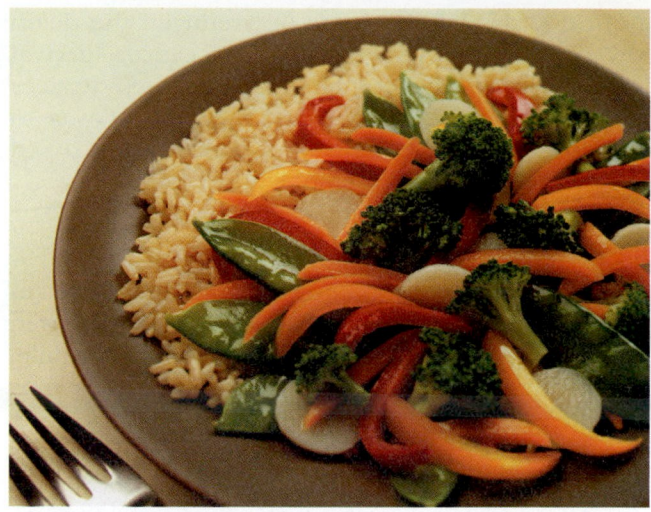

Eating more plant foods and less red meat and processed meats can reduce the risk of colon cancer as much as 75 percent.

colon and rectal cancer at an early, treatable stage, including a fecal occult blood test and digital rectal exam (see Table 13-5). Some cancers can be treated by early detection and removal of polyps. Treatment usually involves surgery if the disease is localized, with chemotherapy and radiation added if it may have spread.

Lung Cancer

Lung cancer is a rare disease except among smokers. Exposure to sidestream cigarette smoke increases the risk for nonsmokers. Lung tissue damage and cellular changes that precede lung cancer have been observed in 93 percent of active smokers but in only 6 percent of ex-smokers and 1 percent of nonsmokers. If a smoker quits, these early precancerous cellular changes are reversible, and the damaged bronchial lining often returns to normal. If the smoker continues, the abnormal cell growth may progress to cancer.

While lung cancer deaths are declining in men due to decreased smoking, they have increased in women and surpassed breast cancer deaths by 80 percent. Lung cancer, the leading cancer killer for both men and women, has a low survival rate because it is seldom discovered in its earliest stages. Symptoms include chronic cough, blood-streaked sputum, chest pain, and recurrent bronchitis or pneumonia. By the time it has grown large enough to produce noticeable symptoms or to be visible on X ray, it is already well advanced. It metastasizes readily through the bloodstream to the brain and other organs and is difficult to treat. Surgery is usually the first treatment option, followed by chemotherapy and radiation. Surgery may extend survival but seldom produces a cure. Early detection has not reduced the death rate either. The 5-year rate for lung cancer survival is 5 percent and has not changed, despite advances in cancer treatment, in 40 years. The best way to prevent lung cancer is to not smoke and to avoid environmental tobacco smoke.

Prostate Cancer

This is the most common cancer (excluding skin cancer) and the second leading cause of cancer deaths in men. It affects about one in six men over a lifetime. The prostate gland produces seminal fluid. It wraps around the urethra, the tube that transports urine from the bladder to outside the body. When it swells from infection or disease, it blocks urinary flow.

These factors increase risk of prostate cancer:

✓ Age over 50 (risk increases with age)
✓ Diet high in saturated fats
✓ Obesity
✓ African American (incidence is far higher than for white men)
✓ Family history of prostate cancer

Preventive behaviors include consuming a diet low in animal fats and high in plant foods (especially those red in lycopenes found in red and pink foods such as tomatoes), and exercising 30 minutes or more most days of the week. Symptoms of prostate cancer include difficulty starting or stopping urination; weak urine flow; blood in the urine; painful urination; need to urinate frequently, particularly at night; and pain in the lower back, pelvis, or thighs. These signs are very general and can be caused by many other conditions. The methods for detecting prostate cancer are the prostate-specific-antigen (PSA) test and the digital rectal exam. These should be done annually starting at age 50 or earlier.

Skin Cancer

Skin cancer accounts for nearly half of all cancers. About one in five Americans will eventually get skin cancer. Sun overexposure during childhood and the teen years accounts for over three-fourths of your lifetime exposure to the sun's ultraviolet radiation. Well-tanned skin is a sign of injury to the skin, not a sign of health. Anyone can get skin cancer, but most susceptible are those who work out in the sun, live in sunny climates, or have blond or red hair, light-colored eyes, or fair skin that doesn't tan easily (Table 13-6).

The three main types of skin cancer that may be caused by UV radiation are basal cell, squamous cell, and malignant melanoma. Basal cell cancers, the most common, are raised pearly nodules that involve the outer layers of skin. Squamous cell

Skin Type	Sunburn and Tanning History	SPF
I	Always burns, never tans	20–30
II	Burns easily, tans minimally	15–20
III	Burns moderately, tans gradually to light brown	15
IV	Burns minimally, tans well to medium brown	15
V	Rarely burns, tans profusely to dark	10–15
VI	Never burns, deeply pigmented	10–15

TABLE 13-6   What Is Your Skin Type?

cancers are either wartlike growths that ulcerate in the center or pinkish, raised, opaque nodules. These cancers are related to cumulative exposure to UV radiation and sensitivity of a person's skin to sun damage. They are highly curable, do not tend to metastasize, and can be removed by a physician. See Figure 13-7 for typical examples.

Over 90 percent of these cancers appear on sun-exposed areas, such as the face, neck, ears, hands, and forearms. A recent study of people under the age of 40 has found that over the last 30 years, basal cell cancer has more than doubled in women and squamous cell cancer has increased fourfold in both sexes. Researchers attributed the increase to increased sun exposure and use of tanning beds. Studies indicate that the risk of melanoma jumps by 75 percent in people who use tanning beds in their teens and twenties. As a result, the World Health Organization has moved tanning beds to its highest cancer risk category.

Malignant **melanoma,** which usually starts as a dark wart or mole, is the most rapidly increasing type of skin cancer in the United States. Rather than cumulative sun exposure, intermittent severe overexposure leading to sunburn, particularly in childhood and adolescence, appears to increase risk for

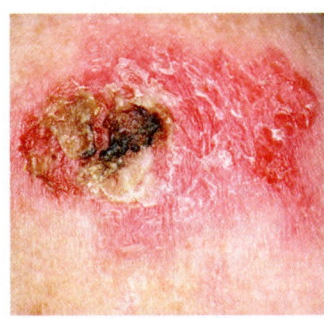 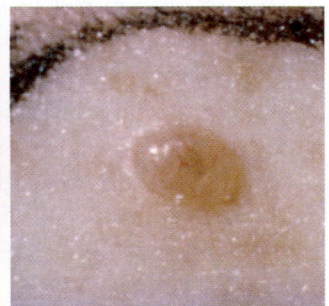

Squamous cell cancer
A flat, red spot that is rough, dry or scaly. A lump that bleeds or develops a crust

Basal cell cancer
Small, smooth, shiny, pale, or waxy lump

FIGURE 13-7   Basal and squamous cell cancers.

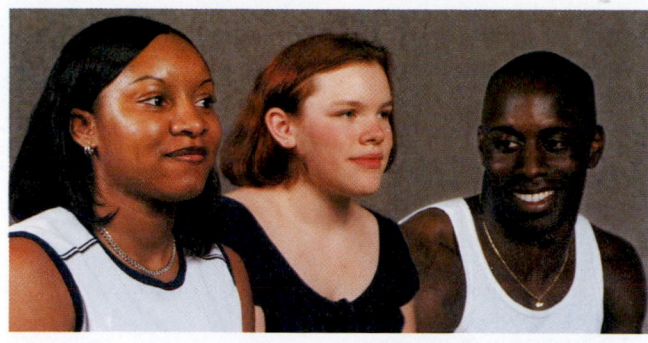

Skin cancer risk is greater in people with fair skin. Melanin in darker skin provides a measure of protection from damaging UV rays.

melanoma in later life. It has a deadly tendency to metastasize and accounts for about 75 percent of skin cancer deaths. The problem is particularly severe for men and whites. Men die of melanoma at twice the rate of women. People with naturally dark skin, type VI, have a built-in measure of protection. About 98 percent of malignant melanoma occurs in whites, though African Americans tend to be diagnosed at a later stage. Malignant melanoma diagnosed at an early stage can be treated, but when it penetrates even one-tenth of an inch into the skin, the survival rate decreases by 50 percent. Contributing to increasing rates of skin cancer is the fact that in the upper atmosphere, the thinning ozone layer allows more of the sun's damaging ultraviolet radiation to reach the skin. As a result, skin cancer rates are increasing by about 3 percent per year, faster than those for any other cancer. Approximately 90 percent of skin cancers can be prevented by protecting the skin from the sun's rays.

While young people often think of themselves as immune to skin cancer, nearly one-third of

melanomas occur in people under age 45. Among 25- to 29-year-old women, melanoma is more common than any other type of non-skin cancer, including breast and colon cancers. The most common sites are the upper back and the back of the legs, but it can occur anywhere from the scalp to the soles of the feet. You don't have to be a dermatologist to recognize a potential melanoma. Know what skin cancer looks like and examine your skin at least once a year using the skin self-exam in Figure 13-8. Learn where your moles are and what they look

If You Can <u>Spot</u> It, You Can <u>Stop</u> It

Coupled with a yearly skin exam by a doctor, *self-examination* of your skin once a month is the best way to detect the early warning signs of basal cell carcinoma, squamous cell carcinoma, and malignant melanoma, the three main types of skin cancer. *Look for a new growth or any skin change.*

What you'll need: a bright light; a full-length mirror; a hand mirror; two chairs or stools; a blow-dryer.

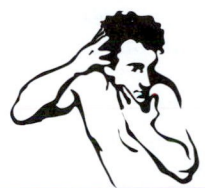

Examine head and face, using one or both mirrors. Use a blow-dryer to inspect scalp.

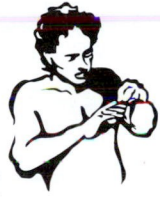

Check hands, including nails. In full-length mirror, examine elbows, arms, underarms.

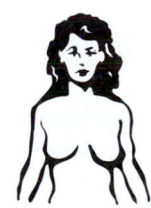

Focus on neck, chest, torso. Women: Check under breasts.

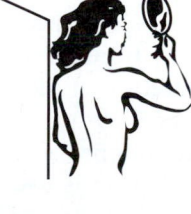

With back to the mirror, use hand mirror to inspect back of neck, shoulders, upper arms, back, buttocks, legs.

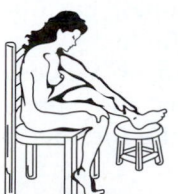

Sitting down, check legs and feet, including soles, heels, and nails. Use hand mirror to examine genitals.

FIGURE 13-8   **Skin self-exam.**

Source: Reprinted by permission of the Skin Cancer Foundation.
© 1992 New York, NY, USA www.skincancer.org

THINK ABOUT IT

Vitamin D is necessary for health. It can be obtained from foods (milk, oily fish), from vitamin pills, and is manufactured in your skin when exposed to sunlight. However, skin cancer risk increases with accumulated exposure to sunlight. What are considerations to keep in mind if you want to reduce cancer risk yet still get a healthy dose of vitamin D?

connect

Go online to Connect to complete this activity.
http://connect.mcgraw-hill.com

- **Asymmetry**—The shape of one half does not match the other.

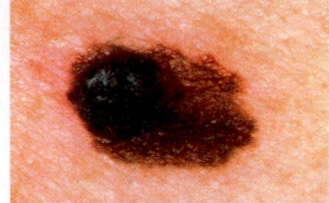

- **Border**—The edges are often ragged, notched, blurred, or irregular in outline; the pigment may spread into the surrounding skin.

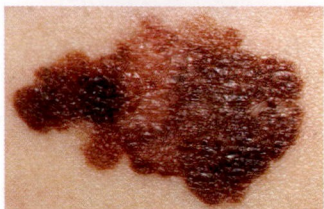

- **Color**—The color is uneven. Shades of black, brown, and tan may be present. Areas of white, gray, red, pink, or blue also may be seen.

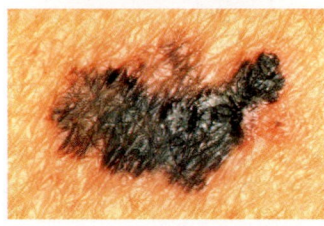

- **Diameter**—There is a change in size, usually an increase. Melanomas are usually larger than the eraser of a pencil (¼ inch or 5 millimeters).

- **Evolving**—growing or changing in shape, size, or color. Or **elevation**—raised or lumpy surface.

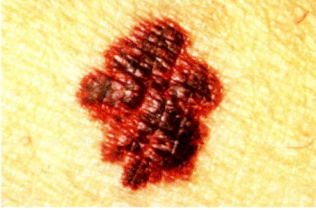

FIGURE 13-9   ABCDE test for malignant melanoma.

like, and then you will notice if there are any changes. If you find unusual moles or skin spots, the American Melanoma Society suggests using the ABCDE test for early detection of malignant melanoma (Figure 13-9). Besides moles, watch for sores that do not heal; unusual bumps; and chronically scaly, red, or pinkish patches of skin. If detected early, skin cancer has an 85 to 99 percent cure rate. Surgery is the usual treatment for basal and squamous cell cancers, and radiation is used occasionally. Malignant melanoma requires not only surgery for the tumor but often removal of adjacent lymph nodes. Table 13-7 summarizes the risk factors for skin cancer. Videos illustrating how melanoma develops and spreads and the ABCD test are included on the Internet Resources list at the end of the chapter.

Testicular Cancer

Most people think that cancer is a disease old people get. Cancer of the testicle is different. It is not one of the most common types of cancer in this

TABLE 13-7	Risk Factors for Skin Cancer

While anyone can get skin cancer, these characteristics indicate higher risk:

- Light skin color
- Family history of skin cancer
- Personal history of skin cancer
- Atypical mole or a large number of moles (over 50)
- Freckles (indicating sun sensitivity and sun damage)
- Severe sunburn in childhood
- Chronic sun overexposure
- Frequent use of tanning beds, especially before age 20.

country, but it is the most common cancer in young men between the ages of 15 and 34. Warning signs include a swelling or hard lump in the testicle, a dull ache in the lower abdomen and groin, a sensation of heaviness, and pain in the testes. Your risk of getting testicular cancer is 40 times higher if you have a testicle that never descended into the scrotum or descended after age 6. World-renowned cyclist Lance Armstrong was diagnosed with testicular cancer at age 25, was treated, and is now cancer free. Before he recovered, he created the Lance Armstrong Foundation, livestrong.com, to advocate for people with cancer.

Lives could be saved if more testicular cancers were detected and treated early. The 5-year survival rate of testicular cancer is 91 percent. Treatment does not mean losing your "manhood" or your ability to have normal sex, and it doesn't mean you can't have children.

Men discover most testicular cancers by learning how to examine their testicles. In doing this once a month, you can greatly increase the chances of finding a testicular cancer early if it does occur. All young men should learn and practice the monthly testicular self-examination, which is detailed in Figure 13-10, from adolescence on.

Uterine and Cervical Cancer

With the widespread use of Pap smears for early detection, the death rate from uterine cancer has declined. Nearly all cases of cervical cancer are linked to the **human papilloma virus (HPV),** which is spread through sexual contact. Risk factors for cervical cancer include

- ✓ Becoming sexually active at an early age
- ✓ Having had several different sex partners
- ✓ Genital infections such as herpes, HPV, and HIV
- ✓ Smoking (it weakens the immune system)

A Pap test, in which cells from the cervix and uterine lining are examined under a microscope, is a simple procedure that can be done at intervals by

Testicular Self-Exam (TSE)

When is the best time to perform the TSE?
- During or right after a warm shower or bath
- Warm water relaxes the skin on the scrotum, making the TSE easier to perform
- Remember to do the TSE once a month

What are the symptoms of testicular cancer?
- A hard, painless lump on the testicle (most common sign)
- Slight enlargement of one of the testicles
- A dull ache or feeling of heaviness in the testicles, groin, or lower abdomen

Who is most at risk?
- White males ages 15-35
- Men with a testicle that did not come down into the scrotum
- Men with a father or brother with testicular cancer

How do I perform the TSE?

1. Check each testicle one at a time.
2. Place your index and middle fingers under the testicle and your thumb on top.
3. Gently roll the testicle between your thumb and fingers. It should feel smooth to the touch.
4. Feel for any hard lumps on the testicle.
5. Repeat the process with the other testicle.
6. If you find a lump, see your doctor immediately.

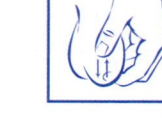

FIGURE 13-10 Testicular self-exam (TSE).

Source: Reproduced with permission from the Oncology Group, New York, New York.

physicians as a part of each pelvic examination. There are usually no symptoms with early-stage cervical cancer. When the cells invade nearby tissue, symptoms include abnormal bleeding, bleeding between periods or after sex, and increased vaginal discharge. Bleeding after menopause may also indicate cervical cancer. If cervical cancer is detected at an early stage, it can easily be removed. Use of the Pap test, along with timely treatment, can prevent nearly all deaths from cervical cancer. Use of condoms can prevent sexual infections that initiate the disease. Also, vaccination against HPV 16 and HPV 18 is effective in preventing HPV infection, thus, cervical cancer. See Chapter 15, Preventing Sexually Transmitted Disease, for more information.

Uterine cancer affects the lining of the uterus and is most common in women over age 50. The risk factors are similar to those for breast cancer, including obesity and increased lifetime estrogen exposure. Symptoms include abnormal uterine bleeding and spotting, especially after menopause. Uterine cancer is usually treated with surgery, radiation, chemotherapy, and/or hormones.

◆ COPING WITH CANCER

What can you do when someone you care about is diagnosed with cancer? Many of us will face this at some time in our lives because cancer affects one in three people. You may have mixed emotions: anger and grief that this could happen to someone close to you, fear of the future, or compassion and sympathy for what that person is facing. You might feel uncomfortable around that person, not knowing what to say or do, and tend to avoid him or her or avoid discussing the illness. What can you do? Plenty. First, you should realize that cancers overall have a 60 percent cure rate. Second, loving support from friends and family members increases the quality of life and survival rate to such an extent that it is a powerful adjunct to medical treatment. A study at Stanford University found that women with advanced breast cancer who participated in weekly support groups doubled their predicted life expectancy and lived an average of 18 months longer than did those who were not in support groups. Here are several things you can do to help a friend or loved one deal with cancer:

1. Share your thoughts and feelings and encourage your friend to do so. Allow your friend to express hopes, fears, and sadness; accept those feelings

Tips for Behavior Change to Fight Cancer

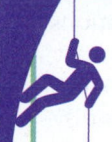

- Eat more plant foods–5 to 9 servings daily.
- Include 1 or 2 fruits and vegetables at each meal and for snacks.
- Reduce refined grains in your diet; eat more whole grains.
- Eat cruciferous vegetables cooked or in salads.
- Include more brightly colored vegetables in your diet.

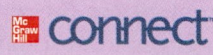

Go online to Connect to complete this activity.
http://connect.mcgraw-hill.com

without trying to change them. Showing your love and concern and discussing mutual fears can bring you closer and provide great comfort. There is no right way to feel about cancer, no right way to react. Being honest and open strengthens relationships.

2. Offer to accompany your friend on a visit to the doctor or hospital. You can provide transportation to and from treatments, take notes while the doctor gives instructions, and provide support.

3. Instead of saying "Call me if you need anything," offer specific help: cook a meal, do the dishes, do laundry, walk the dog, take the kids to the park, pick up medicine from the pharmacy.

4. Encourage your friend to join you in some enjoyable activities: go to a movie or rent some comedy videos, go for a walk together, go on a picnic, or have a potluck dinner with friends.

5. Contact a cancer survivor who can talk to your friend, answer questions, and share the insights of someone who has walked down the same road.

6. Help your friend contact a cancer support group. While you can't know what your friend is going through, other cancer patients do know and can provide the kind of open discussion and empathy that reduces distress and strengthens coping skills. Provide transportation to meetings. Some resources that may help you locate support groups: the American Cancer Society (800-227-2345) and the National Cancer Institute's Cancer Information Service (800-422-6237). Also check with your friend's physician, church, or hospital or on the Internet.

What if *you* are diagnosed with cancer? How can you cope? Here are some suggestions:

1. Take an active role: learn everything you can about the cancer and its treatments.

2. Ask lots of questions so that you understand what is happening to you and what your options are. Think about what you can do to enhance your recovery and discuss it with your doctor.

3. Take care of yourself. Exercise, eat healthfully, get enough sleep, manage stress. Your immune system needs every advantage you can give it. If you don't feel like going for a walk, try stretching or doing yoga. Ask your doctor how long you need to wait after a chemotherapy treatment to exercise.

4. Build a support system. Many studies point to the positive effect of a good support system on health and the immune system. Some friends won't feel comfortable knowing that you have cancer because of their fear of the disease or the fear that you will die. They may not know what to say or do, and as a result you could become socially isolated. Have friends and relatives join you in a walk, a meal, shopping, or going to a movie. Ask friends for help with research, transportation to medical appointments, cooking meals, home maintenance, and so on. Learn to accept help graciously.

5. Talk about your feelings. Sharing your concerns openly and honestly with a friend or family member may bring you closer and help you cope better.

6. Find a cancer support group. Talk to a cancer survivor. We don't know why, but there is something about sharing experiences that helps people in support groups live longer than those who go it alone.

7. Maintain your sense of humor. Do something that makes you laugh every day. Watch a funny video, have a good laugh with a friend. A sense of humor helps you cope with cancer and treatments. Cultivate positive feelings to mobilize your body's healing energies and make yourself feel better.

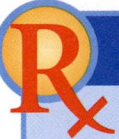

PRESCRIPTION FOR ACTION

You've read the chapter. Now go do one or more of these:

✓ Check the expiration date on your sunscreen.

✓ Do a skin, breast, or testicular self-exam. Schedule a reminder to do one on your calendar for next month too.

✓ Review the "Healthy Changes" table and try one or more of these changes today.

✓ Eat a green, orange, or deep yellow vegetable and a fruit at your next meal.

✓ Show a family member or friend the skin cancer pictures and ABCDE test for malignant melanoma.

✓ If you smoke, cut the number of cigarettes you smoke in half or quit for a day.

✓ Take out the skin map lab in this chapter and map your skin spots.

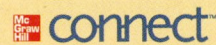   Go online to Connect to complete this activity. http://connect.mcgraw-hill.com

Frequently Asked Questions

Q. Do tanning beds provide a safe tan?

A. Tanning beds used to emit only UVA ("tanning") rays, but now many approximate natural sunlight, emitting a mix of UVA and UVB ("burning") radiation. UVA rays penetrate deeper into the skin than do UVB rays and can cause serious damage to DNA in skin cells. Both kinds injure the skin, collagen, and immune response and encourage wrinkling and skin cancer. It is a myth that tanning beds provide a safe "base" tan before a midwinter vacation. The protection is minimal, and you will still burn unless you apply sunscreen.

Q. Are self-tanning lotions and sprays safe?

A. While many early products turned the skin orange, some newer products contain an FDA-approved dye, dihydroxyacetone (DHA). It stains skin a light brown and is safe to use because it appears to work only on the outermost skin layer. Best results are obtained for people with skin types II and III who have applied the product two to four times within 1 day. Skin darkened with a dye does not provide UV protection, and you still need to wear sunscreen to guard against burns.

Q. I sunburned nearly every summer during childhood. Am I doomed to have skin cancer?

A. While sunburns and sun overexposure during childhood increase your lifetime risk of skin cancer, the skin does have a capacity to heal. Skin cancer isn't inevitable, but if you are at higher risk, it is especially important to know what skin cancer looks like, examine your skin monthly, and use sunscreen when you are outside. What are you doing now to take care of your skin?

Q. My grandfather and father had skin cancer. Does cancer run in families?

A. All cancers are caused by a malfunctioning gene that controls cell growth and replication. The American Cancer Society estimates that about 5 to 10 percent of cancers are related to an inherited gene that predisposes a person to a certain type of cancer, such as certain types of breast cancer. Having an inherited copy of a damaged gene doesn't mean that cancer is inevitable; rather, the risk is higher, and it is more important than ever that a person practice preventive behaviors. Gene malfunctions in most other cancers are initiated by external factors such as sunlight and chemical exposure (e.g., tobacco use) or internal factors such as hormones. Most skin cancers are related to sun overexposure, although if you inherited fair skin that burns easily, you are more susceptible to UV damage than is someone who inherited a darker skin tone.

Q. I smoked two packs of cigarettes a day for 3 years but quit and haven't had one in 5 years. What is my risk of cancer?

A. After 5 smoke-free years, your risk is about half that of a smoker. After 10 smoke-free years, it will be the same as if you never smoked.

Q. I hear blueberries and pomegranates are high in antioxidants. Should I eat them instead of other foods?

A. No. There is no one perfect food. Eating a lot of one food at the expense of others can shortchange you on a balance of nutrients. Your best bet is to eat a variety of fruits and vegetables rather than concentrating on a few.

Q. Does eating more fruits and vegetables decrease risk of breast cancer?

A. Studies comparing cancer rates in different countries have indicated that eating five or more servings daily of fruits and vegetables is associated with reduced risk of several chronic diseases, including heart disease, colon cancer, and several other cancers, particularly if this habit is started young and practiced across a lifetime. This may also help improve diabetes control and in maintaining healthy weight. A recent study of 50,000 postmenopausal women reported no significant benefit of a low-fat diet or increased consumption of fruits and vegetables in reducing risk of breast or colon cancer. However the difference in fruit/vegetable consumption between groups was probably too small (one serving) to show an effect. In addition, few participants met the dietary fat goal of 20 percent, as fat consumption averaged 28 percent! For those who did meet the guidelines, there was a small, but beneficial reduction in breast cancer rates. What this study shows is that we cannot wait until age 50 to start eating healthfully and expect a large reduction in cancer risk. Cancer risk factors build over a lifetime, and dietary habits are most effective if practiced over many years. Other things you can do to prevent breast cancer as well as other chronic diseases include avoiding weight gain in adulthood, no or moderate use of alcohol, and exercising regularly.

Q. The only vegetable I like is corn. Can't I just take a vitamin pill or a few supplements instead of eating fruits and vegetables to reduce cancer risk?

A. In addition to a healthy diet, a daily multivitamin can provide added protection against a number of chronic diseases. However, pills cannot make up for a bad diet. There is good evidence that a diet rich in certain fruits, vegetables, and whole-grain products lowers the risk of some types of cancer, but it is not yet clear whether it is the antioxidants, folic acid, or another of the dozens of phytochemicals in these foods that makes them cancer-protective. A plant may be more than the sum of its nutrients. Taking a vitamin supplement is good, but no one compound, or even a small group of compounds, will replace hundreds of nutrients, many of which we are only beginning to learn about. Don't count on a vitamin pill alone to replace a diet abundant in fruits and vegetables.

Q.   Is it true that air pollution increases lung cancer risk as much as smoking?

A.   No. Being a smoker presents a far greater risk of lung cancer than does air pollution. While breathing polluted air does contribute to increased lung cancer risk, the American Cancer Society estimates the risk to be about 1/100th that of smoking a pack of cigarettes a day. Breathing dirty air presents a greater risk of respiratory problems for people with asthma, bronchitis, and heart disease.

Q.   Do food additives and preservatives cause cancer?

A.   No; this is a common misconception. In fact, preservatives can reduce risk of foodborne illness. Obesity, smoking, and inactivity are far greater risk factors. Check out www.aicr.org for more information on diet and cancer.

Q.   Do underwire bras cause breast cancer? What about antiperspirants? Caffeine? Cell phones?

A.   No on all counts. There have been many large-scale studies of the causes of breast cancer, and none of the causes you've asked about has been linked to increased risk. Risk reducers include limiting alcohol to one drink a day or less, maintaining normal weight, doing daily exercise, and eating five or more daily servings of produce. A study of 420,000 cell phone users over a 20-year period showed no link between cell phones and brain tumors.

Summary

You can significantly increase your chances of living a healthy, active life, free of disabling disease, by making wise daily personal choices. Your risk of cancer can be greatly decreased with awareness of primary and secondary risk factors and appropriate lifestyle changes. These changes involve avoiding tobacco, reducing sun exposure, eating more plant foods and fewer high-fat animal products, doing regular exercise, maintaining a healthy weight, using little or no alcohol, using protective measures against viral infections, and minimizing exposure to radiation, workplace hazards, and some chemicals. Early detection is also important. This includes knowing cancer's seven warning signals, performing regular self-exams, and having regular cancer-related checkups. Cancer is not inevitable. Acting to control risks in your immediate environment is a powerful way to enhance your total wellness.

Terms

- antioxidants
- benign
- cancer
- carcinogens
- crucifera
- free radicals
- human papilloma virus (HPV)
- malignant
- melanoma
- metastasis
- phytochemicals
- precancerous
- tumor

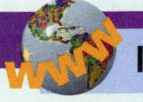

Internet Resources

American Cancer Society

www.cancer.org

Has a wealth of information about different types of cancers, cancer facts and data, prevention, detection, treatment, coping with cancer, and discussion groups. Also has a search engine for information on cancer resources and activities in your area.

American Institute for Cancer Research

www.AICR.org

Provides comprehensive information on diet and health guidelines for cancer prevention for consumers and health professionals.

Cancerfacts.com

www.cancerfacts.com

Contains a cancer profiler with information on specific cancers, including treatment options, side effects, and data on the latest medical research. Also has cancer news, personal stories, support groups, and links to other cancer resources.

Centers for Disease Control and Prevention

www.cdc.gov

Has information and statistics on a wide variety of health concerns, including cancer statistics and fact sheets.

The Harvard Center for Cancer Prevention

www.yourdiseaserisk.harvard.edu

Provides a quiz for estimating your risk of having cancer, as well as tips on prevention.

Lance Armstrong Foundation

www.livestrong.org

Provides information on testicular and breast cancer prevention, detection, and treatment.

Mayo Clinic

www.mayoclinic.com

A comprehensive health information Web site that has a Cancer Center containing basic cancer information, treatments, coping with cancer, alternative care, and a self-test quiz on cancer prevention.

National Cancer Institute

www.cancer.gov

Provides comprehensive information from the National Institutes for Health with cancer fact sheets and information on types of cancer, treatments, prevention, genetics, causes, screening, testing, and coping with cancer. Has links to cancer literature and clinical trials.

Oncolink

www.oncolink.org

A site from the University of Pennsylvania that contains information on types of cancer, statistics, treatment options, clinical trials, coping with cancer, frequently asked questions, latest cancer news articles, and other cancer resources.

Skin Cancer Foundation

www.skincancer.org

Provides information on types of skin cancers, prevention, detection, self-exams, sun safety, treatments, and the latest research articles. Has photos to enable early identification of melanoma.

Susan G. Komen Breast Cancer Foundation

www.komen.org

Contains valuable information about breast cancer prevention, detection, and treatment including a video on how to do a breast self-exam and breast cancer self-test.

Videos

ABCDE Test for Malignant Melanoma
www.mayoclinic.com/health/melanoma/DS00575
Breast Cancer: Screen and Treat
http://tinyurl.com/ch13screen
How to Do a Skin Self-Exam
http://tinyurl.com/ch13sksexam
Five Habits for Healthy Skin
www.mayoclinic.com/health/skin-care/SN00003
How Melanoma Develops and Spreads
http://mayoclinic.com/health/melanoma/min00657
Mammography (an Introduction)
http://tinyurl.com/ch13mamography
Reducing the Chances of Getting Cancer
http://tinyurl.com/ch13mam
Skin Cancer Prevention and Early Detection
http://tinyurl.com/ch13skin
Skin Cancer/Sunscreen: The Dilemma
http://tinyurl.com/ch13spf
Sun Exposure
http://tinyurl.com/ch13sunexposure
Sunless Tanning
www.mayoclinic.com/sunless_tanning/sn00037
Tanning Beds
www.mayoclinic.com/health/tanning/HQ01487
Treating Cervical Cancer
http://video.healthination.com/usnews/hpv-cervical-cancer.html
Vitamin D and Cancer Reduction
http://tinyurl.com/ch13vitd
Vitamin D Prevents Cancer. Is It True?
http://tinyurl.com/ch13vitd2
What Is Breast Cancer?
http://video.healthination.com/usnews/breast-cancer.html
What Is Prostate Cancer?
http://video.healthination.com/usnews/prostate-cancer.html
Why Do a Skin Self-Exam?
http://video.healthination.com/usnews/skin-self-exam.html

LAB Activity 13-1

Name _____ **Class/Activity Section** _____ **Date** _____

What Is Your Cancer Risk?

Cancer isn't always something that "just happens." Behaviors that you practice regularly over a lifetime can increase or decrease your risk of a serious illness, including cancer. Take this test to check your risk related to personal behaviors and then assess what changes you can make to reduce your risk. Scores below 40 indicate an increased risk of cancer due to personal behavior.

		Yes
1.	I do not smoke.	8
2.	I do not use smokeless tobacco.	4
3.	I am rarely exposed to sidestream smoke.	2
4.	I avoid tanning, even in tanning booths.	2
5.	I use at least SPF 15 sunscreen when outside for 20 minutes or longer.	2
6.	I use a hat, long-sleeved shirt, and protective clothing if I must be outside for several hours in the sun.	2
7.	I seldom eat fried foods.	1
8.	I eat red or processed meat, only a couple of times a week.	1
9.	I usually consume low-fat dairy products.	1
10.	I eat five or more servings of fruits and vegetables daily.	1
11.	I eat whole-grain products regularly.	1
12.	I eat cruciferous vegetables two or more times weekly.	1
13.	I often eat deeply colored or leafy green vegetables.	1
14.	I consume fruits and vegetables high in vitamin C five or more times a week.	1
15.	I rarely eat charcoal-grilled or smoked meats.	1
16.	I rarely eat heavily salted or pickled meats.	1
17.	I am physically active 30 minutes or more, 3 to 5 days a week.	4
18.	My physical activity includes 3 or more days of aerobic activity, following the FITT formula.	2
19.	I am within 5 pounds of my ideal weight.	3
20.	My waist measurement is less than 35 inches (female) or 40 inches (male).	3
21.	I use little or no alcohol.	1
22.	I use protective measures to avoid STDs.	1
23.	I limit my exposure to insecticides, X rays, and known carcinogens in the workplace (e.g., asbestos, PCBs).	1

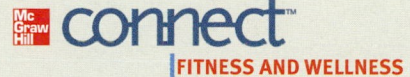

http://connect.mcgraw-hill.com

	Yes
24. I know cancer's seven warning signals.	1
25. I do a monthly breast or testicular self-exam.	1
26. I do a regular skin self-exam.	1
27. I follow the regular cancer checkup schedule.	1

1. Over the next 3 weeks, 3 to 6 months, 1 year, or more, what changes can you make to reduce your cancer risk?

   a. 3 weeks:

   b. 3 to 6 months:

   c. 1 year or more:

LAB Activity 13-2

Lunch Box Guidelines

Cancer risk reduction is as simple as choosing your next meal. Use the six dietary guidelines in Chapter 13 to complete the following items:

1. Give four *different* dietary guidelines for reducing cancer risk and, using the **menu below,** select a food that exemplifies each guideline.

   Guideline

   -
   -
   -
   -

   Food

   -
   -
   -
   -

2. List two dietary habits that increase cancer risk and use the following menu to select a specific food example for each.

RESIDENCE HALL DINING SERVICE MENU

LUNCH

	Salad Bar	Desserts
cream of chicken soup	shredded lettuce	strawberries
lentil soup	fresh spinach	soft-serve frozen yogurt
toasted bacon sandwich	chopped broccoli and cauliflower	sugar cookie
tuna in lettuce cup	soy nuts	
veggie burger	pea, peanut, and cheese salad	
yogurt	canned onion rings	
sliced American cheese	applesauce	
luncheon meats	bacon bits	
dill pickles	tomato slices	
potato chips	cottage cheese	
whole kernel corn	shredded cheddar cheese	
white bread	shredded carrots	
whole-wheat bread	beans	
butter		

McGraw Hill **connect**™
FITNESS AND WELLNESS

http://connect.mcgraw-hill.com

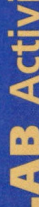

3. Plan your own cancer-reducing 1-day menu using foods available to you in *your* residence hall or home and following the dietary recommendations for reducing cancer risk given in this chapter.

Breakfast:

Lunch:

Dinner:

Snack:

Foods to reduce or eliminate:

CHAPTER 14

Understanding Substance Abuse and Addictive Behavior

STUDY QUESTIONS

You will have successfully mastered this chapter if you can answer the following:

1. What are the three common elements found in addiction?
2. How does addiction start in the brain?
3. What is the most abused legal drug in the United States?
4. What five factors affect alcohol absorption, and what are four reasons women can get drunk faster than men?
5. What is the difference between low-risk alcohol use and high-risk alcohol use?
6. What is binge drinking?
7. What is the blood alcohol concentration (BAC) at which a person is regarded as legally drunk?
8. What is the "Zero . . . One . . . Three Rule for Lower-Risk Drinking"?
9. What are the harmful effects of alcohol on the body, and what should you do if a friend overdoses on alcohol or shows signs of alcohol poisoning?
10. What are five tips/strategies for drinking less or not at all?
11. What is the number one cause of preventable death and health problems in this country?
12. What are the health hazards related to passive smoking?
13. What is the most commonly used illegal drug in the United States? What drug does the government list as its top priority in the war against drugs?
14. What is a psychoactive drug? What categories are discussed in this chapter?
15. What are four common kinds of nonprescription drugs that can lead to physical dependence if overused, and how can prescribed drugs be abused?
16. What are the dangers of using dietary supplements containing ephedra (ephedrine)?

You will find the answers as you read this chapter.

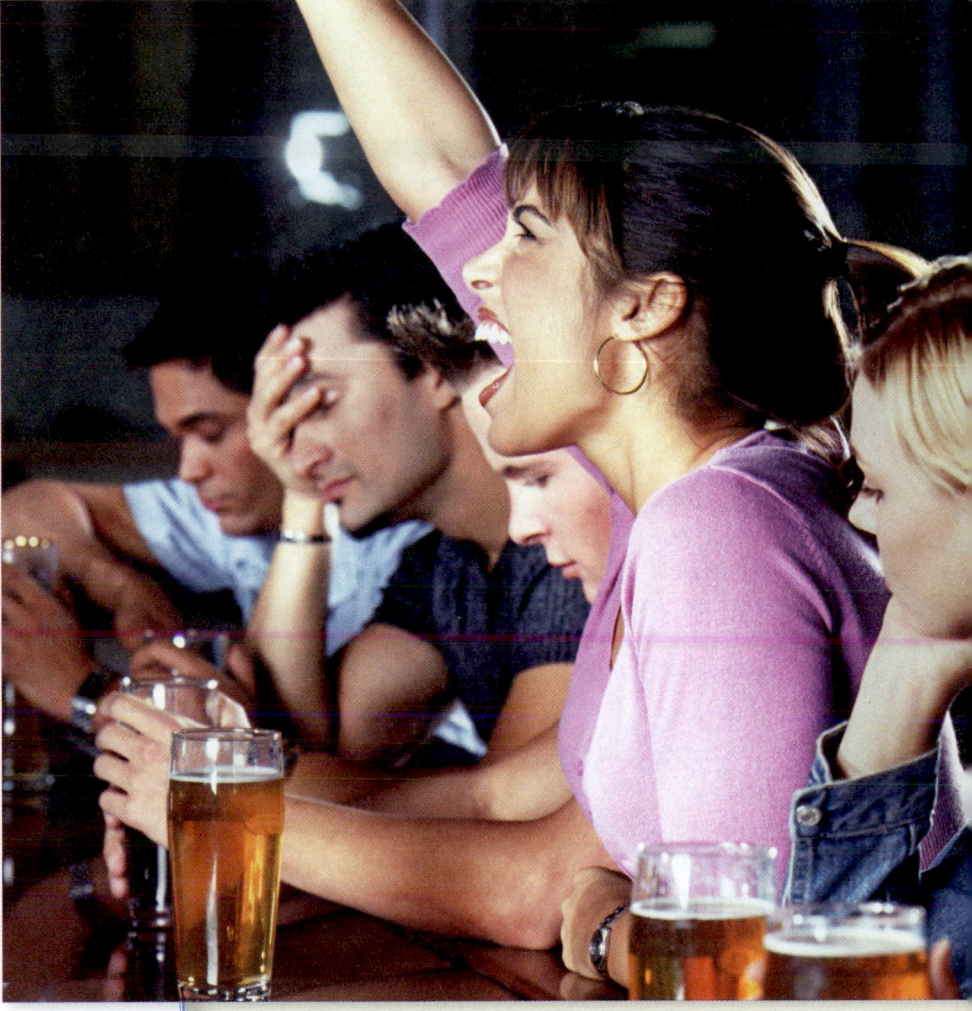

> " *There is a choice you have to make in everything you do. And you must always keep in mind, the choice you make, makes you.* "
>
> —Anonymous

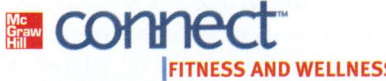

FITNESS AND WELLNESS

http://connect.mcgraw-hill.com

We live in a drug-saturated environment. We have drugs for everything—anxiety, depression, infection, and pain. A **drug** is a chemical that alters a person's physical or mental condition. The question is not whether to use drugs, because most people do, but rather when, where, why, and how much to use them. Most of us use over-the-counter drugs such as aspirin. Others use prescribed drugs for a medical condition. Still others misuse and abuse legal and illegal drugs at the cost of our bankbooks, our relationships, and our lives. In this chapter *alcohol* is addressed first because it is the *most abused legal drug in our* *society and for college students.* Other drugs pose risks for some students. See Table 14-1. This chapter includes alcohol use assessments, responsible drinking guidelines, and strategies for drinking less to help you make decisions and take action about your alcohol use. Other drugs addressed are tobacco and illegal psychoactive recreational drugs: club drugs, depressants (date rape drugs), cannabis (marijuana), stimulants, narcotics, psychedelics, and inhalants. Over-the-counter drugs (including ephedra) and prescription drugs are also discussed. Before we discuss specific drugs, let's examine addiction in general.

◆ ADDICTION

Addiction is a pathological or abnormal relationship with an object or event. It has three common elements:

✓ *Exposure.* Addiction is an illness, not a moral failure, that progresses from a definite beginning toward an end point. It can begin when a person is exposed to a drug (such as alcohol) or a behavior (such as gambling) that he or she finds pleasurable.

✓ *Compulsion.* The person uses a substance or behavior repeatedly despite negative consequences. Defining addiction is difficult because it is often hard to know when the person "crosses the line" between abuse and compulsion.

✓ *Loss of control.* Over time, the search for highs changes to a desire to avoid the effects of withdrawal from the drug or behavior. Addicted people lose their ability to control their behavior.

The most insidious addiction is alcoholism, recognized as a disease by the American Medical Association since 1956. This recognition eliminates notions that the alcoholic is a weak-willed person who could quit drinking if he or she wanted. Recognizing alcoholism and other drug dependence as a disease implies five points:

1. *The disease can be described.* The compulsion to drink (or use other drugs) is manifested in habits that are inappropriate, unpredictable, excessive, and constant.

2. *The course of the disease is predictable and progressive.* It will get worse; it is as simple as that. Sometimes there will be plateaus when the drinking and/or drug behavior seems to remain constant for months or even years. But over time the course of the disease will move

TABLE 14-1   *Annual Prevalence Among College Students: Alcohol and Other Drugs*

Alcohol	85%
Tobacco	42.8%
Marijuana	33%
Amphetamines	8.3%
Cocaine	6.0%
Sedatives	4.8%
Hallucinogens	5%
Designer drugs	3.3%
Opiates	1.5%
Inhalants	1.8%
Steroids	0.9%
Other	2.9%

Statistics were drawn from a sample of 68,000 undergraduate students from 133 colleges in the United States.
SOURCE: CORE Institute: Center for Alcohol and Other Drug Studies. Southern Illinois University at Carbondale. www.siu.edu/departments/coreinst, accessed December 2009.

inevitably toward greater and more serious deterioration. This deterioration can be physical, mental, and spiritual.

3. *The disease is primary.* Alcoholism/drug dependency is a primary disease. Other problems the victim may have cannot be treated until the dependency is treated.

4. *The disease is permanent.* Once you have it, you have it. Trying to learn to use drugs/drink moderately will not work. The chances for successful treatment are much better in the earlier stages of the disease.

5. *The disease is terminal.* If you have a chemical addiction and do not treat and arrest it, you will die from it. Whether the chemical complicates a heart condition, high blood pressure, liver problems, or a bleeding ulcer or precipitates a stroke or suicide, it is still the agent that causes the death.

What Stage of Change Are You In?

Do you refrain from driving every time you drink alcohol?

No

Do you plan to adopt this practice within the next 6 months?

No

Yes

Within the next month?

No

Yes

Yes

Have you done this consistently over the last 6 months?

No

Yes

| Precontemplation | Contemplation | Preparation | | Action | Maintenance |

connect Go online to Connect to report on your stage of change http://connect.mcgraw-hill.com

---

THINK ABOUT IT

Many college sports arenas/stadiums have sponsorship and advertising for alcoholic beverages. Does this occur on your campus? Using glamorized images and messages designed to appeal to younger markets, companies are attempting to associate alcohol usage with athleticism and sporting events. Some groups, including the American Medical Association (AMA), maintain that these ads undermine colleges' efforts to control binge-drinking, alcohol-related incidents, and sexual assaults on campus. Do you believe students are influenced by advertising for alcohol? Do you feel it is appropriate for advertisers to promote alcoholic beverages at school events? Why or why not? What message does the presence of this advertising send?

connect Go online to Connect to complete this activity. http://connect.mcgraw-hill.com

A useful assessment for recognizing any chemical dependency is to ask, *"Is the alcohol (or other drug or behavior) causing* any *continuing disruption in my life—or the lives of those close to me?"* (i.e., physically, mentally, emotionally, socially, or economically). If the answer is yes and you do not stop despite damage to home life, school performance, or career, your chemical usage/behavior constitutes harmful dependence.

Addictive Behaviors Other Than Alcohol or Other Drug Use

In the past, the focus of the term *addiction* centered exclusively on the use of alcohol, tobacco, and other drugs. Recently, a more neutral term, *dependence,* has been substituted for the term *addiction.* Essentially they mean the same thing and are used interchangeably. *Dependencies* or *addiction-like* behaviors may include objects or events such as food, video games (wii, Xbox, etc.), gambling, sex, shoplifting, work, Internet use, spending, exercise, and television. Although these addictive objects or events are different, they produce the desired and pleasurable mood change the addict seeks:

✓ The gambler feels excited when studying a racing form.
✓ The alcoholic feels relaxed and happy when drinking at the neighborhood bar.
✓ The food addict feels rewarded and comforted when eating or shopping for food.
✓ The shoplifter senses a thrill when stealing a magazine from the drugstore.
✓ The sex addict gets aroused when browsing in a pornographic bookstore or searching for a new sex partner.
✓ The addictive spender feels exhilarated during a shopping spree.
✓ The workaholic feels an extreme sense of accomplishment while working 7 days a week.

These objects and events have a normal, socially acceptable function. Food is to nourish, gambling is for fun and excitement, sex is for intimacy, and drugs are to help overcome illness. Most people have a normal, healthy relationship with these things, but dependent behavior results in an abnormal relationship. Dependent individuals seek a pleasurable mood change to fulfill personal needs. The addict turns to the addiction just as someone else may turn to a spouse or best friend for support, nurturing, and intimacy. As the addiction progresses, the addict becomes more preoccupied, withdrawn, and isolated. Table 14-2 illustrates how this type of behavior affects all dimensions of wellness.

We know that chemical addictions produce physiological dependence that results in withdrawal symptoms when the substance is denied. When the object of other dependencies (e.g., food or gambling) is withdrawn, withdrawal symptoms also result (e.g., anxiety, irritability, and moodiness).

Many experts predict that compulsive gambling will soon become a serious national problem. There may be good cause for this concern: Consider the millions of dollars spent in the legal and illegal gambling industries every day. Commercial bingo, dog and horse racing, state and interstate lotteries, and video gambling are on the increase, as is Internet party poker, especially among young adults and women. Gambling casinos are no longer confined to Nevada and New Jersey; they can be found on American Indian reservations and floating up and down our rivers, and they are being built in more states every year. Sports gambling is also booming, especially among college students. As gambling becomes legal in more states, the number of problem gamblers rises proportionally. Gambling is meant for amusement, recreation, and excitement, but it can turn into a devastating addiction in some individuals. Take the self-assessment in Table 14-3 to determine if you or someone you know has a gambling problem.

The glut of credit cards bombarding our mailboxes, as well as online shopping available around the clock and nonstop TV shopping networks, is

TABLE 14-2	*How Addictions Affect the Wellness Dimensions*
Physical	Addicts don't take good care of their bodies. Addictions over time affect various parts of the body—an alcoholic's liver, a bulimic's throat. The added stress of addiction takes its toll on the heart and all other organs of the body; malnourishment is common; the body's immune system breaks down. A body is more accident-prone. Suicidal thoughts may become actions.
Social	Addicts become withdrawn and isolated from others, become loners, and interact only with the object or event of addiction. Their responsibility to family, school, job, and so on diminishes.
Emotional	Feelings of guilt and shame increase; depression is common; unresolved issues increase; mood swings increase; anxiety increases; fits of rage for no reason occur; and paranoia develops (the addict starts to question everyone and everything).
Intellectual	Logic breaks down; the addict's behavior doesn't make sense to him or her; schoolwork falters; he or she loses touch with world events; judgment is impaired.
Spiritual	Addicts are not "connected" in a meaningful way to the world around them; they lose feelings of belonging and being an important part of the world; they lose the sense of knowing themselves; the importance of self drifts farther away; values and priorities shift; addicts begin to rationalize.
Environmental	Addicts show little concern for the health and well-being of the environment, such as conserving natural resources and energy. The addiction (compulsive behavior) consumes the addict's energies.

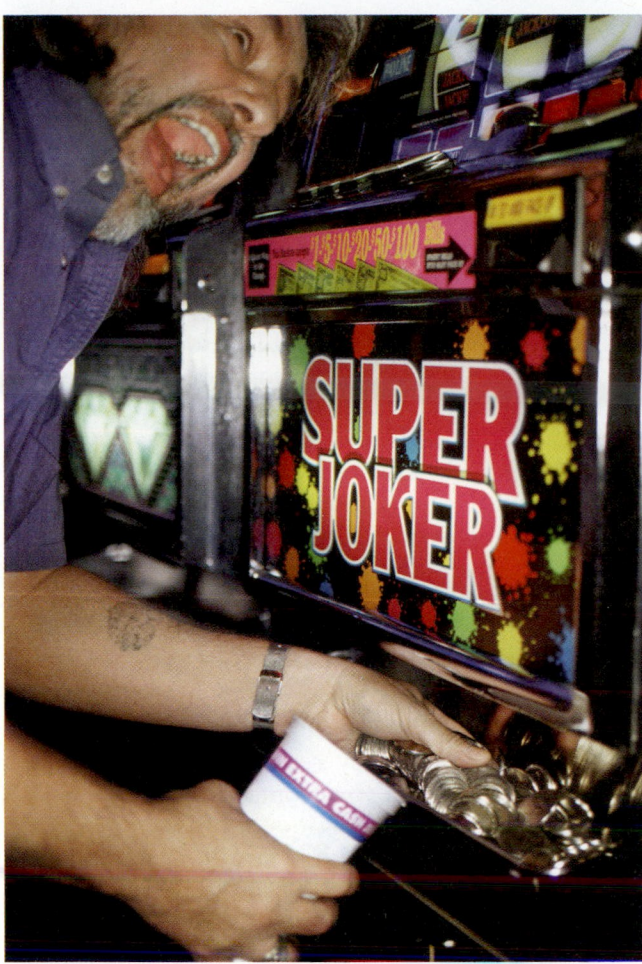

People who live within 50 miles of a casino have twice as much risk of developing a gambling problem as those living farther away. The growing popularity of electronic gambling only increases the problem.

TABLE 14-3   *Do You Have a Gambling Problem?*

Yes	No	
_____	_____	1. Has gambling ever made your home life unhappy or had a negative effect on your relationships with others?
_____	_____	2. Has gambling ever gotten in the way of school or work?
_____	_____	3. Did gambling cause you to have difficulty sleeping?
_____	_____	4. Have you gambled with income or savings while bills went unpaid?
_____	_____	5. Have you made unsuccessful attempts to quit gambling?
_____	_____	6. Have you ever considered breaking the law to pay for your gambling?
_____	_____	7. Have you ever borrowed to finance gambling?
_____	_____	8. Have you ever been depressed or suicidal as a result of your gambling?
_____	_____	9. Have you gambled to get money to meet your financial obligations?
_____	_____	10. Have you ever lied about your gambling?
_____	_____	11. Have you ever been criticized for your gambling or is it affecting your reputation?
_____	_____	12. Do you ever gamble to escape worry or trouble?
_____	_____	13. Do arguments, disappointments, or frustrations create within you an urge to gamble to feel better?
_____	_____	14. Did gambling cause a decrease in your ambition or efficiency?
_____	_____	15. After a win did you have a strong urge to return and win more?
_____	_____	16. Do you ever sell anything to finance gambling?
_____	_____	17. Did you ever have an urge to celebrate good fortune by gambling for a few hours?

Scoring: One "yes" answer indicates you may have a problem. Seven or more "yes" answers indicate that you could be addicted or heading that way.

assisting in the expansion of shopping or spending compulsions. Take the self-assessment in Table 14-4 to determine if shopping or spending is becoming a problem for you.

Individuals with addictions and those who exhibit addictive-like behaviors to substances, objects, or events need professional help. A partial listing of organizations, agencies, and resource centers that give information and assistance with addictions can be found at the end of this chapter.

SCIENCE: ADDICTION STARTS INSIDE THE BRAIN

Addiction is a brain disease with a genetic basis. It is a disruption of the reward mechanism in the brain, which is the part responsible for creating drives. When those drives are powerful enough, it becomes nearly impossible to contain them. A cascade of neurobiological changes, where neurotransmitting chemicals get out of balance, accompanies the transition from voluntary to addictive behavior. One of the most important changes is that addictive behaviors alter the brain's pleasure circuits. Activating this circuit, also called the reward circuit, produces a feel-good sensation. The pleasure circuit communicates in the chemical language of dopamine, a neurotransmitter. Dopamine conveys messages from one brain cell to another (neuron to neuron) in the circuit, affecting the firing of other neurons and producing feelings ranging from mild happiness to euphoria in time. In time, the brain becomes wired in such a way that dopamine pathways

TABLE 14-4   *Do You Have a Shopping or Spending Problem?*

The most prominent symptom of a shopping or spending problem is obvious: *debt!*

Yes	No	
_____	_____	1. Do you shop or spend money when you're disappointed, angry, lonely, or worried?
_____	_____	2. Are your shopping/spending habits causing emotional distress or chaos in your life?
_____	_____	3. Do you find yourself arguing with others about your shopping/spending habits?
_____	_____	4. Do you feel lost without your credit cards?
_____	_____	5. Do you buy items on credit that you wouldn't buy with cash?
_____	_____	6. Do you experience a rush of euphoria and anxiety at the same time when you spend money?
_____	_____	7. Does spending or shopping feel like a reckless or forbidden act?
_____	_____	8. Do you feel guilty, after spending money and perhaps then return the purchased items?
_____	_____	9. Do you lie to others about what you bought or how much money you spend?
_____	_____	10. Do you spend a lot of time juggling accounts and bills to accommodate your spending?

Scoring: If you said "yes" to four of the questions, you might have a shopping or spending problem.

light up at the mere thought of the addictive behavior, and the urge to do it grows insistent.

Almost anything deeply enjoyable can turn into an addiction. Drugs of abuse, alcohol, gambling, shopping, sex, overeating, and other addictive behaviors increase the concentration of dopamine in the brain's reward circuits. The brain starts changing right away as a result of the unnatural flood of dopamine. Because there seems to be more than enough dopamine, the neurons begin to reduce the number of dopamine receptors, make less dopamine, all of which reduces dopamine in the brain. Chronic drug use, alcohol abuse, gambling abuse, and so on initiates this process of destroying dopamine receptors. The consequence of this process is that with fewer dopamine receptors, a "hit" that used to produce pleasure no longer does. This is the molecular basis for tolerance. To get the original high, the person has to increase the dose.

Even worse, the loss of dopamine receptors means that experiences that used to bring pleasure become unable to do so. Nothing ignites the feelings of happiness as it once did. The only escape from chronic dysphoria, irritability, anxiety, and even depression, the user believes, is to take more of the drug or to repeat the behavior. At least one researcher believes everyone could become an addict if sufficiently exposed to drugs or alcohol.

The agony of withdrawal is also a direct result of drugs' resetting of the brain's dopamine system. Withdrawal and abstinence deprive the brain of the only source of dopamine that produces any sense of joy. Without it, life seems not worth living.

Although the biological basis of tolerance, addiction, and withdrawal is yielding some of its secrets, relapse is harder to explain. Why does an addict who has abstained for weeks, months, or longer suddenly seek out the drug? It seems that in the addict's brain even sights, sounds, or smells can trigger chemical or behavior cravings. Brain scans of addicts are helping to explain the complexity of relapse. They reveal enduring changes in areas of the brain (prefrontal cortex) where rational thought can override impulsive behavior. They also show that addicts are less adept at using analytical areas of the brain while performing decision-making tasks. Addiction is a chronic and relapsing brain disease.

Researchers are developing a more detailed understanding of how deeply and completely addiction can affect the brain. Using this knowledge, they have begun to develop new drugs that are showing promise in cutting off the craving that drives an addict irresistibly toward relapse—the greatest risk facing even the most dedicated abstainer. One further and important discovery is that evidence is building to support the *90-day rehabilitation model,* which was stumbled upon by Alcoholics Anonymous (new members are advised to attend a meeting a day for the first 90 days) and is the duration of a typical stint in a drug-treatment program. It turns out that this is just about how long it takes for the brain to reset itself and shake off the immediate influence of the drug. Researchers have documented what they call the sleeper effect, a gradual reengaging of proper decision-making and analytical functions in the brain, after the addict has abstained for at least 90 days. It is thought that a rehabilitated addict is most likely always in recovery. They are not cured, and resuming the drug/activity could be devastating. Complete Lab Activity 14-6 to gain a better understanding of whether addiction is a part of your lifestyle.

◆ ADDICTIVE PERSONALITY

Is there such a thing as an addictive personality? Do some individuals possess such a personality? This controversial topic continues to produce heated debate among scientists. Although the addictive personality type has not been confirmed by research, some experts feel that this personality type does exist. They believe the addictive personality may be found in persons who don't know how to have healthy relationships, have been taught not to trust people, and have never learned to "connect" with others, community, their emotions, and spiritual powers greater than themselves.

These experts believe that early life experiences determine whether a person will live in a state of dependency. They argue that the family environment is the most important determinant because the family is where we learn about relationships. For example, in abusive families, the children are often treated as objects, thus developing low self-esteem and mistrust of people. Also, in neglectful families, children may learn to be passive and to feel dead inside, and they will seek out someone or something that makes them feel alive. This theory reflects the idea that people often form addictions because of the positive feelings (mood change) they experience when using a substance or repeating a behavior.

Experts claim there is no single characteristic or constellation of traits inevitably associated with addiction. So who is vulnerable? Possibly the individual who

- ✓ Has a low sense of self-esteem
- ✓ Likes to try new, exciting, and dangerous things
- ✓ Has a sense of alienation
- ✓ Displays antisocial behavior (is willing to go outside the boundaries of what is normally accepted)
- ✓ Possesses a need for instant gratification
- ✓ Is impulsive
- ✓ Rebels against authority
- ✓ Lies easily
- ✓ Is a perfectionist—a high achiever
- ✓ Seeks approval from others
- ✓ Is overly concerned with how others perceive him or her
- ✓ Tends to be submissive and dependent
- ✓ Has high levels of negative emotionality (a syndrome that includes nervousness, anger, and a tendency to worry and feel victimized)

Many people display these characteristics without becoming addicts. This leads some experts to believe that the personality disorders and antisocial behavior that accompany chemical abuse are the result of this abuse, not the cause of it. They claim there is no way to predict who will become an addict.

◆ ALCOHOL

Alcohol is the most misunderstood drug in America. Some say alcohol is a beverage, and others say it is a drug. They say that it is a mood-altering chemical in liquid form or that it is sinful and dangerous. Some say it is a rite of adulthood and is safe. What conflicting statements! What is alcohol, and what does it do? **Alcohol** (technically known as ethyl alcohol or ethanol) is a central nervous system (CNS) depressant, and it affects the body in many different ways. Alcohol slows brain functions and reaction time, dulls alertness, and impairs body coordination. It intensifies emotions, lowers inhibitions, and increases risk-taking behaviors. It also disrupts judgment and reasoning power. On the positive side, alcohol is a good social lubricant; and, an occasional alcoholic beverage has some health benefits. These health benefits accrue with moderate or low-risk consumption of alcohol. On the negative side, alcohol can be unhealthy and unsafe if abused.

Alcohol Absorption

Most healthy bodies process alcohol in the same manner. Alcohol is water soluble and is transported throughout the body by the blood, which is mostly

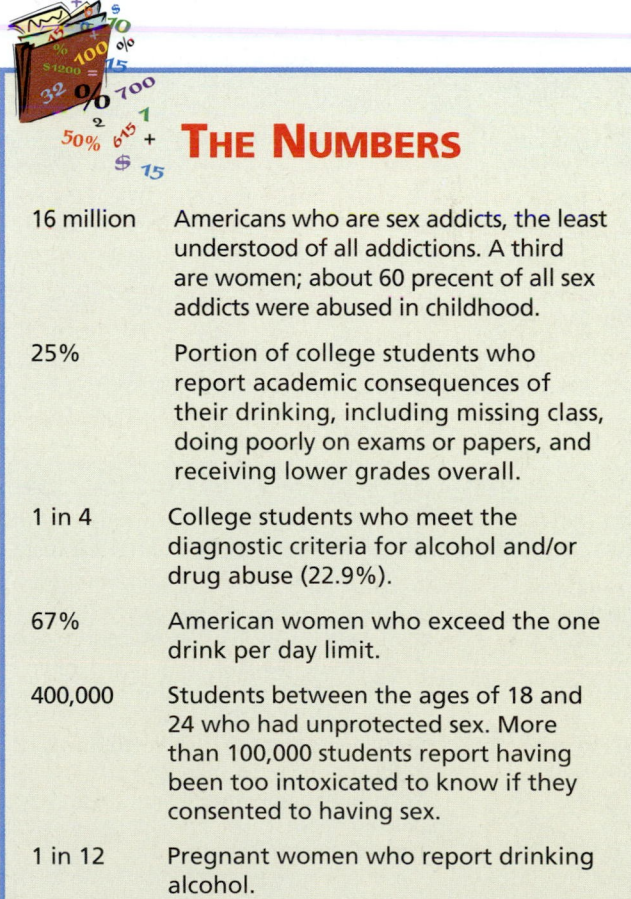

THE NUMBERS

16 million	Americans who are sex addicts, the least understood of all addictions. A third are women; about 60 precent of all sex addicts were abused in childhood.
25%	Portion of college students who report academic consequences of their drinking, including missing class, doing poorly on exams or papers, and receiving lower grades overall.
1 in 4	College students who meet the diagnostic criteria for alcohol and/or drug abuse (22.9%).
67%	American women who exceed the one drink per day limit.
400,000	Students between the ages of 18 and 24 who had unprotected sex. More than 100,000 students report having been too intoxicated to know if they consented to having sex.
1 in 12	Pregnant women who report drinking alcohol.

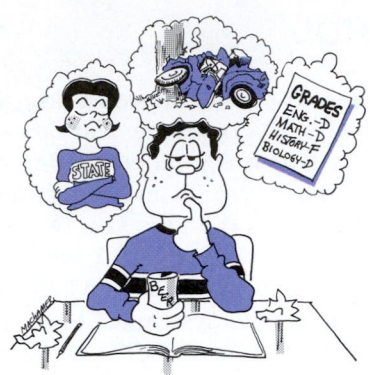

High-risk drinking has many consequences.

water. The amount of alcohol in the blood is expressed as a percentage—for example, 0.08 percent **blood alcohol concentration (BAC)** or blood alcohol level (BAL). With the first sip, alcohol briefly irritates tissues in the mouth and esophagus. Alcohol rapidly enters the bloodstream through the small intestine and, to a small degree, through the stomach. A fraction exits in breath, sweat, and urine. Alcohol is chiefly metabolized (i.e., chemically broken down) in the liver, through which the entire blood supply circulates every 4 minutes. Enzymes in the liver metabolize alcohol into acetaldehyde, a highly toxic chemical. This is converted into acetate and finally into carbon dioxide and water. The process is slow, taking roughly *an hour for each ounce of pure alcohol*. Despite folklore, nothing will speed up liver function or sober up the intoxicated. A person who is drunk and drinks coffee or takes a cold shower does not become sober, only cold, wet, and wide awake. Time, and only time can sober a person up.

The mind-altering effects of alcohol begin soon after it hits the bloodstream. Within minutes, alcohol enters the brain, numbing nerve cells and slowing their messages to the body. In the heart, cardiac muscles strain to cope with alcohol's depressive action, and the pulse quickens. If drinking continues, alcohol builds in the bloodstream and disrupts the centers in the brain that govern speech, vision, balance, and judgment. As more alcohol is ingested, the drinker may lose consciousness. Alcohol is a hazardous anesthetic, with a narrow range between impairment and dead. At a BAC of 0.3 to 0.4 percent, the drinker is comatose and in danger of dying from respiratory failure. See Table 14-5.

TABLE 14-5   *Percentage of Blood Alcohol Concentration (BAC)*

Drinks*	BAC for Men (body weight in pounds)								Drinks	BAC for Women (body weight in pounds)							
	100	120	140	160	180	200	220	240		90	100	120	140	160	180	200	220
1	.04	.03	.02	.02	.02	.02	.02	.02	1	.05	.05	.04	.03	.03	.03	.02	.02
2	.08	.06	.05	.05	.04	.04	.03	.03	2	.10	.09	.08	.07	.06	.05	.05	.04
3	.11	.09	.08	.07	.06	.06	.05	.05	3	.15	.14	.11	.10	.09	.08	.07	.06
4	.15	.12	.11	.09	.08	.08	.07	.06	4	.20	.18	.15	.13	.11	.10	.09	.08
5	.19	.16	.13	.12	.11	.09	.09	.09	5	.25	.23	.19	.16	.14	.13	.11	.10
6	.23	.19	.16	.14	.13	.11	.10	.09	6	.30	.27	.23	.19	.17	.15	.14	.12
7	.26	.22	.19	.16	.15	.13	.12	.11	7	.35	.32	.27	.23	.20	.18	.16	.14
8	.30	.25	.21	.19	.17	.15	.14	.13	8	.40	.36	.30	.26	.23	.20	.18	.17
9	.34	.28	.24	.21	.19	.17	.15	.14	9	.45	.41	.34	.29	.26	.23	.20	.19
10	.38	.31	.27	.23	.21	.19	.17	.16	10	.51	.45	.38	.32	.28	.25	.23	.21

Effects Related to Blood Alcohol Concentration (BAC)

BAC%	Effect
0.02	Impairment begins with first drink
0.03	Relaxation, mood change
0.04	Reduced visual acuity (as much as wearing dark glasses), slight euphoria, and loss of shyness
0.05	Decrease in motor skills, judgment impaired, caution reduced
0.08	**Legally intoxicated; inhibitions lowered; unexpected behavior; slight impairment of balance, speech, vision, and reaction time**
0.10	Movements and speech impaired
0.18	Difficulty staying awake
0.20	Very drunk; loud and difficult to understand; emotions unstable, staggering/muscular coordination reduced; has the appearance of a "sloppy" drunk; may vomit (and can choke)
0.30	Loss of consciousness
0.40+	Onset of coma; possible death due to respiratory arrest

*One drink equals 1½ oz. of 80-proof alcohol, 12 oz. beer, or 4 oz. wine. 0.40% is the accepted level that is lethal for 50% of adults.
Source: Mothers Against Drunk Driving and PRIDE.

Speed of Alcohol Absorption

How quickly alcohol is absorbed into the bloodstream depends on five factors:

1. *Body weight:* Smaller people are affected more quickly by alcohol than larger people.
2. *Gender:* It is not a myth that a man can drink the same amount of alcohol as a woman of equal weight and have a lower BAC. That means a woman can get drunk faster than a man does. There are several explanations for this:
   a. Women metabolize alcohol differently than men. Females have less alcohol dehydrogenase, the first enzyme in the stomach lining that starts to break down the ethanol in alcohol. This phenomenon has more serious long-term consequences for women. They are more likely to develop damage to the liver, heart muscle, and brain at lower levels of alcohol intake. Alcohol may also put them at increased risk of osteoporosis and breast cancer.
   b. Even at the same weight, women typically have a higher percentage of body fat and less body water than men do (alcohol is diluted in body water). Because alcohol is more soluble in water than fat, a given dose becomes more concentrated in a female's body water than in a male's.
   c. Women generally weigh less than men do, so the same amount of alcohol is concentrated in a smaller body mass.
   d. Together with estrogen, these factors have a net concentrating effect on the alcohol in the blood, giving women a more intense hit with each drink. For years, researchers have documented the way females tend to progress more rapidly to alcoholism than do men.
3. *Food intake:* A full stomach slows the absorption of alcohol into the bloodstream.
4. *Beverage imbibed:* Drinks can have different effects based on their composition (e.g., straight, carbonated, or juice mixer). Carbonated drinks such as champagne, rum and Coke, and whisky and soda are absorbed faster than are water-diluted drinks.
5. *Speed of consumption:* Gulping or "chugging" drinks will increase the amount of alcohol taken into the system. One drink, such as a 12-ounce can of beer sipped over an hour's time is not absorbed into the bloodstream as quickly as one that is gulped rapidly.

There are three major types of alcoholic beverages: beer, wine, and distilled spirits (i.e., hard liquor

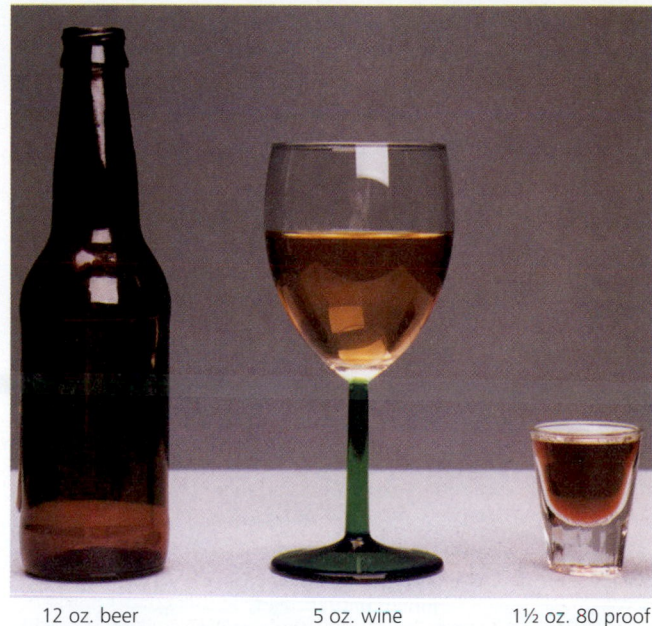

12 oz. beer   5 oz. wine   1½ oz. 80 proof
                                         distilled spirits

All standard-size drinks provide the same amount of alcohol.

such as whiskey, vodka, gin, and brandy). A standard serving of any one beverage contains approximately the same amount of alcohol. Thus, one 5-ounce glass of wine, one 12-ounce beer, one 12-ounce wine cooler, and one shot glass (1.5 oz.) of liquor provide approximately the same amount of alcohol. One person's wine glass is another person's beer mug, so always measure your drinks. See the photo of the three servings of alcohol.

Often wine coolers are not perceived as alcoholic beverages because of their fruit juice base and sweet taste. Beware. They contain the same amount of alcohol as beer or any other alcoholic beverage. These drinks may provide the bridge from soft drinks to other alcoholic beverages for many young people.

Your alcohol history determines how quickly you feel the effects of this drug. It is based on your lifetime alcohol consumption, the frequency of your drinking, and the tolerance you have acquired. The number of drinks it takes for you to feel a "buzz" increases as your tolerance to alcohol increases. **Tolerance** is the body's physical adjustment to the habitual use of a chemical. Due to alcohol tolerance, an experienced drinker with a BAC of 0.08 percent may not feel drunk. In contrast, an inexperienced drinker may feel intoxicated at the same BAC because a tolerance has not developed (Table 14-5). Unless a person has developed a high tolerance for alcohol, a BAC rating of 0.2 percent represents very serious intoxication. Most first-time drinkers would be unconscious by about 0.15 percent and 0.35 to 0.40 percent represents potentially fatal alcohol poisoning.

TABLE 14-6 *Consequences of College Drinking*

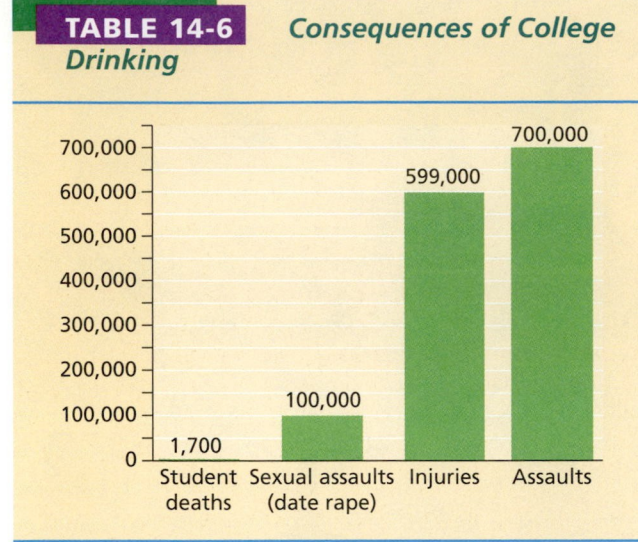

Note: Recent studies suggest that alcohol negatively impacts brain development, which continues until the early twenties.
SOURCE: National Institute on Alcohol Abuse and Alcoholism, accessed December 2009.

Some college students participate in "chugging" contests or other drinking games such as beer pong, quarters, TV/movie theme games, flippy cup, and century club. Research shows that these often lead to higher levels of alcohol consumption and dangerous BAC levels. Because drinking games produce an unpredictable atmosphere, many college organizations are banning them. Drinking games are not proof of maturity or a route to social acceptance. They will only make you drunk, incoherent, and accident-prone, and may lead to the consequences depicted in Table 14-6.

Considering all the factors that affect the alcohol absorption rate, is your level of alcohol use a low- or high-risk behavior?

Impact of Alcohol

Alcohol is by far the most devastating drug—wrecking families and friendships, impairing health, jeopardizing careers, and filling jails, hospitals, and morgues. Alcohol accounts for 50 percent of deaths from motor vehicle crashes, one-third of drownings, and about half of deaths caused by fire. Alcohol is linked to half of homicides, a third of suicides, and two-thirds of assaults. Social workers report that alcohol is a factor in nearly 50 percent of their domestic violence cases. Over 36 percent of the male population in prison report that they were under the influence of alcohol at the time of committing their crimes. The greatest tragedy is that the *number one killer* of teenagers is *drinking and driving*. The majority of these drinkers started early, before they had turned 13. As you can see in Table 14-7, over 80 percent of college

TABLE 14-7 *College Binge Drinking*

Binge drinking is defined as a pattern of drinking that brings BAC to 0.08 percent or above. It is *five* drinks for men and *four* for women in about 2 hours.

What is the extent of binge drinking on campus? (Also see Diversity Issues.)
- 84% drink alcoholic beverages (4 out of 5 students)
- 40% (2 out of 5 students) binge
- 48.6% of males binge
- 40.9% of females binge
- 64% live in a fraternity/sorority house
- 38% live off-campus
- 29% of athletes are frequent binge drinkers compared to 22% of nonathletes

Students least likely to binge are
- African American or Asian
- Aged 24 years or older or married
- Students who put a high priority on their studies
- Students who devote time to special interests
- Students who participate in volunteer activities

Students who drink the least attend
- 2-year institutions
- Religious schools
- Commuter schools
- Historically black colleges/universities

Sober students are affected in many ways: sober students were twice as likely as those at the lowest-drinking-level schools to be insulted or humiliated; to be pushed, hit, or assaulted; and to experience unwanted sexual advances from drinking students. They were two and one-half times as likely to sustain property damage, to end up taking care of a drunken student, and to have their study or sleep time interrupted by classmates drinking.

SOURCE: Henry Wechsler et al. "Trends in College Binge Drinking During a Period of Increased Prevention Efforts: Findings from 4 Harvard School or Public Health College Alcohol Study Surveys: 1993–2005." *Journal of American College Health* (2006). The latest year for which data are available. Over 14,000 students at 119 colleges in 39 states participated.

students report some drinking, ranging from occasional to heavy. Alcohol consumption is one of the major reasons for absenteeism among college students. It is involved in 90 percent of campus rapes, 25 percent of student deaths, and 40 percent of academic problems, and it is the major contributor to campus violence, property damage, and the disruption of sleep and study time. Alcohol is implicated in over 400,000 students having unprotected sex and thousands of unwanted pregnancies and cases of sexually transmitted diseases, including AIDS. Thousands of college students drop out because of drinking. Even nondrinking college students are affected by the drinking of their classmates (see Table 14-7). The single most dangerous consequence of alcohol

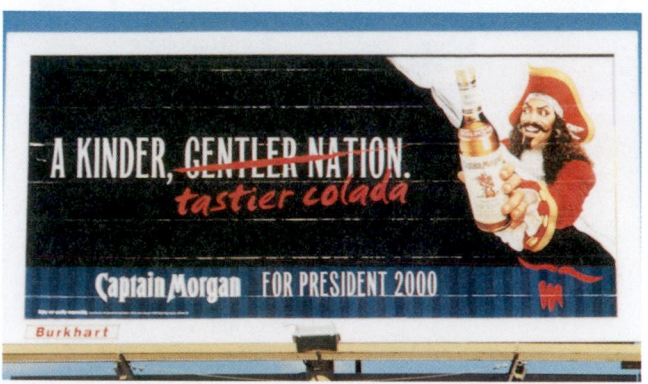

Drinking and driving kills a human being every 31 minutes. Some say billboards advertising alcohol should be banned. Do you think they should?

use may be that it produces a false sense of confidence, even invulnerability, that often leads to disregard for the health, safety, and welfare of oneself and others.

Health and Long-Term Effects of Alcohol

Alcohol is a toxin, and its harmful effects on the body are great. A few drinks may make you drowsy and can interrupt patterns of sleep. Over time, heavy drinking can cause brain damage (it speeds the death of brain cells) and damage nerve endings. It also weakens the bones. It can depress the immune system and cause gastritis, pancreatitis, anxiety, delirium tremens (DTs), and malnutrition. Alcohol is a primary cause of liver failure. When alcohol is present in the liver, it preempts the breakdown of fats, which then accumulate within the liver cells. As fatty cells enlarge, they can rupture or grow into cysts that replace normal cells. After years of heavy drinking, fibrous scar tissue, or cirrhosis, impedes the normal flow of arterial and venous blood through the organ, resulting in liver failure and death.

Another hazard of alcohol consumption is the increased risk of cancer. Women who imbibe more than three drinks a day boost breast cancer risk by 30 percent; one to two drinks a day poses a 10 percent risk. Men and women who drink more than three drinks a day have a 26 percent increased risk of colon cancer. Alcohol also increases the risk of uterine, mouth, throat, stomach, pancreatic, and liver cancer.

Does drinking alcoholic beverages guard against heart disease? Recent studies suggest that consuming no more than one drink per day for women and no more than two drinks for men per day is the amount associated with a reduction in mortality mainly among men over age 45 and women over age 55. This is due to a reduced risk of coronary artery disease because of an increased HDL level. Alcohol also protects the heart by reducing the tendency of

the blood to form clots. *But aspirin does the same thing.* Red wine, because it contains antioxidant phytochemicals, has received some attention as a heart disease protector. But studies show that the crucial element is alcohol itself. Light intake of alcohol appears to reduce mortality risk only in some women who are at high risk for coronary heart disease in the first place. Also, while light alcohol consumption may reduce coronary artery disease, it has destructive effects on the heart muscle. This is especially true in women who appear to be more susceptible to cardiomyopathy (or heart muscle destruction)—even when they drink less than men. Also, alcohol may boost high blood pressure, risk of bleeding and stroke, and promote abnormal heart rhythms.

So this one bit of HDL information about the "protective" relationship of alcohol consumption and heart disease should not be perceived as a "green light" to drink. Keep in mind that the cons overwhelmingly outweigh the pros of drinking alcoholic beverages. For coronary heart disease protection, not smoking, following a proper diet, and staying physically active are far superior methods to the consumption of alcohol.

FETAL ALCOHOL SYNDROME (FAS) AND FETAL ALCOHOL EFFECT (FAE)

Fetal alcohol syndrome (FAS) is a condition acquired by the unborn fetus and caused by the mother drinking alcohol during pregnancy. The alcohol passes through the placenta (within minutes) and affects the unborn child. These infants may suffer from mental retardation and other irreversible physical abnormalities. FAS is the leading known cause of mental retardation in the Western world. Women need to understand that the placenta does not keep unwanted chemicals away from the fetus. Humans are supposed to be the wisest of creatures, yet it is not uncommon to see pregnant women drinking alcoholic beverages, smoking, and taking drugs they would never consider giving to their children. How can they expect their babies to come into the world unaffected?

The expectant mother who drinks is denying her child development of his or her full potential. Alcohol use during pregnancy may cause the child to have learning problems and behavioral difficulties. No one is certain how much alcohol it takes to cause damage to the fetus. Some women drink very little and their babies are still affected.

A far greater number of babies have more subtle symptoms that are sometimes—mistakenly—not attributed to their mothers' alcohol consumption. This less severe manifestation of FAS is called fetal alcohol effect (FAE). The mother of a child diagnosed with FAE did not necessarily drink less during pregnancy than did the mother of a child with FAS, but for some biological reason, the FAE child is not as damaged physically. The FAE child shows traits of impaired memory, poor judgment, and reduced capacity to learn from experience. Reports indicate an increasing frequency of FAS and FAE. Drinking while pregnant is like playing Russian roulette with your baby's life. Why take chances with your baby's future? The message is this: There is no known safe level of alcohol consumption during pregnancy. FAS and FAE are preventable, but abstinence is the only way to guarantee that a baby will suffer no ill effects from alcohol.

Low-Risk and High-Risk Alcohol Consumption

About two-thirds of Americans use alcohol. Some of these individuals exhibit low-risk alcohol use and others exhibit high-risk alcohol use. What is the difference between the two? **Low-risk alcohol use** is defined as drinking no more than *one drink per day for women* and no more than *two drinks per day for men*. This is sometimes called *moderate use of alcohol*. See Table 14-8. This level of drinking generally does not cause problems, either for the drinker or for society. Keep in mind that any use of alcohol involves some risk and that the lowest risk of all is zero consumption.

Who is the **high-risk user?** It is the alcohol abuser who doesn't follow the guidelines for low-risk

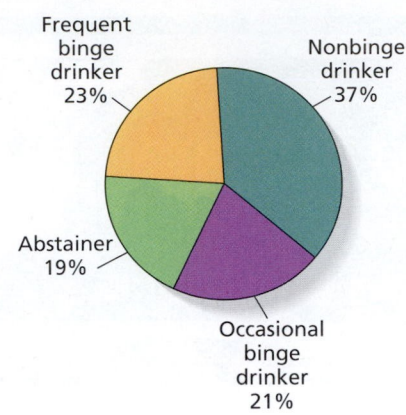

Frequent binge drinker 23%

Nonbinge drinker 37%

Abstainer 19%

Occasional binge drinker 21%

FIGURE 14-1   When it comes to college alcohol use, 84 percent of college students drink, but nonbinge drinkers and abstainers (when totaled together) are the majority.

use or the individual guilty of bingeing. **Binge drinking** is a pattern of drinking alcohol that brings blood alcohol concentration (BAC) to 0.08 percent or above. For the typical adult this equates to *five* drinks for a man and *four* drinks for a woman in about *2 hours*. This is called problem or heavy drinking. Binge drinking is clearly dangerous for the drinker and for society. Consuming fourteen drinks in a week for men (seven for women) is also considered high-risk or heavy drinking.

Binge drinkers on college campuses experience and cause more problems than students who do not binge. An occasional binger is a student who binged once or twice in a 2-week period. A frequent binger is a student who binged three or more times in a 2-week period. See Figure 14-1.

Compared to nonbinge drinkers, frequent bingers are 17 times more likely to miss a class, 10 times more likely to vandalize property, and 8 times more likely to get hurt or injured as a result of their drinking. Furthermore, the secondhand effects of binge drinking harm and violate the rights of others on campus. These range from automobile-related fatalities to serious injuries, from vandalism and physical assaults, to problems of everyday life such as losing sleep and study time.

Binge drinking is also a women's health issue. Heavy alcohol use coupled with inexperience with drinking puts young women in serious jeopardy for sexual assault. About 10 percent of female students who are frequent binge drinkers report being raped or subjected to nonconsensual sex, compared to only 3 percent of nonbingeing female students. Also, most campus rapes occur after heavy drinking.

The abuse of alcohol involves drinkers who consider alcohol something other than a beverage to be consumed with meals or to celebrate special occasions. These drinkers include not only bingers but also individuals who use alcohol as a medication

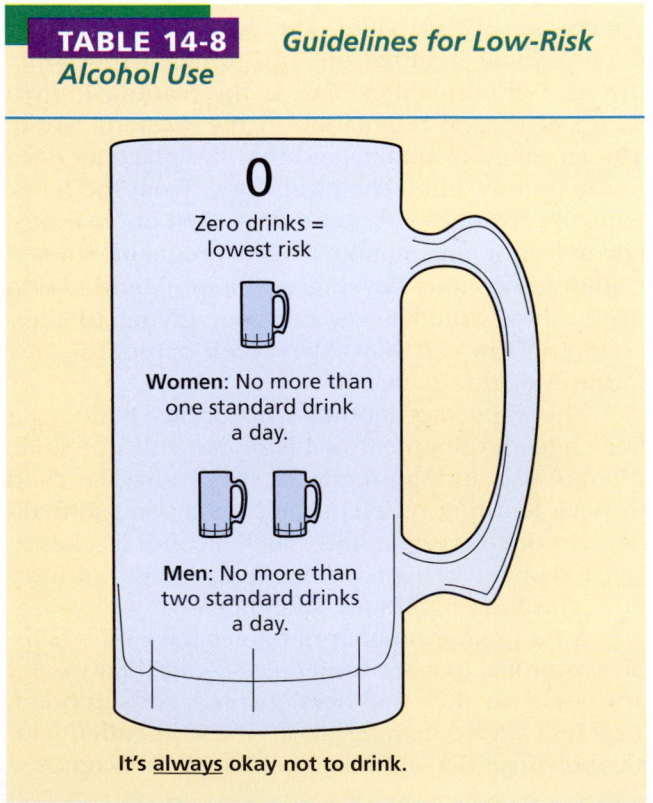

TABLE 14-8   *Guidelines for Low-Risk Alcohol Use*

0

Zero drinks = lowest risk

Women: No more than one standard drink a day.

Men: No more than two standard drinks a day.

It's <u>always</u> okay not to drink.

TABLE 14-9   *Michigan Guidelines: The Zero . . . One . . . Three Rule for Lower-Risk Drinking*

0 =	No level of drinking is recommended. Never drink and drive—even one block.
1 =	Drink only one alcoholic beverage per hour if you do drink.
3 =	Never drink more than three alcoholic beverages per day (or more than five per week).

SOURCE: Concept partially developed by Enjoy Michigan Safety Coalition. Furnished by Michigan Office of Highway Safety Planning.

to kill pain, to alter emotions (when mad or depressed), to help them sleep, or to cope with life. If you drink when pregnant or drink and drive, you are abusing alcohol. See Lab Activity 14-1, and list the pros and cons for low-risk and high-risk alcohol use.

To lower your risk of negative consequences, follow the Zero . . . One . . . Three Rule for Lower-Risk Drinking in Table 14-9, which was developed in Michigan, or the Guidelines for Low-Risk Use (Table 14-8).

Strategies for Dealing with Alcohol

Alcohol is an accepted drug in today's society, but you don't have to go along with the crowd. Who controls and makes decisions about your life—you or others? Take charge. One voice can make a difference; that voice is yours.

Review the Top 10 "Tips for a Safer Party" for avoiding the chaos of intoxication and, more important, avoiding alcohol poisoning. Here are additional strategies for drinking less or not at all:

✓ Let your waistline be your incentive. Alcoholic beverages are loaded with "empty" calories (high in calories, low in nutrients). There is some evidence that alcohol not only adds calories to the diet but also keeps the body from burning dietary fat properly. Alcohol in the bloodstream slows down fat metabolism more than 30 percent while speeding up the burning of carbohydrates. This unused fat is deposited on the thighs, hips, and stomach.
✓ Switch to juice or soft drinks after the three-drink maximum.
✓ At restaurants, order food first, not an alcoholic beverage. That way you will have less time to drink.
✓ After exercise or when extra thirsty, avoid carbonated alcoholic drinks. They are absorbed too fast, and you may be tempted to gulp them down. Drink a glass of cold water first.
✓ Don't hold the drink in your hand. Put it down somewhere—this will help slow down consumption.

TOP 10 LIST

Tips for a Safer Party

1. Follow the Guidelines for Low-Risk Alcohol Use (Table 14-7) or the Michigan Zero . . . One . . . Three Rule (Table 14-9) and remember, "It's always okay not to drink."
2. Confine alcohol use to leisure activities, eating, and social functions.
3. If you plan to drink alcohol, be sure to eat first or eat while drinking.
4. Always use a buddy system when going to parties.
5. Always know the source of your drink (alcoholic beverage or not). Never take an open drink from a common container or unknown source.
6. Never drink alcohol if you are under the age to do so.
7. Never drive after drinking or get into a vehicle with someone who has. Remember, impairment starts with the first drink.
8. Cover your drink at all times.
9. Do not drink fast! Pace your consumption by sipping and take your second drink no sooner than 1 hour after the first.
10. Learn what to do if a friend passes out from drinking alcohol or displays signs of alcohol poisoning.

Remember, if you need a drink to be social, that is *not* social drinking!

✓ Try cocktails without the alcohol (e.g., a Bloody Mary without the vodka) or nonalcoholic beer.
✓ Dilute your drinks with water, ice, or extra fruit juice to slow alcohol absorption; beware of unfamiliar drinks with unknown alcohol content.
✓ Make sure your drinks are accurately measured.
✓ Volunteer to be the designated driver (you may even get free soft drinks).

Alcohol Poisoning

It is important, and potentially life-saving, to know what to do if friend passes out from drinking alcohol or shows signs of alcohol poisoning.

First, know the critical signs of alcohol poisoning, they are:

✓ Mental confusion, stupor, coma, or person cannot be roused
✓ Vomiting (Do not give them anything to eat or drink. Put them on their side—so they don't choke.)
✓ Seizures
✓ Slow breathing (fewer than 8 breaths, per minute)
✓ Irregular breathing (10 seconds or more between breaths)

Tips for Behavior Change: for Alcohol Use

Refer to the Stage of Change flowchart on page 473. What is your stage of change after answering the questions and tracing the flowchart?

Refer to Figure 2.2 (page 36) to see which processes of change are most effective for facilitating your transition from your current stage to the next stage (or *maintaining* your behavior if you are already in the maintenance stage). Here are some behavioral examples for selected processes of change:

- Consciousness-raising: Collect media accounts of drinking and driving accidents in your area.
- Social liberation: Identify campus transportation services/options for students who have been out drinking at night.
- Emotional arousal: Spend a Saturday night in a hospital emergency room observing the consequences of drinking and driving.
- Self-liberation: Publicly announce to your friends that you are making a commitment to never drive after drinking.
- Countering: Arrange for a designated driver for the social events you plan to attend when you may be drinking alcohol.

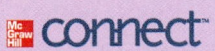 **Go online to Connect to complete this activity.**
http://connect.mcgraw-hill.com

✓ Hypothermia (low body temperature), bluish skin color, paleness (Cover them only with a light sheet, not a blanket. If they have overdosed on alcohol, their internal body temperature has fallen. Shivering is good, it stimulates them and helps keep them alive.)

Second, know what you should do:

✓ Know the danger signs.
✓ Do not wait for all symptoms to be present.
✓ Be aware that a person who has passed out may die.
✓ If there is *any* suspicion of an alcohol overdose, call 911 for help. Don't try to guess the level of drunkenness.

Finally, do you know what can happen to someone with alcohol poisoning that goes untreated? Here are the possibilities: the victim chokes on his or her own vomit; breathing slows, becomes irregular, or

stops; heart beats irregularly or stops; hypothermia; hypoglycemia (too little blood sugar) leads to seizures; and untreated severe dehydration from vomiting can cause seizures, permanent brain damage, or death.

Even if the victim lives, an alcohol overdose can lead to irreversible brain damage. Rapid binge drinking (which often happens on a bet or a dare or at a 21st birthday celebration) is especially dangerous because the victim can ingest a fatal dose before becoming unconscious. Always be safe, not sorry—call for help. What BAC is the recognized level that is lethal for 50 percent of adults? How many drinks does it take to reach this deadly level? See Table 14-5 for BAC information.

Party Schools

Several universities regularly listed among the nation's top "party schools" are joining with city officials and bar owners to try to curb the supply of the biggest contributor to binge drinking on and off campus: abundant, cheap beer. Two factors drive drinking on campus, according to Harvard's School of Public Health:

1. *Price.* The lower the cost of pitchers, kegs, and cases of beer, the higher the rates of heavy drinking among students. Aggressive advertising in campus newspapers feeds the problem.
2. *Prevalence.* The higher the number of bars and liquor stores around campus, the higher the percentage of binge drinkers.

Researchers concluded that college towns that discourage drink discounts, toughen ID checks, and banish beer from campus buildings endure slightly fewer problems. Many college towns are working with bar owners, beer distributors, and city officials to discourage drink-til-you-drop specials and to start police "party patrols" to clamp down on rowdy keggers and students violating the national legal drinking age of 21.

Colleges serious about curbing campus drinking and changing the alcohol-drinking culture are implementing additional efforts:

✓ *Set clear substance-abuse policies and consequences of violations.*
✓ *Screen:* Screen all students for substance-abuse problems. Target high-risk students and times, and provide needed interventions and treatment.
✓ *General alcohol education programs.* There is an increased effort to direct these programs toward Greek-affiliated students and athletes because these students represent above-average alcohol consumption and alcohol-related problem levels on many campuses.

✓ *Restrictions on the supply of alcohol.* These measures include prohibiting keg delivery to dormitories and fraternity and sorority houses, restrictions on alcohol sales at intercollegiate sports events, and tailgate parties.

✓ *Restricting alcohol advertisements.* Some schools restrict alcohol advertising at home sporting events, and a few prohibit advertisements for off-campus bars or clubs in campus newspapers or bulletin boards.

✓ *Living environment.* Some schools offer alcohol-free dormitories and living spaces and substance-free recreational opportunities.

✓ *Provide full-time education.* Schools are returning to the practice of holding classes and exams Mondays through Fridays. A college should not enable students to drink from Thursday to Sunday.

✓ *Start freshman orientation before students arrive on campus.* Schools are sending the message "No binge drinking major offered here." They are using alumni, high school counselors, and the admissions office to get the message out.

✓ *Other measures.* These include efforts in providing an infrastructure to monitor and respond to students' problem drinking, engaging students in service learning courses and community service and including information in the academic curricula about substance-abuse education. Some schools are conducting social norms campaigns to inform students about actual levels of drinking on campus. Use Lab Activity 14-2 to examine the alcohol culture on your campus.

College Binge Drinking and Positive Norming and Harm Reduction

Studies such as the Harvard School of Public Health College Alcohol Study indicate that students who drink at the binge level create enormous problems for themselves and for other students at their colleges

(Table 14-7). As Table 14-10 reveals, frequent binge drinkers consumed more than 72 percent of the alcohol students drank. They also accounted for more than three-fifths of the more serious alcohol-related problems on campus. But only 23 percent of college students are the worst bingers—a minority on our campuses. No doubt about it, a great deal of alcohol is being consumed on our college campuses. However, most students who consume alcohol are not causing a lot of problems. It's the minority, the frequent bingers, who are visible and the ones who are creating most of the havoc. See Figure 14-1.

The perception on most campuses is that all students are consuming vast amounts of alcohol and causing numerous problems for themselves and everyone else. Studies indicate that this is not the true picture (Table 14-10 and Figure 14-1). These studies suggest that students tend to overestimate the acceptability and the actual drinking behavior of their peers. This creates a *false perception* and cements beliefs that such extreme norms exist and may serve to justify and explain extreme behavior. This in turn may influence students to engage in heavy drinking: the "everyone is doing it, so I'm a nerd if I don't, too!" mentality. The reality is, as the Harvard data revealed, that nondrinkers or non-binge drinkers are the majority. The study further revealed that the median number of drinks consumed per week by all students, regardless of drinking status, was 1.5. When students were divided by drinking pattern, the median number of drinks per week was 0.8 for those who did not binge drink. This is the reality on most campuses. So not everyone is getting into trouble with alcohol. It's the highly visible minority. How many drinks per week do frequent bingers consume? See Table 14-10.

So what can be done to bring reality to the forefront and diminish false perceptions? One alcohol intervention technique is to challenge and attempt to correct these inaccurate perceptions. It is frequently

TABLE 14-10	*The Worst Bingers Consume the Most Alcohol on Campus*		
	Campus Drinkers	Mean Number of Drinks per Week	Percent of Total Alcohol Consumed on Campus
• Frequent binge drinkers (the worst bingers)— binged three or more times in 1 week	23% (about 1/2 the total bingers)	14.5	72
• Occasional bingers	22%	4.8	24
• Other (nonbinge drinkers)	36%	0.8	14

As this table illustrates, the worst bingers drink most of the alcohol consumed on our college campuses (about 72 percent) even though they represent just 23 percent of the total of 44 percent on campus who binge. This minority of college drinkers gets far too much attention!

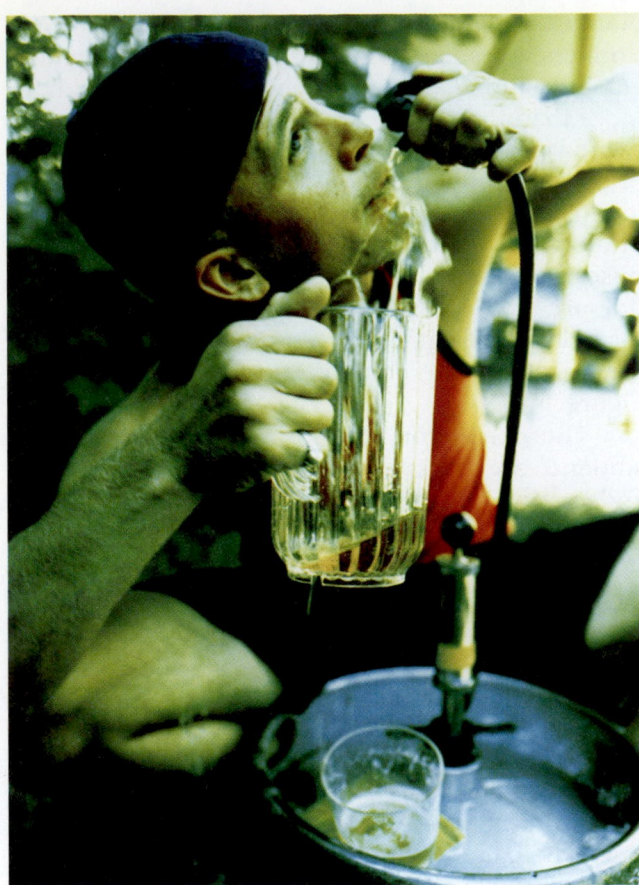

Beer kegs and bar specials make alcohol one of the cheapest forms of entertainment on campus (one glass of beer from a keg is about 25¢). The lower the cost of alcohol, the more heavily students drink.

newborn infants may be addicted if the mother abused alcohol during pregnancy. Most alcoholism is a result of abusive or high-risk drinking. The difference between the alcohol abuser and the alcoholic is control over drinking. The abusive drinker can stop. The addict cannot. Ask yourself, "Do I *want* it, or do I *need* it?"

Alcoholism is a drug (chemical) dependence. It involves progressive preoccupation with drinking, leading to physical, mental, or social dysfunction. Each year more than 100,000 Americans die of alcohol-related causes. Approximately 1 in 13 Americans is an alcoholic. The point where heavy drinking merges into alcohol dependence is blurry. The behaviors may appear to be the same. For example, both the abuser and the addict may suffer from blackouts, passing out, arrests, hangovers, absenteeism, accidents, violence, poor job or school performance, and poor relationships.

The way in which you were introduced to alcohol as a child strongly influences your attitudes and drinking behavior as an adult. Table 14-11 lists factors indicative of those who would experience the fewest problems with alcohol in adulthood. How do you stack up with these factors?

The *binger* and the *alcohol abuser* need to change their drinking behavior by quitting or following the Guidelines for Low-Risk Drinking or the Michigan Guidelines: The Zero . . . One . . . Three Rule for Lower-Risk Drinking. The *alcoholic* must quit. No alcoholic should quit "cold turkey" (abruptly)

called **positive norming** (or "social norming") and is coupled with **risk/harm reduction.** This technique uses a variety of strategies to help students internalize accurate norming information. Positive norming programs are designed to reduce campus drinking by emphasizing the "norm" of moderate drinking among students. The accurate norms help students deal with peer pressure and not succumb to that pressure to drink when they may not wish to or not consume more than they want. Read "Strategies for Dealing with Alcohol" and "Harm Reduction" ideas in "Frequently Asked Questions" later in this chapter for more information. Complete Lab Activities 14-3 and 14-4 to gain a better understanding of how alcohol affects your life.

Alcoholism

No one plans to become an alcoholic, yet alcoholism is on the rise. Currently, nearly 14 million Americans—1 in 13—are alcoholics. Risky drinking that could lead to becoming an alcoholic includes binge drinking and heavy drinking on a regular basis. Even

TABLE 14-11	Social Self-Assessment

You are least likely to have problems with alcohol if

1. You were exposed to alcohol in relatively small quantities early in life by your family or in the context of a religious or cultural group.
2. Your family members viewed alcohol as a food and consumed small quantities, primarily at mealtime.
3. Your parents set a good example by practicing lower-risk drinking behaviors.
4. Your family did not view drinking alcoholic beverages as a means of demonstrating maturity, adulthood, or masculinity/femininity.
5. Abstinence with respect to the consumption of alcoholic beverages was accepted as a legitimate choice.
6. Drunkenness was not an acceptable form of behavior.
7. Alcohol was viewed as a beverage and not as the central focus of a group activity.
8. Rules and rituals associated with drinking were known and understood by all group members and were reasonable and agreeable to those members.

SOURCE: National Institute on Alcohol Abuse and Alcoholism.

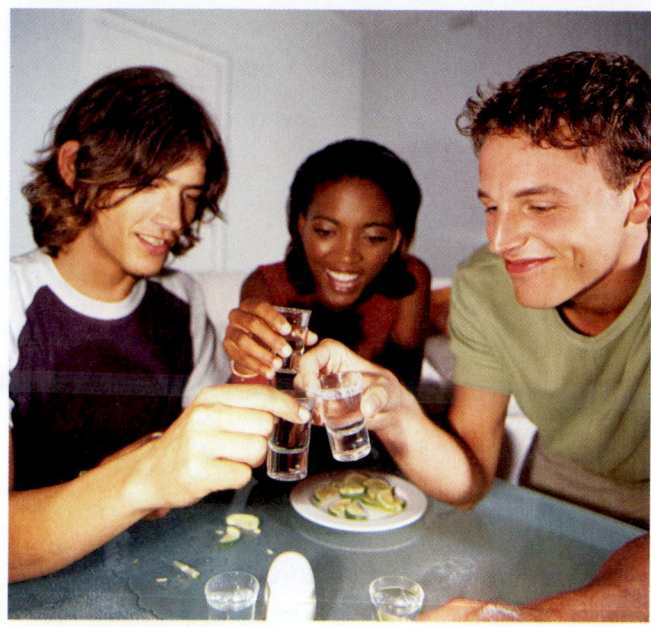

Fifty to 80 percent of college-age students take part in drinking games (Joe Califano—CASA, Columbia University). Are you a high-risk alcohol user? Why? Why not?

these risk factors is suggestive of an increased risk of alcoholism:

1. Family history of alcoholism or other drug use.
2. Heavy alcohol abuse for more than 1 year.
3. Drinking to intoxication before the age of 15.
4. More than two drinking incidents per year that result in serious adverse consequences, such as an arrest, a fight, a blackout, etc.
5. Consumption of tobacco in any form.
6. Seeking out events at which alcohol will be served.
7. Most of your friends are heavy drinkers.

If you have even *one* of these risk factors, consider getting a professional assessment. Take the quiz in Table 14-12 to find out if you have a drinking problem. See Table 14-13 for tips on how to make behavior changes in relation to controlling your consumption of alcohol.

For those with an alcohol problem, help is available. There is hope. Many people have gone to treatment centers, hospitals, clinics, and self-help groups for assistance in dealing with drinking problems.

One popular group that offers assistance to alcoholics of all ages is Alcoholics Anonymous (AA). AA was founded in 1935 by two alcoholics: a stockbroker and a surgeon who met in Akron, Ohio. They discovered that leaning on each other for emotional

without proper supervision, however, as the body has become dependent on alcohol.

Anyone who drinks should carefully examine the following list because the presence of one of

TABLE 14-12   *Do You Have a Drinking Problem?*

Yes	No	
____	____	1. Do you occasionally drink heavily after a disappointment or a quarrel, or after someone gives you a hard time?
____	____	2. When you have trouble or feel under pressure, do you drink more than usual?
____	____	3. Have you noticed that you are able to handle more alcohol than you did when you first started drinking?
____	____	4. Do you sometimes forget what happened while you were drinking?
____	____	5. When drinking with other people, do you try to have a few extra drinks when others will not know it?
____	____	6. Are there times when you feel uncomfortable if alcohol is not available?
____	____	7. Do you sometimes gulp your drinks?
____	____	8. Do you sometimes feel a little guilty about your drinking?
____	____	9. Are you a binger?
____	____	10. Do you often take a drink to help you relax?
____	____	11. Do you often drink when you are alone?
____	____	12. Are you untruthful about how much you have had to drink when questioned on the subject?
____	____	13. Are you secretly irritated when family or friends discuss your drinking?
____	____	14. Do you often find that you wish to continue drinking after your friends say they have had enough?
____	____	15. Has your drinking ever created problems between you and your friends, between you and your parents, or with the law?
____	____	16. Have you ever injured yourself or another person after drinking?
____	____	17. Have you often failed to keep promises you have made to yourself about controlling or cutting down on your drinking?
____	____	18. Does drinking ever cause you to take time off work or to miss class, scheduled meetings, or appointments?
____	____	19. Do you sometimes have the shakes (or a hangover) in the morning and find it helps to have a little drink?
____	____	20. Do you ever become frightened after you have been drinking heavily?

Scoring: You should regard a "yes" answer to any one of the questions as a warning sign. Questions 1–12 relate to early alcoholism. Questions 13–20 relate to more advanced alcoholism. Seek professional help if you are concerned that you may have an alcohol problem.

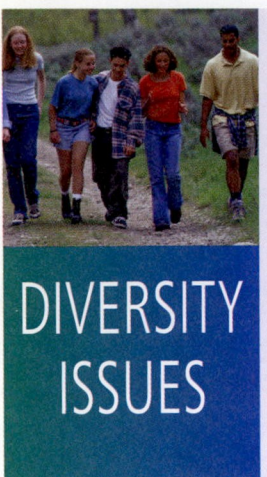

DIVERSITY ISSUES

Racial and Ethnic Differences in College Alcohol Use

Percentages of Students Who Drank Alcohol in the Previous Year

Asian/Pacific Islanders	71%
African Americans	72%
Native Americans	83%
Hispanics	85%
Caucasians (whites)	87%

A national study found the largest number of abstainers to be among Asian/Pacific Islander and African American college students.

Percentages of Students Who Are Binge Drinkers

African Americans	21%
Asian/Pacific Islanders	26.2%
Hispanics	34.4%
Native Americans	40%
Caucasians (whites)	50.2%

White and Native American college students reported the highest percentage of frequent binge drinking in a national survey. African American women were the least likely to binge drink, while white males were the most likely to binge.

---

support was crucial to keeping them on the wagon. The group they started had only 100 members during the first 4 years. It now has a worldwide membership of over 2 million. AA is a fellowship of mutual and spiritual support that has endured in simplicity.

TABLE 14-13 *Tips for Behavior Change: Controlling Alcohol*

Stages of Change: In What Stage Are You?

1. Precontemplation: "Contrary to what others say, I don't have a problem with alcohol."
2. Contemplation: "I would probably be better off if I cut back on alcohol consumption."
3. Preparation: "I am preparing to cut back on my alcohol consumption."
4. Action: "I drink very little alcohol anymore and am hosting alcohol-free parties."
5. Maintenance: "I socialize regularly without thinking of alcohol as a necessary component."

Processes of Change

After identifying your current stage, try using some of the following selected processes and behavior strategies that are appropriate for your particular stage to facilitate your transition into the next stage (refer to Figure 2-2).

- Consciousness-raising: Pay attention to media accounts of violent behavior or tragic consequences of alcohol consumption. Study strategies for dealing with alcohol in this chapter.
- Social liberation: Identify nondrinking social functions on campus.
- Emotional arousal: Spend a Saturday night in the hospital emergency room observing the consequences of too much alcohol.
- Commitment: Publicly announce to your social group your nonalcoholic intentions.
- Countering: Develop exotic nonalcoholic drinks for your next party.
- Helping relationships: Support and encourage others to sponsor social events without alcohol.

There are no dues and no minutes; the only condition for membership is *a desire to stop drinking*.

While AA is astonishingly effective for some people, it does not work for everyone; studies suggest it succeeds about 20 percent of the time. However, researchers have made extraordinary progress in understanding the physical basis of addiction. They know now that the 20 percent success rate can shoot up to 40 percent if treatment is ongoing—members continue to attend meetings long after their last drink. Also, AA works better when combined with other forms of treatment, including counseling and medical care.

Alcohol and the Law

Society has responded to the alcohol problem with legislation. All 50 states have a drinking age of 21 years. More and more studies are confirming the logic behind keeping the legal age at 21. Science is telling us that alcohol use in youth has serious ramifications for both mental health and long-term physical health. You are breaking the law if you are under age 21 and are using, possessing, or transporting alcohol. These laws partly discourage some students from drinking, which lowers the potential for accidents. Drinking to *any* extent reduces the ability of any driver. In most states, an individual can be arrested for driving under the influence if demonstrating impairment (driving erratically, etc.) even if their BAC is below 0.08 percent.

A tough new standard for drunken driving has become federal law. All states had to comply with this new law by 2004. This law defines driving under the influence of alcohol as driving with a blood alcohol content (BAC) of 0.08 percent. Whether a person feels intoxicated is not the point; the point is whether he or she registers 0.08 on a breathalyzer (see Table 14-5). The rationale for the law is that it may act as a deterrent to drinking and driving. Some states have dropped the figure to 0.05 percent as

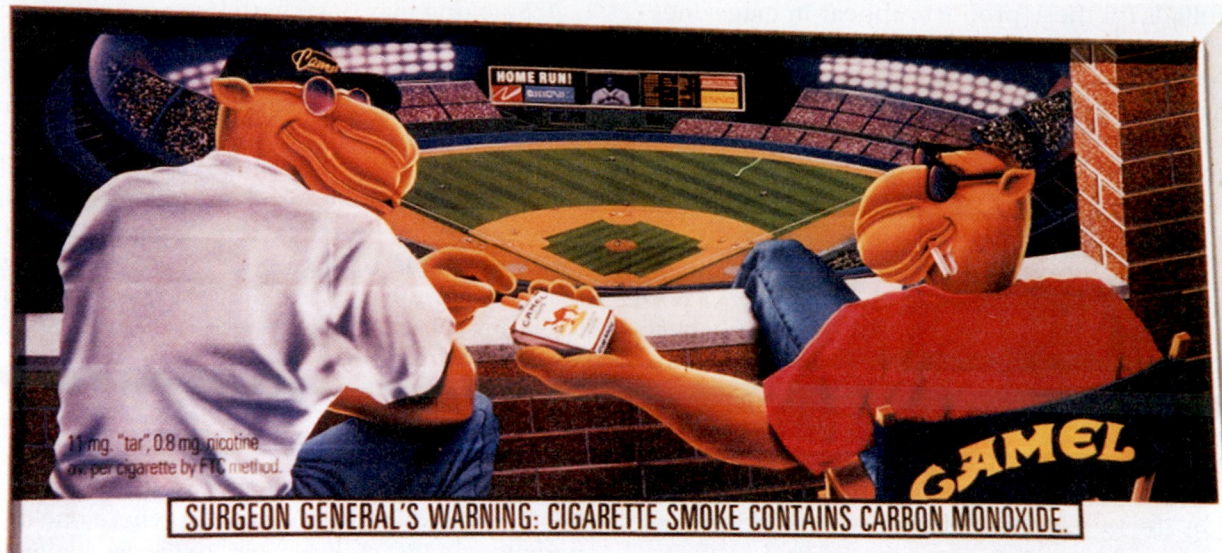

The courts have ruled that tobacco companies conspired since the 1960s to hide the dangers of smoking. At least one tobacco company admits that "smoking causes lung cancer, heart disease, and emphysema; is addictive; and that the industry markets to young people." Tobacco companies know that if people are not smokers by the time they turn 18, they will probably never light up.

presumption of intoxication. The point is, there is no safe drinking BAC.

Here is the message: You could be one of the persons who die in the next 20 minutes due to alcohol-related accidents. Or you could be crippled or permanently injured for life. Do not let it be you. Most people think it won't happen to them.

◆ TOBACCO

If you are a regular smoker, you may be losing about 6 minutes of life expectancy for every cigarette you smoke. For most smokers that means a life expectancy reduced by 5 to 7 years. The U.S. surgeon general has described cigarette smoking as "the number one preventable cause of death and health problems in our society." To put things in perspective, more people die from smoking-related diseases than from alcohol, cocaine, heroin, suicide, homicide, car accidents, and AIDS combined. Over 400,000 people die each year because they smoked cigarettes. That is more than seven times the total U.S. battle fatalities during the Vietnam War. Every day in this country 3,000 children become regular smokers. More than one-third of these individuals will die prematurely of smoking-related diseases. For years the Food and Drug Administration and the American Medical Association have pushed for nicotine to be declared an addictive drug that should be regulated.

The government has also recently banned the sale of tobacco products to anyone under age 18. But still tobacco manufacturers find ways to tempt young users. Cigarettes, small cigars, and smokeless

products are now created in various candy, fruit, and alcohol flavors to entice young people. New cigarette product names include Kauai Kolada, Warm Winter Toffee, and Winter Mocha Mint. Alcohol flavor names include Screw Driver Slots and Snake Eyes Scotch.

THE NUMBERS

101 poisons	Number found in cigarettes; that's 100 more than in rat poison.
1	A body bag is generated every 72 seconds by tobacco. That is 1,200 every day.
15.1 million	Americans who abuse controlled prescription drugs, nearly doubling the 7.8 million in 2003 (e.g., OxyContin, Vicodin, painkillers, tranquilizers, sedatives, stimulants).
1 in 5	Teens who abused prescription drugs in 2005, tripling the previous rate.
16.6%	Number of 18- to 25-year-olds who use marijuana.
68%	Increased risk for nonsmoking young premenopausal women of developing breast cancer from long-term exposure to secondhand smoke. It is 29% increased risk in nonsmoking post-menopausal women.

Colorful ads for these products appear in magazines with a large youth readership.

Despite the frightening statistics, the warnings, and the publicity given to the health risks of smoking, each year thousands of young people still start smoking.

Smoking Is Becoming Socially Unacceptable

Little was known about the health consequences of smoking until 1964, when the first surgeon general's report on smoking and health was published. At that time, nearly half of our population smoked. In the years since, millions of people have quit, and now smokers constitute less than a quarter of the population. The decline in smoking has been influenced by the proliferation of restrictive worksite and public smoking policies. Once considered sophisticated, smoking now seems to be most prevalent in the lower socioeconomic and the least-educated groups. Studies reveal that smoking is twice as high among those with less than a high school education than it is among those with a college education. Smoking by college students climbed but has recently declined to about where it was decade ago—23.8 percent. Overall, just under 21 percent smoke in this country.

Before World War II, smoking was considered a masculine activity, and few women smoked. After World War II, with increasing emancipation, women began smoking in ever-increasing numbers. As a result, lung cancer deaths for women tripled. While the proportions of adult men and women smokers have dropped since 1964, surveys indicate that men have given up smoking more often than have women.

Smoking may once have been considered glamorous, but today attitudes are changing. Smoking commercials have been banned from radio and television since 1971. Cigarette advertisements and packages carry health warnings. Over 70 percent of adult smokers have tried to quit smoking or would like to try. Nonsmokers are tired of passive smoking—breathing air polluted by tobacco smoke—and are insisting on the right to breathe clean air in workplaces and public areas. Nationwide, colleges are responding to nonsmokers by increasing smoke-free zones on campuses.

Why Do People Smoke?

The most important influences in starting to smoke are family and friends. In families where one or both parents smoke, children are twice as likely to be smokers as are children of parents who are nonsmokers. Many teenagers start smoking because they think everybody else does, and they want to be like their friends or appear more adult. They don't think much about the costs or health risks of smoking. Powerful advertising directed at young people (e.g., Joe Camel) de-emphasizes the harmful factors. The tobacco industry spends billions on advertising to convince young people that they should take up smoking. For young people, cigarettes are considered a gateway drug—the first drug many use as a stepping stone to illicit drugs and heavy drinking.

Nicotine, a drug in tobacco, is addicting, as anyone who has tried to quit smoking has quickly discovered. It causes the release of the "feel good" chemical dopamine when it reaches the brain. Nicotine is an

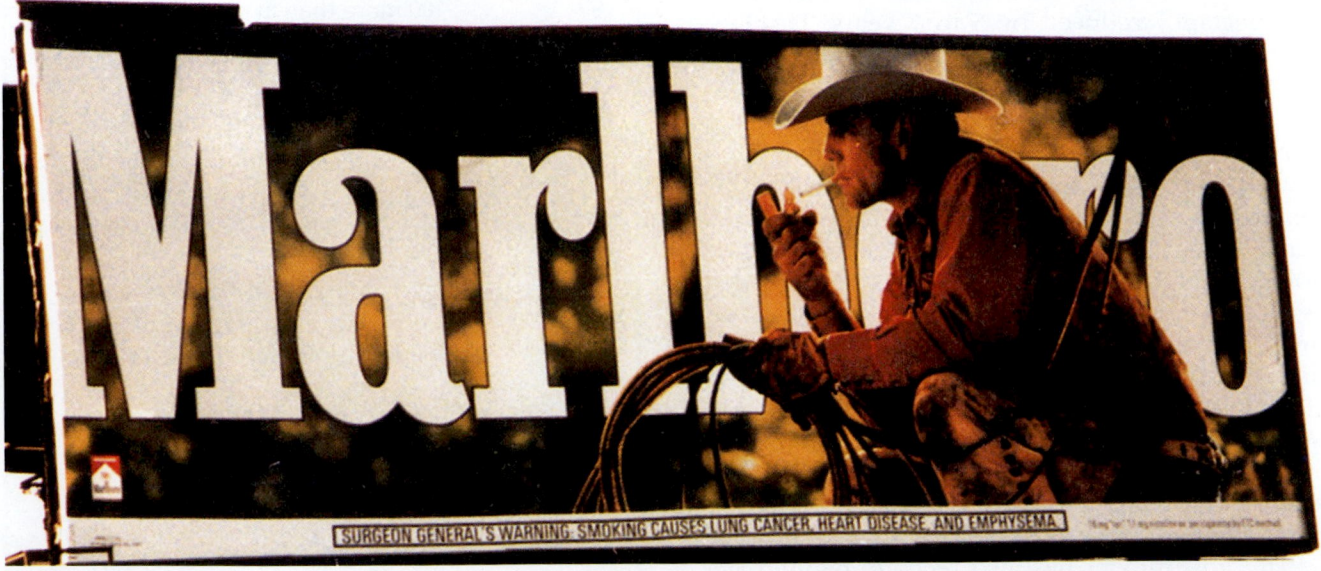

The Marlboro man and Joe Camel billboards advertising tobacco products are past history. Since 1998 tobacco companies have agreed to stop billboard advertising and stop marketing to young people.

alkaloid drug synthesized by the tobacco plant in the same fashion that the opium poppy (the source of heroin) and the coca plant (the source of cocaine) synthesize their addictive substances. Habituation to nicotine may occur after smoking only three packs of cigarettes. Once hooked on nicotine, a person can find it difficult to quit. Indeed, experts say that addiction to nicotine can be as strong as addiction to cocaine or heroin. Without a steady supply of nicotine, withdrawal symptoms may occur. (See Lab Activity 9-5, *Are You Addicted to Tobacco?* on the book's Web site, and Lab Activity 14-5, *Tobacco Use Values Clarification.*) Although 70 percent of smokers want to stop smoking, only 6 to 8 percent successfully do so each year. The high rate of relapse is a consequence of the effect of nicotine dependence. Smokers' families and friends should be more aware that smoking is not only a nasty habit but a form of drug dependence.

Health Risks of Smoking

Among the 4,000 potentially toxic chemicals in cigarette smoke, the three major toxic substances are nicotine, carbon monoxide, and tar. Nicotine stimulates the cardiovascular system. Increased heart rate and blood pressure place a burden on the heart muscle, which then needs more oxygen. Carbon monoxide, a toxic gas, immediately reduces the blood's ability to carry oxygen and ultimately damages the inner surface of coronary arteries, increasing the rate of atherosclerosis. When combined with vasoconstriction, a narrowing of the arteries, atherosclerosis can cause ischemia (lack of oxygen) and coronary tissue damage. Smoking also increases arrhythmias, increases stickiness and clotting of blood cells, and decreases levels of HDL. This is why twice as many smokers as nonsmokers die from heart attacks. Also, smoking contributes to peripheral vascular disease, which is hardening of the arteries in the lower legs. This condition can affect the ability to walk and may eventually lead to amputation of the legs.

Tar contains potent carcinogens. It also contains chemicals that irritate lung tissue and may promote chronic bronchitis and emphysema. These substances can paralyze and destroy the cilia that line the bronchi, allowing tar and other particles to accumulate in the lungs. This causes *smoker's cough,* the body's attempt to rid itself of the buildup of particulate matter. Long-term contact between lung tissue and tar can cause cellular changes that lead to the development of cancer.

The reduction in a person's life expectancy due to smoking parallels increasing cigarette use. Mortality is higher the younger a person started smoking, the longer a person has smoked, the deeper a smoker

inhales, and the higher the tar and nicotine content of the tobacco used. If a smoker is overweight, has moderately elevated blood pressure, or has a high cholesterol level, the risk of having a heart attack skyrockets.

If you've smoked for many years, does it do any good to quit? Yes. Heart attack risk declines by about half in the first year after quitting. The risk continues to decrease with each year of abstinence until, after 10 to 15 years, an ex-smoker has almost the same risk of dying as if he or she had never smoked (Figure 14-2). People who quit smoking may gain weight (men gain about 10 pounds, and women about 11); of course there is no comparison between the health risks of being 10 or 11 pounds overweight and the hazards of smoking. Regardless of how long or how much a person has smoked, quitting is beneficial.

Smokeless Tobacco

Cigarette smoking is not the only form of tobacco that presents health risks. Smokeless tobacco—snuff and chewing tobacco—is surging in popularity among young adult males. Often used by athletes, smokeless tobacco seems to be viewed as a safe alternative to cigarette smoking, which is forbidden by coaches of athletic teams. The tobacco industry wants you to believe that snuff and chewing tobacco provide all the pleasure of cigarettes without the risks. But the evidence shows otherwise. Highly carcinogenic tobacco nitrosamines are released in concentrations 1,000 times higher in smokeless tobacco–saliva mixtures than in cigarette smoke. Snuff and chewing tobacco cause many problems, ranging from bad breath to cardiovascular disease and cancer. A decrease in the ability to taste and smell, stained teeth,

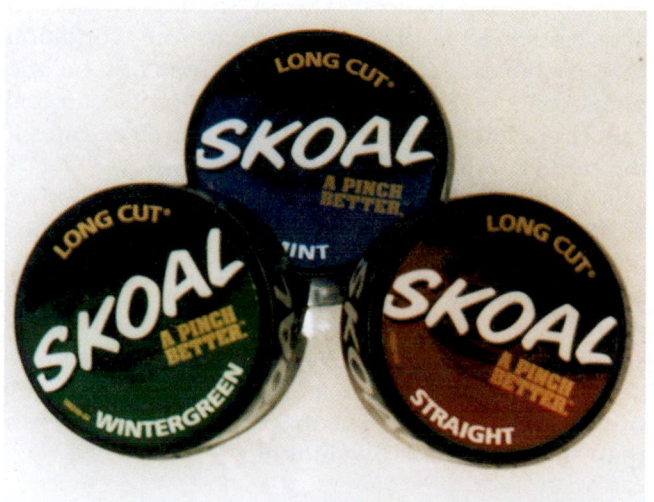

Nicotine from smokeless tobacco is absorbed directly into the bloodstream from the mouth (one of the most efficient delivery systems known) and eventually produces dependency.

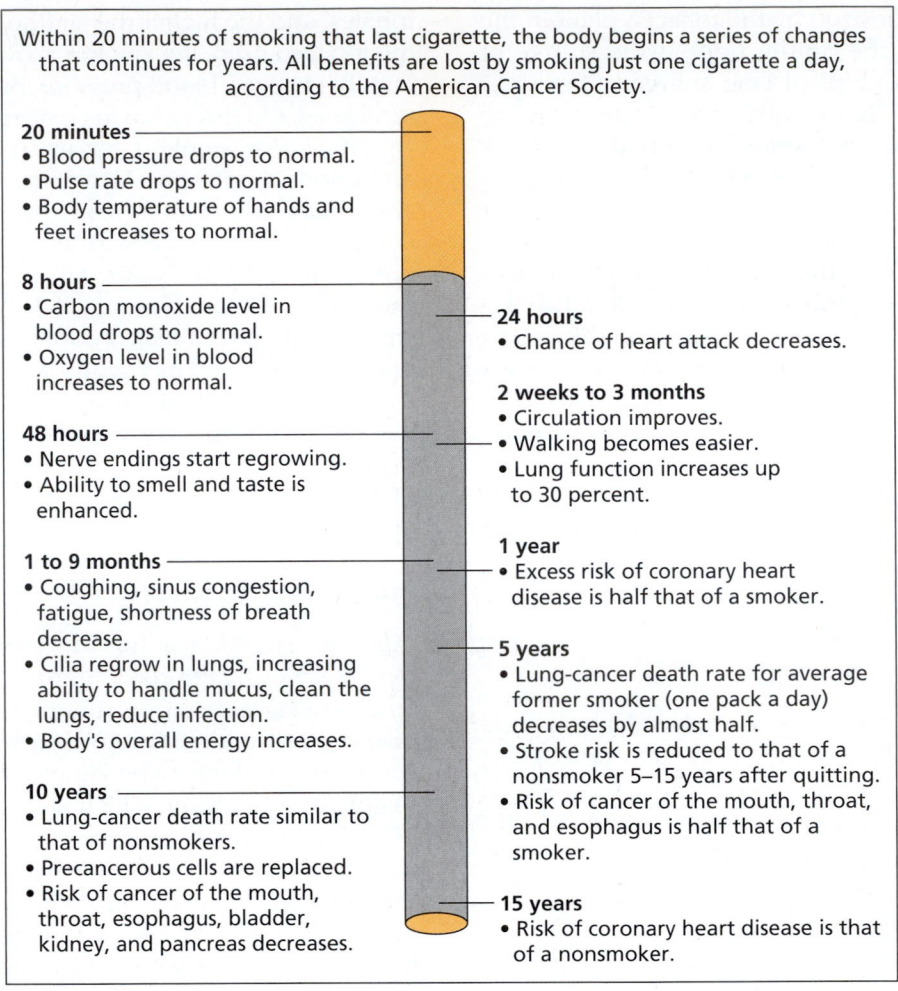

Within 20 minutes of smoking that last cigarette, the body begins a series of changes that continues for years. All benefits are lost by smoking just one cigarette a day, according to the American Cancer Society.

20 minutes
- Blood pressure drops to normal.
- Pulse rate drops to normal.
- Body temperature of hands and feet increases to normal.

8 hours
- Carbon monoxide level in blood drops to normal.
- Oxygen level in blood increases to normal.

48 hours
- Nerve endings start regrowing.
- Ability to smell and taste is enhanced.

1 to 9 months
- Coughing, sinus congestion, fatigue, shortness of breath decrease.
- Cilia regrow in lungs, increasing ability to handle mucus, clean the lungs, reduce infection.
- Body's overall energy increases.

10 years
- Lung-cancer death rate similar to that of nonsmokers.
- Precancerous cells are replaced.
- Risk of cancer of the mouth, throat, esophagus, bladder, kidney, and pancreas decreases.

24 hours
- Chance of heart attack decreases.

2 weeks to 3 months
- Circulation improves.
- Walking becomes easier.
- Lung function increases up to 30 percent.

1 year
- Excess risk of coronary heart disease is half that of a smoker.

5 years
- Lung-cancer death rate for average former smoker (one pack a day) decreases by almost half.
- Stroke risk is reduced to that of a nonsmoker 5–15 years after quitting.
- Risk of cancer of the mouth, throat, and esophagus is half that of a smoker.

15 years
- Risk of coronary heart disease is that of a nonsmoker.

FIGURE 14-2 When smokers quit.

gum damage, tooth loss, and wear on the chewing surfaces of the teeth caused by grit in the tobacco are commonly experienced. Use of smokeless tobacco also causes leukoplakia, a precancerous condition that produces thick, rough, white patches on the gums, tongue, or inner cheek. Experts predict an oral cancer epidemic beginning in two or three decades if the trend continues.

In addition, smokeless tobacco is addictive. Evidence has revealed that tobacco companies manipulated the chemical recipes of their products. These chemical changes supposedly allow more nicotine to be absorbed into the bloodstream, thus making the product gradually more addictive. Many people feel that the dependency produced by smokeless tobacco is harder to break than that produced by smoking.

Are You a Passive Smoker?

The U.S. surgeon general's new report provides conclusive scientific evidence of the alarming public health threat posed by secondhand smoke. It declares that smoking bans are the only way to protect nonsmokers. Nonsmokers, who outnumber smokers 4 to 1, want to stop **passive smoking** (secondhand smoke)—breathing air polluted by tobacco smoke—especially when they hear the findings from this new report. Reports state that passive smoking causes more than 60,000 deaths per year, including breast and lung cancer, plus heart disease and strokes.

The decision to smoke can no longer be considered a private matter. Past solutions such as separating smokers and nonsmokers in the same room are inadequate. The AHA concludes that "the only sure way to protect nonsmokers from environmental tobacco smoke is to eliminate smoking from areas that smokers share with nonsmokers." This once radical step is now scientifically proven—indoor smoking may soon be a thing of the past. And a more recent extreme step involves many businesses, colleges, and public buildings moving the smokers 30 feet or more from the entrances of

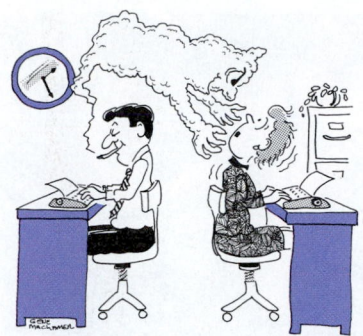

Smoking is everybody's business. Some employers are firing and not hiring workers who smoke—even in their own homes.

buildings so that nonsmokers don't have to walk through smoke-filled air to enter.

It does not make sense to strengthen your heart and lungs with regular exercise only to be at the mercy of smokers when you venture into public. Get involved and start campaigning for eliminating exposure to secondhand smoke.

Here are some tips to keep others from smoking around you:

✓ Speak up. Make others aware of the dangers of secondhand smoke and let them know *you don't like it*.
✓ Suggest alternative places for others to smoke—outside.
✓ Display reminders. Hang "Thank you for not smoking!" signs in your home, car, office, and so on.
✓ Get rid of ashtrays.
✓ Discuss smoking cessation strategies. Many new products and strategies are available to help smokers quit. Bringing these up in conversation makes your antismoking concerns clear. It may save your life and that of someone close to you.

How to Quit Smoking

Millions of Americans have quit smoking. Some try to reduce the number of cigarettes they smoke. Others quit "cold turkey." The vast majority try to stop on their own, but only 6 to 8 percent manage to do it. Research confirms that when smokers combine the use of health coaching (or counseling) with some type of stop-smoking medication, the rate of quitting jumps to more than 20 percent.

See the Web sites at the end of this chapter for further assistance if you would like to stop smoking. If you are a nonsmoker wishing to help a smoker who is trying to quit, you should know that the support of family and friends is the second

most important factor in breaking the grip of the nicotine habit.

Giving up smoking can be a long-term process, and some people must try several times before they quit for good. It is not easy. Smokers have about the same success rate as those trying to break an alcohol or heroin addiction, but this doesn't mean that a person can't quit. Every year thousands of people quit smoking, but it takes effort, desire, support, and a firm commitment. If a person stops smoking for a while and then starts again, he or she should not be considered weak. Some former smokers say they still crave cigarettes long after they quit smoking. The smoker who does not succeed in quitting on the first try should try and try again. Mark Twain said it best: "It's easy to *quit* smoking. I should know—I've done it dozens of times."

If you're ready to toss those cigarettes, *Clearing the Air: A Guide to Quitting Smoking,* available from the American Cancer Society, gives these recommendations:

✓ *Identify your reasons* for quitting.
✓ *Set a target date for quitting.* Then list the reasons you want to quit. Review them whenever you crave tobacco.
✓ *Identify your barriers to quitting* (e.g., your spouse smokes or you have relapsed before due to stress or weight gain).
✓ *Make specific plans ahead of time for dealing with temptations.* Identify two or three coping strategies that work for you (such as taking a walk or calling a friend).
✓ Before you quit, *change to a brand you find distasteful* and then taper off a little more each day. Smoke only half of each cigarette. Smoke only during even hours of the day.
✓ *Involve friends and family.* Tell them when and why you are going to quit and ask for their support.
✓ *On the day you quit,* toss out all cigarettes and matches. Go to the dentist to have your teeth cleaned. Keep busy and concentrate on getting through that 1 day without tobacco.
✓ After quitting, *change your normal routine.* Spend as much time as possible away from places and situations you associate with smoking. Go jogging, drink more fluids, get plenty of rest.
✓ When you get the "crazies," *chew on carrots, pickles, sunflower seeds, or sugarless gum.* Take a shower. Never allow yourself to think, "One won't hurt."
✓ *Mark progress.* Each month, celebrate the anniversary of your quit date. Put aside the money you've saved by not smoking and treat yourself to something special. You deserve it.

The Clock Strategy

Another strategy for quitting smoking is to let the clock tell you when to smoke. The clock strategy was reported to be twice as successful in the long term as quitting cold turkey. This is how it works:

Step 1: Assign yourself specific times of the day to light up.

Step 2: Gradually lengthen the intervals between cigarettes.

Step 3: Cut back progressively on the number of cigarettes per week (decreasing cigarettes by one-third each week).

The key to why the clock strategy seems to work so well lies in breaking the link between everyday smoking cues and the habit of lighting up. That is, smokers don't smoke when they want to. They smoke on cue. By repeatedly putting nicotine urges on hold for manageable periods, smokers gain practice and self-confidence for when they finally stop. If you wish to quit smoking, try this new strategy. We wish you success!

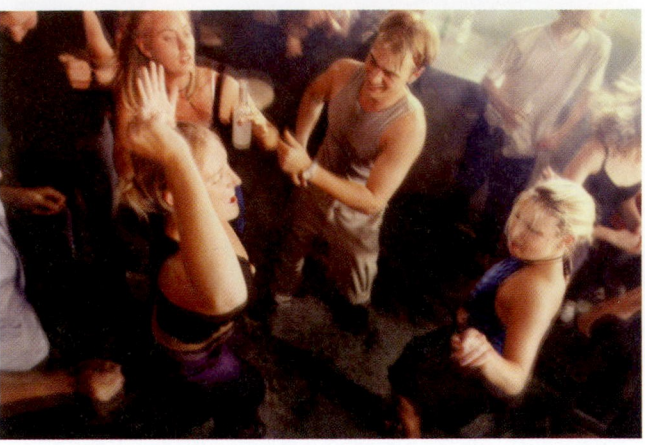

Raves are high-energy, all-night dance facilities that feature hard-pounding technomusic and flashing laser lights.

PSYCHOACTIVE DRUGS

A **psychoactive drug** is any substance capable of altering feelings, moods, perceptions, and behaviors. These mind-affecting or mind-altering changes result from the drug's action on the brain. Psychoactive drugs are classified in this text by their effect on the CNS. The classification includes (1) depressants, (2) cannabis (marijuana), (3) stimulants, (4) narcotics or opiates, (5) psychedelics, and (6) inhalants. See Table 14-1 for how prevalent these are among college students and Table 14-14 for the effects, medical uses, and street or common names of drugs in each classification.

While students use illegal drugs at much lower rates than they use alcohol, illicit drug use has led to tragedies, including violence, sexual assault and rape, hospitalization for overdoses, and premature death.

Before we discuss the specific classifications of psychoactive drugs, let's look at club drugs. This group includes both depressants and stimulants.

Club Drugs

The term **club drugs** (also called "party drugs") refers to a wide variety of drugs that are being used at bars, college hangouts, dance clubs, and all-night dance parties called "raves" or "trances." Club drugs are attractive because they are inexpensive, produce increased stamina, and produce intoxicating highs. The National Institute on Drug Abuse has supported

research that shows the use of club drugs can cause serious health problems and, in some cases, death. When used in combination with alcohol, these drugs can be even more dangerous. The club drug category includes both stimulants such as MDMA (Ecstasy)—the most popular club drug—and depressants such as GHB, Rohypnol, and ketamine. Sponsors of raves promote them with flyers distributed at record shops, clothing stores, college campuses, and other rave clubs and over the Internet. Raves can be held at either permanent dance clubs or temporary clubs set up in abandoned warehouses, open fields, or

TOP 10 LIST

Warning Signs of Substance Abuse

1. Change in attendance patterns at school/work.
2. Change in behavior—previously happy individual becomes withdrawn, rebellious, depressed, tired, or aggressive.
3. Forms different friendships and associates with known drug users.
4. Loss of interest in hobbies, sports, and school.
5. Eating and sleeping habits are altered.
6. Weight loss and other physical complaints.
7. Poor physical appearance (e.g., clothes, personal hygiene).
8. Increased borrowing of money from friends or family members; stealing from home, school, or employer.
9. Heightened secrecy about actions and possessions.
10. Change from typical capabilities, such as work habits, efficiency, self-discipline, mood, and attitude expression.

TABLE 14-14   *Psychoactive Drugs*

Drugs	Street or Common Names	Legal	Medical Uses	Effects
Depressants (Date Rape Drugs)				
GHB (Gamma-hydroxybutyrate)	G, liquid ecstasy, Georgia Home Boy, salty water, Easy lay	No	None	Unconsciousness, seizures, amnesia, vomiting, coma
Rohypnol	Roofies, roach, rope, the forget pill, date rape drug	No	None	Euphoria, reduced inhibitions, unconsciousness, amnesia, vomiting, coma
Ketamine (Ketamine hydrochloride)	K, Special K, Ket, Kit kat, Vitamin K, cat valium	No, only in veterinary use	Veterinary anesthetic	Unconsciousness, paralysis, amnesia, vomiting, delirium, coma
Cannabis				
Marijuana	Pot, grass, weed, Mary Jane, Acapulco Gold, Black Bart, reefer, joints, herb	No	Under investigation	Euphoria, relaxed inhibitions, increased appetite, disoriented behavior, lowers resistance to bacterial and viral infections, impairs memory and concentration, increased heart rate and blood pressure, red eyes, slow reaction time, impairs learning and problem solving, sleeplessness, damages lungs and reproductive function; addiction
Stimulants				
Cocaine	Crack, Coke, Blow, C, candy, Charlie, Girl, double bubble, California cornflakes, flake, snow, nose candy	No	Local anesthetic	Increased alertness, relieves fatigue, euphoria, depresses appetite, insomnia, excitation, increased pulse rate and blood pressure; causes emotional problems, mood surges, lack of dependability, damage to respiratory and immune systems, heart attack, stroke, seizures, death; addiction
Methamphetamine	Ice, speed, meth, crystal, crystal meth, crank, Poorman's cocaine, glass	No	None	Euphoria, hallucinations, decreased appetite, rapid weight loss, increased wakefulness and physical activity, hyperthermia, irritability, anxiety, increased heart rate and blood pressure, strokes, severe tooth and gum damage ("meth mouth"), rapid aging in appearance, acne, cardiovascular problems that can lead to death, paranoia or violent behavior, kidney problems, liver and brain damage; addiction; death
MDMA (Ecstasy)	E, XTC, love drug, lover's speed, Disco biscuits, Adam	No	None	Increased blood pressure and heart rate, involuntary teeth clenching, nausea, tremors, dehydration, decreases brain serotonin levels, increased energy, hallucinations, insomnia, liver damage, seizures, heat stroke, death
Amphetamines (Dexadrine, etc.)	Bennies, black beauties, crosses, LA turnaround, speed, truck drivers, uppers	Yes	None	Increased heart rate, blood pressure, metabolism; feelings of exhilaration, energy; increased mental alertness, insomnia, aggressiveness; tremor, irritability; tolerance; addiction; psychosis; heart failure

(continued)

TABLE 14-14   *Psychoactive Drugs (continued)*

Drugs	Street or Common Names	Legal	Medical Uses	Effects
Narcotics or Opiates				
Heroin	Horse, smack, dead-on-arrival (DOA), junk, H, hardstuff, brown sugar	No	Under investigation	Euphoria, drowsiness, depressed respiration, constricted pupils, clouded mental functioning, slowed slurred speech, watery eyes, runny nose, loss of appetite, insomnia, suppression of pain, nausea and vomiting, cold and clammy skin, convulsions, coma, costs lead to crime, death, addiction
Psychedelics				
LSD (lysergic acid diethylamide)	Acid, sugar cubes, trips, microdot, cap, California sunshine, brown bomber, windowpanes, blotter acid	No	None	Delusions and hallucinations, poor perception of time and distance, emotional swings, bizarre changes in behavior, loss of concentration and memory, panic attacks, bad trips, flashbacks, depression
"Mushrooms" (Psilocybin and Psilocyn-Tryptamines)	Magic mushrooms, mushroom, shroom, businessman's trip, silly putty, simple Simon, purple passion	No	None	Hallucinations, inability to discern fantasy from reality, panic reactions, psychosis, nausea, vomiting, muscle weakness, drowsiness, lack of coordination, dilation of pupils
Inhalants				
Commercial solvents	Airplane glue, plastic cement, paint thinner, gasoline, cleaning fluids, nail polish remover, marking pens, typewriter correction fluid	Yes	None	Slow CNS function, temporary mild euphoria, produces a dreamlike high resembling drunkenness, damages nerves that control breathing leading to coma or death; bone, marrow, liver, and kidney damage; even one use may be lethal causing cardiac arrest called "sudden sniffing death"
Aerosols	Cooking sprays, glass chillers, spray paints, computer sprays, fire extinguishers, deodorizers, hair sprays, Freon gas	Yes	None	
Also: Nitrites (Nitrite room odorizers)				
Amyl nitrate	Snappers, Poppers	Yes	Treating heart disease patients	
Butyl nitrite	Rush, locker room, and super bullet	Yes	None	
Gas Anesthetics	Nitrous oxide (laughing gas) and canned whipped cream Chloroform, ether, halothane, cyclopropane	Yes	Surgical anesthetic	

empty buildings for a single weekend event. Club drugs can also be found at rock concerts, nightclubs, schools, and private homes. A recent resurgence in the availability of some hallucinogens, such as LSD (lysergic acid diethylamide) and PCP (phencyclidine), at raves and dance clubs may necessitate their inclusion in the club drug category as well. Even methamphetamine is increasingly being used as a club drug.

Depressants

Depressants are drugs known as sedatives. They slow down the CNS, relax or tranquilize, and produce sleep. This category includes the "date rape drugs": gamma-hydroxybutyric acid (GHB), Rohypnol ("roofies"), and ketamine. See Table 14-14. Alcohol, discussed earlier in this chapter, is also a CNS depressant.

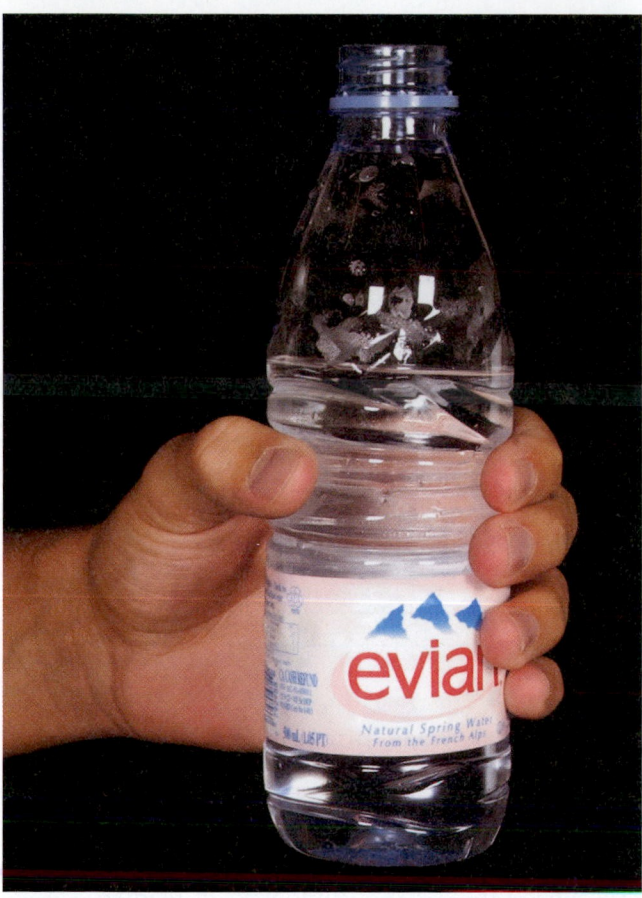

The "date rape drug" GHB can easily be slipped into water bottles and offered to unsuspecting females at raves, bars, clubs, and parties. Be aware!

All three **date rape drugs** are used to cause women (and sometimes men) to become overly relaxed or pass out and yield unknowingly in a sexual way. They are powerful sedatives and become extremely dangerous when mixed with other CNS depressants, such as alcohol or narcotic drugs. This combination is potentially life-threatening and can be fatal. To reduce the risk of substance-related rape, practice the following suggestions:

1. Do not leave beverages unattended.
2. Do not take any beverages, including alcohol, from someone you do not know well or trust.
3. At a bar or club, accept drinks only from the bartender, waiter, or waitress.
4. At parties, do not accept open container drinks from anyone.
5. Do not drink anything that has an unusual taste or appearance, such as a salty taste, excessive foam, or unexplained residue or color.
6. Watch out for your friends. Anyone appearing disproportionately inebriated in relation to the amount of alcohol he or she has consumed may be in danger.

7. Anyone who believes he or she has consumed a sedative-like substance should be driven to a hospital emergency room or someone should call 911 for an ambulance. Try to keep a sample of the beverage for analysis.

Cannabis (Marijuana)

Marijuana is an intoxicating psychoactive drug that may produce both depressant and psychedelic effects. *It is the United States' most widely used illegal drug* and trails only alcohol and tobacco in popularity as a social or recreational drug. The availability and popularity of marijuana renders the drug a significant threat to the country.

The prevalence of the drug has contributed to both an acceptance of its use among some adults (young and old) and a perception that marijuana use is not harmful.

Although marijuana contains at least 421 ingredients, delta-9-tetrahydrocannabinol (THC) is the principal psychoactive ingredient. Overall potency, as characterized by THC content, has continually risen over the last decade, potentially exposing users to a higher risk of dependence. THC is fat soluble and is stored in fatty tissues of the body, brain, and reproductive organs. Due to this, complete elimination of a single dose is slow and may require 1 month or more before the body is drug free. During this time, marijuana residuals can be detected in the urine.

Marijuana use causes brain cell damage and lowered sperm count. THC changes the cell membrane, causing it to be less efficient with less energy, particularly in the brain and testicles. Additionally, it can result in **amotivational syndrome** due to changes in the brain cell membranes. A person with this syndrome experiences low energy, apathy, and little drive to do anything. Students exhibit this syndrome by not going to class, not completing assignments,

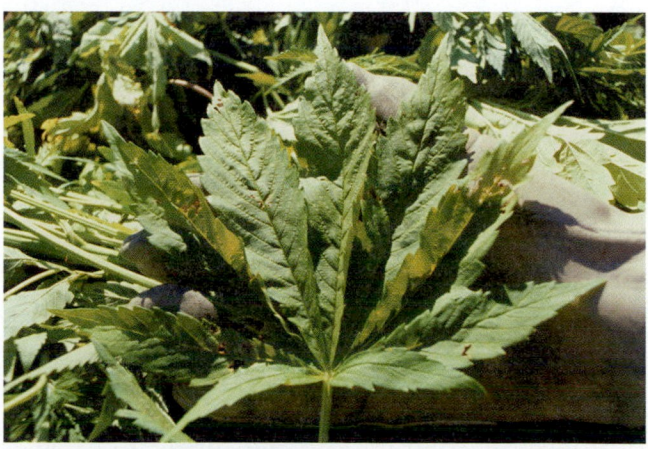

If you think "everybody's doing it," you're wrong.

TABLE 14-15	Do You Have a Marijuana Problem?

Yes	No	
_____	_____	1. Is it hard to imagine your life without marijuana?
_____	_____	2. Do you find yourself using marijuana more now than you have in the past?
_____	_____	3 Do you think marijuana is safe and not addictive?
_____	_____	4. Do you use marijuana to escape from problems, cope with stress, or to relax?
_____	_____	5. Do you hang out with people who get high and know where to get marijuana?
_____	_____	6. Do you do things under the influence of marijuana that you wouldn't normally do?
_____	_____	7. Do you worry that you will run out of marijuana?
_____	_____	8. Have you started to lose interest in things that used to mean a lot—schoolwork, sports, hobbies, or friends who don't drink or use drugs?
_____	_____	9. Has a friend or relative expressed concern about your use of marijuana and suggested that you cut down?
_____	_____	10. Are you finding it more difficult to remember things that recently happened?
_____	_____	11. Do you feel tired more often?
_____	_____	12. Have you noticed that you react more slowly to situations, even if they are serious?
_____	_____	13. Do you find you are getting more colds, flus, or other infections?
_____	_____	14. Have you promised yourself to slow down or stop using but find that you are unable to keep the promise for a few days or weeks at a time?

Scoring: Did you answer "yes" to one or more questions? If so, you may have a problem with marijuana.

"vegetating" on a chair, or appearing not to care about anything.

Smoking marijuana increases risk of cancer. Research reveals that one joint can deliver four times as much cancer-causing tar as one cigarette. See the Frequently Asked Questions for more information.

Drinking alcohol while smoking marijuana is dangerous. Marijuana inhibits vomiting, causing the alcohol to remain in your system. This increases the chance of alcohol poisoning. Use of marijuana severely reduces the ability to drive a car. It impairs motor coordination, impairs judgment and perception, and decreases awareness of external stimuli (such as flashing lights). Take the self-assessment in Table 14-15; also see Table 14-16.

Stimulants

Stimulants are chemical substances that speed up the central nervous system, resulting in alertness and excitability. This category includes cocaine and crack, methamphetamine, MDMA (Ecstasy), and amphetamines. See Table 14-14. Caffeine is discussed in Chapter 7 in "Drugs Affecting Physical Performance."

COCAINE AND CRACK

Cocaine, in both powdered and crack forms, is one of the top three drug threats to the United States (along with methamphetamine and heroin). High demand for and availability of the drug, expansion of cocaine distribution markets, and high rates of overdose all contribute to the threat. Cocaine is transported to the United States and distributed at the wholesale level primarily by Colombian and Mexican drug-trafficking organizations.

Cocaine is extracted from the coca plant, mainly harvested in Central and South America. It is usually used in powder form. **Crack,** a cocaine derivative, is crystallized free-base cocaine sold in ready-to-smoke "rocks."

METHAMPHETAMINE

The U.S. government has targeted methamphetamine as its number *one* priority in the war against drugs

TABLE 14-16	Marijuana Use

One in four college students reported using marijuana within the last year.

Characteristics Predicting Marijuana Use

- Higher among students at noncommuter colleges and colleges with pubs on campus

Student Characteristics Associated with Marijuana Use

- Being single.
- Being Caucasian (white).
- Being male.
- Spending more time at parties and socializing with friends and less time studying. Participating in high-risk behaviors such as binge drinking; cigarette smoking; having multiple sexual partners; and perceiving parties as important and religion and community service as not important.

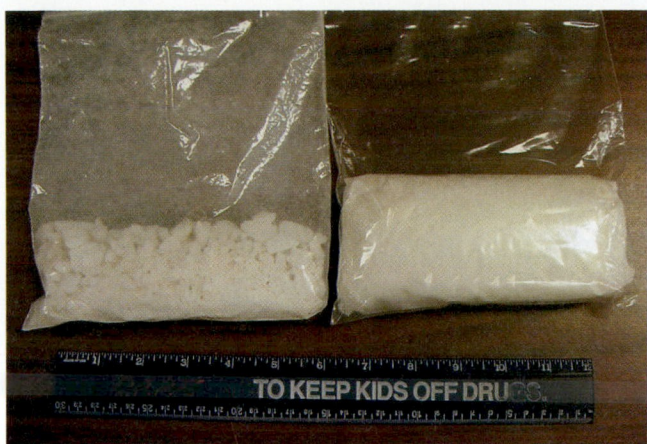

Cocaine in both the crack form (left) and the powdered form (right) can be found on college campuses. Users are 24 times more likely to have a heart attack during the first hour after taking the drug.

and tags it as the top drug threat in the United States. The threats posed to the United States by **methamphetamine** (a synthetic form of amphetamine) include these issues:

✓ High rate of addiction with its use.
✓ Severe physiological effects associated with its use
✓ Violence and environmental damage associated with the production, distribution, and use of the drug
✓ Involvement of international drug-trafficking organizations (especially Mexican)

Meth is produced using ephedrine or pseudoephedrine (found in over-the-counter allergy, cold, and diet medications).

Ice is the street name for crystallized methamphetamine and is sometimes called **crystal meth.** It resembles glass fragments or ice shavings. Ice is to meth what crack is to cocaine, but meth is more addictive than cocaine.

What makes methamphetamine such an attractive high? Meth users report that after taking the drug they experience a sudden "rush" of pleasure or a prolonged sense of euphoria, as well as increased energy, focus, confidence, sexual prowess, and feelings of desirability. However, after that first try, users require more and more of the drug to get that feeling and maintain it. Because of increased sex drive, a lowering of sexual inhibitions, and impaired judgment, users' risk of sexually transmitted disease escalates.

The signs of methamphetamine use include

✓ Carelessness about personal appearance and living conditions (noticeable aging of face)
✓ Unusual periods of sleep or sleeplessness
✓ Excessive secretiveness
✓ Dilated and nonreactive pupils
✓ Weight loss
✓ Nervousness
✓ Profuse sweating
✓ Loss of teeth and extreme tooth decay
✓ Sleeping disorders
✓ Paranoia
✓ Skin sores that don't heal, caused by scratching at imaginary insects called "crank bugs"

Both the main ingredient for manufacture of the drug (ephedrine) and the international trafficking originates in Asia and Europe. It is then shipped to Mexico. Next, it is smuggled across the U.S. border and resold to the operators of stove-top labs throughout the country. Methamphetamine can easily be manufactured in stove-top labs in homes, rural shacks, motel rooms, and even backs of trucks and campers by a "cook" with a few hundred dollars' worth of equipment by extracting ephedrine from over-the-counter allergy, cold, and diet pills or from pseudoephedrine. The recipe is on the Internet, available to those who know where to look.

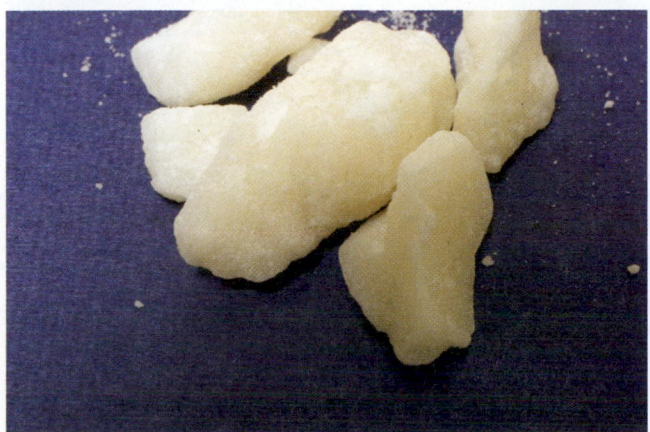

Meth (a.k.a. crack or ice) is one of the world's most addictive drugs.

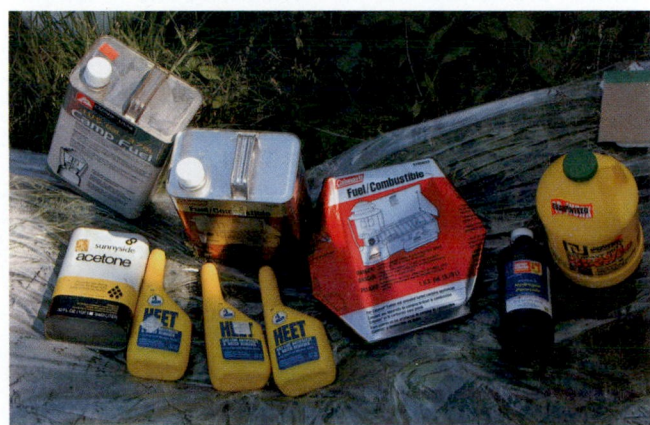

Common, easy-to-purchase chemicals are used to make meth. When meth is smoked, an ammonia-like residue is left that eats away the teeth at the gum line.

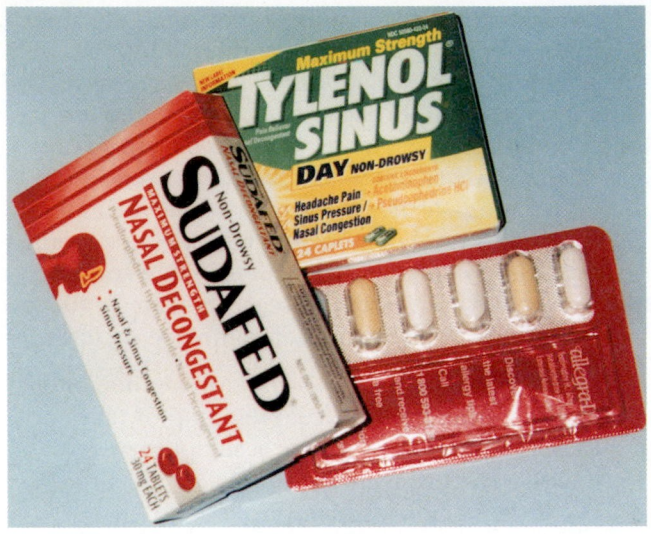

Many legal items, including cold and diet pills containing the key ingredient, ephedrine (or pseudoephedrine); lithium from rechargeable batteries; coffee filters; drain cleaners; lye; plastic tubing; and anhydrous ammonia, are used to produce methamphetamine illegally in home labs.

A new method of making meth, called "shake and bake," has contributed to a recent spike in the number of meth arrests. This cheaper, faster, and simpler method produces smaller batches using ingredients that can be carried in a backpack. Less pseudoephedrine is required for smaller batches, so the purchase of ingredients goes undetected. The whole process is done in 1- to 2-liter soda bottles. The chemicals are mixed and shaken, and this can be done even while driving. Every method of making meth is dangerous, but more extreme burns are occurring because in this process bottles are held by the drug maker. Lately, drug task force agents have noticed an increase in the use of instant cold ice packs (or dry ice packs) by meth producers. Meth "cooks" are buying the packs (which contain ammonia nitrate) to extract the ammonia needed for their recipes. Meth cooks are constantly adapting, making labs smaller and smarter and finding new recipes with common ingredients to produce meth.

Methamphetamine is dangerous, not only to the meth user but to society at large and to the environment. It is estimated that every pound of methamphetamine produced leaves behind 5 to 7 pounds of toxic waste.

MDMA (ECSTASY)

The most popular club drug is **MDMA (Ecstasy)** (3,4-methylenedioxymethamphetamine). It has enjoyed popularity because it combines the "rush," or stimulating effects, of cocaine with the hallucinogenic qualities of psychedelics.

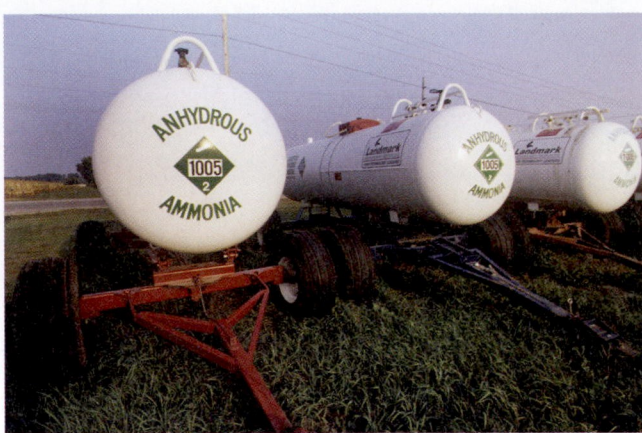

"Meth cookers" sometimes get anhydrous ammonia, a liquid agricultural fertilizer, by siphoning it from farm and co-op tanks.

MDMA is taken orally in tablet or capsule form. The user begins to feel the effects within 1 hour of ingestion. The effects may last up to 6 hours, depending on the dose, the purity, and the environment in which it is taken. Some users take multiple doses in order to prolong the effect, sometimes consuming as many as 10 tablets in a single night.

Many problems that users encounter with MDMA are similar to those found with the use of amphetamines and cocaine. The main physiological problems with Ecstasy use are

✓ Use can result in heart failure or heat stroke because it greatly increases blood pressure and heart rate. Body temperature can increase to 109 degrees if it is taken at a club or rave where there is physical exertion.

✓ Dehydration among novice users who don't drink enough water and dance themselves into

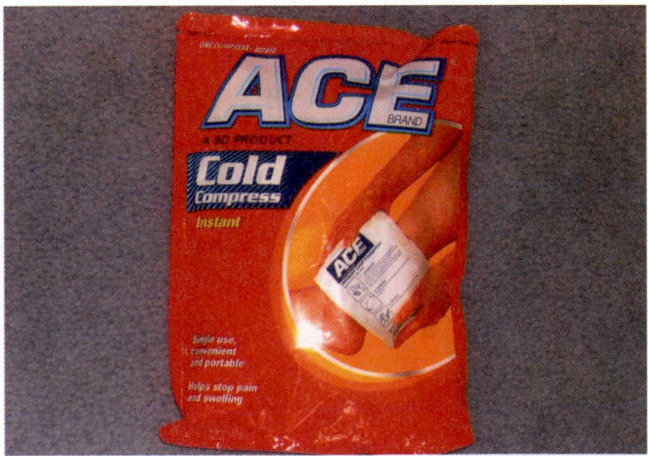

A new recipe has hit the meth scene. "Cooks" are extracting ammonia from instant cold ice packs for the "shake and bake" method. The packets can be easily purchased at Walmart, Target, or any drug store.

severe dehydration and overexertion. Rave promoters often provide bottled water and sports drinks to manage hyperthermia and dehydration; pacifiers to prevent involuntary teeth clenching; and menthol nasal inhalers, chemical lights, neon glow sticks, necklaces, and bracelets to enhance the effects of MDMA.

Narcotics or Opiates

Narcotics are powerful painkillers. The narcotic analgesics, often referred to as opioids, also produce pleasurable feelings (euphoria), induce sleep, and depress breathing. This category includes heroin.

HEROIN

Heroin is a psychoactive drug that depresses the CNS. It is the most abused and the most rapidly acting of the opiates.

Users are seldom aware of precisely what they are buying on the street from pushers. It may be mixed or cut with substances such as powdered milk, sugar, starch, quinine, and even strychnine and arsenic. A cheaper and more potent form of heroin, originating in Mexico and known as "black tar" or "tootsie roll," is being widely used in the United States.

A sign of increased purity is the increasing rate of fatal overdoses. Some pushers, to be more competitive, are offering superpure heroin (90 percent pure) to users. This too-potent heroin is known as "Poison," "People's Choice," "China Cat," and "Red Sun" and has been linked to a string of overdose deaths.

Any drug-abusing lifestyle may depress the strength of the immune system and the body's ability to withstand infection. Using needles to inject any drug may also increase the risk of infections and diseases (e.g., HIV/AIDS and hepatitis B and C from sharing or using unsterile equipment).

Psychedelics

Psychedelic drugs are known as mind-expanders or hallucinogens. These drugs affect an individual's perception, awareness, and emotions and can also cause *hallucinations*, completely groundless false perceptions. They can also cause *illusions,* misinterpretations of reality or something imagined. This category includes LSD and psilocybin and psilocyn (mushrooms).

LSD

LSD (lysergic acid diethylamide) is a dangerous and unpredictable hallucinogenic drug. It is a liquid drug, usually dropped onto paper or pills and sold as individual hits. LSD is the most available and popular hallucinogen in the United States. It induces hallucinations more powerful than those of any other drug, adding to its appeal among those at raves and dance clubs seeking enhanced auditory and visual experiences.

Users refer to their experience with LSD as a *trip* and to acute adverse reactions as a *bad trip*. Some fatal accidents and suicides have occurred during states of LSD intoxication because of the user's highly suggestive state and feelings of invulnerability. Examples of this include users walking out in front of fast-moving automobiles and jumping out of high windows.

Many LSD users experience **flashbacks,** a recurrence of certain aspects of a person's drug experience without the user having repeated use of the drug. A flashback occurs suddenly, often without warning, and may occur within a few days or well over a year after LSD use.

"MUSHROOMS" (PSILOCYBIN AND PSILOCYN)

A **mushroom** is the street name for psilocybin and psilocyn, two drugs classified chemically as tryptamines. Both drugs are obtained from certain mushrooms that are indigenous to tropical and subtropical regions of South America, Mexico, and the United States.

Psilocybin mushrooms are popular at raves and clubs, and increasingly on college campuses. They are ingested orally, brewed as a tea, or added to other foods (or coated with chocolate) to mask their bitter flavor. In addition to the risks associated with ingestion of psilocybin, individuals also risk poisoning if one of the many varieties of poisonous mushrooms is incorrectly identified as a psilocybin mushroom.

Inhalants

Inhalants, like marijuana, are considered a step-up drug. Young people start with inhalants, get hooked, and move on to more powerful drugs. The abuse of inhalants is called **huffing. Inhalants** are volatile nondrug substances (often ordinary household products) that have druglike effects when inhaled. A few of these substances have some medical uses, specifically, amyl nitrite and nitrous oxide. Inhalants are a diverse group of breathable chemicals that produce mind-altering vapors.

Inhalants are classified into three major groups, all potentially hazardous to users. See Table 14-14.

Be alert to obvious signs of inhalant abuse:

✓ Slow, thick, slurred speech; disorientation; general drunken appearance
✓ Complaints of headaches

✓ Signs of paint or other products where they would not normally be (face, fingers)
✓ Chemical odors on breath, clothing, or rags
✓ Rapid disappearance of household aerosol or cleaning products
✓ Red or runny eyes or nose (can have nosebleeds)
✓ Spots and/or sores around the mouth
✓ Nausea and/or loss of appetite
✓ Stockpiling cases of computer cleaner, or using up cans of air freshener rapidly

◆ OVER-THE-COUNTER AND PRESCRIPTION DRUGS

Legal drugs are often subdivided into over-the-counter drugs (OTCs) and prescription drugs. More than 300,000 OTCs are available in the United States. Aspirin is the most common OTC, but most cold medicines, cough syrups, and laxatives also fall into this category. OTCs are not addictive if used correctly, and they must have clear warnings and instructions printed on their labels for consumer use and protection. Still, there is a difference between *safe* and *harmless*. OTCs can do damage if used incorrectly, and some can lead to physical dependence if overused.

Five common kinds of nonprescription drugs are especially likely to produce adverse side effects or dependence:

1. *Nasal sprays*. After several days' use, these can produce a "rebound" effect, making your nose more congested than ever. The rebound effect is the result of increased swelling of the nasal tissues. If you use a spray, limit use to 1 or 2 days.
2. *Laxatives*. The most habit-forming laxatives are the so-called stimulants, which work by stimulating the walls of the intestines. A diet high in fruits, vegetables, and grains, plus 2 quarts of fluids a day, will almost always eliminate constipation. Laxatives should not be used to induce weight loss.
3. *Eyedrops*. These blood vessel constrictors will whiten bloodshot eyes, but like nasal sprays, they can produce a rebound effect.
4. *Alcohol/codeine cough syrups*. Codeine, a narcotic, works directly on the part of the brain that controls coughing. In many drugstores, you can obtain codeine-containing cough suppressants by signing at the cash register. Some of these medications contain substantial amounts of alcohol, dangerous for anyone with an alcohol problem.
5. *Stimulants such as herbal energizers, food supplements, fatigue reducers, antihistamines, cold medications, asthma relievers, and diet and exercise aids*. Caffeine, ephedrine, pseudoephedrine, and phenylpropanolamine (PPA) are the most common types of stimulants used in these drugs.

Pseudoephedrine, a drug used to treat nasal and sinus congestion, although not requiring a prescription, now by law must be kept behind the counter. Those who need the medicine must show photo I.D. and may purchase only a limited supply. This is because pseudoephedrine is a key ingredient used to make methamphetamine.

Drugs in this group can cause an increase in physical tolerance with repeated use. Physical tolerance and prolonged use will be followed by withdrawal symptoms upon cessation of use. For additional information see the ephedrine and methamphetamine sections in this chapter.

Phenylpropanolamine (PPA) has been found to increase the risk of hemorrhagic stroke. The Food and Drug Administration is taking steps to remove PPA from all drug products and recommends that consumers not use any products that contain PPA.

OTC stimulants, frequently sold at convenience stores and truck stops or even out-of-the-home businesses, are advertised using descriptions such as "herbal," "natural," "performance enhancing," and "nutritional supplement." This gives the impression that they are healthful and harmless substances. However, most of these products contain powerful stimulants such as ephedrine and megadoses of caffeine and have dangerous side effects if used excessively or improperly.

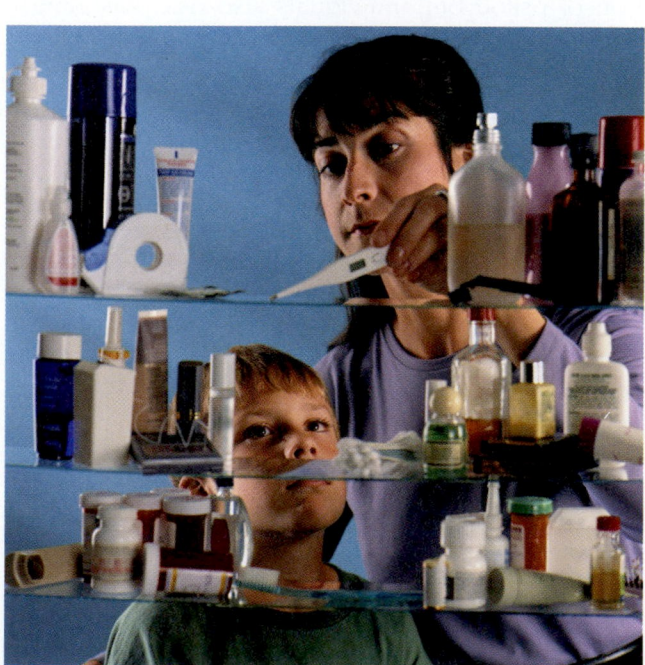

Over-the-counter drugs should be used with caution.

Most prescription drugs are put to good use (for example, antibiotics used for treating infection), but many are abused. Prescription drugs that are sometimes abused include amphetamines, barbiturates, narcotics, and tranquilizers. These drugs are used for a wide range of purposes, such as to stimulate and/or depress the CNS, overcome fatigue, suppress hunger, induce sleep, deaden the senses, relieve pain, and control anxiety.

There seems to be a pill for every need. Unfortunately, once prescribed, drugs are often taken in amounts and combinations not anticipated by the prescribing physician. Some physicians prescribe drugs more readily than do others, and some fail to stress the importance of reading labels carefully and taking drugs only as directed. Drugs prescribed to diminish physical or mental anguish are sometimes used for social purposes, leading to drug abuse.

Synergistic reaction, a major problem with drug use, is a phenomenon that occurs when drugs are taken in combination, where the cumulative effect is greater than the effects of the drugs when taken separately. This results in an exaggerated drug effect or a prolonged drug reaction. Used alone, alcohol and tobacco are linked to oral cancer. Used together, the risk escalates. The same is true for alcohol and oral contraceptives in connection to an increased risk of stroke and coronary heart disease. The combined effects of OTC stimulants and caffeine can be fatal.

Ephedrine

Ephedrine is an amphetamine-like drug extracted from an Asian herb called **ephedra.** It is also known as *ma huang* and is commonly found in OTC herbal supplements. It is used in an array of products sold as weight-loss aids, asthma products, energy boosters, and body-building aids. Ephedrine can be especially dangerous for people with hypertension or other cardiovascular disease. It should not be taken by persons who have anxiety disorders (panic attacks), glaucoma, thyroid disease, or diabetes. The drug's side effects (even in healthy people) include raised blood pressure, irregularities in heart rate, insomnia, tremors and headaches, seizures, heart attacks, strokes, and death. It can also have effects similar to bipolar disorder. In supplements, it is commonly combined with caffeine (or other stimulating herbs such as guarana), which may compound its effects and can cause blood vessel constriction, a rapid heart rate, and a sudden rise in blood pressure. The drug is best avoided altogether, and this combination should never be used. The main danger, experts say, is associated with heat stroke that results from increased heart rate and blood pressure. Despite this it remains available without prescription in many products. In 2004 the FDA banned the herb due to links to heart attacks, strokes, seizures, and death. This ban came too late to prevent the high-profile heat stroke death of the Baltimore Orioles' 23-year-old pitcher Steve Bechler. Bechler was taking the supplement to lose weight during spring training when he collapsed on February 16, 2003. He died the next day after his temperature rose to 108 degrees.

It is available in capsule, drink, and chewing gum forms and is sold in nutrition stores, gyms, supermarkets, service stations, and on the Internet. Products that contain ephedrine may or may not list it on their label. Products with any of the following contain ephedrine:

- ✓ ma huang
- ✓ ephedra sinica
- ✓ sida cordifolia
- ✓ pinellia

℞ PRESCRIPTION FOR ACTION

You've read the chapter. Now go do one or more of these:

✓ Count how many bars/clubs are within 1 mile of campus.

✓ Find out how many calories and nutrients are in a 12-ounce can of beer, in a margarita, in a wine cooler, and/or in other popular alcoholic drinks.

✓ List the OTC (over-the-counter) drugs you take in 1 week.

✓ List the prescription drugs you take in a week.

✓ Investigate where you can get help to stop smoking (or where you can send a friend who smokes).

✓ Check to see if alcoholic drink specials (and bars) are advertised on your campus newspaper. What percentage of students at your college are 21 or older?

✓ Find out if alcoholic beverage companies sponsor athletic events or help fund buildings on your campus. Which companies?

✓ Have you been affected by someone's alcohol/drug use? How? (e.g., interrupted sleep, disrupted study time, physical harm.) Find out where can you report drug/alcohol problems.

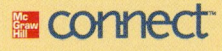 **connect**

Go online to Connect to complete this activity.
http://connect.mcgraw-hill.com

Frequently Asked Questions

Q.   Is Spice, or K₂, safe to use?

A.   No. Spice is a slang term used to describe a host of dried herbal products that are sprayed with chemicals and when used mimics the high of marijuana. K_2 is synthetic marijuana and cannot be detected in most drug screens. It is marketed as incense (or "aromatherapy") and "not for human consumption," but most users buy the product and smoke it in pipes, joints, or bongs like pot. Some users report elevated heart rates, anxiety, panic attacks, and shortness of breath.

Q.   Are smokeless e-cigarettes safe?

A.   Electronic cigarettes (cigars and pipes), while becoming quite popular, *are not safe.* They look like ordinary smokes, but there is no burning and no secondhand smoke. They produce a nicotine infused mist that is absorbed directly into the lungs. The cigarette is actually a battery-powered cartridge in which the nicotine is dissolved. According to the National Institutes of Health, regular cigarettes contain about 10 milligrams of nicotine and e-cigarettes contain 16 milligrams.

Q.   Is marijuana legal for certain medical conditions?

A.   No. The U.S. Supreme Court ruled marijuana use for medicinal purposes to be illegal. This ruling allows the federal government to prosecute individuals for the manufacture and distribution of marijuana even though some state laws have allowed its use.

Proponents of medical marijuana argue that it can treat the following conditions:

- Nausea resulting from cancer treatment
- Appetite loss in persons with AIDS
- Pain resulting from the spread of cancer and migraine headaches
- Spasticity resulting from multiple sclerosis, epilepsy, and spinal cord injury
- Eye pressure and pain resulting from glaucoma

However, the medical marijuana business is booming in the states that have legalized the drug. The Federal government can prosecute users in the states where it is legal and employers are not obligated to accommodate use the use of medical marijuana even outside of work in the these states.

Q.   During final exams my roommate used Ritalin as a "study aid" to stay awake and study for final exams. Is this a safe drug?

A.   No. The abuse of Ritalin (and Adderall), an ADHD drug, on college campuses is rising. About one in every five college students has used the drug illegally. Students take Ritalin and Adderall to increase concentration during late-night study sessions, to snort it for a cocaine-like high, or to suppress their appetites. Illegally taking these drugs can result in serious side effects such as revving up the cardiovascular system (increased heart and respiratory rates, nervousness), insomnia, loss of appetite, headaches, dilated pupils, dry mouth, and feelings of superiority. Abusing the drugs at higher doses can result in tremors, convulsions, paranoia, and death. Health risks are increased when Ritalin is snorted. Although these drugs are not physically addictive, students tend to begin to believe they need them.

Q.   I saw a warning about "extreme Ecstasy" on the 6:00 news. What is it?

A.   It is a new turbo-charged form of Ecstasy that is mixed with methamphetamine. The combination of the two drugs could easily lead to overdoses and death, much like the wave of similar fatalities from heroin laced with fentanyl. It is produced in Canada and illegally crosses the border into the United States. Fifty-five percent of Ecstasy samples seized in the United States in 2007 contained methamphetamine. Dealers are aggressively targeting young people.

Q.   True or False: Smoking one joint is the same as smoking one cigarette.

A.   False. Smoking one joint is the same as smoking five cigarettes—smoking four joints is the same as smoking one entire pack. Because marijuana smokers tend to take longer, deeper drags and hold smoke in their lungs longer, they end up with three to five times the tar and carbon monoxide in their bodies. Plus, marijuana is smoked unfiltered (in joints, blunts, and pipes) and burns at a higher temperature, which is more damaging to the lungs.

Q.   What is the definition of "risk reduction" or "harm reduction"? What does it involve?

A.   The simplest definition: A lower-risk drinker does not harm anyone including himself or herself. Also, a lower-risk drinker limits the amount of alcohol consumed in order to maintain sound judgment. This involves six steps:

1. Deciding why you want to reduce your risk. Some possible motivations are
   - To avoid acting stupid.
   - Family history of alcohol problems (your chances of having problems are three to four times greater than those of people without a family history).
   - Commitment to a healthy lifestyle.
   - Cost—alcohol is expensive.
   - Excessive drinking can be a roadblock to achieving life goals.
2. Deciding what your limits are: The more you consume, the more your judgment is impaired. Remember, your body can process only one drink per hour!

3. Determining what places you at risk for exceeding your limits:
   - Emotions—if you are angry/anxious, you may drink too much.
   - Environments—certain places or people may lead you to drink too much.
   - Events—recent problems/losses/stressors contribute to overdrinking.
   - Activities—drinking games/chugging/keg parties are associated with overdrinking.
4. Developing strategies for every risk situation in Step 3:
   - Drink only if YOU want to.
   - Drink only as much as YOU want to.
   - Drink only the type of drink YOU want to.
   - Do not drink if YOU feel negative emotions or the urge to "get drunk."
   - Be assertive—YOU can say no and not be rejected.
5. Evaluating and improving on your strategies: If you make a mistake and act irresponsibly, consider it a learning experience. Explore why it happened and change your strategies accordingly.
6. Rewarding yourself for making responsible choices: Buy fun stuff with some of the money you save.

Q. Are the nicotine replacement products as bad as smoking cigarettes?

A. No, they do not have all the tars and poisonous gases found in cigarettes. Furthermore, they provide less nicotine than a smoker gets from cigarettes. These products should not be used by pregnant or nursing women. People with other medical conditions should check with their doctor before using a nicotine replacement product. Most important is that smokers quit completely before starting to use these products.

Q. Cigars are so popular now. Are they safe?

A. No! Cigars, and pipes too, may be considered more glamorous and acceptable than cigarettes, but they still kill. Research reveals that cigar smokers are twice as likely as nonsmokers to get cancer of the mouth, throat, and lung. They also run about one and a half times the risk of all smoking-related cancers and are more likely to develop heart disease or chronic obstructive pulmonary disease. The rates for cigar and pipe smokers are lower than those among people who smoke cigarettes only because those smokers consume less tobacco on average, not because cigar and pipe tobacco is less harmful. Flavored cigars are deadly too!

Q. Are the nearly nicotine-free cigarettes safe?

A. No. The nicotine level may be low, but the danger remains high. These cigarettes still contain everything that is bad in tobacco. Four thousand potentially toxic compounds, including chemicals that cause cancer and damage the cardiovascular system, are still present.

Q. Are "bidis" and clove cigarettes safer than regular cigarettes?

A. No. Bidis are thin, flavored, unfiltered tobacco cigarettes from India. They are popular because they are cheaper, come in attractive flavors (chocolate, strawberry, licorice, and grape), and are perceived as safer and more natural than cigarettes. Actually, they release more nicotine and other toxic chemicals than do ordinary smokes. Clove cigarettes also are no safer than regular cigarettes despite the claims. Known as kreteks and imported chiefly from Indonesia, they are about 60 percent tobacco and 40 percent ground cloves. Some have filters; some do not. Clove smoke adds its own harmful substances to tobacco smoke, and these cigarettes deliver more tar than regular cigarettes do.

Q. Is there a connection between high school binge drinking and college binge drinking?

A. Yes. Very few high school binge drinkers stop binge drinking in college. More than half of all college binge drinkers first binged in high school. However, many students who did not binge in high school begin binge drinking in college. Some aspects of the college environment may promote binge drinking. Colleges should develop strategies to prevent this . . . some are doing so.

Q. I am worried about my brother's drinking. Other family members are concerned too. How can I tell if he is becoming an alcoholic?

A. Take the quiz in Table 14-12, "Do You Have a Drinking Problem?" for your brother. Also, the presence of even one of the seven risk factors listed on page 487 is suggestive of an increased risk of alcoholism.

   If you answered "yes" to several of the questions for your brother on the quiz or checked off even one of the risk factors for alcoholism, it is time to seek professional help for your brother. Call the Federal Center For Substance Abuse Treatment for information about local treatment. (800-662-4357). Good luck.

Q. What causes hangovers, and can anything help ease or prevent them?

A. A hangover is a combination of alcohol withdrawal, sleep deprivation, dehydration, and nervous shock (nerves are in a hypersensitive state). The best remedies are the time-tested ones: drink lots of fluids (nonalcoholic), sleep it off (expose the nervous system to as little stimulation as possible), and take nonsteroid anti-inflammatory drugs (aspirin or ibuprofen).

   The amount needed to trigger a hangover depends partly on how much you're used to drinking. As little as one or two drinks, for example, can leave some people feeling wiped out if they seldom drink. Do not to drink on an empty stomach or when you're worn out from exercise or lack of sleep.

Q. Ephedra-free weight-loss aids are flooding the market. Are they any safer?

A. No. Some of the most hyped diet pills have basically replaced ephedra with another traditional Chinese remedy, citrus aurantium. It is called bitter orange and is derived from Seville oranges. This extract contains synephrine, a member of the amphetamine family. Some call it "ephedra's little brother." Bitter orange is commonly combined in a cocktail of ingredients that may intensify its effects. Hundreds of different ingredients are combined in dietary supplements, and little research on how they all interact has been done. If you are sensitive to caffeine or have signs of high blood pressure, you should avoid bitter orange until more studies have been done.

Q. Is it true that OxyContin abuse is increasing? Is it associated with heroin use?

A. Yes and yes. OxyContin, a time-release tablet, is a trade name product for the generic narcotic oxycodone hydrochloride, an opiate agonist. OxyContin, sometimes referred to as "poor man's heroin" or "hillbilly heroin," is a high-powered prescription painkiller and is often prescribed to cancer and surgery patients and those with injuries, arthritis, and lower back conditions. The drug is popular among abusers because of its heroin-like effects. OxyContin tablets can be ingested several ways: by chewing, by crushing them and then snorting the powder, or by dissolving them in water and injecting the solution. When OxyContin is not taken in tablet form, the controlled-release is cancelled and the user has a high risk of receiving a lethal dose due to the drug being released immediately into one's system. As initiatives to curb the abuse of OxyContin are implemented, abusers of the drug may begin to use other oxycodones, such as Percocet and Percodan. Abusers may also begin to use heroin, especially if it continues to be readily available, pure, and relatively inexpensive.

Summary

The wellness journey does not include substance abuse. Before drinking alcohol, smoking, or using other drugs, consider what these substances do to you. Your mind and body are capable of handling stress and emotional and physical pain without the help of drugs. You can feel happy, sexy, sad, angry, and joyous and experience love without artificial chemicals to enhance your feelings or help you cope with life's challenges. The fact is, these substances magnify your problems. The single biggest killer of young adults is not heart disease, stroke, or cancer. It is accidents. Over half of all fatal accidents are alcohol- or drug-related. Use of many substances leads to tolerance or addiction as well as health problems. No other drug, not even alcohol, comes close to nicotine in terms of deaths, illness, and other economic costs, such as fires.

Before using any substance, whether over the counter, illegal, or prescribed, remember that you have choices. What you do now will affect your future. Be responsible and choose wisely.

Terms

- addiction
- alcohol
- alcoholism
- amotivational syndrome
- binge drinking
- blood alcohol concentration (BAC)
- club drugs
- cocaine
- crack
- crystal meth (ice)
- date rape drugs
- depressants
- drug
- ephedrine (ephedra)
- fetal alcohol syndrome (FAS)
- flashbacks
- heroin
- high-risk alcohol use
- huffing
- ice
- inhalants
- low-risk alcohol use
- LSD
- Marijuana
- MDMA (Ecstasy)
- methamphetamine
- mushrooms
- narcotics
- passive smoking
- positive norming
- psychedelic drugs
- psychoactive drug
- risk/harm reduction
- stimulants
- synergistic reaction
- tolerance

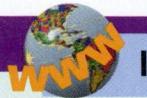 ## Internet Resources

Al-Anon/Alateen

www.al-anon.alateen.org

Provides information to family members of alcoholics and young people affected by alcoholism.

Alcoholics Anonymous

www.aa.org

Contains information about alcoholism and Alcoholics Anonymous programs.

American Lung Association Fact Sheet

www.lungusa.org

Contains information on the health risks of smoking.

CDC's Tobacco Information and Prevention Source Page

www.cdc.gov/tobacco

Contains surgeon general's reports, research, educational materials, and tips on how to quit smoking.

Club Drugs

www.clubdrugs.gov

Provides information and resources on treatment and prevention strategies.

Cocaine Anonymous

www.ca.org

Includes literature for cocaine addicts and contact information for CA support groups.

College Drinking: Changing the Culture

www.collegedrinkingprevention.gov

Provides links to alcohol policies at colleges across the country; an interactive diagram of the human body and how alcohol affects it.

Core Institute

www.siu.edu/~coreinst

Southern Illinois University's Core Institute is the leading research assessment and development organization for alcohol and drug prevention programs.

Debtors Anonymous

www.debtorsanonymous.org

Provides strategies for dealing with this addiction.

Facts on Tap

www.factsontap.org

Has the latest information on the college alcohol and drug scene, including links, quizzes, activities, and relationship tips.

Gam-Anon

www.gam-anon.org

Has information and support for young people with a gambling addiction.

Gamblers Anonymous

www.gamblersanonymous.org

Provides information and support for gambling addiction.

MedlinePlus

www.nim.nih.gov/medlineplus

National Library of Medicine site with detailed information on all drugs.

Mothers Against Drunk Driving

www.madd.org

Provides news, statistics, and information on MADD's activities to stop drunk driving and underage drinking.

Narcotics Anonymous

www.na.org

Contains readings on drugs and addiction.

National Clearinghouse for Alcohol and Drug Information

www.health.org

Has information about alcohol and drugs.

National Council on Alcoholism and Drug Dependence

www.ncadd.org

Includes facts and advocacy information.

National Inhalant Prevention Coalition

www.inhalants.org

Provides information about inhalants.

National Institute on Alcohol Abuse and Alcoholism

www.drugabuse.gov

Government site focuses on research and education related to alcohol use and abuse; has FAQ section.

National Institute on Drug Abuse

www.nida.nih.gov

Provides information on drugs and drug abuse and statistics.

Overeaters Anonymous

www.oa.org

Includes information and help strategies.

Sexaholics and Sex Addicts Anonymous

www.sa.org

Contains information on this addiction. Both practice the basic principles of recovery found in "Twelve Steps and Twelve Traditions of Alcoholics Anonymous."

Street Drugs

www.streetdrugs.org

Contains topics, information, and reports on drugs and drug use.

U.S. Drug Enforcement Administration

www.dea.gov

Good resource and information on all drugs.

LAB Activity 14-1

Alcohol: High-Risk vs. Low-Risk

Directions: List as many pros and cons for high-risk and low-risk alcohol use as you can. Ask friends for their input. Read about high-risk and low-risk alcohol use in this chapter.

A. High-Risk Use	
Pro	Con
(Examples: I get to be with friends who drink; get to drink away my problems.)	(Examples: I won't get to go out with my friends; will have to find another group of friends; may have to study on Thursday through Saturday nights; need to find another way to unwind.)
•	•
•	•
•	•
•	•
•	•

B. Low-Risk Use	
Pro	Con
(Examples: I won't do something I'll regret the next morning; will save money, will avoid a hangover; do better in school/work.)	(Examples: I can still have a beer and not get drunk; may have to find new friends; may not feel at ease socially.)
•	•
•	•
•	•
•	•
•	•

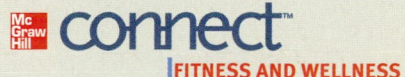

Mc Graw Hill **connect**
|FITNESS AND WELLNESS

http://connect.mcgraw-hill.com

Discussion

1. Was it harder to list the pros for high-risk use or low-risk use? _____ Why?

2. Was it harder to list the cons for high-risk use or low-risk use? _____ Why?

LAB Activity 14-2

Name _____ Class/Activity Section _____ Date _____

What Is the Alcohol Culture on Your Campus?

Directions: Answer or address the following questions to examine the alcohol culture on your campus.

1. Is your college known as a "party school"? Yes _____ No _____ Discuss why or why not.

2. If your college is a party school, do you know of any efforts of your campus to curb this reputation? Or of the community and/or local police? If so, describe.

3. Does your college have an alcohol awareness program? Yes _____ No _____ If so, describe.

4. How many bars/liquor stores are within a mile of campus? _____

5. Can off-campus bars and clubs advertise in the campus newspaper and bulletin boards? Yes _____ No _____ List and discuss.

6. Do you think advertisements can influence students' drinking behavior? Yes _____ No _____ How?

7. Are alcohol-free residence halls and living spaces available at your school? Yes _____ No _____

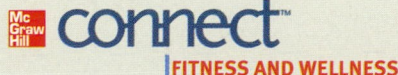

http://connect.mcgraw-hill.com

LAB Activity ■ CHAPTER 14

8. Are alcohol signs allowed in residence hall rooms and/or windows? Yes _____ No _____

9. Do you know of efforts to help students who have drinking problems? Or who are arrested for DUI or for underage drinking? Yes _____ No _____ Describe.

10. Is alcohol restricted at intercollegiate sporting events and at tailgate parties? Yes _____ No _____

11. Does your school provide social norming information? Yes _____ No _____

12. Does your school provide alcohol-free dances, social events, etc.? Describe.

13. Does your campus bookstore sell shot glasses, beer mugs with the school's crest or logo on them, or tee shirts/sweatshirts with references to drinking alcohol? Describe.

14. Does your school have alcohol restrictions/rules to deal with sporting event tailgate parties? What are they?

15. Is your school a "dry campus" (no alcohol allowed)? Yes _____ No _____ If so, do some students use alcohol on or near campus anyway? Yes _____ No _____ How do you feel about this situation?

LAB Activity 14-3

Name _____ Class/Activity Section _____ Date _____

Substance Abuse Values Clarification and Critical Thinking

1. Complete each of the following value clarification statements according to your feelings. Discuss each response in a few sentences:

   a. I view substance abuse as . . .

   b. The thought that alcohol, tobacco, and caffeine are drugs . . .

   c. If my sister continued to smoke while pregnant, I would . . .

   d. If my 16-year-old brother asked me to get him some beer, I would . . .

   e. If the police picked me up for driving while intoxicated, I would . . .

   f. The next time my roommate comes in drunk and disturbs my study time (or sleep), I'm going to . . .

   g. How serious is alcohol/substance abuse (on a scale of 1 to 5, with 5 being most serious)?
      • In the United States: _____
      • At this university: _____
      • In my residence hall (fraternity/sorority house, apartment): _____
      • In my home: _____
      • Defend your ratings. What substances are being abused; what can/should be done to curb the abuse?

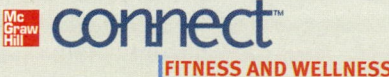

http://connect.mcgraw-hill.com

2. Discuss the pros and cons of each of the following statements:
    a. A mother should be charged with murder if she takes illegal drugs during pregnancy and her baby dies of addiction at birth.

    b. A nursing mother should be charged with child abuse if she drinks alcohol or uses illegal drugs.

    c. Any pregnant woman has a right to drink alcohol.

3. Almost 40 percent of top country songs feature references to drugs or alcohol; a whopping 70 percent of rap music and 14 percent of rock music contain drug or alcohol references in their titles and/or lyrics.
    Look over this list of songs that reference alcohol, drugs, or cigarettes in their titles or lyrics: "Gin and Juice" (Snoop Dogg), "I Wanna Get High" (Cypress Hill), "Cigarettes and Alcohol" (Oasis), "Rehab" (Amy Winehouse), "Whiskey River" (Willie Nelson), "Cocaine" (Eric Clapton), "Beer" (Reel Big Fish), "High Time" (Grateful Dead), "Heroin Girl" (Everclear), "Purple Haze" (Jimi Hendrix), "Beer Can" (Beck), "Now I Wanna Sniff Some Glue" (Ramones), "Let's Go Get Stoned" (Sublime).
    a. Is there a link between song content and behavior? Yes _____ No _____ Explain:

    b. Do references to drugs and alcohol reflect society's values? Yes _____ No _____ Explain:

    c. Do they reflect your values? Yes _____ No _____ Explain:

    d. Which substances (alcohol/drugs) are most often mentioned?

    e. Think about current music that depicts substance use. See examples above. Give three additional examples and name the substance mentioned:

        •

        •

        •

    f. How do music/videos/TV/movies influence the use of drugs in our society?

LAB Activity 14-4

Name _____ Class/Activity Section _____ Date _____

Alcohol/Substance Abuse Harm Reduction

Use the text (Chapter 14) to respond to the following 11 items:

1. Complete the "Do You Have a Drinking Problem?" self-assessment (Table 14-12). Are you concerned about or surprised at your score?

   Yes _____ No _____ Discuss:

2. While leaving a party, you see a girl passed out on the lawn. What should you do? List six actions you should take.

3. Use five factors that affect alcohol absorption to give a profile of the person who will get drunk fastest.

4. How does alcohol change people's behavior? Give five examples from your observations.

5. You want to plan a safe party. List five ways you can help those attempting to reduce their use of or abstain from using alcohol (or drugs).

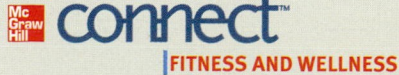

http://connect.mcgraw-hill.com

6. How can you reduce your risk of intoxication and/or alcoholism? List seven strategies.

7. What is "risk reduction" or "harm reduction"? Describe the six steps involved.

8. George can drink two six-packs before he feels drunk. Susan feels tipsy after two drinks. Should both be considered legally drunk at the same BAC? Discuss the reasons for your response.

9. Why do women get drunk faster then men?

10. Describe low-risk alcohol use. What is considered high-risk alcohol use?

11. Define binge drinking.

12. What is the BAC of someone who has consumed a potentially fatal overdose of alcohol? Approximately how many drinks would this be for a female/male? What are the signs of alcohol poisoning? What should you do if you suspect a friend has overdosed on alcohol?

LAB Activity 14-5

Tobacco Use Values Clarification and Critical Thinking

1. Tobacco companies spend thousands of dollars *an hour* to convince people that smoking is fun and exciting. List five ways they do this:

   a.

   b.

   c.

   d.

   e.

   How can you resist these tactics? How can you help others resist these tactics?

   a.

   b.

2. Young people should be angered by the overt efforts of tobacco industry advertising campaigns to entice them to use tobacco. Yes _____ No _____ Defend your response.

3. Recent tobacco advertising trends target women and young people. Have you noticed this trend?
   Yes _____ No _____
   a. How do the tobacco companies design cigarettes to appeal to the female consumer?

4. Discuss the pros and cons of each of the following statements. Label your *pro* and *con* remarks:
   a. The tobacco *industry* should be made to compensate the cost of physical damage of the smoker (i.e., pay for the health care/medical costs due to tobacco use).

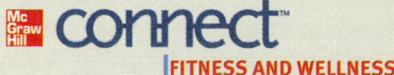

http://connect.mcgraw-hill.com

LAB Activity ■ CHAPTER 14

b. The tobacco *consumer* should be made to compensate the cost of physical damage of other smokers (i.e., pay for the health care/medical costs due to using tobacco).

c. Nonsmokers should help pay the health care costs (lung cancer treatments, bypass surgeries, etc.) of coworkers who smoke when both groups share group health insurance plans.

d. Insurance companies should drop the policies of people who smoke.

e. The age of 18 is the ideal age to be allowed to purchase tobacco products legally.

f. Tobacco farmers should continue to be subsidized by the federal government.

g. Congress should legislate tobacco to be an illegal drug, and its manufacture and use should be controlled by the FDA.

h. Secondhand smoke should be outlawed—no smoking inside any building.

i. No smoking inside any home.

j. Cigarette packages should require labeling such as "cigarettes kill," "cigarettes cause cancer," or "this product is addictive."

k. Businesses/companies have the right to fire and ban the hiring of workers who smoke—even in their own homes.

5. How much should a pack of cigarettes cost? _____ Why?

6. Complete the following statement:
   I won't smoke today because . . .

7. List the new tobacco/nicotine products that you have seen recently. Where have you seen them? What is your opinion of them?

LAB Activity 14-6

Addiction: Part of Your Lifestyle?

1. Assess your lifestyle for addictive behaviors that do not involve drugs (e.g., gambling, Table 14-3; shopping or spending, Table 14-4; overexercising, Chapter 7, Table 7-3; or maybe you are watching too much TV). Develop a plan to reduce these activities and create more balance in your life.

2. Which self-assessments did you use?

3. What was/were your score(s)? _____ _____ _____ What was your reaction to each?

4. What strategies can you initiate to reduce your involvement in these activities? List at least six strategies.

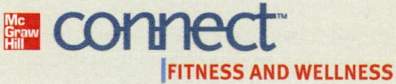

http://connect.mcgraw-hill.com

FITNESS AND WELLNESS

CHAPTER 15

Preventing Sexually Transmitted Disease

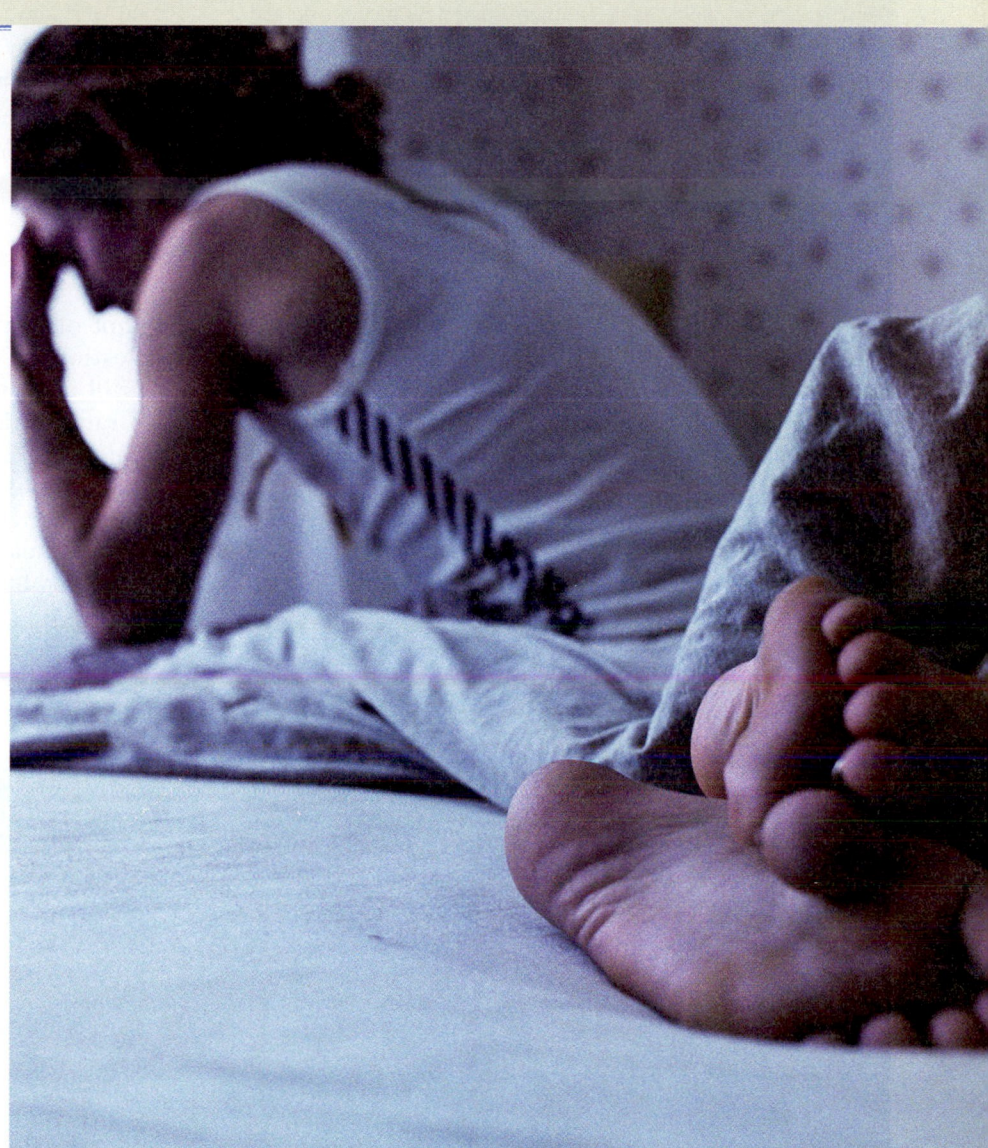

STUDY QUESTIONS

You will have successfully mastered this chapter if you can answer the following:

1. What are the symptoms of AIDS and the most common sexually transmitted diseases?
2. What are three curable and four incurable sexually transmitted diseases?
3. What are four ways HIV is transmitted?
4. What is the latency period for AIDS?
5. What are three high-risk and three low-risk sexual activities?
6. What are five ways to deter unwanted sexual pressure?
7. What are three actions you can take to decrease the risk of acquiring a sexually transmitted disease?

You will find the answers as you read this chapter.

" *You make your own luck.* "
—Unknown

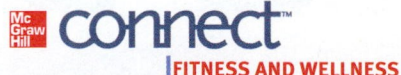
FITNESS AND WELLNESS

http://connect.mcgraw-hill.com

Diseases spread through sexual contact were once called *venereal diseases (VD)*, named for Venus, the Greek goddess of love, mother of Cupid. The terms sexually transmitted infection or **sexually transmitted disease (STD)** refer to diseases spread primarily through sexual intercourse but also through other intimate behavior; sex play; and, occasionally, nonsexually. Understanding their symptoms and how they are spread and treated are important steps in risk reduction.

Wellness implies taking responsibility for one's well-being and reducing health risks through personal behaviors. Unprotected sex can put you at risk for acquiring sexually transmitted diseases, some of which are incurable, even fatal. The risk of acquiring an STD, however, can be low to zero, depending on the behavioral choices you make. The purpose of this chapter is to increase your awareness of sexually transmitted diseases, how they are transmitted, their symptoms, and how to protect yourself through lower-risk activities that include abstinence, mutual monogamy, and barrier protection. You will also learn about coping with unwanted sexual pressure, recognizing and avoiding sexually risky situations, and dealing with the trauma of sexual assault. With this knowledge, you will be able to make informed choices to maintain high-level wellness by avoiding the risk of acquiring an STD with its physical, social, and emotional costs.

◆ SEXUALLY TRANSMITTED DISEASE

While **acquired immune deficiency syndrome (AIDS)** claims the spotlight as the most deadly and feared STD, we are experiencing a silent epidemic of other STDs in the United States. As a group, STDs are the number one communicable disease problem, but many people are unaware of this because of our cultural reluctance to discuss STDs and fear of public embarrassment. Only colds and flu, not officially reported, occur more frequently. It is estimated that one in two sexually active people will acquire an STD by age 24. Estimated annual rates of infection of the most common STDs are shown in Figure 15-1.

Changing mores appear to be a major factor in the increasing rate of STDs. Young people are becoming sexually active earlier yet marrying later, and divorce has become more common. As a result, people often have more sexual partners. Increasing

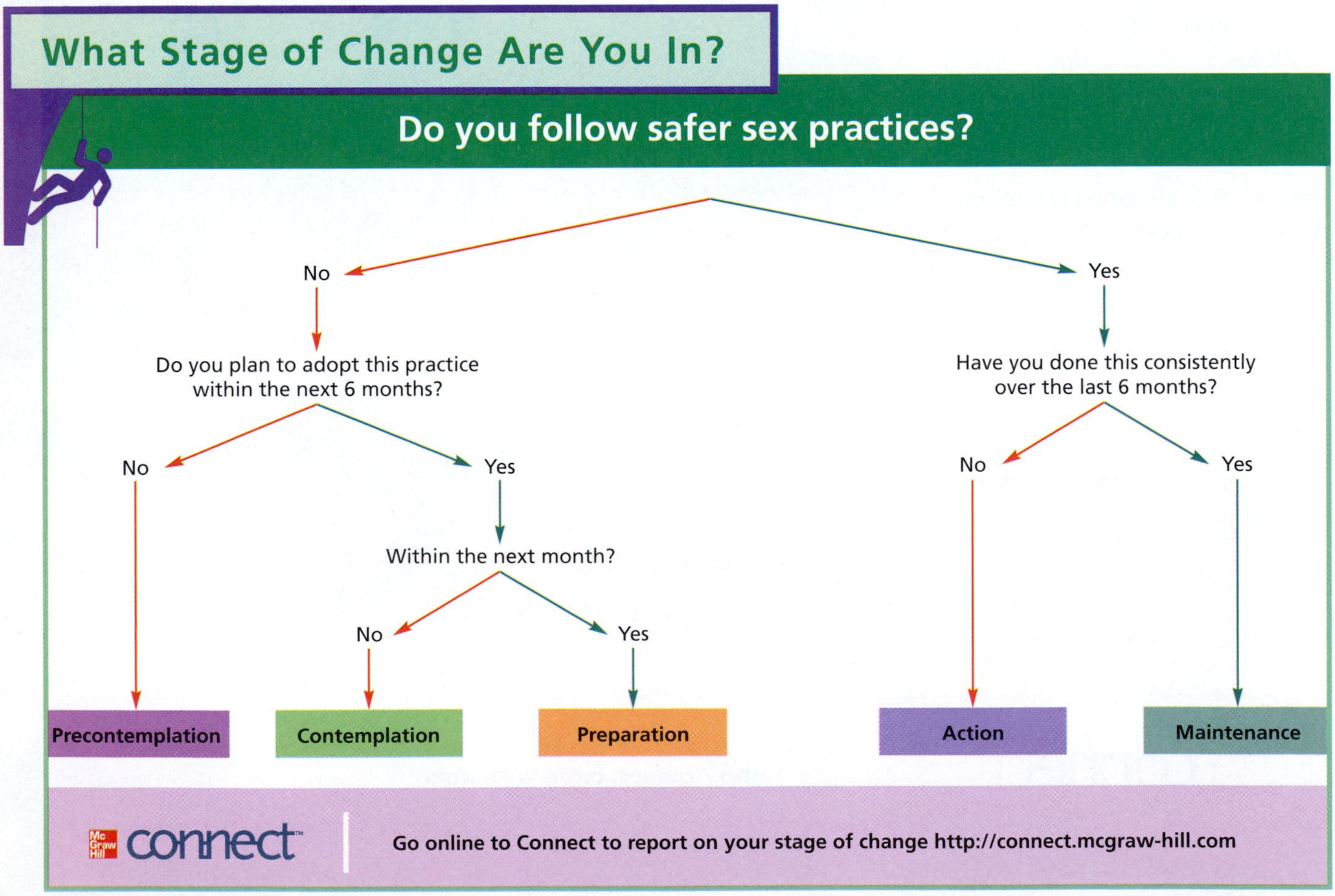

What Stage of Change Are You In?

Do you follow safer sex practices?

- No
  - Do you plan to adopt this practice within the next 6 months?
    - No → **Precontemplation**
    - Yes
      - Within the next month?
        - No → **Contemplation**
        - Yes → **Preparation**
- Yes
  - Have you done this consistently over the last 6 months?
    - No → **Action**
    - Yes → **Maintenance**

 connect™   Go online to Connect to report on your stage of change http://connect.mcgraw-hill.com

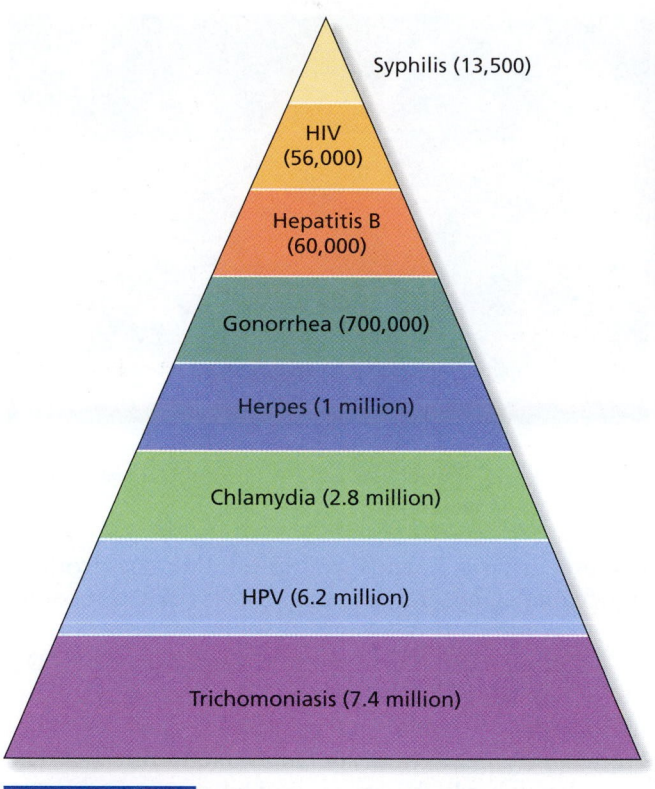

Syphilis (13,500)

HIV (56,000)

Hepatitis B (60,000)

Gonorrhea (700,000)

Herpes (1 million)

Chlamydia (2.8 million)

HPV (6.2 million)

Trichomoniasis (7.4 million)

FIGURE 15-1   **Estimated annual new cases of sexually transmitted diseases.**

SOURCE: Centers for Disease Control, National Center for HIV, STD, and TB Prevention www.cdc.gov/STD/Nov. 2009.

Tips for Behavior Change for Safer Sex

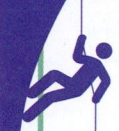

- Practice abstinence or mutual monogamy with an uninfected sexual partner.
- Do not mix drinking and sex. Even if you have a condom, you may be too drunk to put it on correctly.
- Use lower-risk sexual activities such as hugging, kissing, touching, and holding hands.
- Practice barrier protection; use latex condoms to prevent transmission of infection.
- If you are sexually active, have an STD check-up with every health exam, or every 6 months if you have more than one partner.

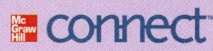 connect   Go online to Connect to complete this activity. http://connect.mcgraw-hill.com

rates of premarital sexual intercourse among young people offer more opportunity for the spread of disease. Involvement with alcohol, a concern on many college campuses, is tied to increased sexual activity and lack of commitment to one's sex partner, which increase STD risk. Another factor may be the development of the birth control pill, which resulted in decreasing use of the condom. With concern over AIDS, however, this is changing. Both male and female condoms not only prevent conception but serve as barriers to the transmission of STDs.

STDs affect people of all backgrounds and economic levels but are most common in people in their late teens to twenties: 90 percent of reported STDs occur among persons age 15 to 29. Nevertheless, your risk of acquiring an STD is determined by your behavior, not by your age or sexual orientation. Risk can be reduced or increased by personal choices that you control. If you choose to be sexually active, you are at risk. Your chances of exposure to an STD increase with multiple sexual partners and with increased frequency of sexual activity. The risk of infection is low to zero in a mutually monogamous relationship or if you abstain from sex. The benefits of preventing STDs are given in Table 15-1.

Unfortunately, many people, especially young people, believe that STDs aren't serious or that "STDs only happen to others," and they fail to take precautions. A person may think, "If I get one, I'll just go get it taken care of." Many college students misjudge the risks of their sexual behavior. They think they are at "extremely low risk" for STDs even though they were previously diagnosed with an STD, have had numerous sexual partners, and inconsistently use condoms. Some STDs are curable,

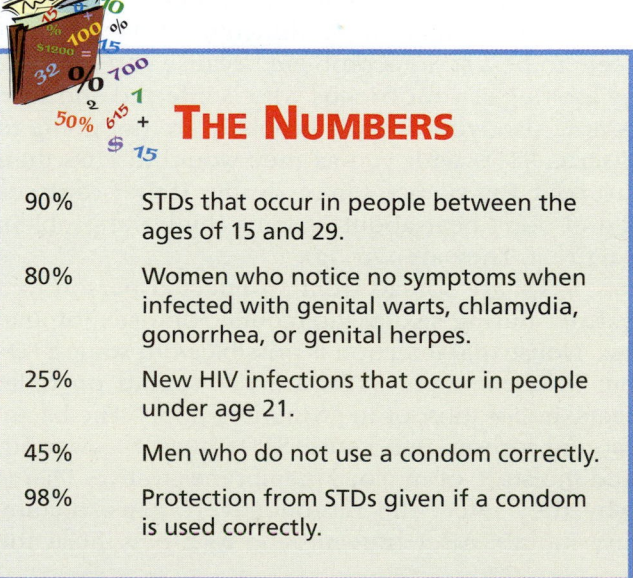

THE NUMBERS

90%	STDs that occur in people between the ages of 15 and 29.
80%	Women who notice no symptoms when infected with genital warts, chlamydia, gonorrhea, or genital herpes.
25%	New HIV infections that occur in people under age 21.
45%	Men who do not use a condom correctly.
98%	Protection from STDs given if a condom is used correctly.

TABLE 15-1 Benefits of Preventing STDs on Wellness Dimensions

Dimension	Benefits
Physical	• Protect your health by avoiding diseases—some of which are incurable • Enhanced appreciation for the wisdom of self-care and prevention
Emotional	• Peace of mind knowing you are protected from STDs • Avoid anxiety and distress of worrying you might have an STD or worrying about a flare-up
Social	• Enhances your relationship, knowing that an STD is one thing you will NOT share • Shows caring to protect yourself and your partner
Intellectual	• Knowledge of how STDs are spread enables you to use preventive measures
Occupational	• Decreased absenteeism—no need to miss work due to STD-related illness or treatments • Decreased medical care costs and days of disability
Spiritual	• Experience the satisfaction of living in accordance with your values and sharing *them* with your partner
Environmental	• You are making the world a better, safer place to live now and for future generations by preventing the spread of STDs

but some are not. Even some of the traditionally curable STDs are becoming antibiotic resistant, making treatment more difficult. STDs may not seem to be a serious problem because you can't tell by looking at your friends who is infected and who is not. Also, your friends probably are not going to discuss STDs with you as they would discuss their last cold. But silence can be deadly. If they can't see it and don't hear about it, some think the problem isn't real. They are wrong.

STDs are spread from an infected person to a partner during sexual intercourse, oral sex, or anal sex. Nonsexual infection is possible with some STDs but is uncommon. STDs are not spread on toilet seats, in hot tubs, or in swimming pools. The bacteria and viruses that cause STDs need the warmth and moisture of mucous membranes to live. That is why they infect the reproductive organs, rectum, and mouth. After transmission to a new host, the

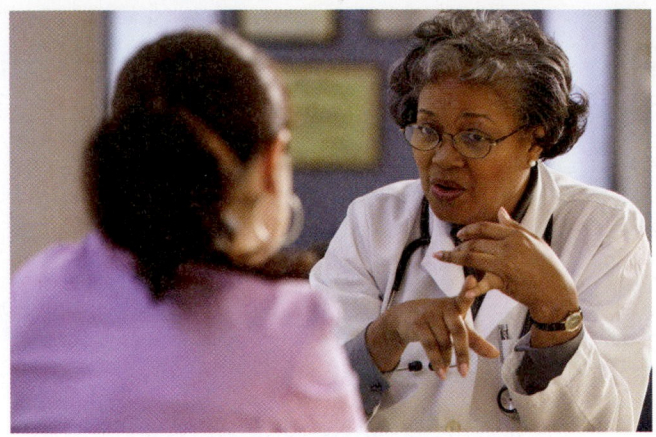

If you think you might have an STD, abstain from sex and see a doctor immediately.

bacteria or virus quickly multiplies and may produce noticeable symptoms in 2 days to 4 weeks, but sometimes an infected person notices no symptoms.

Women are particularly vulnerable to STDs, including AIDS, because they have more mucous membranes in their genital tissue than men do. Vaginal and cervical tissue can sustain microscopic tears through which viruses, and bacteria, often transmitted by semen, can enter. In addition, women experience early warning signs of STDs much less frequently than men do, resulting in more advanced disease before treatment is sought. STDs are serious and, if left untreated, can cause permanent damage.

If you are sexually active, it is important to get a yearly screening for STDs. Early diagnosis and treatment may prevent serious physical harm and prevent spread of the disease to other sexual partners. Symptoms of STDs vary with the type of infection and may differ between males and females. Be aware of the warning signs that may indicate the presence of an STD (Table 15-2).

TABLE 15-2 Symptoms of Sexually Transmitted Disease

Women	Women and Man
• Pelvic pain • Bleeding from the vagina between periods • Burning or itching around the vagina • Pain deep inside the vagina during sexual intercourse	• Abnormal discharge from the penis or vagina • A burning sensation during urination or bowel movements • Sores, bumps, or blisters near the mouth, rectum, or genitals • Flulike feelings with fever, chills, or aches • Redness and swelling in the throat • Swelling in the groin

If you notice a symptom, see your doctor!

TABLE 15-3	Curable and Incurable STDs
Bacterial (Curable)	**Viral (Incurable)**
• Chlamydia • Gonorrhea • Syphilis	• Genital herpes • Genital warts • Hepatitis B • AIDS

Diagnosis and treatment of STDs are confidential. *Contact the STD clinic of your local county health department or see a doctor immediately if you suspect that you may have an STD.* Your local family planning clinic can also give information on where to go for help, or you can call one of the hotlines at the end of this chapter. Wherever you are treated, your case will be kept private.

There are over 25 known STDs, some of which are incurable. Most STDs are either bacterial or viral. The most common bacterial STDs, which are treatable, are chlamydia, gonorrhea, and syphilis. Viral STDs, which are incurable, include genital herpes, genital warts, hepatitis B, and AIDS (Table 15-3). A person can have more than one STD at a time. Although less prevalent than other STDs, AIDS is causing much concern because it is not only incurable but fatal. *Common STDs, their symptoms, and their treatments are discussed in alphabetical order* and are summarized in Table 15-4.

TABLE 15-4	Common STDs, Symptoms, and Treatments	
STD	**Symptoms**	**Treatment**
AIDS	HIV: flulike or no symptoms AIDS: night sweats, pneumonia, fatigue, swollen lymph nodes, frequent infections, other symptoms of immunodeficiency	Antiviral medications to treat symptoms; there is no cure
Bacterial vaginosis	Itching, foul-smelling vaginal discharge	Antibiotics
Chancroid	Soft, painful sore on genitals	Antibiotics
Chlamydia	Vaginal or penile discharge, pain or burning during urination; women may be asymptomatic	Antibiotics
Genital herpes	Painful genital blisters that break open and scab over; may be internal or asymptomatic	Antiviral medications to treat symptoms; there is no cure
Gonorrhea	Vaginal or penile discharge, pain or burning during urination; women may be asymptomatic	Antibiotics
Hepatitis B	Fatigue, jaundice, nausea, loss of appetite, dark or brownish urine, abdominal pain	Vaccine before infection and antiviral medication after infection; there is no cure
HPV	Genital warts, cervical cancer, or no symptoms Increased risk of penile cancer in men Body may clear infection over time	Warts may be frozen, burned off, cut off, or treated with medication. Cancer treated with surgery, radiation, and/or chemotherapy
Pubic lice	Intense itching in pubic area, nits on pub hairs	Insecticidal shampoo
Scabies	Intense itching in pubic area	Insecticidal shampoo
Syphilis	A chancre (painless sore) on area of contact, usually within 3 weeks; later, if untreated, flulike symptoms and a rash	Antibiotics
Trichomonas	Itching, foul-smelling discharge in women; men asymptomatic	Antibiotics

◆ ACQUIRED IMMUNE DEFICIENCY SYNDROME (AIDS) AND HIV

AIDS is a threat to everyone, heterosexual and homosexual. Since AIDS first appeared in 1981, over 1 million cases have been reported and more than half a million people have died after developing AIDS. Around two-thirds of these people did not live to the age of 45. AIDS remains a leading cause of death in young people age 25 to 44. While AIDS cases have dropped among gay and bisexual men, they have increased among women, children, teens, heterosexuals, African Americans, and Hispanics. See Figure 15-2 for the estimated rates of new HIV infections by race/ethnicity in the United States reported by the CDC. One in four new HIV infections in the United States occurs in people under age 21. Teens and young adults are particularly vulnerable to AIDS because they take risks when they may not appreciate the risks—of sex or drug use, for example.

What Is AIDS? What Is HIV?

AIDS is a syndrome or group of symptoms caused by the **human immunodeficiency virus (HIV).** The virus is not alive but is an infectious agent. It does not kill a person directly but attacks a particular type of **lymphocytes** (white blood cells) called **T-cells.** Lymphocytes control cell growth, transport nutrients to cells, and produce antibodies that protect the body against infection. They travel under their own power throughout the body and body fluids. When T-cells sense the presence of a disease, they send messages to other white cells to resist the infection. The virus penetrates T-cells and forces them to make copies of the virus. Then the cells die. Gradually, over a period of years, when enough lymphocytes are destroyed, symptoms of AIDS appear. Victims

Estimated Rates of New HIV Infections by Race/Ethnicity

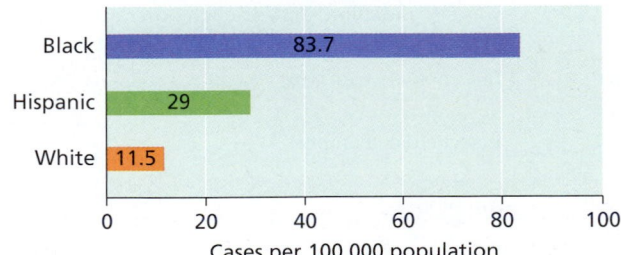

Cases per 100,000 population

FIGURE 15-2   **Estimated Number of Person Living with HIV/AIDS by Race/Ethnicity, 2001–2005—33 States.** Source: Centers for Disease Control and Prevention, 2009.

suffer from an impaired immune system, poor control of cell growth, and poor cell nutrition. A weakened immune system reduces the body's ability to defend itself against **opportunistic diseases** produced by common bacteria, viruses, parasites, and fungi that surround but do not usually have the opportunity to infect people with healthy immune systems. A person suffers infection after miserable infection, is susceptible to unusual cancers, and may become emaciated (slim disease). Another risk is tuberculosis, a contagious lung disease that has increased, mainly because of the AIDS epidemic. Other STD infections, especially those that cause genital lesions, such as herpes and syphilis, may occur concurrently with HIV and may speed the acquisition and transmission of HIV.

What Are Symptoms of an HIV Infection?

Many HIV carriers feel well and have no symptoms for up to 10 to 12 years before the immune system is suppressed enough to cause problems. That is the difference between someone who tests HIV positive and someone who is diagnosed with AIDS. The Centers for Disease Control and Prevention defines AIDS as the syndrome of having fewer than 200 T-cells or of testing HIV positive and having one or more specific opportunistic infections. Early warning signs that may indicate a weakened immune system include chronic fatigue, swollen lymph glands, unexplained weight loss, fevers, and night sweats. Poor appetite; persistent diarrhea; an itchy, spreading skin rash; and thrush (a white fungus) in the mouth are also common. (These symptoms are shared by many diseases and do not necessarily mean that you have HIV.) The body's immune system eventually becomes so weak that otherwise rare opportunistic infections may infect an AIDS victim, causing life-threatening illness.

AIDS symptoms include a persistent cough and fever associated with shortness of breath, which may be related to pneumocystis carinii pneumonia, a parasitic lung infection, and tuberculosis. Kaposi's sarcoma, a cancer of the blood vessels, causes pink or purplish lesions on the skin and elsewhere. Women may suffer from persistent vaginal infections, severe pelvic inflammatory disease, and recurrent cervical cancers. In advanced stages of the disease, the virus may also damage the brain and spinal cord, causing memory loss, partial paralysis, or AIDS-related dementia.

You can't tell by looking if someone has HIV. There are many HIV carriers who look and feel fine and don't even know they are infected. A blood test is necessary to detect the presence of the HIV virus. It is not known whether 100 percent of HIV-infected

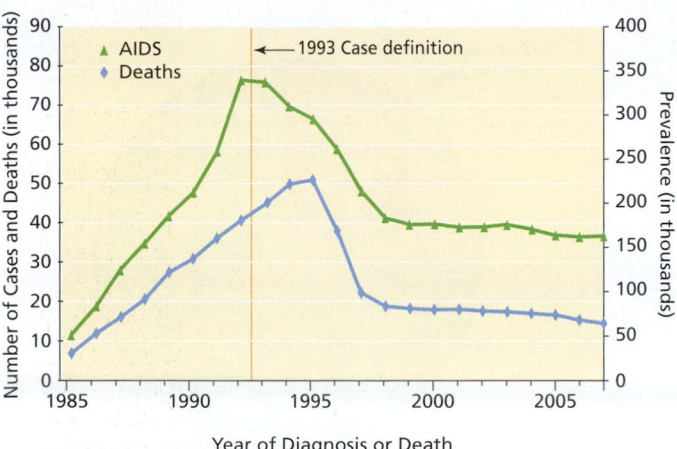

FIGURE 15-3   Estimated Number of AIDS Cases and Deaths among Adults and Adolescents with AIDS, 1985–2005—United States.

SOURCE: Centers for Disease Control & Prevention 2008.

individuals will develop AIDS. You can carry HIV in your body for years and experience no symptoms as it gradually destroys your immune system. When enough of the immune system has been destroyed, you may develop AIDS. Some people with AIDS alternate between periods of illness and periods of relatively good health. It is thought that, given time, probably all HIV-infected individuals will develop AIDS. There is hope, however, that new drug treatments may turn HIV into a chronic treatable, if not curable, infection rather than a death sentence. The biggest drop in AIDS deaths began in 1996 with the use of combination antiretroviral therapy, which has slowed the progression of HIV in infected individuals and contributed to a decline in AIDS incidence (Figure 15-3).

How Does HIV Spread?

HIV is transmitted in body fluids such as blood, semen, vaginal fluid, and breast milk. The risk of acquiring HIV is increased by the presence of other STDs, particularly inflammation from chlamydia or gonorrhea, or open sores such as those from syphilis and herpes. It is most often spread in one of the four ways shown in Table 15-5.

TABLE 15-5   *How HIV Is Transmitted*

- Through sexual intercourse with an AIDS carrier
- Through sharing of hypodermic needles
- By pregnant women to the fetuses they carry
- Rarely through a transfusion of blood

Some cases of AIDS from tainted blood and blood products occurred before 1985. Today, blood donors are screened and blood is tested for HIV antibodies to ensure the safety of our blood supply.

HIV: What Is Safe?

AIDS is an infectious disease, but it is not spread through casual social contact with the general public or HIV carriers. You can share a classroom, dining area, or locker room with an HIV-infected individual without risk of transmission. HIV cannot be "caught" like a cold. It is not spread by insects. You cannot get HIV by shaking hands or by touching the clothes of a person infected with HIV. HIV is not spread through eating utensils, dishes, or food handled by a person with HIV. It is not spread through sweat or tears. It is impossible to get HIV by donating blood because a clean needle is used for each donor. In studies of households where people with HIV were present, HIV was rarely spread except through sexual contact or from infected mothers to their infants. You cannot get HIV from hugging, body massages, masturbation, or nonsexual contact. The AIDS virus is fragile. It cannot long survive outside the human body and is easily killed by common household bleach or disinfectant. Can a person get HIV from kissing? There is no risk in a kiss on the cheek. However, small amounts of the virus are present in saliva and could possibly be transferred to another person during deep kissing, especially if bleeding gums, oral sores, or cuts exist. To be safe, the Department of Health and Human Services recommends that you avoid deep or prolonged French kissing with someone who may be infected with HIV. And what about blood-sucking insects? If mosquitoes can spread malaria, can they spread HIV? There has been no recorded case of transmission of HIV from mosquitoes. While a mosquito can pick up and carry HIV in its gut, the virus cannot reproduce there or travel to its saliva. Flies, lice, ticks, and other insects also cannot spread the virus.

Should I Be Tested for AIDS?

The Public Health Service recommends that you be counseled and tested if you have had any STD, shared drug needles, had sex with a prostitute, or had sex with a man who has had sex with other men. Anyone who has had unprotected sex with three or more partners is also at risk. People who have always practiced safe behavior do not need to be tested. See Figure 15-4 for the proportion of HIV/AIDS cases by sex and exposure category.

Realize that a first test doesn't always detect HIV because the test doesn't react to the HIV virus

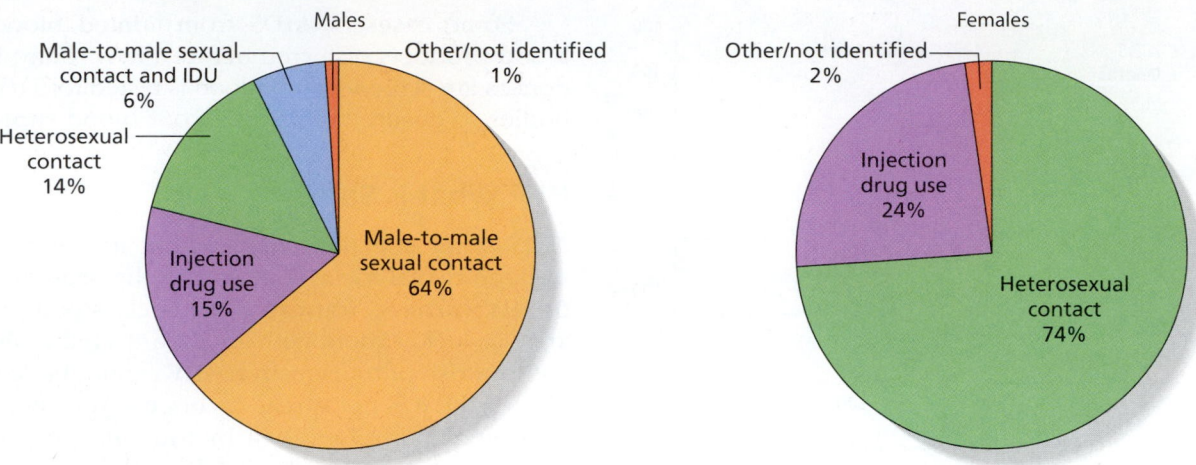

Note. Data adjusted for reporting delays and missing risk-factor information.

FIGURE 15-4   **Percentages of AIDS Cases among Adults and Adolescents, by Sex and Transmission Category 2007—50 States.**
SOURCE: Centers for Disease Control and Prevention, 2009.

itself but to antibodies the body produces to the virus. The time from when a person is exposed to HIV to the time when antibodies to the virus appear in the blood is 3 to 6 months. A person taking the test shortly after being infected may test negative, but that person can still spread HIV. Several months later, a test will show the infection. For more information, call your local public health agency or the AIDS hotline at the end of this chapter.

What About an AIDS Vaccine?

Vaccines are being developed and tested, but there is still no effective vaccine to prevent AIDS, and there is no cure. Results may not be available for several years due to the long incubation period and slow progress of the disease. Another problem is that the virus rapidly mutates to produce new forms. A vaccine might be effective for only one viral strain.

It will take several years to test the effectiveness of any vaccine developed to prevent HIV infection. There is hope that new treatments will be found and that HIV will eventually be treated as a chronic infection rather than a fatal disease. Still, avoiding exposure to the virus is the best way to prevent infection. We cannot depend on technology for a cure. Behavioral change to prevent infection is the only answer (Table 15-6).

Why Should I Be Concerned About AIDS?

Too many young people think that AIDS can't happen to them. They think that it isn't in their peer group or neighborhood. But when you have sex

TABLE 15-6	*Tips for Behavior Change: Safer Sex*

Stages of Change: In What Stage Are You?

1. Precontemplation: "I am not concerned about pregnancy or contracting an STD, and I do not use safer sex practices."
2. Contemplation: "It would probably be a good idea to start practicing safer sex."
3. Preparation: "I am currently making plans to use safer sex practices."
4. Action: "I have begun practicing safer sex."
5. Maintenance: "I always practice safer sex."

Processes of Change

After identifying your current stage, try using some of the following selected processes and behavior strategies that are appropriate for your particular stage to facilitate your transition into the next stage.

- Consciousness-raising: Learn/read about the risks of unsafe sex
- Social liberation: Investigate whether there are HIV awareness/support groups in your area
- Reward: Reflect on the emotional responsibility and turmoil that would occur as a result of an unwanted pregnancy, STD, or AIDS
- Self-liberation: Carry latex condoms
- Countering: Practice responses (polite and direct refusals) if someone tries to pressure you into a sexual encounter
- Helping relationships: Join a campus group that promotes awareness of HIV and STDs

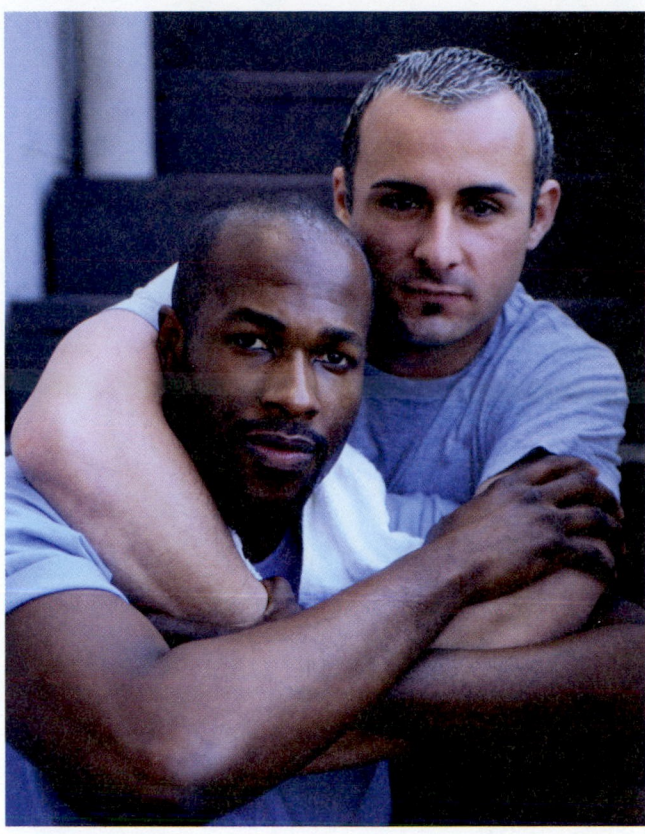

STD infection is related to behavior, not ethnic group or sexual orientation. If this couple is sexually active, using condoms will reduce STD risk.

with someone, you are in a sense having sex with all that person's past partners. There are students on campus who are HIV positive and are having sex. According to Dr. Richard P. Keeling of the American College Health Association Task Force on AIDS, blood samples tested from colleges across the United States revealed that 2 to 3 students per 1,000 tested HIV positive. In a university of 20,000 this means 40 to 60 people may carry the virus. Keeling says, "AIDS is a young person's disease. The average age of diagnosis is 32. The incubation period to diagnosis averages 10 to 12 years, so the highest risk time is ages 16 to 28. The problem doesn't seem real on most college campuses because people silently infected with HIV are not likely to appear ill." Many students who carry HIV look fine and have no symptoms. They may not even know they are infected. However, during intercourse, they can spread the disease to others.

Among gay men, the group with the highest HIV infection rate, significant behavioral change is already dropping the rate of infection and diagnosis. There has been insufficient behavioral change among the next two most frequently infected groups: IV drug users and their partners and young heterosexuals with multiple partners. Heterosexual contact accounts for 75 percent of HIV diagnoses among women and 15 percent among men. Surveys of young people show that while most know how to prevent spread of HIV, over 50 percent report having sexual intercourse with more than one partner and sporadic or no use of condoms. Most students know the facts about AIDS, but many do not use condoms or know their sexual partners. Why? Keeling states six reasons:

1. *They feel invincible.* They think, "Things like that don't happen to people like me."
2. *They lack social skills and have low self-esteem.* Many people don't feel comfortable with sexual feelings or behavior and don't feel comfortable talking about these matters or negotiating with a sexual partner to take precautions.
3. *They engage in unwanted sexual behavior.* They become involved in sex without really wanting to—due to peer pressure, role expectations, or alcohol. Alcohol is involved in a tremendous amount of risky sexual behavior on campus. Alcohol increases risk taking and decreases ambivalence and judgment. It is impossible for sex under the influence of alcohol to be safe in terms of prevention of STDs.
4. *They are victims of sexual assault.* Date rape is a common unreported campus problem. If there is no consent, no precautions can be taken.
5. *Society sends mixed messages.* Our society may say, "Just say no," but in advertising and media it screams, "Just say yes. It will be okay. Just try it."
6. *They share needles.* On campus, this is less a problem of recreational drugs than of anabolic steroids. If needles are shared, it doesn't matter what's in them; they can still spread HIV.

It doesn't matter who you are. It is not who you are that causes AIDS, but what you do. If you do things that can spread HIV, consider the risks. The problem with HIV is that if you make a mistake in judgment, it's irreversible. When you risk AIDS and lose, you lose it all.

◆ CHLAMYDIA

Chlamydia is caused by the bacterium *Chlamydia trachomatis.* It is one of the most widespread and damaging STDs. The Centers for Disease Control and Prevention estimate that 3 million cases occur annually. The rate of infection in women was reported as 543 per 100,000 people, and in men it was 190 per 100,000. The lower rate reported among men probably indicates that the partners of many women with chlamydia remain untreated. Young women have the highest rate of infection, with 46 percent of infections reported in 15- to 19-year-olds and another 33 percent in 20- to 24-year-old women. An estimated 1 in 10 college-age women is infected. Chlamydia is spread mainly through sexual intercourse but can be spread by the fingers from one body area to another, such as from the genitals to the eyes. It affects twice as many people as gonorrhea, although it mimics its symptoms, and both diseases often occur together. For this reason, physicians usually treat both infections if one is diagnosed. Early symptoms are usually mild, and if they occur, they appear within 1 to 3 weeks of exposure. Chlamydia causes an abnormal genital discharge and **urethritis,** an inflammation of the urethra, which produces a burning sensation during urination. In women, it can also cause lower abdominal pain. In men, chlamydia can infect the epididymis, causing painful scrotal swelling. About 80 percent of women and 50 percent of men have no noticeable symptoms and may not know they are infected. This makes the disease more difficult to diagnose and cure. As a result, the disease is often not diagnosed until it has done permanent damage.

Untreated chlamydia in women can produce a serious inflammation of the sexual organs called **pelvic inflammatory disease (PID).** PID is extremely damaging and can infect the lining of the uterus, fallopian tubes, and ovaries. This may cause fever and pain in the lower abdomen and scarring and blockage of the fallopian tubes and leave a woman unable to bear children. Of those with PID, 9 percent will have a life-threatening tubal pregnancy, 18 percent will experience chronic pelvic pain, and 20 percent will become infertile. A new urine screening test for chlamydia makes detection easier. The preferred treatment for chlamydia is tetracycline.

While anyone who is sexually active can get a chlamydial infection, the highest rates occur among those who have had more than one sexual partner, have had a new sexual partner in the last 2 months, are African American, are between 15 and 24 years old, are of lower socioeconomic status, or are living in an inner-city neighborhood.

◆ GENITAL HERPES

Genital herpes, a viral infection, is another major contributor to human misery. It has no cure and thus often brings feelings of shame, depression, regret, anxiety, and personal anguish as well as physical pain. Once you have it, you have it for life. Symptoms

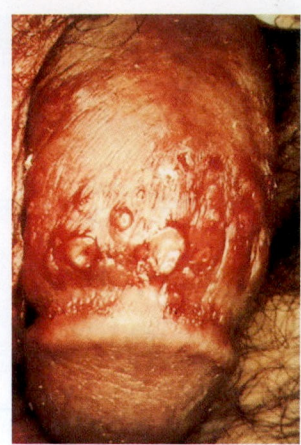

Genital herpes.

usually occur within 2 to 30 days of having sex. Early signs include itching, tingling, or burning on the legs, buttocks, or genitals. This is followed by small, painful genital sores or blisters that break open and crust over, causing intense itching and extreme pain. In addition, active herpes may be accompanied by fever, swollen glands, and general flulike feelings. Herpes virus is shed from the sores, which are highly contagious. After the blisters appear, they last from 1 to 3 weeks and then heal and disappear. The first episode is usually the most painful, and most people can expect to have four or five recurrences a year. Once established, the herpes virus migrates into nerve cells, where it may lie dormant or reactivate to cause recurring outbreaks of sores from time to time. New attacks of the disease appear at intervals, triggered by lowered resistance, fever, sunburn, or stress.

Genital herpes is caused by the **herpes simplex virus.** A virus invades body cells to live and reproduce. Nearly all herpes infections are caused by Herpes Simplex Type II, transmitted from one infected individual to another by direct contact, including kissing, sexual contact (vaginal, oral, or anal sex), and skin-to-skin contact. This is different from the common Herpes Simplex Type I, which causes cold sores to appear on or around the mouth. However, it is possible to spread Type I to the genitals or Type II to the mouth by touching the sores and scratching or rubbing somewhere else. You can also become infected by both types of herpes at the same time. Consistent use of latex condoms provides the best protection against infection. However, they *do not* provide complete protection because herpes is spread by skin-to-skin contact rather than blood or body fluids. A herpes lesion may not be covered by a condom. It is important to avoid letting the lesions contact someone else's body through touching, kissing, or sexual contact. Touching an eye after touching a sore can cause a severe eye infection called *ocular herpes*. Washing the hands thoroughly after touching a sore can prevent transmission of the virus.

At least 80 percent of infected individuals are unaware that they have genital herpes—their symptoms are so mild that they go unnoticed. Because many unreported cases exist, experts estimate that the nationwide infected population may be as large as one in five, or 45 million Americans. Infections are most common between ages 18 and 25 years. Risk factors for genital herpes include having more than one sexual partner, being sexually active for a number of years, exposure to other genital infections, and lower socioeconomic level. While infection is more common in nonwhites, symptomatic infections occur more frequently in whites. In women, herpes sores can occur internally and cause no discomfort. However, these infected individuals can still spread the virus to others, and a mother with herpes can give it to her baby. Babies born to infected mothers can become infected with herpes at birth. In infants, the virus can cause blindness, brain damage, and death. For this reason, babies are usually delivered by caesarean section if the mother has genital herpes.

While a person was once thought to be contagious only during herpes outbreaks, studies indicate that herpes can be spread, particularly from men to women, even if a person does not have symptoms. Women are four times as likely to get herpes from men as men are to get it from women, perhaps because of the greater exposure of vaginal and cervical mucous membranes to the virus during sexual contact.

The severity and duration of symptoms can be decreased with prescription antiviral drugs such as valacyclovir (Valtrex). These medications can also be taken to prevent recurrence of symptoms, although they cannot cure the disease. Thus, the joke "What is the difference between love and herpes?" Answer: "Only herpes is forever."

GENITAL WARTS AND OTHER HUMAN PAPILLOMA VIRUS INFECTIONS

Genital warts are caused by the **human papilloma virus (HPV),** which is related to the virus that causes skin warts. HPV infections are epidemic among young people of college age. Not all of them cause

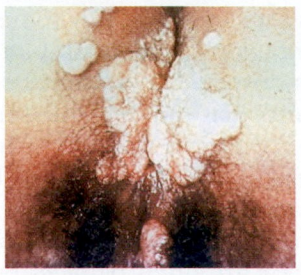

Genital warts on a female.

visible warts. More than 40 types of HPV infections infect the genital tract, and a person can have more than one type of HPV at a time. Once HPV has invaded cells, depending on its type, it may produce genital warts; cancer of the cervix, vulva, anus, mouth, or penis; or there may be no symptoms. Both cervical cancer in women and penile cancer in men are associated with HPV, and these cancers all too often occur in sexually active young adults. HPV 16 and HPV 18, the most common types in cervical cancer patients, increase risk 200 percent. Vaccination against HPV 16 and HPV 18 can effectively prevent HPV infection from these two strains.

Most people who have had two or more sex partners have been exposed to HPV. Like herpes, HPV is passed through direct skin-to-skin contact through sexual activity. Though rare, nonsexual transmission is possible because HPV can remain alive for several hours on wet towels or undergarments. HPV infections are more common in women than in men, probably because the warmth and moisture of a woman's vagina provide ideal conditions for viral growth.

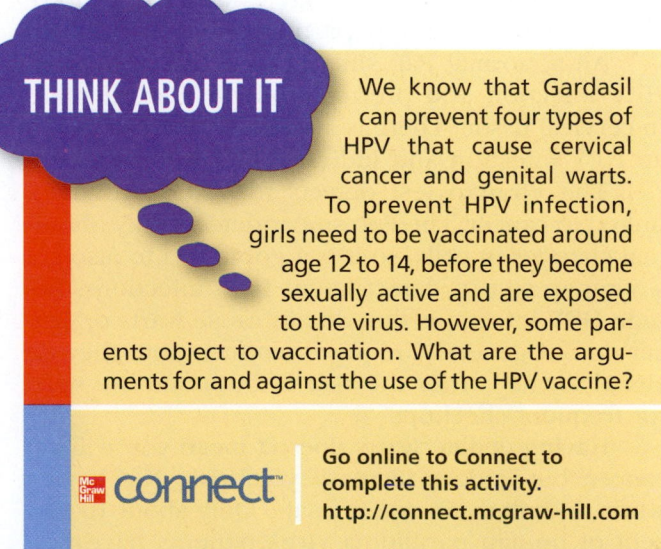

THINK ABOUT IT

We know that Gardasil can prevent four types of HPV that cause cervical cancer and genital warts. To prevent HPV infection, girls need to be vaccinated around age 12 to 14, before they become sexually active and are exposed to the virus. However, some parents object to vaccination. What are the arguments for and against the use of the HPV vaccine?

connect

Go online to Connect to complete this activity.
http://connect.mcgraw-hill.com

Genital warts are caused by some types of HPV, are highly contagious, and take 1 to 8 months to appear after exposure. Until the warts appear, there are no symptoms that indicate presence of the HPV virus. Between the time of exposure and the appearance of warts, either partner can have the virus unknowingly and give it to the other. Genital warts may be flat or rounded bumps with a cauliflower-like appearance. They are often painless but may itch or burn. In men, most genital warts occur on the outside of the penis. In women, they may appear around the vulva and inside the vagina and cervix. They may also appear in the mouth, in the throat, or around the anus, and they do not go away.

Warts can grow and spread, so they should be removed. Warts can be frozen with liquid nitrogen, burned off with an electric needle or laser, or removed surgically or chemically. While these methods can eliminate the external lesions, they do not eradicate the virus, which may become dormant and reappear later or may be destroyed by the body's immune system.

You can detect some genital warts by self-examination. Men should check the penis regularly. Women should use a mirror to examine the vulva and anus. Warts inside the vagina can be found by a doctor.

Genital warts, the most common symptom of HPV, can also lead to cervical cancer, one of the leading cancer killers of women. In some cases, warts turn into precancerous growths called *dysplasia* and later become cancerous. Cervical cancer is thus considered a sexually transmitted disease. This cancer infects far too many young women of childbearing age and is not just a disease of the elderly. Other risk factors for HPV include initiating sexual activity at an early age and having unprotected sex with multiple partners.

An abnormal Pap smear can detect an unseen HPV infection and precancerous cellular changes in cervical tissue. There is also a test that can detect an HPV infection and indicate the strain of the virus. The Virapap test detects five strains of HPV linked to cancer. The Pap smear detects only abnormal changes in cells, so it is a good idea to also get a Virapap test to detect latent HPV infections. Benign HPV infections that do not cause warts or cancer do not generally require treatment, but they do signal to the carrier the risk of both and the need for frequent checkups.

Having genital warts doesn't mean you will get cancer, but it does increase your risk. Not having warts doesn't mean you are safe. Only about 10 percent of human papilloma virus patients have visible warts, so it is possible to be infected and unaware of it. The good news is that most HPV infections are cleared by the body in 2 to 4 years and only a small percentage progress to cancer.

The HPV Vaccine

The best way to prevent getting an HPV infection is to take protective measures to avoid direct skin-to-skin genital contact with the virus. The 3-shot HPV vaccine Gardasil is another aid in preventing infection with HPV types 16 and 18, which cause most (70 percent) cervical cancers, and types 6 and 11, which cause about 90 percent of genital warts. However, Gardasil does not provide complete protection against all types of HPV, so protective measures are still necessary, and women should still be screened for cervical cancer. Gardasil will not cure a preexisting HPV infection, genital warts, or cervical cancer. It is most effective for women ages 9 to 26 who have not been exposed to the virus; and since it targets four strains, even if a person has an infection with one strain, it can protect against the other three strains. Another vaccine, Cervarix, is undergoing testing for women up to age 45.

GONORRHEA

Gonorrhea, the second most common bacterial STD, was named by Galen in 150 B.C. from Greek words meaning "flow of seed." At that time, the penile discharge of men infected with gonorrhea was thought to be semen. Actually, the discharge was pus produced from inflammation of the urethra. The gonorrhea bacteria grow and multiply quickly in mucous membranes such as in the cervix, mouth, rectum, and urinary tract. In women, the most common site of infection is the cervix, but it can spread to the ovaries and fallopian tubes, causing PID. It can be spread directly through sexual intercourse or from the genitals to the mouth with the fingers.

As with chlamydia, gonorrhea often has no symptoms, or the symptoms go undetected as the

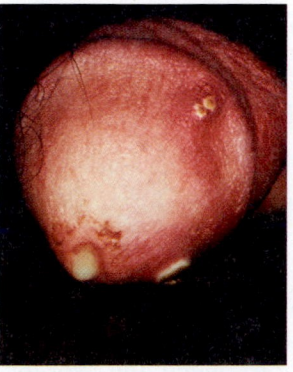

Gonorrhea.

infected individual continues to spread the disease. Men are much more likely to notice the symptoms than are women. Up to 80 percent of women infected have no symptoms, compared with 20 percent of men. If symptoms occur, they usually appear within 2 to 14 days of infection. Gonorrhea often strikes the urethra, causing a burning sensation during urination. Males may notice an unusual penile discharge, as well as swollen lymph glands in the groin. Women may experience an abnormal vaginal discharge, abdominal pain, or vaginal bleeding. A rectal infection may produce anal itching or discharge. Oral infections usually produce no symptoms, though a few victims may get a sore throat. Early symptoms may clear up on their own, but a person can still be infected and spread the disease to others.

If not treated, gonorrhea may cause permanent damage to the reproductive organs and cause sterility. In men, it may damage the penis, making urination difficult and erection impossible. It can also infect the epididymis, leaving scar tissue that can block the flow of semen from the infected testicle. In women, it can scar the fallopian tubes, making it impossible to bear children. In both sexes, the bacteria can spread to the bloodstream, producing a generalized bacterial infection. It can infect joints with gonococcal arthritis and irreversibly damage heart valves, the spinal cord, or the brain. It can be spread from an infected mother via the birth canal to her baby, causing eye infection and blindness if not treated immediately.

Gonorrhea is usually treated with penicillin and antibiotics, although penicillin-resistant strains have developed. Up to 75 percent of cases in some regions are penicillin-resistant, making treatment more difficult. This increasing occurrence of penicillin-resistant gonorrhea underscores the need for taking protective measures during sexual activity and for being tested once or twice a year even if there are no symptoms.

While overall rates of infection have declined, infection rates for minority adolescents and young adults remain high, especially in high-density urban areas among those who have unprotected sex or multiple sexual partners.

◆ HEPATITIS B

Hepatitis B, formerly called *serum hepatitis*, is an inflammatory disease that destroys liver tissue. It is caused by a virus spread during vaginal, anal, and oral sex with an infected partner. It spreads through contact with saliva, nasal mucus, sperm, and menstrual blood. It is also spread through the sharing of contaminated needles (drugs, tattooing, acupuncture) and direct blood contact. Additionally,

a mother with hepatitis B can give it to her baby during childbirth. A person infected with the virus can be an asymptomatic carrier and can spread it even though there is no active infection. The incubation period ranges from 1 to 9 months. Many people have no symptoms or mild symptoms, which can include lingering flulike feelings: weakness, fatigue, loss of appetite, nausea, vomiting, and fever. This may be accompanied by itching, hives, and joint pain. In a few days, this is followed by brownish urine; loose, light yellow stools; yellowing of the eyes and skin; abdominal discomfort; liver enlargement; and, in severe cases, liver failure. While many people recover, about 10 percent of people with hepatitis B develop a chronic form of the disease, which may produce only mild or no obvious symptoms. Chronic hepatitis may lead to a progressive destruction of liver cells, cirrhosis, or liver cancer. There is an effective vaccine for hepatitis B that is recommended for people at high risk for infection.

◆ SYPHILIS

Syphilis was rampant in Europe in the late 1400s, spread during times of war by soldiers who frequented prostitutes and then returned home to their wives and mistresses. It was also reportedly spread by soldiers who sailed with Columbus to the New World and by many Renaissance explorers who took it beyond the boundaries of Europe. It was first known as the "great pox," in contrast to which "smallpox" was later named, and was at first thought to be a special divine punishment for sexual transgressions. In the eighteenth century, syphilitics wore wigs and high collars to hide hair loss and throat lesions. Many early treatments used mercury or arsenic, which produced side effects as bad as the disease. Although syphilis has been a serious health problem during all major wars, it was not until after World War II began that the U.S. Public Health Service started using penicillin to combat it.

Some social problems, such as poverty, lack of access to health care, and lack of education, are associated with high levels of syphilis in some populations. The infection rate among African Americans,

> *For when it has once been received into the body, it does not immediately declare itself; rather it lies dormant for a certain time and gradually gains strength as it feeds.*
>
> —Fracastoro (1483–1553),
> Syphilis, the "French Disease"

particularly those living in inner cities, is seven times higher than the rate for whites, according to the Centers for Disease Control and Prevention. Nevertheless, the risk of acquiring any STD is determined by behavior, not by racial or ethnic factors. Avoiding risky behavior and making responsible choices are the keys to reducing STD rates even in high-risk groups. Like other bacterial STDs, syphilis is easily spread because its symptoms are often unnoticed or confused with other diseases. Syphilis is known as "the great imitator" because it mimics so many other diseases.

Syphilis occurs in four stages—primary, secondary, latent, and tertiary—depending on how long a person has had it and how far it has progressed.

Primary Syphilis

The first sign of syphilis is a **chancre,** or small painless sore, which appears within 1 to 12 weeks of sexual contact. It may appear on the penis, in the vagina, in the mouth, or in any other area that contacted the bacteria, and it lasts 1 to 5 weeks. It is often accompanied by painless swelling of the lymph nodes in the groin. The initial sore may go unnoticed and will disappear if left untreated. The disease then enters a secondary stage 2 weeks to 6 months later.

Secondary Syphilis

In the secondary stage, skin rash, fever, headache, sore throat, swollen lymph glands, flulike symptoms, and patchy hair loss may occur. The symptoms are so general that the disease can be misdiagnosed even if medical help is sought. The rash may appear as pink spots or small raised bumps on the palms, soles of the feet, back, chest, arms, legs, face, or abdomen. Small, moist sores may appear in the mouth, and lesions may appear in the genital area. Secondary symptoms, if they occur,

may clear up in 2 to 6 weeks without treatment but may recur for up to 2 years. During this time, an infected individual can still spread the disease. If untreated, although the initial symptoms may subside and a person can feel normal, the disease progresses.

Latent Syphilis

In latent syphilis, the third stage, a person is generally no longer infectious to others unless there is a relapse of moist lesions or unless the disease is passed to a baby during pregnancy. This stage can last for several years with no symptoms, but the infecting bacteria can continue to multiply.

Tertiary Syphilis

While two-thirds of untreated people have no more symptoms, the one-third who are affected may suffer permanent damage to the cardiovascular or nervous system. Tertiary syphilis can occur anywhere from 3 to 40 years after initial infection. Complications include heart disease, blindness, brain damage, paralysis, insanity, and death.

Penicillin was found to be effective against syphilis in the 1940s. It is still considered the treatment of choice.

◆ OTHER SEXUALLY TRANSMITTED INFECTIONS

Trichomonas is caused by a microscopic parasite, and **bacterial vaginosis** is caused by an imbalance in the bacteria that normally populate the vagina. The symptoms—vaginal itching and a foul-smelling, cheesy discharge—tend to affect only women, but the infective organisms may be harbored in a man's urethra or penile foreskin and may be spread to others. Both are treated with medication to cure the infection. **Chancroid** infection causes soft, painful genital sores and is treated with antibiotics. Chancroids may

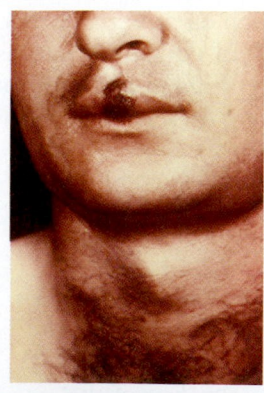

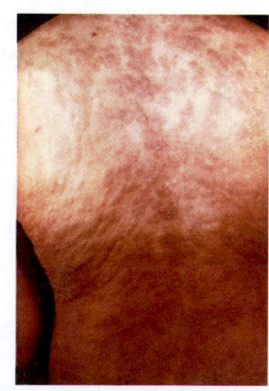

Oral chancre, primary syphilis.   Rash from secondary syphilis.

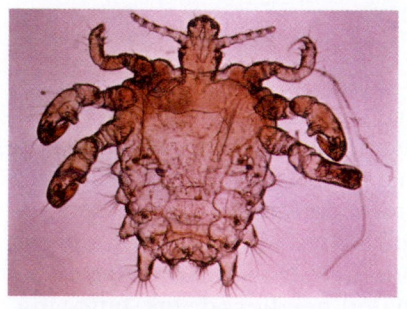

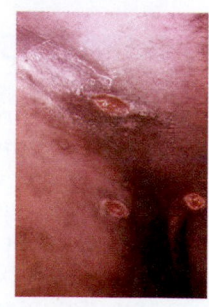

Pubic louse.   Chancroid.

increase susceptibility to HIV. Pubic lice and scabies, a mite, may be transmitted sexually or nonsexually. **Pubic lice** (crabs) are usually found in the pubic hairs, and **scabies** burrow under the skin in the pubic area to lay eggs. Both cause intense itching, are highly contagious, and are treated with several applications of an insecticidal shampoo.

HOW CAN I PROTECT MYSELF FROM STDs?

While the facts about AIDS and other STDs are sobering, the good news is that you can reduce your risk of exposure to zero through personal choices. The best prevention for any STD is sexual abstinence or a mutually monogamous sexual relationship with an uninfected partner. *There is no safe sex, only less risky sex.* No orgasm is worth dying for. Unless you are willing to throw away your future, you must weigh the choices and consequences. If you are sexually active with more than one partner, take steps to avoid becoming a victim of AIDS and other sexually transmitted diseases.

ABSTINENCE

Sexual abstinence is the choice to refrain from sexual activity. The choice of abstinence is a personal decision based on what you feel is right for you. People abstain for different reasons, including religious, social, moral, health, or that they

✓ Do not feel ready for a sexual relationship.
✓ Want time to develop friendship and trust in a relationship before having sex.
✓ Feel that sex belongs only in marriage or a close, committed relationship.
✓ Do not have the time or energy to put into a sexual relationship.
✓ Do not have to deal with feelings of guilt, hurt, or confusion if the relationship ends.
✓ Want to avoid the risk of pregnancy.
✓ Want to avoid the risk of contracting a sexually transmitted disease.
✓ Have a sexual health concern or infection that needs to be addressed.

Abstinence can mean different things to different people. To some it means "Just say no" or "Wait until marriage," and these choices should be respected. To others it means waiting for the right person, place, and time to have sex. Discuss sexual values and beliefs with your partner before you find yourself in

TOP 10 LIST

Ways to Reduce the Risk of STDs

1. Abstain from sexual contact with others or have a mutually monogamous relationship with an uninfected sexual partner.
2. Communicate assertively about sexual feelings, activities, sexual history, and STDs.
3. Choose lower-risk sexual activities that have less likelihood of transmitting STDs.
4. Separate alcohol and drugs from sexual activity. Drunk sex can't be safe sex. Do not use intravenous drugs. If you do, do not share drug needles and syringes. Don't have sex with people who shoot drugs.
5. Protect yourself. Use latex condoms or dental dams.
6. Be selective. Limit the number of partners you have sex with. The fewer partners you have, the lower your risk is.
7. Do not have sex with someone who has several sex partners or with prostitutes. Prostitutes may also use IV drugs, increasing their chances of exposure to HIV.
8. Immunize for HPV and hepatitis B.
9. Observe a partner discreetly for discharge, sores, or a rash. While it may not seem romantic, if you see anything that concerns you, don't have sex!
10. If you are sexually active, have an STD checkup every time you have a health exam. This is especially important for women, who often have no signs of an STD. Have an STD checkup every 6 months if you have more than one partner.

In addition: Know the symptoms of STDs, and if you notice a symptom that concerns you, abstain from sex and see a physician. If you do acquire an infection, make sure that all partners are notified and treated. To prevent infecting others, don't have sex until you have completed treatment and the doctor says you are cured.

a sexual situation, especially in a new relationship. Here are some questions you might ask yourself to clarify your feelings and values:

✓ Why am I choosing to be abstinent?
✓ What does abstinence mean to me? What are my "dos and don'ts"?
✓ Am I comfortable with my current level of involvement and intimacy with my partner?
✓ Do I feel pressured into having a sexual relationship?
✓ Do I feel physically and emotionally ready for a sexual relationship?
✓ Am I comfortable talking with my partner about sex? If not, am I ready to have sex?

TABLE 15-7	*Levels of Risk of Contracting an STD*
High Risk	Wet kissing with the mouth open Oral or vaginal sex without a condom Anal sex with or without a condom, especially receptive anal sex
Low Risk	Oral sex using a condom Vaginal sex using a condom Masturbating a partner using a latex barrier
No Risk	Kissing with the mouth closed Hugging, touching, holding hands Massage, fantasy, masturbation

✓ What do I want from this relationship? How will I feel if I have sex and the relationship ends?

✓ Are my partner and I ready and willing to use protective measures against STDs and unplanned pregnancy?

You can choose to be abstinent at any time, even if you have had sex in the past. The choice of abstinence may be for a short time or for years, but being abstinent does not mean that you give up being loving or sensual. There are many ways to express affection physically besides sexual intercourse (see "No Risk" activities in Table 15-7). Many people enjoy dating even more when they have agreed sexual intercourse is off limits. It gives partners a chance to develop creative ways to show love for each other, to focus more on feelings, shared interests, values, and goals and less on sex. Sex isn't an emergency. Abstinence is an important and personal choice and an excellent way to avoid exposure to sexually transmitted diseases.

◆ CHOOSING LOWER-RISK SEXUAL ACTIVITIES

There are many ways to show someone you care besides having sex: respect, sharing, trust, commitment. Lasting relationships are built on alternative ways of expressing love and affection. Even if you have decided to have sex, there are lower-risk sex techniques you can use to protect yourself from STDs. Keep in mind that your skin is your largest sexual organ and your imagination is your most important sexual asset. Consider the options in Table 15-7.

◆ PLANNING AHEAD FOR SAFER SEX

When you are in the middle of a passionate embrace, it may not seem convenient to discuss safer sex or how to use a condom, and using condoms takes practice. Before beginning a sexual relationship, plan ahead. Think about what you'll say to your partner about using condoms. It may help to use a news story about AIDS to bring up the subject of safer sex. Make your feelings about condom use clear. Tell your partner you want to take precautions because you care about both of you. If your partner won't agree to use condoms, don't have sex.

And what about STD testing? If you see that your relationship is headed toward sex, pick a time that you won't be interrupted to talk about getting tested. Do *not* text your partner, as abbreviations might be misunderstood. Do not talk about names or numbers of past partners, as this is not the point. This is about both partners being tested so that if either has an infection it can be medically managed. You can go to a clinic together or go to your own doctor. You and your partner can share copies of the test results and make sure you were tested for the same things. If your partner doesn't want to be tested, then he or she isn't worth the risk.

◆ HOW TO USE CONDOMS

If abstinence or a mutually faithful, single-partner relationship is not your choice, the next best way to protect yourself from sexually transmitted diseases, including AIDS, is to use a latex condom during sex. While condoms are not 100 percent effective in preventing STDs, if used correctly, it is estimated that they can reduce risk by up to 98 percent. Condom breakage rates are low, around 2 in 100. Most condom failures are due to incorrect or inconsistent use. Unfortunately, few people know how to use condoms correctly, resulting in a failure rate of 40 percent or more. If you are a woman, carry condoms even if you don't plan to have sex (few young adults who have sex plan it). Do not store condoms in a hot place such as a glove compartment or carry them in a wallet for more than 1 week (they need to be fresh). Use a condom every time, including for oral or anal sex. Avoid skin condoms (lambskin)—they do not provide protection from all STDs, though they do prevent pregnancy.

To maximize condom effectiveness, follow these steps (Figure 15-5):

1. Be careful when opening the package. Be especially careful not to tear the condom with a fingernail or teeth.

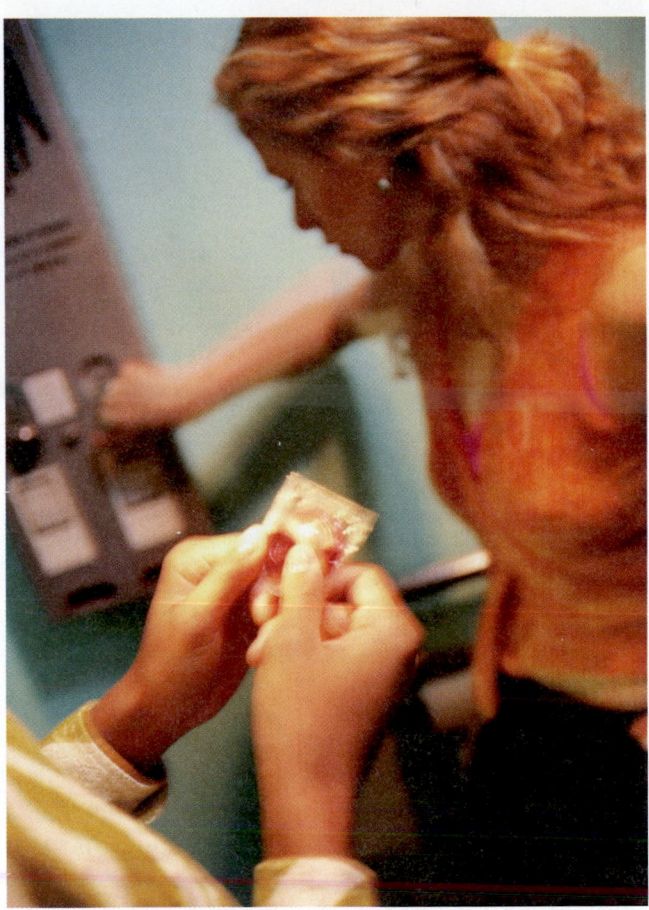

If you are sexually active, carry your own condoms even if you don't plan to have sex.

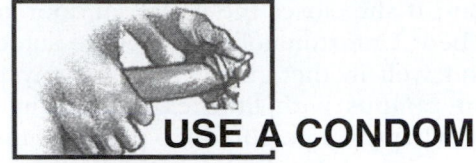

USE A CONDOM

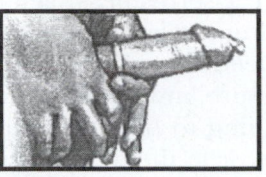

USE A LUBRICANT

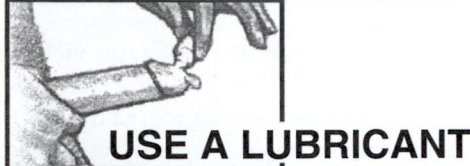

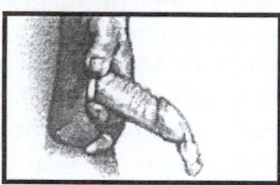

FIGURE 15-5   How to use a condom.

2. Put the condom on before penetration, even if ejaculation is not planned. Withdrawal is not effective in preventing STDs. Unroll the condom on the erect penis. Hold the tip as you unroll the condom, making sure there is no air inside. Leave about 1/2-inch space for semen at the tip. If there is no space at the tip, the force of semen coming out of the penis can break the condom.

3. Apply a water-based lubricant onto the tip of the condom. Do not use an oil-based lubricant. Vaseline or baby oil quickly deteriorates latex. A few people have reactions to spermicides containing nonoxylynol-9. Do not use a spermicide that causes a rash or irritation, as this could increase the chance of infection.

4. Withdraw while the penis is still erect. Hold the rim of the condom to avoid spilling semen. Throw the used condom away. Do not reuse it.

If you and your partner don't like male condoms, you can try a female condom, which works like an extra large male condom inserted into a woman's vagina. It consists of a 6½-inch-long plastic tube with a large ring on each end. One ring holds it in the vagina, and the other ring fits outside the vaginal lips. It is as effective in preventing conception and STDs as the male condom, and it gives a woman the ability to protect herself and her partner; however, it is more expensive, is somewhat unwieldy, and has not proved popular.

COPING WITH UNWANTED SEXUAL PRESSURE AND AVOIDING SEXUAL ASSAULT

Maria met Carlos at a football game and invited him to a party at an off-campus apartment. Carlos doesn't know anyone at the party but doesn't want to miss the fun. The music is lively and the drinks are free, so he has a few drinks and starts feeling relaxed. Maria shows up and invites him to go to her room so they can talk. He agrees. They take their drinks and head toward the bedroom.

Is a woman "asking for it" if she has been drinking? Is consent implied if Maria invites Carlos into her room? If she closes the bedroom door and sits on the bed? Unfortunately, the double standard is alive and well in the United States. Many people come to campus with little experience in sexual matters. What can a person do to prevent unwanted sexual behavior? Dr. Richard Keeling says, "We need to build skills in assertiveness, self-esteem, decision making, running a relationship, and dealing with intimacy. We need a personal commitment that says my life, my future, my potential are more valuable than what's going to happen in this relationship or on this date or in the next 10 minutes." What do you do when he or she wants to have sex and you don't?

An estimated 80 percent of rape victims are attacked by someone they know: a date, a former partner, or a casual acquaintance. Many people with active social lives involve themselves in parties and activities with the expectation of meeting new friends and dating partners. There is a tendency to assume that this is a safe way to meet people, but placing trust in someone you know only casually can put you in an unsafe situation, particularly if alcohol is involved. Some people have trouble understanding how a person can be raped by someone known. Date rape has been characterized as a four-stage process, and while these stages do not always occur, they show how sexual assault can happen even to someone who exercises caution:

1. *Intrusion.* The offender begins by violating the victim's space in one way or another. He (men can also be raped, but most rapes involve men assaulting women, so we'll use that scenario here) may start by interrupting while she is talking, talking about personal topics she feels uncomfortable with, or touching her unnecessarily or inappropriately.
2. *Desensitization.* The victim lets down her guard. While the intrusion makes her uncomfortable, she ignores the feelings and thinks, "That's just the way he is" or "He doesn't mean anything by it."
3. *Isolation.* The offender tries to get the victim alone, for example, in a car or her home, where she might think she is safe, and uses tactics that put her at greater risk, such as encouraging her to drink alcohol.
4. *Offender denial.* The offender justifies his actions to himself and others by insisting that the victim gave consent and encouraged his behavior. This also increases the victim's feelings of confusion and guilt.

It might happen like this: Marcus and Kari were introduced by mutual friends. Marcus has invited

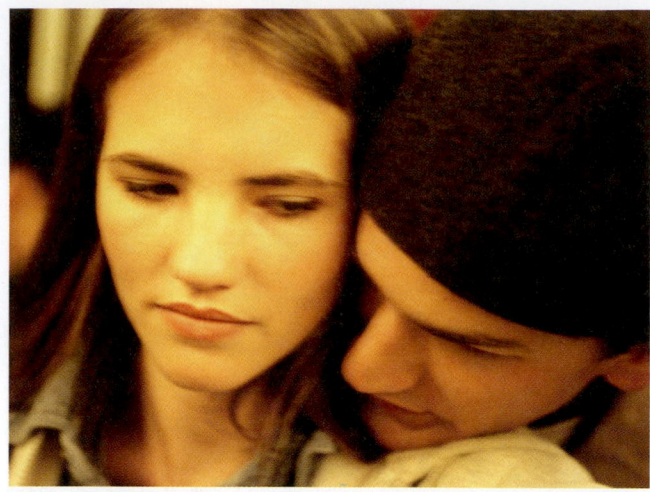

To avoid coercive sexual situations, communicate clearly your feelings, limits, and intentions.

Kari to go out to a movie with him. He seems to be a nice guy, so she accepts. They go to the movie and have a couple of beers afterward. Then Marcus takes Kari home. Parked by her home, Marcus engages Kari in a conversation that grows increasingly personal, and he begins making advances that make Kari uncomfortable (intrusion). Assuming that this is typical behavior for him (desensitization), she puts up with it for a while and gently tries to discourage him. She had intended to go to her apartment alone, but Marcus has a long drive home and asks for a cup of coffee. This seems reasonable, so Kari accepts and Marcus accompanies her to her apartment (isolation). Her belief that she can control the situation and her desire to spare his feelings put her at risk. As soon as they are inside the door, Marcus pins her to the wall with a kiss and becomes increasingly aggressive. When she finally tells him to stop, he becomes verbally abusive, calling her a "tease" and a "bitch." Then he forces himself on her. Afterward, he asks her why she invited him to her apartment if she didn't want sex and insists that it was consensual sex (offender denial).

Unfortunately, these scenes are too common, and the victim is left feeling somehow responsible for the rape and wondering what she did to cause it or why she didn't head it off. Men can be raped too—about 10 percent of reported rapes are of men. Many go unreported because of homophobia (in men-on-men rape) and the myth that rape is a crime of desire rather than of violence.

If you are sexually assaulted, follow these steps:

✓ Once out of immediate danger, call the police.
✓ Do not change clothes, shower, urinate, defecate, gargle, take medication, drink alcohol, or do anything else that might destroy evidence.

✓ Go with a trusted friend to a hospital emergency room, where a doctor will ask for information about the assault, conduct a rape exam, and collect physical evidence to be used in court.

If a friend of yours is a victim of date rape, remember the following:

✓ Rape is not a result of uncontrolled passion. It is a violent assault using sex as a weapon.
✓ No one wants to be forced to have sex. No matter what happened, no one wants to be a victim of a crime. A person has handled the situation right if he or she is alive.
✓ You can't control what others think or say about it. Do not isolate yourself or the victim from friends who know about the rape. Neither you nor the victim has any reason to feel shame, embarrassment, or guilt. Your understanding and support are important.
✓ If the assault is reported to the police, the victim is not responsible for what happens to the rapist, regardless of what pressure is brought by the family or friends of the assailant. The courts are responsible for the outcome, and the rapist is responsible for the rape.

To avoid coercive sexual pressure or sexual assault, you must break the chain of circumstances that lead to these outcomes. Here are some tips from the Santa Monica Rape Treatment Center.

Men

✓ *Don't fall for the stereotype* that when a woman says no, she means yes. If she says no to sexual contact, believe her and stop.

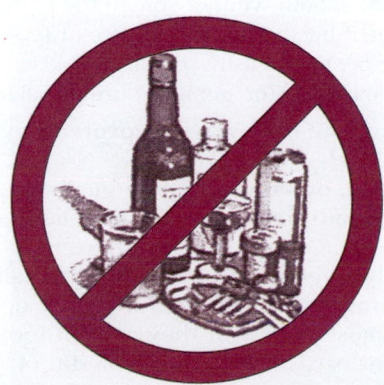

Consider the risks and consequences of sex under the influence.

✓ *Don't make assumptions about a person's behavior.* Just because a woman drinks heavily, dresses provocatively, or goes with you to your room, don't assume she wants sex. Just because she had sex with you once, don't assume she is willing now. Also, don't assume that because she willingly engages in kissing or other intimate behavior she wants sexual intercourse.
✓ *Don't assume that silence is consent.* Having sex with someone who is intoxicated, unconscious, drugged, or otherwise incapable of giving consent is rape.

Women and Men

✓ *Attend parties with friends you can trust.* Look out for each other. Leave together rather than alone or with a new acquaintance. If you are attracted to someone you'd like to get to know better, agree to meet for lunch the next day.
✓ *Be selective.* Even if a person you just met seems nice, find out about him or her from friends and family.
✓ *Avoid isolation.* Don't go to a secluded place or a wild party with a new acquaintance. Go to concerts, movies, lectures, or restaurants; double date; and stay around people. When you get to know the person well, you can relax the rules.
✓ *Communicate.* Don't lead someone on. Don't expect a person to know how you feel unless you speak up. Make your feelings, limits, and intentions clear. You have a right to say no to any unwanted sexual contact. If you are being pressured and feel uncertain, ask the person to respect your feelings.
✓ *Listen closely to what a person is saying.* If you think she or he is giving you a mixed message, ask for clarification. On a date when neither person stops to check out what the other person is feeling, the situation can get out of hand.
✓ *Make sure* how *you say something agrees with what you say.* Your body language may come across louder than your words. If you say no with downcast eyes and a smile to soften the refusal, you may end up giving the other person a mixed message. You are more likely to get your message across if you look a person directly in the eye and say no assertively.
✓ *Be aware.* Pay attention to what is happening. Rely on your gut instinct. If a situation

doesn't feel right, exit as quickly as you can and go to a safe place.

✓ *Speak up if you believe someone is at risk.* If you see a friend in trouble at a party or if someone is using force and pressuring a friend, don't be afraid to intervene. You may save your friend from the trauma of sexual assault and that person from criminal prosecution.

✓ *Stay sober.* You'll be more likely to make wise decisions if you are sober.

✓ *At parties, keep your drink in your sight.* If you forget, pour it out and buy a new one. No drink is worth the risk of consuming a date rape drug.

Both men and women must be especially careful in situations involving drinking or drugs. They decrease reasoning ability and your ability to make a decision and communicate effectively. They increase willingness to take risks you wouldn't normally take. Alcohol, a social lubricant par excellence, sets you up for unwanted sexual behavior and STDs. It is involved in approximately half the incidents of coercive sexual behavior. It decreases the ability to recognize an unsafe situation and react appropriately. It also decreases the likelihood that you will use a condom. Even if you have one, you may be too drunk to put it on.

℞ PRESCRIPTION FOR ACTION

You've read the chapter. Now go do one or more of these:

✓ If you are sexually active and have not been screened for STDs in the last year, call to schedule a checkup with your physician or health clinic.

✓ Plan how you will deal with unwanted sexual pressure, and what you can do to avoid an unsafe situation.

✓ Think about how you will bring up the subject of safer sex or abstinence to a potential partner.

✓ Consider ways to express affection physically without sexual intercourse.

✓ If you have questions about STDs, write them down and phone an appropriate STD hotline listed at the end of this chapter.

✓ Download a fact sheet on STDs at www.cdc.gov/std/

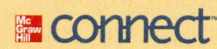 Go online to Connect to complete this activity. http://connect.mcgraw-hill.com

---

Frequently Asked Questions

Q. Does spermicide protect against STDs?

A. No. Spermicide is used to kill sperm, so it protects against pregnancy. When used frequently or in excess, it can actually increase the risk of STDs. Most spermicides contain nonoxlynol-9 (N-9), which can cause inflammation of the vagina and cervix. This makes a woman more susceptible to infection by STDs and makes it easier to transmit STDs to a partner. Consider unlubricated condoms or use spermicides that do not contain N-9.

Q. Can I get an STD from oral sex?

A. STDs are spread through vaginal, anal, and oral sex. One exposure is enough to put you at risk for an STD. To reduce your risk, use an unlubricated condom or dental dam.

Q. Can I get an STD from a public restroom?

A. Not likely. Most pathogens that cause STDs cannot survive away from the human body, and are only spread though exchange of body fluids or skin-to-skin contact during sex. Pubic lice can survive outside the human body for 24 hours, so while their spread is possible, it is unlikely.

Q. Can I get an STD from kissing?

A. If your partner's mouth is infected with an STD, it is possible, though rare, that an STD could be spread. If your partner has a genital infection, kissing on the mouth will not spread the pathogen. However, if he/she has a cold sore or fever blister (oral herpes), it is easily spread by a kiss, and can be transmitted to the genitals during oral sex.

Q. What are the best ways to protect myself from STDs?

A. Abstinence provides the only guarantee. Mutual monogamy with an uninfected partner is also safe. Other than this, there is no safe sex, only *safer* sex. Latex male or female condoms provide protection and greatly decrease risk of most STDs, but they are not foolproof. Condoms occasionally break or slip off, are less effective if used incorrectly, and do not protect against lesions that they do not cover.

Q. My partner has herpes, but we never have sex during an outbreak, so I can't get infected with the herpes virus, can I?

A. Even though a person may not have visible signs of herpes, he or she can still shed the virus and infect a partner in the earliest stages, several days before an outbreak. While condoms can protect against many STDs, and they reduce risk of exposure through skin-to-skin contact, they may not cover all the areas where the herpes virus is present.

Q. My partner had genital warts, but they were removed. Is he cured? Can he still infect me?

A. Genital warts are caused by a human papilloma virus. While the external warts can be treated and removed, the virus can still be present and cause a recurrence. There is no cure for HPV infection, so it is important to use condoms during any sexual activity to prevent becoming infected.

Q. I was just diagnosed with genital herpes. I always use a condom. My partner has never had these symptoms. How is that possible?

A. A woman may be asymptomatic, or the herpes lesions may appear internally, so a person may be infected and not know it. While it does greatly reduce the risk of STDs, a condom may not totally cover all the herpes lesions, so infection may be spread.

Q. Does the pill protect a person from STDs?

A. No. While oral contraceptives and other birth control measures reduce risk of pregnancy, they do not give protection from STDs. Use of male or female condoms does offer protection from STDs.

Q. Can warts on the hands or feet be spread to the genitals?

A. No. These warts are caused by different types of HPV and do not spread to the genitals or mouth.

Q. I once had pelvic inflammatory disease. I was treated for chlamydia and cured. How does PID affect a person's chances to have children?

A. The risks of pelvic inflammatory disease include scarring, constriction, and blockage of the fallopian tubes. Complete blockage results in sterility. Partial blockage increases the risk of an ectopic (tubal) pregnancy. This occurs when a fertilized egg implants in an area other than the uterus, such as a fallopian tube. This is a serious complication that can rupture a fallopian tube, causing internal bleeding and even death. However, PID affects people differently, so it is important to consult your physician.

Q. If a person is in the latency period for HIV and gives blood, can it infect another person?

A. All blood donors are screened for risk factors and all blood donations are tested for several viruses, including HIV. If a virus is found, the blood is discarded and the donor is notified. If a blood donor became infected with HIV in the 2 weeks before donating blood, tests for the HIV antigen may not detect the virus in the blood. While there is a slight chance that a blood transfusion might infect a person receiving blood, the risk has been estimated to be from 1 in 675,000 to 1 in 1 million. If you are planning to have surgery, it is possible to donate your own blood for use during the operation as a sure way to avoid infection.

Q. Where can a person go to be tested for HIV?

A. Confidential testing is available at several places. Check with your family doctor, the university health center, or your local public health agency or call the AIDS hotline listed at the end of this chapter under "Additional Information Resources."

Q. Are STDs more common among African Americans, Hispanics, and other minorities? If so, why?

A. All racial and ethnic groups are affected by STDs, but there are persistent racial disparities in STD rates, with African Americans disproportionately affected. Although African Americans account for only about 13 percent of the population, the CDC reports that they account for 51 percent of HIV/AIDS cases diagnosed, 70 percent of the total number of gonorrhea cases, and nearly 50 percent of all chlamydia and syphilis cases. Hispanics have infection rates three times higher than whites for HIV and chlamydia. Some of this may be due to the fact that people of color may be more likely to go to public clinics that report the statistics better than private physicians do. But higher rates of STDs may also be due to poverty, disparities in access to health care, and/or lack of information about STDs. Regardless, it is behaviors, not racial or ethnic status, that affect health risk. Access to prevention, screening, and treatment is critical to addressing these disparities.

Q. What should I do if I think I might have an STD?

A. You may feel angry, embarrassed, or fearful. Don't let this stop you from doing the right thing.
- **See your doctor.** Only a physician can correctly diagnose and treat an STD.
- Take your medicine as prescribed.
- Inform your sexual contact(s). They might not be aware that they have been infected.
- If you have an STD, do not hide it from a potential sexual partner. Discuss it frankly before you are in the throes of a passionate embrace. Make sure your partner understands about risks of infection and protective measures and *use them* every time.
- If you are having an outbreak, abstain from sex.

Summary

Sexually transmitted diseases are a serious problem, especially among young adults. Chlamydia, gonorrhea, syphilis, genital herpes, and human papilloma virus are the most common STDs. HIV/AIDS, a deadly STD, makes preventive measures more important than ever for those who are sexually active. To reduce the risk of STDs, people must take responsibility for their sexual behavior and take protective measures, for themselves and their partners. It is also important to learn skills in communication, assertiveness, negotiation, and relating to others. Awareness of the risk of sexual assault and guidelines for recognizing and preventing it can make dating relationships safer for all.

Terms

- acquired immune deficiency syndrome (AIDS)
- bacterial vaginosis
- chancre
- chancroid
- chlamydia
- genital herpes
- genital warts
- gonorrhea
- hepatitis B
- herpes simplex virus
- human immunodeficiency virus (HIV)
- human papilloma virus (HPV)
- lymphocytes
- opportunistic diseases
- pelvic inflammatory disease (PID)
- pubic lice
- scabies
- sexual abstinence
- sexually transmitted disease (STD)
- syphilis
- T-cells
- trichomonas
- urethritis

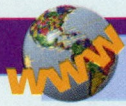

Internet Resources

Advocates for Youth

www.advocatesforyouth.org

Provides information about reproductive and sexual health. Has publications, news stories, statistics, and more.

American Academy of Family Physicians

www.familydoctor.org

Provides basic information on STDs, symptoms, and prevention.

American Social Health Association

www.ashastd.org

Provides information on prevention, screening, and disease management; a glossary of terms related to sexual health and disease; instructions for condom use; and fact sheets on STDs. Has good links to other sites.

Australia Ministry for Health: Child and Youth Health

www.cyh.com/

A good site for people who want to learn more about health relationships and sexual health. Click on "Young Adult Health" and "Sexual Health."

AVERT

http://www.avert.org

AVERT is an international HIV and AIDS charity, based in the U.K., working to avert HIV and AIDS worldwide through education, treatment, and care.

Centers for Disease Control and Prevention

www.cdc.gov

Has information and statistics on sexually transmitted diseases.

Columbia University's Q&A Internet Service

www.goaskalice.com

Click on "Sexual Health" for answers to your questions about STDs.

Medline Plus: Teen Sexual Health

www.nim.nih.gov/medlineplus/teensexualhealth.html

Contains news relating to sexual health and links to basic information sources (infections, condom use, abstinence, etc.).

National Institute of Allergy and Infectious Diseases, National Institutes of Health

www.niaid.nih.gov

Has fact sheets on sexually transmitted infections.

Planned Parenthood

www.plannedparenthood.org

Call 800-230-PLAN. Provides information about the diagnosis and treatment of STDs. Click on "Health Info," then "Sexually Transmitted Infections."

Videos

STD Awareness http://tinyurl.com/ch15stdaware

STD Documentary http://tinyurl.com/ch15stddoc

Types of Sexually Transmitted Infections
http://tinyurl.com/ch15sti

What Is HPV?
http://tinyurl.com/ch15hpv

Preventing HPV
http://tinyurl.com/ch15hpv

Syphilis, Chlamydia, Gonorrhea, Genital Warts, About
HIV and AIDS, Hepatitis B Vaccine, AIDS and Pregnancy
www.healthyroadsmedia.org/english/index.html

Two People Getting Tested for Chlamydia
http://tinyurl.com/ch15chlamidtest

The Process of HIV Cell Entry
http://tinyurl.com/ch15hiv

How to Use a Condom
www.ashastd.org/condom_use.cfm

How to Use a Female Condom
http://tinyurl.com/ch15female

Additional Information Resources

Division of STD Prevention (DSTDP)
Centers for Disease Control and Prevention
www.cdc.gov/std
Order Publications Online at www.cdc.gov/std/pubs/

STD information and referrals to STD Clinics
CDC-INFO
1-800-CDC-INFO (800-232-4636)
TTY: 1-888-232-6348
In English, en Español

National Herpes Hotline
1-919-361-8488

National STD Hotline
1-800-227-8922

CDC National Prevention Information Network (NPIN)
P.O. Box 6003
Rockville, MD 20849-6003
1-800-458-5231
1-888-282-7681 Fax

1-800-243-7012 TTY
E-mail: info@cdcnpin.org
www.cdcnpin.org

American Social Health Association (ASHA)
P.O. Box 13827
Research Triangle Park, NC 27709-3827
1-800-783-9877
www.ashastd.org

National AIDS Hotline
1-800-CDC-INFO (1-800-232-4636)
TTY: 1-888-232-6348
Hours: 24 hours a day, 7 days a week
E-mail: cdcinfo@cdc.gov

Project Inform
National HIV/AIDS Treatment Infoline: 1-800-822-7422
International: 1-415-558-9051
Hours: Monday through Friday 10:00 am to 4:00 pm
(Pacific Time)

LAB Activity 15-1

Name _____ Class/Activity Section _____ Date _____

Values Clarification Statements

Complete or respond to the following statements. They may be used for class discussion.

1. AIDS is _____

2. STDs are _____

3. If I found out I had an STD, I would _____

4. If I found out my partner had an STD, I would _____

5. Five ways to show someone you care about him or her without having sex are _____

   _____

   _____

   _____

   _____

   _____

6. Money for AIDS research should be cut because people get AIDS due to immoral lifestyles. Agree or disagree? Explain. _____

   _____

   _____

   _____

7. HIV infection is not a significant risk for college students. Agree or disagree? Explain. _____

   _____

   _____

   _____

   _____

8. My peers are changing their sexual behavior because of AIDS. Agree or disagree? Explain. ____

   _____

   _____

   _____

   _____

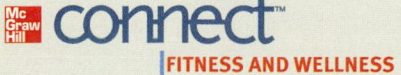

9. Condoms are not used much to prevent STDs on this campus. Agree or disagree? Explain _____

_____

_____

_____

10. Because of AIDS, it is easier to talk to my peers about sex. Agree or disagree? Explain. _____

_____

_____

_____

11. Both men and women should share responsibility for safer sex. Agree or disagree? Explain. _____

_____

_____

_____

12. "Just say no" is the right message to give young people about how to prevent STDs. Agree or disagree? Explain. _____

_____

_____

_____

13. Schools should distribute condoms to students. Agree or disagree? Explain. _____

_____

_____

_____

14. Sexual intercourse improves a relationship. Agree or disagree? Explain. _____

_____

_____

_____

15. Condom ads should be allowed on television. Agree or disagree? Explain. _____

_____

_____

_____

16. The media responsibly portray sex. Agree or disagree? Explain. _____

_____

_____

_____

LAB Activity 15-2

Name _____   Class/Activity Section _____   Date _____

Discussing Safer Sex

1. A person you know from class walks you home from a party and starts pressuring you for sex. You want to keep the friendship, but you don't want sex. What do you say?

2. At a party, a friend of yours has been drinking a lot and is being pressured to leave with a new acquaintance. Your friend is drunk and in no shape to make a decision. What do you say?

3. How would you lead into a discussion of condom use with a potential partner?

4. You want to use a condom, but your partner doesn't. How would you persuade your partner to use one?

5. How would you bring up the topic of STDs or previous risky sexual behavior with someone with whom you have a serious relationship?

6. You are in a long-term dating relationship and need to tell your partner that you have genital herpes. How do you begin this discussion?

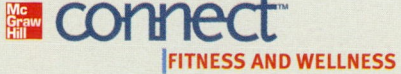

http://connect.mcgraw-hill.com

LAB Activity 15-3

Name _____ Class/Activity Section _____ Date _____

STD Discussion

1. Why is it often difficult for people to talk about STDs openly? Is it important to talk more openly about it? What would make it easier to discuss?

2. How do advertising, music, TV, and movies affect the decisions people make about engaging in risky or protective sexual behaviors?

3. If you could have the media give young adults one really important message about STDs, what would it be?

4. Has HIV affected your life? How?

5. Most people in college know about HIV and know how to protect themselves from STDs. But many don't follow through and have unprotected sex. What can be done to reduce risky behaviors (other than passing out condoms)?

6. What are the most important parts of a healthy romantic relationship?

7. You are in a new relationship and want to talk to your partner about testing for STDs, but you don't know how to bring it up. How do you get started?

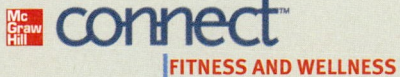

http://connect.mcgraw-hill.com

8. You have tested positive for an STD and need to tell your partner. What are some important points to bring up in your discussion?

9. How does each of the following factors affect the way you have or will make decisions about protecting yourself from STDs? Rate each factor from most to least important.

_____ friends

_____ parents

_____ media

_____ celebrities

_____ religious beliefs

_____ drugs or alcohol

_____ physical feelings

_____ person you are with

_____ your own values

10. Add your own STD question or issue here for discussion.

Exploring Lifetime Wellness Issues

STUDY QUESTIONS

You will have successfully mastered this chapter if you can answer the following:

1. Can you identify the four premises on which workplace wellness programs are based and give examples of wellness programs that corporations might offer their employees?

2. What are three ways parents can foster wellness habits in their children? Give two examples of behaviors within each dimension of wellness that parents can develop in a child.

3. What are two responsible precautions you can take to minimize your risk of injury/trouble in each of the following situations?
   a. While driving
   b. Walking alone on campus at night
   c. Living in an apartment or house

4. Can you describe five responsible precautions you can take to minimize your risk of being attacked, assaulted, or robbed?

5. Can you identify three trends and describe how they will affect wellness in the future?

6. Can you identify and describe three future challenges we face in regard to wellness?

7. What are six environmental concerns that may affect our wellness?

8. Can you define *quackery* and list six of its common characteristics?

You will find the answers as you read this chapter.

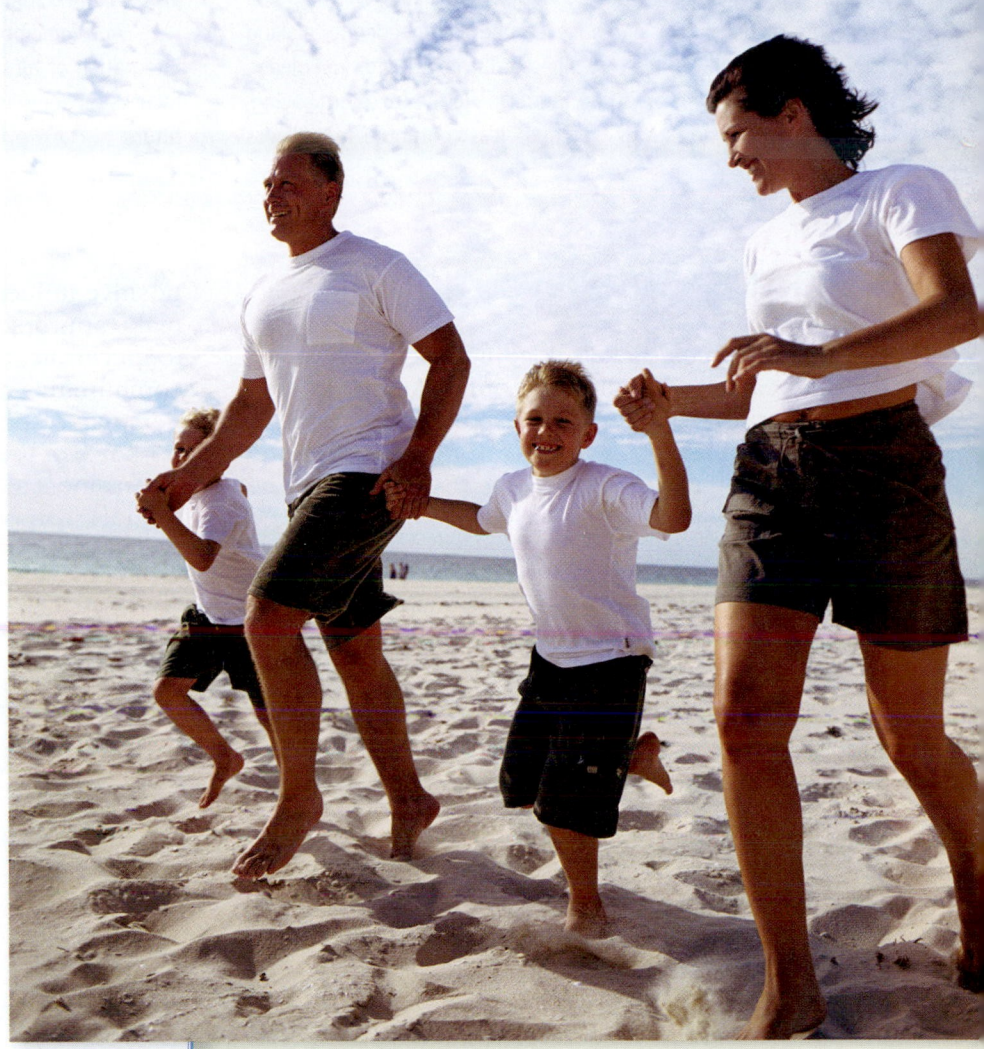

> " *Don't tell me what your priorities are. Instead, tell me what you did today and then I'll tell you what your priorities are.* "
> —Anonymous

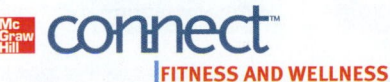

FITNESS AND WELLNESS

http://connect.mcgraw-hill.com

The purpose of this book is to present wellness as a lifestyle where positive choices result in optimal functioning and enhanced living. Of course, everyone has the same mortality: 100 percent. Nevertheless, the goal of wellness is to maintain health and vitality for as long as possible. While we cannot control everything that happens to us, we must all strive to accept personal responsibility for, and make informed decisions about, things that we can control. You now have the knowledge that will help you make informed decisions and have learned skills needed for making behavioral change. You are "wellness educated." With knowledge comes responsibility, so you no longer have the luxury of saying, "I didn't know!" You know which choices contribute to wellness and which ones do not. You can choose to eat right, exercise, and manage stress or choose not to. You know the possible consequences of such choices. The challenge of wellness is ongoing, whereas college coursework eventually comes to an end. A new career, different living environments, and family responsibilities will bring many changes to your life. During these changes, the wellness lifestyle can prevail. We hope it will grow for you. Wellness is a process, not a solution. It is a journey, not a destination.

And remember that wellness involves a balance among and integration of *all* seven dimensions of wellness. This final chapter focuses on some important issues to consider as you plan for the future.

◆ PARTNERS IN PREVENTION

The *Healthy People 2020* document sets high goals for the health and well-being of the American people. It emphasizes personal responsibility and self-empowerment as the means for increasing the quality and quantity of life. Some people need to be educated to make informed decisions. Others need positive influences and social support to help them make appropriate choices. For the wellness lifestyle to permeate our culture, support systems within communities must be available. While emphasizing personal responsibility, we cannot overlook the importance of the collective burden of responsibility of government policies, a wellness curriculum in the schools, corporate action, and the American family.

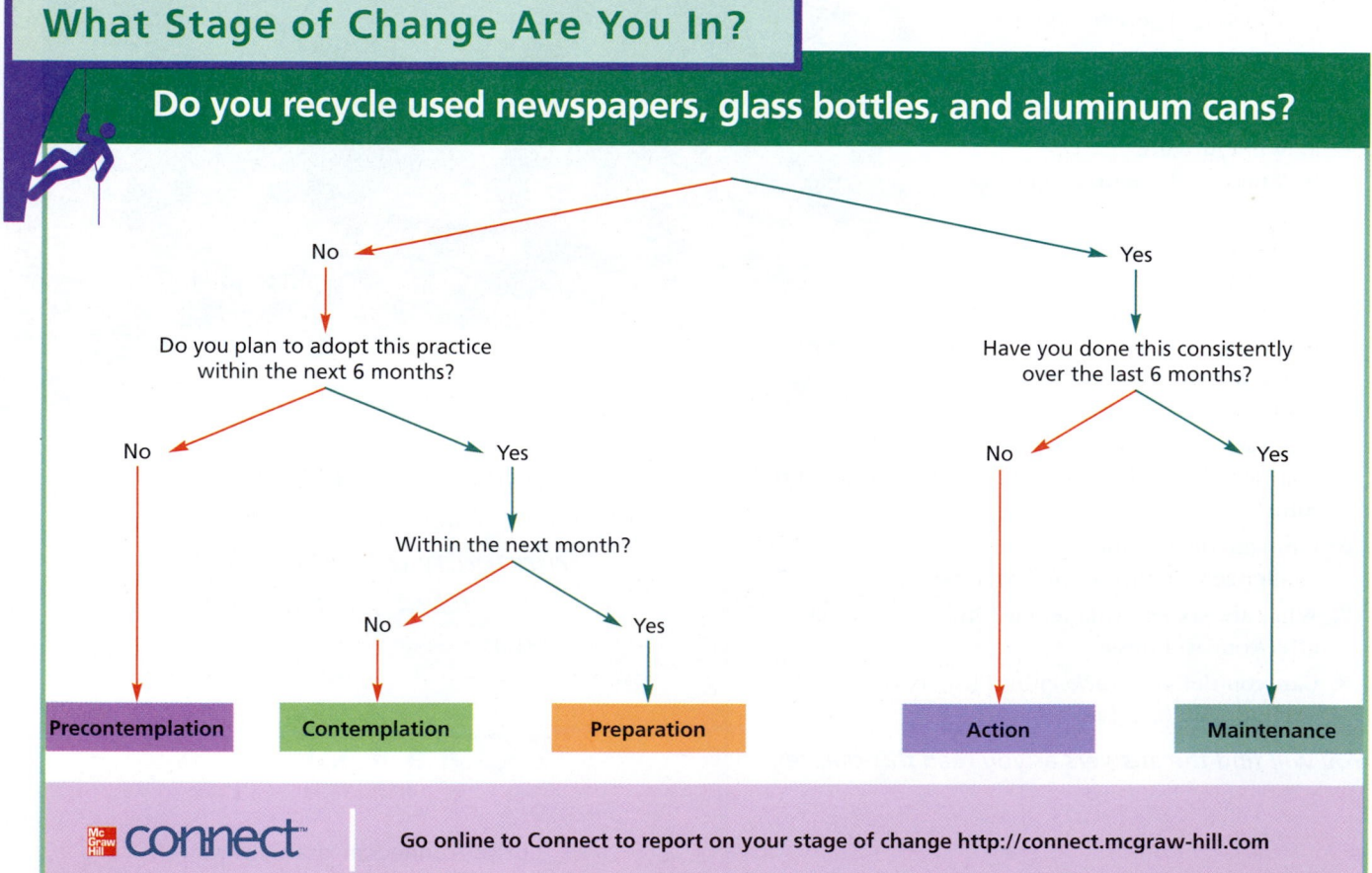

What Stage of Change Are You In?

Do you recycle used newspapers, glass bottles, and aluminum cans?

No

Do you plan to adopt this practice within the next 6 months?

No — Yes

Within the next month?

No — Yes

Yes

Have you done this consistently over the last 6 months?

No — Yes

| Precontemplation | Contemplation | Preparation | Action | Maintenance |

Go online to Connect to report on your stage of change http://connect.mcgraw-hill.com

Although personal behaviors contribute to the leading causes of death, behaviors occur in and are influenced by the environment. Various media and popular songs that glamorize drinking, violence, sex, and immoral behavior undermine our nation's health and well-being. For example, cigarette ads show likable young people in upscale settings enjoying smoking. The subliminal message is that cigarettes must not be so bad if such bright, attractive people are not afraid to smoke. In these ads, though, there are never dirty ashtrays, nicotine-stained teeth, or anyone coughing or getting chemotherapy. There is no dangerously underweight baby lying in intensive care. There is no one dying. An important part of wellness education is deciphering these messages and knowing what truly promotes well-being. Unfortunately our society sometimes makes it easy to do things we know are not good for us. It is easy to cocoon ourselves in our cars—driving through the ATM, fast-food restaurant, drugstore, and dry cleaner; in our offices—e-mailing, faxing, and telephoning; in our homes—watching movies, playing video games, and surfing the Internet. It is easy to overeat, underexercise, and feel stressed.

Individuals, families, communities, corporations, and the government share the task of enhancing the well-being of Americans. You are wellness educated, so part of this challenge of culture change rests with you. We must all work for changes in society that make it easier for everyone to stay healthy. How will you effect this change? Are you ready to become a leader and an example of wellness to those around you?

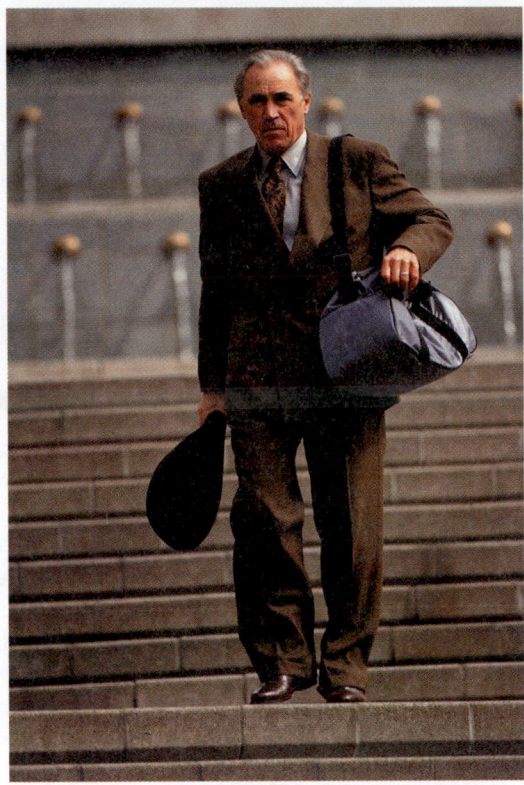

Many companies support employee wellness.

◆ WELLNESS IN THE WORKPLACE

Your job will be a prominent facet of your adult life. You will spend at least 50 percent of your waking hours at work if you maintain a full-time job or career. Cell phones, computers, e-mail, and fax machines have altered the complexion of American work. Twenty-four-hour manufacturing and retail shopping, the Internet, home-based businesses, voice mail, and telemarketing have revolutionized the business place. Even with enhanced technology and conveniences, the working hours of most Americans are longer than they were 50 years ago. These realities make the workplace a likely place to receive information and support regarding personal health improvement and wellness living. Leaders in business and industry are beginning to see employee wellness as an asset to be maintained and enhanced. When employees are happy and healthy, productivity increases. The promotion of

wellness programs in business and industry is based on four related premises:

1. Prevention is preferable to curing.
2. Teaching people to stay healthy is generally less expensive than treating them when they are ill.
3. Healthful lifestyles offer a better quality of life, higher morale, increased productivity, and possibly increased longevity.
4. Health promotion programs promote a favorable corporate image and help attract healthy, capable employees who see these programs as a valuable employee benefit.

Rising medical insurance costs, employee absenteeism, and sick leaves cut deeply into profits and lead to increases in the cost of doing business. On average, U.S. *Fortune* 500 corporations spend 61.2 percent of after-tax profits on medical care for employees, dependents, and retirees. As a result, corporate officials are finding ways to incorporate wellness into the workplace. This exciting avenue for health promotion can bring about changes in behavior for an improved lifestyle and enhance personal relationships. Wellness in the workplace can be promoted in a variety of ways. Programs can involve

✓ Diagnosis (assessment of current health and habits). Examples: blood pressure screenings, cholesterol and glucose testing.

✓ Education (give information about health enhancement). Examples: brochures on stress management, newsletters with back care information or healthy recipes.

✓ Behavior Modification (give on-site help and support in making a specific behavior change). Examples: healthy food choices in the cafeteria, employee workout center, smoking cessation classes, walking paths on the grounds.

Regardless of how they are organized, most corporate health promotion programs aim to facilitate behavior change. Employers realize that the work and nonwork parts of our lives are interactive. That is, job satisfaction is also dependent on family happiness, leisure pursuits, and feelings of worth. Knowing this, employers are actively pursuing a multidimensional approach to supporting employee wellness. Examples are flexible work hours, child care, on-the-job retraining, sports team participation, job sharing, smoke-free work sites, parental leaves, family hikes and picnics, and children's fitness classes. Several forward-thinking companies are responding to the needs of employees with elderly parents by providing elder care as well as providing substance abuse and marital counseling. Spouses and children of employees account for 40 to 60 percent of a company's health care expenditures, so such multidimensional programs can be cost-effective.

Due to the growing interest in and emphasis on wellness in business and industry, many employers prefer hiring personnel who have already adopted a wellness lifestyle. This should be added incentive for you to continue healthy living. As a potential employee, your confirmed dedication to wellness may also influence your final selection of a job and your chances of getting hired. You may favor a company that is highly supportive of wellness and provides wellness programs for employees, and that company may favor you. Remember how important a supportive environment is in the maintenance of positive lifestyle choices.

Many college students, pressured by school demands, believe they will have more time to exercise and eat right once they graduate. Your life will most likely be as busy, if not more so, once you begin your career. Time restraints and demands will always be with you. Making wellness living an important part of your current lifestyle will help you maintain it after graduation, as a habit.

◆ FAMILY ISSUES

In all cultures, the family unit is the primary transmitter of values and attitudes in the society. Each partner in a relationship comes with values, norms, and expectations derived from his or her family. Couples continue to grow, interact, and develop a value framework. If there are children in the family, the parental role of maintaining the culture from generation to generation is created. The interacting dynamics of a family unit promote the spiritual, physical, psychological, and social growth of each member.

The family units in today's society are not identical. Single parents, divorce, combined families, nontraditional relationships, and joint custody are realities that have changed the American family structure. Dual careers have altered the role of women within the family. Such changes affect the balance between work life and family life, often creating role conflicts, stress, and changing values. Regardless of the makeup of the family unit, nurturance remains essential for all members to strive toward full potential.

The Well Relationship

Many romantic fairy tales conclude with "and they lived happily ever after." Whereas these words *end* the story, marriage is most often the *beginning* of the story of a relationship in real life. Choosing someone to marry or to spend your life with is possibly the most important decision you will make in your life. Much of your happiness and life satisfaction will be based on the success of this relationship. Like the wellness lifestyle, a relationship demands conscious effort, commitment, and sacrifice. It is a partnership that involves change and growth. Many factors influence the success of such a relationship. Look at the Top 10 "Elements for Building a Strong and Lasting Relationship."

As in wellness growth, partner growth is a process. It doesn't happen all at once. Enjoy each step along the path.

The Well Child

If you become a parent, it will be your challenge to initiate wellness living in your child. All dimensions (emotional, social, physical, intellectual, spiritual, environmental, and occupational) demand your attention. If you favor behaviors that promote wellness, your children will follow your example. Family wellness patterns can set the stage for a lifelong pattern of self-responsibility. Self-responsibility relies on learning and practicing skills; therefore, you can be the master teacher of wellness and help your child grow as a decision maker. Children do not learn just in school. They learn by watching you too. If you exercise, eat nutritiously, read instead of watch television, handle stress, communicate your feelings, and display attitudes of cooperation and

TOP 10 LIST

Elements for Building a Strong and Lasting Relationship

1. *Communication:* Partners must be able to share their true feelings and really listen to each other (without being judged).
2. *Compromise:* Each partner must be willing to give a little. Sometimes it's 50:50, sometimes 100:0.
3. *Common values:* Common values and shared goals help maintain focus during tension-filled times.
4. *Likability and respect:* Enjoying each other's company and respecting each other's needs are essential.
5. *Shared responsibilities:* In a world where the two-parent career is the norm, each partner must be willing to share the responsibilities of home and child care.
6. *Finances:* Having a common financial philosophy or strategy for handling money can prevent many emotional confrontations.
7. *Trust:* Partners need to feel secure in their commitment and devotion to one another—without deception, secrets, or lies.
8. *Space:* Each partner needs to have his or her identity and be allowed to grow individually.
9. *Sense of humor:* Laughing and having fun are ways to keep daily problems in proper perspective.
10. *Love:* Unselfish love and devotion to each other will stand the test of time!

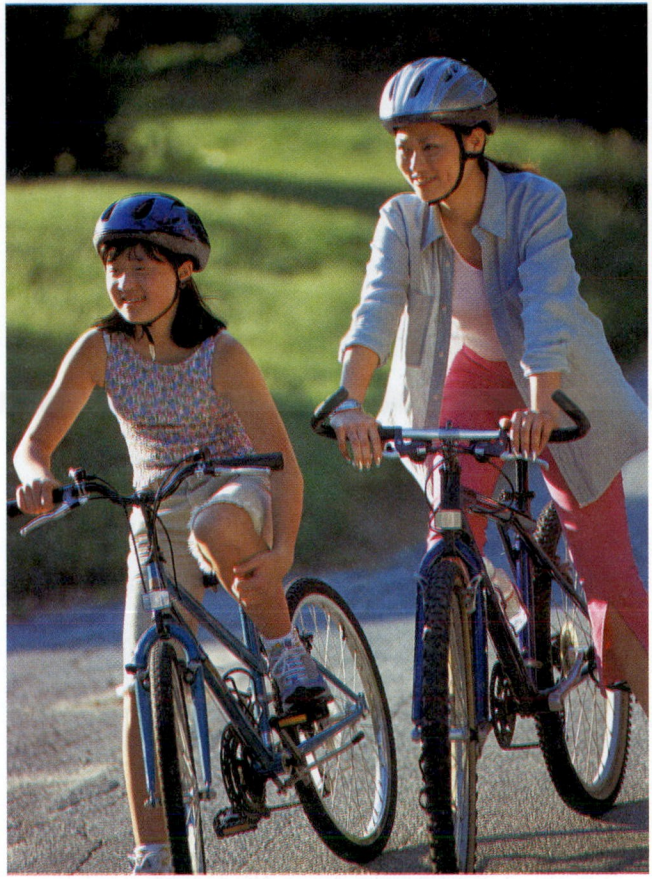

Parents are important role models for wellness.

respect, your child will too. Studies show that the strongest predictors of lifetime exercise activity in children are enjoyment of physical activity, family support of physical activity, and direct parental modeling of physical activity.

Nearly half of youths age 10 to 18 do not engage in enough physical activity to derive any aerobic or endurance benefit. Forty percent of children age 5 to 8 have at least one major heart disease risk factor. Obesity in children and teens is rising rapidly, and because of budget problems and more emphasis on academics, many schools are eliminating physical education. Thirty-eight percent of school-age children watch 3 or more hours of television on an average school day. Children with unhealthy habits have a greater likelihood of growing up to be unhealthy adults, so part of every parent's responsibility should be to create an environment for children that is conducive to optimum health and wellness. This includes being a positive role model. Aristotle expressed it best: "Good habits formed at youth make all the difference."

The self-concept of most children is formed by the time they start kindergarten; therefore, you as parents will be prime molders of that self-concept. Positive self-esteem is an important foundation as a child moves into larger social spheres beyond the family. A child with a high degree of self-worth is able to confront life's situations with confidence and optimism. Optimism and self-confidence are the building blocks for wellness living.

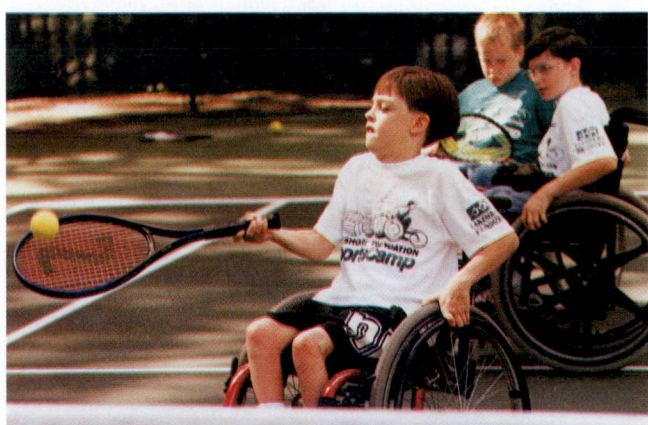

Every child deserves an opportunity to grow in all dimensions of wellness. (Photo courtesy of The Lakeshore Foundation, Birmingham, AL.)

TABLE 16-1 *Wellness Behaviors That Can Be Developed by a Child*

Physical Dimension

- Forms habits of regular, vigorous exercise
- Establishes healthy eating habits and preferences
- Forms self-care habits (seat belts, fire, bike riding, etc.)
- Establishes attitudes about smoking, drug use, and alcohol

Social Dimension

- Seeks companionship with others
- Senses responsibility for behavior
- Shows concern and respect for others
- Displays willingness to share work responsibilities with others

Emotional Dimension

- Forms feelings of self-worth and self-confidence
- Talks freely about feelings
- Develops appropriate coping behaviors for a variety of situations
- Displays the capacity to give and receive love

Spiritual Dimension

- Develops an awareness of life versus death
- Develops a sense of the importance and expanse of life
- Begins establishing a value system; can distinguish right from wrong
- Begins showing compassion and forgiveness

Intellectual Dimension

- Develops creativity and curiosity
- Establishes listening skills
- Learns cause-and-effect concepts
- Recognizes the expanse of the world through a variety of experiences

Occupational Dimension

- Identifies a variety of jobs/careers
- Understands the importance of work and effort
- Begins developing work habits
- Begins understanding the importance of money

Environmental Dimension

- Develops habits of recycling bottles, papers, cans, and so on
- Displays habits of energy conservation (water, electricity, etc.)
- Develops an appreciation for nature (plants, wildlife, etc.)
- Learns to maintain a clean environment by not littering

Although it is popularly believed that risk-taking behavior among teenagers and preteens is most strongly influenced by peer pressure, research by adolescent medicine specialists has shown that family closeness plays a key role. Young people who have a balance of strong attachment to family and parental encouragement to be involved in positive extracurricular activities are least likely to take part in high-risk activities (alcohol and drug use, sexual activities, cigarette experimentation) that could seriously affect their well-being.

Although the broad concept of wellness is difficult for young children to understand, they can become aware and learn the value of specific wellness choices. Their capacity to understand the cause and effect of certain choices depends on their age and maturity level. Can children learn to habitually fasten their seat belts? Select fruits for snacks? Show respect for others? Appreciate nature? Enjoy vigorous exercise? Of course, they can. Look at Table 16-1 for examples of wellness behaviors that parents are instrumental in developing in their children.

◆ PERSONAL SAFETY ISSUES

Throughout this book we have tried to increase your awareness of risks and personal choices that affect your wellness. Injuries and illnesses stemming from accidents and environmental hazards sometimes seem to be beyond the average person's control. Especially accidents—which are the fifth overall cause of death in the United States (but the number one cause of death among 15- to 44-year-olds)—often appear to be a matter of chance. You can substantially reduce the risks you are exposed to while driving, traveling, getting around campus, and working around your apartment or house by heeding basic safety precautions. Some of these precautions seem like common sense, yet for whatever reason, many people fail to follow even commonsense precautions. Federal, state, and local regulations have been established to help protect us from a variety of traffic, fire, water, and air travel tragedies. But laws and regulations cannot *make* people act. When you strive for high-level wellness, you must take seriously *all* lifestyle choices. The wellness concept is centered on an ongoing personal commitment to positive choices, so safety awareness and responsibility cannot be excluded.

We tend to focus solely on the impact an accident has on the physical dimension of wellness. The truth is, such a trauma can equally affect the emotional, social, occupational, and even spiritual dimensions. The following personal safety issues focus on choices that can help you control risks in your immediate environment.

Automobile Seat Belts

Motor vehicle crashes are the leading cause of death every year for Americans age 3 through 33. In

TABLE 16-2	*Why I Don't Buckle Up*

1. *"Seat belts are uncomfortable."* Unlike the original floor-anchored belts, new belts are designed to let you move freely until a collision occurs. And they are a lot more comfortable than a body cast or traction!

2. *"I'm only going to the store down the street."* Seventy percent of crashes occur within 25 miles of home, and 80 percent occur at speeds less than 40 mph. People not wearing seat belts have been killed at speeds less than 12 mph!

3. *"The belt will prevent me from being thrown clear of the accident."* Exactly! Your chances of being killed are 25 times greater if you're thrown out of the car.

4. *"The seat belt will trap me in a burning or submerged car."* Only one-half of 1 percent of crashes result in fire or submergence. Unfortunately, television action shows capitalize on such scenes. If you find yourself in this terrifying predicament, wouldn't it be better to have been restrained and thus be conscious enough to get out of the vehicle rather than to have had your head smashed into the windshield, leaving you unconscious and incapable of escaping?

talking about motor vehicle collisions, we deliberately chose not to use the word *accident,* which would imply a luck/fate approach to the topic. Instead, we use *crash* because it is well understood what specific actions you can take to reduce risks. Drunk-driving laws, child car-restraint regulations, seat belt laws, availability of air bags, and designated driver programs have done much to curtail traffic fatalities. Still, according to the National Highway Traffic Safety Administration (NHTSA), almost 40,000 Americans died in 2008 in car crashes (over 2 million were injured).

The importance of using seat belts cannot be overstated. Even if you practice all the other advice in this book (exercise regularly, eat a nutritious diet, don't smoke, etc.), *one* crash without a seat belt could immediately and irrevocably end your wellness program. It does not make sense, if we care about health and wellness, not to buckle up. Table 16-2 lists

the most common excuses people give for choosing not to use their seat belts. We hope you do not use the same flimsy excuses. Overall seat belt compliance is around 84 percent, but younger drivers are the least compliant. Sixty-five percent of 16- to 20-year-olds killed in nighttime crashes were unbelted at the time. Even though newer model cars include air bags, your seat belt is still your first line of defense in all crashes.

Driving Safety

The best driver is a defensive driver—one who can anticipate potential danger and respond appropriately. Attitude is a key ingredient in defensive driving. Speeding, following too closely, and improper lane changing are the most common traffic infractions leading to crashes. Driver inattention has also become a major contributor to crashes. The National Highway Traffic Safety Administration (NHTSA) has estimated that driver inattention or distraction is responsible for nearly 80 percent of traffic crashes.

Drivers focusing on newspapers, eating, cell phones, grooming, iPods, and navigation devices cause an estimated 1.2 million crashes every year. Cars have become mobile offices and living rooms, causing driver inattention to be the fourth most serious detriment to safe driving, behind drunken driving, aggressive driving, and speeding. One of the most common distractions for a driver is using a cell phone. According to the NHTSA, in the United States 974,000 vehicles on the road at any given daylight moment are being driven by someone who is using a handheld cell phone. Research indicates that whether it is a hands-free or handheld cell phone, the cognitive distraction is significant enough to degrade a driver's performance. This can cause a

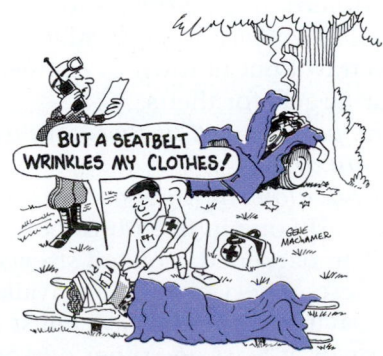

What is your excuse for not wearing a seat belt?

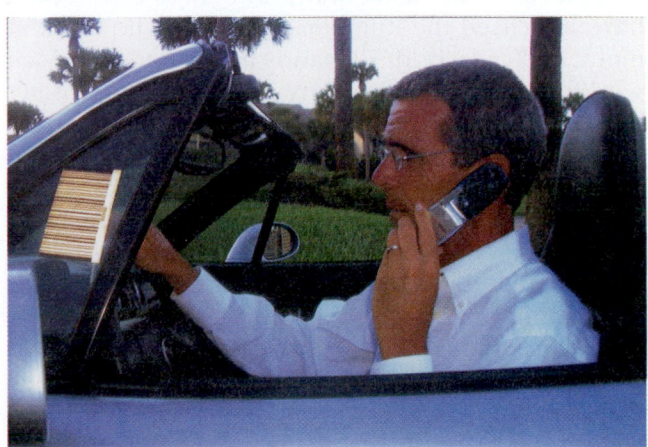

In some parts of the country it is illegal to talk on a cell phone while driving, because talking on a phone while driving quadruples the risk of having a crash. Texting while driving is even worse.

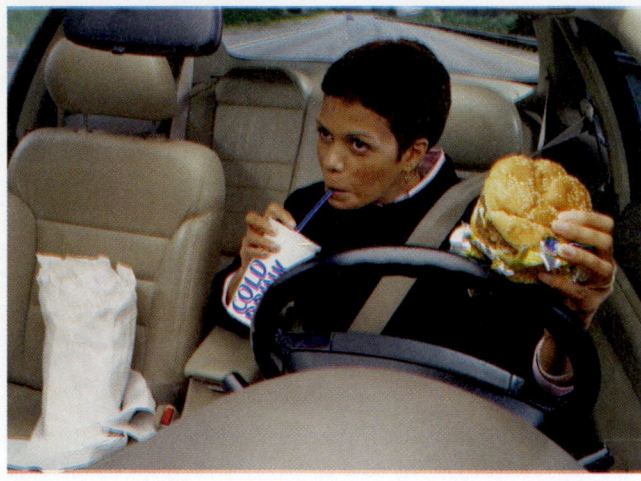

Distractions have become a large part of everyday driving and contribute to nearly 80 percent of crashes.

driver to miss key visual and audio cues needed to avoid a crash. A recent surge in fatal accidents caused by text-messaging on cell phones by drivers has resulted in legislation in several states to make it illegal to use cell phones while driving.

A driving risk causing new concern is *driving while drowsy (DWD)*. DWD has been an underrated risk factor in crashes and accounts for as many as 100,000 car crashes annually in the United States. A *Sleep in America* survey found that 60 percent of drivers admit to driving while drowsy. Furthermore, 37 percent of drivers have admitted to actually falling asleep at the wheel! And the greatest incidence of drowsy driving crashes occurs among drivers under the age of 25. For a variety of reasons, more people are juggling jobs (sometimes more than one), school, and family responsibilities. Loss of sleep and driving at odd hours have become commonplace. Today's economy and high-tech boom have increased the number of people who work at night. A "24/7 world" demands an around-the-clock workforce. As a result, many Americans do not get enough sleep. Sleep deprivation affects many aspects of personal well-being, including driving safety. Getting 6 to 8 hours less sleep than usual over a week not only impairs mental efficiency and reaction time but also weakens the immune system and causes depression, anxiety, and irritability. Combining drowsiness with the comforts in modern vehicles, it is easy to lose sight of the fact that driving a powerful automobile carries tremendous responsibility and demands constant attention.

Crime Prevention

As much as we hate to admit it, crime and violence are a real part of contemporary U.S. life. Whether

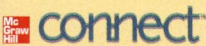
you are at school, traveling, at work, or going about daily living routines, you can become a victim. Even in the idyllic setting of a college campus, assaults, sexual attacks, and thefts occur. You can help protect yourself from being a victim by taking some basic precautions. A constant awareness of your environment is the best weapon for guarding your personal safety. Always be alert to your surroundings whether in your car, on the street, in a campus building, or at home. There is nothing extraordinary about the following personal safety tips. They are simple examples of assuming self-responsibility for your wellness.

1. *Always lock your house, apartment, residence hall room, and car—even when you are there.*
2. *Take extra precautions (i.e., informing a friend or neighbor, securing valuables, leaving lights and/or a radio on, etc.) when leaving for an extended vacation, attending a publicized family funeral or wedding, or attending a graduation activity.* College athletes who have to travel out of town to competitions are popular targets for thefts.
3. *At night, park in well-lit spots and walk in brightly lit areas.*
4. *Never walk alone at night or in unpopulated areas.* Nearly one in five rapes occurs on unfamiliar, darkened, isolated streets. Use a campus escort service if one is available. Even during daylight hours, always enlist the company of at least one other person when jogging or exercising outside.

5. *Beware of suspicious persons in buildings, hallways, parking areas, elevators, stairwells, and rest rooms.* Note their description and contact the police or security.

6. *Don't let strangers know when you are home alone.*

7. *Glance into your car, checking the seats and floor, before getting in.*

8. *Never hitchhike or pick up hitchhikers.*

9. *If you are being harassed, turn and proceed toward lights and people.* If someone accosts you, yell "fire" instead of "help," because more people are likely to respond.

10. *Watch your alcohol consumption.* Drinking puts you at risk and makes you vulnerable to assault, robbery, and rape.

11. *Secure all valuables and don't flaunt expensive possessions.*

12. *When you are walking alone, walk with your shoulders back and your head held high.* Keep a strong and steady pace. Remain alert and be aware of your surroundings. Muggers and rapists rarely attack those who appear assured and confident. Also, walk facing traffic, even if you're on the sidewalk. This prevents an assailant in a car from sneaking up on you from the rear.

13. *Don't wear headphones or other devices that would make it difficult to predict and avoid a confrontation.*

14. *Let a roommate or a friend know where you are going and how long you might be gone when you leave.*

Too often after an accident or tragic event someone says, "I wish I would have. . . ." Always have a plan of action. Play a mental game of "what if"—where you would go and what you would do should a dangerous situation occur. Trust your instincts. Research shows that a large percentage of people who have been assaulted had a feeling something was wrong just before being attacked. Being careful may seem boring to some, but it *is* the wellness way.

◆ WELLNESS TRENDS AND CHALLENGES FOR THE FUTURE

In his 1982 highly acclaimed book *Megatrends,* John Naisbitt predicted, "The focus of health care is shifting from the short-term treatment of illness to the long-term attainment of wellness. No longer regarded as a passing fad, wellness is a trend that is here to stay." We have already seen the wellness trend give impetus to societal changes. Smoking bans in restaurants, seat belt laws, shopping mall

wellness screenings, community walking clubs, and healthier food choices in groceries and restaurants are examples of positive wellness changes. What else is down the road for wellness? What other changes and trends will you see in your lifetime? Also, what are the challenges that will continue to demand attention? The remainder of this chapter addresses these questions as well as consumer issues.

Trend 1: Changes in Health Care

One of the biggest trends is the changing focus in hospitals and the health care profession. Medical care is beginning to shift from strictly a sickness business to a wellness business. Many community hospitals offer a variety of wellness programs with the intention of preventing individuals from becoming ill and needing hospitalization. Cholesterol testing, nutrition workshops, family counseling, drug rehabilitation, weight-management classes, and exercise prescription are examples of such programs. Some hospitals offer support services for a variety of specific groups (cancer survivors, families with Alzheimer members, diabetes education, etc.).

Prevention is finally being acknowledged as a cornerstone of the health care system, rather then an afterthought. Health promotion efforts that change behaviors can have a profound impact on the health of the nation because lifestyle behaviors account for 75 percent of chronic diseases. Community-based programs that provide screenings, immunizations, and education cost less than paying for illness. Many medical schools are expanding physician training to include studying lifestyle and preventive influences on health and

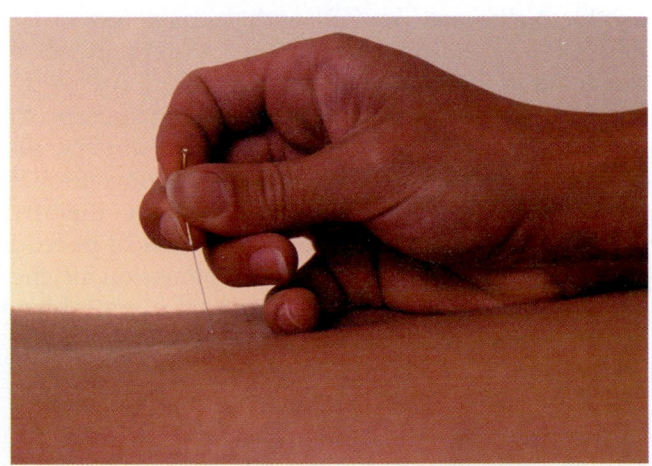

Alternative therapies such as acupuncture are gaining respectability as emerging research supports their effectiveness.

disease rather than solely learning to identify and cure illness. There is compelling evidence showing that physicians exert a strong influence on their patients' behavior patterns. By incorporating preventive services and counseling into their patient encounters, physicians can dramatically affect the well-being of the nation. In this way, physicians can become a prime force in advocating a wellness lifestyle.

One of the most interesting evolutions occurring in health care is the emergence and acceptance of more natural medical therapies. "Alternative," "complementary," "holistic," "integrative," or "naturopathic" medicine, with treatments involving acupuncture, nutritional and herbal supplementation, massage, homeopathy, hypnosis, aromatherapy, and biofeedback, are being introduced into hospitals and medical research centers across the country. Many of these therapies are ancient medical traditions from Oriental, Native American, Asian, and European cultures. With or without the doctor's blessing, Americans are flocking to these therapies. According to a national government survey released in May 2007, 38 percent of U.S. adults age 18 and over use some form of alternative therapy. Women were more likely than men to use these therapies, and persons with higher educational attainment were more likely than persons with lower educational levels. In addition, annual expenditures on these therapies accounts for approximately $33.9 billion of total out-of-pocket health care expenditures.

As evidence that the medical and scientific communities are recognizing these previously unorthodox methods, the National Institutes of Health (NIH) established the National Center for Complementary and Alternative Medicine (NCCAM). NCCAM has defined **complementary medicine** and **alternative medicine** (CAM) as "a group of diverse medical and health care systems, practices, and products that are not presently considered to be part of conventional medicine." Complementary medicine is used *together with* conventional medicine. An example would be to use aromatherapy to help lessen a patient's discomfort after surgery. Alternative medicine is used *in place of* conventional medicine. An example of an alternative therapy would be using a special diet to treat cancer instead of using radiation. The overriding mission of the NCCAM is to support rigorous research and objective inquiry into which complementary and alternative practices work, which do not, and why they work or don't work. There are current ongoing studies involving CAM practices for arthritis, asthma, cardiovascular diseases, cancer, immunology, digestive diseases, osteoporosis, diabetes, and more. This is providing Americans with reliable information about the safety and effectiveness of

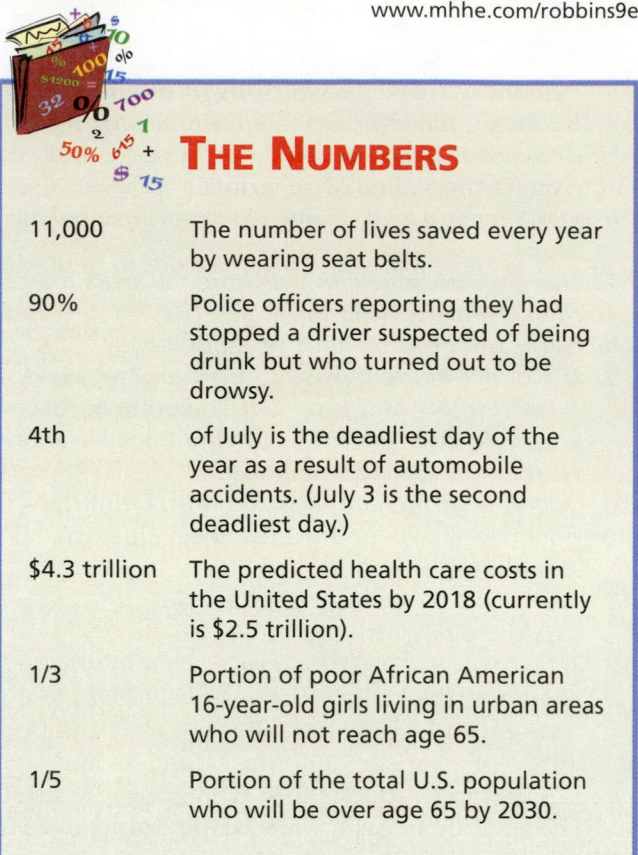

THE NUMBERS

11,000	The number of lives saved every year by wearing seat belts.
90%	Police officers reporting they had stopped a driver suspected of being drunk but who turned out to be drowsy.
4th	of July is the deadliest day of the year as a result of automobile accidents. (July 3 is the second deadliest day.)
$4.3 trillion	The predicted health care costs in the United States by 2018 (currently is $2.5 trillion).
1/3	Portion of poor African American 16-year-old girls living in urban areas who will not reach age 65.
1/5	Portion of the total U.S. population who will be over age 65 by 2030.

these practices. As a result of the emerging research, many of these therapies are gaining a more mainstream image among a multitude of skeptical medical doctors.

Why are people attracted to alternative therapies? The reasons vary, but may include the availability of information via the Internet relevant to alternative therapies, dissatisfaction with conventional medical practices, and the desire of patients to become active partners in their healing process. One-half of CAM users initially try these therapies out of interest and curiosity. Many express a strong belief that such therapies help.

Results from many studies are validating these natural therapies. Because most of these alternative treatments are far less expensive and less physically invasive than standard medical procedures, their use and popularity will continue to grow dramatically. With scientific journals covering complementary therapies now appearing, it is evident that science is beginning to direct medicine back toward the principles of enabling the body to heal itself with more natural and preventive practices—*including* personal lifestyle changes. These visionary words by Thomas Alva Edison represent this wellness trend: "The doctor of the future will give no medicine, but will interest his patients in the care of the human frame, in diet and in the cause and prevention of disease."

The high cost of medical care and the rising cost of health insurance have initiated another related trend. Insurance companies are beginning to provide incentives for staying well. Insurance benefits are being expanded and costs are being lowered for those who actively strive for optimal well-being by refraining from smoking, participating in periodic health screenings, maintaining a healthy weight, and exercising regularly. Some health insurance companies now cover the costs of the new, emerging complementary therapies such as acupuncture and massage therapy. Group health benefits at reduced rates will be sought by companies that promote wellness in their workplaces and have predominantly healthy employees.

The underlying theme is that *preventing* ill health is more efficient and effective than *treating* illness. Prevention saves money, lives, and suffering, and, most important, it enhances human vitality and potential.

Trend 2: Aging America

All demographic studies document that the population of the United States is getting older. In January 2011, the first baby boomer will turn 65. Baby boomers (those born after World War II between 1946 and 1964) make up the largest segment of our population. In 2000, 13 percent of the U.S. population was 65 years of age or over. It is estimated that by 2030, this percentage will almost double, resulting in 71 million citizens, or one in five Americans. It is estimated that the population 85 years of age and older will more than double to nearly 10 million persons! This oldest of the old is the fastest growing segment of our population, and women constitute the majority of this older group.

It is well understood that poor health and loss of independence are not inevitable consequences of aging. Research has shown that healthy lifestyles are more influential than genetic factors in helping older people avoid the deterioration traditionally associated with aging. Therefore, many people are living longer because of healthier habits as well as modern medical treatments for heart disease and cancer. Death rates from heart disease among persons age 65 to 84 have been reduced by half. This is all good news as far as your life expectancy is concerned but could lead to huge shortfalls in available health care, pensions, and social services. Nevertheless, diabetes and other obesity-related conditions are on the rise. As a result, the nation's health care spending is projected to increase by 25 percent due to these demographic shifts and anticipated health needs.

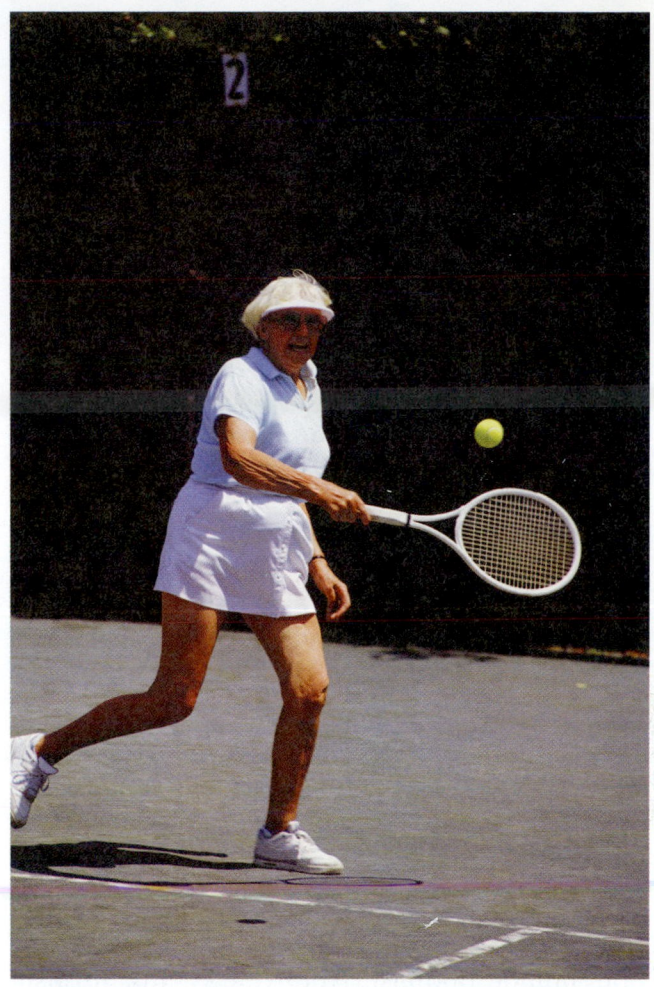

The older population is growing at a faster rate than is the population as a whole. And many seniors are healthy, self-sufficient, and physically capable.

Many older people are healthier, wealthier, and better educated than previous generations, but these gains have not been equal among today's older Americans. As a result, describing the 60-plus age group is not an easy task. This diverse group is not one unified consumer group with similar needs and attitudes. Much of this population is not, as many would think, senile or confined to nursing homes. A study released by the National Academy of Sciences found a 14.5 percent decline in the proportion of older people who cannot take care of themselves. Yet some groups of older Americans are disproportionately disadvantaged, especially women and minorities. Many senior citizens have money to spend and a desire to continue being active contributors to society. Some have retired, remarried, and begun second careers. A recent AARP survey revealed that 80 percent of retirees plan to continue working in some capacity. Consider the impact this will have in the working world! These people want and need programs for nutrition education, exercise, personal enrichment, and financial management. They want housing alternatives and socialization opportunities. It is apparent that an aging population will dramatically affect both the health and the economic facets of our society.

Trend 3: The Mind–Body Connection

There has been an explosion of research in **psychoneuroimmunology (PNI),** the study of how emotions, behavior, and mental attitudes affect the immune system and the onset and course of illness. At one time, physiologists thought the immune system functioned independently from the central nervous and endocrine systems. Now it is clear that emotional states affect us right down to our cells. Researchers have shown that nerve cells connect directly to organs of the immune system, that hormones responsive to stressful experiences affect the immune response, and that psychological and social factors can affect the immune system's responsiveness. Additional research into the chemicals produced by the brain has shown that the immune system and the brain communicate chemically. Mental states such as loneliness, depression, fear, and pessimism alter the responses in the immune system. Stress is considered one of the top contributors to a lowered immune system. In contrast, experiencing close relationships, hope, compassion, humor, optimism, forgiveness, and altruism enhance the body's ability to fight diseases. Owning a pet has even been found to have a positive effect on health! The immune system is most active during sleep. During your deepest states of sleep, your body releases immune system moderators that promote resistance to viral infections. Therefore, sleep deprivation is harmful to your immune system. Look at the Top 10 "Immune System Boosters." How many of these traits do you possess?

One of the first studies in support of psychoneuroimmunology was conducted by Dr. David Spiegel, a psychiatrist at the Stanford University School of Medicine. He and his colleagues demonstrated the power of group support for cancer patients. Patients with advanced breast cancer who participated in weekly group sessions had significantly enhanced survival times and a much better quality of life—less anxiety, less depression, and half as much pain. Spiegel's research continues to support the impact of social support and the mind on the physical body. Mental outlook is not a fixed quality. People can learn optimism and happiness at any age! Dr. Spiegel's words say it all: "It is not simply mind over matter, but it is clear that mind matters."

TOP 10 LIST

Immune System Boosters

1. *Optimism.* Health can be a self-fulfilling prophecy. Good things happen to people who expect them. Pessimism, fatalism, and resignation are linked to poorer health.
2. *An unsinkable spirit.* Belief in the ability to make it through any crisis is essential.
3. *Taking charge.* Whereas a fighting spirit provides motivation, a take-charge attitude (also termed *active coping*) puts that spirit into action.
4. *Stress reduction.* By using exercise, relaxation, meditation, and other personal coping strategies, you give your immune system a big boost.
5. *Altruism.* Giving to others and making the world a better place have physical and mental benefits.
6. *A sense of humor.* Being able to laugh at yourself— as opposed to ridiculing others—is health enhancing.
7. *Absence of malice.* Those who have a lot of hostility are especially susceptible to disease.
8. *Social connectedness.* How would you answer the question, "Can you count on anyone to provide you with emotional support?" A yes means your relationships with people make a real difference in your health.
9. *Sleep.* Getting 7 to 9 hours of sleep every night allows your immune system to function optimally.
10. *Nutritional support.* The immune system is a voracious user of vitamins and minerals. Just as a Ferrari can't run on kerosene, your system needs good fuel to function adequately.

This area of research brings a fascinating approach to health care. Mind–body interventions, including relaxation techniques, meditation, biofeedback, autogenic training, and visualization, are being given credibility thanks to sophisticated research. In fact, the National Institutes of Health plans to spend $3.5 million over the next several years on "mind/body" medicine. Clinical applications of these techniques have shown promise in arresting the development of heart disease, cancer, AIDS, gastrointestinal problems, asthma, and chronic pain. Pioneers in this emerging area—Dr. Dean Ornish, Dr. Herbert Benson, and Dr. Andrew Weil— view mind–body therapies as mainstream medicine (rather than "alternative") that provide as much symptom relief as drugs or any other modern medical treatment has to offer. This exciting news clearly solidifies the strong connection between emotions, spirit, spirituality, and physical well-being. The future looks bright in this important area of medical research.

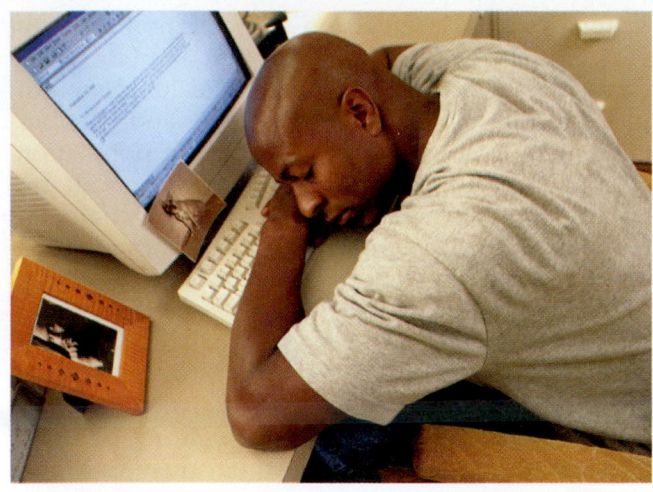

Sleep deprivation not only affects your productivity and driving safety, it weakens your immune system.

Challenge 1: Rising Health Care Costs

Since 1960 health care spending has grown significantly faster than the economy, meaning that we are spending an even larger portion of our incomes on this care. In 1960, health care constituted 5.1 percent of the total U.S. economy. Today it constitutes 17.6 percent and is expected to skyrocket an average of 7 percent per year. What is causing this escalating cost? Technological advances, new medical procedures, an aging population, and an ever-expanding list of new drugs have created a culture where curing diseases, eliminating discomforts, and staving off aging is growing faster than the ability of many Americans to pay. Replacement hips, vision correction surgery, liposuction, and a vast array of drugs like Viagra have changed the definition of old age. The root of the crisis is unmanageable costs in a system that focuses on "disease management" rather than true "health care." Costly tests and procedures are often ordered by physicians because they are worried about lawsuits. Billions are spent on tests, treatments, and hospitalizations that do little or nothing to improve our health. Chronic diseases like type 2 diabetes are on the rise. The doubling of obesity since 1987 accounts for nearly 30 percent of the rise in health care spending. Drug companies spend millions to advertise the benefits of their drugs, increasing drug costs, and nearly one-third of our health care dollars go to the administrative costs of health insurance companies. It is no wonder that spiraling health care costs are bankrupting some employers. Ironically, although there is excess care for some, millions have no health care insurance for even basic care.

It is a complex problem, but the bottom line is that more health expenditures do not always equal better health. For example, a middle-aged attorney with health care coverage of 100 percent hospitalization, 100 percent coverage of physician's visits, and a prescription drug plan may take two medicines for diabetes, one for high blood pressure, two for high cholesterol, and one for anxiety. He may have already had two angioplasties for clogged arteries, and has a good chance of having future heart bypass surgery. This person has wonderful health insurance and an abundance of health care. What he doesn't have is *health!* According to David Cutler, a health economist at Harvard, one problem in medicine is that "we pay for what's done, not what's accomplished." There is no clear answer for curbing these escalating costs other than promoting prevention, because preventing illness is far cheaper than treating it.

Challenge 2: Diversity

One of the biggest challenges we face is making wellness information and services available to *everyone*—and making wellness a priority in *all* people's lives despite our many differences. The racial and ethnic composition of the United States is changing dramatically. According to the U.S. census, America is becoming more racially diverse. Roughly one-third of the U.S. population are minorities, with the Hispanic population growing the fastest. Hispanic Americans outnumber African Americans for the first time in history, making them the largest minority group in the United States. The Asian American population is also rising rapidly. These facts make the United States one of the most multiracial countries in the world.

Our diversity should be celebrated and recognized as a basis for national strength; it also presents challenges in meeting the health and wellness needs of everyone. Ideally, wellness has no race, class, or income. However, the gulf is widening between the haves and the have-nots, the insured and the uninsured, and whites and minorities. Despite widespread efforts to promote a population-wide adoption of healthy lifestyles, little progress has been made in decreasing the incidence of—and the racial/ethnic disparities in—chronic diseases over the past decade. The death rate for chronic diseases is more than twice as high among adults with fewer than 12 years of education than among those with more than 12 years of education. And blue-collar workers, low-socioeconomic and low-education groups, and persons with the highest risk for coronary heart disease (particularly smokers) are the individuals most resistant to public health promotion. These people cannot afford health club memberships and specialized medical screenings. Many are more concerned about maintaining decent housing and feeding their families than about their cholesterol levels.

Generalizations about various subgroups from local studies can be misleading because of the disparities among subgroups in different geographic locations. Nevertheless, the most striking aspect of health comparison rates is the tremendous gap between low-income people and all other groups. Nearly one of every eight Americans lives in a family with an income below the federal poverty level; and for virtually all the chronic diseases that lead the nation's list of killers, low income is a special risk factor. Poor urban neighborhoods are unhealthy *not* because of drugs or violence, as some would guess, but because of chronic diseases like heart disease, type 2 diabetes, and obesity. Social factors and physical environments have a huge impact on lifestyle choices.

Everyone deserves a high level of functioning and well-being. Showing how small lifestyle changes can enhance well-being, providing wellness information, and changing attitudes toward self-responsibility in our diverse population are difficult. But making wellness available to all Americans is a wellness issue.

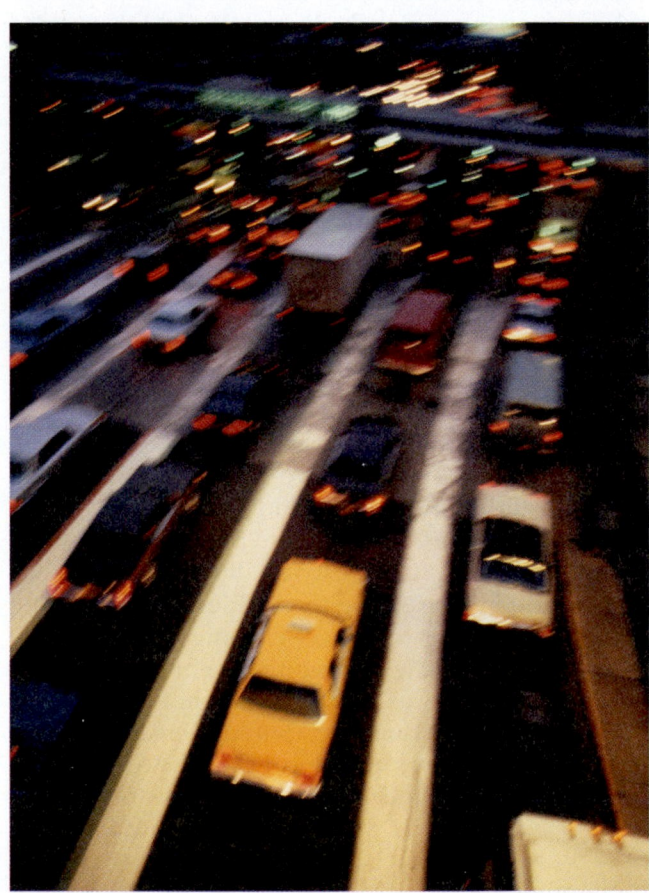

Carbon dioxide emissions from fossil fuels are a huge contributor to world pollution.

In today's world, television is a common learning environment, especially for the uneducated. While there is a considerable amount of health-related information in television programming and commercials, many times, for our vastly diverse population, the suggestions seem impersonal, impractical, and unrealistic. This presents a considerable challenge to those in health promotion. Perhaps the biggest payoff would be to integrate wellness information, behaviors, and attitudes into all segments of primary and secondary school curricula, reaching all youth before unhealthy life habits develop. Schools are increasingly challenged to deliver an educational experience that meets the cultural needs of a diverse student body. Wellness information should also be integrated into America's workplaces and community centers.

In *Healthy People 2020,* the U.S. government prioritized "eliminating health disparities and improving health for all groups" as one of its foremost goals. However, it is not enough to ask or expect every individual to accept responsibility for health and well-being without communities, businesses, health organizations, families, and civic organizations joining *with the government* to bring about national wellness. This would be a good time to review the "Diversity Issues" box in Chapter 1. Are there any actions that you can take to help eliminate health disparities?

Challenge 3: The Environment

Environmental policy has long been an important part of public health. Throughout history, regulations regarding safe food, water, and sewage management have substantially improved our well-being. However, rapid technological changes have resulted in new environmental hazards, including many whose effects on the body may remain unrecognized for years. Worldwide consumption has had a tremendous effect on the world's resources and energy supplies. Cartoon character Pogo's insightful quip "We have met the enemy and he is us" is particularly appropriate in addressing the challenge we face in saving and protecting the environment. This opens new opportunities for you to make an impact on your wellness—and that of others.

Being apathetic or becoming accustomed to environmental pollution is a serious matter. That you cannot do everything is no excuse for doing nothing. There is a lot you can do to limit, or at least minimize, the pollution and overconsumption in your "little world." As in all areas of wellness improvement, form a personal plan to combat environmental hazards. Look at the following list of environmental concerns, and consider ways you could make

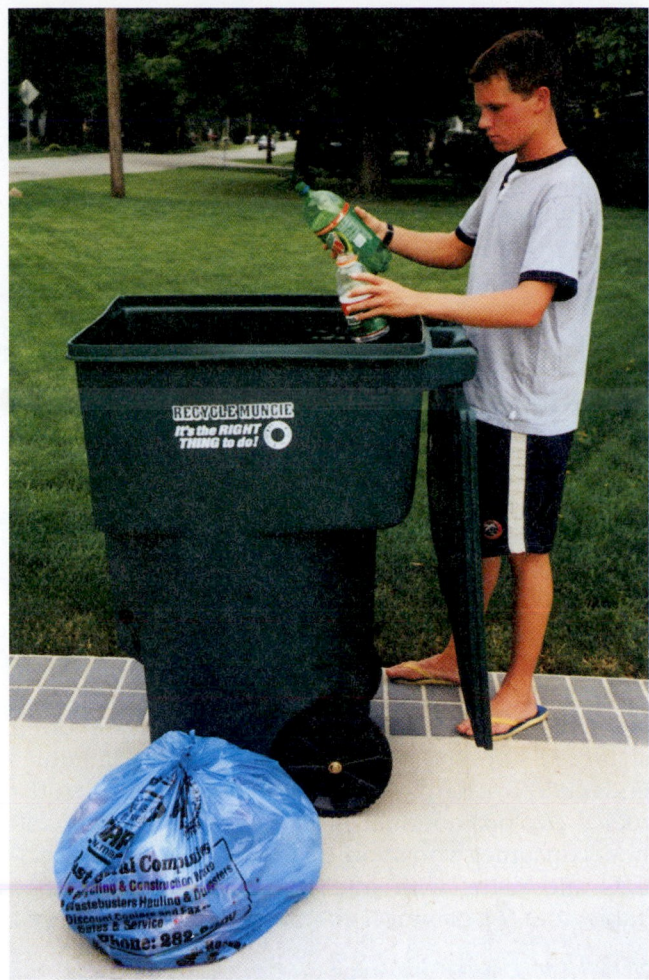

Recycling conserves natural resources, lowers demand for energy, reduces air and water pollution, and saves landfill space. You *can* make a difference!

3. Making new paper out of recycled paper uses only 10 to 40 percent of the energy required to make new paper from virgin materials. Also, fewer chemicals are needed in the manufacturing process.
4. Residues of harmful pesticides can be found in the air, on crops, in the ground, and in water supplies. Lawn and garden chemicals are significant contributors to this.
5. Water and air, essential for life, face increasing contamination. Fish caught in polluted waters may be contaminated.
6. Loud rock music is associated with hearing loss.
7. Traffic sounds, aircraft noise, and noisy industrial areas are associated with stress and stress-related physical symptoms.
8. Radon gas and asbestos have been linked to cancer. Radon is a naturally occurring radioactive gas emitted by soil and rocks. Radon is diluted to safe levels outdoors but can be dangerously concentrated if trapped in poorly ventilated basements, houses, and buildings. Asbestos, a commonly used insulating material, has been linked to a variety of lung diseases. By order of the U.S. government, no asbestos has been manufactured since 1997.
9. Exposure to high levels of lead is toxic to the central nervous system and can be fatal. House paints used before 1980 often contained lead. Also, people who live near airports, battery factories, and landfills are at risk.
10. Plastic bags, bottles, and cups often wind up in the world's oceans, eventually killing marine mammals and fish who mistakenly think this trash is food.

We often take too many things for granted. Part of your challenge in wellness living will be to assume some responsibility for preserving the environment. Lab Activity 16-2 is intended to help you evaluate your habits. This personal challenge must then progress to the next level: more social and political action nationwide. Remember the 3 R's: reduce, reuse, and recycle.

changes in your daily living to make the world a better place in which to live.

1. The earth's protective ozone layer—our shield against the sun's hazardous ultraviolet rays—is being eaten away by human-made chemicals. The result is damaged food crops and ocean plants, increased skin cancer and cataracts, and changes in weather systems. The United States accounts for 25 percent of the world's annual global warming pollution, yet we make up only 4 percent of the world's population. Aerosol sprays, refrigerants, plastic foam, and cleaning fluids contain chlorofluorocarbons (CFCs)—also agents of ozone destruction.
2. Our excessive use of paper, plastic, glass, and aluminum contributes to our landfills. We are improving in this area, however. Forty-five percent of all paper, 40 percent of all plastic soft drink bottles, and 55 percent of aluminum cans are now recycled. But we can do better!

◆ CONSUMER ISSUES

Today's consumers are taking a more active role in their own medical research, self-diagnosis, and self-care, thanks partly to the Internet and the availability of medical research in popular magazines. As we live longer, our need grows to become better informed about self-care. Drug companies now advertise and have made many drugs available over the counter (OTC) that were formerly attained only with

Tips for Behavior Change for Recycling

Refer to the Stage of Change flowchart on page 552. What is your stage of change after answering the questions and tracing the flowchart?

Refer to Figure 2.2 (p. 36) to see which processes of change are most effective for facilitating your transition from your current stage to the next stage (or *maintaining* your behavior if you are already in the maintenance stage). Here are some behavioral examples for selected processes of change:

- Consciousness-raising: Investigate the impact on the environment of excessive trash in landfills, rivers, and oceans.
- Social liberation: Search out places near your residence where recyclables are collected.
- Emotional arousal: Watch a documentary on the physical impact of trash on wildlife (plastic bags swallowed by sea turtles, etc.).
- Self-liberation: Post a sign on the refrigerator as a reminder of items in your residence that can be recycled.
- Environment control: Organize an area in your residence with bins or bags for easy separation of recyclable papers, cans, glass, and so forth.

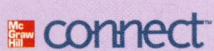 Go online to Connect to complete this activity. http://connect.mcgraw-hill.com

deliberately deceive potential buyers, others sincerely believe in what they are promoting. Most quackery products are foods, drugs, gadgets, or cosmetics that promote physical change—baldness cures, bust enhancers, wrinkle removers, miracle cancer treatments, instant-weight-loss schemes, youth elixirs, arthritis cures, and sexual enhancements. These products and schemes are usually developed for the purpose of financial gain. However, quackery is not an all-or-nothing phenomenon. For example, vitamin B_{12} pills can be lifesaving for those suffering from some forms of anemia, but advertising them for everyone as "pep pills" is fraudulent. Health fraud is big business in the United States. Americans spend billions of dollars each year on quack products and treatments.

Many people erroneously believe that product advertisements are screened by government agencies and that claims on television, on the Internet, or in print must be true. This is not so. It is hard to resist the "promise" of effortless, quick shortcuts to health and wellness. Many promoters are wealthy as a result of our willingness to spend money for miracle solutions. Unfortunately, the results are often shattered hopes and wasted money and sometimes endangered health. Misconceptions and half-truths fuel these promotional fires. As an educated wellness consumer, you should be able to evaluate products and plans with intelligence and realism. See Table 16-3 for common characteristics of quackery.

TABLE 16-3   *How to Recognize Quackery*
Some products use scientific jargon and carry professional-looking logos and endorsements (many are bogus). Watch for the following characteristics common in quackery:
1. It sounds too good to be true.
2. It is quick and painless.
3. It has a "secret," "special," "foreign," "magical," "exclusive," or "ancient" formula.
4. It is available only through the mail (most often through a P.O. box number) or telephone and only from one supplier.
5. It is a scientific "breakthrough" or "miracle cure" that has been overlooked by the medical community.
6. It uses testimonials or case histories from "satisfied customers" as the only proof of its effectiveness.
7. It is a single product effective for a wide variety of ailments.
8. It uses pseudoscientific languages: "detoxifies," "revitalizes immunities," "offers enzymatic protection," and so on.
9. It displays degrees, credentials, or titles from unaccredited or unknown schools.

a doctor's prescription. A vast array of OTC drugs are available to self-directed patients for numerous health conditions like arthritis, insomnia, asthma, headaches, and so on. But along with advantages and benefits come new opportunities for improper use, "shotgun" remedies, and misinformation. Some of the health information online is unreliable, or is simply incorrect. Similarly, some home and self-referred tests and remedies have little value or accuracy. Some users may overlook or disregard directions and warnings.

Hopes and promises of self-diagnosis and self-care open up opportunities for quackery. **Quackery** is the promotion of a misleading health claim that is unproven. The word *quack* derives from "quacksalver," a Dutch word meaning "someone who boasts about his salves." "Health fraud" is often used as a synonym for quackery, but this use can be problematic because quackery can exist without fraud, a word that implies deliberate deception. Whereas some promoters

Remember, if it sounds too good to be true, it probably is. Sometimes, television personalities or well-known celebrities write books, represent products in advertisements, or are portrayed as experts in the field of health and fitness. Be wary of the credibility of this type of product/information marketing.

Even health news reported on television should be regarded with healthy skepticism. An overeager journalist may report the results of one isolated study that found that "your electric toaster can cause cancer!" News reports may oversimplify or exaggerate the results from a single research study. Remember, a single study should never be regarded as fact. Scientific evidence accumulates bit by bit until many well-designed studies point to a similar conclusion.

The Internet is a potential medium for confusion and quackery. Millions search the Internet for answers, cures, and information on a variety of medical conditions. Typing "hair loss" into a general search engine can produce ads for a hair-growth cream, a link to "Bob's Hair Site," a message board with testimonials, or a wig manufacturer. It is hard to know whether you can trust the accuracy of the information on some commercial Web sites. As a general rule, Web addresses ending with .net, .gov, .org, or .edu and those associated with well-known medical centers such as the Mayo Clinic, Harvard Medical School, and the like are reliable.

There are several reasons quackery continues to be a part of health care. Just remember that the thirst for health information is complicated by

✓ Americans' hunger for quick solutions
✓ Ignorance on the part of uneducated consumers
✓ Desperation by people with serious or terminal diseases
✓ Entrepreneurs and companies looking for profits
✓ Journalists looking for headlines
✓ Scientists pursuing fame
✓ Costs of some of these products being less expensive than conventional treatments
✓ Distrust of conventional medicine

As an educated and wise wellness consumer, maintain a spirit of inquiry and guarded caution as you read current health news.

Many hospitals, schools, corporations, community wellness centers, and health organizations offer legitimate programs that can assist you in pursuing a wellness lifestyle. Investigate references and sources before falling for any fly-by-night scheme. Your physician, the Better Business Bureau, the local consumer office, or the nearest office of the Food and Drug Administration (FDA) can offer professional advice if you suspect a product or company is making untrue claims.

◆ A PARTING THOUGHT

Suppose you are the owner of a fine show dog. To make this dog a champion, you handle her in special ways: You make sure she gets proper exercise every day, her coat is brushed and groomed, and her diet is carefully monitored (at the grocery store you walk past the doggie treats and junk food to buy Be Lean and Win Dog Food). Her living environment is regulated to make her the best show dog possible. Do you treat yourself as you would a champion show dog? Do you walk past the treats and junk food to the "be lean and win" food? Are you managing your environment in such a way that it makes you the best you can be? You have 24 hours a day 365 days a year to make choices. Our society provides you with the opportunity to make many positive choices. Our society also allows for choices that are not in your best interest. You now have the knowledge and skills to make choices that enhance your well-being.

Remember, wellness is a journey in which the benefits are gained along the way. It is not a life of self-sacrifice and delayed gratification. It is being the most you can be every day of your life. It is reveling that you have considerable control over your well-being and happiness. Go to it! We wish you well.

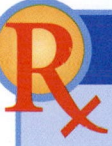
PRESCRIPTION FOR ACTION

You've read the chapter. Now go do one or more of these:

✓ Fasten your seat belt.
✓ Lock your room, apartment, or house each time you leave.
✓ Check the battery in your smoke detector.
✓ Recycle all used cans, paper, and bottles.
✓ Turn off the lights when you leave a room.
✓ Turn off the faucet while brushing your teeth and the shower when soaping up.
✓ Think positive thoughts to enhance your immune system.

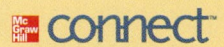 Go online to Connect to complete this activity. http://connect.mcgraw-hill.com

 **Frequently Asked Questions**

Q. Is talking on a cell phone while driving any worse than having a conversation with someone in the car while driving?

A. Any activity a driver engages in while driving has the potential to distract him or her from the primary task of driving. Manually dialing a cell phone can be especially distracting, similar to eating food or changing a CD. A significant difference is the fact that a passenger in a car can help monitor the driving situation along with the driver and pause for, or alert the driver to, potential hazards (e.g., stop talking at a busy intersection or when you're merging on the freeway). In contrast, a person on the other end of the phone line is unaware of the roadway situation.

Q. I am interested in trying complementary and alternative therapies, especially acupuncture. How can I find more information about such practices or find a practitioner in my area?

A. The NCCAM's online database (www.nccam. nih.gov) includes research and information on various disease conditions and links directly to MEDLINE's alternative medicine information. When looking for a qualified practitioner, you may want to contact medical regulatory and licensing agencies in your state. Many states license acupuncture, naturopathy, herbal medicine, homeopathy, and massage therapy. Many CAM specialties have professional associations with Web sites that provide information about a specialty and listings for licensed practitioners close to your locale.

Q. Are discarded cell phones a problem for the environment?

A. Great question! Cell phones are a rapidly growing segment of e-waste. (It used to be just computers!) Since most cell phones are replaced by users every 18 months, by 2005 about 130 million of these devices (weighing about 65,000 tons) will have been retired. Other wireless devices, such as personal digital assistants, pagers, game players, pocket PCs, and portable MP3 music players, will add to the load. All these devices contain similar electronic components and plastic housings. Because these devices are small, consumers may think it's OK to toss them in the trash. However, most of these wireless devices contain toxic materials, including lead and brominated flame retardants, which cause air and water pollution. Also, many have rechargeable batteries that contain potentially toxic heavy metals.

To cut down on this waste, try to select wireless products that are durable and can be upgraded or expanded instead of being replaced. Give away, trade in, or sell usable products. Check out donation or retailer reuse and recycling programs.

Q. I am confident that I can distinguish quackery or bogus health products from legitimate ones. What confuses me are the health reports that emerge almost daily that often contradict a previous report. One day coffee is good for you; the next day it is linked to heart attacks. Beta-carotene supplements prevent cancer in one report. Another report shows that they increase cancer risk in smokers. How do I know what to believe?

A. Part of well-informed wellness is distinguishing high-quality health research from flimsy or biased data. However, it can be confusing because the modern media often sensationalize, misinterpret, overgeneralize, or give only partial results from research studies. The more you know about the economics, politics, and methodology of research, the better able you are to form a sound opinion. Ask yourself the following questions as you weigh the evidence:

- Where is the work published? In a supermarket tabloid? In a homemaker's magazine? In a scientific journal that uses a board of experts to review the article?
- Who paid for the research? (Some companies and foundations might profit from certain outcomes, e.g., a ginseng manufacturer touting the researched benefits of ginseng.)
- Do my biases lead me to want to believe this information?
- Are advertisers using this information to sell a product?
- Is this only a preliminary finding that has not been fully tested?
- Are the researchers from respectable institutions?
- Was good scientific methodology used? What was the number of subjects involved in the study? Was there a control group?

Remember, it takes more than headlines to draw a sound conclusion. Many repeated studies are often necessary. Only after weighing *all* the scientific evidence can sound public health policy be recommended. Unfortunately, you cannot believe everything you read and hear.

Summary

Everyone is born with a genetic blueprint. However, personal lifestyle choices have a great impact on whether you maximize your potential. The business world has also discovered the value of wellness in the workplace in terms of increased productivity, lower health insurance costs, and enhanced employee morale. Knowing how important a supportive environment is in pursuing wellness, you may want to consider working for a company that supports and values employee wellness. After all, you will spend at least one-third of your life at work.

Wellness is an integral part of a productive family life. Family wellness involves meeting the various physical, psychological, and social needs of all members, regardless of age, as they strive toward their full potential. If you are a parent, you will be the master teacher of lifestyle habits to your children. Your example will have a strong influence on your children's ability to make responsible wellness choices.

Accidents are the fifth most common cause of death in the United States. However, accidents (especially automobile crashes) are the number one cause of death among young people. All accidents and crime are not simply a matter of chance. You can substantially reduce your risks of being a victim by heeding basic precautions. Acting to control risks in your immediate environment is a powerful way to enhance your total wellness.

Wellness is not a passing craze. The wellness trend is revolutionizing the medical care system. The broad scope of wellness creates opportunities for life enhancement for *everyone*. New research on the mind–body relationship, including how attitudes, beliefs, and emotional states can affect the immune system, is creating increased interest in the *total* wellness concept of health. An aging population and rising health care costs create unprecedented challenges for us all. Wellness becomes a global issue as we work together to protect the environment, and as an informed wellness consumer, you must be able to evaluate wellness products and programs. The ultimate challenge is to get the word to all people (especially to those who need wellness the most) and get it to them while they are young. Empowering people to have a mind-set of self-responsibility is the only guaranteed way to perpetuate wellness as the undisputed way of life for everyone.

Terms

- alternative medicine
- complementary medicine
- psychoneuroimmunology (PNI)
- quackery

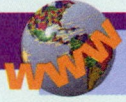 Internet Resources

American Association of Retired Persons

www.aarp.org

Offers information and resources affecting adults over age 50.

Environmental Protection Agency

www.epa.gov

Provides laws, regulations, and resources on environmental issues for the purpose of protecting human health and safeguarding the environment.

Federal Trade Commission

www.ftc.gov

Features consumer information from the federal government about diets, drugs, fitness, consumer fraud, aging concerns, smart buying, and much more.

Healthy Aging

www.cdc.gov/aging/

Information for promoting health, preventing disease, and enhancing the quality of life among older Americans.

Internet Consumer Recycling Guide

www.obviously.com/recycle

A comprehensive guide for consumers about recycling common household items—from plastics to junk mail.

Leadership for Healthy Communities

www.leadershipforhealthycommunities.org

Provides information that can help create and support policies, programs, and initiatives that enable active living in communities. Various strategies and resources for implementation are included.

National Center for Complementary and Alternative Medicine (NCCAM)

www.nccam.nih.gov

A government site with research, clinical trials, alerts and advisories, and current news from the NCCAM.

National Highway Traffic Safety Administration

www.nhtsa.dot.gov

Gives a multitude of information, facts, and statistics on all types of traffic and vehicle safety concerns.

National Institute on Aging (NIA)

www.nia.nih.gov

Has health information, research, and other resources regarding the aging process, diseases, and other lifestyle issues associated with aging.

National Resources Defense Council

www.nrdc.org

Offers information about air, energy, water, global warming, forests, chemicals, and wildlife.

National Safety Council

www.nsc.org

Has information on highway, workplace, recreation, and home safety. Offers facts, resources, and links to a multitude of safety topics.

Office of Minority Health

www.omhrc.gov

A government site with research, health concerns, initiatives, news, and reports about minority health issues.

Quackwatch

www.quackwatch.org

Is somewhat controversial but seeks to expose and attack unproven medical treatments, unsafe medical practices, and health fraud.

Sleep Foundation

www.sleepfoundation.org

Has facts, information, and statistics regarding all aspects of sleep and sleep-related problems.

U.S. Food and Drug Administration

www.fda.gov

Provides information about the safety and effectiveness of food, drugs, cosmetics, weight-loss products, and any medical devices intended for human use.

The Wellness Councils of America

www.welcoa.org

Promotes healthy lifestyles in the workplace by providing information on building sound wellness programs and services.

Whole Health MD

www.wholehealthmd.com

Provides consumers with professional guidance on the many benefits of integrative medicine, including food, therapies, supplements, and medical conditions.

LAB Activity 16-1

Look to the Future

Imagine that you are 5 years older, in a committed relationship with a partner, raising a child, and working in your chosen field.

1. Describe four wellness programs that you want your employer/company to offer. (If you plan to be self-employed or involved in a small business, describe the wellness programs you would want your hospital or community to offer.)

   a.

   b.

   c.

   d.

2. List five family activities that are important to you to promote family wellness.

   a.

   b.

   c.

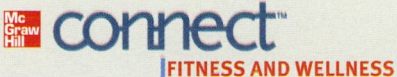
http://connect.mcgraw-hill.com

CHAPTER 16 ■ LAB Activity

    d.

    e.

3.   Describe how you manage your own regular fitness program. (Where? When? What type of activity? etc.)

4.   Not including fitness, what lifestyle and wellness habits are you committed to for your lifetime? (Your answer may involve the entire wellness spectrum.)

LAB Activity 16-2

Name _____ **Class/Activity Section** _____ **Date** _____

The Environment: "One Man's Trash . . ."

We know we are supposed to conserve, save, sustain, and support the environment. However, many people don't know where to begin! The following questionnaire will help you evaluate your current efforts and show you many ways *you can make a difference*.

Circle the statement number if you can say "yes" to it. Do not circle it if you say "no."

ENERGY ON THE ROAD

1. Fuel efficiency is a primary factor I consider when purchasing a vehicle.
2. My vehicle has a manual transmission.
3. I keep my vehicle tuned regularly, including regular oil changes and properly inflated tires.
4. I carpool whenever possible.
5. I use public transportation, ride a bike, or walk whenever I can.

ENERGY AT HOME

1. When purchasing appliances, I consciously buy the most energy-efficient model even if it may cost a bit more.
2. I have switched from using incandescent lightbulbs to using compact fluorescent bulbs wherever possible.
3. I consciously turn off lights, TVs, and radios when I leave a room or am not using them.
4. I limit my use of the clothes dryer by combining loads or hanging clothes to dry.
5. The windows and doors of my residence have good seals and caulking.
6. I turn off the water when soaping in the shower, brushing my teeth, and shaving.
7. I take showers rather than baths.
8. My shower has a low-flow head.
9. I have energy-efficient heating and cooling in my residence.
10. I keep the thermostat/air conditioning at 68 degrees in the winter and 78 degrees in the summer.
11. I open my dishwasher to let dishes air-dry rather than heat-dry.
12. I make sure faucets and toilets are not leaking.
13. I run the dishwasher and the washing machine only when they have full loads.
14. I often hand-wash dishes rather than use the dishwasher.
15. I dispose of household hazardous waste according to the instructions.

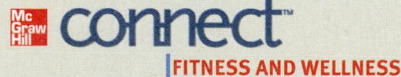

http://connect.mcgraw-hill.com

16.   I close off rooms in my residence that do not need to be heated/air-conditioned.

17.   I use sunlight wisely by closing blinds/curtains in the summer when the air conditioner is in use and open blinds/curtains on cold, sunny days.

RECYCLING

1.   I separate and recycle plastic, paper, aluminum, and glass.

2.   I buy recycled products even when they cost a little more.

3.   I compost yard trimmings, fruit and vegetable scraps, and coffee grounds.

4.   I consciously buy products with the least amount of packaging.

5.   I regularly use reusable dishes and utensils rather than plastic or Styrofoam.

GENERAL

1.   I am thrifty with paper by not printing out unnecessary e-mails, articles, ads, and so on.

2.   I reuse paper by using scraps or blank sides of used sheets.

3.   In storing food or taking my lunch, I use reusable containers rather than foil or plastic wrap.

4.   I limit my use of pesticides, chemicals, and aerosols.

5.   I purchase organic produce whenever possible.

6.   I take a canvas bag with me when I shop instead of using paper and plastic ones from stores.

7.   I have joined or financially supported groups working on environmental causes.

8.   I vote for political candidates who support environmental issues.

How many statement numbers did you circle by answering "yes"? _____

How many are not circled because you answered "no"? _____

After reading this list, state five actions that you could personally start doing *today* to contribute to a better environment.

1.

2.

3.

4.

5.

LAB Activity 16-3

Quackery Detection

Doctors Accidentally Discover "Lazy Way" to Remove Cellulite

Discovery Astounds Scientific Community

Swedish researchers at the University of Pelento have discovered (accidentally) a secret formula that ACTUALLY SHRINKS CELLULITE! This astounding discovery has virtually *eliminated the need for dieting or torturous exercise!* This miracle formula is being marketed exclusively under the trade name SHRINK-IT 5000.

Clinically Tested

Exhaustive medical tests at a world-famous medical center in Burgess, Australia, have proven that **SHRINK-IT 5000** has no harmful side effects and is the most effective cellulite-reducing formula of all time. Like a magnet, the chemical molecules in **SHRINK-IT 5000** tie up and trap undigested fat particles many times their size. And it begins happening almost instantly! In fact, it is so effective that some people tend to overdo it and become too thin—within days!!

1 Month Supply (Was $79.90) NOW ONLY

$49.90 SAVE $30!

Eat All You Want and Keep Losing Cellulite

This amazing formula was discovered by scientists searching for a compound to shrink varicose veins. Researchers were amazed to find the test group actually lost a considerable amount of cellulite fat— all while eating anything they wanted. Dr. Garth Robbins stated in the *Universal Journal of Clinical Science:* "This formula will virtually revolutionize the way people typically try to lose fat (with deprivating diets and exhaustive exercise)."

Act Now

This is a limited time offer. Since news of this product is sweeping the country, send in your order today. Don't let this golden opportunity get away. Imagine being the thin, attractive person you've dreamed about! **SHRINK-IT 5000** is available only from Powers Pharmaceuticals, which holds exclusive North American rights. Call now. Orders accepted by phone only.

1-800-987-6543 ALL CREDIT CARDS ACCEPTED

Testimonials from Satisfied Customers

"I couldn't believe how quickly **SHRINK-IT 5000** worked. I lost 10 pounds in the first 3 days."

Ann, Cadillac, MI

"I love to eat, so I changed absolutely nothing in my diet and still lost 20 pounds thanks to **SHRINK-IT 5000.**"

Tim, S. Augustine, FL

"Exercise? No way! I lost all of my weight by just taking **SHRINK-IT 5000** and never exercising."

Gayle, North Webster, IN

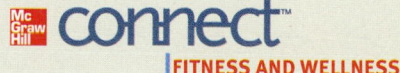 **connect** FITNESS AND WELLNESS

http://connect.mcgraw-hill.com

Answer the following questions:

1. List indications of quackery in the advertisement for SHRINK-IT 5000.

2. What makes this advertisement attractive or seem legitimate to the uninformed consumer?

3. If your sister were ready to send away for this product with the hope of reducing fat thighs, what would you tell her? How would you advise anyone wanting to spot reduce the fat on his or her thighs?

BIBLIOGRAPHY

Chapter 1

Ardell, D. B. "Definition of Wellness." *Ardell Wellness Report* 37 (Winter 1995): 1.

Centers for Disease Control and Prevention. National Center for Chronic Disease Prevention and Health Promotion. *Behavioral Risk Factor Surveillance—United States, 2008*. www.cdc.gov/brfss

Centers for Disease Control and Prevention. National Center for Chronic Disease Prevention and Health Promotion. *Chronic Disease Overview,* December 2009. www.cdc.gov/chronicdisease

Centers for Disease Control and Prevention. National Center for Chronic Disease Prevention and Health Promotion. *The Burden of Chronic Diseases and Their Risk Factors: National and State Perspectives 2004,* February 2004. www.cdc.gov/nccdphp

Centers for Disease Control and Prevention. National Center for Chronic Disease Prevention and Health Promotion. *The Power of Prevention: Chronic Disease . . . the Public Health Challenge of the 21st Century, 2009.* www.cdc.gov/chronicdisease

Centers for Disease Control and Prevention. National Center for Chronic Disease Prevention and Health Promotion. *Youth Risk Behavior Surveillance—United States, 2007,* June 6, 2008. www.cdc.gov/yrbss

Centers for Disease Control and Prevention. National Center for Health Statistics. *Health, United States, 2008,* March 2009. www.cdc.gov/nchs

Centers for Disease Control and Prevention. National Center for Health Statistics. *National Vital Statistics Report, 58* (August 2009). www.cdc.gov/nchs

Dunn, H. "High-Level Wellness for Man and Society." *American Journal of Public Health* 49 (June 1959): 786–792.

Eyre, H., et al. "Preventing Cancer, Cardiovascular Disease, and Diabetes." *Circulation* 109 (June 29, 2004): 3244–3255.

Farley, T., and D. A. Cohen. *Prescription for a Healthy Nation*. Boston: Beacon Press, 2005.

Foust, C. D. "Wellness and Psychosocial Spiritual Health" in *Wellness for Life,* Johnson, W. E., et al. Peosta, IA: Eddie Bowers publishing co., 2002.

Frieden, T. R. "Asleep at the Switch: Local Public Health and Chronic Disease." *American Journal of Public Health* 94 (December 2004): 2059–2061.

Hammermeister, J., and M. Peterson. "Does Spirituality Make a Difference? Psychosocial and Health-Related Characteristics of Spiritual Well-Being." *American Journal of Health Education* 32 (September/October 2001): 293–297.

Heffler, S., et al. "Health Spending Projections for 2002–2012." *Health Affairs* 22 (March/April 2003).

McGinnis, J. M. "A Vision for Health in Our New Century." *American Journal of Health Promotion* 18 (November/December 2003): 146–150.

Mokdad, A. H., et al. "Actual Causes of Death in the United States, 2000." *Journal of the American Medical Association* 291 (March 10, 2004): 1238–1245.

Mokdad, A. H., et al. "Correction: Actual Causes of Death in the United States, 2000." *Journal of the American Medical Association* 293 (January 19, 2005): 293–294.

O'Donnell, M. P. "What Works Best? Knowledge, Skills, Motivation, and Opportunity." *American Journal of Health Promotion* 19 (May/June 2004): IV.

Olshansky, S. J., et al. "A Potential Decline in Life Expectancy in the United States in the 21st Century." *The New England Journal of Medicine* 352 (March 17, 2005): 1138–1145.

Peel, N. M., R. J. McClure, and H. P. Bartlett. "Behavioral Determinants of Healthy Aging." *American Journal of Preventive Medicine* 28 (April 2005): 298–304.

Roberts, C. K., and R. J. Barnard. "Effects of Exercise and Diet on Chronic Disease." *Journal of Applied Physiology* 98 (January 2005): 3–30.

Trust for America's Health. *A Healthier America: A New Vision and Agenda,* September 2007. www.healthyamericans.org

Trust for America's Health. *Our Vision for a Healthier America,* October 2008. www.healthyamericans.org

U.S. Department of Health and Human Services. *Healthy People 2020: National Health Promotion and Disease Prevention Objectives*, 2010. www.healthypeople.gov

U.S. Department of Health and Human Services. *The Health Consequences of Smoking: A Report of the Surgeon General.* May 27, 2004. www.surgeongeneral.gov

Weil, Andrew. *Why Our Health Matters: A Vision of Medicine That Can Transform Our Future*. New York: Hudson Street Press, 2009.

Winkleby, M. A., and C. Cubbin. "Changing Patterns in Health Behaviors and Risk Factors Related to Chronic Diseases, 1990–2000." *American Journal of Health Promotion* 19 (September/October 2004): 19–27.

World Health Organization. *Move for Health 2005*. www.who.int

World Health Organization. "Preamble to the Constitution of the World Health Organization." April 7, 1948. www.who.int

World Health Organization. *World Health Report 2002–Reducing Risks, Promoting Healthy Life*. www.who.int

World Health Organization. *World Health Report 2004–Healthy Life Expectancy*. www.who.int

Chapter 2

Barry, T. R., and B. L. Howe. "The Effects of Exercise Advertising on Self-Efficacy and Decisional Balance." *American Journal of Health Behavior* 29 (March/April 2005): 117–126.

Bedford, P. "Watch Old Habits Disappear." *IDEA Health & Fitness Source* (May 2004): 46–50.

Brown, S. "Measuring Perceived Benefits and Perceived Barriers for Physical Activity." *American Journal of Health Behavior* 29 (March/April 2005): 107–116.

Chapman, M. A. "Bad Choices: Why We Make Them, How to Stop." *Psychology Today* 32 (September/October 1999): 36–39, 71.

Evers, K. E., J. O. Prochaska, J. L. Johnson, L. M. Mauriello, J. A. Padula, and J. M. Prochaska. "A Randomized Clinical Trial of a Population and Transtheoretical-Based Stress Management Intervention." *Health Psychology* 25 (July 2006): 521–529.

Gallagher, K. I., and J. M. Jakicic. "Overcoming Barriers to Effective Exercise Programming." *ACSM's Health & Fitness Journal* 6 (November/December 2002): 6–12.

Goldberg, S. "The 10 Rules of Change." *Psychology Today* 35 (September/October 2002): 38–44.

"How to Banish a Bad Habit." *Consumer Reports on Health* (March 2003): 8–9.

Jakicic, J. M., and A. D. Otto. "Motivating Change: Modifying Eating and Exercise Behaviors for Weight Management." *ACSM's Health & Fitness Journal* 9 (January/February 2005): 6–12.

Johnson, S. S., A. L. Paiva, C. O. Cummins, J. L. Johnson, S. J. Dyment, J. A. Wright, J. O. Prochaska, J. M. Prochaska., and K. Sherman. "Transtheoretical Model-Based Multiple Behavior Intervention for Weight Management: Effectiveness on a Population Basis." *Preventive Medicine* 46 (March 2008): 238–246.

King, A. C., J. E. Martin, and C. Castro. "Behavioral Strategies to Enhance Physical Activity Participation." In L. A. Kaminsky et al., eds. *ACSM's Resource Manual for Guidelines for Exercise Testing and Participation,* 5th ed. Philadelphia: Lippincott Williams & Wilkins, 2006.

Kottler, J. A. *Making Changes Last*. Philadelphia: Brunner-Routledge, 2001.

Marano, H. E. "Reinvention: How to Be Perfect." *Psychology Today,* February 3, 2004. www.psychologytoday.com

Mellin, L. *The Pathway*. New York: Regan Books, 2003.

Napolitano, M. A., et al. "Principles of Health Behavior Change." In L. A. Kaminsky et al., eds. *ACSM's Resource Manual for Guidelines for Exercise Testing and Participation,* 5th ed. Philadelphia: Lippincott Williams & Wilkins, 2006.

Prochaska, J. O., J. C. Norcross, and C. C. DiClemente. *Changing for Good*. New York: William Morrow, 1994.

Prochaska, J. O., and W. F. Velicer. "The Transtheoretical Model of Health Behavior Change." *American Journal of Health Promotion* 12 (September/October 1997): 38–44.

Seligman, M.E.P. *Authentic Happiness*. New York: Free Press, 2002.

Seligman, M.E.P. *Learned Optimism*. New York: Simon & Schuster, 1998.

Shilts, M. K., M. Horowitz, and M. S. Townsend. "Goal Setting as a Strategy for Dietary and Physical Activity Behavior Change: A Review of the Literature." *American Journal of Health Promotion* 19 (November/December 2004): 81–93.

Wallace, L. S., and J. Buckworth. "Application of the Transtheoretical Model to Exercise Behavior among Nontraditional College Students." *American Journal of Health Education* 32 (January/February 2001): 39–47.

Chapter 3

Aberg, Maria, et al. "Cardiovascular Fitness is Associated with Cognition in Young Adulthood." *Proceedings of the National Academy of Sciences* 106 (December 8, 2009): 20906–20911.

American College of Sports Medicine. *ACSM Issue Position Stand on Exercise and Older Adults,* July 20, 2009. www.acsm.org

American College of Sports Medicine. *ACSM's Guidelines for Exercise Testing and Prescription,* 8th ed. Philadelphia, PA: Lippincott Williams & Wilkins. 2009.

American College of Sports Medicine. *ACSM's Health-Related Physical Fitness Assessment Manual*. 3rd ed. Philadelphia, PA: Lippincott Williams & Wilkins, 2009.

Blair, S. N., et al. "Influences of Cardiorespiratory Fitness and Other Precursors on Cardiovascular Disease and All-Cause Mortality in Men and Women." *Journal of the American Medical Association* 276, no. 3 (July 17, 1996): 205–210.

Blair, S. N., et al. "Physical Fitness and All-Cause Mortality: A Prospective Study of Healthy Men and Women." *Journal of the American Medical Association* 262, no. 17 (November 3, 1989): 2395–2401.

Blair, S. N., Y. Cheng, and J. S. Holder. "Is Physical Activity or Physical Fitness More Important in Defining Health Benefits?" *Medicine and Science in Sports and Exercise* 33 (6Suppl) (June 2001): S379–399.

Borg, G. "Psychophysical Bases of Physical Exertion." *Medicine and Science in Sports and Exercise* 14 (1982): 707.

Church, T. S., C. P. Earnest, J. S. Skinner, and S. N. Blair. "Effects of Different Doses of Physical Activity on Cardiorespiratory Fitness Among Sedentary, Overweight, or Obese Postmenopausal Women with Elevated Blood Pressure." *Journal of the American Medical Association* 297 (May 16, 2007): 2081–2091.

Cooper, K. H. "A Means of Assessing Maximal Oxygen Intake: Correlation between Field and Treadmill Testing." *Journal of the American Medical Association* 203 (January 1968): 201–204.

Dohoney, P., J. A. Chromiak, D. Lemire, B. R. Abadie, and C. Kovacs. "Prediction of One Repetition Maximum (1-RM) Strength from a 4–6 and a 7–10 RM Submaximal Strength Test in Healthy Young Adult Males." *Journal of Exercise Physiology Online* 5 (August 2002): 54–59. http://faculty.css.edu/tboone2/asep/Dohoney.doc

Ford, E. S., et al. "Healthy Living Is the Best Revenge." *Archives of Internal Medicine* 169 (August 2009): 1355–1362. www.asahq.org/hwa/HealthyLivingIsTheBestRevenge.pdf

Haskell, W. L., et al. "Physical Activity and Public Health: Updated Recommendation for Adults from the American College of Sports Medicine and the American Heart Association." *Medicine and Science in Sports and Exercise* 39 (August 2007): 1423–1434.

Kaminsky, L. A., et al. "Evaluation of a Shallow Water Running Test for the Estimation of Peak Aerobic Power." *Medicine and Science in Sport and Exercise* 25 (November 1993): 1287–1292.

Keener, E., et al. "Undergraduate Student Physical Fitness Assessment." Muncie, IN: Ball State University, Spring 1989.

Lieberman, J. A., W. L. Bockenek, and G. Stendig. *Therapeutic Exercise,* Medscape.com (January 20, 2009).

Liu-Ambrose, T., et al. "Resistance Training and Executive Functions." *Archives of Internal Medicine* 170 (January 2010): 170–178.

Mandic, S., et al. "Characterizing Differences in Mortality at the Low End of the Fitness Spectrum." *Medicine & Science in Sports & Exercise* 41 (August 2009): 1573–1579.

Martin, C. K., et al. "Exercise Dose and Quality of Life." *Archives of Internal Medicine* 169 (February 2009): 269–278.

Penedo, F. J, and J. R. Dahn. "Exercise and Well-Being: A Review of Mental and Physical Health Benefits Associated with Physical Activity." *Current Opinion in Psychiatry* 18 (February 2005): 189–193.

Medline Plus. *Exercise May Help Stave Off Mental Decline.* National Institutes of Health (January 11, 2010). www.nlm.nih.gov/medlineplus/news/fullstory_93948.html

Sloan, A. W., and J. Weir. "Nomograms for Prediction of Bone Density and Total Body Fat from Skinfold Measurements." *Journal of Applied Physiology* 28 (1970): 221–222.

Sun, Qui, et al. "Physical Activity at Midlife in Relation to Successful Survival in Women at Age 70 Years or Older." *Archives of Internal Medicine* 170 (January 2010): 194–201.

U.S. Department of Health and Human Services. *2008 Physical Activity Guidelines for Americans,* October 2008. www.health.gov/paguidelines/guidelines/default.aspx

U.S. Department of Health and Human Services. *Healthy People 2020.* www.healthypeople.gov/HP2020/

Williamson, J., and Pahor, M. "Evidence Regarding the Benefits of Physical Exercise." *Archives of Internal Medicine* 170 (January 2010): 124–125.

Chapter 4

American College of Sports Medicine. *ACSM's Guidelines for Exercises Testing and Prescription,* 8th ed. Philadelphia: Lippincott, Williams, & Wilkins, 2009.

Bassett Jr., D. L., P. L. Schneider, and G. E. Huntington. "Physical Activity in an Old Amish Community." *Medicine and Science in Sports and Exercise* 36, no. 1 (January 2004): 79–86.

Bennett, G., K. Wolin, E. Puleo, et al. "Awareness of the National Physical Activity Guidelines for Health Promotion Among U.S. Adults." *Medicine & Science in Sports & Exercise* 41, no. 10 (October 2009): 1849–1855.

Blair, S. N., et al. "Influences of Cardiorespiratory Fitness and Other Precursors on Cardiovascular Disease and All Cause Mortality in Men and Women." *Journal of the American Medical Association* 276, no. 3 (July 17, 1996): 205–210.

"Boosting Your Immunity: What Helps and What Harms Your Body's Ability to Defend Itself." *Consumer Reports on Health* 20, no. 12 (December 2008): 8–9.

Borg, G. "Psychophysical Bases of Physical Exertion." *Medicine and Science in Sports and Exercise* 14 (1982): 344–386.

Brady, J. F. "Exercising the Brain." *ACSM's Health & Fitness Journal* 13, no. 2 (April 2009): 27–31.

Bravata, Dena M., Chrystal Smith-Spangler, et al. "Using Pedometers to Increase Physical Activity and Improve Health: A Systematic Review." *Journal of the American Medical Association* 298, no. 19 (November 27, 2007): 2296–2304.

Castelli, D. M., C. H. Hillman, M. Buck, et al. "Physical Fitness and Academic Achievement in Third and Fifth Grade Students." *Journal of Sport Exercise Psychology* 29 (2007): 239–252.

Corbin, C. "Helping Clients Understand National Physical Activity Guidelines." *ACSM's Health & Fitness Journal* 13, no. 5 (September/October 2009): 17–22.

Cuddihy, T. F., R. P. Pangrazi, and L. M. Tomson. "Pedometers: Answers to FAQs from Teachers." *Journal of Physical Education, Recreation, and Dance* 76, no. 2 (February 2005): 36–40.

"Depression, Physical Inactivity Linked." American College of Sports Medicine. May 31, 2007. www.acsm.org/AM/Template.cfm?Section=News

Harvey, J., R. Eime, W. Payne. "Effectiveness of the 2006 Commonwealth Games 10,000 Steps Walking Challenge." *Medicine & Science in Sports & Exercise* 41, no. 8 (August 2009): 167–1681.

Helgerud, J., K. Hoydal, E. Wang, et al. "Aerobic High-Intensity Intervals Improve VO2max More than Moderate Training." *Medicine & Science in Sports & Exercise* 39, no. 4 (2007): 665–671.

Hoeger, W. K., L. Bond, L. Ransdell, et al. "One-Mile Step Count at Walking and Running Speeds." *ACSM's Health & Fitness Journal* 12, no. 1 (January/February 2008): 14–19.

Hultquist, C. N., et al. "Comparison of Walking Recommendations in Previously Inactive Women." *Medicine and Science in Sports and Exercise* 37, no. 4 (April 2005): 676–683.

Karvonen, M., K. Kentala, and O. Mustala. "The Effects of Training on Heart Rate: A Longitudinal Study." *Annals of Medicine and Experimental Biology* 35 (1957): 307–315.

Kilpatrick, M. "Exercise, Mood, and Psychological Well-Being: A Practitioner's Guide to Theory, Research, and Application." *ACSM's Health & Fitness Journal* 12, no. 5 (September/October 2008): 14–20.

Klein, D. A., L. Burr, and W. J. Stone. "Making Physical Activity Stick: What Can We Learn from Regular Exercisers?" *ACSM's Health & Fitness Journal* 9, no. 4 (January/February 2005).

Lee, I-Min. "Dose-Response Relation Between Physical Activity and Fitness: Even a Little Is Good, More Is Better." *Journal of the American Medical Association* 297, no. 19 (May 16, 2007): 2137–2139.

Le Maurier, G. C. "Walk Which Way?" *ACSM's Health & Fitness Journal* 8, no. 1 (January/February 2004): 7–10.

Loupias, J., and L. Golding. "Deep Water Running: A Conditioning Alternative." *ACSM's Health & Fitness Journal* 8, no. 5 (September/October 2004): 5–8.

Melanson, E., J. R. Knoll, M. L. Bell, et al. "Commercially Available Pedometers: Considerations for Accurate Step Counting." *Preventive Medicine* 39 (2004): 361–368.

Nieman, D. C. "How Do the 2008 Physical Activity Guidelines for Americans Differ from Previous Recommendations? There Seems to Be So Many of Them and I Am Definitely Confused." *ACSM's Health & Fitness Journal* 13, no. 3 (May/June 2009): 5–7.

Neiman, D. C. "Marathon Training and Immune Function." *ACSM's Health & Fitness Journal* 13, no. 2 (April 2009): 6–7.

Persinger, R., C. Foster, M. Gibson, et al. "Consistency of the Talk Test for Exercise Prescription." *Medicine and Science in Sports and Exercise* 36, no. 9 (September 2004): 1632–1636.

Saunders, M. J., H. G. Ryan, D. L. Wenos, et al. "Trekking Poles Increase Physiological Responses to Hiking Without Perceived Exertion." *Journal of Strength Conditioning Research* 22, no. 5 (2008): 1468–1474.

Schneider, Patrick L., J. R. Bassett, D. L. Thompson, et al. "Effects of 10,000 Steps Per Day Goal in Overweight Adults." *Journal of Health Promotion* 21, no. 2 (2006): 85–89.

Schneider, P. L., S. E. Crouter, and D. R. Bassett Jr. "Pedometer Measures of Free-Living Physical Activity: Comparison of 13 Models." *Medicine and Science in Sports and Exercise* 36, no. 2 (2004): 331–335.

Stanforth, D. and M. Mackert. "Social Undermining of Healthy Eating and Exercise Behaviors." *ACSM's Health & Fitness Journal* 13, no. 3 (May/June 2009): 14–20.

"Step-Based Guidelines in New Pair of Studies: Steps to Meet ACSM/CDC Recommendation." American College of Sports Medicine. June 1, 2007. www.acsm.org/AM/Template.cfm?Section=News

Swain, D. P. "Exercise Equipment: Assessing the Advertised Claims." *ACSM's Health & Fitness Journal* 13, no. 5 (September/October 2009): 8–11.

Swain, David P. "Moderate- or Vigorous-Intensity Exercise: What Should We Prescribe?" *ACSM's Health & Fitness Journal* 10, no. 5 (September 2006): 7–11.

Thompson, D. L. "Cancer and Exercise." *ACSM's Health & Fitness Journal* 13, no. 2 (March/April 2009): 5.

Thompson, D. L. "Improving VO2max." *ACSM's Health & Fitness Journal* 9, no. 5 (September/October 2005): 4.

Thompson, D. L. "VO2max: The Basics: Part I." *ACSM's Health & Fitness Journal* 9, no. 3 (May/June 2005): 5.

Thompson, D. L. "VO2max: Links to Health and Performance." *ACSM's Health & Fitness Journal* 9, no. 4 (July/August 2005): 5.

U.S. Department of Health and Human Services. *2008 Physical Activity Guidelines for Americans*. ODPHP Publication No. U0036, October 2008. www.health.gov/paguidelines

Van Der Horst, Klazine, Maijke J. Pau, et al. "A Brief Review on Correlates of Physical Activity and Sedentariness in Youth." *Medicine & Science in Sports & Exercise* 39, no. 8 (August 2007): 1241–1250.

Voelker, Rebecca. "Studies Suggest Dog Walking a Good Strategy for Fostering Fitness." *Journal of the American Medical Association* 296, no. 6 (August 9, 2006): 643.

Chapter 5

Alter, M. *Science of Flexibility,* 3rd ed. Champaign, IL: Human Kinetics, 2004.

Bacurau, R. F., et al. "Acute Effect of a Ballistic and a Static Stretching Exercise Bout on Flexibility and Maximal Strength." *Journal of Strength and Conditioning Research* 23 (January 2009): 304–308.

Bradley, P. S., P. D. Olsen, and M. D. Portas. "The Effect of Static, Ballistic and PNF Stretching on Vertical Jump Performance." *Journal of Strength & Conditioning Research* 21 (February 2007): 223–226.

Bumgardner, W. *Stretching Principles and Guidelines,* December 2007. http://walking.about.com/od/stretching/a/blexstretch.htm

Costa, P. B., B. S. Graves, M. Whitehurst, P. L. Jacobs. "The Acute Effects of Different Durations of Static Stretching on Dynamic Balance Performance." *Journal of Strength and Conditioning Research* 23 (January 2009): 141–147.

Godsey, C. *Ten Good Reasons to Try Yoga,* February 2008. http://meriter.staywellsolutionsonline.com/Library/Wellness/Fitness/1,2767

Herman. S., and D. T. Smith. "Four-Week Dynamic Stretching Warm-Up Intervention Elicits Longer-Term Performance Benefits." *Journal of Strength and Conditioning Research* 22 (January 2008): 1286–1297.

Humphries, B. E., L. Dugan, and T.L.A. Doyle. "Muscular Fitness." In Kaminsky, L., ed., *ACSM's Resource Manual for Guidelines for Exercise Testing and Prescription,* 5th ed. Philadelphia: Lippincott, Williams & Wilkins, 2006.

Inverarity, L. *Stretching 101,* November 8, 2007. http://physicaltherapy.about.com/od/flexibilityexercises/a/stretchbasics.htm

Kurz, T. *Stretching Scientifically: A Guide to Flexibility Training,* 4th ed. Island Pond, VT: Stadion Publishing Co., 2003.

Mayo Clinic, "Stretching: Focus on Flexibility," February 21, 2009. www.mayoclinic.com/health/stretching/HO01447

Quinn, E. *When to Stretch—Why Experts Recommend Athletes Stretch After Exercise,* April 3, 2009, http://sportsmedicine.about.com/cs/flexibility/a/aa022102a.htm

Rubini, E. C., A.L.L. Costa, and P.S.C. Comes. "The Effects of Stretching on Strength Performance." *Sports Medicine* 37 (March 2007): 213–224.

Samuel, M. N., W. R. Holcomb, M. A. Guadagnoli, M. D. Rubley, and H. Wallmann. "Acute Effects of Static and Ballistic Stretching on Measures of Strength and Power." *Journal of*

Strength and Conditioning Research 22 (September 2008): 1422–1428.

The Stretching Institute. *PNF Stretching Explained Proprioceptive Neuromuscular Facilitation.* www.thestretchinghandbook.com/archives/pnf-stretching.php

Thacker, S. B., et al. "The Impact of Stretching on Sports Injury Risk: A Systematic Review of the Literature." *Medicine & Science in Sports & Exercise* 36, no. 3 (March 2004): 371–378.

Young, W. B. "The Use of Static Stretching in Warm-Up for Training and Competition." *International Journal of Sports Physiology & Performance* 2 (June 2007): 212–216.

Chapter 6

American College of Sports Medicine. *ACSM's Guidelines for Exercise Testing and Prescription,* 5th ed. Philadelphia: Lippincott, Williams & Wilkins, 2006.

Barclay, L. "Progressive Resistance Strength Training May Help Improve Physical Function in Older Adult." *Medscape Orthopaedics* (July 28, 2009). www.medscape.com/viewarticle/706561

Barclay, L. "Resistance Plus Aerobic Exercise May Be Best for Sedentary, Abdominally Obese Older Adults." *Medscape Orthopaedics* (February 5, 2009). www.medscape.com/viewarticle/587921

Consumer Reports. "A Safer, Livelier Way to Strengthen Your Body's Core Muscles." *Consumer Reports on Health* (April 2005): 8–10.

Evetovich, T., and K. Eversole. "Adaptations to Resistance Training." In Kaminsky, L., ed., *ACSM's Resource Manual for Guidelines for Exercise Testing and Prescription,* 5th ed. Philadelphia: Lippincott, Williams & Wilkins, 2006.

Hartman, M. M., et al. "Resistance Training Improves Metabolic Economy During Functional Tasks in Older Adults." *Journal of Strength and Conditioning Research* 21 (January 2007): 91–95.

Haskell, W. L., et al. "Physical Activity and Public Health: Updated Recommendation for Adults from the American College of Sports Medicine and the American Heart Association." *Medicine & Science in Sports & Exercise* 39 (August 2007): 1423–1434.

Hoffman, J. *ACSM Current Comment. Resistance Training and Injury Prevention,* November 2009. www.acsm.org/AM/Template.cfm?Section=Current_Comments1&Template=/CM/ContentDisplay.cfm&ContentID=8625

Kraemer, W. J., and M. S. Fragala. "Personalize It: Program Design in Resistance Training." *ACSM's Health and Fitness Journal* 4 (July/August 2006): 7–17.

Kraemer, W. J., and N. A. Ratamess. "Fundamentals of Resistance Training: Progression and Exercise Prescription." *Medicine & Science in Sports & Exercise* 36 (April 2004): 674–688.

Kraemer W. I., J. S. Volek, and C. Dunn-Lewis. "L-carnitine Supplementation: Influence upon Physiological Function." *Current Sports Medicine Reports* (July August 2008): 218–223.

Mayo Clinic. *Strength Training,* March 19, 2009. http://mayoclinic.com/health/fitness/MY00396/DSECTION=strength-training

Medscape Orthopaedics. "Pumping Iron Improves Heart Health and May Help Tighten Waistline." *Medscape* (February 22, 2000). www.medscape.com/viewarticle/411663

Ogura, Y., et al. "Duration of Static Stretching Influences Muscle Force Production in Hamstring Muscles." *Journal of Strength and Conditioning Research* 21 (March 2007): 788–792.

Powers, S., and E. T. Hurley. *Exercise Physiology.* New York: McGraw-Hill, 2007.

Sanders, S. "Core Stability and Exercise Prescription: A Research Update: Implications for Physiotherapists." *Sport Health* 25 (Autumn 2007): 16–17, 20.

Sillanpää, E., et al. "Body Composition and Fitness During Strength and/or Endurance Training in Older Men." *Medicine and Science in Sports and Exercise* (May 2008): 950–958.

Sternlicht, E., et al. "Electromyographic Comparison of a Stability Ball Crunch with a Traditional Crunch." *Journal of Strength and Conditioning Research* 21 (February 2007): 506–509.

Wallace, J. "Principles of Musculoskeletal Exercise Programming." In Kaminsky, L., ed., *ACSM's Resource Manual for Guidelines for Exercise Testing and Prescription,* 5th ed. Philadelphia: Lippincott, Williams & Wilkins, 2006.

Yamamoto, L. M., R. M. Lopez, J. F. Klau, D. J. Casa, W. J. Kraemer, and C. M. Maresh. "The Effects of Resistance Training on Endurance Distance Running Performance Among Highly trained runners: A Systematic Review. *Journal of Strength Conditioning Research* 6 (November 22, 2008): 2036–2044.

Chapter 7

American College of Sports Medicine Round Table Consensus Statement: "Impact of Physical Activity During Pregnancy and Postpartum." American College of Sports Medicine. June 1, 2006. www.acsm.org

"Anabolic Steroid Abuse." National Institute on Drug Abuse Research Report Series. August, 2006. www.drugabuse.gov

"Brain Health: What to Keep in Mind." *Wellness Letter, University of California, Berkeley* 25, no. 8 (May 2009): 1–2.

Brandon, J. L., L. W. Boyette, A. Lloyd, et al. "Resistive Training and Long-Term Function in Older Adults." *Journal of Aging and Physical Activity* 12, no. 1 (January 2004): 10–28.

Cassilhas, Ricardo C., Valter A. Viana, et al. "The Impact of Resistance Exercise on the Cognitive Function of the Elderly." *Medicine & Science in Sports & Exercise* 39, no. 8 (August 2007): 1401–1407.

Del Caso, J., E. Estevez, and R. Mora-Rodriques. "Caffeine During Exercise in the Heat." *Medicine & Science in Sports & Exercise* 41, no. (January 2009): 164–173.

"Exercise During Pregnancy." The American College of Obstetricians and Gynecologists. July, 2007. www.acog.org

Fern, A. K. "Benefits of Physical Activity in Older Adults: Programming Modifications to Enhance the Exercise Experience." *ACSM's Health & Fitness Journal* 13, no. 5 (September/October 2009): 12–16.

Hobson, R., E. Clapp, P. Watson, et al. "Exercise Capacity in the Heat Is Greater in the Morning Than in the Evening in Men." *Medicine & Science in Sports & Exercise* 41, no. 1 (January 2009): 174–180.

Kalapotharakos, V., M. Michalopoulou, et al. "The Effects of High- and Moderate-Resistive Training on Muscle Function in the Elderly." *Journal of Aging & Physical Activity* 12, no. 2 (April 2004): 131–143.

Kemmler, W., S. Von Stengel, K. Engelke, et al. "Exercise Decreases the Risk of Metabolic Syndrome in Elderly Females." *Medicine & Science in Sports & Exercise* 41, no. 2 (February 2009): 297–305.

Kruskall F. I., and A. Meracle. "Coffeine and Ex Perfi What's all the Buy about?" *ACSM's Health & Fitness Journal* 13, no. 6 (November/December 2009): 17–23.

Lee, I., M. C. Hsieh, and R. S. Paffenbarger. "Exercise Intensity and Longevity in Men: The Harvard Alumni Health Study." *Journal of American Medical Association* 273, no. 15 (April 19, 1995): 1179–1184.

Leibman, B. "Breaking Up. Strong Bones Need More Than Calcium." *Nutrition Action, Center for Science in the Public Interest* 32, no. 3 (April 2005): 1–8.

Leibman, B. "You Must Remember This: How to Keep Your Brain Younger." *Nutrition Action Health Letter, Center for Science in the Public Interest* (April 2009): 1–7. Lemere, B., D. Gagnon, O. Jay, et al. "Differences Between Sexes in Rectal Cooling Rates After Exercise-Induced Hyperthermia." *Medicine & Science in Sports & Exercise* 41, no. 8 (August 2009): 1633–1639.

Loland, N. "Exercise, Health, and Aging." *Journal of Aging & Physical Activity* 12, no. 2 (April 2004): 170–184.

Manore, M. A. "Feeding the Active Female: Part II." *ACSM's Health & Fitness Journal* 9, no. 5 (September/October 2005): 26–28.

Marino, F., and T. Noakes. "Cold Fluids Improve Exercise Performance in the Heat by Slowing the Rate of Heat Gain." *Medicine & Science in Sports & Exercise* 41, no. 8 (August 2009): 1682–1683.

Mottola, M. F., I. Jiroux, R. Gratton, et al. "Nutrition and Exercise Prevent Excess Weight Jain in Overweight Pregnant Women." *Medicine and Science in Sports and Exercise* 42, no. 2 (February 2010): 265–272.

Neiman, David C. "What Can I Do to Prevent Osteoarthritis?" *ACSM's Health & Fitness Journal* 10, no. 6 (November/December 2006): 5–7.

Plvarnik, J. M., and L. Mudd. "Oh Baby! Exercise During Pregnancy and the Postpartum Period." *ACSM's Health & Fitness Journal* 13, no. 3 (May/June 2009): 8–13.

Popkin, Barry. "Pour Better or Pour Worse: How Beverages Stack Up." *Nutrition Action Health Letter* 33, no. 5 (June 2006): 1–7.

Slawta, J. N., and R. Ross. "Exercise for Osteoporosis Prevention." *ACSM's Health & Fitness Journal* 8, no. 6 (November/December 2004): 12–19.

Scott, Shelby. "Exercise in the Postpartum Period." *ACSM's Health & Fitness Journal* 10, no. 4 (July/August 2006): 30–41.

Smekal, Gerhard, Serge P. Von Duvillard, et al. "Menstrual Cycle: No Effect on Exercise Cardiorespiratory Variables or Blood Lactate Concentration." *Medicine & Science in Sports & Exercise* 39, no. 7 (July 2007): 1098–1106.

Sorace, P., P. Ronai, and J. Churilla. "Resistance Training for Cardiac Patients." *ACSM's Health & Fitness Journal* 12, no. 6 (November/December 2008): 22–28.

Stover, Beth, and Bob Murray. "Drink Up! The Science of Hydration." *ACSM's Health & Fitness Journal* 11, no. 2 (March/April 2007): 7–11.

"Taking Performance-Enhancing Drugs: Are You Risking Your Health?" December, 2006. www.mayoclinic.com

U.S. Department of Health and Human Services. *2008 Physical Activity Guidelines for America*. ODPHP Publication No. U0036, October 2008. Accessed December 2009. www.health.gov/phguidelines

Chapter 8

American Orthopedic Foot and Ankle Society. "Ankle Sprain Strengthening Exercises." January 2008. www.aofas.org/Scripts/4Disapi.dll/4DCGI/cms/review.html?Action=CMSDocument&DocID=57

American Orthopedic Foot and Ankle Society. "Ankle Sprain Stretching Exercises." January 2008. www.aofas.org/Scripts/4Disapi.dll/4DCGI/cms/review.html?Action=CMS_Document&DocID=58

American Orthopedic Foot and Ankle Society. "Achilles Tendinitis." January 2008. www.aofas.org/scripts/4disapi.dll/4DCGI/cms/review.html?Action=CMS_Document&DocID=26

American Orthopedic Foot and Ankle Society. "Plantar Fasciitis." January 2009. www.aofas.org/scripts/4disapi.dll/4DCGI/cms/review.html?Action=CMS_Document&DocID=51

American Orthopedic Foot and Ankle Society. "Stress Fractures," January 2008. www.aofas.org/scripts/4disapi.dll/4DCGI/cms/review.html?Action=CMS_Document&DocID=54

Bumgardner, W. "Blister Prevention and Treatment—How to Stop Blisters." About.com: Walking. Accessed December 2009. http://walking.about.com/cs/blisterschafing/a/aablisterprev.htm

Cluett, J. "Bursitis." Orthopedics.about.com, December 2009. http://orthopedics.about.com/cs/sportsmedicine/a/blbursitis_2.htm

Cluett, J. "Iliotibial Band Syndrome." Orthopedics.about.com. Accessed December 2009. http://orthopedics.about.com/cs/sportsmedicine/a/itbs.htm

Collins N., K. Crossley, E. Beller, R. Darnell, T. McPoil, and B. Vicenzino. "Foot Orthoses and Physiotherapy in the Treatment of Patellofemoral Pain Syndrome: Randomised Clinical Trial." *British Medical Journal* 337 (October 2008): a1735.

Hanson, R., and D. J. Petron. "Differentiating Common Causes of Chronic Leg Pain in Athletes." *Athletic Therapy Today* 12 (January 2007): 21–23.

Kedlaya, D., and T. Kuang. "Post-Exercise Muscle Soreness." April 6, 2007. www.emedicine.com

Kenucan, D., and L. Kravitz. "Overtraining: Undermining Success?" *ACSM's Health & Fitness Journal* 11 (April 2007): 8–12.

Kumar, S., V. Sharma, P. Vijai, and M. Negi. "Efficacy of Dynamic Muscular Stabilization Techniques (DMST) over Conventional Techniques in Rehabilitation of Chronic Low Back Pain." *Journal of Strength and Conditioning Research* 23 (October 2009). Epub ahead of print. www.ncbi.nlm.nih.gov/pubmed/19858754

Luke, A. "Q&A" *ACSM Fit Society Page* (Summer 2009): 2, 6. www.acsm.org

Mayo Clinic. "Ankle Pain." April 22, 2008. www.mayoclinic.com/health/ankle-pain/MY00083

Mayo Clinic. "Back Pain at Work: Preventing Aches, Pains and Injuries." February 2009. http://mayoclinic.com/health/back-pain/hq00955/method=print

Medline Plus. "Heel Injuries and Disorders." August 2009. www.nlm.nih.gov/medlineplus/heelinjuriesanddisorders.html

Medline Plus. "Bursitis." November 2009. www.nlm.nih.gov/medlineplus/bursitis.html

Medline Plus. "Muscle Cramps" October 2009. www.nlm.nih.gov/medlineplus/musclecramps.html

Quinn, E. "The Side Stitch." About.com:Sportsmedicine. Accessed December 2009. http://sportsmedicine.about.com/cs/injuries/a/aa053100a.htm

Quinn E. "Shin Splints—Prevent and Treat the Pain of Shin Splints." Accessed December 2009. http://sportsmedicine.about.com/cs/leg_injuries/a/leg2.htm

Quinn E. "What Is the Difference Between a Strain and a Sprain." Accessed December 2009. http://sportsmedicine.about.com/cs/injuries/a/sprains.htm

Quinn, E. "Weight Training Best for Easing Back Pain." Accessed December 2009. http://sportsmedicine.about.com/b/2009/06/10/weight-training-best-for-easing-back-pain.htm

Ruiz, B., and S. M. Zaffer. "Hamstring Injury." emedicine from WebMD (June 16, 2008). http://emedicine.medscape.com/article/90881-print

Witvrouw, E. "The Role of Stretching in Tendon Injuries." *British Journal of Sports Medicine* 41 (April 2007): 224–226.

Chapter 9

American Heart Association. "Heart Disease and Stroke Statistics—2010 Update." National Center, 7272 Greenville Avenue, Dallas, TX 75231-4596. 2006.

"Are You an Apple or a Pear?" *University of California, Berkeley Wellness Letter* 24, no. 9 (June 2008): 1–2.

The BARI 2 D Study Group. "A Randomized Trial of Therapies for Type 2 Diabetes and Coronary Artery Disease." *New England Journal of Medicine* 360, no. 24 (June 11, 2009): 2503–2515.

Blair, S. N., and T. S. Church. "The Fitness, Obesity, and Health Equation." *Journal of the American Medical Association* 292, no. 10 (September 8, 2004): 1232–1234.

Brubaker, P. M., and C. Ozemek. "Exercise Therapy for the failing Heart, Harmful or Helpful?" *ACSM's Health & Fitness Journal* 14, no. 2 (March/April 2010): 9–15.

Case, P. E., et al. "Stemming the Tide: Are You Prepared for the Diabetes Epidemic?" *ACSM's Health & Fitness Journal* 10, no. 1 (January/February 2006): 7–13.

Centers for Disease Control and Prevention/National Center for Health Statistics (CDC/NCHS). *CVD Statistics.* Accessed January 2010.

Christou, D. D., C. L. Gentile, et al. "Fatness Is a Better Predictor of Cardiovascular Disease Risk Factor Profile than Aerobic Fitness in Healthy Men." *Circulation* 11 (April 18, 2005): 1904–1914.

Churilla, J. R. "The Metabolic Syndrome: The Crucial Role of Exercise Prescription and Diet." *ACSM's Health & Fitness Journal* 13, no. 1 (January/February 2009): 20–25.

Danesh, M. B., et al. "C-Reactive Protein and Other Circulation Markers of Inflammation in the Prediction of Coronary Heart Disease." *New England Journal of Medicine* 350, no. 14 (April 1, 2004): 1387–1097.

De Jong, A. "Peripheral Artery Disease: Impact on Lifestyle and Rehabilitation Opportunities." *ACSM's Health & Fitness Journal* 14, no. 2 (March/April 2010): 42–44.

Denollet, J. "DS14: Standard Assessment of Negative Affectivity, Social Inhibition, and Type D Personality." *Psychosomatic Medicine* 67 (2005): 89–97.

Dietz, W. H., and T. N. Robinson. "Overweight Children and Adolescents." *New England Journal of Medicine* 352, no. 20 (May 19, 2005): 2100–2109.

Donovan, Elizabeth, and Amy Olson. American Heart Association News Release: "Drinking Heavily in College May Lead to Heart Disease Later in Life." Accessed April 19, 2007. www.americanheart.org.

"Don't Be a Diagnostic Error." *Consumer Reports On Health* 21, no. 9 (September 2009): 1–5.

Flegal, K. M., et al. "Excess Deaths Associated with Underweight, Overweight, and Obesity." *Journal of the American Medical Association* 293, no. 15 (April 20, 2005): 1861–1867.

Ford, Earl S., Umed A. Ajani, Janet B. Croft, et al. "Explaining the Decrease in U.S. Deaths from Coronary Disease, 1980–2000." *New England Journal of Medicine* 356, no. 23 (June 7, 2007): 2388–2398.

Gaglione, M. "Obesity and Risk of Death." *New England Journal of Medicine* 360, no. 10 (March 5, 2009): 1042–1044.

Hansson, G. K. "Inflammation, Atherosclerosis, and Coronary Artery Disease." *New England Journal of Medicine* 352, no. 16 (April 21, 2005): 1685–1695.

Haskell, William L., I-MIN Lee, Russel R. Pate, Kenneth E. Powell, Steven N. Blain, et al. "Physical Activity and Public Health: Updated Recommendation for Adults from the American College of Sports Medicine and the American Heart Association." *Special Reports: Medicine & Science in Sport & Exercise* 39, no. 8 (August 2007): 1423–1434.

Hittel, D. S., W. E. Kraus, et al. "Exercise in Muscles of Overweight Men and Women with Metabolic Syndrome." *Journal of Applied Physiology* 98 (January 2005): 168–179.

Hu, F. B., et al. "Adiposity and Physical Activity as Predictors of Mortality." *New England Journal of Medicine* 352, no. 13 (March 31, 2005): 1381–1384.

Keys, A. "Coronary Heart Disease in Seven Countries." *Circulation* 41 (Suppl. 1, 1970): 1.

Krause, W. E., and P. S. Douglas. "Where Does Fitness Fit In?" *New England Journal of Medicine* 353, no. 5 (August 4, 2005): 517–519.

Kress, Jeff, Jan M. Schroeder, et al. "Learning the Ropes: Challenging Children with Diabetes." *ACSM's Health & Fitness Journal* 10, no. 5 (September/October 2007): 19–23.

La Fontaine, T., and J. Roitman. "Contemporary Cardiovascular Rehabilitation In the New Millennium."

ACSM's Health & Fitness Journal 12, no. 5 (September/ October 2008): 21–27.

LaRocca, T., D. Seals, A. E. Walker, et al. [Abstract 5081.] "Leukocyte Telomere Length Preserved with Age in Adults Who Exercise and Is Related to Vascular Endothelial Function." *Circulation* 118 (October 2008): 1141.

"Managing Your Blood Sugar." *Consumer Reports on Health* 21, no. 4 (April 2009): 1–5.

Mell, M. M. "New York City's War on Fat." *New England Journal of Medicine* 360, no. 19 (May 7, 2009): 2015–2020.

Miller, G. E., K. E. Freedland, et al. "Cynical Hostility, Depressive Symptoms, and the Expression of Inflammatory Risk Markers for Heart Disease." *Journal of Behavioral Medicine* 26, no. 6 (December 2003): 501–515.

Parr, Richard, and Shara Haught. "Abdominal Visceral Fat: The New Direction in Body Composition." *ACSM's Health & Fitness Journal* 10, no. 4 (July/August 2006): 26–29.

Pescatello, L. S., W. R. Thompson, and N. F. Gordon. "A Preview of ACSM's Guidelines for Exercise Testing and Prescription, Eight Edition." *ACSM's Health & Fitness Journal* 13, no. 4 (July/August 2009): 23–26.

Pilolla, K., and M. Manore. "Gestational Diabetes Mellitus." *ACSM's Health & Fitness Journal* 12, no. 5 (September/ October 2008): 8–13.

Pischon, T., H. Boeing, and K. Hoffman, "General and Abdominal Adiposity and Risk of Death in Europe." *New England Journal of Medicine* 359, no. 20 (November 13, 2008): 2105–2120.

Preston, S. "Deadweight?—The Influence of Obesity on Longevity." *New England Journal of Medicine* 352, no. 13 (March 31, 2005): 1135–1137.

Pronk, Nico. "The Metabolic Syndrome—The 'Syndrome X Factor'—at Work." *ACSM's Health & Fitness Journal* 10, no. 5 (October 2006): 38–42.

Ribisl, P. "Exercise—the New Penicillin: Inflammation and Chronic Disease." *ACSM's Health & Fitness Journal* 7, no. 4 (July/August 2003): 28–30.

Ridker, P. M., J. E. Buring, et al. "C-Reactive Protein, the Metabolic Syndrome and Risk of Incident Cardiovascular Events: An 8-Year Follow-up of 14,719 Initially Healthy American Women." *Circulation* 107, no. 3 (2003): 391–397.

Roberts, C. K., and J. R. Barnard. "Effects of Exercise and Diet on Chronic Disease." *Journal of Applied Physiology* 98 (January 2005): 3–30.

Sacks, F., M., G. A. Bray, V. J. Carey, et al. "Comparisons of Weight Loss Diets with Different Compositions of Fat, Protein, and Carbohydrates." *New England Journal of Medicine* 360, no. 9 (February 26, 2009): 859–873.

Schardt, D. "Menopause, Reducing Symptoms: What Works: What Doesn't?" *Nurtition Action Health Letter* (November 2008): 9–11.

Schum, J. L., R. S. Jorgensen, et al. "Trait Anger, Anger Expression, and Ambulatory Blood Pressure: A Meta-Analytic Review." *Journal of Behavioral Medicine* 26, no. 5 (October 2003): 395–415.

Scott, Shelby. "Essential Hypertension: Lifestyle Intervention Treatments." *ACSM's Health & Fitness Journal* 11, no. 4 (July/August 2007): 37–38.

"Slow Burn: How Inflammation Can Trigger a Heart Attack." *Nutrition Action Health Letter* (January/February 2009): 1–7

Sorace, Paul, Thomas LaFontaine, and Tom R. Thomas. "Know the Risks: Lifestyle Management of Dyslipidemia." *ACSM's Health & Fitness Journal* 10, no. 4 (July/August 2006): 18–24.

Stanforth, D. and M. Mackert. "Social Undermining of Healthy Eating and Exercise Behaviors." *ACSM's Health & Fitness Journal* 13, no. 3 (May/June 2009): 14–19.

"Step-Based Guidelines in New Pair of Studies: Steps to Meet ACSM/CDC Recommendation." American College of Sports Medicine. New Release. Accessed June 1, 2007. http://www.acsm.org

Stewart, S. T., D. M. Cutter, and A. B. Rosen. "Forecasting the Effects of Obesity and Smoking on U.S. Life Expectancy." *New England Journal of Medicine* 361, no. 23 (December 3, 2009): 2252–2260.

Telford, Richard D. "Low Physical Activity and Obesity: Causes of Chronic Disease or Simply Predictors?" *Medicine & Science in Sports & Exercise* 39, no. 8 (August 2007): 1193–1199.

"The Hidden Factor in Disease." *Consumer Reports on Health* 19, no. 1 (January 2007): 1–4.

Thompson, Dixie. "Women and Cardiovascular Disease." *ACSM's Health & Fitness Journal* 11, no. 4 (July/August 2007): 5.

Thompson, W. R. *ACSM's Guidelines for Exercise Testing and Prescription,* 8th ed. Philadelphia: Lippencott, Williams, & Wilkins, 2009.

Toole, J. F., and M. R. Malinow. "Lowering Homocysteine in Patients with Ischemic Stroke to Prevent Recurrent Stroke, Myocardial Infarction, and Death." *Journal of the American Medical Association* 291, no. 5 (February 4, 2004): 565–755.

Weiss, R. J., J. Dziura, et al. "Obesity and the Metabolic Syndrome in Children and Adolescents." *New England Journal of Medicine* 350, no. 23 (June 3, 2004): 2362–2374.

Werner, C., T. Furster, C. Roggia, et al. "Beneficial Effects of Long-Term Edurance Exercise on Leukocyte Telomere Biology." *Circulation* 120, no. 18 (November 3, 2009): s492.

Werner, C. T. Furster, T. Widmann, et al. "Physical Exercise Prevents Cellular Senescence in Circulating Leukocytes in the Vessel Wall." *Circulation* 120, no. 24 (December 15, 2009): 2438–2447.

"Well and Informed." *University of California, Berkeley Wellness Letter, The Newsletter of Nutrition, Fitness, and Self-care* 26, no. 7 (April 2010): 8.

Chapter 10

Barnes, V. A., et al. "Impact of Meditation on Resting and Ambulatory Blood Pressure and Heart Rate in Youth." *Psychosomatic Medicine* 66, no. 6 (November/December 2004): 909–914.

Benson, H. *The Relaxation Response.* New York: Avon Books, 1976.

Bertisch, S. M., C. C. Wee, and R. S. Phillips. "Alternative Mind–Body Therapies Used by Adults With Medical Conditions." *Journal of Psychosomatic Research* 66, no. 6 (June 2009): 511–519.

Biobehavioral Approaches to Pain, Rhonda J. Moore, ed. *New England Journal of Medicine* 361, no. 2 (July 9, 2009): 215.

Bluementhal, J. A., et al. "Effects of Exercise and Stress Management Training on Markers of Cardiovascular Risk in Patients with Ischemic Heart Disease." *Journal of American Medical Association* 293, no. 13 (April 13, 2005): 1626–1634.

Blumenthal, James A., et al. "Exercise Pharmacotherapy in the Treatment of Major Depressive Disorder." *Psychosomatic Medicine* 69, no. 7 (September 2007): 587–596.

Blumenthal, James A., et al. "Spirituality, Religion, and Clinical Outcomes in Patients Recovering from an Acute Myocardial Infarction." *Psychosomatic Medicine* 69, no. 6 (July/August 2007): 501–508.

Brydon, L., P. C. Strike, C. Bhatta, R. Mimi, et al. "Hostility and Physiological Responses to Laboratory Stress in Acute Coronary Syndrome Patients." *Journal of Psychosomatic Research* 68, no. 2, (February 2010): 109–116.

Calado, R. T., and N. S. Young. "Telomere Diseases." *New England Journal of Medicine* 361, no. 24 (December 19, 2009): 2353–2365.

Crady, T. "College of the Overwhelmed: The Campus Mental Health Crisis and What to Do About It." *Journal of College Student Development* 46, no. 5 (September/October 2005): 556–558.

Davidson, R. J., J. Kabat-Zinn, et al. "Alterations in Brain and Immune Function Produced by Mindfulness Meditation." *Pychosomatic Medicine* 65 (2003): 564–570.

Denollet, J. "DS14: Standard Assessment of Negative Affectivity, Social Inhibition and Type D Personality." *Psychosomatic Medicine* 67, no. 1 (2005): 89–97.

Eaker, Elaine D., et al. "Marital Status, Marital Strain, and Risk of Coronary Heart Disease or Total Mortality: The Framingham Offspring Study." *Psychosomatic Medicine* 69, no. 6 (July/August 2007): 509–513.

Fliege, H., M. Rose, P. Arch, et al. "The Perceived Stress Questionnaire (PSQ) Reconsidered: Validation and Reference Values from Different Clinical and Healthy Adult Samples." *Psychosomatic Medicine* 67 (January 1, 2005): 78–88.

Frey, B. B., T. P. Daaleman, et al. "Measuring a Dimension of Spirituality for Health Research: Validity of the Spirituality Index of Well-Being." *Research on Aging* 27, no. 5 (September 1, 2005): 556–577.

Galper, D. I., et al. "Inverse Association between Physical Inactivity and Mental Health in Men and Women." *Medicine and Science in Sports & Exercise* 38, no. 1 (January 2006): 173–178.

Gerber, M., and U. Puhse. "Don't Crack Under Pressure— Do Leisure-Time Physical Activity and Self-Esteem Moderate the Relationship Between School-Based Stress and Psychosomatic Complaints?" *Journal of Psychosomatic Research* 65, no. 4 (October 2008): 363–369.

Hammer, Mark, and Andrew Steptoe. "Association Between Physical Fitness, Parasympathetic Control, and Proinflammatory Responses to Mental Stress." *Psychosomatic Medicine* 69, no. 7 (September 2007): 660–666.

Hausteiner, C., D. Klupsch, R. Emeny, et al. "Clustering of Negative Affectivity and Social Inhibition in the Community: Prevalence of Type D Personality as a Cardiovascular Risk Marker." *Psychosomatic Medicine* (January 25, 2010), 10.1097/PSY.0b013e3181cb8bae.

Holmes, T. E., and R. H. Rahe. "The Social Readjustment Rating Scale." *Journal of Psychosomatic Research* 11 (1967): 213–219.

Hummer, R. A. "Commentary: Understanding Religious Involvements and Mortality Risk in the United States." *International Journal of Epidemiology* 34, no. 2 (April 1, 2005): 452–453.

Kiecolt-Glaser, J., L. Christian, H. Preston, et al. "Stress, Inflammation and Yoga Practice." *Psychosomatic Medicine* (January 11, 2010), 10.1097/PSY.0b013e3181cb9377.

Kobasa, S. C. "The Hardy Personality: Toward a Social Psychology of Stress and Health." In R. S. Sanders, and J. Suls, eds., *Social Psychology of Health and Illness.* Hillsdale, NJ: Erlbaum, 1982.

Kupper, Nina, Johan Denollet, et al. "Heritability of Type-D Personality." *Psychosomatic Medicine* 69, no. 7 (September 2007): 675–681.

La Forge, R. "Aligning Mind and Body: Exploring the Disciplines of Mindful Exercise." *ACSM's Health & Fitness Journal* 9, no. 5 (September/October 2005): 7–14.

Largo-Wright, E., et al. "Perceived Problem Solving, Stress, and Health Among College Students." *American Journal of Health Behavior* 29, no. 4 (July/August 2005): 360–370.

Loponen, M., C. Hublin, R. Kalimo, et al. "Joint Effect of Self-Reported Sleep Problems and Three Components of the Metabolic Syndrome on Risk of Coronary Heart Disease." *Journal of Psychosomatic Research* 68, no. 2 (February 2010): 149–158.

Low, C., K. Salomon, and K. A. Mathews. "Chronic Life Stress, Cardiovascular Reactivity, and Subclinical Cardiovascular Disease in Adolescents." *Psychosomatic Medicine* 71, no. 9 (November/December 2009): 927–931.

Maglione-Garves, C. A., et al. "Cortisol Connection: Tips on Managing Stress and Weight." *ACSM's Health & Fitness Journal* 9, no. 5 (September/October 2005): 20–23.

Mykletum, Arnstein, et al. "Anxiety, Depression, and Cause-Specific Mortality: The HUNT Study." *Psychosomatic Medicine* 69, no. 1 (January 2007): 47–53.

Peterson, J. "Ten (Lame) Reasons People Commonly Give for Not Exercising." *ACSM's Health & Fitness Journal* 10, no. 1 (January/February 2006): 44.

Roberts, R. E. "Positive Well-Being and Sleep." *Journal of Psychosomatic Research* 68, no. 4 (April 2008): 417–418.

Rosch, P. J., editor in chief. "Can Laughter and Humor Help You Live Longer?" *Health and Stress, The Newsletter of the American Institute of Stress* (November 2005): 1–13.

Rosenzeig, S., J. M. Greeson, D. Reibel, et al. "Mindfulness-Based Stress Reduction for Chronic Pain Conditions: Variation in Treatment Outcomes and Role of Home

Meditation Practice." *Journal of Psychosomatic Research* 68, no. 1 (January 2010): 29–36.

Scott, S. "Combating Depression with Exercise." *ACSM's Health & Fitness Journal* 9, no. 4 (July/August 2005): 3–33.

Seeman, T. E., et al. "Religiosity/Spirituality and Health, A Critic's Review of the Evidence for Biological Pathways." *American Psychology* 58, no. 1 (January 2003): 53–63.

Selye, Hans. *Stress without Distress.* New York: Lippincott, 1984.

Sheps, David S., et al. "Psychological Stress and Myocardial Ischemia: Understanding the Link and the Implications." *Psychosomatic Medicine* 69, no. 6 (July/August 2007): 491–492.

Sloan, R. P., P. A. Shapiro, E. E. Gorenstein, et al. "Cardiac Autonomic Control and Treatment of Hostility." *Psychosomatic Medicine* 72, no. 1 (January 2010): 1–8.

Tacon, A. M., et al. "Mindfulness Meditation, Anxiety Reduction, and Heart Disease: A Pilot Study." *Family and Community Health* 26, no. 1 (January 2003): 25–33.

Torpy, J. M., A. E. Burke, and R. M. Glass. "Acute Emotional Stress and the Heart." *Journal of American Medical Association* 298, no. 3 (July 18, 2007): 360.

Vlachopoulos, C., et al. "Divergent Effects of Laughter and Mental Stress on Arterial Stiffness and Central Hemodynamics." *Psychosomatic Medicine* 71 (February 27, 2009): 446–453.

Voelker, R., "Stress, Sleep Loss, and Substance Abuse Create Potent Recipe for College Depression." *Journal of the American Medical Association* 291, no. 18 (May 12, 2004): 2177–2179.

White, Victoria M., et al. "Is Cancer Risk Associated with Anger Control and Negative Effect? Findings from a Prospective Cohort Study." *Psychosomatic Medicine* 69, no. 7 (September 2007): 667–681.

Wilson, G., and M. Prithard. "Comparing Sources of Stress in College Student Athletes and Non-Athletes." *Athletic Insight, The Online Journal of Sport Psychology* 7, no. 1 (March 2005).

Wittstein, I. S., D. R. Thiemann, J. Lima, et al. "Neurohumoral Features of Myocardial Stunning Due to Sudden Emotional Stress." *New England Journal of Medicine* 352, no. 6 (February 10, 2005): 539–548.

Winterowd, C. "The Relationship of Spiritual Beliefs and Involvement with the Experience of Anger and Stress in College Students." *Journal of College Student Development* 46, no. 5 (September/October 2005): 515–529.

Ziegelstein, Roy C. "Acute Emotional Stress and Cardiac Arrhythmias." *Journal of the American Medical Association* 298, no. 3 (July 18, 2007): 324–329.

Chapter 11

Brand-Miller, J., et al. *The New Glucose Revolution: The Authoritative Guide to the Glycemic Index—The Dietary Solution for Lifelong Health,* 3rd ed. New York: Marlow and Co., 2007.

Centers for Disease Control and Prevention. National Center for Chronic Disease Prevention and Health Promotion.

Behavioral Risk Factor Surveillance—United States, 2007. www.cdc.gov/brfss

"Does Glycemic Index Really Make a Difference?" *Tufts University Health & Nutrition Letter* 27 (March 2009): 4–5.

"Eat Like a Mediterranean to Protect Your Aging Brain." *Tufts Health & Nutrition Letter* 27 (November 2009): 1–2.

"Eating for Total Health." *Tufts University Health & Nutrition Letter* 28 (May 2010): special suppl.

"Five New Reasons to Get Whole Grains." *Tufts University Health & Nutrition Letters* 25 (August 2007): 1–2.

"How Omega-3 Fats May Protect Against Cancer." *American Institute for Cancer Research Newsletter* 84 (Summer 2004): 1, 3–4.

Lang, T., and M. Heasman. *Food Wars: The Global Battle for Mouths, Minds and Markets.* London: Earthscan, 2004.

Lappe, J., et al. "Vitamin D and Calcium Supplementation Reduces Cancer Risk: Results of a Randomized Trial." *American Journal of Clinical Nutrition* 85 (June 2007): 1586–1591.

Liebman, B. "From Sun & Sea: A New Study Puts Vitamin D and Omega-3's to the Test." *Nutrition Action Healthletter* 36 (November 2009): 1, 3–7.

Liebman, B. "Sugar Overload: Curbing America's Sweet Tooth." *Nutrition Action Healthletter* 37 (January/February 2010): 1, 3–8.

Liebman, B. "What Should I Eat?" *Nutrition Action Healthletter* 36 (October 2009): 1, 3–6.

Liebman, B. "Whole Grains: The Inside Story." *Nutrition Action Healthletter* 33 (May 2006): 1, 3–5.

Mitrou, P. "Mediterranean Dietary Pattern and Prediction of All-Cause Mortality in a U.S. Population." *Archives of Internal Medicine* 167 (December 10/24, 2007): 2461–2468.

National Osteoporosis Foundation. *Take Action: Healthy Bones, Build Them for Life!* Washington, D.C., 2004. www.nof.org

"New Labeling Helps You Avoid Trans Fats." *Tufts University Health & Nutrition Letter* 23 (January 2006): 1–2.

Roberts, C. K., and R. J. Barnard. "Effects of Exercise and Diet on Chronic Disease." *Journal of Applied Physiology* 98 (January 2005): 3–30.

U.S. Department of Agriculture. Center for Nutrition Policy and Promotion. "Diet Quality of Americans in 1994–96 and 2001–02 as Measured by the Healthy Eating Index—2005." *Nutrition Insights* 37 (December 2007).

U.S. Department of Agriculture. Center for Nutrition Policy and Promotion. "The Food Supply and Dietary Fiber: Its Availability and Effect on Health." *Nutrition Insights* 36 (November 2007).

U.S. Department of Agriculture. Center for Nutrition Policy and Promotion. *The Healthy Eating Index.* Washington, D.C., June 2008.

U.S. Department of Agriculture. Center for Nutrition Policy and Promotion. *MyPyramid.* Washington, D.C., March 2010. www.MyPyramid.gov

U.S. Department of Agriculture. Center for Nutrition Policy and Promotion. "Nutrient Content of the U.S. Food Supply." March 2008.

U.S. Department of Agriculture. U.S. Department of Health and Human Services. *What We Eat in America*. Washington, D.C., 2009.

U.S. Department of Health and Human Services. *Bone Health and Osteoporosis: A Report of the Surgeon General*. Washington, D.C., 2004.

U.S. Department of Health and Human Services. National Heart, Lung, and Blood Institute. *The DASH Eating Plan*. April 2006.

World Cancer Research Fund/American Institute for Cancer Research. *Food, Nutrition, Physical Activity, and the Prevention of Cancer: A Global Perspective*. Washington, D.C.: American Institute for Cancer Research, 2007. www.dietandcancerreport.org

Chapter 12

American Psychiatric Association. *Diagnostic and Statistical Manual of Mental Disorders,* 4th ed. Washington, D.C., 2000.

Blair, S. N., and E. A. Leermakers. "Exercise and Weight Management." In T. A. Wadden and A. J. Stunkard (eds.), *Handbook of Obesity Treatment*. New York: The Guilford Press, 2002.

"Boosting Metabolism to Lose Weight: What Works, What Doesn't *Environmental Nutrition* 31 (January 2010): 1, 4.

Bouchard, C., et al. "The Response to Long-Term Overfeeding in Identical Twins." *New England Journal of Medicine* 322 (May 24, 1990): 1477–1482.

Braveman, P. "A Health Disparities Perspective on Obesity Research." *Preventing Chronic Disease* 6 (July 9, 2009).

"Build Muscle to Speed Fat-Burning." *American Institute for Cancer Research Newsletter* 94 (Winter 2007): 4.

Calle, E. E., et al. "Overweight, Obesity, and Mortality from Cancer in a Prospectively Studied Cohort of U.S. Adults." *New England Journal of Medicine* 348 (April 24, 2003): 1625–1638.

Centers for Disease Control and Prevention. National Center for Chronic Disease Prevention and Health Promotion. *Behavioral Risk Factor Surveillance—United States, 2008*. www.cdc.gov/brfss

Centers for Disease Control and Prevention. National Center for Chronic Disease Prevention and Health Promotion. *Health, United States, 2008*. March 2009. www.cdc.gov/nchs

Centers for Disease Control and Prevention. National Center for Chronic Disease Prevention and Health Promotion. *Obesity: Halting the Epidemic by Making Health Easier*. February 2009.

"Differences in Prevalence of Obesity Among Black, White, and Hispanic Adults—United States, 2006–2008." *Morbidity and Mortality Weekly Report,* July 17, 2009.

Ewing, R., et al. "Relationship Between Urban Sprawl and Physical Activity, Obesity, and Morbidity." *American Journal of Health Promotion* 18 (September/October 2003): 47–57.

"F as in Fat: How Obesity Policies Are Failing in America 2009." Trust for America's Health and Robert Wood Johnson Foundation, July 2009. www.healthyamericans.org

Flegal, K. M., et al. "Excess Deaths Associated with Underweight, Overweight, and Obesity." *Journal of the American Medical Association* 293 (April 20, 2005): 1861–1867.

Fletcher, A. M. *Thin for Life: 10 Keys to Success from People Who Have Lost Weight and Kept It Off*. New York: Houghton Mifflin Co., 2003.

Horgen, K. B., and K. D. Brownell. "Confronting the Toxic Environment: Environmental and Public Health Actions in a World Crisis." In T. A. Wadden and A. J. Stunkard (eds.), *Handbook of Obesity Treatment*. New York: The Guilford Press, 2002.

Howard, B. V., et al. "Low-Fat Dietary Pattern and Weight Change over 7 Years: The Women's Health Initiative Dietary Modification Trial." *Journal of the American Medical Association* 295 (January 4, 2006): 39–49.

Klein, S., et al. "Absence of an Effect of Liposuction on Insulin Action and Risk Factors for Coronary Heart Disease." *New England Journal of Medicine* 350 (June 17, 2004): 2549–2557.

LaVeist, T. A., et al. "Environmental and Socio-Economic Factors as Contributors to Racial Disparities in Diabetes Prevalence." *Journal of General Internal Medicine* 24 (October 2009): 1144–1148.

Liebman, B. "Cancer: How Extra Pounds Boost Your Risk." *Nutrition Action Healthletter* 34 (September 2007): 1, 3–7.

"Lose Belly Fat to Lower Colon Cancer Risk." *Tufts University Health & Nutrition Letter* 24 (October 2006): 8.

Mark, D. H. "Deaths Attributable to Obesity." *Journal of the American Medical Association* 293 (April 20, 2005): 1918–1919.

Pescatello, L. S., S. L. Volpe, and N. Clark. "Which Is More Effective for Maintaining a Healthy Body Weight: Diet or Exercise?" *ACSM's Health & Fitness Journal* 8 (September/October 2004): 9–14.

Preston, S. H. "Deadweight?—The Influence of Obesity on Longevity." *New England Journal of Medicine* 352 (March 17, 2005): 1135–1137.

"Racial Disparities in Diabetes Prevalence Linked to Living Conditions." *Science Daily*. Johns Hopkins University Bloomberg School of Public Health, September 30, 2009.

Rolls, B. J., L. S. Roe, and J. S. Meengs. "Reduction in Portion Size and Energy Density of Foods Are Additive and Lead to Sustained Decreases in Energy Intake." *American Journal of Clinical Nutrition* 83 (January 2006): 11–17.

Schardt, D. "Secrets of Successful Losers." *Nutrition Action Healthletter* 35 (January/February 2008): 8.

Somer, E. *10 Habits That Mess Up a Woman's Diet*. New York: McGraw-Hill, 2006.

Stein, C. J., and G. A. Colditz. "The Epidemic of Obesity." *Journal of Clinical Endocrinology and Metabolism* 89 (June 2004): 2522–2525.

Stunkard, A. J., et al. "The Body-Mass Index of Twins Who Have Been Reared Apart." *New England Journal of Medicine* 322 (May 24, 1990): 1483–1487.

"The Skinny on Popular Diets." *Harvard Heart Letter* 16 (February 2005): 4–6.

Wadden, T. A., and A. J. Stunkard (eds.). *Handbook of Obesity Treatment*. New York: The Guilford Press, 2002.

"Waist-to-Hip Ratio Predicts Heart Risk Better Than BMI." *Tufts University Health & Nutrition Letter* 23 (January 2006): 1–2.

Weinbrenner, T., et al. "Circulating Oxidized LDL Is Associated with Increased Waist Circumference Independent of Body Mass Index in Men and Women." *American Journal of Clinical Nutrition* 83 (January 2006): 30–35.

Williams, P. T., and P. D. Wood. "The Effects of Changing Exercise Levels on Weight and Age-Related Weight Gain." *International Journal of Obesity* 30 (March 2006): 543–551.

World Cancer Research Fund/American Institute for Cancer Research. *Food, Nutrition, Physical Activity, and the Prevention of Cancer: A Global Perspective*. Washington, D.C.: American Institute for Cancer Research, 2007. www.dietandcancerreport.org

Young, L., and Nestle, M. "The Contribution of Expanding Portion Sizes to the U.S. Obesity Epidemic." *American Journal of Public Health* 92 (February 2002): 246–249.

Yusuf, S., et al. "Obesity and the Risk of Myocardial Infarction in 27,000 Participants from 52 Countries: A Case-Control Study." *Lancet* 366 (November 5, 2005): 1640–1649.

Chapter 13

American Cancer Society. *Cancer Facts and Figures 2010*. Atlanta: American Cancer Society 2010. www.cancer.org

American Institute for Cancer Research/World Cancer Research Fund. *Food, Nutrition, Physical Activity, and the Prevention of Cancer: A Global Perspective*. Washington, D.C: AICR, 2007.

Autier P., and S. Gandini. "Vitamin D supplementation and Total Mortality." *Archives of Internal Medicine* (September 2007): 1730–1737.

Barclay, L. "Medscape Medical News: American Academy of Dermatology Issues Updated Position Statement on Vitamin D." July 16, 2009. www.medscpe.com/viewarticle/706024?src=rss

Barclay, L. "Weight Gain in Adulthood Linked to Increased Postmenopausal Breast Cancer Risk." October, 2007. www.medscape.com

Bataille, V. "Risk Factors for Melanoma Development." *Expert Review of Dermatology,* December 2009. www.medscape.com/viewarticle/713727

Bikle, D. D. "UV Radiation, Vitamin D and Epidermal Carcinogenesis: Can Vitamin D Production in the Skin Serve as a Protective Barrier Against Nonmelanoma Skin Cancer?" *Expert Review of Dermatology* (December 2009): 557–566. www.medscape.com/viewarticle/713649

Blair, S. N., et al. "Physical Fitness and All-Cause Mortality: A Prospective Study of Healthy Men and Women." *Journal of the American Medical Association* 262 (November 3, 1989): 2395–2401.

Centers for Disease Control and Prevention. *The State Indicator Report on Fruits and Vegetables, 2009*. September 2009. www.fruitsandveggiesmatter.gov/indicatorreport/

Harvard Center for Cancer Prevention. "Harvard Report on Cancer Prevention Vol. 1: Causes of Human Cancer." *Cancer Causes and Control* 7 (Suppl): 1996.

International Agency for Research on Cancer. "Exposure to Artificial UV Radiation and Skin Cancer." World Health Organization, July 2009. www.iarc.fr/en/publications/pdfs-online/wrk/wrkl/index.php

Koushik, A., et al. "Fruits, Vegetables, and Colon Cancer Risk in a Pooled Analysis of 14 Cohort Studies." *Journal of the National Cancer Institute* 99 (November 2007): 1471–1483.

Lappe, J. M., et al. "Vitamin D and Calcium Supplementation Reduces Cancer Risk: The Results of a Randomized Trial." *American Journal of Clinical Nutrition* (June 2007): 1586–1591.

Lenz, T. L. "Vitamin D Supplementation and Cancer Prevention." *American Journal of Lifestyle Medicine* (December 2009): 365–368. www.medscape.com/viewarticle/712529

Mayo Clinic. "Cancer Prevention: 7 Steps to Reduce Your Risk." September 2008. www.mayoclinic.com/health/cancer-prevention/CA00024

Mayo Clinic. "Sunless Tanning: A Safe Alternative to Sunbathing." Accessed January 2010. http://mayoclinic.com/health/sunless-tanning/SN00037

McDonald, R. "Nutrition and Cancer Prevention." *ACSM Fit Society Page* (Spring 2009): 1–2.

Meyerhardt, J. A., et al. "Physical Activity and Male Colorectal Cancer Survival." *Archives of Internal Medicine* (December 2009): 2102–2108.

National Cancer Institute. "Cancer: Questions and Answer." U.S. National Institutes of Health. Accessed January 29, 2010. www.cancer.gov/cancertopics/factsheet/Sites-Types/general

National Cancer Institute. "Cancer Trends Progress Report—2007 Update." December, 2007. www.cancer.gov

National Cancer Institute. "Cellular Telephone Use and Cancer Risk." U.S. National Institutes of Health. Accessed January 29, 2010. www.cancer.gov/cancertopics/factsheet/Risk/cellphones

National Cancer Institute. "HumanPapilloma Virus (HPV) Vaccine." U.S. National Institutes of Health. October 22, 2009. www.cancer.gov/cancertopics/factsheet/Prevention/HPV-vaccine

National Institutes of Health. "Dietary Supplement Fact Sheet: Vitamin D, Office of Dietary Supplements." Accessed January 28, 2010. http://dietarysupplements.info.nih.gov/factsheets/vitamind.asp

Servan-Schreiber, D. *Anticancer: A New Way of Life*. New York: Penguin Group, 2008.

Speck, R., and Kathryn Schmitz. "Cancer Prevention: Lifestyle Change." *ACSM Fit Society Page* (Spring 2009): 4.

World Cancer Research Fund/American Institute for Cancer Research. *The Second Expert Report, Food, Nutrition, Physical Activity, and the Prevention of Cancer: A Global Perspective*. Washington, DC: American Institute for Cancer Research, 2009.

Chapter 14

"Big Differences in Why Girls vs. Boys Use Cigarettes, Alcohol, and Drugs." A Report from the National Center on Addiction and Substance Abuse. Columbia University, New York (February 2003).

CORE Institute: Center for Alcohol and Other Drugs Studies. Southern Illinois University at Carbondale. Accessed October, 2005. www.siu.edu/departments/coreinst/public

Friedman, R. A. "The Changing Face of Drug Abuse—The Trend Toward Prescription Drugs." *New England Journal of Medicine* 354 (April 6, 2006): 1448.

Hampton, Tracy. "Genes Harbor Clues to Addiction Recovery." *Journal of the American Medical Association* 292, no. 3 (July 21, 2004): 321–322.

Hingston, R., et al. "Magnitude of Alcohol-Related Mortality and Morbidity among U.S. College Students Ages 18–24: Changes from 1998 to 2005." *Annual Review of Public Health* 26 (2005): 259–279.

Kuehn, Bridget M. "Brain Scans, Genes Provide Addiction Clues." *Journal of the American Medical Association* 297, no. 13 (April 4, 2007): 1419–1421.

Kuehn, Bridget M. "Genome Provides Clues on Addiction." *Journal of the American Medical Association* 295, no. 20 (May 24/31, 2006): 2345–2346.

Johnston, L. D., P. M. O'Malley, and J. G. Bachman. *Monitoring the Future National Survey Results on Drug Use, 1975–2001. Vol. II: College Students and Adults Ages 14–40.* Bethesda, MD: National Institute on Drug Abuse, 2002.

Mallett, K. A., R. Turrisi, M. E. Larimer, et al. 'Have I Had One Too Many?' Assessing Gender Differences in Misperceptions of Intoxication Among College Students." *Journal of Studies on Alcohol & Drugs* 70, no. 6 (November 2009): 964.

McGinn, C. B. "Close Calls with Club Drugs." *New England Journal of Medicine* 352 (June 30, 2005): 2671.

Mendelson, J. H. "Alcohol Problems in Adolescents and Young Adults: Epidemiology, Neurobiology, Prevention, and Treatment." *New England Journal of Medicine* 354 (May 25, 2006): 2299.

"Methamphetamine." Wikipedia, The Free Encyclopedia. July 18, 2007. www.wikipedia.org

National Drug Intelligence Center, U.S. Department of Justice. *Psilocybin Fast Facts* (August 2003).

National Institute on Alcohol Abuse and Alcoholism. "A Call to Action: Changing the Culture of Drinking at U.S. Colleges." Co-chairs: E. A. Malloy (University of Notre Dame) and M. Goldman (University of South Florida), April 2002.

National Institute on Drug Abuse. "Research Report: Methamphetamine Abuse." September 9, 2006. www.nida.nih.gov

National Institute on Drug Abuse. "Drugs, Brains, and Behavior: The Science of Addiction." For release February 13, 2007. Accessed October 8, 2007. www.nida.nih.gov.newsroom

Neiman, David C. "You Asked for It: A Question Authority Examines the Pros and Cons of Moderate Alcohol Absorption for Healthy Active Men and Women." *ACSM's Health & Fitness Journal* 11, no. 4 (July/August 2007): 6–7.

Nelson, T. F., R. A. LaBrie, D. A. LaPlante, et al. "Sports Betting and Other Gambling in Athletes, Fans, and Other College Students." *Research Quarterly in Exercise and Sport* 78, no. 4 (2007): 271–283.

O'Connor, P. G. "The Science of Addiction: From Neurology to Treatment." *New England Journal of Medicine* 354 (May 25, 2006): 1671.

Public Broadcasting Service: Frontline. "The Meth Epidemic: How Meth Destroys the Body." (February 14, 2006.)

Rutledge, P. C., A. Park and K. J. Sher. "21st Birthday Drinking: Extremely Extreme." *Journal of Consulting Clinical Psychology* 76, no. 3 (2008): 514–515.

Saitz, R. "Unhealthy Alcohol Use." *New England Journal of Medicine* 352 (February 10, 2005): 596.

"Steroids and Sports: A Dangerous Mix?" Mayo Clinic. March 6, 2004. www.mayoclinic.com

"Trends in College Binge Drinking during a Period of Increased Prevention Efforts: Findings from 4 Harvard School of Public Health College Alcohol Study Surveys, 1993–2001." 2005. www.hsph.harvard.edu.cas

Volpe, Stella Lucia. "Alcohol and Athletic Performance." *ACSM's Health & Fitness Journal* 14, no. 3 (May/June 2010): 28–30.

Wechsler, H., and L. Nelson. "What We Have Learned from the Harvard School of Public Health College Alcohol Study: Focusing Attention on College Student Alcohol Consumption and the Environmental Conditions That Promote It." *Journal of Studies on Alcohol and Drugs* 69, no. 4 (July 2008): 481–490.

Wechsler, H., T. F. Nelson, J. E. Lee, et al. "Perception and Reality: A National Evaluation of Social Norms Marketing Interventions to Reduce College Students' Heavy Alcohol Use." *Journal of Studies on Alcohol* 64, no. 4 (2003): 484–494.

Wechsler, H., M. Seibring, I. C. Liu, et al. "Colleges Respond to Student Binge Drinking: Reducing Student Demand or Limiting Access." *Journal of American College Health* 52, no. 4 (2004): 159–168.

Weitzman, E. R., and T. F. Nelson. "College Student Binge Drinking and the Prevention Paradox: Implications for Prevention and Harm Reduction." *Journal of Drug Education* 30, no. 3 (2004): 247–266.

Weitzman, E. R., T. F. Nelson, H. Lee, et al. "Reducing Drinking and Related Harms in College: Evaluation of the 'A Matter of Degree' Program."*American Journal of Preventive Medicine* 27, no. 3 (2004): 150–168.

Wollschaeger, Bernd. "The Science of Addiction: From Neurobiology to Treatment." Review: *Journal of the American Medical Association* 298, no. 7 (August 15, 2007): 809–810.

Chapter 15

"Auntie Jessie's Journal. "Help! How to Talk to Your Partner About STDs." MedHelp (July 5, 2008). www.medhelp.org/user_journals/show/15788?personal_page_id=2329

Centers for Disease Control and Prevention. "Bacterial vaginosis." February 2008. http://www.cdc.gov/std/BV/STDFact-Bacterial-Vaginosis.htm

Centers for Disease Control and Prevention. *Cases of HIV Infection and AIDS in the United States and Dependent Areas, 2007,* 19 (February 18, 2009). www.cdc.gov/hiv/topics/surveillance/resources/reports/2007report/

Centers for Disease Control and Prevention. "Chlamydia and LGV." November 2009. http://www.cdc.gov/std/chlamydia/default.htm

Centers for Disease Control and Prevention. "Common Questions about HPV and Cervical Cancer." August 2007. www.cdc.gov/std/hpv/common-question.htm

Centers for Disease Control and Prevention. "Genital Herpes." January 2008. http://www.cdc.gov/std/Herpes/default.htm

Centers for Disease Control and Prevention. "Gonorrhea." February 2008. http://www.cdc.gov/std/Gonorrhea/default.htm

Centers for Disease Control and Prevention. "A Glance at the HIV/AIDS Epidemic." April 2008. http://www.cdc.gov/hivdefalt.htm/resources/factsheets/At-A-Glance.htm

Centers for Disease Control and Prevention. "Hepatitis." November 2009. http://www.cdc.gov/std/hepatitis/

Centers for Disease Control and Prevention. "Hepatitis B." March 2009. www.cdc.gov/hepatitis/B/index.htm

Centers for Disease Control and Prevention. "HPV—Human Papillomavirus Infection." November 2009. http://www.cdc.gov/std/hpv/default.htm

Centers for Disease Control and Prevention. "PID—Pelvic Inflammatory Disease." April 2008. http://www.cdc.gov/std/PID/STDFact-PID.htm

Centers for Disease Control and Prevention. "Sexually Transmitted Diseases—General Information." January 2008. http://www.cdc.gov/std/general

Centers for Disease Control and Prevention. "Sexually Transmitted Diseases: General Information." March 2009. www.cdc.gov/std/general/

Centers for Disease Control and Prevention. "Sexually Transmitted Disease Surveillance 2007." January 20, 2009. www.cdc.gov/std/stats07/toc.htm

Centers for Disease Control and Prevention. "Syphilis." November 2009. http://www.cdc.gov/std/syphilis/default.htm

Centers for Disease Control and Prevention. "STD Clinical Slides." www.cdc.gov/std/training/clinicalslides/slides-dl.htm

Centers for Disease Control and Prevention. "Trichomoniasis." November 2009. http://www.cdc.gov/std/trichomonas/default.htm

Chapter 16

Barnes, P. M., B. Bloom, and R. L. Nahin. "Complementary and Alternative Medicine Use Among Adults and Children: United States, 2007." *National Health Statistics Report #12*. Hyattsville, MD: National Center for Health Statistics, 2008.

Beattie, B. L., et al. "A Vision for Older Adults and Health Promotion." *American Journal of Health Promotion* 18 (November/December 2004): 200–203.

Centers for Disease Control and Prevention. National Center for Health Statistics. *Health, United States, 2006*, November 2006. www.cdc.gov/nchs

Centers for Disease Control and Prevention. National Center for Chronic Disease Prevention and Health Promotion. *Healthy Aging: Improving and Extending Quality of Life Among Older Americans 2009*, January 2009. www.cdc.gov/nccdphp

Centers for Disease Control and Prevention and The Merck Company Foundation. *The State of Aging and Health in America 2007*. Whitehouse Station, NJ: The Merck Company Foundation, 2007.

Centers for Disease Control and Prevention. National Center for Chronic Disease Prevention and Promotion. *Youth Risk Behavior Surveillance—United States, 2007*, June 6, 2008. www.cdc.gov/yrbss

Eckel, R. H., et al. "America's Children: A Critical Time for Prevention." *Circulation* 111 (April 19, 2005): 1866–1868.

"Exploring the Alternatives." *Tufts University Health & Nutrition Letter* 26 (September 2008): 4–5.

Farley, T., and D. A. Cohen. *Prescription for a Healthy Nation*. Boston: Beacon Press, 2005.

Federal Interagency Forum on Aging-Related Statistics. *Older Americans 2008: Key Indicators of Well-Being*. Washington, D.C., March 2008.

Nahin, R. L., P. M. Barnes, B. J. Stussman, and B. Bloom. "Costs of Complementary and Alternative Medicine (CAM) and Frequency of Visits to CAM Practitioners: United States, 2007." *National Health Statistics Report #18*. Hyattsville, MD: National Center for Health Statistics, 2009.

National Highway Traffic Safety Administration. "Overall Traffic Fatalities Reach Record Low." July 2009.

National Highway Traffic Safety Administration. U.S. Department of Transportation. *The Impact of Driver Inattention on Near-Crash/Crash Risk*, April 20, 2006.

National Sleep Foundation. *2009 Sleep in America Poll*. March 2009. www.sleepfoundation.org

Pinzon-Perez, H. "Complementary and Alternative Medicine, Holistic Health, and Integrative Healing: Applications in Health Education." *American Journal of Health Education* 36 (May/June 2005): 174–178.

Schulz, A. J., and L. Mullings (eds.). *Gender, Race, Class and Health: Intersectional Approaches*. San Francisco: Wiley, Jossey-Bass, 2005.

Seligman, M. E. P. *Authentic Happiness*. New York: Free Press, 2002.

Spiegel, D., and C. Classen. *Group Therapy for Cancer Patients*. New York: Basic Books, 1999.

"The Bad News About Products 'Too Good to Be True': How to Be a Savvy—and Safe—Consumer." *Tufts University Health & Nutrition Letter* 27 (September 2009): 4–5.

"Trends in Health Care Costs and Spending." The Kaiser Family Foundation. March 2009.

U.S. Census Bureau. U.S. Department of Commerce. "An Older and More Diverse Nation by Midcentury." Washington, DC, August 2008. www.census.gov

Weil, A. *Why Our Health Matters: A Vision of Medicine That Can Transform Our Future*. New York: Hudson Street Press, 2009.

Winkleby, M. A., and C. Cubbin. "Changing Patterns in Health Behaviors and Risk Factors Related to Chronic Diseases, 1990–2000."*American Journal of Health Promotion* 19 (September/October 2004): 19–27.

PHOTO CREDITS

INDEX